Stedman's

GI & GU
WORDS

INCLUDES
NEPHROLOGY
Fifth Edition

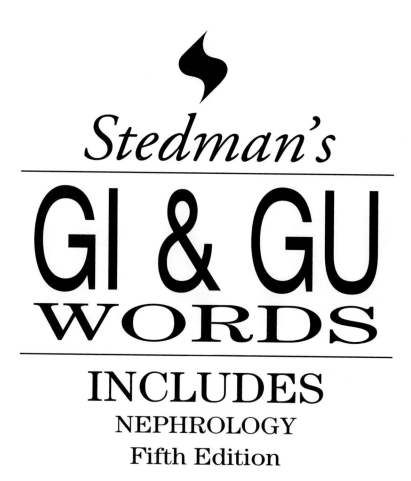

Stedman's

GI & GU
WORDS

INCLUDES
NEPHROLOGY
Fifth Edition

 Wolters Kluwer | Lippincott Williams & Wilkins
Health

Philadelphia · Baltimore · New York · London
Buenos Aires · Hong Kong · Sydney · Tokyo

Publisher: Julie K. Stegman
Editorial Manager: Eric Branger
Associate Managing Editor: Erin M. Cosyn
Manufacturing Coordinator: Margie Orzech-Zeranko
Typesetter: Aptara, Inc.
Printer & Binder: Data Reproductions Corporation

Copyright © 2008 Lippincott Williams & Wilkins
351 West Camden Street
Baltimore, Maryland 21201-2436

Printed in the United States of America

Fifth Edition, 2008

Library of Congress Cataloging-in-Publication Data

Stedman's GI & GU words : includes nephrology. – 5th ed.
    p. ; cm. – (Stedman's word books)
Includes bibliographical references.
ISBN 978-0-7817-7613-4
1. Gastroenterology–Terminology.   2. Urology–Terminology.   I. Stedman, Thomas Lathrop,
1853–1938.   II. Title: GI and GU words.   III. Title: Stedman's GI and GU words.   IV. Series.
[DNLM: 1. Gastrointestinal Diseases–Terminology–English.   2. Female Urogenital
Diseases–Terminology–English.   3. Gastroenterology–Terminology–English.   4. Male
Urogenital Diseases–Terminology–English.   5. Nephrology–Terminology–English.
6. Urology–Terminology–English.
WI 15 S812 2008]
RC802.S68 2008
616.3'30014–dc22   2008000904

08 09 10 11
1 2 3 4 5 6 7 8 9 10

Contents

Acknowledgments

An important part of our editorial process is the involvement of medical transcriptionists—as advisors, reviewers, and/or editors.

We extend special thanks to Kathy Hess, CMT, and Patricia Lee White, CMT, for editing the manuscript, helping resolve many difficult questions, and contributing material for the appendix sections. We are grateful to our MT Editorial Advisory Board members Marty Cantu; Shemah Fletcher; Tina Whitecotton, RMT, FAAMT; Robin Koza; Kathy Kranz; and Diana Krahenbuhl, CMT, who were instrumental in the development of this reference. They recommended sources and shared their valuable judgment, insight, and perspective.

We also extend thanks to Janet West for working on the appendices. Additional thanks to Helen Littrell, IMT for performing the final prepublication review. Other important contributors to this edition include Beverly S. Oberline, CMT and Jo-Ann Clarke.

As with all our *Stedman's* word references, this resource incorporates the suggestions and expertise of our many contacts in the medical transcriptionist community. Thanks to all of our advisory board participants, reviewers, and editors; AAMT meeting attendees; and others who have written us with requests and comments—keep talking, and we'll keep listening.

Editor's Preface

As an affluent nation, the US has indulged itself right into a state of obesity of epidemic proportions along with its consequent illnesses—diabetes, heart disease, etc. In this latest edition of *Stedman's GI & GU Words, Includes Nephrology, Fifth Edition*, you will find a number of new terms related to obesity and obesity-related conditions as well as procedures and treatments designed to conquer this epidemic.

During my many years of editing for LWW, I have been fortunate to work with many fine co-editors. This time was no different. I was pleased to work with Patty White, CMT, on this project. Working together on this edition of *Stedman's GI & GU Words* allowed us to become reacquainted with each other after a number of years of absence. In addition, it has been my pleasure to work with Erin Cosyn, a managing editor whom I now consider my new e-mail "friend." Her insight and guidance have been invaluable in navigating the implementation of a new Word Book process. Of course, I would expect nothing less from *Stedman's*, the finest publisher of medical word books around!

Kathy Hess, CMT

Publisher's Preface

Stedman's GI & GU Words, Includes Nephrology, Fifth Edition, offers an authoritative assurance of quality and exactness to the wordsmiths of the healthcare professions—medical transcriptionists, medical editors and copyeditors, health information management personnel, court reporters, and the many other users and producers of medical documentation.

The specialties of gastroenterology, urology, and nephrology have evolved significantly over the past several years. Gastroenterology-related terminology includes: GI endoscopy, hepatology, and clinical nutrition. Urology-related terminology includes: genitourinary surgery, laparoscopic urology, endourology, urolithology and lithotripsy, renography, ultrasonography, male infertility, urogynecology, and fluorodynamics.

In *Stedman's GI & GU Words, Includes Nephrology, Fifth Edition*, users will find thousands of words that relate to the specialties of gastroenterology, urology, and nephrology. Users will also find terms for protocols, diagnostic and therapeutic procedures, new techniques, lab tests, clinical research terms, as well as equipment names, and abbreviations with their expansions. The appendix sections provide anatomical illustrations with useful captions and labels, sample reports, and common terms by procedure.

This compilation of more than 100,000 entries, fully cross-indexed for quick access, was built from a base vocabulary of approximately 66,000 medical words, phrases, abbreviations, and acronyms. The extensive A-Z list was developed from the database of *Stedman's Medical Dictionary, 28th Edition,* and supplemented by terminology found in current medical literature (please see list of References on page xvii).

We at Lippincott Williams & Wilkins strive to provide you with the most up-to-date and accurate word references available. Your use of this word book will prompt new editions, which we will publish as often as updates and revisions justify. We welcome your suggestions for improvements, changes, corrections, and additions—whatever will make this *Stedman's* product more useful to you. Please complete the postage-paid card in this book for future suggestions and recommendations, or visit us online at www.stedmans.com.

Explanatory Notes

Medical transcription is an art as well as a science. Both approaches are needed to correctly interpret the dictation of a physician, whose language is a product of education, training, and experience. This variety in medical language means that there are several acceptable ways to express certain terms, including jargon. *Stedman's GI & GU Words, Includes Nephrology, Fifth Edition*, provides variant spellings and phrasings for many terms. These elements, in addition to complete cross-indexing, make *Stedman's GI & GU Words, Includes Nephrology, Fifth Edition*, a valuable resource for determining the validity of terms as they are encountered.

Alphabetical Organization

Alphabetization of main entries is letter by letter as spelled, ignoring punctuation, spaces, prefixed numbers, or other characters. For example:

cesium
cesium-137 wire
CE-SM gastric lesion staging by endoscopy
***Cestoda* tapeworm**

In subentry alphabetization, the abbreviated singular form or the spelled-out plural form of the noun main entry word is ignored.

Format and Style

All main entries are in **boldface** to expedite locating a sought-after term, to enhance distinction between main entries and subentries, and to relieve the textual density of the pages.

Irregular plurals and variant spellings are shown on the same line as the singular or preferred form of the word. For example:

diagnosis, pl. diagnoses
CA-125, CA125

Hyphenation

As a rule of style, multiple eponyms (e.g., Cantwell-Ransley technique) are hyphenated. Also, hyphens have been added between a manufacturer and one or more eponyms (e.g., Vital-Metzenbaum dissecting scissors).

Please note that in many cases, hyphenation is a question of style, not of accuracy, and thus is a matter of choice.

Possessives

Possessive forms have been dropped in this reference for the sake of consistency and conformance with the guidelines of the American Association for Medical Transcription (AAMT) and other groups. Please note, however, that in many cases, retaining the possessive, like hyphenating, is a question of style, not of accuracy, and thus is a matter of choice. To form the possessive of a word, simply add the apostrophe or apostrophe "s" to the end of the word.

Cross-indexing

The word list is in an index-like main entry-subentry format that contains two combined alphabetical listings:

(1) A *noun* main entry-subentry organization, which is typical of the A-Z section of medical dictionaries like *Stedman's*:

fibroblast
    human synovial f.
    interstitial f.
    perivascular f.

muscle
    circular m.
    pelvis m.
    smooth m.

(2) An *adjective* main entry-subentry organization, which lists words and phrases as you hear them. The main entries are the adjectives or modifiers in a multiword term. The subentries are the nouns around which the terms are constructed and to which the adjectives or modifiers pertain:

anterior
    a. abdominal wall
    a. axillary line
    a. nephrectomy

intestinal
    i. decompression
    i. endoscopy
    i. hemorrhage

This format provides the user with more than one way to locate and identify a multiword term. For example:

Ellik
    E. kidney stone basket

basket
    Ellik kidney stone b.

cautery
    blind c.
    Bovie c.

Bovie
    B. cautery
    B. holder

It also allows the user to see together all terms that contain a particular descriptor, as well as all types, kinds, or variations of a noun entity. For example:

lavage
    l. bowel preparation
    colonic l.
    l. cytology
    gastric l.

treatment
    t. morbidity
    Murphy t.
    t. protocol
    suppression t.

Wherever possible, abbreviations are separately defined and cross-referenced. For example:

IBD
    inflammatory bowel disease

inflammatory
    i. bowel disease (IBD)

disease
    inflammatory bowel d. (IBD)

References

In addition to the manufacturers' literature we gather at various medical meetings, scientific reports from hospitals, and the lists of our MT Editorial Advisory Board members (from their daily transcription work), we used the following sources for new terms in *Stedman's GI & GU Words, Includes Nephrology, Fifth Edition.*

Books

Agur AMR, Lee MJ. *Grant's Atlas of Anatomy, 10th Edition.* Baltimore: Lippincott Williams & Wilkins, 1999.

Andriole GL, Coplen D. *The Year Book of Urology 2005.* Philadelphia: Elsevier, 2005.

Blaser MJ. *Infections of the Gastrointestinal Tract, 2nd Edition.* Philadelphia: Lippincott Williams & Wilkins, 2002.

Blumenthal M, Goldberg A, Brinckmann J. *Herbal Medicine: Expanded Commission E Monographs.* Newton, MA: Integrative Medicine Communications, 2000.

Drake E. *Sloane's Medical Word Book, 4th Edition.* Philadelphia: Saunders, 2001.

Eastwood G, Avunduk C. *Manual of Gastroenterology, 2nd Edition.* Baltimore: Lippincott Williams & Wilkins, 1994.

Eisenberg RL. *Gastrointestinal Radiology: A Pattern Approach, 4th Edition.* Philadelphia: Lippincott Williams & Wilkins, 2003.

Gartner H. *Color Atlas of Histology, 3rd Edition.* Philadelphia: Lippincott Williams & Wilkins, 2001.

GI Words and Phrases. Modesto, CA: Health Professions Institute, 1989.

Gilinsky NH, Forbes A. *Self-Assessment Color Review of Gastroenterology.* Baltimore: Lippincott Williams & Wilkins, 1999.

Gomella LG. *The 5-Minute Urology Consult.* Baltimore: Lippincott Williams & Wilkins, 2000.

Graham SD, Jr. Glenn JF, Keane TE, Glenn JF. *Glenn's Urologic Surgery, 6th Edition.* Philadelphia: Lippincott Williams & Wilkins, 2004.

Hardy NO, Westport CT. From *Stedman's Medical Dictionary, 28th Edition.* Baltimore: Lippincott Williams & Wilkins, 2005.

Thomas HC, Lemon S, Zuckerman AJ. *Viral Hepatitis, 3rd Edition.* Malden, MA: Blackwell Publishing, Ltd., 2005.

Kelsen DP. *Gastrointestinal Oncology: Principles and Practices.* Charlottesville, VA: Lippincott, Williams & Wilkins, 2002.

Lance LL. *2006 Quick Look Drug Book.* Baltimore: Lippincott Williams & Wilkins, 2006.

Lichtenstein G. *Year Book of Gastroenterology 2005*. Philadelphia: Elsevier, 2005.

Massry SG, Glassock RJ. *Massry and Glassock's Textbook of Nephrology, 4th Edition*. Baltimore: Lippincott Williams & Wilkins, 2000.

Moore KL and Agur A. *Essential Clinical Anatomy, 2nd Edition*. Philadelphia: Lippincott Williams & Wilkins, 2002.

Moore KL and Dalley AF II. *Clinical Oriented Anatomy, 4th Edition*. Baltimore: Lippincott Williams & Wilkins, 1999.

Nettina, SM. *The Lippincott Manual of Nursing Practice, 7th Edition*. Philadelphia: Lippincott Williams & Wilkins, 2001.

Peters DC. *Treatment Options in Gastroenterology*. Baltimore: Lippincott Williams & Wilkins, 2000.

Prakash C. *A Therapeutic Guide to Common Problems in Gastroenterology*. Philadelphia: Lippincott Williams & Wilkins, 2003.

Premkumar K. *The Massage Connection Anatomy and Physiology*. Baltimore: Lippincott Williams & Wilkins, 2004.

Vera Pyle's Current Medical Terminology, 9th Edition. Modesto, CA: Health Professions Institute, 2003.

Sauerland, E. *Grant's Dissector, 12th Edition*. Baltimore: Lippincott Williams & Wilkins, 1999.

Schiff ER, Sorrell MF, Maddrey WC. *Schiff's Diseases of the Liver, 10th Edition*. Philadelphia: Lippincott Williams & Wilkins, 2006.

Schrier RW. *Diseases of the Kidney and Urinary Tract, 7th Edition*. Philadelphia: Lippincott Williams & Wilkins, 2001.

Schrier RW. *Essential Atlas of Nephrology*. Philadelphia: Lippincott Williams & Wilkins, 2001.

Schrier RW. *Manual of Nephrology, 5th Edition*. Baltimore: Lippincott Williams & Wilkins, 1999.

Seldin DW, Giebisch G. *The Kidney: Physiology and Pathophysiology, 3rd Edition*. Baltimore: Lippincott Williams & Wilkins, 2000.

Siorky MD. *Handbook of Urology*. Philadelphia: Lippincott Williams & Wilkins, 2004.

Tessier C. *The AAMT Book of Style for Medical Transcription, 2nd Edition*. Modesto, CA: AAMT, 2002.

Walsh PC, Retik AB, Vaughan ED, Wein AJ. *Campbell's Urology, 7th Edition*. Philadelphia: Saunders, 1998.

Yamada T. *Atlas of Gastroenterology, 3rd Edition*. Philadelphia: Lippincott Williams & Wilkins, 2003.

Images

LifeART Nursing 2, CD-ROM. Baltimore: Lippincott Williams & Wilkins.

LifeART Pediatrics 1, CD-ROM. Baltimore: Lippincott Williams & Wilkins.

LifeART Super Anatomy Collection 3, CD-ROM. Baltimore: Lippincott Williams & Wilkins.

LifeART Super Anatomy Collection 4, CD-ROM. Baltimore: Lippincott Williams & Wilkins.

UpToDate Clinical Reference Library on CD, Version 8:3. Wellesley, MA: UpToDate, 2000.

Yamada T, Alpers DH, Laine L, Owyang C, Powell DW. *Textbook of Gastroenterology, 3rd Edition on CD-ROM*. Philadelphia: Lippincott Williams & Wilkins, 1999.

Journals

American Journal of Gastroenterology. Baltimore: Lippincott Williams & Wilkins, 1998, 2000–2006.

AUA News. Baltimore: Lippincott Williams & Wilkins, 1996–2000.

Contemporary Dialysis and Nephrology. Philadelphia: Lippincott Williams & Wilkins, 1996.

Contemporary Gastroenterology. Philadelphia: Lippincott Williams & Wilkins, 1999–2000.

Contemporary Urology. Philadelphia: Lippincott Williams & Wilkins, 1996, 1999–2000.

Current Opinion in Gastroenterology. Philadelphia: Lippincott Williams & Wilkins, 1999–2006.

Current Opinion in Nephrology and Hypertension. Philadelphia: Lippincott Williams & Wilkins, 1999–2006.

Current Opinion in Urology. Philadelphia: Lippincott Williams & Wilkins, 1999–2006.

Dialysis & Transplantation. Van Nuys, CA: Creative Age Publications, Inc., 1996.

Diseases of the Colon & Rectum. Philadelphia: Lippincott Williams & Wilkins, 1999–2001.

Gastroenterology Nursing. Philadelphia: Lippincott Williams & Wilkins, 1996.

Gastrointestinal Endoscopy. St. Louis: Mosby-Yearbook, Inc., 1996–2006.

Inflammatory Bowel Disease. Philadelphia: Lippincott Williams & Wilkins, 1999–2001.

Journal of Clinical Gastroenterology. Philadelphia: Lippincott Williams & Wilkins, 1999–2006.

Journal of the American Society of Nephrology. Philadelphia: Lippincott Williams & Wilkins, 1996–2004.

Journal of Urology. Baltimore: Lippincott Williams & Wilkins, 1997–2001.

Latest Word. Philadelphia: Saunders, 1999–2001.

Ostomy/Wound Management. Wayne, PA: HMP Communications, 1999–2006.

Techniques in Urology. Philadelphia: Lippincott Williams & Wilkins, 1999–2000.

Urology Times. Cleveland: Advanstar Communications, 1996.

Websites

http://gastroenterology.medscape.com/Home/Topics/gastroenterology/gastroenterology.html

http://urology.medscape.com/Home/Topics/urology/urology.html

http://www.acg.gi.org/

http://www.asge.org/index.jsp

http://www.asn-online.com/

http://www.betterworld.com/BWZ/9608/act.htm#Gas

http://www.centerwatch.com

http://www.duj.com

http://www.fascrs.org

http://www.fda.gov

http://www.gastro.org

http://www.herbalremedies.com/cinnamon1.html

http://www.hort.purdue.edu/newcrop/med-aro/factsheets/DILL.html

http://www.hpisum.com

http://www.kcweb.com/herb/goldenseal.htm

http://www.kidney.org

http://www.mtdaily.com

http://www.mtdesk.com/newterms.shtml

http://www.niddk.nih.gov

http://www.observations.org/Healing2/Articles/GastIntestHerbs.html

http://www.pdrhealth.com/drug_info/nmdrugprofiles/herbaldrugs/100620.shtml

http://www.physci.org/1/herb/urgen.html#Ap

http://www.spwb.saunders.net

http://www.virtualdrugstore.com/druglist.html

A
  adenine
    A antigen
    A Bayesian nomogram
    A bile
    A ring
    A ring of esophagus
A4
  androstenedione
AA
  alcohol abuse
    AA amyloid
AAA
  abdominal aortic aneurysm
AAC
  acute acalculous cholecystitis
  antibiotic-associated colitis
AAD
  acid-ash diet
  antibiotic-associated diarrhea
AAG
  antral atrophic gastritis
Aagenaes syndrome
A-a gradient
AAH
  acute alcoholic hepatitis
  atypical adenomatous hyperplasia
AAL
  anterior axillary line
AAPC, AAPMC
  antibiotic-associated pseudomembranous
  colitis
Aaron sign
Aarskog-Scott syndrome
Aarskog syndrome
AAS
  acute abdominal series
AASK
  African-American Study of Kidney
  Disease and Hypertension
AASLD
  American Association for the Study of
  Liver Diseases
AAV
  adenoassociated virus
abacterial pyuria
Abadie enterostomy clamp
abarelix
abate
Abbe
    A. intestinal anastomosis
    A. small-bowel operation
**Abbe-McIndoe vaginal
 construction**
Abbott

    A. AxSYM antibody to hepatitis C
    virus lab test
  enzimoimmunoassay MEIA A.
    A. esophagogastroscopy
    A. esophagogastrostomy
    A. HCV EIA 2nd generation kit
    A. HCV test kit
    A. IMx PSA assay
    A. LifeCare pump
    A. Lifeshield needleless system
    A. TDx monoclonal fluorescence
    polarization immunoassay
    A. tube
Abbott-Miller tube
**Abbott-Rawson double-lumen
 gastrointestinal tube**
ABC
  avidin-biotin complex
  alkaline phosphatase Vectastain ABC
  ABC reagent
ABCB4 gene
abdomen
    acute surgical a.
    boardlike rigidity of a.
    boat-shaped a.
    carinate a.
    diffusely tender a.
    distended a.
    doughy a.
    dull to percussion a.
    exquisitely tender a.
    flabby a.
    flat plate of a.
    hyperresonant a.
    navicular a.
    nondistended a.
    a. obstipum
    pendulous a.
    plain film of a.
    protuberant a.
    resonant a.
    rigid a.
    rotund a.
    scaphoid a.
    silent a.
    soft a.
    splinting of a.
    surgical a.
    tight a.
    tympanitic a.
abdominal
    a. abscess
    a. angina
    a. aorta
    a. aortic aneurysm (AAA)

abdominal (*continued*)
  a. aortography
  a. apoplexy
  a. apron
  a. ballottement
  a. bruit
  a. canal
  a. cavity
  a. circumference (AC)
  a. colectomy
  a. compartment syndrome (ACS)
  a. compression (AC)
  a. compression belt
  a. contents
  a. crisis
  a. cryptorchidism
  a. cutaneous nerve entrapment syndrome
  a. decompression
  a. desmoid tumor
  a. distention
  a. dropsy
  a. ectopic pregnancy
  a. fasciocutaneous flap
  a. fat
  a. fat pad
  a. fistula
  a. fluid wave
  a. fullness
  a. ganglion block
  a. girth
  a. guarding
  a. incision dehiscence
  a. inguinal ring
  a. kidney
  a. laparotomy pad
  a. lavage
  a. leak-point pressure (ALPP)
  a. membrane
  a. migraine
  a. muscle deficiency syndrome
  a. nephrectomy
  a. nephrotomy
  a. pain
  a. paracentesis
  a. partitioning
  a. part of esophagus
  a. patch electrode
  a. peritoneum
  a. pool
  a. pressure technique
  a. procedure
  a. pulse
  a. radiography
  a. rectopexy
  a. region
  a. retropexy
  a. rigidity
  a. sacrocolpopexy
  a. section
  a. situs inversus
  a. stoma
  a. surgery
  a. tap
  a. testis
  a. tomodensitometric examination
  a. tympany (AT)
  a. typhoid
  a. ultrasonography
  a. ultrasound
  a. ureter
  a. vascular accident
  a. viscus
  a. wall
  a. wall hernia
  a. wall lift technique
  a. wall mass
  a. wall venous pattern
  a. zone

abdominalgia
  periodic a.

abdominalis
  angina a.
  facies a.
  pulsus a.
  purpura a.

abdominis
  angina a.
  diastasis rectus a.
  hydrops a.
  rectus a.

abdominocentesis
abdominocystic
abdominogenital
abdominopelvic
  a. cavity
  a. orocecal transit time

abdomino-Peña pullthrough procedure
abdominoperineal
  a. excision
  a. resection (APR)

abdominoplasty
  Ehrlich a.
  Monfort a.
  Randolph a.

abdominosacral resection
abdominoscopy
abdominoscrotal hydrocele
abdominothoracic
abdominovaginal
abdominovesical pouch
abenteric
Aberdeen knot
aberrans
  vas a.
  vasculum a.

aberrant
    a. crypt focus (ACF)
    a. mRNA splicing
    a. obturator vein
    a. pancreas
    a. suprarenal cortex
    a. umbilical stomach
    a. ureter
aberrantes
    ductuli a.
aberration
    a. by scintigraphy
    genetic a.
aberratio testis
abetalipoproteinemia
ABG
    arterial blood gas
ABGII hemodialysis machine
ABH blood group
ability
    impaired urinary concentrating a.
    a. of glucocorticoid receptor
    renal autoregulatory a.
    a. to form solid stool
abiraterone acetate
Ablaser laser delivery catheter
ablate-and-chip method
Ablatherm HIFU system
ablation
    androgen a.
    carbon dioxide laser plaque a.
    cold forceps a.
    cold snare a.
    cryogenic a.
    cryosurgical a.
    endoscopic thermal a.
    endoscopic ultrasound-guided alcohol a.
    homogeneous a.
    laser a.
    microwave a.
    a. model
    needle a.
    neoadjuvant total androgen a.
    percutaneous radiofrequency a.
    photochemical a.
    photothermal laser a.
    prostate gland needle a.
    radiofrequency a.
    radiofrequency interstitial tissue a.
    sphincter of Oddi a.
    thermal a.
    transurethral needle a. (TUNA)
    tumor a.
    ultrasound a.
    valve a.
    visual laser a.

ablative
    a. adrenalectomy
    a. laser therapy
abluminal
ABM
    adjusted body mass
abnormal
    a. bowel wall enhancement
    a. esophageal test
abnormality
    amino acid a.
    atherosclerotic a.
    chromosomal a.
    clotting a.
    coloboma, heart disease, atresia choanae, retarded growth, genital hypoplasia, and ear a.'s (CHARGE)
    congenital urologic a.
    crystallization a.
    diminished branching a.
    electrolyte a.
    hematologic a.
    hepatic a.
    immunologic a.
    laboratory a.
    metabolic a.
    mucosal a.
    ocular a.
    a. of hepatic artery
    omphalocele, exstrophy of bladder, imperforate anus, and spinal a. (OEIS)
    platelet a.
    pruning a.
    rectosphincteric a.
    spinal cord injury without radiographic a. (SCIWORA)
    urogenital a.
    vascular a.
ABO
    ABO barrier
    ABO blood group
    ABO incompatible
Abocide disinfectant
ABO-incompatible living donor kidney transplantation
aboral migration
AB/PAS
    Alcian blue and periodic acid-Schiff
Abrams-Griffith nomogram
abrasion
    mucosal a.
Abrikosov tumor
abrupt pulse
abscess
    abdominal a.
    amebic liver a.
    anal a.
    anorectal a.

abscess (*continued*)
    appendiceal a.
    bile duct a.
    biliary a.
    cavernosal a.
    cholangitic a.
    cortical a.
    crypt a.
    cuff a.
    deep interloop a.
    diaphragmatic a.
    distant a.
    diverticular a.
    Douglas a.
    echinococcal liver a.
    endoscopic transpapillary drainage of
      pancreatic a.
    entamebic a.
    Entamoeba histolytica a.
    enteroperitoneal a.
    epididymal a.
    epiploic a.
    fecal a.
    filarial a.
    a. formation
    fungal liver a.
    gallbladder wall a.
    gas a.
    gas-forming liver a.
    helmintic a.
    hepatic a.
    high intermuscular a.
    horseshoe a.
    interloop a.
    intermesenteric a.
    intersphincteric perirectal a.
    intraabdominal a.
    intrahepatic a.
    intramesenteric a.
    intraperitoneal a.
    ischiorectal a.
    kidney a.
    lacunar a.
    liver a.
    midabdominal a.
    nongas-forming liver a.
    pancreatic pseudocyst a.
    paracolic a.
    parafrenal a.
    paranephric a.
    pararectal a.
    pelvic a.
    pelvirectal a.
    percutaneous drainage of
      epididymal a.
    perianal fistula a.
    pericecal a.
    pericholecystic a.
    pericolic a.

    perineal a.
    perinephric a.
    perirectal a.
    perirenal a.
    peritoneal cavity a.
    periureteral a.
    periurethral a.
    phlegmonous a.
    pilonidal perirectal a.
    postcecal a.
    postoperative a.
    preperitoneal a.
    prostatic a.
    protozoan a.
    psoas a.
    pylephlebitic a.
    pyogenic liver a.
    rectal a.
    renocortical a.
    retrocecal a.
    retroesophageal a.
    retroperitoneal a.
    retroperitoneal iliopsoas a.
    root a.
    seminal vesicle a.
    spermatic a.
    splenic a.
    stercoraceous a.
    sterile a.
    subacute a.
    subaponeurotic a.
    subcapsular hepatic a.
    subdiaphragmatic a.
    subhepatic a.
    subperitoneal a.
    subphrenic a.
    suprahepatic a.
    supralevator perirectal a.
    testicular a.
    tympanitic a.
    urachal a.
    urethral a.
    urinary a.
    urinous a.

Abscession biliary drainage catheter

absence
    enuretic a.
    a. of comorbid disorders
    a. of diluted duct
    protein in vitamin K a. (PIVKA)

absent
    a. bowel sounds
    a. gag reflex
    a. peristalsis

Absidia
    A. capillata
    A. coerulea
    A. corymbifera
    A. ramosum

absolute
    a. alcohol
    a. alcohol sclerosant
    a. dehydration
    a. diet
    a. erythrocytosis
    a. sterility
absorbable
    a. clip
    a. gelatin sponge
    a. staple
    a. suture
absorbent padding
absorptiometer
absorptiometry
    dual-energy x-ray a. (DEXA, DXA)
    dual-photon a.
absorption
    alcohol a.
    antibiotic a.
    DEXA a.
    dual-energy x-ray a.
    enteral a.
    fluorescent treponemal antibody a.
      (FTA-ABS)
    fractionated plasma separation and
      a. (FPSA)
    gastrointestinal a.
    impaired gastric a.
    internal a.
    intestinal a.
    oxalate intestinal a.
    paracetamol a.
    reservoir mucosal a.
    transcellular a.
    xenobiotic a.
absorptive
    a. cell
    a. hypercalciuria
    a. hyperoxaluria
abstinence
abuse
    alcohol a.
    ethanol a.
    intravenous drug a.
    ipecac a.
    laxative a.
    phencyclidine a.
    salicylate a.
    sexual a.
    substance a.
ABV
    doxorubicin, bleomycin sulfate,
      vinblastine
ABVD
    doxorubicin, bleomycin sulfate,
      vinblastine, dacarbazine
ABW
    actual body weight

AC
    Acinetobacter calcoaceticus
    activated charcoal
      Pepcid AC
ACA
    aminocaproic acid
    anticentromere antibody
acalculous
    a. cholecystitis
    a. gallbladder disease
Acanthocephala
acanthocytosis
acanthosis
    glycogenic a.
    a. nigricans
acarbose
acathectic
acathexia
Acationox
ACBE
    air-contrast barium enema
accelerated
    a. fibrinolysis
    a. hypertension
    a. senescence
    a. transplant rejection
acceleration
    cavernous artery blood flow a.
accelerator
    serum thrombotic a.
    a. urinae
Accellon Combi cervical biosampler
access
    arteriovenous a.
    endoscopic a.
    hemodialysis vascular a.
    intravenous a. (IVAC)
    a. papillotomy
    percutaneous renal a.
    peritoneal a.
    reliable percutaneous renal a.
    vascular a.
    venovenous a.
accessorium
    pancreas a.
accessorius
    ductus pancreaticus a.
    lien a.
accessory
    a. adrenal
    a. adrenal gland
    Assura irrigation a.
    a. diaphragm
    a. digestive organ
    a. duct of Luschka
    a. duct of Santorini
    a. obturator artery
    a. pancreas
    a. pancreatic duct

A

accessory (*continued*)
a. parotid gland
a. phallic urethra
a. portal system of Sappey
a. saphenous vein
a. sex gland
a. spleen
a. superior colic artery
a. thyroid gland
a. trocar
a. vessel
accident
abdominal vascular a.
accordion-like bunching
accordion sign
Accu-Chek III
Accu-Dx test
AccuMeter
ChemTrak A.
accumulation
gamma-aminobutyric acid a.
glomerular a.
glycoprotein a.
lysosomal a.
tubular iron a.
Accu-Prep
Fleet A.-P.
accurate
A. catheter
A. Surgical and Scientific
Instruments (ASSI)
Accuratome precurved papillotome
AccuSharp endoscope
Accutorr oscillometric device
ACD
adult celiac disease
ACE
angiotensin-converting enzyme
BICAP silver ACE
ACE gene polymorphism
ACE inhibitor
ACE procedure
ACEI
angiotensin-converting enzyme inhibitor
aceruloplasminemia
hereditary a.
acetaldehyde
acetaminophen (APAP)
a. hepatotoxicity
a. overdose
a. toxicity
acetate
abiraterone a.
anaritide a.
buserelin a.
calcium a.
cellulose a.
chlormadinone a.

cortisone a.
Cortone A.
cyproterone a. (CPA)
desmopressin a.
free a.
goserelin a.
hydrocortisone a.
Hydrocortone A.
leuprolide a.
mafenide a.
medroxyprogesterone a. (MPA)
megestrol a.
methylprednisolone a.
octreotide a.
phorbol myristate a. (PMA)
roxatidine a.
uranyl a.
acetazolamide
acetic
a. acid
a. acid chromoendoscopy
a. acid-enhanced magnifying
endoscopy
a. acid-guided biopsy
acetohydroxamic
a. acid
a. acid irrigation
acetomorphine
acetonemic
acetonitrile eluate
acetonuria
acetowhite lesion
acetyl
a. coenzyme hypoglycin A
a. triglycine renal scan
acetylation
acetylcholine (Ach, ACh)
acetylcholinesterase
acetylcysteine, *N*-acetylcysteine
acetylsalicylic acid (ASA)
5-acetylsalicylic acid
acetylsulfadiazine
acetylsulfaguanidine
acetylsulfathiazole
acetyltransferase
choline a. (ChAT)
ACG
American College of Gastroenterology
Ach, ACh
acetylcholine
achalasia
a. balloon dilation
a. cardia
classic a.
cricopharyngeal a.
a. dilator
esophageal a.
idiopathic a.

pelvirectal a.
secondary a.
sphincteral a.
vigorous a.
achalasia-like esophagus
ache
stomach a.
Achiever
A. balloon dilation catheter
A. balloon dilator
achlorhydria
a. apepsia
gastric a.
histamine-resistant a.
medically induced a.
watery diarrhea, hypokalemia, and
a. (WDHA)
achlorhydric
acholangic
a. biliary cirrhosis
a. biliary fibrosis
acholia
acholic stool
acholuria
acholuric jaundice
achoresis
achromaturia
Achromycin V
achylia
a. gastrica
a. gastrica haemorrhagica
a. pancreatica
achylous
achymia
achymosis
acid
acetic a.
acetohydroxamic a.
5-acetylsalicylic a.
acetylsalicylic a. (ASA)
amino a.
aminocaproic a. (ACA)
aminolevulinic a. (ALA)
5-aminolevulinic a. (5-ALA)
4-aminosalicylic a. (4-ASA)
5-aminosalicylic a. (5-ASA)
amoxicillin and clavulanic a.
arachidonic a.
aromatic amino a.
ascorbic a.
benzoic a.
benzoyl-tyrosyl-paraaminobenzoic a.
(BT-PABA)
7-beta-epimer of chenodeoxycholic a.
bile a.
bile acid-ethylenediaminetetraacetic a.
(BA-EDTA)
branched-chain amino a. (BCAA)

caustic a.
a. cell
chenodeoxycholic a. (CDA, CDCA)
cholic a. (CA)
cinnamic a.
citric a.
clavulanic a.
a. clearance test (ACT)
cocarcinogenic fecal bile a.
complementary deoxyribonucleic a.
(cDNA)
conjugated bile a.
conjugated linoleic a. (CLA)
cyclooxygenase messenger
ribonucleoprotein a. (COX mRNA)
cysteine sulfinic a.
delta-aminolevulinic a. (d-ALA)
deoxycholic a.
deoxyribonucleic a. (DNA)
Diagnex Blue test for gastric a.
diatrizoic a.
diethylenetriamine pentaacetic a.
(DTPA)
dihydroxyeicosatrienoic a.
diisopropyliminodiacetic a. (DISDA,
DISIDA)
dimercaptosuccinic a. (DMSA)
a. dyspepsia
eicosapentaenoic a. (EPA)
epoxyeicosatrienoic a. (EET)
epsilon aminocaproic a.
essential amino a.
essential fatty a. (EFA)
esterified fecal a.
ethacrynic a.
ethylenediaminetetraacetic a. (EDTA)
ethyleneglycoltetraacetic a. (EGTA)
fatty a.
fecal bile a. (FBA)
folic a.
folinic a.
free fatty a. (FFA)
free fecal bile a.
gamma aminobutyric a. (GABA)
gastric a.
genomic deoxyribonucleic a. (gDNA)
a. gland
glutamic a.
a. guanidine
thiocyanate-phenol-chloroform
method
guanidinosuccinic a. (GSA)
a. hematin method
a. hemolysis test
hepatoiminodiacetic a. (HIDA)
HETE a.
hippuric a.
homovanillic a. (HVA)

acid (*continued*)
hyaluronic a.
hydrochloric a. (HCl)
hydroxyeicosatetraenoic a. (HETE)
20-hydroxyeicosatetraenoic a.
  (20-HETE)
5-hydroxyindoleacetic a.
  (5-HIAA)
hydroxyindoleacetic a. (HIAA)
a. hypersecretion
hypervariable deoxyribonucleic a.
ibotenic a.
iminodiacetic a. (IDA)
a. indigestion
a. infusion
a. ingestion
a. inhibitory factor
a. injury
intravesical hyaluronic a.
iocetamic a.
iopanoic a.
iothalamic a.
[131]I paraaminohippuric a.
isovaleric a.
keto a.
a. labile
lactic a.
Lewis a.
linoleic a.
lithocholic a. (LCA)
lithocholic acid-deoxycholic a.
  (LCA-DCA)
long-chain fatty a. (LCFA)
luminal a.
mandelic a.
medium-chain fatty a. (MCFA)
mefenamic a.
2-mercaptoethanesulfonic a.
  (MESNA)
messenger ribonucleic a. (mRNA)
methylaminoisobutyric a.
  (MeAIB)
2-methylcitric a.
methylmalonic a.
a. microclimate
mucosal fatty a.
nalidixic a.
N-benzoyl-L-tyrosyl-P-aminobenzoic
  a.
N-2-hydroxyethyl-piperazine-N-2-
  ethane-sulfonic a. (HEPES)
nitroblue tetrazolium-
  paraaminobenzoic a. (NBT-PABA)
nonsulfated bile a.
Novamine amino a.
nucleic a.
okadaic a.
oleic a.
oral bile a. (OBA)

oxalic a. (OA)
PAH a.
pantothenic a.
paraaminobenzoic a. (PABA)
paraaminohippuric a.
paraisopropyliminodiacetic a.
  (PIPIDA)
a. perfusion test
phenazopyridine hydrochloric a.
a. phosphate osteoclast
polyglycolic a. (PGA)
polyprenoic a.
pteroylglutamic a.
a. pump
a. reflux
a. reflux test
a. regurgitation
renal excretion of a.
renal messenger ribonucleic a.
renal messenger ribonucleoprotein a.
reptilase a.
a. resistance assay
retinoic a.
ribonucleic a. (RNA)
saponifiable fecal bile a.
saturated fatty a. (SFA)
secondary bile a.
a. secretion
a. secretory disorder
seminal plasma citric a.
serum hyaluronic a.
serum uric a.
short-chain fatty a. (SCFA)
sialic a.
small interfering ribonucleic a.
a. sphingomyelinase
sulfuric a.
a. suppression
a. suppression therapy (AST)
a. suppressive agent
tannic a.
taurocholic a.
technetium-99m diethylenetriamine
  pentaacetic a. (^{99m}Tc-DTPA)
technetium-99m diisopropyl
  iminodiacetic a.
total bile a. (TBA)
tranexamic a.
Travasol amino a.
tricarboxylic a. (TCA)
trichloroacetic a. (TCA)
trihydrocoprostanic a. (TCA)
unsaturated fatty a.
uric a.
ursodeoxycholic a. (UDCA)
valproic a.
vanillacetic a. (VLA)
vanillylmandelic a. (VMA)
zoledronic a.

acid-ash diet (AAD)
acid-base
    a.-b. balance
    a.-b. disorder
    a.-b. disturbance
    a.-b. equilibrium
    a.-b. imbalance
acidemia
    a. defect
    isovaleric a.
    a. of stool test
acid-fast bacillus (AFB)
acidic
    a. environment
    a. epididymal glycoprotein
    a. fibroblast growth factor
    a. sialomucin
    a. sulfomucin
acidification
    a. defect
    duodenal a.
    a. of stool test
    urine a.
acidity
    circadian gastric a.
    gastric a.
    intracellular a.
    intragastric a.
    titratable a.
    urinary a.
acid-neutralizing capacity (ANC)
acidopathy
    specific organic a.
acidophilic
    a. body
    a. degeneration
    a. PAS-positive granule
acidophilus
    a. capsule
    Lactobacillus a.
    a. milk
acidosis
    acute a.
    a. after urinary intestinal
      diversion
    anion gap a.
    bicarbonate wastage renal
      tubular a.
    carbon dioxide a.
    chronic metabolic a. (CMA)
    congenital lactic a.
    distal renal tubular a. (dRTA)
    generalized distal renal
      tubular a.
    high anion gap metabolic a.
    hyperchloremic metabolic a.
    hypokalemic renal tubular a.
    lactic a.
    long-term effect of metabolic a.

    metabolic a.
    nonanion gap metabolic a.
    proximal renal tubular a.
    Rector-Gordon-Healey-Mendoza-
      Spitzer type IV renal tubular
      a.
    renal hyperchloremia a.
    renal tubular a. (RTA)
    renal tubular metabolic a.
    renal tubular a. type I-IV
    respiratory a.
    uremic a.
    winter a.
acidotic
acid-pepsin reflux esophagitis
acid-peptic
    a.-p. condition
    a.-p. disease
    a.-p. esophagitis
    a.-p. juice
    a.-p. ulcer
acid-provoked spasm
acid-related disorder (ARD)
acid-Schiff
    Alcian blue and periodic a.-S.
      (AB/PAS)
    periodic a.-S. (PAS)
    a.-S. stain
acid-suppressed stomach
Acidulin
aciduria
    aminoisobutyric a.
    beta aminoisobutyric a.
    3-hydroxy-3-methylglutaric a.
    l-glyceric a.
acification
    intracellular a.
acinar
    a. adenocarcinoma
    a. agglomerate
    a. cell
    a. cell carcinoma
    a. defect
    a. gradient
    a. hepatocellular carcinoma
    a. tissue
acinarization of pancreas
Acinetobacter **(A)**
    A. calcoaceticus (AC)
    A. lwoffii
acini (*pl. of* acinus)
acinic cell
aciniform
acinitis
acinose (*var. of* acinous)
acinotubular
acinous, acinose
    a. adenoma
    a. cell

acinus, *pl.* **acini**
    liver a.
    pancreatic a.
    a. renalis malpighii
    a. renis malpighii
AcipHex
acipimox
acivicin
ACKD
    acquired cystic kidney disease
ackee fruit poisoning
ACL
    anal canal length
ACLA
    anticardiolipin antibody
aclacinomycin A
Acme One Time enteral feeding bag
ACMI
    American College of Medical
    Informatics
        ACMI cystourethroscope
        ACMI endoscope
        ACMI fiberoptic colonoscope
        ACMI fiberoptic esophagoscope
        ACMI fiberoptic
          proctosigmoidoscope
        ACMI gastroscope
        ACMI Martin endoscopy forceps
        ACMI monopolar electrode
        ACMI fiberoptic sigmoidoscope
        ACMI ulcer measuring device
acnes
    Propionibacterium a.
acne vulgaris
aconitine
acontractile detrusor
acontractility
    bladder a.
    detrusor a.
aconuresis
acoprosis
acoprous
acorn-tipped
    a.-t. bougie
    a.-t. catheter
acorn treatment
acoustically transparent cradle
ACP-ASIM
    American College of
    Physicians-American Society of
    Internal Medicine
ACPO
    acute colonic pseudoobstruction
acquired
    a. chordee
    a. cystic kidney disease
      (ACKD)
    a. diverticulosis
    a. functional megacolon

    a. gastric ectopia
    a. hernia
    a. hyperlipoproteinemia
    a. hyperoxaluria
    a. immunity
    a. immunodeficiency
    a. immunodeficiency syndrome
      (AIDS)
    a. lactose deficiency
    a. neutrophil chemotaxis defect
    a. pancreatitis
    a. renal artery aneurysm
    a. renal cystic disease (ARCD)
    a. ureteropelvic junction
      obstruction
acquisita
    epidermolysis bullosa a.
    hypertrichosis lanuginosa a.
acquisition
    endoscopic data a.
acraturesis
acrobystia
acrobystiolith
acrobystitis
acrocephalopolydactylous dysplasia
acrochordon
acrocyanosis
acrodermatitis enteropathica
acrolein
acromphalus
acrophase
acroposthitis
acrosin
acrosomal granule
acrosome
    a. reaction
    a. reaction assay
acrosome-reacted spermatozoon
acrylate
ACS
    abdominal compartment syndrome
ACT
    acid clearance test
ACTH
    adrenocorticotropic hormone
Acticoat
    A. composite dressing
    A. foam dressing
Acticon neosphincter
Actidose-Aqua
Actigall
Actilon
actin
    a. filament
    smooth muscle isoform a.
acting
    long a. (LA, L.A.)
Actinomyces naeslundii
actinomycin C, D

actinomycosis
    biliary a.
    gastric a.
    intraabdominal a.
actinomycotic
    a. appendicitis
    a. esophageal disease
actinomycotica
    perityphlitis a.
action
    cytolytic a.
    immunomodulatory a.
    snake venom-converting
      enzyme-inhibiting a.
    viruslike a. (VLA)
Action-II
Actis venous flow controller
ActiTest
activated
    a. alkaline glutaraldehyde
    a. capsule endoscope
    a. charcoal (AC)
    a. partial thromboplastin time
      (aPTT, APTT)
    a. protein C resistance (APCR)
    a. thromboplastin time
activation
    antibody-independent complement a.
    B-lymphocyte a.
    complement a.
    nuclear transcriptional a.
    a. of programmed cell death
      pathway
    platelet a.
    selective bladder a.
    T-cell a.
    T-lymphocyte a.
    very late a. (VLA)
activator
    continuous erythropoiesis receptor a.
      (CERA)
    plasminogen a. (PA)
    tissue plasminogen a. (TPA, tPA)
    tissue-type plasminogen a.
    urokinase plasminogen a.
    vascular plasminogen a. (v-PA)
active
    a. bowel sounds
    bowel sounds normal and a.
      (BSNA)
    a. chronic gastritis
    a. chronic hepatitis
    a. congestion
    a. duodenal ulcer
    A. Living incontinence pad
    A. Living incontinence shield
    a. renin
    a. schistosomiasis
    a. source of bleeding
    a. systemic bacterial infection
    a. transport
actively bleeding varix
Activia yogurt
activin A
activity
    adenosine deaminase a.
    antiandrogenic a.
    antiproliferative a.
    a. assay
    ATPase a.
    beta galactosidase a.
    brush-border disaccharidase
      specific a.
    brush-border enzyme a.
    brush-border hydrolase a.
    cavitation bubble a.
    clinical a.
    complement hemolytic a.
    disaccharidase enzyme a.
    efferent renal sympathetic nerve a.
      (ERSNA)
    endogenous peroxidase a.
    fibrinolytic a.
    gastric myoelectrical a.
    gastric urease a.
    hepatic uroporphyrinogen
      decarboxylase a.
    hourly scratching a. (HSA)
    hyaluronidase a.
    intrinsic enzymatic a.
    Knodell criteria for histology a.
    mitotic a.
    motor a.
    muscarinic a.
    myoelectric a.
    Na+/H+ antiporter a.
    Na/K-ATPase a.
    necroinflammatory a.
    nonstrenuous a.
    opsonic a.
    oxidoreductase a.
    phasic contractile a.
    phospholipase A2 catalytic a.
    plasma renin a.
    postheparin lipolytic a. (PHLA)
    protein serine/threonine kinase a.
    PyNPase a.
    renal sympathetic a.
    renal vein renin a. (RVRA)
    renal xanthine oxidase-xanthine
      dehydrogenase a.
    respiratory burst a.
    a. score
    serum cholinesterase a.
    single potential analysis of
      cavernous electrical a.
    specific a.
    spermidine uptake a.

activity (*continued*)
    spike-burst electrical a.
    sympathetic nervous system a.
    thermic effect of physical a.
     (TEPA)
    tumorigenesis a.
    tyrosine kinase a.
    xanthine oxidoreductase a.
Actril disinfectant
actual
    a. body weight (ABW)
    a. gastric myoelectric uncoupling
    a. intraprostatic temperature
    a. weight (AW)
Acucise
    A. access sheath
    A. balloon
    A. balloon catheter
    A. balloon cutting device
    A. endopyelotomy
    A. endopyelotomy catheter
    A. retrograde procedure
    A. RP outpatient procedure
AcuDiet
    Diastate A.
acuity
acuminata (*pl. of* acuminatum)
acuminatum, *pl.* **acuminata**
    condyloma a.
    Dinophysis a.
    esophageal condyloma a.
    giant anorectal condyloma a.
AcuNav steerable phased vector-array
  ultrasound catheter probe
acupuncture
AcuSnare polypectomy device
Acuson-128 color flow Doppler machine
acute
    a. abdominal series (AAS)
    a. abdominal vascular disease
    a. acalculous cholecystitis (AAC)
    a. acidosis
    a. alcoholic hepatitis (AAH)
    a. appendicitis
    a. cellular rejection
    a. cholecystitis
    a. colonic pseudoobstruction
     (ACPO)
    a. corrosive esophagitis
    a. diverticulitis
    a. drug-induced cholestasia
    a. edematous pancreatitis (AEP)
    a. epididymitis
    a. erosive gastritis (AEG)
    a. esophageal food impaction
     (AEFI)
    a. extrarenal obstruction
    a. fatty liver
    a. fatty liver of pregnancy (AFLP)

a. febrile neutrophilic dermatosis
 (AFND)
a. flank pain
a. flank pain syndrome
a. focal bacterial nephritis (AFBN)
a. gallstone pancreatitis (AGP)
a. gastric anisakiasis
a. gastric ischemia
a. gastric mucosal lesion
a. gastroenteritis (AGE)
a. glomerulonephritis (AGN)
a. graft-versus-host disease
a. hemorrhagic cystitis (AHC)
a. hemorrhagic gastritis
a. hemorrhagic pancreatitis (AHP)
a. hepatic coma
a. hepatic failure
a. hepatic rupture
a. hepatic toxicity
a. hepatitis
a. hepatocellular degeneration
a. humoral renal allograft rejection
a. hydramnios
a. hypokalemic nephropathy
a. idiopathic inflammatory bowel
 disease
a. idiopathic scrotal edema
a. infectious colitis
a. infectious diarrhea
a. infectious nonbacterial
 gastroenteritis
a. infundibulopelvic angle
a. intermittent porphyria (AIP)
a. interstitial nephritis (AIN)
a. intrinsic renal failure
a. juvenile cirrhosis
a. lead poisoning
a. leukopenia
a. liver failure (ALF)
a. lobular hepatitis
a. lymphoblastic leukemia (ALL)
a. lymphocytic leukemia (ALL)
a. megacolon
a. mercury poisoning
a. mesangial proliferative
 glomerulonephritis
a. methanol intoxication
a. mononucleosis-like hepatitis
a. MVT
a. myelomonocytic leukemia
a. necrotizing esophagitis
a. nephritic syndrome
a. nephrosis
a. nonobstructive pyelonephritis
a. nonocclusive bowel infarction
a. nonvariceal upper gastrointestinal
 hemorrhage
a. obstructive suppurative cholangitis
 (AOSC)

a. occlusive mesenteric ischemia
a. on chronic liver disease
(AOCLD)
a. on chronic liver failure
a. pancreatitis prevention
a. parenchymatous hepatitis
a. phase of neurogenic bladder
a. phase protein
A. Physiology and Chronic Health
Evaluation (APACHE)
a. polycystic disease
a. poststreptococcal
glomerulonephritis (APSGN)
a. proctitis
a. recurrent pancreatitis (ARP)
a. rejection of liver transplant
a. relapsing pancreatitis
a. renal failure (ARF)
a. renal insufficiency (ARI)
a. renal transplant vasculopathy
a. schistosomiasis
a. sclerosing hyaline necrosis
(ASHN)
a. scrotum
a. self-limited colitis (ASLC)
a. self-limited hepatitis
a. serum sickness nephritis
a. suppurative cholangitis (ASC)
a. suppurative nephritis
a. surgical abdomen
a. tubular necrosis (ATN)
a. tubular necrosis backleak
a. urate nephropathy
a. ureteric colic
a. urethral syndrome
a. urethritis
a. uric acid nephropathy
a. urinary retention (AUR)
a. variceal bleeding
a. vascular rejection
a. viral hepatitis (AVH)
a. yellow atrophy
a. yellow atrophy of liver
acute-phase response element
(APRE)
AcuTrainer handheld electronic device
Acutrim
acyclic retinoid
acyclovir sodium
acylation stimulating protein
acyltransferase
lecithin-cholesterol a. (LCAT)
acystia
A-D
antidiarrheal
Imodium A-D
A/D
arthritic dose
Ascriptin A/D

ADA
American Diabetes Association
ADA diet
Adacolumn Apheresis System
Adair-Allis forceps
Adalat CC
adalimumab
Adamantiades-Behçet syndrome
Adams Needle yucca
Adapin
adaptation
failed a.
intestinal a.
adapter, adaptor
camera a.
C-mount a.
Cook plastic Luer-Lok a.
friction-fit a.
Olympus camera with enlarging a.
Polaroid with ACMI a.
Ralks a.
swivel a.
Tuohy-Borst a.
Y a.
adaptic
A. dressing
A. packing
adaptive
a. colitis
a. gastroprotection
a. immunity
a. relaxation
a. thermogenesis (AT)
adaptor (*var. of* adapter)
ADC
antral diverticulum of colon
ADCC
antibody-dependent cell-mediated
cytotoxicity
antibody-dependent cellular cytotoxicity
Adcon-P adhesion barrier solution
ADD
angled delivery device
Add-A-Cath
Lawrence A.-A-C.
add-back treatment
Addis
A. count
A. method
Addison
A. clinical planes
A. crisis
A. disease
A. point
A. syndrome
addisonian syndrome
addisonii
melasma a.
additional unproven role

addressin
ADD'Stat laser
adducin
    alpha a.
adduct
    MAA a.
    malondialdehyde-acetaldehyde a.
adduction
    arytenoid a.
adductor
    a. brevis muscle
    a. longus muscle
ADE
    apparent digestive energy
adefovir
adelomorphous cell
adenasthenia gastrica
adenemphraxis
Aden fever
adenine
    a. phosphoribosyltransferase (APRT)
    a. phosphoribosyltransferase
      deficiency
adenitis
    mesenteric a.
    phlegmonous a.
    syphilitic inguinal a.
adenoacanthoma
adenoassociated virus (AAV)
adenocarcinoma (ACA)
    acinar a.
    anular a.
    appendiceal a.
    bladder mesonephric a.
    clear cell a.
    colloid-producing a.
    colonic a.
    colorectal a.
    duodenal a.
    esophageal a.
    exophytic a.
    flat rectal a.
    gastric a.
    giant cell a.
    hepatoid a.
    infiltrating a.
    a. in situ
    invasive a.
    metachronous small-bowel a.
    metastatic a.
    mucinous a.
    mucin-producing a.
    mucosal a.
    a. of infantile testis
    papillary a.
    Paris renal a.
    peritoneal a.
    prostatic a.

    renal a.
    rete testis a.
    scirrhous a.
    seminal vesicle a.
    testicular a.
    ulcerating a.
    urachal a.
adenofibromyoma
    testicular a.
adenoid cystic carcinoma
adenoleiomyofibroma
adenolysis
adenoma, *pl.* **adenomas, adenomata**
    acinous a.
    adrenal cortex a.
    adrenocortical a.
    aggressive a.
    aldosterone a.
    bile duct a. (BDA)
    bladder nephrogenic a.
    Brunner gland a.
    carcinoma ex pleomorphic a.
    chromophobe a.
    colonic a.
    colonoscopic view of a.
    colorectal villous a.
    cortical a.
    depressed a.
    duodenal a.
    embryonal a.
    flat a.
    gastric a.
    hepatic a.
    hepatocellular a. (HCA)
    a. hyperplastic polyp ratio
    incidental a.
    islet cell a.
    kidney a.
    Leydig cell a.
    liver cell a. (LCA)
    mesonephric a.
    metachronous a.
    moderately differentiated a.
    monopolypoid a.
    mucinous a.
    nephrogenic a.
    nonhyperfunctioning adrenocortical a.
    nonpolypoid a.
    papillary a.
    periampullary a. (PAA)
    Pick testicular a.
    Pick tubular a.
    pituitary a.
    poorly differentiated a.
    prostatic a.
    rectal villous a.
    renocortical a.
    a. sebaceum

serrated a.
sessile a.
sheetlike a.
synchronous a.
testicular tubular a.
a. to nonadenoma ratio
tubulovillous a.
undifferentiated a.
villoglandular a.
villous colorectal a.
well-differentiated a.
adenoma-associated antigen
adenoma-carcinoma sequence
adenomas (*pl. of* adenoma)
adenomata (*pl. of* adenoma)
adenomatoid tumor
adenomatosis
multiple endocrine a. type I, II
(MEA-I, −II)
adenomatous
a. colorectal polyp
a. epithelium
a. gastric polyp
a. hyperplasia
a. polyp (AP)
a. polyp-cancer sequence
a. polyp of colon (APC)
a. polyp of stomach
a. polyposis
a. polyposis coli (APC)
a. polyposis coli gene
adenomucinosis
disseminated peritoneal a.
adenomyoepithelioma of stomach
adenomyoma of gallbladder
adenomyomatosis
gallbladder a.
adenomyosarcoma
embryonal a.
adenomyosis
adenopapillomatosis
gastric a.
adenopathy
axillary a.
inguinal a.
lymph node a.
palpable a.
periductal a.
posterior mediastinal a.
adenosarcoma
embryonal a.
adenosine
a. deaminase
a. deaminase activity
a. diphosphatase (ADPase)
a. diphosphate (ADP)
a. monophosphate (AMP)
a. nucleotide

a. signal
a. triphosphatase (ATPase)
a. triphosphate (ATP)
adenosis
sclerosing a.
adenosquamous cell carcinoma
adenovirus
a. colitis
enteric a.
human a. 12
a. infection
subgroup F a.
adenovirus-12 viral protein
adenylate
a. cyclase
a. cyclase complex
adenyl cyclase stimulation
adequacy
dialysis a.
urea a.
ADF
aortoduodenal fistula
ADH
alcohol dehydrogenase
antidiuretic hormone
adherence
a. assay
bacterial a.
adherent
a. clot
a. invasive *Escherichia coli*
adhesin
bacterial a.
adhesion
antigen-independent a.
attic a.
bacterial a.
banjo-string a.
cell-cell a.
coronal a.
dense a.
a. dyspepsia
fibrous a.
filmy a.
a. formation
freeing up of a.'s
hard a.
hepatic a.
intraabdominal a.
intraperitoneal a.
lysis of a.'s
mannose-specific a.
a. molecule
omental a.
pelvic a.
perihepatic a.
peritoneal a.
postcholecystitis a.

adhesion (*continued*)
    postoperative a.
    preputial a.
    taking down of a.'s
    T-cell a.
    thick a.
    thin a.
    tight perirectal a.
    tuft a.
    violin-string a.
adhesive
    a. band
    a. base
    Comfeel skin a.
    a. dressing
    fibrin tissue a.
    a. ileus
    Indermil a.
    Mastisol liquid surgical a.
    a. peritonitis
    a. protein receptor
    a. tape
    tissue a.
    Uro-Bond skin a.
ADHF
    American Digestive Health
    Foundation
Adipex-P
adiphenine
adipocele
adipohepatic
adipolytic
adiponectin
adipopectic
adipopexis
AdipoR1
AdipoR2
adipose
    a. artery of kidney
    a. capsule of kidney
    a. tissue
adiposogenital dystrophy
adiposum
    hepar a.
adiposuria
adiposus
    ascites a.
adjacent hepatic artery
adjunctive nephrectomy
adjustable silicone gastric banding (ASGB)
adjusted body mass (ABM)
adjustment
    risk a.
adjuvant
    a. alpha blockade
    anesthesia a.
    a. drug therapy
    Freund a.

    a. hepatic arterial infusion chemotherapy
    a. nephrectomy
    a. treatment
Adlone
adminicula (*pl. of* adminiculum)
adminiculum, *pl.* **adminicula**
    a. lineae albae
administration
    intravesical electromotive drug a.
    percutaneous bacille Calmette-Gúerin a.
adnexa
    hepatocellular a.
adnexal
    a. fullness
    a. mass
    a. tenderness
    a. torsion
    a. tumor
adolescent
    a. genitalia
    a. genitourinary examination
    a. incontinence
    a. penis
    a. spina bifida
    a. stress hematuria
    a. urologic evaluation
adonis
adoptive immunotherapy
ADP
    adenosine diphosphate
ADPase
    adenosine diphosphatase
ADPKD
    autosomal-dominant polycystic kidney disease
        oligosymptomatic ADPKD
ADPKD1
    autosomal-dominant polycystic kidney disease 1
    A. gene
    A. genotype
ADPKD2
    autosomal-dominant polycystic kidney disease 2
    A. genotype
adrenal
    accessory a.
    a. artery
    a. catecholamine
    a. cortex
    a. cortex adenoma
    a. cortex androgen
    a. cortex carcinoma
    a. cortex estrogen-secreting tumor
    a. cortex fine-needle biopsy
    a. cortex ganglioneuroma
    a. cortex hyperfunction

a. cortex testosterone-secreting tumor
a. cortex zone
a. corticoadenoma
a. crisis
a. cryptococcosis
a. disease
a. gland
a. gland atrophy
a. gland composition
a. gland cyst
a. gland incidentaloma
a. gland innervation
a. gland laparoscopic excision
a. gland mass
a. gland melanoma
a. gland metastatic tumor
a. gland microscopic section
a. gland myelolipoma
a. hemorrhage
a. hirsutism
a. insufficiency
Marchand a.'s
a. medulla
a. rest
a. rest tumor
a. scintigraphy
a. steroid
a. tuberculosis
a. vein
a. vein aldosterone sampling
a. venography
a. virilism
a. zona glomerulosa hyperplasia

adrenalectomy
ablative a.
endoscopic a.
flank approach a.
ipsilateral a.
laparoscopic a.
needlescopic laparoscopic a.
open a.
partial a.
retroperitoneoscopic a.
thoracoscopic transdiaphragmatic a.
transperitoneal laparoscopic a. (TLA)

adrenalin
a. chloride
a. injection
a. injection therapy

adrenalinuria
adrenal-sparing surgery
adrenergic
alpha a.
a. neuron
a. receptor
a. signal

adrenergic-cholinergic agonist
adrenoceptive

adrenocortical
a. adenoma
a. carcinoma
a. macrocyst

adrenocorticohyperplasia
adrenocorticotrophic (*var. of* adrenocorticotropic)
adrenocorticotropic, adrenocorticotrophic
a. hormone (ACTH)
a. hormone infusion test

adrenogenital syndrome
adrenomedullin 52-amino acid peptide
adrenoreceptor
alpha-1 a.

adrenostatic
adrenotoxin
adrenotrophic (*var. of* adrenotropic)
adrenotropic, adrenotrophic
adrenotropin
adrenotropism
Adriamycin
cisplatin, cyclophosphamide, A. (CisCA, CISCA)
A. glomerulopathy
A. nephropathy
A. PFS

Adriamycin-induced nephrosis
Adrucil
Adson
A. clamp
A. dissecting hook
A. needle holder
A. suction tube
A. tissue forceps

Adson-Brown tissue forceps
adsorption
ADT
adenosine triphosphate

adult
a. celiac disease (ACD)
a. familial hyaline membrane disease
a. hypolactasia
a. intersexual
a. lactase deficiency
a. phimosis
a. polycystic kidney disease (APKD)
a. polycystic liver disease (APLD)
a. sigmoidoscope

adult-onset
a.-o. nocturnal enuresis
a.-o. obesity

advance
A. formula
A. male sling
postoperative a.
preoperative a.
technical a.
a. to regular diet

advanced
> A. Care cholesterol test
> a. glycation end (AGE)
> Imodium A.
> A. surgical suture applier
> A. Systems Integration (ASI)
> a. therapeutic endoscopy

Advanced-RF Natal Care

advancement
> Duckett meatal a.
> Glenn-Anderson a.
> meatal a.
> a. of rectal flap
> sleeve a.
> a. sleeve flap

Advanta bed

advantage
> A. midurethral sling
> GE RT 3200 A. II

Advantx digital system

adventitia
> fibrofatty a.
> tunica a.

adventitial fibroplasia

adventitious
> a. albuminuria
> a. cyst

adverse prognostic factor

Advia
> A. Centaur HAV IgM immunoassay
> A. Centaur HBc Total
> immunoassay

Advicor

adynamic
> a. bone
> a. bone disease (ABD)
> a. ileus
> a. intestinal obstruction

adysplasia
> kidney a.

Adzorbstar

AEC
> American Endosonography Club
> AEC Study

AEFI
> acute esophageal food impaction

AEG
> acute erosive gastritis

AELT
> ascites euglobulin lysis time

Aeo-O-Scope colonoscope

AEP
> acute edematous pancreatitis

AER
> albumin excretion rate
> alcohol elimination rate
> automatic endoscopic reprocessor

AERD
> atheroembolic renal disease

aerobic
> a. culture
> a. glycolysis

Aerococcus

aerocystography

aerocystoscope

aerocystoscopy

aerodigestive tract

aerogastria
> blocked a.

aerogenes
> *Enterobacter a.*

Aeromonas
> *A. bestiarum*
> *A. caviae*
> *A. diarrhea*
> *A. hydrophila*
> *A. liquefaciens*
> *A. media*
> *A. punctata*
> *A. salmonicida*
> *A. sobria*
> *A. trota*

***Aeromonas*-associated enterocolitis**

aeroperitonia

aerophagia, aerophagy

aerophagy (*var. of* aerophagia)

aerosialophagy

aerosis

aerosol
> hydrocortisone acetate rectal a.
> inhalation a.
> ^{99m}Tc DTPA a.

aerourethroscope

aerourethroscopy

aeruginosa
> *Pseudomonas a.*

aeruginosum
> sputum a.

AES
> anal endosonography
> anterior esophageal sensor

AESOP
> automated endoscopic system for
> optimal positioning

aethoxysclerol

AFB
> acid-fast bacillus

AFBN
> acute focal bacterial nephritis

afferent
> a. arteriolar vasoconstriction
> a. glomerular arteriole
> a. ileal limb
> a. innervation
> a. jejunal limb
> a. limb nipple stenosis
> a. loop
> a. loop syndrome

a. nerve fiber
a. neuron
a. projection
a. renal nerve
a. terminal
a. tubular isoperistaltic segment
a. vessel of glomerulus

afferentia
vasa a.

affinity-avidity hypothesis
aflatoxin
AFLP
acute fatty liver of pregnancy
AFP
alpha fetoprotein
African
A. hemochromatosis
A. iron overload
A. potato
African-American
A.-A. Study of Kidney Disease
A.-A. Study of Kidney Disease and
Hypertension (AASK)
africanum
Pygeum a.
AFTP
ascitic fluid total protein
AFUD
American Foundation for Urologic
Diseases
A/G
albumin-globulin ratio
AG
albumin-globulin
Trial AG
AGA
American Gastroenterological
Association
antigliadin antibody
IgG AGA
agalactiae
Streptococcus a.
agalactosuria
agammaglobulinemia
Bruton-type a.
X-linked infantile a.
aganglionic
a. bowel
a. megacolon
a. segment of colon
aganglionosis
congenital intestinal a. (CIA)
agar
brain-heart infusion a.
a. bridge
a. dilution
EMB a.
eosin-methylene blue a.
a. gel

MacConkey a.
phenylethyl alcohol a.
Sabouraud glucose a.
sorbitol-MacConkey a.
thiosulfate-citrate-bile salts-sucrose a.
(TCBS)
vancomycin/nalidixic acid a.
Wilkins-Chalgren a.

agarose
a. gel
a. gel electrophoresis
agastria
agastric
AGE
acute gastroenteritis
advanced glycation end
agency
Regional Organ Procurement A.
(ROPA)
agenesis
bladder a.
corpus callosum a.
kidney a.
pancreatic a.
renal a.
sacral a.
scrotal a.
seminal vesicle a.
agenitalism
agenosomia
agent
acid suppressive a.
Albunex imaging/contrast a.
antiadhesive a.
anticholinergic a.
antidiarrheal a.
antidiuretic hormonelike a.
antifungal a.
antihypertensive a.
antimicrobial a.
antimotility a.
antimuscarinic a.
antisecretory a.
antispasmodic a.
5-ASA a.
azole antifungal a.
benzamide prokinetic a.
beta sympathomimetic tocolytic a.
bulk a.
bulking a.
carbon dioxide trapping a.
central adrenergic a.
chemotherapeutic a.
contrast a.
cyanocobalamin radioactive a.
cytotoxic a.
distal tubular acting a.
Durasphere injectable bulking a.
embolic a.

agent (*continued*)
    gadolinium EOB-DTPA contrast a.
    gallstone solubilizing a.
    gastrokinetic a.
    Hawaii a.
    hemostatic a.
    imidoacetic acid radioactive a.
    immunosuppressive a.
    interleukin-2 receptor-blocking a.
    iodinated contrast a.
    iopamidol contrast imaging a.
    Levovist contrast a.
    Macroplastique soft tissue synthetic
      bulking a.
    motility a.
    mucolytic a.
    nonsteroidal antiinflammatory a.
      (NSAIA)
    Norwalk a.
    paramagnetic contrast a.
    parasympathomimetic a.
    peripheral adrenergic a.
    periurethral bulking a.
    pharmacologic a.
    progestational a.
    progesteronal a.
    prokinetic a.
    renoprotective a.
    rose bengal sodium [131]I
      radioactive a.
    Rubratope-57 radioactive a.
    sclerosing a.
    selenomethionine radioactive a.
    Sethotope radioactive a.
    test-yolk buffer
      cryopreservation a.
    thrombolytic a.
    vanilloid a.
    virucidal a.
    Yoshi-864 antineoplastic
      alkylating a.
age-related nocturia
ageusia, ageustia
ageusic
ageustia (*var. of* ageusia)
agglomerate
    acinar a.
agglutination
    Ames semiquantitative a.
    a. test
agglutinin
    febrile a.'s
    peanut a.
aggregate
    lymphoid a.
aggregated lymphatic follicles
  of Peyer
aggregati
    folliculi lymphatici a.

aggregation
    bile salt a.
    erythrocyte a.
    familial a.
aggressive
    a. adenoma
    a. fibromatosis
    a. therapeutic trial
Agile patency system
agilis
    Lactobacillus a.
aglomerular
AGN
    acute glomerulonephritis
agnogenic myeloid metaplasia
agona
    Salmonella a.
agonadal
agonadism
agonic intussusception
agonist
    adrenergic-cholinergic a.
    alpha-1 a.
    alpha-adrenergic a.
    alpha-2 adrenergic a.
    Bay K 8644 channel a.
    beta-2 a.
    beta-3 a.
    beta adrenergic a.
    cholinergic a.
    dopamine a.
    dopaminergic a.
    farnesoid X receptor a.
    5-HT4 a.
    kappa receptor opioid a.
    motilin a.
    muscarinic cholinergic a.
    nicotinic a.
    nonpeptidyl a.
    opioid receptor a. (ORA)
Agoral
agouti-related protein
AGP
    acute gallstone pancreatitis
agranulocytic ulcer
agrimony
AGUS
    atypical glandular cells of unknown
      significance
ahaustral
AHC
    acute hemorrhagic cystitis
AHD
    arteriohepatic dysplasia
AHLT
    auxiliary heterotopic liver
      transplantation
AHP
    acute hemorrhagic pancreatitis

A-Hydrocort
Aichi virus
AID
    artificial insemination donor
AIDS
    acquired immunodeficiency
    syndrome
AIDS-related complex (ARC)
AIH
    artificial insemination husband
    autoimmune hepatitis
A28 immunologic study
AIN
    acute interstitial nephritis
    anal intraepithelial neoplasia
AIO
    all-in-one
        AIO parenteral solution
AIP
    acute intermittent porphyria
    aldosterone-induced protein
AIPRI
    angiotensin-converting enzyme
        inhibition in progressive renal
        insufficiency
        AIPRI trial
air
    biliary a.
    blood gas on room a.
    a. cushion
    a. cyst
    a. cystogram
    a. embolism
    free a.
    a. insufflation
    intramural colonic a.
    intraperitoneal a.
    a. pressure enema reduction
    a. pyelography
    a. swallowing
    a. thermometer
    a. tightness test
air-contrast barium enema (ACBE)
air-filled
    a.-f. balloon
    a.-f. loop
airflow obstruction
air-fluid level
airfuge
    Beckman a.
Airlift balloon retractor
airway
    double-lumen gastric laryngeal
      mask a.
    a. epithelium
    esophageal gastric tube a.
      (EGTA)
    esophageal obturator a. (EOA)
    gastric laryngeal mask a. (GLMA)

    a. obstruction
    patent a.
airway-arterial fistula
AJCC
    American Joint Committee on Cancer
    AJCC TNM tumor classification
AJCC/UICC
    American Joint Committee on
      Cancer/International Union Against
      Cancer
    AJCC/UICC staging system
Ajmalin
    A. liver disease
    A. liver injury
AJPBD
    anomalous junction of
      pancreaticobiliary ducts
Akerlund
    A. deformity
    diverticulum of A.
akinesia, akinesis
    rectal a.
akinesis (*var. of* akinesia)
Aksys PHD system
5-ALA
    5-aminolevulinic acid
ALA
    aminolevulinic acid
    antilymphocyte antibody
alactasia
Alagille syndrome
Alagille-Watson syndrome
AL amyloid
alanine aminotransferase (ALT)
alanine-glyoxylate aminotransferase
alarm
    bed-wetting a.
    a. clock voiding
    enuresis a.
    glutaraldehyde a.
    a. symptom
    a. therapy
alascence
    Diphyllobothrium a.
Alaxin
Alazide
alba
    linea a.
albae
    adminiculum lineae a.
Albarran
    A. deflecting level
    A. disease
    A. gland
    A. laser cystoscope
    A. mechanism
    A. reflecting bridge
    A. test
    A. tubule

albendazole
albensis
    Vibrio cholerae biotype *a.*
Albert-Lembert
    A.-L. method
    A.-L. suture
Albert suture
albicans
    Candida a.
albiduria, albinuria
albinuria (*var. of* albiduria)
Albright
    A. hereditary osteodystrophy
    A. solution
Albuferon
albuginea
    a. penis
    a. testis
    tunica a.
albugineotomy
albugineous
albuginitis
albumin
    Bence Jones a.
    bovine serum a. (BSA)
    a. dialysis
    diethylenetriamine-pentaacetic acid-galactosyl-human serum a.
    a. excretion rate (AER)
    fatty acid-free bovine serum a.
    glycated a.
    a. gradient
    human serum a.
    ^{125}I a.
    intravenous a.
    macroaggregated a. (MAA)
    a. messenger RNA
    a. metabolism
    nonglycated a.
    plasma a.
    a. plasma concentration
    serum a. (SAB)
    sonicated a.
    a. synthesis
    technetium-99m galactosyl-human serum a. (^{99m}Tc-GSA)
    technetium-99m macroaggregated a. (^{99m}Tc-MAA)
albuminaturia
albumin-bound toxin
albumin-coated resin hemoperfusion
albumin-globulin (AG)
    albumin-globulin ratio (A/G)
albuminocholia
albuminoid liver
albuminorrhea (*var. of* albuminuria)
albuminous nephritis
albuminuria, albuminorrhea

    adventitious a.
    Bamberger hematogenic a.
    globular a.
    nephrogenous a.
    postrenal a.
    residual a.
albuminuric retinitis
albumosuria
    Bence Jones a.
Albunex
    A. imaging/contrast agent
    A. injection
albus
    Staphylococcus a.
Albustix test
alcalifaciens
    Providencia a.
Alcian
    A. blue
    A. blue and periodic acid-Schiff (AB/PAS)
    A. blue dye
    A. blue stain
Alcock
    A. canal
    A. syndrome
Alcock-Timberlake obturator
alcohol
    absolute a.
    a. absorption
    a. abuse
    a. consumption
    a. cooling bath
    a. dehydrogenase (ADH)
    a. dehydrogenase inhibition
    a. diuresis
    a. elimination rate (AER)
    ethyl a. (EtOH)
    ethylene-vinyl a.
    graded a.
    a. injection of tumor
    a. intoxication
    isoamyl a.
    polyvinyl a.
    a. potentiation
    a. sclerosis
    a. thermometer
alcohol-fixed gastric biopsy
alcoholic
    a. cirrhosis
    a. diarrhea
    a. fatty liver
    a. fibrosis
    a. foamy degeneration
    a. hemorrhagic gastritis
    a. hepatitis
    a. hyalin
    a. liver disease (ALD)

a. pancreatitis
a. prognostic factor
a. varix
alcohol-induced
a.-i. extracellular volume
contraction
a.-i. gastric injury
a.-i. gastrointestinal symptom
a.-i. hypoglycemia
a.-i. pancreatitis
alcoholism
American Medical Society on A.
(AMSA)
alcoholuria
**alcohol-use disorders identification test
(AUDIT)**
Alconefrin
ALD
alcoholic liver disease
Aldactazide
Aldactone
Aldara
aldehyde dehydrogenase (ALDH)
Alden loop gastric bypass
alder
black a.
aldesleukin
ALDH
aldehyde dehydrogenase
Aldoclor
aldolase
fructose a.
Aldomet
Aldoril
aldose reductase (AR)
aldosterone
a. adenoma
a. blockade
a. deficiency
a. synthase
a. synthase polymorphism
aldosterone-induced protein (AIP)
**aldosterone-sensitive distal
nephron**
aldosterone-to-renin ratio
aldosteronism
aldosteronoma
aldosteronopenia
aldosteronuria
Aldrich-Mees line
Aldridge operation
alemtuzumab
alendronate
Aleo meter
Alequel
alert
Sears Wee A.
aletris

Alexander-Adams operation
Alexander elevator
alexandrite
a. and rhodamine
a. laser
a. laser lithotripsy
alexithymia
aleydigism
ALF
acute liver failure
American Liver Foundation
alfa
darbepoetin a.
epoetin a.
IFN a.
interferon a. (IFNa)
a. interferon
a. interferon therapy
a. interferon treatment
lymphoblastoid interferon a.
recombinant interferon a. (rIFN-A,
rIFN-alfa)
alfa-2a
interferon a.-2a (IFNa-2a)
PEG-interferon a.-2a
recombinant interferon a.-2a
teceleukin and interferon a.-2a
alfacon-1
interferon a.-1
Alfa-gliatest
ELISA Kit A.-g.
alfa-n1
interferon a.-n1
alfa-n3
interferon a.-n3
alfaxalone
alfentanil
Alferon N
alfuzosin HCl
Algenic Alka
algesimeter
Boas a.
Al-Ghorab
A.-G. modification
A.-G. modification shunt
A.-G. procedure
Algicon
Algidex Ag Silver dressing
algidicarnis
Clostridium a.
algid malaria
alginate spray
alginolyticus
Vibrio a.
alginuresis
Alglucerase
algoid cell
Alibra

alicaforsen
Alimaxx-E esophageal stent system
alimentary
>a. apparatus
>a. bolus
>a. canal
>a. diabetes
>a. edema
>a. glycosuria
>a. hyperinsulinism
>a. obesity
>a. system
>a. therapy
>a. tract
>a. tract duplication

alimentation
>central venous a.
>enteral a.
>forced a.
>parenteral a.
>peripheral intravenous a.
>rectal a.
>total parenteral a.

Alimentum
A-line
>arterial line

aliquot
AlitraQ
Alka
>Algenic A.

alkali
>caustic a.
>a. ingestion

alkaline
>a. citrate therapy
>a. injury
>a. milk drip
>a. phosphatase (ALP, AP)
>a. phosphatase-antialkaline phosphatase (APAAP)
>a. phosphatase isoenzyme
>a. phosphatase test
>a. phosphatase Vectastain ABC
>a. protease inhibitor (API)
>a. reflux esophagitis
>a. reflux gastritis (ARG)

alkaline-ash diet
alkalinity
alkalinization
>oral a.
>a. test
>urinary a.

alkalitherapy
alkaloid
>ergot a.
>indolalkylamine a.
>*Veratrum* a.

alkalosis
>hypochloremic-hypokalemic metabolic a.
>hypokalemic metabolic a.
>metabolic a.
>respiratory a.
>watery diarrhea with hypokalemic a. (WDHA)

Alka-Mints
alkane
>breath a.

alkanet
alkaptonuria
Alka-Seltzer
Alken renal stone approach
Alkets
ALL
>acute lymphoblastic leukemia
>acute lymphocytic leukemia

allantoic
>a. cyst
>a. tract

allantois
allele
>carrier of a.
>HLA-DP a.
>I1307K a.
>IK a.

allelic
allelotyping
>p53 a.

Allemann syndrome
Allen
>A. anastomosis clamp
>A. intestinal clamp
>A. intestinal forceps
>A. stirrup
>A. strap
>A. test

Allen-Brown shunt
Allen-Kocher clamp
Allen-Masters syndrome
allergen
>food a.

allergic
>a. colitis
>a. cystitis
>a. dermatitis
>a. enteropathy
>a. eosinophilic esophagitis
>a. interstitial nephritis (AIN)
>a. proctitis
>a. reaction
>a. vasculitis

allergy
>cow's milk a. (CMA)
>cow's milk protein a.
>food a.
>gastrointestinal a.

latex a.
medication a.
ALLHAT
    antihypertensive and lipid-lowering
      treatment to prevent heart attack trial
Alliance
    A. II inflation system
    A. integrated inflation system
Allient Sorbent hemodialysis system
alligator jaws Olympus grasping forceps
alligator-type grasping forceps
Allingham
    A. colotomy
    A. fissure
    A. operation
    A. rectum excision
    A. ulcer
all-in-one (AIO)
Allis
    A. catheter
    A. clamp
    A. forceps
    A. inhaler
    A. tooth grasper
Alliston GE reflux repair
allium vegetable
alloantibody
    donor-specific a.
alloantigen-dependent
    postoperative a.-d.
alloantigen response
alloantigen-specific
allocating cadaveric kidney
allocation
    Eurotransplant kidney a.
allochezia
allodynia
allogeneic (*var. of* allogenic)
allogenic, allogeneic
    a. hepatocyte
    a. kidney transplant
    a. liver perfusion
    a. mixed leukocyte culture
    a. MLC
allograft
    clinically stable human renal a.
    hepatic a.
    human leukocyte antigen renal a.
    injured a.
    kidney a.
    long-term survival of renal a.
    nephrectomy a.
    outcome of cadaveric renal a.
    a. parenchyma
    a. rejection
    renal a.
    Repliform dermal a.
    a. survival
    a. survival rate

allograft-mediated hypertension
AlloMune system
alloplast
    bioactive antimicrobial coated solid
      a.
alloplastic
    a. biomaterial
    a. prostatic bladder
    a. spermatocele
allopurinol
allorecognition
allotransplantation
    pediatric renal a.
    renal a.
allowance
    recommended daily a. (RDA)
all-purpose capsule (APC)
All-Silicone Side-Eye EPT feeding tube
allylamine
Almacone II
aloe
    cascara sagrada and a.
Aloka MP-PN ultrasound probe
alopecia
alosetron
    a. HCl
    a. HCl tablet
    a. hydrochloride
Aloxi
ALP
    alkaline phosphatase
alpha
    a. adducin
    a. adrenergic
    a. blockade
    a. chain disease
    a. dextrinase
    ER a.
    estrogen receptor a. (ER alpha)
    a. fetoprotein (AFP)
    a. fetoprotein level
    a. gene
    a. glycerylphosphorylcholine
    a. heavy-chain disease
    a. hemolytic streptococcus
    a. hydroxylase
    A. I inflatable penile prosthesis
    A. I penile implant
    a. ketoacid dehydrogenase
    a. ketoglutaramate
    a. methylparatyrosine
    a. motor neuron
    a. receptor antagonist
    a. receptor blockade therapy
    a. *Streptococcus viridans*
    a. sympathetic blockade
    transforming growth factor a.
      (TGF-alpha)
    tumor necrosis factor a.

alpha-1
    a.-1 acid glycoprotein
    a.-1 adrenergic receptor
    a.-1 adrenoceptor antagonist
    a.-1 adrenoreceptor
    a.-1 agonist
    a.-1 antitrypsin
    a.-1 antitrypsin globulin
    a.-1 antitrypsin level
    a.-1 blocker
    a.-1 globulin
    a.-1 glycero-monooctanoin

alpha-2
    a.-2 adrenergic agonist
    a.-2 adrenergic receptor
    a.-2 beta-1 integrin cell-surface
       c.

alpha-3
    a.-3 beta-1 integrin
    alpha-3, -4, -5 chain

alpha-adrenergic
    a.-a. agonist
    a.-a. antagonist
    a.-a. receptor

alpha-2a interferon
alpha-amylase
    pancreatic a.-a.

5-alpha-androstane-3-alpha 17-beta-diol
5-alpha-androstane-3-beta 17-beta-diol
alpha-21 antiplasmin
alpha-1-antitrypsin
    a.-1-a. deficiency
    a.-1-a. deficiency disease
    a.-1-a. disease (AATD)
    a.-1-a. disease-related
       emphysema

alpha-2b
alpha-5 beta-1 integrin
alpha-blocker
    a.-b. therapy
    a.-b. treatment

7-alpha-dehydroxylation
alpha-delta mannosidase
9-alpha-fluorohydrocortisone
alpha-galactosidase A
alpha-gliadin fraction
alpha-glucosidase inhibitor
17-alpha-hydroxylase deficiency
alpha-KG
alpha-KGDH
alpha-KGM
alpha-loop maneuver
Alphamul
alphaprodine
alpha-receptor
5-alpha-reductase
    5-a.-r. inhibition
    5-a.-r. inhibitor

alpha-sigmoid loop
alpha-TGI
alpine cranberry
Alport syndrome
ALPP
    abdominal leak-point pressure
alprazolam
alprostadil/prazosin HCl
alprostadil urethral suppository
Alprox-TD
ALR cystoresectoscope
Alstrom disease
Alstrom-Edwards syndrome
ALT
    alanine aminotransferase
    ALT test
Altace
Altemeier
    A. perineal rectal pullthrough
      procedure
    A. perineal rectosigmoidectomy
    A. repair
alteration
    genetic a.
    molecular genetic a.
    nuclear matrix a.
altered sperm motility
ALternaGEL
alternate-day treatment
alternate mRNA splicing
alternating calculi
alternative
    a. cell attachment domain
    a. endourological procedure
Altertome
    Microvasive A.
Althausen test
Altmann pulse
Altracin
Altra-Flux hemodialyzer
Altra Nova hemodialyzer
ALT-RCC
    autolymphocyte-based treatment for
      renal cell carcinoma
altretamine
Altrex hemodialyzer
Alu-Cap
Aludrox
alum
    a. curd
    intravesical a.
aluminum
    a. carbonate
    a. hydroxide
    a. hydroxide and magnesium
      trisilicate
    a. hydroxide, magnesium hydroxide,
      and simethicone

A

a. phosphate
a. toxicity
Alupent
Alutabs
alvei
    Hafnia a.
alveolar
    a. echinococcosis
    a. hydatid cyst
    a. hydatid disease
    a. rhabdomyosarcoma
AlveoSampler
    QuinTron A.
alverine citrate
alvi
    incontinentia a.
alvimopan
alvine calculus
alvus
Alzer osmotic minipump
AMA
    antimitochondrial antibody
    AMA inflatable cylinder
Amadori product
AMAG
    autoimmune metaplastic atrophic
    gastritis
amalonaticus
    Citrobacter a.
Amanita
    A. mushroom
    A. mushroom hepatotoxicity
    A. *phalloides* mushroom
    poisoning
amantadine
amaranth, amaranthum
amaranthum (*var. of* amaranth)
Amaryl
amasesis
amastigote
amatoxin
amaurosis
    Leber a.
AmB
    amphotericin B
ambenonium chloride
Ambicor penile prosthesis
ambigua
    Shigella a.
ambiguous external genitalia
ambiguus
    nucleus a.
Ambilhar
AmB-induced reduction GFR
ambiothermic
AmBisome
amblygeustia
ambulant (*var. of* ambulatory)

ambulation
ambulatory, ambulant
    a. blood pressure
    a. hemorrhoidectomy
    a. intraesophageal bilirubin
    monitoring
    a. intraesophageal pH monitoring
    a. manometry
    a. probe
    a. urodynamic monitoring (AUM)
    a. urodynamics
ameba, *pl.* **amebae,** *pl.* **amebas**
amebae (*pl. of* ameba)
amebas (*pl. of* ameba)
amebiasis
    hepatic a.
    indigenous a.
    intestinal a.
    a. of bladder
amebic
    a. appendicitis
    a. colitis
    a. dysentery
    a. granuloma
    a. hepatitis
    a. lectin antigen
    a. liver abscess
    a. trophozoite
    a. ulcer
amebicidal
amebism
ameboma mimicking carcinoma
ameliorated vasodilating response
America
    Crohn and Colitis Foundation of A.
    (CCFA)
American
    A. ACMI flexible fiberoptic
    sigmoidoscope
    A. Anorexia/Bulimia Association
    A. Association for the Study of
    Liver Diseases (AASLD)
    A. Association of Kidney
    Patients
    A. Board of Colon and Rectal
    Surgery
    A. College of Gastroenterology
    (ACG)
    A. College of Medical Informatics
    (ACMI)
    A. College of Physicians-American
    Society of Internal Medicine
    (ACP-ASIM)
    A. Diabetes Association (ADA)
    A. Digestive Health Foundation
    (ADHF)
    A. Endoscopy automatic reprocessor
    A. Endoscopy dilator

American (*continued*)
A. Endoscopy mechanical lithotriptor
A. Endosonography Club (AEC)
A. Endosonography Club study
A. Foundation for Urologic Diseases (AFUD)
A. Gastroenterological Association (AGA)
A. Joint Committee on Cancer (AJCC)
A. Joint Committee on Cancer/International Union Against Cancer (AJCC/UICC)
A. Kidney Fund
A. Liver Foundation (ALF)
A. liverwort
A. Medical Society on Alcoholism (AMSA)
A. Medical Systems (AMS)
A. Society for Gastrointestinal Endoscopy (ASGE)
A. Society of Nephrology
A. trypanosomiasis
A. Urological Association (AUA)
A. Urological Association symptom index
A. white pond lily
American-type culture collection
americanus
    Necator a.
Amerigel dressing
Amerlex-M second antibody
Ames
A. Hemastix reagent strip
A. semiquantitative agglutination
A. test
A-Methapred
AMF
    autocrine motility factor
Amicar
Amicon filter
amicrobic cystitis
amicrofilaremic filariasis
amidation
    carboxyl-terminal a.
amidolytic assay
amifloxacin
amifostine
amikacin
Amikin
amiloride hydrochloride
Amin-Aid powdered feeding
amine
    aromatic a.
    biogenic a.
    a. precursor uptake and decarboxylation (APUD)
    a. precursor uptake and decarboxylation cell

primary a.
secondary a.
tertiary a.
amino
a. acid
a. acid abnormality
a. acid-based dialysate solution
a. acid excretion in neonate
a. acid-glucose mixture
A. Mel Hepa
a. terminus
aminoacetate
dihydroxyaluminum a.
aminoacidopathy
dibasic a.
28-amino acid peptide
aminoaciduria
hyperdibasic a.
imidazole a.
a. in neonate
overflow a.
renal a.
transport a.
aminobenzoate
butyl a.
a. potassium
4-aminobiphenyl
aminobisphosphonate gastrotoxic drug
aminocaproic acid (ACA)
Aminofusin L Forte amino acid solution
aminoglutethimide
aminoglycoside
aminoguanidine
aminoisobutyric aciduria
5-aminolevulinic
5-a. acid (5-ALA)
5-a. acid-induced fluorescence endoscopy
5-a. acid-induced fluorescence laparoscopy
aminolevulinic acid (ALA)
aminonucleoside
glomerular epithelial cell toxin puromycin a.
puromycin a.
aminopenicillin
aminopeptidase
leucine a. (LAP)
aminophylline
aminopromazine
aminopropionitrile
beta a.
aminopropylation
aminopyrine
a. breath test
a. clearance
aminorex

aminosalicylate
5-aminosalicylic
    5-a. acid (5-ASA)
    5-a. acid enema
4-aminosalicylic acid (4-ASA)
amino-terminal undecapeptide
aminothiol concentration
aminotransferase
    alanine a. (ALT)
    alanine-glyoxylate a.
    aspartate a. (AST)
amiodarone
Amipaque
Amitiza
Amitone
amitriptyline hydrochloride
amlodipine besylate
ammonemia, ammoniemia,
 hyperammonemia
    idiopathic a.
ammonia
    arterial a.
    blood a.
    a. level
    plasma a.
    a. production
    serum a.
    a. toxicity
ammonia-13 (^{13}N)
ammoniagenesis
ammoniagenic coma
ammoniemia (*var. of* ammonemia)
ammonium
    a. acid urate calculus
    a. acid urate urolithiasis
    a. hydroxide
amnion
amodiaquine
Amoeba
Amogel PG
amorphous filling defect
amoxicillin
    a. and clavulanic acid
    luminal a.
    a. trihydrate
amoxicillin-clavulanate treatment
amoxicillin-omeprazole treatment
amoxicillin-tinidazole-ranitidine therapy
Amoxil
amp
    amperage
AMP
    adenosine monophosphate
      AMP level
      urinary cyclic AMP
AMP-c
    cyclic adenosine monophosphate
amperage (amp)
amphetamine

amphibolic, amphibolous
    a. fistula
amphipathic bile salt
amphiregulin (AR)
Amphocin
Amphojel
Amphotec
amphotericin
    a. B (AmB)
    a. B-induced reduction glomerular
      filtration rate
    a. B nephropathy
    a. B resistance
    a. B therapy
    liposomal a. B (L-Amb)
ampicillin
Ampicin
Amplatz
    A. catheter
    A. fascial dilator
    A. sheath
    A. Super Stiff guidewire
    A. TractMaster system
Amplicor
    A. HBV monitor test
    A. HCV RNA test
amplification
    a. refractory mutation
      system-polymerase chain reaction
      (ARMS-PCR)
    transcription-mediated a. (TMA)
amplitude
    esophageal body contraction a.
    high-energy a.
    mean distal contraction a.
      (MDCA)
amplitude-acrophase vector
amplitude-coded color Doppler
 sonography
ampulla, *pl.* **ampullae**
    a. ductus deferentis
    duodenal a.
    Henle a.
    a. hepatopancreatica
    invagination of a.
    Lieberkühn a.
    a. of rectum
    a. of vas deferens
    a. of Vater
    rectal a.
    a. recti
ampullae (*pl. of* ampulla)
ampullary
    a. ablative therapy
    a. carcinoma
    a. granulation tissue
    a. hamartoma
    a. lesion
    a. stenosis

ampullary (*continued*)
    a. stone
    a. tumor
ampullectomy
    endoscopic snare a.
    mucosectomy cap-assisted a.
ampulloma
ampullopancreatic carcinoma
amputation
    penile a.
AMS
    American Medical Systems
    AMS controlled-expansion penile
      prosthesis
    AMS double-cuff Silastic artificial
      urinary sphincter
    AMS Hydroflex penile prosthesis
    AMS inflatable penile prosthesis
    AMS malleable penile prosthesis
    AMS penile prosthesis cylinder
    AMS 3-piece inflatable penile
      prosthesis
    AMS ProstaJect ethanol injection
      system
    AMS Sphincter urinary prosthesis
    AMS Ultrex penile prosthesis
AMSA
    American Medical Society on
    Alcoholism
    amsacrine
amsacrine (AMSA)
Amsterdam
    A. biliary stent
    A. criteria
    A. criteria for hereditary
      nonpolyposis colorectal cancer
Amsterdam-type prosthesis
Amussat
    A. incision
    A. operation
    A. valve
    A. valvula
amygdala, *pl.* **amygdalae**
amygdalae (*pl. of* amygdala)
amylacea
    corpora a.
amylase
    ascitic a.
    a. concentration
    pancreatic alpha a.
    P-type a.
    salivary a.
    serum a.
    S-type a.
    a. unit
    urinary a.
amylase/creatinine clearance ratio
amylase-resistant starch (ARS)
amylin

amyl nitrite
amyloglucosidase
amylo-1,6-glucosidase deficiency
amyloid
    AA a.
    AL a.
    a. kidney
    a. nephropathy
    a. nephrosis
    serum a. A (SAA)
    serum a. P (SAP)
amyloidlike glomerulopathy
amyloidoma
amyloidosis
    cutaneous lichen a.
    hepatic a.
    kidney a.
    localized a.
    a. of bladder
    rectal a.
    renal a.
    secondary a.
    systemic a.
    type IV a.
amyloidosis-associated kidney disease
amyloidotic glomerulus
amylopectinosis
amylorrhea
amylosuria, amyluria
amyluria (*var. of* amylosuria)
ANA
    antinuclear antibody
anabolic
    a. steroid
    a. steroid spermatogenesis
      impairment
    a. steroid treatment
***Anacardium occidentale* L**
anacidic stomach
anacidity
ANAD
    anorexia nervosa and associated
    disorders
anadenia ventriculi
anaerobe
    obligate a.
anaerobic
    a. culture
    a. glycolysis
anaerobiotic
anal
    a. abscess
    a. anastomosis
    a. atresia
    a. bag
    a. bulging
    a. canal
    a. canal hypertonia
    a. canal length (ACL)

A

a. column
a. condyloma
a. crypt
a. dilation
a. dilator
a. discharge
a. disk
a. effluent
a. electrical stimulation
a. EMG PerryMeter sensor
a. encirclement
a. endoscopy
a. endosonography (AES)
a. epidermoid carcinoma
a. fascia
a. fibrosis
a. fissure
a. fistula
a. foreign body
a. ileostomy with preservation of sphincter
a. incontinence
a. intersphincteric groove
a. intraepithelial neoplasia (AIN)
a. intramuscular gland
a. mapping
a. margin
a. neoplasm
a. pecten
a. pit
a. pitting
a. plate
a. pouch
a. procidentia
a. prolapse
a. protrusion
a. reflex
a. sepsis
a. sinus
a. sphincter
a. sphincter contraction
a. sphincter dysfunction
a. sphincter function
a. sphincter reconstruction
a. sphincter repair
a. sphincter squeeze pressure
a. sphincter tone
a. squamous dysplasia
a. squamous intraepithelial lesion (ASIL)
a. stenosis
a. stricture
a. surgery
a. transitional zone (ATZ)
a. transitional zone dysplasia
a. triangle
a. ulceration
a. valve
a. vector manometry

a. verge
a. wart
a. wink
a. wound
analeptic enema
anales
columnae a.
sinus a.
valvulae a.
analgesia
patient a.
patient-controlled a. (PCA)
analgesic, analgetic
a. effect
narcotic a.
a. nephropathy
a. requirement
analgesic-antipyretic
analgetic (*var. of* analgesic)
analgosedation
analis
pecten a.
analog (*var. of* analogue)
analogue, analog
arginine a.
prostaglandin a.
somatostatin a.
Analpram-HC anorectal cream
analyses (*pl. of* analysis)
analysis, *pl.* **analyses**
anthropometric a.
bioelectrical impedance a. (BIA)
Bland-Altman a.
body composition a.
CFTR gene a.
cineradiographic a.
contexture a.
cosinor a.
cytogenetic a.
cytometric a.
Diacyte DNA ploidy a.
2-dimensional flow cytometric a.
DNA ploidy a.
electrophoresis immunoblot a.
enzymatic spectrophotometric a.
fecal a.
flow cytometric a.
flow cytometry a.
fluid a.
fluorescent image a.
Fourier transform a.
gastric a.
gene-linkage a. (GLA)
heteroduplex a.
histochemical-ultrastructural a.
image a.
incrustation a.
Kaplan-Meier a.
logistic regression a.

analysis (*continued*)
    monoclonality by genetic a.
    multivariable logistic regression a.
    multivariate a.
    Northern blot a.
    a. of virulence factor
    ploidy a.
    prefreeze semen a.
    pressure flow a.
    p53 tumor-suppressor gene a.
    pulse-width a.
    real-time spectral a.
    reflectance a.
    regression a.
    renal morphometric a.
    retrospective a.
    semen a.
    sequencing a.
    serum cytokine a.
    single-parameter DNA a.
    single-strand conformation
     polymorphism a.
    Southern blot a.
    spectral a.
    spectrophotometric a.
    stepwise regression a.
    survival a.
    trace-gas a.
    univariate a.
    urine cytokine a.
    Vindelov method flow cytometry
     a.
    Western blot a.
    x-ray a.
analyzer, analyzor
    automatic chemical a.
    Beckman ion-selective a.
    Cell Soft semen a.
    C-Trak a.
    GastrograpH Mark III pH a.
    Hamilton-Thorn motility a.
    Hitachi a.
    iChem urine chemistry a.
    Immulite 2000 anti-HBc IgM a.
    Immulite HBsAg immunoassay a.
    MicroLyzer gas a.
    Olympus SP-series image a.
    Orion ion a.
    Packard Auto-Gamma a.
    reflectance spectrum a.
    RJL bioelectrical impedance a.
    sequential multiple a. (SMA)
    Siemens Somatom DRH CT a.
    Synchron automated a.
    tissue spectrum a. TS-200
    ultrasound bone a.
    wave a.
analyzor (*var. of* analyzer)
AnaMantle HC

Anandron
anaphylactica
    enteritis a.
anaphylactic reaction
anaphylactoid
    a. food sensitivity
    a. purpura
    a. purpura nephritis
anaphylaxis
anaplasia
anaplastic
    a. malignant teratoma
    a. seminoma
    a. Wilms tumor
Anaprox
anaritide acetate
anasarca
anascitic
Anasept skin and wound antiseptic
Anaspaz
anastalsis
anastomose
anastomoses (*pl. of* anastomosis)
anastomosis, *pl.* **anastomoses**
    Abbe intestinal a.
    anal a.
    antecolic a.
    antiperistaltic a.
    aseptic a.
    bilioenteric a.
    Billroth I, II a.
    bladder neck-to-urethra a.
    Brackin ureterointestinal a.
    Braun a.
    Carrel aortic patch a.
    cervical esophagogastric a.
     (CEGA)
    circular stapled a.
    a. clamp
    Coffey ureterointestinal a.
    coloanal a. (CAA)
    colocolonic a.
    colorectal a. (CRA)
    Cordonnier technique ureterocolonic
     a.
    Couvelaire ileourethral a.
    crunch stick a.
    curved end-to-end a. (CEEA)
    delayed a.
    diseased organileal pouch-anal a.
    dismembered a.
    dog-ear of a.
    double-stapled ileal pouch-anal a.
    Duhamel laparoscopic
     pullthrough a.
    end-to-end a. (EEA)
    end-to-side a. (ESA)
    enteroenteric a.
    esophagocolic a.

esophagojejunal a.
extracorporeal a.
extravesical a.
fishmouth a.
Furniss ureterointestinal a.
Gambee a.
Goodwin technique ureterocolonic a.
Halsted a.
handsewn a.
hepaticojejunal a.
Hofmeister a.
Hofmeister-Pólya a.
homocladic a.
Horsley a.
H-shaped ileal pouch-anal a.
ileal pouch-anal a. (IPAA)
ileal pouch-distal rectal a.
ileoanal a. (IAA)
ileocolic a. (ICA)
ileorectal a. (IRA)
ileosigmoid a.
ileotransverse colon a.
ileovesical a.
intestinal a.
intracorporeal a.
intravesical a.
isoperistaltic a.
J-shaped ileal pouch-anal a.
Kocher a.
Lane ileorectal a.
2-layer interrupted intestinal a.
Leadbetter and Clarke ureteral a.
LeDuc ureteral a.
Lich-Gregoire a.
low anterior resection in
  combination with coloanal a.
  (LAR/CAA)
low coloanal a.
magnetic compression a.
Maunsell-Weir coloanal a.
mechanical a.
mesocaval a.
microvascular a.
mucosa-to-mucosa a.
Navy single-layer everting a.
neobladder-urethra a.
Nesbit technique ureterocolonic a.
nondismembered a.
Pagano technique ureterocolonic a.
Pagano ureteral a.
pancreaticogastric a.
Parks ileoanal a.
peristaltic a.
Politano-Leadbetter a.
Pólya a.
portacaval a. (PCA)
pouch-anal a.
primary a.
pyeloileal a.

pyeloileocutaneous a.
rectosigmoid a.
refluxing ileourethral a.
reniportal a.
restorative proctocolectomy and ileal
  pouch anal a. (RP/IPAA)
retrocolic a.
right-angle end-to-side a.
Roux-en-Y a.
Roux-type gastroduodenal a.
Schoemaker a.
side-to-side a.
single-layer continuous intestinal a.
small-bowel a.
spatulated overlap a.
splenorenal venous a.
S-shaped ileal pouch-anal a.
stapled end-to-end ileoanal a.
stapled intestinal a.
stapled pouch-anal a.
State end-to-end a.
Strickler technique
  ureterocolonic a.
Strickler ureteral a.
sutureless bowel a.
tension-free a.
transanal a.
transureteroureteral a.
ultralow a.
ureteral a.
ureterocolonic a.
ureteroileal a.
ureterointestinal a.
ureterosigmoid a.
ureterotubal a.
ureteroureteral a.
urethrovesical a.
vascular a.
vesicourethral a.
von Haberer-Finney a.
Wallace a.
wide elliptical a.
wide-lumen stapled a.
W-shaped ileal pouch-anal a.
Z-plasty a.
anastomotic
  a. complication
  a. leak
  a. leakage
  a. material
  a. recurrence
  a. repair
  a. stoma
  a. stricture
  a. suture
  a. ulcer
  a. ulceration
  a. urethroplasty
anastomotic-stomal ulcer

anatomic, anatomical
    a. anomaly
    a. approach
    a. characteristic
    a. finding
    a. fundoplication failure
    a. radical retropubic prostatectomy
    a. stress incontinence
anatomical (*var. of* anatomic)
anatomically correct fundoplication
anatomy
    anomalous a.
    aortoiliac a.
    Billroth II a.
    congenitally altered a.
    distal ureteral a.
    normal a.
    pelvic a.
    peritoneal a.
Anatrast barium sulfate paste
anatrophic
    a. nephrolithotomy
    a. nephroscopy
    a. nephrotomy
ANC
    acid-neutralizing capacity
ANCA
    antineutrophil cytoplasmic antibody
ANCA-associated systemic vasculitis
Ancalixir
ANCA-SVV
    antineutrophilic cytoplasmic
    autoantibody-small vessel vasculitis
Ancef
anchor
    Cope viscerotomy a.
    esophageal Z stent with a.'s
    Mainstay urologic soft tissue a.
    Mitek bone a.
    transvaginal bone a.
anchoring
    a. balloon
    a. suture
Ancobon
Ancure abdominal aortic aneurysm system
Ancylostoma, Ankylostoma
    A. duodenale
ancylostomiasis
Andersen
    A. disease
    A. syndrome
    A. triad
Anderson
    A. classification
    A. gastric tube
Anderson-Hynes dismembered pyeloplasty
Andractim
Andresen diet

Andrews
    A. operation
    A. suction tip
androblastoma
Androderm testosterone transdermal patch
AndroGel
androgen
    a. ablation
    a. ablation therapy (AAT)
    a. ablative monotherapy
    adrenal cortex a.
    a. blockade
    a. deficiency
    a. deprivation
    a. deprivation therapy
    exogenous a.
    a. gonadotropin feedback control
    a. insensitivity syndrome
    plasma a.
    a. precursor
    a. priming
    a. receptor
    a. receptor element
    a. suppression
    a. withdrawal endocrine therapy
androgen-binding protein
androgen-independent prostate cancer
androgenital syndrome
androgenization
androgenize
androgen-presenting cell
androgyny
    infertility a.
    sexual dysfunction a.
andrologist
andrology
andropause
androstenedione
    basal a.
androstenedione-to-testosterone ratio
androsterone
anechoic
anejaculation
Anemagen OB gelcaps
anemia
    autoimmune hemolytic a.
    B_{12} a.
    Banti splenic a.
    copper deficiency a.
    Faber a.
    febrile pleomorphic a.
    folate a.
    hemodialysis-associated a.
    hemolytic a.
    homozygous sickle cell a.
    hypochromic microcytic a.
    hypovolemic a.

iron deficiency a.
macroangiopathic hemolytic a.
megaloblastic a.
a. of chronic renal failure
pernicious a.
posthepatitis aplastic a.
refractory sideroblastic a.
ribavirin-induced a.
sickle cell a.

AnemiaPro anemia screening test
anemic urine
anephric
anepiploic
Anergan
anergy
clonal a.
aneroid manometry
Anestacon 2% lidocaine hydrochloride jelly
anesthesia
a. adjuvant
general endotracheal a. (GETA)
local a.
methoxyflurane a.
pharyngeal a.
Ponka technique for herniorrhaphy a.
Ponka technique for local a.
preperitoneal a.
spinal a.
topical oropharyngeal a. (TOPA)
anesthetic
Cetacaine topical a.
EMLA a.
eutectic mixture of local a.'s (EMLA)
a. hepatitis
a. hepatotoxicity
lidocaine topical a.
topical a.
Xylocaine topical a.
aneuploid cell
aneuploidy
DNA a.
mucosal a.
AneuRx stent graft system
aneurysm
abdominal aortic a. (AAA)
acquired renal artery a.
aortic a.
arterial a.
arteriosclerotic a.
berry a.
bilobate false a.
cirsoid a.
congenital renal artery a.
cricoid a.
Dieulafoy cirsoid a.
dissecting abdominal a.

dissecting renal artery a.
embolization of a.
extravisceral a.
false a.
fusiform renal artery a.
gastric a.
GDA a.
hepatic artery a.
hypogastric artery a.
iliac artery a.
intramural a.
intrarenal renal artery a.
mycotic a.
perforating a.
renal artery a.
ruptured abdominal aortic a. (RAAA)
saccular a.
splenic artery a. (SAA)
thoracoabdominal aortic a. (TAAA)
aneurysmal, aneurysmatic
a. dilation
aneurysmatic (*var. of* aneurysmal)
aneurysmectomy
ANF
atrial natriuretic factor
Angelchik
A. antireflux prosthesis
A. ring prosthesis
Angeles
Los A. (LA)
University of California at Los A. (UCLA)
angelica root
Anger scintillation camera
angiectasia, angiectasis
angiectasis (*var. of* angiectasia)
angiitis, angitis
hypersensitivity a.
angina
abdominal a.
a. abdominalis
a. abdominis
a. dyspeptica
intestinal a.
Schultz a.
anginal attack
anginiform
anginose, anginous
anginous (*var. of* anginose)
angioarchitecture of arterial supply of diverticulum
angioblast
angiocatheter
Angiocath PRN catheter
angiocholecystitis
angiocholitis proliferans
Angiocol

angiodysplasia
    bleeding colonic a.
    diffuse a.
    gastric a.
    gastroduodenal a.
    pedunculated a.
    submucosal endothelial a.
    submucosal fibromuscular a.
angiodysplastic lesion
angioedema
    hereditary a. (HAE)
angiofibroma
    nasopharyngeal a.
    a. of penis
angiogenesis
    tumor a.
angiogenic factor
Angiografin
angiogram
    celiac a.
    cystic duct a.
    mesenteric a.
    splenic a.
angiographic
    a. assessment
    a. endhole catheter
    a. intervention
    a. portacaval shunt
    a. variceal embolization
angiographically
angiography
    biliary a.
    a. catheter
    celiac a.
    computed tomographic a. (CTA)
    computerized tomographic hepatic a.
      (CTHA)
    3D gadolinium-enhanced MR a.
    diagnostic a.
    digital venous subtraction a.
      (DVSA)
    dynamic fluorescein a.
    fluorescence a.
    intraarterial digital subtraction a.
    intraoperative a.
    intravenous renal a.
    magnetic resonance a. (MRA)
    mucosal a.
    quantitative a.
    renal a.
    selective mesenteric a.
    subtraction a.
    superior mesenteric a.
    therapeutic a.
    visceral a.
    Wilms tumor a.
angioinfarction
AngioJet
    A. rapid thrombectomy system

A. Rheolytic thrombectomy system
A. Xpeedior catheter
angiokeratoma
    a. corporis diffusum
    a. corporis diffusum universale
    diffuse a.
    a. of Fordyce
    a. of scrotum
    scrotal a.
angioma, *pl.* **angiomata,** *pl.* **angiomas**
    bleeding a.
    cherry a.
    gastric a.
    littoral cell a.
    petechial a.
    spider a.
    telangiectatic a.
    testicular a.
    umbilicated a.
    upper gastrointestinal a.
angiomas (*pl. of* angioma)
angiomata (*pl. of* angioma)
angiomatoid tumor
angiomatosis
    bacillary a.
    hepatic a.
angiomatous lymphoid hamartoma
Angiomed
    A. blue stent
    A. Puroflex stent
angiomyolipoma
    gastric a.
    kidney a.
    renal a.
    tuberous sclerosis a.
angioneurectomy
angioneurotic
    a. anuria
    a. edema
    a. hematuria
angioplasia
angioplasty
    a. balloon
    a. balloon catheter
    balloon percutaneous
      transluminal a.
    percutaneous transluminal a.
      (PTA)
    percutaneous transluminal
      balloon a.
    percutaneous transluminal renal a.
      (PTRA)
    renal percutaneous transluminal a.
angiosarcoma
    bladder a.
    hepatic a.
    radiation-induced a.
angiosclerosis
    radiation-induced a.

angiostatin
AngioStent
angiostrongyliasis
angiotensin
 a. I-converting enzyme
  insertion/deletion polymorphism
 a. I, II, III
 a. II infusion test
 a. II receptor
 proximal tubular secretion of a.
 a. receptor blocker (ARB)
angiotensin-converting
 a.-c. enzyme (ACE)
 a.-c. enzyme gene
 a.-c. enzyme gene polymorphism
 a.-c. enzyme inhibition in
  progressive renal insufficiency
  (AIPRI)
 a.-c. enzyme inhibition in
  progressive renal insufficiency
  trial
 a.-c. enzyme inhibitor
  (ACEI)
angiotensin-dependent hypertension
angiotensinogen
Angiovist
Angiozyme
angitis (*var. of* angiitis)
angle
 acute infundibulopelvic a.
 anorectal a.
 Camper a.
 cardiohepatic a.
 duodenojejunal a.
 epigastric a.
 hepatorenal a.
 inferolateral a. (ILA)
 infundibulopelvic a.
 mesangial a.
 a. of His
 a. of incidence
 splenorenal a.
angled
 a. delivery device (ADD)
 a. dissecting forceps
angle-tip glidewire
angostura
angular
 a. notch of stomach
 a. velocity
angularis
 a. body
 incisura a.
angulation
anguli (*pl. of* angulus)
angulus, *pl.* **anguli**
 a. of stomach
 a. on lesser curve
anhaustral colonic gas pattern

anhemolytic streptococcus
anhepatic stage of liver transplantation
anhydrase
 carbonic a. (CA)
 carbonic a. II (CA II)
anhydrosis
anhydrous
 sodium phosphate dibasic a.
ani (*pl. of* anus)
anicteric
 a. sclerae
 a. skin
 a. viral hepatitis
anidulafungin
anileridine
anion
 a. exchange
 a. exchange resin
 a. gap
 a. gap acidosis
anion-cation secretory curve
anionic
 a. ferritin
 a. IgG 4 fraction
aniridia
anisakiasis
 acute gastric a.
 gastric a.
anisakid larva
Anisakis
 A. marina
 A. simplex
anise
 star a.
anismus
anisocoria
anisocytosis
anisokaryosis
anisonucleosis
anisotropine methylbromide
anisoylated plasminogen-streptokinase
 activator complex
anistreplase
anitidine
ankle jerk
ankyloproctia
Ankylostoma (*var. of Ancylostoma*)
ankylostomiasis
ankylurethria
anlage, *pl.* **anlagen**
 a. of pancreas
 prepancreatic a.
 splenic a.
anlagen (*pl. of* anlage)
AN69 membrane dialyzer
Ann
 A. Arbor cancer staging
 A. Arbor Hodgkin disease
  classification

ANNA
  antineuronal nuclear antibody
annexin
annular (*var. of* anular)
annuli (*pl. of* annulus)
annulus (*var. of* anulus), *pl.* annuli
ano
  fissure in a.
  fistula in a.
anococcygeal raphe
anococcygeus
anocutaneous
  a. line
  a. reflex
  a. stimulation
anoderm
Anodyne therapy system
Anogesic
anomalies (*pl. of* anomaly)
anomalotrophy
anomalous
  a. anatomy
  a. arrangement of pancreaticobiliary
    ductal system
  a. calyx
  a. genitalia
  a. junction of pancreaticobiliary
    ducts (AJPBD)
  a. pancreaticobiliary communication
  a. pancreaticobiliary duct (APBD)
  a. pancreaticobiliary ductal union
    (APBDU)
  a. pancreaticobiliary union (APBU)
  a. pancreatobiliary duct junction
    (APBDJ)
anomaly, *pl.* **anomalies**
  anatomic a.
  cloacal a.
  Cruveilhier-Baumgarten a.
  Dieulafoy a.
  DiGeorge a.
  duplication a.
  fixation a.
  a. of Zahn
  pan-bud a.
  penile a.
  urachal a.
  ureter duplication a.
  urinary tract a.
  urogenital sinus a.
  vitelline duct a.
anoplasty
  cutback a.
  dermal island-flap a.
  House advancement a.
  Martin a.
  posterior sagittal and 3-flap a.
  a. treatment
  Y-V a.

anorchia (*var. of* anorchism)
anorchism, anorchia
  bilateral a.
anorectal
  a. abscess
  a. angle
  a. atresia
  a. band
  a. carcinoma
  a. disease
  a. dressing
  a. dysgenesis
  a. endosonography
  a. examination
  a. fistula
  a. flexure
  a. foreign body
  a. function test
  a. herpes
  a. imaging
  a. junction
  a. line
  a. malformation
  a. manometry
  a. measurement
  a. mobilization
  a. myectomy
  a. nomenclature
  a. physiology
  a. physiology testing
  a. ring
  a. sensorimotor
    dysfunction
  a. sepsis
  a. space
  a. sphincter
  a. stenosis
  a. surgery
  a. syphilis
  a. varix
anorectic, anoretic, anorexic
  a. drug
anorectitis
anorectocolonic
anorectoplasty
  Laird-McMahon a.
  posterior sagittal a. (PSARP)
anorectum
anoretic (*var. of* anorectic)
anorexia
  a. nervosa
  a. nervosa and associated disorders
    (ANAD)
anorexia-cachexia syndrome
anorexiant
anorexic (*var. of* anorectic)
anorexigenic
anorgasmia (*var. of* anorgasmy)
anorgasmy, anorgasmia

anoscope
  Bacon a.
  Boehm a.
  Brinkerhoff a.
  Buie-Hirschman a.
  Ferguson a.
  Hirschmann a.
  Otis a.
  Pratt a.
  Pruitt a.
  Sims a.
  slotted a.
anoscopic
anoscopy
anosigmoidoscopy
anospinal center
anovaginal fistula
anovesical
anoxia
  chemical a.
  gastric a.
ANP
  atrial natriuretic peptide
  ANP receptor
ANS
  autonomic nervous system
Ansaid Oral
ansa pancreaticus
Anson-McVay femoral herniorrhaphy
antacid
  liquid a.
  Remegel soft chewable a.
  trial a.
AntaGel liquid
antagonist
  alpha-adrenergic a.
  alpha-1 adrenoceptor a.
  alpha receptor a.
  beta-adrenergic a.
  BQ123 receptor a.
  calcium channel a. (CCA)
  CCK a.
  cholecystokinin a.
  cytokine a.
  dopamine a.
  endothelin a.
  EtA a.
  EtB a.
  histamine a.
  histamine-2 receptor a. (H2RA)
  hormone a.
  H2-receptor a. (H2RA)
  5-HT$_3$, 5-HT$_4$ a.
  5HTM3 receptor a.
  interleukin-1 receptor a.
  intravenous H2 receptor a.
    (IVH2RA)
  luteinizing hormone-releasing
    hormone a.
  opiate a.
  opioid a.
  PIVKA-II a.
  platelet glycoprotein 2b3a receptor
    a.
  potassium-canrenoate a.
  serotonin receptor a.
  TxA2 receptor a.
  type 3 serotonin receptor a.
antagonistic drug
antagonist-II
  prothrombin induced by vitamin K
    absence or a.-II (PIVKA-II)
antecedent pancreatic injury
antecolic
  a. anastomosis
  a. gastrectomy
  a. long-loop isoperistaltic
    gastrojejunostomy
antecubital arteriovenous fistula
anteflexed uterus
antegrade
  a. approach
  a. colonic enema (ACE)
  a. continence enema (ACE)
  a. continence enema, in situ
    appendix
  a. continence enema procedure
  a. contrast study
  a. cystography
  a. double-balloon enteroscopy
  a. ejaculation
  a. endopyelotomy
  a. nephroscopy
  a. peristalsis
  a. pyelogram
  a. pyelography
  a. scrotal sclerotherapy
  a. stent replacement
  a. ureteral drainage
  a. ureteroscopic manipulation
  a. urography
Antegren
antepartum constipation
anterior
  a. abdominal wall
  a. abdominal wall syndrome
  a. and posterior (A&P)
  arteria caecalis a.
  arteria pancreaticoduodenalis superior
    a.
  a. axillary line (AAL)
  a. band of colon
  a. cecal artery
  a. cord syndrome
  a. duodenal ulcer
  a. esophageal sensor (AES)
  a. extremity
  a. fecal incontinence

anterior (*continued*)
a. fissure
a. fistula
a. hemiblock
a. horn
a. hypospadias
a. innominate osteotomy
a. nephrectomy
a. oblique position
a. pelvic exenteration
a. perineum
a. rectopexy
a. rectus fascia
a. rectus sheath
a. renal fascia
a. resection
a. rib impingement syndrome
a. scrotal nerve
a. spinal artery syndrome
a. transabdominal approach
a. urethra
a. urethral valve
a. vaginal wall sling (AVWS)
a. wall antral ulcer
anterolateral thoracotomy incision
anteroposterior (AP)
a. cystoresectoscope
anterosuperior
a. pancreaticoduodenal (ASPD)
a. pancreaticoduodenal artery
anteverted uterus
antevesical hernia
anthelminthic (*var. of* anthelmintic)
anthelmintic, anthelminthic
anthelone E, U
Anthos ht II automatic photometer
anthracene glycoside
anthracene-type laxative
anthraquinone laxative
anthrax
intestinal a.
anthrone
a. colorimetric technique
a. method
Rhein a.
anthropometric
a. analysis
a. calculation
a. marker
a. measurement
anthropometry
anthropomorphic parameter
anti-ABO antibody
antiactin antibody
antiadhesive agent
anti-alpha fetoprotein
antiandrogenic activity
antiandrogen withdrawal syndrome
antiasialoglycoprotein receptor

antibacterial personal catheter
antibasement membrane antibody
antibiotic
a. absorption
beta-lactam a.
broad-spectrum a.
a. enterocolitis
a. group
long-term a.
macrolide a.
a. management
perioperative a.
preoperative a.
prophylactic a.
a. prophylaxis
a. therapy
topical a.
antibiotic-associated
a.-a. colitis (AAC)
a.-a. diarrhea (AAD)
a.-a. pseudomembranous colitis
(AAPC, AAPMC)
antibiotic-coated stent
antibiotic-induced
a.-i. diarrhea
a.-i. enterocolitis
antibody
Amerlex-M second a.
anti-ABO a.
antiactin a.
antibasement membrane a.
antibrush border a.
anticardiolipin a. (ACA, ACLA)
anticentromere a. (ACA)
anticolonic a.
anticytokeratin monoclonal a.
anti-DCP monoclonal a.
antidelta IgM a.
antidesmin monoclonal a.
antiendomysial a. (anti-EMA)
antiendomysium a.
antiendothelial a.
antienterocyte a.
antiepithelial membrane antigen a.
antiextractable nuclear a. (anti-ENA)
anti-GBM a.
antigliadin a. (AGA)
antiglomerular basement membrane
a.
anti-HA a.
anti-HAV IgM a.
anti-HB a.
anti-HBc IgM a.
anti-HBs a.
anti-HCV core a.
anti-HD a.
anti-HGF a.
antihuman leukocyte antigen a.
antiidiotype a.

antiinterleukin-2 receptor alpha
  monoclonal a.
antilymphocyte a. (ALA)
antimicrosomal a.
antimitochondrial a. (AMA)
antimyeloperoxidase a.
antineuronal nuclear a. (ANNA)
antineutrophil cytoplasmic a.
  (ANCA)
antineutrophil cytoplasmic IgG a.
antinuclear a. (ANA)
anti-PCNA/cyclin monoclonal a.
antiphospholipid a. (APA)
antiphospholipid-anticardiolipin a.
anti-RAP a.
anti-RAP-GST a.
antireticulin a.
anti-RNA polymerase a.
antirotavirus a.
anti-*Saccharomyces cerevisiae* a.
  (ASCA)
antismooth muscle a.
antisomatostatin a.
antisperm a.
anti-TBM a.
anti-Thy-1 a.
antithyroglobulin a. (ATA)
anti-TNF alpha a.
anti-TrkC a.
antivimentin a.
assay for neutrophil a.'s
ATGAM polyclonal a.
basal cell-specific anticytokeratin a.
bladder a.
4B4 monoclonal a.
19B7 monoclonal a.
B72.3 murine monoclonal a.
cagA a.
CD14 monoclonal a.
celiac disease-specific EMA a.
CM1 polyclonal a.
cytophilic a.
cytotoxic a.
Das-1 monoclonal a.
eluted a.
endomysial a. (EMA)
endomysium a.
endotoxin a.
enzyme-conjugated anti-IgA a.
fibronectin monoclonal a.
FlexSure anti-*H. pylori* IgG a.
fluorescein isothiocyanate conjugated
  a.
fluorescein isothiocyanate-labeled
  monoclonal a.
fluorescent antinuclear a. (FANA)
Fx1A a.
HBe a.
HBeAb a.

HCV a.
hepatitis B core a. (HBcAb)
hepatitis Be a. (HBeAb)
hepatitis B early a. (HBeAb)
hepatitis B surface a. (HBsAb)
heterologous anti-GBM a.
Heymann a.
HMB-45 monoclonal a.
humanized anti-CD3 monoclonal a.
hybridoma-derived monoclonal a.
IgG2a a.
IgG alpha gliadin a.
IgG reticulin a.
IgM anti-HAV a.
IgM anti-HBc a.
IgM-HA a.
immune rabbit a.
immunoglobulin A endomysial a.
immunoglobulin A transglutaminase
  a.
immunoglobulin G2a a.
immunoglobulin G antigliadin a.
indium-111 murine anti-CEA
  monoclonal a.
infectious mononucleosis heterophil
  a.
islet cell a. (ICA)
LDP-02 a.
liver-kidney microsomal a.
lymphocytotoxic a.
M a.
microsome a. (MCHA)
milk protein a.
mitochondrial a.
monoclonal a. (MAb)
monoclonal anti-DNA a.
monoclonal a. BR96
MU-3 monoclonal a.
mycelial a.
mycobacterial a.
p53 a.
panel-reactive a.
para-ANC a.
PBC-associated a.
PC10 monoclonal a.
perinuclear antineutrophil cytoplasmic
  a. (p-ANCA)
phosphotyrosine a.
polyclonal epidermal growth factor
  a.
protein a. (PAb)
rabbit polyclonal a.
recipient-derived anti-HLA a.
serum virus a.
smooth muscle a. (SMA)
thyroglobulin a. (TGHA)
thyroid microsomal a.
thyroid-specific a.
a. to bromodeoxyuridine

antibody (*continued*)
    a. to c100 (anti-c100)
    a. to core peptide 9 (anti-CP9)
    a. to core peptide 10 (anti-CP10)
    a. to c100 protein
    a. to EMA
    a. to GOR (anti-GOR)
    a. to GOR epitope
    a. to hepatitis-associated antigen
      (anti-HAA) (HBsAb)
    a. to hepatitis A virus (anti-HAV)
    a. to hepatitis Be antigen
    a. to hepatitis Be antigen (HBeAb)
    a. to hepatitis B surface antigen
      (anti-HBsAg, HBsAb)
    a. to hepatitis C virus (anti-HCV)
    a. to hepatitis D virus
      (anti-HDV)
    a. to HTLV-I (anti-HTLV-I)
    a. to keratin
    a. to Leu M1
    UCHL-1 monoclonal a.
    xenoreactive a.
antibody-dependent
    a.-d. cell-mediated cytotoxicity
      (ADCC)
    a.-d. cellular cytotoxicity (ADCC)
antibody-directed cytotoxic response
antibody-independent complement
  activation
antibody-mediated protection
antibrush border antibody
anti-c100
    antibody to c100
anticardiolipin
    a. antibody (ACA, ACLA)
    a. antibody syndrome
anti-CD3
    SMART a.-CD3
anti-CD45
anticentromere
    a. antibody
    a. autoantibody (ACA)
anticholinergic
    a. agent
    a. drug
    a. medication
    a. medicine therapy
anticholinesterase
    parasympathomimetic a.
antichymotrypsin
    prostate-specific antigen bound to
      alpha-1 a. (PSA-ACT)
anticlass II MAb
anti-claudin-7
anti-CMV antiserum
anticoagulant
    lupus a. (LA)
anticoagulant-induced hematuria

anticoagulation therapy
anticodon
anticolonic antibody
anticonvulsant agent hepatotoxicity
anti-CP9
    antibody to core peptide 9
anti-CP10
    antibody to core peptide 10
anticytokeratin monoclonal antibody
anticytokine
anti-DCP monoclonal antibody
antidelta IgM antibody
antidepressant
    a. drug hepatotoxicity
    tricyclic a.
antidesmin monoclonal antibody
antidiabetic agent hepatotoxicity
antidiarrheal, antidiarrhetic (A-D)
    a. agent
    opioid a.
antidiarrhetic (*var. of* antidiarrheal)
antidiuretic
    a. arginine vasopressin V2 receptor
      (AVPR2)
    a. hormone (ADH)
    a. hormonelike agent
anti-DNA
    a.-DNA binding
    a.-DNA immunologic study
antidopaminergic
antidote
    opium a.
antidysenteric
anti-E2
    envelope 2 antigen
antielastase
anti-EMA
    antiendomysial antibody
antiemetic drug
anti-ENA
    antiextractable nuclear antibody
      anti-ENA immunologic study
antiendomysial
    a. antibody (anti-EMA)
    a. antibody test
antiendomysium antibody
antiendothelial antibody
antiendotoxin measure
antienterocyte antibody
antiepileptic drug hypersensitivity
antiepithelial membrane antigen antibody
antiestrogen
antiextractable nuclear antibody
  (anti-ENA)
antifilarial
antifol
    Baker a.
antifolate
    multitargeted a.

antifungal
    a. agent
    a. esophageal infection
antifungal-resistant opportunistic infection
anti-GBM
    antiglomerular basement membrane
    a.-GBM antibody
    a.-GBM disease
    a.-GBM glomerulonephritis
antigen
    A a.
    adenoma-associated a.
    amebic lectin a.
    antibody to hepatitis-associated a.
     (anti-HAA)
    antibody to hepatitis Be a.
    antibody to hepatitis Be a.
     (HBeAb)
    antibody to hepatitis B surface a.
     (anti-HBsAg, HBsAb)
    anti-40 kDa colonic a.
    antineutrophil cytoplasmic a.
    antismooth muscle a. (ASMA)
    antiviral capsid a.
    Australian a.
    B a.
    basement membrane a.
    bladder cancer a. 4 (BLCA4)
    bladder tumor a. (BTA)
    blood group a.
    C100-3 a.
    C22-3 a.
    CA-50 a.
    cancer a. 125 (CA-125, CA 125)
    cancer-associated sialyl-Lea a.
    carbohydrate a. 19-9 (CA-19-9)
    carcinoembryonic a. (CEA)
    CD25 a.
    cell membrane epithelial a.
    circulating tumor-associated a.
    class I, II a.
    a. DD23
    DD23 a.
    delta a.
    endogenous renal a.
    endomysium a.
    enterobacterial common a. (ECA)
    envelope 2 a. (anti-E2)
    epithelial membrane a.
    ethylchlorformate polymerized a.
    extracted nuclear a. (ENA)
    extrarenal a.
    factor VIII a.
    fetal sulfoglycoprotein a. (FSA)
    free prostate-specific a.
    free-to-total prostate-specific a.
     (FTPSA)
    gastrointestinal cancer-associated a.
     (GICA)

Helicobacter pylori stool a.
  (HpSA)
hepatitis-associated a. (HAA)
hepatitis B a. (HBAg)
hepatitis B core a. (HBcAg)
hepatitis Be a.
hepatitis B early a. (HBeAg)
hepatitis B surface a. (HBsAg)
hepatitis B virus-encoded a.
hepatitis D a. (HDAg)
hepatitis E virus a. (HEVAg)
hidden a.
histocompatibility a.
HIV P24 a.
HLA-DR a.
human leukocyte a. (HLA)
immunobead reacting a.
K a.
40-kDa colonic a.
leukocyte common a.
Lewis A blood group a.
Lewis B, X, Y a.
liver membrane a.
liver-specific a.
a. M344
a. marker
MHC class I, II a.
monoclonal a.
nephritogenic a.
nuclear protein cyclin proliferating
  cell nuclear a.
O a.
pancreatic oncofetal a. (POA)
polysaccharide a.
a. positive
ProstaMark early prostate cancer a.
  (ProstaMark EPCA)
prostate gland prostate-specific
  membrane a.
prostate-specific a. (PSA)
prostate-specific membrane a.
  (PSMA)
recombinant hepatitis C a.
reticulin a.
sialosyl-Tn a.
sialyl Lewis A a.
sialyl-Tn a.
solubilized human leukocyte a.
soluble egg a. (SEA)
soluble liver a. (SLA)
a. specific
squamous cell carcinoma a.
stage-specific embryonic a.
a. stimulation
a. stool detection test
T a.
T138 a.
Thomsen-Friedenreich a.
tissue polypeptide a.

antigen (*continued*)
    transplantation a.
    tumor-associated a. (TAA)
    tumor-rejection a.
    Ulex europeus I a.
    voiding dysfunction role of prostate
      stem cell a.
antigen-antibody system
antigen-dependent pathway
antigenemia
    pp65 a.
antigenic
    a. determinant
    a. modulation
    a. phenotype
antigen-independent
    a.-i. adhesion
    a.-i. pathway
antigen-matched donor
antigen-presenting cell (APC)
antigen-specific
    nucleocapsid a.-s.
antigliadin
    a. antibody (AGA)
    IgA a.
    IgM a.
    luminal a.
antiglobulin (AG)
antiglomerular
    a. basement membrane (anti-GBM)
    a. basement membrane antibody
    a. basement membrane antibody
      nephritis
    a. basement membrane disease
    a. basement membrane
      glomerulonephritis
    a. basement membrane-negative
      crescentic glomerular nephritis
anti-GOR
    antibody to GOR
anti-gp330 immunoglobulin G
anti-HAA
    antibody to hepatitis-associated antigen
anti-HA antibody
anti-HAV
    antibody to hepatitis A virus
    IgM anti-HAV
    anti-HAV IgM antibody
anti-HAV-positive
    IgG anti-HAV-p.
anti-HB antibody
anti-HBc
    hepatitis B surface antibody
      anti-HBC IgM antibody
      monoclonal anti-HBC
anti-HBe
    hepatitis B early antibody
anti-HBs
    hepatitis B surface antibody

    anti-HBs antibody
    Elecsys PreciControl anti-HBs
anti-HBsAg
    antibody to hepatitis B surface antigen
anti-HCV
    antibody to hepatitis C virus
      anti-HCV antibody third generation
      anti-HCV core antibody
anti-HD antibody
anti-HDV
    antibody to hepatitis D virus
anti-*Helicobacter*
    a.-*H. pylori* IgM
    a.-*H. pylori* treatment
antihepatitis A-IgM immunologic study
anti-HGF antibody
antihistamine
anti-HSV IgM Ab titer
anti-HTLV-I
    antibody to HTLV-I
antihuman leukocyte antigen antibody
anti-Hu test
antihydropic
antihypertensive
    a. agent
    a. and lipid-lowering treatment to
      prevent heart attack trial
      (ALLHAT)
    a. treatment
antiicteric
antiidiotype antibody
antiincontinence procedure
antiinfective biomaterial
antiinflammatory cytokine
antiinhibin
**antiinterleukin-2 receptor alpha
  monoclonal antibody**
anti-40 kDa colonic antigen
antilipemic drug
antilithic
antiliver
    a. kidney microsome (anti-LKM)
    a. microsomal antibody detection
anti-LKM
    antiliver kidney microsome
antilymphocyte
    a. antibody (ALA)
    a. globulin (ATGAM)
    a. heteroconjugate
    a. therapy
antimajor histocompatibility complex
anti-M2 antimitochondrial antibody level
antimegalin antiserum
antimesenteric
    a. border
    a. border of distal ileum
    a. enterotomy
    a. fat pad
    a. surface

antimesocolic side of cecum
antimicrobial
    a. agent
    macrolide a.
    a. prophylaxis
    a. resistance
    a. therapy
antimicrosomal antibody
Antiminth
antimitochondrial antibody (AMA)
antimony
    a. monocrystalline electrode
    a. pH electrode
    a. sodium tartrate
    a. trioxide
antimotility
    a. agent
    a. drug
antimüllerian derivative syndrome
antimuscarinic
    a. agent
    a. drug
antimycobacterial drug
antimyeloperoxidase antibody
antinatriuresis
antinauseant
antineoplastic drug hepatotoxicity
antineuronal
    a. enteric antibody test
    a. nuclear antibody (ANNA)
antineutrophil
    a. cytoplasmic antibody (ANCA)
    a. cytoplasmic antibody titer
    a. cytoplasmic antigen
    a. cytoplasmic autoantibody
    (ANCA)
    a. cytoplasmic IgG antibody
antineutrophilic cytoplasmic
  autoantibody-small vessel vasculitis
  (ANCA-SVV)
antinociceptive effect
antinuclear
    a. antibody (ANA)
    a. antibody immunologic study
antiobesity compound
antioncogene therapy
antioxidant
    endogenous lipophilic a.
    A. Polyp Prevention Trial
anti-PCNA/cyclin monoclonal antibody
antiperistalsis
antiperistaltic
    a. anastomosis
    a. reflux
    a. technique
antiphospholipid
    a. antibody (APA)
    a. syndrome (APS)
antiphospholipid-anticardiolipin antibody

antiplasmin
    alpha-21 a.
antiporter
    Na+/H+ a.
antiproliferative
    a. activity
    a. effect
    a. immunosuppressant
antiproteinuric effect
antiprotozoal
antipsychotic drug hepatotoxicity
antipyrine clearance
anti-RAP antibody
anti-RAP-GST antibody
antireflux
    a. double-J stent
    a. flap-valve mechanism
    a. nipple
    a. operation
    a. procedure
    a. prosthesis
    a. regimen
    a. surgery
    a. therapy
    a. ureteral implantation technique
    a. valve
    a. wrap
antirefluxing
    a. colonic conduit
    a. nipple
antireticulin antibody
anti-RNA polymerase antibody
antirotavirus antibody
antiruminant
anti-*Saccharomyces cerevisiae* antibody
  (ASCA)
antisarcoma chemotherapy
anti-Schiff stain
antischistosomal
antisecretory
    a. agent
    a. drug
    a. opioid
    a. therapy
antisense
    a. DNA inhibition
    a. oligonucleotide
    a. RNA probe
    a. strategy
antiseptic
    Anasept skin and wound a.
    Avagard instant hand a.
    a. dressing
antiseptic-impregnated central venous
  catheter
antiserum
    anti-CMV a.
    antimegalin a.
    galanin a.

antiserum (*continued*)
    nephrotoxic a.
    VIP a.
anti-SLA test
antismooth
    a. muscle antibody
    a. muscle antigen (ASMA)
antisomatostatin antibody
Antispas
antispasmodic
    a. agent
    a. drug
antisperm antibody
anti-SSA immunologic study
anti-SSB immunologic study
antistreptolysin-O titer
anti-Tamm-Horsfall protein
anti-TBM antibody
antithrombin III deficiency
anti-Thy-1
    a.-T.-1 antibody
    a.-T.-1 nephritis
antithymocyte
    a. antibody-induced
       glomerulonephritis
    a. gammaglobulin (ATGAM)
    a. globulin (ATG, ATGAM)
antithyroglobulin antibody (ATA)
antithyroid
    a. autoantibody
    a. drug hepatotoxicity
anti-TNF alpha antibody
antitopoisomerase-I autoantibody
antitoxin
    dysentery a.
anti-TrkC antibody
antitrypsin
    alpha-1 a.
antitubular basement membrane
antitumor necrosis factor therapy
antiulcer
Antivert
antivimentin antibody
antiviral
    a. capsid antigen
    a. chemotherapy
Antizol for injection
Antopol-Goldman lesion
antral
    a. atrophic gastritis (AAG)
    a. biopsy
    a. cancer
    a. D, EC cell
    a. diverticulum of colon (ADC)
    a. edema
    a. gastric cell
    a. gastrin
    a. gastrin cell hyperfunction
    a. gastritis

    a. G-cell hyperplasia
    a. manometry
    a. membrane
    a. mucosa
    a. nodularity
    a. peptide
    a. peristalsis
    a. polyp
    a. pressure transducer
    a. resection
    a. scintigraphy
    a. somatostatin
    a. stasis
    a. stenosis
    a. stricture
    a. ulcer
    a. vascular ectasia
    a. web
antralization
antral-predominant gastritis
antral-type mucosa
antrectomy
    Roux-en-Y biliary bypass with a.
Antrenyl
Antrocol
antroduodenal
    a. manometry
    a. ulcer
antroduodenectomy
antroduodenojejunal manometry
antrofundal mucosa
antropyloric
antropyloroduodenal
    a. common chamber (APDCC)
    a. motility
    a. region
antrostomy
antrotomy
antrum
    cardiac a.
    duodenal a.
    gastric a.
    a. of stomach
    a. of Willis
    prepyloric a.
    a. pyloricum
    retained a.
Anturol
anucleate fragment
anular, annular
    a. adenocarcinoma
    a. esophageal stricture
    a. pancreas
anuli (*pl. of* anulus)
anulus, annulus, *pl.* **anuli**
    a. urethralis
anum
    per a.
anuresis

anuretic
anuria
> angioneurotic a.
> calculous a.
> compression a.
> flash pulmonary edema with a.
> obstructive a.
> postrenal a.
> prerenal a.
> renal a.
> suppressive a.

anuric
anus, *pl.* **ani**
> arcus tendineus musculi levatoris ani
> artificial a.
> atresia ani
> ectopic a.
> imperforate a.
> levator ani
> a. malformation
> patulous a.
> preternatural a.
> pruritus ani
> rosette appearance of a.
> Rusconi a.
> a. vesicalis
> a. vestibularis
> vulvovaginal a.

anusitis
Anusol HC, HC-1
anvil portion of EEA stapler
Anxanil
anxiety-related diarrhea
anxiolytic sedative
Anzemet
AOCLD
> acute on chronic liver disease

aorta, *pl.* **aortae**
> abdominal a.
> supraceliac a.

aortae (*pl. of* aorta)
aortic
> a. aneurysm
> a. dissection
> a. hiatus
> a. patch
> a. punch
> a. superior mesenteric artery bypass
> a. valvular stenosis

aortica
> dysphagia a.

aortoduodenal fistula (ADF)
aortoenteric
> a. fistula
> a. graft

aortoesophageal fistula
aortogastric fistula
aortograft duodenal fistula

aortography
> abdominal a.
> biplanar a.

aortohepatic arterial graft
aortoiliac anatomy
aortoostial lesion
aortorenal
> a. bypass
> a. bypass graft
> a. reimplantation

aortosigmoid fistula
aortotomy
AOSC
> acute obstructive suppurative cholangitis

A&P
> anterior and posterior

AP
> adenomatous polyp
> alkaline phosphatase
> anteroposterior
> AP marker enzyme

APA
> antiphospholipid antibody

APAAP
> alkaline phosphatase-antialkaline phosphatase

APACHE
> Acute Physiology and Chronic Health Evaluation
> APACHE-II, -III scoring system
> APACHE-II point
> APACHE-II score

apancreatic
APAP
> acetaminophen

apatite
> a. calculus
> carbonate a.

APBD
> anomalous pancreaticobiliary duct

APBDJ
> anomalous pancreatobiliary duct junction

APBDU
> anomalous pancreaticobiliary ductal union

APBU
> anomalous pancreaticobiliary union

APC
> adenomatous polyp of colon
> adenomatous polyposis coli
> all-purpose capsule
> antigen-presenting cell
> argon plasma coagulation
> argon plasma coagulator
> APC 300
> APC stool test
> APC tumor suppressor gene

APCR
> activated protein C resistance

APD
> automated peritoneal dialysis

APDCC
> antropyloroduodenal common chamber

ape diet

apellous

apenteric

apepsia
> achlorhydria a.

apepsinia

aperistalsis

aperistaltic esophagus

aperture
> stomal a.

apex *pl.* **apices**
> a. of duodenal bulb
> a. of external ring

aphallia

aphasia

apheresis

Aphrodyne

aphtha, *pl.* **aphthae**

aphthae (*pl. of* aphtha)

aphthoid
> a. proctocolitis
> a. ulcer

aphthosa
> cachexia a.

aphthous
> a. erosion
> a. gastropathy
> a. stomatitis
> a. ulcer

aphthous-type lesion

API
> alkaline protease inhibitor
> transcription factor API

apical
> a. biopsy status
> a. canaliculus
> a. duodenal ulcer
> a. membrane
> a. polar nephrectomy
> a. sound
> a. thickening

apices (*pl. of* apex)

APKD
> adult polycystic kidney disease

aplasia
> bone marrow a.
> kidney a.
> pure red cell a. (PRCA)
> seminal vesicle a.

aplastic bone disease

APLD
> adult polycystic liver disease

apo, Apo
> apolipoprotein
> > apo A-I
> > apo A-IV
> > apo B-48

Apo-Amitriptyline

Apo-Amoxi

APOB **gene**

Apo-Chlorax

Apo-Chlordiazepoxide

Apo-Cimetidine

Apo-Erythro

Apo-Erythro-ES

apoferritin

Apo-Hydroxyzine

apolipoprotein (apo, Apo)
> a. B-48
> a. B-containing lipoprotein
> a. B gene
> a. CII/CIII ratio
> a. synthesis

APOLT
> auxiliary partial orthotopic liver transplantation

Apo-Metronidazole

apomorphine

aponeurosis
> buccopharyngeal a.
> external oblique a.
> ischiorectal a.
> a. of external oblique
> a. of internal oblique
> superficial perineal a.

apoplexy
> abdominal a.
> mesenteric a.
> urethral a.

apoprotein

apoptosis
> crypt cell a.
> detachment-induced a.
> enterocyte a.
> a. in cell line

apoptotic
> a. cell death
> a. index
> a. response

Apo-Ranitidine

Apo-Sulfatrim

Apo-Tetra

Apo-Tolbutamide

Apo-Trimip

apparatus, *pl.* **apparatus**
> alimentary a.
> biliary a.
> contractile a.
> digestive a.
> a. digestorius
> GIA autosuture a.

Golgi a.
juxtaglomerular a.
Manifold II slot-blot a.
von Petz suturing a.
Wangensteen suction a.
apparent
a. digestive energy (ADE)
a. mineral corticoid excess
syndrome
appearance
beaklike a.
bird-beak a.
bull's-eye a.
cloverleaf a.
cobblestone a.
coiled spring a.
corkscrew a.
ground-glass a.
lead-pipe a.
leafless tree a.
mushroom-and-stem a.
normalized protein nitrogen a.
(nPNA)
a. of normal colon vasculature
picket fence a.
pinwheel a.
pseudo-Billroth I a.
pseudotumor a.
sausagelike a.
sawtoothed a.
soap-sudsy a.
spiculated a.
spiderweb a.
stack-of-coins a.
string-of-beads a.
tadpolelike a.
target a.
through-and-through a.
tigroid a.
toxic a.
wind sock a.
Appedrine
appendage
cecal a.
epiploic a.
torsion of a.
vermicular a.
appendectomy (appy), appendicectomy
colonoscopic a.
emergency a.
emergent a.
incidental a.
interval a.
inversion a.
inversion-ligation a.
laparoscopic a.
a. tape
uncomplicated a.
appendical (*var. of* appendiceal)

appendiceal, appendical
a. abscess
a. adenocarcinoma
a. intussusception
a. Kaposi sarcoma
a. mass
a. mucocele
a. opening
a. orifice
a. perforation (AP)
a. stump
appendicectasis
appendicectomy (*var. of* appendectomy)
appendices (*pl. of* appendix)
appendicism
appendicitis
actinomycotic a.
acute a.
amebic a.
bilharzial a.
a. by contiguity
chronic a.
foreign body a.
fulminating a.
gangrenous a.
a. granulosa
helmintic a.
left-sided a.
lumbar a.
myxoglobulosis a.
necropurulent a.
nonperforated a.
a. obliterans
obstructive a.
pelvic a.
perforated a.
purulent a.
recurrent a.
relapsing a.
retrocecal a.
retroileal a.
segmental a.
skip a.
stercoraceous a.
subperitoneal a.
suppurative a.
traumatic a.
verminous a.
appendicocecostomy
appendicocele
appendicocystostomy
continent cutaneous a.
dismembered reimplanted a.
nonplicated a.
orthotopic a.
plicated a.
reversed reimplanted a.
appendicoenterostomy
appendicolith

appendicolysis
appendicopathy
appendicostomy
    Malone continent a.
appendicoumbilical stoma
appendicovesicostomy
    Mitrofanoff a.
appendicular
    a. artery
    a. colic
    a. dyspepsia
appendicularis
    arteria a.
appendix, *pl.* **appendices**
    antegrade continence enema, in situ
     a.
    base of a.
    cecal a.
    divided a.
    a. dyspepsia
    a. epididymidis
    epiploic a.
    a. fibrosa
    gangrenous a.
    hot a.
    indurated a.
    inflamed a.
    Morgagni a.
    nonperforated a.
    normal a.
    paracecal a.
    perforated a.
    retrocecal a.
    retroileal a.
    ruptured a.
    simultaneous Malone antegrade
     continent enema and Mitrofanoff
     procedure using divided a.
    subcecal a.
    suppurative a.
    a. testis
    a. testis torsion
    vermiform a.
    xiphoid a.
appetite
    a. disorder
    perverted a.
    voracious a.
apple
    bitter a.
    cashew a.
    a. tree
apple-core lesion
apple-peel bowel syndrome
appliance
    external cooling a.
    Gentle Touch colostomy a.
    Karaya ring ileostomy a.
    ostomy a.

application
    laparoscopic clip a.
    research a.
    ultrathin needle brachytherapy-style
     delivery renal a.
applicator
    Betadine PrepStick Plus a.
    Mick a.
    microwave a.
    Multifire clip a.
    multiload occlusive clip a.
    resorbable thread clip a.
    Stabiliplan orthovolt a.
Applied Biosystems nucleic acid extractor
applier
    Advanced surgical suture a.
    clip a.
    cotton-tipped a.
    Endoclip a.
    multiloaded clip a.
    Stone clamp a.
Appolito suture
approach
    Alken renal stone a.
    anatomic a.
    antegrade a.
    anterior transabdominal a.
    Bianchi a.
    case-by-case a.
    choledochofiberscopic a.
    consortial a.
    detailed stepwise a.
    extrasphincteric a.
    fascial sling a.
    flank a.
    Framingham risk-factor a.
    gasless laparoscopic a.
    Henry a.
    invasive transvaginal a.
    Kraske parasacral a.
    laparoscopic-assisted a.
    microbial a.
    minilaparotomy a.
    minimally invasive a.
    Palomo a.
    percutaneous transhepatic a.
    perineal a.
    peroral a.
    posterior lumbar a.
    preperitoneal a.
    Redman a.
    retrograde a.
    retroperitoneal a.
    supraduodenal a.
    surgical a.
    thoracoabdominal extrapleural a.
    thoracoabdominal intrapleural a.
    transduodenal a.
    transmural a.

transpapillary a.
transvesical laparoscopic a.
ureteroscopic a.
vaginal wall a.
ventral transperitoneal laparoscopic a.
wait-and-see a.
Appropriate Use of Gastrointestinal Endoscopy guidelines
approximation
a. suture
tissue a.
wound a.
approximator clamp
appy
appendectomy
APR
abdominoperineal resection
apraxia
constructional a.
swallow a.
aprepitant
Apresoline
aprindine
aproctia
apron
abdominal a.
fatty omental a.
a. skin incision
A-4 protein
aprotinin
APRT
adenine phosphoribosyltransferase
APRT deficiency
APS-1
autoimmune polyglandular syndrome type 1
APSGN
acute poststreptococcal glomerulonephritis
APT-Downey alkali denaturation test
Aptima
A. Combo2 assay
A. CT assay
Aptosyn
aPTT, APTT
activated partial thromboplastin time
APUD
amine precursor uptake and decarboxylation
apudoma
Aquacel Ag dressing
Aquachloral
AquaMEPHYTON
aquaporin-1
aquaporin water channel
aquaretic drug
AquaSens fluid monitoring system
aquaticus
Thermus a.

Aquazide-H
aqueous
A. Charcodote
a. phenol
AR
aldose reductase
autoradiography
AR mRNA
arabic
gum a.
arabinotarda
Shigella a. type A, B
Ara-C, ara-C
cytarabine
arachidonic
a. acid
a. acid metabolite
a. acid oxidation
arachis oil
arachnoid fibrosis
Aralen
Aramine
Arandel cell harvester
Aranesp
Arantius ligament
ARB
angiotensin receptor blocker
arbaprostil
arbitrary unit
arborization of ducts
arc
sacral reflex a.
a. shadow
ARC
AIDS-related complex
arcade
gastroepiploic a.
ARCD
acquired renal cystic disease
arch
arterial a.
cortical a.
fallopian a.
pubic a.
tendinous a.
Treitz a.
archaea
methanogenic a.
architecture
crypt a.
distorted crypt a.
hepatic a.
intestinal villous a.
lobular a.
Arcobacter
A. butzleri
A. cryaerophilus
A. nitrofigilis
A. skirrowii

Arctic Omega fish oil supplement
arcuate
- a. artery
- a. line
- a. vein

arcus
- a. tendineus fasciae pelvis
- a. tendineus musculi levatoris ani

ARD
- acid-related disorder

ardeparin
ardor urinae
area, *pl.* **areae, areas**
- cell surface a.
- choledochoduodenal a.
- a. gastrica
- gastrohepatic bare a.
- high-echoic a.
- intermicrovillar a.
- Killian-Jamieson a.
- medial preoptic a.
- midepigastric a.
- midrectal a.
- mycophenolate a.
- a. nuda hepatis
- Paget disease of perianal a.
- perianal a.
- pericolostomy a.
- peripancreatic a.
- periportal a.
- peristomal a.
- postcricoid a.
- a. postrema
- punctate a.
- retroperitoneal a.
- skip a.
- subhepatic a.
- target a.
- watershed a.

areae (*pl. of* area)
areflexia
- detrusor a.

areflexic bladder
Arena hemodialysis device
Arenaria rubra
areas (*pl. of* area)
ARF
- acute renal failure
- mercuric chloride-induced ARF

ARG
- alkaline reflux gastritis

argentaffin, argentaffine
- a. cell
- a. reaction test
- a. stain

argentaffine (*var. of* argentaffin)
Arginaid dietary supplement
arginase deficiency

arginine
- a. analogue
- a. vasopressin (AVP)

arginosuccinate
Arglaes powder dressing
argon
- a. beam coagulator
- A. Beamer 2 device
- a. ion laser
- a. ion plasma coagulation
- a. laser therapy
- a. plasma coagulation (APC)
- a. plasma coagulator (APC)
- a. pumped-dye laser

Argyle
- A. chest tube
- A. Ingram trocar catheter
- A. Medicut R catheter

Argyle-Salem sump tube
argyrophilia
- cytoplasmic a.

argyrophilic
- a. and argyrophobic neurons
- a. cell

ARI
- acute renal insufficiency

Arias syndrome
Aristocort
Aristospan
arm
- cell-mediated a.
- humoral a.
- Leonard A.

armamentarium
- contemporary urologic a.

Armanni-Ebstein lesion
Armanni-Ehrlich degeneration
3-armed basket forceps
ARMS-PCR
- amplification refractory mutation system-polymerase chain reaction

Army-Navy retractor
Arndorfer
- A. capillary perfusion system
- A. pneumohydraulic capillary infusion system

aromatase inhibitor
aromatic
- a. amine
- a. amino acid (AAA)

Aronson esophageal retractor
aroylhydrazone chelator
ARP
- acute recurrent pancreatitis

ARPKD
- autosomal-recessive polycystic kidney disease

array
- curved linear a.

DNA a.

sensory a.

arrest

spermatogenic a.

arrestin

arrhythmic frequency range

arrhythmogenicity

Arrow

A. Raulerson syringe

A. UserGard injection cap system

ARROWgard Blue hemodialysis catheter

arrowhead sign

ARS

amylase-resistant starch

arsenical polyneuropathy

Artane

artefact (*var. of* artifact)

artefacta

dermatitis a.

arteria (*var. of* artery), *pl.*

arteriae

a. appendicularis

a. caecalis anterior

a. caecalis posterior

a. caudae pancreatis

a. colica dextra

a. colica media

a. epigastrica inferior

a. epigastrica superficialis

a. epigastrica superior

a. gastrica dextra

a. gastrica posterior

a. gastrica sinistra

a. gastroomentalis dextra

a. gastroomentalis sinistra

a. hepatica communis

a. hepatica propria

a. ileocolica

a. lienalis

a. lusoria

a. mesenterica inferior

a. mesenterica superior

a. pancreatica dorsalis

a. pancreatica inferior

a. pancreatica magna

a. pancreaticoduodenalis superior anterior

a. pancreaticoduodenalis superior posterior

a. rectalis inferior

a. rectalis media

a. rectalis superior

a. splenica

arteriae (*pl. of* arteria)

a. gastricae breves

a. ileales

a. intestinales

a. jejunales

a. pancreaticoduodenales inferiores

a. sigmoideae

arterial

a. ammonia

a. aneurysm

a. arch

a. blood gas (ABG)

a. blood sample

a. buffer response

a. circulation

a. embolization

a. line

a. oxygen desaturation

a. portography

a. priapism

a. saturation

a. spider

a. steal

a. stimulation venous sampling (ASVS)

a. thrombosis

a. underfilling

a. wall necrosis

arterial-enteric fistula

arterialization of portal vein

arteriogenic impotence

arteriogram

hepatic a.

superior mesenteric a.

arteriographic embolization

arteriography

celiac a.

celiomesenteric a.

gastric a.

hepatic a.

mesenteric a.

pancreaticoduodenal a.

penile a.

renal a.

selective left gastric a.

superselective a.

visceral a.

arteriohepatic dysplasia (AHD)

arteriola (*var. of* arteriole)

arteriolar

a. hyalinosis

a. nephrosclerosis

arteriole, arteriola

afferent glomerular a.

efferent glomerular a.

glomerular a.

Isaacs-Ludwig a.

juxtamedullary a.

postglomerular a.

preglomerular a.

renal a.

arteriolopathy

cyclosporine a.

arterioportal
a. fistula
a. vein shunting
a. venous shunt
arterioportographical examination
arterioportography
arteriosclerosis obliterans
arteriosclerotic
a. aneurysm
a. renal artery disease
arteriotomy
end-to-side a.
arteriovenous (AV)
a. access
a. catheter
a. fistula (AVF)
a. hemofiltration
a. malformation (AVM)
a. shunt
arteritis
radiation-induced obliterative a.
Takayasu a.
villous a.
artery, arteria
abnormality of hepatic a.
accessory obturator a.
accessory superior colic a.
adjacent hepatic a.
adrenal a.
anterior cecal a.
anterosuperior pancreaticoduodenal a.
appendicular a.
arcuate a.
ascending ileocolic a.
ASPD a.
atherosclerotic renal a.
bladder a.
bulbar a.
bulbourethral a.
caliber-persistent a.
capsular a.
carotid a.
caudal pancreatic a.
cavernosal a.
colic a.
common hepatic a. (CHA)
common iliac a.
common penile a.
cremasteric a.
cystic a.
deep a.
deferential a.
dorsal pancreatic a.
dorsal penile a.
epigastric a.
external iliac a.
femoral a.
gastric a.

gastroduodenal a. (GDA)
gastroepiploic a. (GEA, GEPA)
gluteal a.
gonadal a.
great pancreatic a.
helicine a.
hepatic a.
high transection of inferior mesenteric a.
hypogastric a.
ileal a.
ileocolic a.
iliac a.
inferior hemorrhoidal a.
inferior mesenteric a. (IMA)
inferior pancreatic a.
inferior pancreaticoduodenal a.
inferior phrenic a.
interlobar renal a.
internal iliac a.
internal pudendal a.
left gastroomental a.
lienal a.
lumbar a.
lusorian a.
mesenteric a.
middle adrenal a.
middle colic a. (MCA)
middle hemorrhoidal a.
obturator a.
a. of Drummond
ovarian a.
pancreatica magna a.
penile a.
phrenic a.
piriformis a.
polar a.
posterorsuperior pancreaticoduodenal a.
preureteral iliac a.
proper hepatic a.
prostatic a.
proximal superior mesenteric a.
pudendal a.
rectal a.
renal a.
retroduodenal a.
retrograde vascularization of superior mesenteric a.
right gastroomental a.
sacral a.
scrotal-perineal a.
spermatic a.
splenic a.
submucosal a.
superior hemorrhoidal a.
superior mesenteric a. (SMA)
superior vesical a.
testicular a.

umbilical a.
urethral a.
uterine a.
vesical a.
vesiculodeferential a.
a. weld strength
arthralgia
arthritic dose (A/D)
arthritis
colitic a.
dysenteric a.
enteropathic reactive a.
peripheral a.
reactive a.
rheumatoid a. (RA)
temporomandibular a.
urethral a.
villous a.
arthropathy
psoriatic a.
arthroplasty
arthrosia
exanthesis a.
artichoke
Articulator injection needle
artifact, artefact
barium a.
mirror-image a.
pellet a.
reverberation a.
artificial
a. anus
a. bezoar
a. Carlsbad salt
a. cystine stone
a. erection
a. erection test
a. genitourinary sphincter
a. genitourinary sphincter
implantation
a. gut
a. hepatic support
a. insemination donor (AID)
a. insemination husband
(AIH)
a. kidney (AK)
a. Kissingen salt
a. organ
a. urethral sphincter (AUS)
a. urinary sphincter (AUS)
a. urinary sphincter implantation
a. urinary sphincter
pressure-regulating balloon
a. Vichy salt
aryepiglottic
a. fold
a. muscle
arylamine
arytenoepiglottidean fold

arytenoid
a. adduction
a. cartilage
AS-800
AS-8. artificial sphincter
AS-8. balloon
AS-8. cuff
AS-8. male bulbous urethra
AS-8. pump
4-ASA
4-aminosalicylic acid
5-ASA
5-aminosalicylic acid
5-ASA agent
5-ASA enema
ASA
acetylsalicylic acid
Asacol delayed-release tablet
asa foetida
Asahi dialyzer
ASA-induced gastric ulceration
ASAP
atypical small acinar proliferation of
prostate
ASAP channel-cut automated biopsy
needle
Microvasive ASAP 18
ASAP prostate biopsy needle
ASAP Stacker automated
multisample biopsy system
ASC
acute suppurative cholangitis
ASCA
anti-*Saccharomyces cerevisiae*
antibody
ascariasis
biliary a.
endobiliary a.
intrahepatic a.
pancreatic a.
ascaricidal
ascaricide
ascarid
ascaris
A. infestation
A. lumbricoides
A. suum
ascendens
colon a.
ascending
a. cholangitis
a. colon
a. ileocolic artery
a. limb
a. pyelography
a. pyelonephritis
a. urethrogram
ascent
kidney a.

ascites
    a. adiposus
    bile a.
    biliary a.
    blood-tinged a.
    bloody a.
    chyliform a.
    a. chylosus
    chylous a.
    cirrhotic a.
    cloudy a.
    culture-negative neutrocytic a. (CNNA)
    demeclocycline-induced a.
    dialysis-related a.
    a. drainage tube
    eosinophilic a.
    a. euglobulin lysis time (AELT)
    exudative a.
    fatty a.
    gelatinous a.
    hemodialysis-associated a.
    hemorrhagic a.
    hydremic a.
    idiopathic a.
    malignant a.
    milky a.
    myxedema a.
    narrow albumin gradient a.
    nephrogenic a.
    nephrogenous dialysis a.
    neutrocytic a.
    nonchylous a.
    pancreatic a.
    pseudochylous a.
    refractory a.
    resistant a.
    straw-colored a.
    tense a.
    transudative a.
    urinary a.
    urine a.
    wide albumin gradient a.
ascitic
    a. amylase
    a. fluid total protein (AFTP)
    a. tumor fluid (ATF)
ascitogenous
ascorbic acid
Ascriptin A/D
ASCUS
    atypical squamous cells of undetermined significance
asecretory
Aselli pancreas
aseptic
    a. anastomosis
    a. intermittent catheterization

    a. technique
    a. wound
Asepti-steryl disinfectant
Asepto irrigation syringe
ASGB
    adjustable silicone gastric banding
ASGE
    American Society for Gastrointestinal Endoscopy
ash
    A. Split Cath
    A. Split Cath XL
    wafer a.
Asherson syndrome
Ashkenazi Jewish community
ASHN
    acute sclerosing hyaline necrosis
Ashton
    A. briefs
    A. pants
ASI
    Advanced Systems Integration
    ASI prostatic stent
    ASI Titan stent
asialism
asialoglycoprotein receptor
Asiatic
    A. cholera
    A. dogwood
    A. schistosomiasis
Asid Bonz PP infusion pump
ASIL
    anal squamous intraepithelial lesion
asitia
Askina Derm film dressing
Ask-Upmark
    A.-U. kidney
    A.-U. renal segment
ASLC
    acute self-limited colitis
ASMA
    antismooth muscle antigen
Asopa
    A. hypospadias repair
    A. procedure
asparaginase
asparagine
aspartate
    a. aminotransferase (AST)
    ornithine a.
    a. transferase
aspartyl protease-mediated cleavage
A-Spas
ASPD
    anterosuperior pancreaticoduodenal
    ASPD artery
aspect
    paraspinous a.

spinous a.
urologic a.
aspergillosis esophagitis
aspergillus
A. bezoar
A. *flavus*
A. *fumigatus*
A. infection
A. *niger*
Aspergum
aspermatism
aspermatogenesis
aspermatogenic sterility
aspermia
asphyxiating thoracic dystrophy
aspidium
aspirate
gastric a.
heme-positive NG a.
nasogastric a.
aspirated sample
aspirating needle
aspiration
a. and dissection tube
a. biopsy
a. biopsy cytology (ABC)
a. catheter
corporeal a.
CT-guided fine-needle a.
diagnostic a.
endoscopic transesophageal
fine-needle a.
endoscopic ultrasound-guided
fine-needle a. (EUS-FNA)
epididymal sperm a. (ESA)
EUS-guided fine-needle a.
fetal bladder a.
fine-needle a. (FNA)
gastric a.
Iglesias method of a.
Levin tube a.
lymphocele a.
microepididymal sperm a.
(MESA)
microscopic epididymal sperm a.
microsurgical epididymal sperm a.
(MESA)
a. mucosectomy
percutaneous balloon a.
percutaneous CT-guided a.
percutaneous epididymal sperm a.
(PESA)
percutaneous needle a.
peritoneal a.
a. pneumonia
pulmonary a.
real-time endoscopic
ultrasound-guided fine-needle a.
real-time fine-needle a. (RTFNA)

seminal vesicle a.
silent a.
sonography-guided a.
sperm a.
suprapubic a.
a. syringe
tracheobronchial a.
aspirator
Cavitron ultrasonic surgical a. (CUSA)
Thorek gallbladder a.
aspirin
enteric-coated a.
aspirin-induced gastritis
Aspisafe nasogastric tube
asplenia syndrome
Assam fever
assay
Abbott IMx PSA a.
acid resistance a.
acrosome reaction a.
activity a.
adherence a.
amidolytic a.
Aptima Combo2 a.
Aptima CT a.
Aura-Tek FDP a.
Ausab EIA a.
Behring OPUS Plus
immunofluorescence a.
Bioclot protein S a.
Bio-Rad protein a.
BioWhittaker a.
bladder tumor a.
branched DNA a.
calprotectin a.
^{14}C glucose uptake a.
Ciba-Corning ACS PSA a.
Clostridium difficile toxin a.
competitive protein-binding a.
cytotoxin a.
disaccharidase a.
electroimmunodiffusion a.
electrophoretic mobility shift a.
ELISA-like a.
enhanced reverse transcriptase
polymerase chain reaction a.
enzyme-linked immunosorbent a.
(ELISA)
enzyme-linked immunosorbent a. I
(ELISA-I)
enzyme-linked immunosorbent a. II
(ELISA-II)
enzyme-linked immunosorbent a. III
(ELISA-III)
erythrocyte lysis a.
estrogen receptor a. (ERA)
fibroblast ECM adhesion a.
fibroblast PMN adhesion a.
a. for neutrophil antibodies

assay (*continued*)
Galacto-Light a.
gastric juice ammonia a.
granzyme B ELISPOT a.
Helicobacter pylori stool a.
heme-porphyrin a.
hemizona a.
HemoQuant a.
hepatitis A virus antigen reduction a.
high-throughput screening a.
HPLC fluorescence a.
Hybritech Tandem prostate-pecific antigen a.
Hybritech Tandem-R PSA a.
IgA tTG a.
Immulite 2000 free PSA a.
Immulite 2000 third-generation PSA a.
immunobead a.
immunoradiometric a. (IRMA)
IMx Hg a.
indirect immunofluorescence a.
inhibition a.
Inno-LiPA a.
intact hormone a.
latex agglutination a.
limiting dilution a.
liquid chromatographic a.
p53 a.
PMN chemotaxis a.
pp65 antigenemia a.
Prometheus First Step inflammatory bowel disease screening a.
Pros-Check PSA a.
protein-protein a.
Pyrilinks-D urinary a.
qualitative microculture a.
radioenzymatic a.
radioimmunoinhibition a.
radioimmunoprecipitation modified a.
recombinant immunoblot a. (RIBA)
recombinant tissue transglutaminase radioligand a.
recombinant tTG radioligand a.
renal vein renin a. (RVRA)
representative electrophoretic mobility shift a.
Roche Elecsys free prostate-specific antigen a.
second-generation recombinant immunoblot a.
solution hybridization RNAse protection a.
sperm penetration a. (SPA)
stool antigen a.
stool toxin a.
Tandem-E PSA immunoenzymetric a.
Tandem-ERA PSA immunoenzymetric a.
Tandem-R PSA a.
tissue culture a.
TNF-alpha a.
Tosoh a.
toxin a.
transcriptase polymerase chain reaction a.
tumor necrosis factor-alpha a.
urine-based enzyme-linked immunosorbent a.
UroVysion a.
Versant HCV RNA qualitative a.
Vysis UroVysion DNA probe a.
Yang polyclonal a.
Yang Pros-Check PSA a.

assay-2
recombinant immunoblot a.-2

assembly
Dentsleeve extruded silastic perfused manometric a.
dilating catheter-gastrostomy tube a.
Konigsberg 5-channel solid-state catheter a.
8-lumen catheter a.
multiple-sidehole manometric a.
purpose-built silicone rubber multilumen manometric a.
standard silicone manometric a.

assessment
angiographic a.
blood flow a.
endoscopic color Doppler a.
extrapyramidal function a.
integrated a.
nutritional a.
a. of bowel preparation quality
outcome and process a.
penile vascular function a.
Sepsis-Related Organ Failure A. (SOFA)
Severity of Dyspepsia A. (SODA)
urodynamic a.

ASSI
Accurate Surgical and Scientific Instruments
ASSI end-to-end vasoepididymostomy
ASSI laparoscopic electrode
ASSI Microspike approximator clamp

assistance
Doppler a.

assistant
gastrointestinal a. (GIA)

assisted
a. reproduction
a. reproductive technique

association
American Anorexia/Bulimia A.
American Diabetes A. (ADA)
American Gastroenterological A.
(AGA)
American Urological A. (AUA)
Dystrophic Epidermolysis Bullosa
Research A. (DEBRA)
Internal Ostomy A. (IOA)
megacystis-megaureter a.
MURCS a.
RESOLVE: The National Infertility
A.
strong a.
United Ostomy A. (UOA)
assumption of homogeneity
Assura
A. AC closure device
A. closed minipouch
A. convex drainable pouch
A. convex urostomy pouch
A. deluxe irrigation set
A. EasiClose device
A. economy irrigation set
A. irrigation accessory
A. irrigation sleeve
A. ostomy belt
A. pediatric pouch
A. pediatric skin barrier flange
A. standard drainable pouch
A. stoma cap
AST
acid suppression therapy
aspartate aminotransferase
AST test
19A2 stain
AST/ALT ratio
asterixis
asteroid body
asthenospermia
asthenospermic
asthenoteratospermia
asthenozoospermia
Astler-Coller
A.-C. classification A, B1, B2, C1,
C2
A.-C. modification of Dukes
classification
Astra
A. profile
A. profile test
Astra/Merck Group
Astramorph
AstraZeneca Pharmaceuticals LP
astrovirus
a. gastroenteritis
human *A.* (HAstV)
**Astwood-Coller staging system for
carcinoma**

ASVS
arterial stimulation venous
sampling
asymmetric, asymmetrical
a. pupils
asymmetrical (*var. of* asymmetric)
asymmetry
asymptomatic
a. bacterium
a. bacteriuria
a. calculus
a. gallstone
a. hemodialysis patient
a. hypocalcemia
a. mass
a. proteinuria
a. pyelonephritis
a. urinary tract infection
(AUTI)
a. urolithiasis
asystole, asystolia
lavage-induced cardiac a.
asystolia (*var. of* asystole)
ATA
antithyroglobulin antibody
Atabrine
Atarax
atazanavir
ATF
ascitic tumor fluid
ATG
antithymocyte globulin
ATGAM
antilymphocyte globulin
antithymocyte globulin
ATGAM polyclonal antibody
atheroembolic renal disease (AERD)
atheroembolism
atheroembolus
atherogenesis
atheromatous
atherosclerosis
graft a.
ostial artery a.
**atherosclerosis-induced cavernosal
ischemia**
atherosclerotic
a. abnormality
a. plaque
a. renal artery
a. renal artery stenosis
a. renovascular disease
Ativan
Atkins diet
Atkinson
A. introducer
A. prosthesis
A. scoring system for dysphagia
A. silicone rubber tube

Atlantic ileostomy catheter
ATN
    acute tubular necrosis
atomic
    a. absorbance spectrophotometer
    a. force microscopy
atonia (*var. of* atony)
atonic
    a. bladder
    a. colon
    a. constipation
    a. dyspepsia
    a. esophagus
atony, atonia
    chronic intestinal a.
    gastric a.
    intestinal a.
    sphincter a.
    ureteral a.
atopic dermatitis
atorvastatin
atovaquone
ATP
    adenosine triphosphate
ATP7A **gene**
ATPase
    adenosine triphosphatase
    ATPase activity
    ATPase inhibitor
atracurium
atrasentan HCl
atraumatic
    a. clamp
    a. grasper
    a. locking/grasping forceps
    a. suture
    a. tip
atresia
    anal a.
    a. ani
    anorectal a.
    bile duct a.
    biliary a.
    congenital biliary a.
    congenital duodenal a.
    duodenal a.
    esophageal a.
    extrahepatic bile duct a.
      (EHBDA)
    extrahepatic biliary a. (EBA)
    follicular a.
    gastric a.
    ileal a.
    intestinal a.
    intrahepatic a. (IHA)
    jejunoileal a.
    Kasai classification for extrahepatic
      bile duct a.

    meatal a.
    prepyloric a.
    pyloric a.
    suprapubic cystotomy tract urethral a.
    urethral a.
    vaginal a.
atretogastria
atrial
    a. liver pulse
    a. natriuretic factor (ANF)
    a. natriuretic peptide (ANP)
Atrigel
Atrocholin
atrophia (*var. of* atrophy)
atrophic
    a. cirrhosis
    a. gastritis
    a. pangastritis
    a. urethritis
    a. vagina
atrophicus
    lichen sclerosus et a.
atrophied
atrophy, atrophia
    acute yellow a.
    adrenal gland a.
    crypt a.
    familial microvillus a.
    fundic gland a.
    gastric mucosal a.
    healed yellow a.
    intestinal a.
    lobar a.
    mucosal a.
    multiple-system a.
    muscle a.
    parenchymatous a.
    partial villous a. (PVA)
    proliferative inflammatory a.
    sclerotic a.
    seminal vesicle a.
    skin a.
    splenic a.
    subtotal villous a. (SVA)
    Sudeck a.
    tubular a.
    villous a.
    white a.
atropine
    a. derivative
    a. infusion
    a. methylnitrate
    a. sulfate
ATS
    autotransfusion
    ATS canister
attachment
    crystal a.

mesenteric a.
peritoneal a.
attack
anginal a.
Gowers a.
Attain tube-feeding formula
attapulgite
attenuated adenomatous polyposis coli
attenuation
attic adhesion
atubular glomerulus
atypia
cellular a.
hepatocellular a.
atypical
a. adenomatous hyperplasia (AAH)
a. distribution of disease
a. ductular cell
a. gallbladder disease
a. glandular cells of unknown significance (AGUS)
a. small acinar proliferation of prostate (ASAP)
a. squamous cells of undetermined significance (ASCUS)
ATZ
anal transitional zone
AUA
American Urological Association
AUA symptom index
Aub-Dubois
A.-D. standard
A.-D. table
AUDIT
alcohol-use disorders identification test
Auerbach
A. and Meissner plexus
A. mesenteric plexus
augmentation
bladder a.
a. cystoplasty
a. enterocystoplasty
gastroileac a.
hemi-T a.
ileocecocystoplasty bladder a.
Mainz pouch a.
orthotopic bladder a.
a. plaque
rectal a.
ureteral bladder a.
urothelial a.
augmented
a. anastomotic urethroplasty
a. biofeedback
a. bladder
a. valved rectum
Augmentin

AUM
ambulatory urodynamic monitoring
AUR
acute urinary retention
auranofin
Aura-Tek
A.-T. FDP assay
A.-T. FDP test
aureus
methicillin-resistant *Staphylococcus a.* (MRSA)
Staphylococcus a.
Auriculin
AUS
artificial urethral sphincter
artificial urinary sphincter
Ausab EIA assay
auscultation of bowel sounds
auscultatory
a. sign
a. sound
Ausonics Opus 1
Australian antigen
australis
Pseudo-nitzschia a.
autacoid (*var. of* autocoid)
autemesia
authority
United Kingdom Transplant Support Service A. (UKTSSA)
AUTI
asymptomatic urinary tract infection
auto
A. Suture Multifire Endo GIA stapler
A. Suture Premium CEEA stapler
autoanalyzer
Beckman 2 a.
Coulter automated a.
Hitachi 737 a.
autoantibody
anticentromere a. (ACA)
antineutrophil cytoplasmic a.
antithyroid a.
antitopoisomerase-I a.
circulating a.
a. production
ScI-70 a.
autoaugmentation
bladder a.
a. cystoplasty
laparoscopic laser-assisted a.
autocholecystectomy
autoclave
heat-sterilized by a.
steam a.
a. sterilized

autoclaved India ink
autoclaving
autocoid, autacoid
autocrine
    a. motility factor (AMF)
    a. regulation
    a. reinforcing loop
autocystoplasty
autodigestion
autoerotic rectal trauma
autofluorescence
    a. and reflectance imaging
    a. endoscopy
autofluorescent endoscopic system
autogenous
    a. spermatocele
    a. tunica vaginalis graft
autografting
autoimmune
    a. cholangitis
    a. cirrhosis
    a. connective tissue disorder
    a. deficiency syndrome
    a. hemolytic anemia
    a. hepatitis (AIH)
    a. immunoglobulin mediation
    a. interstitial nephritis
    a. metaplastic atrophic gastritis (AMAG)
    a. polyglandular syndrome type 1 (APS-1)
    a. sensorineural hearing loss
    a. thyroid disease
    a. thyroiditis
autoimmunity
    thyroid a.
autointoxicant
autointoxication
autolavage
autologous
    a. chondrocyte
    a. fascia lata sling cystourethropexy
    a. fat
    a. HBcAg-specific CD4+
    a. liver cell
    a. rectus fascia
    a. rectus fascia sling
    a. transfusion
autolymphocyte-based treatment for renal cell carcinoma (ALT-RCC)
autolymphocyte therapy
automated
    a. anastomotic instrument
    a. counter Technicon RTX
    a. endoscopic system for optimal positioning (AESOP)
    a. peritoneal dialysis (APD)
automatic

    a. chemical analyzer
    a. endoscopic reprocessor (AER)
    a. needle driver
    a. titration system
automatically sequenced
autonephrectomy
    silent a.
autonomic
    a. dysfunction
    a. dysreflexia
    a. hyperreflexia
    a. nerve fiber
    a. nerve-preserving 3-space dissection
    a. nervous system (ANS)
    a. neurogenic bladder
    a. neuropathy
    a. seizure
autopepsia
autophosphorylation
autoplasty
    peritoneal a.
autopoisonous
autoradiogram
autoradiography (AR)
autoreactivity
    liver-directed a.
autoregressive
autoregulation
    renal a.
autosomal-dominant
    a.-d. disorder
    a.-d. polycystic kidney disease (ADPKD)
    a.-d. polycystic kidney disease 1 (ADPKD1)
    a.-d. polycystic kidney disease 2 (ADPKD2)
autosomally
    a. inherited form of nephrolithiasis
    a. recessive inherited disease
autosomal-recessive
    a.-r. Alport syndrome
    a.-r. mode
    a.-r. polycystic kidney disease (ARPKD)
autosplenectomy
autostapling device
autosuture technique
Autotome
    DomeTip A.
    A. rotatable sphincterotome
autotoxic
autotoxicosis
autotoxin
autotransfusion (ATS)
autotransplantation
    a. of splenic fragment
    posttraumatic a.

pyloric a.
renal a.
auxiliary
  a. heterotopic liver transplantation
    (AHLT)
  a. partial orthotopic liver
    transplantation (APOLT)
  a. partial orthotopic living donor
    transplantation
  a. procedure
  a. transplant
AV
  arteriovenous
  AV fistula
Avagard instant hand antiseptic
avascular
  a. cuff technique
  a. necrosis
  a. stricture
Avastin IV infusion
avenolith
avens
  water a.
Aventyl
average flow rate
aversion therapy
AVF
  arteriovenous fistula
AVF-induced renal ischemia
AVH
  acute viral hepatitis
avian myeloblastosis virus reverse
  transcriptase
avidin-biotin complex (ABC)
avidin-biotin-peroxidase
  a.-b.-p. complex
  a.-b.-p. complex method
Avihepadnavirus
Avitene
avium
  Mycobacterium a.
avium-intracellulare
  Mycobacterium a.-i.
    (MAI)
AVM
  arteriovenous malformation
avoidance maneuver
AVP
  arginine vasopressin
AVPR2
  antidiuretic arginine vasopressin V2
  receptor
A-V shunt
avulsion
  splenic a.
AVWS
  anterior vaginal wall sling
AW
  actual weight

axes (*pl. of* axis)
axial
  a. flap
  a. hiatal hernia
  a. image
Axid
axillary adenopathy
Axiom double sump tube
axis, *pl.* **axes**
  bowel a.
  brain-gut a.
  cardiopyloric a.
  celiac a.
  crypt-villus a.
  a. deviation
  enteroinsular a.
  gut-liver a.
  hypertension resistance a.
  hypothalamic-pituitary a. (HPA)
  hypothalamic-pituitary-testicular-penile
    a.
  macrophage-TGF-beta a.
  neurohumoral-immune a.
  pituitary-gonadal a.
  renin-angiotensin-aldosterone a.
  reproductive a.
axoaxonic synapse
Axokine
axonopathy
axon reflex
axoplasmic
AxSYM free PSA test
Aylett operation
Ayre brush
Azactam
azamethonium
azan stain
azapetine
Aza-Pred therapy
azar
  kala a.
Azasan
azasteroid inhibitor
azathioprine
azide
  sodium a.
azidothymidine (AZT)
azithromycin
azlocillin
azole
  a. antifungal agent
  a. therapy
azoospermatism (*var. of* azoospermia)
azoospermia, azoospermatism
  excretory a.
  occlusive a.
  steroid-induced a.
  unreconstructable obstructive a.
Azo-Standard

azotemia
    extrarenal a.
    prerenal a.
azotemic osteodystrophy
azoturia
azoturic
azoxymethane
AZQ
    diaziquone

AZT
    azidothymidine
Aztec 2-step
aztreonam
Azulfidine EN-tabs
azygos
    a. blood flow
    a. vein
azygous

B

B antigen
B bile
B cellular phenotype
B lymphocyte
B ring
B ring of esophagus

B-1

Dukes B-1

B$_{12}$

B$_{12}$ anemia
B$_{12}$ immunologic study
vitamin B$_{12}$

B2

bromobenzene

B-48

apo B-48
apolipoprotein B-48
plasma apo B-48

B$_6$

vitamin B$_6$

B72.3 murine monoclonal antibody
Babcock

B. clamp
B. intestinal forceps

Babinski reflex
baby

b. Balfour retractor
b. scope
b. soft diet (BSD)

BabyBIG powder for IV infusion
BAC

benzalkonium chloride

bacampicillin
bacillary

b. angiomatosis
b. dysentery

bacille Calmette-Guérin (BCG, bCG)
bacilli (*pl. of* bacillus)
bacillus, *pl.* **bacilli**

acid-fast b. (AFB)
Calmette-Guérin b.
B. cereus
coliform b.
curved b.
dysentery b.
Friedländer b.
Schmitz b.
Shiga b.
Sonne-Duval b.
Stanley b.
Whipple b.

bacitracin zinc
backflow

pyelolymphatic b.

pyelorenal b.
pyelosinus b.
pyelotubular b.
pyelovenous b.

background

experimental b.
mucosal b.

Backhaus

B. dilator
B. towel clamp
B. towel forceps

backleak

acute tubular necrosis b.

backwash ileitis
baclofen
Bacon anoscope
Bacon-Babcock rectovaginal fistula operation
bacterascites

monomicrobial nonneutrocytic
b. (MNB)
polymicrobial b.

bacteremia, bacteriemia

incidence of b.
percentage frequency of b.
risk of b.
Streptococcus bovis b.

bacteria (*pl. of* bacterium)
bacterial

b. adherence
b. adhesin
b. adhesion
b. biofilm
b. biofilm formation
b. cast
b. cholangitis
b. cirrhosis
b. cleavage
b. colitis
b. complication
b. culture
b. cystitis
b. endotoxin
b. enterocolitis
b. esophagitis
b. flora
b. food poisoning
b. host interaction
b. infection
b. interference
b. metabolism in intestine
b. mucosal infiltration
b. nephritis
b. overgrowth
b. overgrowth syndrome

bacterial (*continued*)
  b. pathogenesis
  b. peritonitis
  b. prostatitis
  b. toxigenic diarrhea
  b. translocation
  b. vaginosis
  b. vector
  b. virulence factor
bactericholia, bacteriocholia
bactericidal
  b. function of phagocyte
  b. stomach environment
bactericidal/permeability-increasing protein
bactericide
bacteriemia (*var. of* bacteremia)
bacteriocidal (*var. of* bactericidal)
bacteriology
bacteriospermia
bacteriostatically
bacteriostatic barrier
bacterium, *pl.* **bacteria**
  asymptomatic b.
  Chauveau b.
  coliform b.
  colonic b.
  commensal b.
  gram-negative b.
  gram-positive b.
  human gut b.
  intestinal b.
  mesophilic b.
  pathogenic b.
  planktonic b.
  pyogenic b.
  spiral b.
  sulfate-reducing b.
  toxigenic b.
  urease-positive b.
  urease-producing b.
  uropathogenic b.
bacteriuria
  asymptomatic b.
  catheter-associated b.
Bacteroidaceae
Bacteroides
  B. distasonis
  B. eggerthii
  B. fragilis
  B. melaninogenicus
  B. ovatus
  B. praeacutus
  B. putredinis
  B. splanchnicus
  B. thetaiotaomicron
  B. uniformis
  B. ureolyticus
  B. vulgatus

bactibilia
Bactocill
Bactrim DS
baculovirus
baculum
BAD
  benign anorectal disease
BA-EDTA
  bile acid-ethylenediaminetetraacetic acid
    BA-EDTA solution
Baehr-Lohlein lesion
Baermann
  B. stool filter
  B. stool test
bag
  Acme One Time enteral feeding b.
  anal b.
  Belly b.
  bile b.
  biohazard b.
  Bogota b.
  bowel b.
  breath b.
  Coloplast b.
  colostomy b.
  Davol feeding b.
  DeRoyal Surgical grab b.
  Dobbhoff enteral feeding b.
  Endo Catch b.
  EndoMate grab b.
  Entri-Pak enteral feeding b.
  Extract specimen b.
  gavage b.
  Hollister urostomy b.
  ileostomy b.
  intestinal b.
  Keofeed enteral feeding b.
  Lahey liver transplant b.
  Le B.
  Mikulicz b.
  Mosher b.
  Moveen bedside night b.
  nylon tissue biopsy b.
  ostomy b.
  perfusate b.
  Perry b.
  Petersen b.
  Plummer b.
  pneumatic b.
  Polar enteral feeding b.
  Rutzen ileostomy b.
  stomal b.
  Technoline anal b.
  Top-Fill enteral feeding b.
  Vacutainer b.
  Whitmore b.
BAGF
  brachioaxillary bridge graft fistula
Bagley helical basket

BAIBF
    bile acid-independent bile formation
Bainbridge
    B. intestinal clamp
    B. intestinal forceps
Bakamjian flap
Baker
    B. antifol
    B. intestinal decompression tube
    B. jejunostomy tube
Bakes
    B. common duct dilator
    B. probe
BAL
    blood alcohol level
balance
    acid-base b.
    chloride b.
    electrolyte b.
    equal fluid b.
    glomerulotubular b.
    B. lavage solution
    metabolic b.
    negative nitrogen b.
    nitrogen b.
    positive nitrogen b.
    potassium b.
    sodium b.
    vagosympathetic b.
    water b.
balanced
    b. diet
    b. electrolyte solution
    b. salt solution (BSS)
    b. voiding dysfunction
balanic hypospadias
balanitic epispadias
balanitis
    b. circinata
    circinate b.
    b. circumscripta plasmacellularis
    b. diabetica
    Follmann b.
    b. gangraenosa
    gangrenous b.
    keratotic pseudoepitheliomatous b.
    b. of Zoon
    plasma cell b.
    trichomonal b.
    b. xerotica
    b. xerotica obliterans (BXO)
    yeast b.
balanoblennorrhea
balanocele
balanoplasty
**balanoposthitis chronica circumscripta
  plasma cellularis**
balanoposthomycosis
balanopreputial

balanorrhagia
balanorrhea
balantidial
    b. colitis
    b. dysentery
balantidiasis, balantidosis
Balantidium
    B. coli
    B. coli colitis
balantidosis (*var. of* balantidiasis)
balanus
Balch 1 broth medium
bald gastric fundus
Baldwin perineum needle
Baldy-Webster operation
Balfour
    B. abdominal retractor
    B. gastroenterostomy
    B. self-retaining retractor
Balkan
    B. nephrectomy
    B. nephritis
    B. nephropathy
ball
    b. electrode
    food b.
    fungal b.
    gastrointestinal fungal b.
    hair b.
    b. myoma
    B. operation
    B. procedure
    ureteropelvic fungus b.
    B. valve
    wool b.
Ballance sign
Ballenger forceps
Ballobes gastric balloon
balloon
    Acucise b.
    air-filled b.
    anchoring b.
    angioplasty b.
    artificial urinary sphincter
      pressure-regulating b.
    AS-800 b.
    Ballobes gastric b.
    banana-shaped b.
    barostat b.
    barostatic b.
    Brandt cytology b.
    b. catheter and basket retrieval
      technique
    b. catheter-assisted endoscopic snare
      papillectomy
    centering b.
    b. cholangiogram
    cylindrical b.
    b. cystoscope

B

balloon (*continued*)
  b. cytology
  DASH extraction b.
  b. decompression
  b. defecation
  b. dilating catheter
  b. dilation
  b. dilation of papilla
  b. dilator
  dissecting b.
  doughnut-shaped b.
  esophageal single b.
  b. expulsion test
  extraction b.
  Extractor XL triple-lumen retrieval b.
  fluid-filled b.
  Fogarty b.
  French Swan-Ganz b.
  Garren b.
  Garren-Edwards b.
  gastric b.
  Gau gastric b.
  Grüntzig b.
  Helmstein b.
  high-compliance latex b.
  hot wire b.
  hydrostatic b.
  intragastric b.
  Kaye nephrostomy tamponade b.
  b. kymography
  b. laser
  latex b.
  low-compliance b.
  mercury-containing b.
  Microvasive retrieval b.
  Microvasive Rigiflex through-the-scope b.
  occlusion b.
  b. occlusion cholangiography
  Percival gastric b.
  b. percutaneous transluminal angioplasty
  b. photodynamic therapy
  preperitoneal distention b. (PDB)
  b. proctogram
  Provocative sensitivity b.
  Quantum TTC biliary b.
  rectal b.
  b. reflex manometry
  retrieval b.
  Riepe-Bard gastric b.
  Rigiflex achalasia b.
  Rigiflex TTS b.
  scintigraphic b.
  Sengstaken-Blakemore esophageal b.
  silicone b.
  stone retrieval b.
  b. tamponade prosthesis
  Taylor gastric b.
  through-the-scope b.
  b. topogram
  treatment b.
  b. tube tamponade
  b. ureteral occlusion
  water-displacing b.
  Wilson-Cook dilating b.
  Wilson-Cook esophageal b.
  Wilson-Cook gastric b.
  windowed esophageal b.
  wire-guided hydrostatic b.
balloon-assisted intubation
ballooned hepatocyte
ballooning
  b. degeneration
  b. degeneration of hepatocyte
  eosinophilic b.
  b. esophagoscope
  hepatocellular b.
  b. of cell
  b. of papilla
balloon-occluded retrograde transvenous obliteration (B-RTO)
ballottable liver
ballottement
  abdominal b.
  kidney b.
  b. tenderness
balm
Balneol
BALP
  bone-specific alkaline phosphatase
balsalazide disodium
balsam
  copaiba b.
Balser fatty necrosis
BALT
  bronchus-associated lymphoepithelial tissue
Balthazar grading system
BAM
  bile acid malabsorption
Bamberger hematogenic albuminuria
bamboo jointlike appearance of gastric body
Bamethan
banana
  b. peel effect
  b. plug dipolar generator
  b.'s, rice, cereal, applesauce, and toast (BRAT)
  b.'s, rice, cereal, applesauce, tea, and toast (BRATT)
banana-shaped balloon
bancrofti
  Wuchereria b.

B

band
    adhesive b.
    anorectal b.
    cholecystoduodenal b.
    dysgenetic fibrous b.
    EasyBand adjustable gastric b.
    b. form
    genitomesenteric b.
    Harris b.
    Henle b.
    hymenal b.
    Ladd b.
    Lane b.
    b. ligation
    Lyon ring constrictive b.
    Marlex b.
    mesocolic b.
    omental b.
    pecten b.
    peritoneal b.
    b. placement
    b. 3 protein
    retention b.
    silicone elastomer b.
    snap gauge b.
    Swedish adjustable gastric b.
        (SAGB)
    WBC b.
    Wilson-Cook ligator b.
bandage
    Sureseal pressure b.
    suspensory b.
    T b.
band-and-snare technique
banded gastroplasty with divided pouch
banding
    adjustable silicone gastric b.
        (ASGB)
    crural b.
    b. cylinder
    esophageal b.
    hemorrhoidal b.
    laparoscopic adjustable gastric b.
    Lap-Band adjustable gastric b.
        (LAGB)
    laser adjustable silicone gastric b.
        (LASGB)
    mucosal b.
    suction b.
    variceal b.
Bandito single-band ligator
band-ligator device
band-snare technique
Banff renal allograft rejection classification
banjo-string adhesion
Bannayan-Ruvalcaba-Riley syndrome
Bannayan-Zonana syndrome
Banocide

Banthine
Banti
    B. disease
    B. splenic anemia
    B. syndrome
BAO
    basal acid output
BAP
    bone alkaline phosphatase
BAR
    biofragmentable anastomotic ring
        Valtrac BAR
bar
    cricopharyngeal b.
    intersymphysial b.
    leading b.
    Mercier b.
    symphysial b.
Baraclude
barbed snare
barber pole sign
barberry
Barbidonna No. 2
Barbita
barbital-acetate buffer
barbotage
Barcat
    B. distal hypospadias repair
        technique
    B. procedure
Barcat-Redman hypospadias repair
Barcoo
    B. vomit
    B. vomitus
Bard
    B. alligator cup
    B. automatic reprocessor
    B. Biopty gun
    B. Biopty instrument
    B. BladderScan
    B. BladderScan bladder volume
        instrument
    B. BTA test
    B. button
    B. closed-end adhesive pouch
    B. Companion papillotome
    B. Director guidewire
    B. drainage adhesive pouch
    B. EndoCinch endoscopic suturing
        system
    B. endoscope transesophageal
        endoscopic plication
    B. Extra Ileo B pouch
    B. gastrostomy catheter
    B. gastrostomy feeding tube
    B. irrigation sleeve
    B. Memotherm colorectal stent
    B. oval cup
    B. PEG

Bard (*continued*)
    B. PEG tube
    B. Precisor direct bite forceps
    B. protective barrier
    B. protective barrier film
    B. security pouch
    B. Urolase
    B. Urolase fiber laser system
    B. Visilex mesh
Bardet-Biedl syndrome
Bardex-Foley catheter
Bard-Parker
    B.-P. blade
    B.-P. knife
BardPort implanted port
Bard-Stiegmann-Goff variceal ligation kit
bare area of liver
bariatric
    b. operation
    b. surgery
bariatrics
Baricon contrast medium
barium
    b. artifact
    b. bezoar
    b. burger
    b. contrast hypotonic duodenography
    b. contrast radiography
    double tracking of b.
    b. enema (BE)
    b. enema reduction
    b. enema with air contrast
    b. esophagram
    b. GI series
    b. granuloma
    b. meal
    b. paste
    b. peritonitis
    residual b.
    retained b.
    b. retention
    b. sediment in urine
    b. study
    b. sulfate
    b. sulfate for suspension
    b. sulfate solution
    b. swallow
barium-coated marshmallow
barium-impregnated marshmallow
bark
    elm b.
    pinus b.
barley
Barnes common duct dilator
Barnett pouch
Baro-CAT
baroceptor (*var. of* baroreceptor)
Baroflave contrast medium

barogenic perforation
Barophen
baroreceptor, baroceptor
    high-pressure arterial b.
    low-pressure cardiopulmonary b.
    renal b.
    sinoaortic b.
baroreceptor-mediated mesenteric arterial vasoconstriction
baroreflex
    cardiopulmonary b.
Barosperse contrast medium
barostat
    b. balloon
    electronic b.
    gastric b.
    b. method
    rectal b.
    Synectics visceral stimulator electronic b.
barostatic balloon
barotrauma
    cecal b.
Barr
    B. fistula hook
    B. fistula probe
    B. rectal retractor
    B. rectal speculum
barrel
    b. chest
    Opti-Vue plastic b.
Barrett
    B. carcinoma
    B. disease
    B. dysplasia
    B. epithelium
    B. esophagitis
    B. esophagus (BE)
    B. esophagus-associated adenocarcinoma cell
    B. intestinal forceps
    B. metaplasia
    B. segment
    B. syndrome
    B. ulcer
Barrett-Clagett esophagogastrostomy
Barrett-Donovan-Mayo artificial bladder
Barrett-Murphy intestinal thumb forceps
barrier
    ABO b.
    bacteriostatic b.
    Bard protective b.
    bioabsorbable adhesion b.
    blood-epididymis b.
    blood-liquor b.
    blood-testis b.

blood-urine b.
Colly-Seal wafer-type skin b.
Coloplast skin b.
Comfeel skin b.
Dansac skin b.
b. drape
filtration b.
gastric mucosal b. (GMB)
high-pressure antireflux b.
Hollister Guardian F skin b.
Interceed absorbable adhesion b.
Nu-Hope adhesive waterproof skin
   b.
Nu-Hope protective skin b.
pectin-based skin b.
Premium B.
ReliaSeal skin b.
seminiferous tubule blood-testis b.
Soft Guard XL skin b.
Stomahesive skin b.
Sween-A-Peel skin b.
United XL 14 skin b.

Barrington third reflex

Barron

B. ligation
B. rubber band ligator

Barr-Shuford rectal speculum

Barsony-Polgar syndrome

Bartel cytotoxicity

Barth hernia

Bartholin

B. cyst
B. gland

Bartonella henselae

Bartter syndrome

bar-type esophageal varix

baruria

basal

b. acid output (BAO)
b. acid secretion
b. anal canal pressure
b. anal sphincter pressure
b. androstenedione
b. carbohydrate oxidation rate
b. cell carcinoma
b. cell nevus syndrome
b. cell-specific anticytokeratin
   antibody
b. diet
b. ganglia
b. granular cell
b. interferon gamma
b. lamina
b. metabolic rate (BMR)
b. metabolism
b. release of motilin
b. renal excretion
b. renovascular resistance

b. secretory flow rate (BSFR)
b. secretory flow rate test
b. testosterone

Basaljel

basaloid squamous cell carcinoma (BSCC)

bascule

cecal b.

base

adhesive b.
compressive b.
crypt b.
erythromycin b.
b. excess
Interstitial Cystitis Data B. (ICDB)
b. of appendix
b. of renal pyramid
ulcer b.

baseball stitch

baseline

b. recovered control
b. tenting
b. troponin T

basement

b. membrane
b. membrane antigen
b. membrane protein

bas-fond

basic

b. core promoter
b. diet
b. dye
b. fibroblast growth factor (bFGF)
b. fibroblastic growth factor
b. gastrin

basidiobolomycosis

Basidiobolus ranarum

basil

basiliximab

basket

Bagley helical b.
Cook N-Circle tipless stone b.
DASH tipless extraction b.
Dormia stone b.
Eliminator stone extraction b.
Ellik kidney stone b.
Escape nitinol stone basket
   retrieval b.
b. extraction
b. forceps
Gemini paired-wire helical b.
Glassman b.
Helical b.
laser lithotriptor b.
minihelical b.
nitinol b.
Olympus stone retrieval b.
Positrap miniretrieval b.

basket (*continued*)
    b. procedure
    Pursuer CBD helical stone b.
    Pursuer minihelical stone b.
    retrieval b.
    Segura b.
    Segura-Dretler laser b.
    sphincterotomy b.
    spiral b.
    spiral-tip Segura b.
    stone retrieval b.
    Sur-Catch NT stone retrieval b.
    trapped b.
basketing
    ureteral scoping b.
basket-type crushing forceps
baso
    basophil
basolateral
    b. membrane (BLM)
    b. transporter ferroportin 1
basophil, basophile (baso)
    WBC b.
basophile (*var. of* basophil)
Bassen-Kornzweig
    B.-K. disease
    B.-K. syndrome
Bassini
    B. inguinal hernia repair
    B. inguinal herniorrhaphy
    B. needle
    B. operation
BAS-300 transurethral thermotherapy device
Bates-corrected beta
Bates operation
bath
    alcohol cooling b.
    sitz b.
bathroom privilege
battery
    button b.
    b. ingestion
battery-powered endoscope
Battle
    B. incision
    B. operation
    B. sign
Battle-Jalaguier-Kammerer incision
bat-wing catheter
Bauhin
    B. valve
    valve of B.
Baumgarten
    B. cirrhosis
    B. syndrome
Baumrucker urinary incontinence clamp

Baveno portal hypertensive gastropathy grading system
Baxter
    B. filter
    B. hemodialyzer
    B. Interline IV system
Bayer
    B. Plus
    B. Versant HCV RNA assay test kit
BayGam IM injection
Bay K 8644 channel agonist
Baylor bleeding score
bayonet stylet
bayonet-tip electrode
bayonet-type forceps
Baza Cleanse and Protect
Bazex syndrome
BBDS
    benign bile duct stricture
B1, B2 integrin
BBM
    brush-border membrane
BBMV
    brush-border membrane vesicle
BC
    bicarbonate
    BC Cold Powder
BCAA
    branched-chain amino acid
BCAA/AAA plasma ratio
BCAD 2 powder
BCA-1 protein assay kit
B-cell
    B-c. antigen CD20
    B-c. epitope
    B-c. line
    B-c. PHSL
BCG, bCG
    bacille Calmette-Guérin
    BCG immunotherapy
    intravesical BCG
    BCG live
    BCG live intravesical injection
    Mycobacterium bovis BCG
    BCG vaccine
bcl-2
BCM
    body cell mass
BCNU, bCNU
    carmustine
BCO
    biliary cholesterol output
BCR
    bulbocavernosus reflex
BD
    Becton Dickinson

B

BD ProbeTec urine preservative transport

BDA
bile duct adenoma

BDL
bile duct ligation

bDNA
branched-chain DNA

BDNF
brain-derived neurotrophic factor

BDP
beclomethasone dipropionate

B-D Safety-Gard needle

BE
barium enema
Barrett esophagus

Beacon surgical line

bead
Percoll b.
PMMA b.
Septopal b.

bead-chain
b.-c. cystography
b.-c. study

beaded hepatic duct

beading sign

beaker cell

beaklike appearance

Beale
sacculi of B.

Beamer
B. injection stent
B. injection stent system

bean
bog b.
b. pod

bear claw ulcer

Beardsley
B. cecostomy trocar
B. esophageal retractor
B. intestinal clamp
B. intestinal forceps

Bearn-Kunkel-Slater syndrome

bear's garlic

Beasley-Babcock forceps

beaver
B. blade
B. dissector
b. fever

BEB
blind esophageal brushing

BEC
biliary epithelial cell

becatecarin

Beck
B. abdominal scoop
B. aorta forceps
B. gastrostomy

B. method

Beck-Jianu gastrostomy

Beckman
B. airfuge
B. 2 autoanalyzer
B. ion-selective analyzer
B. pH probe

Beckwith-Wiedemann syndrome

Béclard hernia

beclomethasone dipropionate (BDP)

Becton Dickinson (BD, B-D)

BED
binge-eating disorder

bed
Advanta b.
Enterprise hospital b.
gallbladder b.
graft b.
hepatic b.
liver b.
b. pad
portal vascular b.
raw surface of liver b.
stomach b.
suburothelial vascular b.
ulcer b.

Bedge
B. antireflux mattress
B. pillow

bedside drainage (BSD)

bed-wetting alarm

Beebe hemostatic forceps

beef tapeworm

Beelith

Beer nephroureterectomy

BEF
bronchoesophageal fistula

B.E. Glass abdominal retractor

behavior
binge-purge b.

behavioral treatment

Behçet
B. colitis
B. disease
B. syndrome

behen

Behrend cystic duct forceps

Behring OPUS Plus immunofluorescence assay

beigelii
Trichosporon b.

belch
silent b.

belching

Belfield operation

Bell
B. law

Bell (*continued*)
    B. muscle
    B. suture
Belladenal
belladonna
    tincture of b.
Bellafoline
Bellalphen
bell-clapper deformity
Bellergal-S
belli
    Isospora b.
Bellini
    B. duct
    B. duct carcinoma
    B. ligament
    B. tubule
bellow response
bell-shaped orifice
belly
    B. bag
    Crix b.
    wooden b.
bellyache
BELS
    bioartificial extracorporeal liver support
    BELS system
Belsey
    B. Mark IV antireflux operation
    B. Mark IV fundoplication
    B. Mark IV procedure
    B. Mark IV repair
    B. Mark V operation
    B. partial fundoplication
    B. 2/3 wrap fundoplication
belt
    abdominal compression b.
    Assura ostomy b.
    Coloplast ostomy b.
    B. radical prostatectomy technique
    b. test
Belt-Fuqua hypospadias repair
Belzer
    B. machine
    B. UW liver preservation
    solution
Benadryl
benazepril HCl
Bence
    B. Jones albumin
    B. Jones albumosuria
    B. Jones cylinder
    B. Jones globulin
    B. Jones protein
    B. Jones protein method
    B. Jones proteinuria
    B. Jones urine
bench
    b. surgery

    b. surgical technique
Benchekroun
    B. hydraulic ileal valve
    B. pouch
bend
    cautery b.
    iliac b.
bendroflumethiazide
Benedict
    B. and Franke method
    B. gastroscope
Benedict-Talbot body surface area method
Benelux Multicentre Trial Study Group
Benemid
Bengt-Johansson procedure
benign
    b. adenomatous polyp
    b. anorectal disease (BAD)
    b. bile duct stricture (BBDS)
    b. biliary stricture
    b. cystic mesothelioma
    b. cystic teratoma
    b. duodenocolic fistula
    b. familial hematuria
    b. familial icterus
    b. familial pemphigus
    b. gastric ulcer
    b. gastrocolic-pancreatic fistula
    b. hyperplastic gastropathy
    b. lymphoma
    b. lymphoma of rectum
    b. mesenchymoma
    b. mesothelioma of genital tract
    b. mucous membrane pemphigoid
    (BMMP)
    b. neoplastic precursor
    b. nephrosclerosis
    b. papillary stenosis
    b. paroxysmal peritonitis
    b. pneumatic colonoscopy
    complication
    b. pneumoperitoneum
    b. postoperative cholestasia
    b. postoperative jaundice
    b. prostatic enlargement (BPE)
    b. prostatic hyperplasia (BPH)
    b. prostatic hyperplasia transurethral
    vaporization
    b. prostatic hypertrophy (BPH)
    b. prostatic obstruction (BPO)
    b. recurrent intrahepatic cholestasia
    (BRIC)
    b. tumor
Béniqúe sound
Bennet root
Bennett operation
benoxaprofen

benserazide
Benson pylorus separator
bentiromide test
Bentle button
bent nail syndrome
bentonite flocculation test
Bentson floppy-tipped guidewire
Bentson-type Glidewire
  guidewire
Bentyl
Bentylol
Benzacot injection
benzaldehyde dehydrogenase
benzalkonium chloride (BAC)
benzamide prokinetic agent
benzathine penicillin
benzbromarone
benzethonium chloride 0.025%
benzidine
benzimidazole
  substituted b.
benzoate
benzocaine
benzodiazepine conscious sedation
benzodiazepine-induced
  hypoventilation
benzoic acid
benzoin
  tincture of b.
benzoyl-tyrosyl-paraaminobenzoic acid
  (BT-PABA)
benzphetamine
benzquinamide
benzthiazide
benztropine
benzydamine
benzyl chloride
benzylpenicillin, benzyl penicillin
BEP
  bleomycin, etoposide, cisplatin
Beppu score
bepridil
Berci-Shore
  B.-S. choledochoscope
  B.-S. choledochoscopy
Berens esophageal retractor
Bergenhem operation
Berger
  B. disease
  B. nephropathy
Bergkvist grading system
Bergman sign
Beriplast fibrin sealant
Berkeley-Bonney retractor
Berlin
  B. blue
  B. blue staining
Bernard
  B. canal

B. duct
B. glandular layer
Bernard-Sergent syndrome
Bernard-Soulier syndrome
Bernstein
  B. acid perfusion test
  B. gastroscope
berry aneurysm
Bertiella
  B. mucronata
  B. satyri
  B. studeri
Bertin
  hypertrophy of column of B.
Bertrand method
berylliosis
Besnier-Boeck-Schaumann disease
BESP
  Bipolar EndoStasis probe
Bessauds-Hilmand-Augier syndrome
Bessey-Lowry unit for alkaline
  phosphatase
Best
  B. bite block
  B. gallstone forceps
  B. operation
  B. right-angle colon clamp
bestatin
bestiarum
  Aeromonas b.
besylate
  amlodipine b.
2-beta
  interferon alfa 2-b.
3-beta
  3-b. hydroxysteroid
  3-b. hydroxysteroid dehydrogenase
    (3betaHSD, 3-beta-HSD)
  3-b. hydroxysteroid dehydrogenase
    deficiency
beta
  b. adrenergic agonist
  b. aminoisobutyric aciduria
  b. aminopropionitrile
  Bates-corrected b.
  b. chain
  epoetin b.
  ER b.
  estrogen receptor b. (ER beta)
  b. fetoprotein
  b. fibroblastic growth factor
  b. galactose
  b. galactosidase
  b. galactosidase activity
  growth factor b.
  b. hemolytic streptococcus
  b. hydroxyacyl-coenzyme A
    dehydrogenase
  b. hydroxylase

beta (*continued*)
  b. inhibin
  b. interferon
  interferon b. (IFN beta)
  b. microseminoprotein
  b. oxidation pathway
  b. sitosterolemia
  b. subunit
  b. sympathomimetic tocolytic agent
  Thymosin b. 4
  transforming growth factor b.
    (TGF-beta)
beta-1
  b.-1 chain
  b.-1 chain integrin
  factor b.-1
  transforming growth factor b.-1
    (TGF-beta-1)
beta-2
  b.-2 agonist
  factor b.-2
  b.-2 microglobulin
  b.-2 microglobulin control
  b.-2 test
  transforming growth factor b.-2
    (TGF-beta-2)
beta-3
  b.-3 agonist
  factor b.-3
  transforming growth factor b.-3
    (TGF-beta-3)
beta-actin
  b.-a. cDNA probe
  b.-a. mRNA signal
beta-adrenergic
  b.-a. antagonist
  b.-a. blockade
  b.-a. blocker
  b.-a. receptor
beta-blocker therapy
Beta-Cap
  B.-C. catheter closure
  B.-C. II closure
Betadine
  B. gel
  B. PrepStick Plus applicator
  B. scrub
17-beta-diol
  5-alpha-androstane-3-alpha 17-b.-d.
  5-alpha-androstane-3-beta 17-b.-d.
beta-endorphin
  b.-e. peptide YY
7-beta-epimer of chenodeoxycholic acid
Betagan
beta-HCG autocrine motility factor
11-beta-hydroxylase deficiency
betaine anhydrous solution
beta-lactam antibiotic

beta-lactamase-resistant penicillin
beta-lactam-associated diarrhea
betamethasone
  topical b.
beta-pleated sheet formation
betaretrovirus
  human b. (HBRV)
BetaSorb device
beta-thromboglobulin (BTG)
betaxolol
betazole stimulation test
betel nut
bethanechol
  b. chloride
  b. hydrochloride
  b. test
bethanidine
Bethesda System for cervicovaginal sample
Bethune shears
BetterMAN
bevacizumab
Bevan
  B. abdominal incision
  B. gallbladder forceps
  B. operation
  B. orchiopexy
bevel
  Menghini-type coring b.
beveled speculum
beverage
  Resource Fruit B.
bezafibrate
bezoar
  artificial b.
  Aspergillus b.
  barium b.
  fungal b.
  gastric b.
  medication b.
  orange b.
  percutaneous removal of b.
  persimmon b.
bFGF
  basic fibroblast growth factor
BFR
  blood flow rate
B2 glycoprotein I
BGV
  bleeding gastric varix
BHD
  Birt-Hogg-Dube
  BHD syndrome
Bi
  bismuth
BIA
  bioelectrical impedance analysis
Biafine wound dressing emulsion
Bianchi approach

Biatain foam dressing
Biaxin
BIB
    biliointestinal bypass
bibasilar
bicalutamide
    b. monotherapy
    b. withdrawal phenomenon
BICAP
    bipolar circumactive probe
        BICAP bipolar diathermy
        BICAP bipolar hemostasis probe
        BICAP coagulation
        BICAP electrocoagulation probe
        BICAP electrode probe
        BICAP endoscopic probe
        BICAP hemostatic system
        BICAP II cautery
        BICAP monopolar probe
        BICAP silver ACE
Bicarbolyte
bicarbonate (HCO3, HCO)
    b. buffer system
    b. dialysate
    b. electrolyte
    Krebs-Henseleit b. (KHB)
    potassium b.
    saliva b.
    serum b.
    sodium b.
    urinary b.
    b. wastage renal tubular acidosis
bicarotid trunk
BiCart dialysis fluid
biceps femoris musculocutaneous
  unit
bicho
Bicitra
BiCNU
    carmustine
bicolor guaiac
bicornuate uterus
bicoudate catheter
bicoudé
    catheter b.
bicurve needle
bidigital rectal examination
bidirectional ligation
Biebl loop
bieneusi
    Enterocytozoon b.
Biermer disease
Biesiadecki fossa
bifid
    b. branch
    b. clitoris
    b. penis
    b. renal pelvis
    b. scrotum
    b. tongue
    b. ureter
bifida
    adolescent spina b.
    spina b.
Bifidobacterium
    B. bifidum
    B. brevis
    B. infantis
    B. longum
bifidum
    Bifidobacterium b.
bifidus
    Lactobacillus b.
bifocal multiplane rectal transducer
bifurcation
    hepatic b.
    b. of common bile duct
    tracheal b.
    b. tumor
Bigelow
    B. litholapaxy
    B. operation
bigeminy
big liver and spleen disease (BLSD)
biglycan
    proteoglycan b.
biguanides
Bihrle
    B. dorsal clamp
    B. dorsal clamp-T-C needle holder
BII
    BPH impact index
bikunin
bilabe
Bilagog
bilaminar embryonic disk
Bilarcil
bilateral
    b. anorchism
    b. cryptorchidism
    b. hydronephrosis
    b. lithotomies
    b. nephrectomies
    b. nephroureterectomies
    b. pheochromocytomas
    b. pudendal artery embolization
    b. renal tumors
    b. renal vein thromboses
    b. subcostal incisions
    b. transabdominal incisions
    b. ureteral obstruction (BUO)
    b. ureterostomy takedown
    b. vagotomies
    b. Wilms tumors
bilayer
    lipid b.
    phospholipid b.
Bilbao-Dotter tube

B

bilberry
    bog b.
bile
    A b.
    b. acid
    b. acid binder
    b. acid breath test
    b. acid diarrhea type 1, 2
    b. acid-EDTA solution
    b. acid-ethylenediaminetetraacetic
        acid (BA-EDTA)
    b. acid-independent bile formation
        (BAIBF)
    b. acid malabsorption (BAM)
    b. acid pool
    b. acid sequestrant
    b. acid therapy
    b. acid tolerance test
    b. ascites
    B b.
    b. bag
    C b.
    canalicular b.
    b. capillary
    clear b.
    cloudy b.
    b. concretion
    cystic b.
    b. duct
    b. duct abscess
    b. duct adenoma (BDA)
    b. duct atresia
    b. duct brushing
    b. duct canaliculus
    b. duct cancer
    b. duct cannulation
    b. duct carcinoma
    b. duct cyst
    b. duct dyskinesia
    b. duct epithelial cell
    b. duct hypoplasia
    b. duct ligation (BDL)
    b. duct lumen
    b. duct paucity
    b. duct pressure
    b. duct proliferation
    b. duct stenosis
    b. duct stone
    b. duct stricture
    b. duct trauma
    b. duct-type cytokeratin
    b. ductular cholestasia
    extravasated b.
    b. flow
    b. infarct
    inspissated b.
    b. lake
    limy b.
    lithogenic b.

    milk-of-calcium b.
    b. papilla
    b. peritonitis
    b. phospholipid concentration
        (BPC)
    b. phospholipid output (BPO)
    b. pleuritis
    b. plug
    b. pulmonary embolism
    b. reflux
    b. reflux gastritis
    b. salt (BS)
    b. salt aggregation
    b. salt-binding resin
    b. salt concentrate (BSC)
    b. salt deficiency
    b. salt diarrhea
    b. salt export pump (BSEP)
    b. salt injury
    b. salt-losing enteropathy
    b. salt metabolism (BSM)
    b. salt output (BSO)
    b. salt-phospholipid ratio
    b. salt-stimulated lipase (BSSL)
    b. secretory failure
    SI of b.
    b. solubility test
    stagnant b.
    b. stasis
    supersaturated b.
    thick b.
    b. thrombus
    turbid b.
    viscid b.
    viscous b.
    white b.
bile-laden macrophage
bile-stained
    b.-s. fluid
    b.-s. vomitus
bile-tinged fluid
bilharzial
    b. appendicitis
    b. bladder cancer syndrome
    b. dysentery
    b. worm
bilharzial-related cancer
bilharziasis, bilharziosis
bilharzioma
bilharziosis (*var. of* bilharziasis)
bili
    bilirubin
    bili light
    Bili mask
biliaris
    collum vesicae b.
    corpus vesicae b.
    ductus b.
    fossa vesicae b.

fundus vesicae b.
vesica b.
biliary
  b. abscess
  b. actinomycosis
  b. air
  b. angiography
  b. apparatus
  b. ascariasis
  b. ascites
  b. atresia
  b. balloon catheter
  b. balloon dilator
  b. balloon probe
  b. brush cytology
  b. calculus
  b. canaliculus
  b. cannulation
  b. carcinoma
  b. cholangitis
  b. cholesterol output (BCO)
  b. cholesterol secretion
  b. cirrhosis
  b. cirrhotic liver
  b. clonorchiasis
  b. colic
  b. cryptosporidiosis
  b. cycle
  b. cyst
  b. cystadenocarcinoma
  b. cystadenoma
  b. decompression
  b. dilation
  b. dilator catheter
  b. diverticulum
  b. drainage
  b. duct
  b. ductules
  b. dyskinesia
  b. dyspepsia
  b. dyssynergia
  b. echinococcosis
  b. endoprosthesis
  b. endoprosthesis insertion
  b. endoscopic sphincterotomy
  b. epithelial cell (BEC)
  b. epithelial hyperplasia
  b. excretion
  b. fascioliasis
  b. fibroadenomatosis
  b. fibrosis
  b. fistula
  b. gland
  b. hypercholesterolemia
  xanthomatosis
  b. immunoglobulin
  b. infestation
  b. instrumentation
  b. leakage

  b. lipid
  b. lithotripsy
  b. manometry
  b. microhamartoma
  b. mud
  b. orifice
  b. pancreatitis
  b. papillomatosis
  b. passage
  b. piecemeal necrosis
  b. plexus
  b. prosthesis
  b. radicle
  b. reconstruction
  b. saturation index
  b. scintiscan
  b. sclerosis
  b. sepsis
  b. sludge
  b. sphincter
  b. spiral Z stent
  b. stasis
  b. steatorrhea
  b. stenting
  b. stent patency
  b. structure
  B. Symptoms Questionnaire (BSQ)
  b. tract
  b. tract disease
  b. tract obstruction
  b. tract pain (BTP)
  b. tract pressure
  b. tract stone
  b. tract stricture
  b. tract torsion
  b. tract tumor
  b. tree
  b. tree duplication
biliary-bronchial fistula
biliary-cutaneous fistula
biliary-duodenal pressure gradient
biliation
BiliBed
BiliBlanket phototherapy system
BiliBottoms
BiliChek
  B. breath analyzer device
  B. test
bilicyanin
bilifaction, bilification
bilifer
  canaliculus b.
biliferi
  ductuli b.
  ductus b.
biliferous
bilification (*var. of* bilifaction)
bilifuscin
biligenesis

biligenetic
biligenic
Biligrafin contrast medium
bilihumin
bilin, biline
biline (*var. of* bilin)
bilioduodenal
    b. fistula
    b. prosthesis
bilioenteric
    b. anastomosis
    b. bypass
    b. fistula
biliointestinal bypass (BIB)
biliopancreatic
    b. bypass (BPB)
    b. diversion
    b. diversion with duodenal
    stent
    b. fistula
    b. obesity surgery
    b. shunt
bilious
    b. cholera
    b. colic
    b. diarrhea
    b. emesis
    b. flux
    b. leakage
    b. remittent fever
    b. remittent malaria
    b. stool
    b. vomit
    b. vomiting
biliousness
biliprasin
biliptysis
bilirachia
bilirubin (bili)
    conjugated b.
    delta b.
    direct b.
    b. encephalopathy
    b. ester conjugate
    fat-soluble b.
    fractionation of b.
    indirect b.
    b. infarct
    b. pigment gallstone
    b. protein conjugate
    serum b.
    b. test
    total b.
    unconjugated b. (UCB)
    urinary b.
    urine b.
    water-soluble b.
bilirubinate stone
bilirubinemia

bilirubinoid
bilirubinometer
    direct-reading b.
bilirubinuria
bilis
    Helicobacter b.
    vesicula b.
Biliscopin contrast medium
Bilitec
    B. fiberoptic spectrophotometer
    B. intraluminal fiberoptic
    probe
bilitherapy
biliuria
biliverdin, biliverdine
biliverdine (*var. of* biliverdin)
Bilivist contrast medium
Billingham-Bookwalter rectal fenestrated
  blade
Billroth
    B. cord
    B. forceps
    B. gastroduodenoscopy
    B. gastroenterostomy type I, II
    B. gastrojejunostomy type I, II
    B. hypertrophy
    B. I gastroduodenostomy
    B. II anastomotic scar
    B. II anatomy
    B. I, II anastomosis
    B. I, II gastrectomy
    B. I, II gastrointestinal
    reconstruction
    B. I, II operation
    B. strand
    B. venae cavernosae
BILN 2061 protease inhibitor
bilobar
    b. hyperplasia
    b. hypertrophy
bilobate, bilobed
    b. false aneurysm
    b. gallbladder
    b. polypoid lesion
bilobed (*var. of* bilobate)
bilocular stomach
biloma
Bilopaque contrast medium
Biloptin contrast medium
Biltricide
Bimexes
bimucosa
    fistula b.
binary factor
binder
    bile acid b.
    Dale abdominal b.
    T b.
    b. test

B

binding
> anti-DNA b.
> crystal b.
> phosphotyrosine-SH2 b.
> polypyrimidine tract b. (PTB)
> ryanodine b.
> soluble CD44 b.
> sperm-immunobead b.
> vasoactive intestinal polypeptide b.

bindweed
> greater b.

binge
binge-eating disorder (BED)
bingeing and purging
binge-purge behavior
binucleate renal tubule epithelial cell
bioabsorbable adhesion barrier
bioactive antimicrobial coated solid alloplast
bioartificial
> b. extracorporeal liver support (BELS)
> b. extracorporeal liver support system
> b. liver
> b. liver support device

bioassay
> mink cell b.

bioavailability
bioburden
Biocef
biochanin A
biochemical
> b. characterization
> b. marker

Bioclot protein S assay
biocompatibility
biocompatible
> b. material
> b. membrane

Biodan Prostathermer
biodegradable microsphere
biodistribution of N-isopropyl-p-iodoamphetamine
bioeffect
bioelectrical impedance analysis (BIA)
Bio-Enzabead test
biofeedback
> augmented b.
> bladder b.
> cystometric b.
> sensory b.
> b. therapy
> voiding b.

biofilm
> bacterial b.
> b. formation
> microbial b.

> polymicrobial b.
> resistance monomicrobial b.

biofilm-related encrustation
BioFit Herbgels
Biofix stent
Bio-Flex
> B.-F. CS catheter
> B.-F. Tesio catheter

biofragmentable anastomotic ring (BAR)
Bio-Gel HTP
Biogenex antigen retrieval method
biogenic amine
Bio-Gen urine test strip
Bioglass
biohazard bag
bioincompatible membrane
biolab
> Malakit *Helicobacter pylori* B.

biologic, biological
> b. collagen-based tissue-matrix graft
> b. marker
> b. predictor for treatment outcome of transurethral microwave thermotherapy
> b. response modifier (BRM)
> b. response modifier therapy

biological (*var. of* biologic)
BioLogic-DTPF system
BioLogic-DT system
biomarker
> intermediate b.

biomarker-based imaging
biomaterial
> alloplastic b.
> antiinfective b.
> Emerge b.
> incrustation of b.
> Mycromesh b.
> b. surface
> technical b.
> b. type

biomaterial-associated infection
Biomedical Instruments and Products (BIP)
biomembrane
biomodulation
Biomox
biooclusive dressing
Bioplastique
biopolymer injection
biopsy
> acetic acid-guided b.
> adrenal cortex fine-needle b.
> alcohol-fixed gastric b.
> antral b.
> aspiration b.
> bite b.
> bladder b.
> blind percutaneous liver b.

biopsy (*continued*)
    bone marrow b.
    borderline b.
    brush b.
    b. channel
    cholangioscopic forceps b.
    CLO b.
    cold cup b.
    colonic b.
    colonoscopic b.
    colorectal b.
    cone b.
    contralateral testicular b.
    core needle b.
    corporal b.
    corpus cavernosum b.
    Crosby-Kugler capsule for b.
    CT-guided liver b.
    CT-guided needle aspiration b.
    cup bladder b.
    cytologic b.
    diathermic loop b.
    digitally guided b.
    direct-vision liver b.
    double-bite b.
    duodenal b.
    endoluminal ultrasonography-guided fine-needle aspiration b.
    endoscopic small-bowel b.
    endoscopic strip b.
    endoscopic transbronchial real-time ultrasound-guided b.
    endoscopic transpapillary b.
    endourologic b.
    ERCP-guided b.
    esophageal b.
    EUS-guided Tru-Cut needle b.
    fine-needle aspiration b. (FNAB)
    fine-needle capillary b.
    b. forceps
    freehand b.
    full-thickness b.
    fundic b.
    grasp b.
    guided transcutaneous b.
    guillotine needle b.
    b. gun
    hot b.
    ileal b.
    incisional b.
    b. instrument
    intestinal b.
    jejunal drainage and b.
    jumbo b.
    laparoscopic renal b.
    large-forceps b.
    large-particle b.
    laser-guided b.
    lift-and-cut b.

liver b.
Menghini technique for percutaneous liver b.
morphologic study of renal b.
mucosal b.
multiple b.'s
native renal b.
needle aspiration b. (NABX)
needle core b.
b. of gastric mucosa
open testis b.
paracollicular b.
percutaneous fine-needle pancreatic b.
percutaneous liver b. (PLB)
percutaneous native renal b.
percutaneous pancreas b.
percutaneous testis b.
peritoneal b.
peroral jejunal b.
pinch b.
plugged liver b.
pouch b.
prostate gland b.
protocol b.
PTC-guided b.
punch b.
b. punch
4-quadrant jumbo b.
random bladder b.
rectal b.
renal b.
saucerized b.
scan-directed b.
sextant transrectal ultrasound-guided b.
shave b.
skinny-needle b.
small-bowel b.
snap-frozen b.
snare excision b.
snare loop b.
sonoguided b.
strip b.
suction b.
systematic sextant b.
tangential b.
targeted b.
testicular b.
transcutaneous b.
transfemoral liver b.
transgastric fine-needle aspiration b.
transitional zone b.
transjugular liver b. (TLB)
transpapillary b.
transperineal ultrasound-guided template b.
transrectal ultrasonography-guided b.
transvenous liver b.

trephine b.
Tru-Cut needle b.
ultrasound-guided anterior subcostal
  liver b.
ultrasound-guided systematic sextant
  b.
b. urease test
vaginal cone b.
Vim-Silverman technique for
  liver b.
Watson capsule b.
biopsy-verified chronic glomerulonephritis
Biopty
  B. cut needle
  B. gun
Bio-Rad protein assay
bioreactor
  radial-flow b.
bioresorbable stent
Biosafe PSA4 screen
biosampler
  Accellon Combi cervical b.
Biosearch 7000 enteral feeding
pump
BioShield irrigator
BioSling bioabsorbable urethral
sling
BioSorb resorbable urology stent
Biostent biliary stent
biosynthesis
biota
  gastrointestinal b.
Biotel home screening test
biothesiometry
  penile b.
biotin
  b. deficiency
  endogenous b.
biotinylated DNA probe
Bio-Tract proprietary strain
biotransformation
BioWhittaker
  B. assay
  B. assay test
BIP
  Biomedical Instruments and Products
  B. biopsy instrument
  B. high-speed multibiopsy needle
biperiden
biphasic diurnal rhythm
biplanar aortography
biplane sector probe
bipolar
  b. bleeding
  b. cautery probe
  b. circumactive probe (BICAP)
  B. circumactive probe coagulation
  b. coagulating forceps
  b. electrocautery

b. electrocoagulation (BPEC)
B. EndoStasis probe (BESP)
b. esophageal recording
b. glass electrode
b. hemostasis probe
b. neuron
b. sphincterotome
b. TURP
b. urological loop
Birbeck granule
birch
bird-beak
  b.-b. appearance
  b.-b. configuration
  b.-b. narrowing
birefringence
Birt-Hogg-Dube (BHD)
  B.-H.-D. syndrome
birth trauma
birthwort
Bisac-Evac
bisacodyl
  Fleet B.
  b. tannex
bisantrene
Bisco-Lax
Bishop-Koop ileostomy
Biskra button
bismuth (Bi)
  B. benign bile duct stricture
    classification
  B. classification type I-IV
  b. compound
  b., metronidazole, tetracycline
    (BMT)
  b. nephropathy
  b. salt
  b. sclerotherapy
  b. subsalicylate (BSS)
  b. triple monocapsule
  b. triple regimen
  b. triple therapy
  b. tumor
bismuthate
bismuth-free triple therapy
Bisodol
bisoprolol
4,5-bisphosphate
  phosphatidylinositol 4,5-b. (PI4, 5P2)
bisphosphonate
bistable
bistort
bistriazole
bitartrate
  cysteamine b.
bite
  b. biopsy
  b. biopsy forceps
bithionol

Bitome
  B. bipolar sphincterotome
  B. bipolar system
  B. catheter
bitter
  b. apple
  b. blocker
  b. orange
Bittorf reaction
bivalve mollusc
bizarre leiomyoma
black
  b. alder
  B. Beauty ureteral stent
  b. catnep
  b. clot
  b. cohosh
  b. currant
  b. esophagus
  b. faceted stone
  b. hairy tongue
  b. hellebore
  b. jaundice
  b. liver disease
  b. mulberry
  b. nightshade
  b. pigment gallstone
  b. pigment stone
  b. root
  b. sickness
  b. silk suture
  b. tarry stool
  b. urine
  b. vomit
  b. vomitus
Black-Draught Lax-Senna
bladder
  b. acontractility
  acute phase of neurogenic b.
  b. agenesis
  alloplastic prostatic b.
  amebiasis of b.
  amyloidosis of b.
  b. angiosarcoma
  b. antibody
  areflexic b.
  b. artery
  atonic b.
  b. augmentation
  augmented b.
  b. autoaugmentation
  autonomic neurogenic b.
  Barrett-Donovan-Mayo artificial b.
  b. biofeedback
  b. biopsy
  b. calculus
  b. cancer
  b. cancer angiogenic factor
  b. cancer antigen 4 (BLCA4)

b. cancer-specific nuclear matrix protein
b. *Candida* infection
b. capacity
b. carcinoma in situ
b. carcinosarcoma
b. chimney procedure
b. chondrosarcoma
b. choriocarcinoma
color Doppler imaging of ureteral jet into b.
b. compliance
compliance of b.
congenital bifid b.
b. congenital diverticulum
b. congenital megacystis
b. cooling reflex
cord b.
b. cuff
b. decompensation
b. decompression
defunctionalized b.
b. denervation
b. descensus
distended b.
b. diverticulectomy
dome of b.
double b.
dropped b.
b. duplication
b. dysplasia
b. ear
embryonal transitory b.
b. emptying
encysted b.
b. enlargement
b. epithelium
b. erosion
b. examination
b. excision
b. exstrophy
fasciculated b.
b. filling
b. fistula
gastric b.
Gilchrist ileocecal b.
b. granular cell myoblastoma
b. hernia
high-riding b.
b. histology
b. hydrodistention
hyperreflexic b.
hypertonic b.
b. hypoplasia
hypotonic b.
ileal b.
ileocecal b.
ileocolic b.
b. imaging

b. incontinence
b. infusion
b. inhibition
b. injury
b. innervation
b. intravesical pressure
inversion of b.
b. inverted papilloma
b. involuntary contraction
b. irrigation
irritable b.
kidneys, ureters, b. (KUB)
b. leiomyosarcoma
b. leukoplakia
b. liposarcoma
low-compliance b.
b. lymphohemangioma
b. lymphoma
b. malacoplakia
b. malignant melanoma
b. mapping
b. mast cell
Mayo b.
b. mesonephric adenocarcinoma
b. mucosal graft
b. muscarinic receptor
b. neck
b. neck closure (BNC)
b. neck contracture
b. neck detrusor muscle
b. neck dysfunction
b. neck hypermobility
b. neck obstruction
b. neck-preserving technique
b. neck reconstruction
b. neck sphincteric function
b. neck support pessary
b. neck support prosthesis
b. neck suspension (BNS)
b. neck-to-urethra anastomosis
b. neck transurethral resection
b. neck tubularization
b. neck Y-V plasty
b. neoplasm
b. nephrogenic adenoma
nephroureterectomy with en bloc
  removal of cuff of b.
nervous b.
b. neurofibroma
neurogenic b.
neuropathic b.
b. neurosis
b. nonepithelial tumor
nonneurogenic neurogenic b.
orthotopic b.
b. osteosarcoma
b. outflow obstruction
b. outlet
b. outlet closure

b. outlet kinesiologic study
b. outlet obstruction (BOO)
b. outlet reconstruction
overactive b. (OB)
b. overdistention
Padua ileal b.
b. pain
b. palpation
pancreatic b.
b. patch
b. perforation
b. pheochromocytoma
b. pillar block
pine cone appearance of b.
b. plasmacytoma
b. plate
poorly compliant b.
b. postcystourethropexy instability
b., posterior urethral, abdominal
  wall closure
b. preservation
b. pressure
b. pressure sensor
b. prolapse
prosthetic b.
pseudoneurogenic b.
b. pseudosarcoma
psychological nonneuropathic b.
reflex neurogenic b.
reflex neuropathic b.
b. regeneration
b. replacement
b. replacement urinary pouch
b. retraction
b. rhabdomyosarcoma
rugae of urinary b.
b. rupture
sacculated b.
b. sarcoma
b. schistosomiasis
b. sensation
b. small cell carcinoma
b. smooth muscle
b. spasm
spinning-top deformity of b.
b. squamous cell carcinoma
b. squamous metaplasia
stammering b.
b. stone
b. storage function
strangulation of b.
b. stress relaxation
b. substitution
summit of b.
b. support
suprapubic aspiration of b.
teardrop b.
thimble b.
tic douloureux of b.

bladder (*continued*)
  b. tissue engineering
  trabeculated b.
  b. training
  b. transection
  b. transitional cell carcinoma
  transitional cell carcinoma of b. (TCCB)
  transurethral resection of b. (TURB)
  b. trauma
  b. trigone
  b. tuberculosis
  tuberculosis of kidney and b.
  b. tumor (BT)
  b. tumor antigen (BTA)
  b. tumor antigen test
  b. tumor assay
  b. ulcer
  b. ultrasonography
  uninhibited neurogenic b.
  uninhibited overactive b.
  unstable b.
  ureteral jet into b.
  urinary b.
  uvula of b.
  valve b.
  vascular malformation of b.
  b. vein
  vertex of urinary b.
  b. viscoelasticity
  b. volume
  b. washing
  b. worm
  b. xanthoma
  b. yolk sac tumor
BladderChek
BladderManager portable ultrasonic device
BladderScan
  Bard B.
  B. test
  B. ultrasound
  B. ultrasound scanner
blade
  Bard-Parker b.
  Beaver b.
  Billingham-Bookwalter rectal fenestrated b.
  Bookwalter-Cook anorectal b.
  Bookwalter malleable retractor b.
  Bookwalter-Mayo b.
  Bookwalter-Parks anal sphincter b.
  Bovie b.
  Deaver-type b.
  knife b.
  malleable b.
  razor b.
  scalpel b.
Blair silicone drain

Blaivas
  B. classification of urinary incontinence
  B. urinary incontinence classification
Blake gallstone forceps
Blakemore-Sengstaken tube
Blakemore tube
Blalock pulmonary artery forceps
Blanchard hemorrhoid forceps
blanching
  b. of lesion
  b. of mucosa
bland
  B. cholestasia
  b. diet
  b. food
  b. pulmonary hemorrhage
  b. thrombosis
Bland-Altman analysis
blanket
  Gaymar water-circulating b.
blast
  b. cell
  b. injury
  refractory anemia with excess b.'s (RAEB)
  white blood cell b.
blastema
  renal b.
blastocyst hatching
Blastocystis hominis
blastoid transformation
blastomere
Blastomyces dermatitidis
blastomycosis
  peritoneal b.
Blatin
  B. sign
  B. syndrome
BLCA4
  bladder cancer antigen 4
bleb
bleed
  gastrointestinal b.
  GI b.
  herald b.
  postgastrectomy b.
  postpolypectomy b.
bleeder
bleeding, bleed
  b. acid-peptic disease
  active source of b.
  acute variceal b.
  b. angioma
  bipolar b.
  b. colonic angiodysplasia
  colorectal variceal b.
  contact b.
  b. control

diverticular b.
b. diverticulosis
b. diverticulum
duodenal b.
dysfunctional b.
esophageal variceal b.
esophagogastric variceal b.
excessive b.
first variceal b.
functional b.
gastric varix b.
b. gastric varix (BGV)
b. gastritis
gastrointestinal b. (GIB)
GI b.
b. hemorrhoid
b. jejunal metastasis
jetlike b.
b. lesion
lower gastrointestinal b. (LGIB)
lower GI b.
massive colonic diverticular b.
minute b.
mucosal b.
obscure gastrointestinal b.
occult gastrointestinal b.
painless rectal b.
pancreatitis-related b.
peptic ulcer b.
per anum b.
b. per rectum
b. pile
b. point
b. polyp
prevention of first b.
b. proctitis
rectal b.
recurrent b.
severe variceal b.
b. site
b. site localization
b. time
b. tumor
b. ulcer
upper gastrointestinal b. (UGIB)
vaginal b.
variceal b.

blend
b. waveform
b. waveform desiccation

blended
b. current
b. cut
b. electrocautery

blenderized diet
blennemesis
blennorrhagica
keratoderma b.
keratosis b.

blennuria
bleomycin
carboplatin, etoposide, b. (CEB)
b., etoposide, cisplatin (BEP)
platinum, etoposide, b. (PEB)
platinum, Velban, b. (PVB)
b. sulfate
b. toxicity
Velban, actinomycin D, b. (VAB)
vinblastine, actinomycin D, b.
(mini-VAB)

blessed thistle
blind
b. cautery
b. enema
b. esophageal brushing (BEB)
b. fistula
b. intestine
b. limb
b. lithotripsy
b. loop
b. loop syndrome (BLS)
b. percutaneous liver biopsy
b. stump
b. subtotal colectomy
b. technique
b. upper esophageal pouch

blindgut
blinking reflex
BLL
blood lead level
BLM
basolateral membrane
bloat, bloating
bloating (var. of bloat)
bloc
harvesting en b.
Blocadren
Bloch-Paul-Mikulicz extraperitoneal colon resection
block
abdominal ganglion b.
Best bite b.
bladder pillar b.
caudal b.
celiac plexus b.
collision b.
endoscopic ultrasound-guided celiac
plexus b.
Marcaine b.
nerve b.
neurolytic celiac plexus b.
OB-10 Comfort bite b.
periprostatic b.
portal b.
prostatic b.
spermatic cord anesthetic b.
(SCAB)
transitory b.

B

Block-Ace solution
blockade
    adjuvant alpha b.
    aldosterone b.
    alpha sympathetic b.
    androgen b.
    beta-adrenergic b.
    cavernosal alpha b.
    combined androgen b. (CAB)
    differential neuroaxial b.
    lipoxygenase b.
    maximal androgen b. (MAB)
    muscarinic b.
    reversible b.
blockage
    complete hormonal b.
blocked aerogastria
blocker
    alpha-1 b.
    angiotensin receptor b.
    (ARB)
    beta-adrenergic b.
    bitter b.
    calcium channel b.
    calcium entry b.
    H_2 b.
    histamine b. (HB)
    nicotinic receptor b.
    proton pump b.
    RAS b.
    renin-angiotensin system b.
    starch b.
blocking
    electrical b.
    thermal b.
Blocksom vesicostomy
Blom-Singer
    B.-S. esophagoscope
    B.-S. tracheoesophageal fistula
blood
    b. admixed with stool
    b. agar plate
    b. alcohol level (BAL)
    b. ammonia
    bright red b.
    b. calculus
    b. cast
    b. clot
    clotted b.
    b. coagulation
    b. coagulation disorder
    b. collection
    crossmatched b.
    b. culture
    dark burgundy b.
    dragon's b.
    b. flow
    b. flow assessment
    b. flow rate (BFR)

    frank b.
    b. gas on oxygen
    b. gas on room air
    b. group antigen
    b. in stool
    b. lead level (BLL)
    maroon b.
    nonhemolyzed b.
    nostril b.
    occult b.
    b. on surface of stool
    oozing b.
    b. passed with stool
    b. per rectum (BPR)
    b. pH
    b. pressure (BP)
    b. pressure change
    b. sample
    spurting b.
    stool for occult b.
    b. transfusion
    b. type
    typed b.
    b. urea concentration
    b. urea level
    b. urea nitrogen (BUN)
    b. vessel
    whole b.
bloodborne
    b. non-A non-B hepatitis
    b. pathogen
    b. transmission
    b. virus
blood-contactin catheter
blood-epididymis barrier
Bloodgood
    B. operation
    B. procedure
blood-liquor barrier
blood-streaked stool
bloodstream infection (BSI)
blood-testis barrier
blood-testis-epididymis
blood-tinged ascites
blood-type diet
blood-urine barrier
blood-water clearance
bloody
    b. ascites
    b. diarrhea
    b. discharge
    b. peritoneal fluid
    b. stool
    b. vomitus
blooming effect
blot
    ECL Western b.
    enhanced chemiluminescence
    Western b.

Southern b.
Western b.
blotting
Blount disease
blowhole
    b. cecostomy
    b. ileostomy
blown pupil
BLS
    blind loop syndrome
BLSD
    big liver and spleen disease
BLT
    bright light therapy
blue
    Alcian b.
    Berlin b.
    carmine b.
    b. diaper syndrome
    b. dot sign
    eosin-methylene b. (EMB)
    Evans b.
    B. Max balloon catheter
    methylene b.
    b. navel
    periodic acid-Schiff-Alcian b.
      (PAS-AB)
    b. rubber bleb nevus
      syndrome
    toluidine b.
    Urolene B.
    b. varix
Bluemle pump
Blumberg
    inguinal ligament of B.
    B. sign
Blumer rectal shelf
blunt
    b. abdominal trauma
    b. and sharp dissection
    b. liver trauma
    b. needle
    b. pancreatic trauma
    b. probe
    b. testicular injury
blunting
    costophrenic b.
    haustral b.
    b. of valve
blunt-tipped obturator
blush
    delayed b.
    immediate b.
B-lymphocyte
    B-l. activation
    B-l. system
BM
    bowel movement
b558 membrane-bound cytochrome

BMI
    body mass index
BMMP
    benign mucous membrane pemphigoid
B-mode
    B-m. imaging
    B-m. ultrasonography
    B-m. ultrasound image
19B7 monoclonal antibody
4B4 monoclonal antibody
BMR
    basal metabolic rate
BMS
    burning mouth syndrome
BMT
    bismuth, metronidazole, tetracycline
B72.3 murine monoclonal antibody
BNC
    bladder neck closure
BNO
    bowels not open
BNP
    brain natriuretic peptide
BNS
    bladder neck suspension
boardlike
    b. rigidity
    b. rigidity of abdomen
Boari
    B. bladder flap
    B. bladder flap procedure
    B. operation
    B. ureteral flap repair
Boari-Ockerblad
    B.-O. principle
    B.-O. ureteral flap
Boas
    B. algesimeter
    B. point
    B. sign
    B. test meal
boat-shaped abdomen
Bochdalek
    foramen of B.
    B. hernia
Bodansky unit
Boden-Gibb tumor staging
Bodenhammer rectal speculum
body
    acidophilic b.
    anal foreign b.
    angularis b.
    anorectal foreign b.
    asteroid b.
    bamboo jointlike appearance of
      gastric b.
    Call-Exner b.
    b. cell mass (BCM)
    CMV inclusion b.

B

body (*continued*)
cobblestone appearance of gastric b.
coccidian b.
colonic foreign b.
b. composition analysis
compressible cavernous b.
Councilman b.
Cowdry type A inclusion b.
crescentic b.
Cyanobacterium-like b.
Donovan b.
duodenal foreign b.
embryoid b.
epithelial inclusion b.
esophageal foreign b.
esophageal Lewy b.
falciform b.
b. fluid osmolality
foreign b.
B. Fortress Natural Amino
 tablet
gastric foreign b.
b. habitus
Highmore b.
Howell-Jolly b.
inclusion b.
ingested foreign b.
intracytoplasmic CMV inclusion b.
intraepithelial b.
intranuclear CMV inclusion b.
Jaworski b.
juxtaglomerular b.
ketone b. (KB)
Lafora b.
lower GI tract foreign b.
Mallory hyaline b.
malpighian b.
b. mass index (BMI)
Michaelis-Gutmann b.
b. of epididymis
b. of pubis
oval fat b.
penile b.
perineal b.
peritoneal loose b.
polar b.
b. position
rectal foreign b.
renal tumorlike pyonephrosis with
 foreign b.
retained foreign b. (RFB)
Savage perineal b.
Schaumann b.
Schiller-Duval b.
S-shaped b.
string-of-pearls appearance of gastric
 b.
Symington b.
upper GI tract foreign b.

vaginal foreign b.
vermiform b.
viral inclusion b.
b. water
Weibel-Palade b.
b. weight (BW)
zebra b.
Boeck sarcoma
Boehm
 B. anoscope
 B. proctoscope
 B. rectal diagnostic and treatment
  set
 B. sigmoidoscope
Boehringer kit
Boerema
 B. anterior gastropexy
 B. hernia repair
Boerhaave syndrome
Boettcher crystal
bog
 b. bean
 b. bilberry
boggy prostate
Bogota bag
Bogros space
Bohr effect
Bolande tumor
boldus
 Peumus b.
Boley vascular ectasia
bolster
 mesh b.
 b. suture
bolus
 alimentary b.
 b. challenge test
 b. dressing
 b. extraction
 b. feeding
 food b.
 heparin b.
 b. holdup
 marshmallow b.
 b. transit
 b. transport
bombesin receptor
bone
 adynamic b.
 b. alkaline phosphatase (BAP)
 b. disease
 b. formation
 innominate b.
 b. marrow aplasia
 b. marrow biopsy (BMB)
 b. marrow-derived B cell
 b. marrow stem cell
 b. marrow transplantation-related
  problem

b. metastasis (BM)
b. scan (BS)
b. turnover marker
bone-specific alkaline phosphatase (BALP)
Bonine
Bonney test
B&O No. 15A, 16A C-II suppository
bony
b. defect
b. landmark
b. pelvis
b. tenderness
BOO
bladder outlet obstruction
Bookler swivel-ball laparoscope holder
Bookwalter
B. malleable retractor blade
B. retractor system
B. ring retractor
Bookwalter-Cook anorectal blade
Bookwalter-Goulet retractor
Bookwalter-Hill-Ferguson rectal retractor
Bookwalter-Mayo blade
Bookwalter-Parks anal sphincter blade
Bookwalter-St. Mark deep pelvic retractor
Boost nutritional energy drink
borborygmi (*pl. of* borborygmus)
borborygmus, *pl.* **borborygmi**
Borchardt triad
border
antimesenteric b.
brush b.
b. cell
fundopyloric mucosal b.
intestinal brush b. (IBB)
lobulated b.
mucosal b.
scalloped antimesenteric b.
b. zone
borderline biopsy
bore
magnetic b.
Borge clamp
boring pain
Boros esophagoscope
borreliosis
Borrmann
B. gastric cancer
B. gastric cancer classification
B. gastric cancer typing system type I–IV
B. gastric carcinoma type I–IV
B. scirrhous carcinoma
Bors ice water test
bortezomib
bosentan

Bosniak
B. criteria
B. lesion category I-IV
B. renal cystic disease classification
bosselated surface
both
b. lower quadrants
b. upper quadrants
Botkin disease
Botox
botulinum toxin
botryoid
interlabial sarcoma b.
b. sarcoma
sarcoma b.
botryomycosis
cecal b.
Bottini operation
bottle
McGaw plastic b.
Nu-Hope urine collection b.
b. operation
Vacutainer b.
botulinum
Clostridium b.
b. toxin (Botox, BTX)
b. toxin A
b. toxin injection
botulism immune globulin intravenous
Bouchard
B. disease
B. index
bougie
b. à boule
acorn-tipped b.
bulbous b.
Celestin dilator b.
b. dilator
Eder-Puestow b.
elastic b.
elbowed b.
EndoLumina b.
filiform b.
following b.
French b.
Hegar intrarectal b.
Hurst mercury b.
Hurst-type b.
Jackson esophageal b.
Klebanoff common duct b.
large-diameter b.
Maloney b.
mercury-weighted rubber b.
over-the-scope b.
polyvinyl b.
Savary b.
Savary-Gilliard silastic flexible b.
Savary-Gilliard wire-guided b.
tapered rubber b.

bougie (*continued*)
    through-the-scope b.
    Trousseau esophageal b.
    Wales rectal b.
    wax-tipped b.
    wire-guided polyvinyl b.
bougienage
    esophageal b.
    Hurst b.
    peroral b.
    transgastric esophageal b.
bouillon
Bouin fixative solution
boulardii
    Saccharomyces b.
boule
    bougie à b.
bouquet fever
Bourne test
Bourneville disease
bouton en chemise
Bouveret
    B. syndrome
    B. ulcer
Bouveret-Duguet ulcer
Bovie
    B. blade
    B. cautery
    B. coagulation
    B. electrocautery
    B. electrocoagulation unit
    B. GAX collagen injection
    B. holder
bovied
bovine
    b. dermal collagen
    b. graft
    b. serum albumin (BSA)
    b. thrombin
    b. trypsin
bovis
    Cysticercus b.
    Moraxella b.
    Mycobacterium b.
    Streptococcus b.
bowed sternum
bowel
    b. adherent to omentum
    aganglionic b.
    b. axis
    b. bag
    b. bypass
    b. bypass syndrome
    competent b.
    b. contents
    b. continuity
    dead b.
    detubularized small b.
    dilated loop of b.

    b. dilation
    b. disease
    B. Disease Questionnaire
    b. displacement
    entrapment of b.
    fixed segment of b.
    fluid-filled small b.
    b. forceps
    b. function
    gangrenous b.
    b. gas
    b. grasper
    greedy b.
    b. habit
    incarcerated b.
    b. incontinence
    infarcted b.
    b. injury
    b. intussusception
    b. irrigation
    ischemic b.
    kink in b.
    Ladd correction of malrotation of b.
    large b.
    b. loop
    b. lumen
    b. movement (BM)
    b. necrosis
    necrotizing vasculitis of b.
    Noble surgical plication of b.
    b.'s not open (BNO)
    b. obstruction
    b. perforation
    b. plate
    pleating of small b.
    b. preparation
    b. preparation complication
    prolapsed b.
    b. pseudoobstruction
    b. refashioning procedure
    b. resection
    b. rest (BR)
    small b.
    b. sounds normal (BSN)
    b. sounds normal and active (BSNA)
    b. stoma
    strangulated b.
    b. tone
    toxic dilation of b.
    b. wall
    b. wall induration
bowel-emptying regimen
Bowen
    B. disease
    B. papule
    B. patch
bowenoid papulosis
Bower PEG tube

bowler hat sign
Bowman
    B. Birk protease inhibitor
    B. capsule
    B. space
    B. space cyst
Boyarsky
    B. BPH symptom score
    B. symptom scoring system
Boyce
    longitudinal nephrotomy of B.
    B. modification of
      Sengstaken-Blakemore tube
    B. sign
Boyce-Vest bladder exstrophy procedure
Boyden
    B. sphincter
    B. test
    B. test meal
boydii
    Pseudallescheria b.
    Shigella b.
Boyle and Goldstein saline test
Bozeman
    B. forceps
    B. operation
Bozeman-Fritsch catheter
Bozicevich test
BP
    blood pressure
BPB
    biliopancreatic bypass
BPC
    bile phospholipid concentration
BPE
    benign prostatic enlargement
BPEC
    bipolar electrocoagulation
BPH
    benign prostatic hyperplasia
    benign prostatic hypertrophy
      BPH impact index
BPO
    benign prostatic obstruction
    bile phospholipid output
BPR
    blood per rectum
BQ123 receptor antagonist
Braasch
    B. bulb
    B. catheter
    B. direct catheterization cystoscope
Braasch-Kaplan direct-vision cystoscope
brachial pressure index
brachioaxillary bridge graft fistula
  (BAGF)
brachioradialis
brachiosubclavian bridge graft fistula
  (BSGF)

brachyesophagus
BrachySeed
    B. brachytherapy seed
    B. Pd-103 implant
    B. prostate cancer treatment
BrachySil
brachytherapy
    interstitial b.
    intracavitary application b.
    PharmaSeed I-125 b.
    salvage b.
    transperineal interstitial permanent
      prostate b. (TIPPB)
    Varian b.
Brackin
    B. ureterointestinal anastomosis
    B. ureterointestinal anastomosis
      technique
Bradley
    B. classification of voiding
      dysfunction
    B. disease
    B. loop
bradygastria
bradykinin
bradypepsia
bradyphagia
bradyspermatism
bradystalsis
bradytrophia
bradytrophic
bradyuria
brain
    b. metastasis
    b. myoinositol content
    b. natriuretic peptide (BNP)
brain-derived neurotrophic factor
  (BDNF)
Brainerd diarrhea
brain-gut
    b.-g. axis
    b.-g. dysfunction
    b.-g. peptide
brain-heart
    b.-h. infusion agar
    b.-h. infusion plate
brainstem-sacral loop
brain-type glycogen phosphorylase
  (BGP)
brake
    duodenal b.
    ileal b.
bran
branch
    bifid b.
    b. duct-type tumor
    lateral b.
    b. renal artery disease
    side b.

B

branched
 b. crypt
 b. DNA assay
 b. pancreatic duct
 b. renal calculus
 b. stone
 b. vascular graft
branched-chain
 b.-c. alpha ketoacid dehydrogenase
 b.-c. amino acid (BCAA)
 b.-c. DNA (bDNA)
brancher
 b. deficiency
 b. deficiency glycogenosis
 b. enzyme
 b. glycogen storage disease
branching
 b. complex staghorn calculus
 b. tubule formation
branchiogenous cyst
branchiootorenal syndrome
Brandel cell harvester
Brandt cytology balloon
brash
 sour b.
 water b.
 weaning b.
brasiliensis
 Nippostrongylus b.
 Paracoccidioides b.
BRAT
 bananas, rice, cereal, applesauce, and
 toast
 BRAT diet
BRATT
 bananas, rice, cereal, applesauce, tea,
 and toast
 BRATT diet
Braun
 B. anastomosis
 B. enteroenterostomy
 B. stent
Braune
 B. muscle
 B. valve
Braun-Jaboulay gastroenterostomy
Bravo
 B. Catheter-Free pH testing system
 B. pH monitor
 B. pH monitoring
 B. pH probe
BRBPR
 bright red blood per rectum
BrDu, BrDU, BrdUrd
 bromodeoxyuridine
 BrDu staining
break
 b. cluster homology gene
 mucosal b.

breakage
 intracorporeal needle b.
breakbone fever
breakfast
 Ewald b.
 test b.
Breakstone lithotriptor
breakthrough
 b. dose
 nocturnal acid b. (NAB)
breast
 b. cancer
 b. cancer-associated protein pS2
  expression
breath
 b. alkane
 b. alkane testing
 b. bag
 b. ethane level
 b. hydrogen excretion test
 b. isotope bacterial urease
  detection
 liver b.
 b. odor
 b. pentane test
 b. sounds
 uremic b.
breath-hold MR cholangiography
breathing
 deep b.
 diaphragmatic b.
 intermittent positive-pressure b.
  (IPPB)
 Kussmaul b.
 mouth b.
 sleep-disordered b. (SDB)
BreathTek
Breisky-Navratil straight retractor
Brennemann syndrome
Brenner tumor
brequinar sodium
Brescia-Cimino
 B.-C. fistula
 B.-C. shunt
Breslow-Day test
Brethine
**Bretschneider histidine tryptophan
 solution**
bretylium
breve
 Gymnodinium b.
breves
 arteriae gastricae b.
Brevibloc
brevis
 Bifidobacterium b.
Brewer
 B. infarct
 B. point

brewer's yeast
BRIC
  benign recurrent intrahepatic cholestasia
Bricanyl
Bricker
  B. ileal conduit
  B. operation
  B. pouch
  B. technique
  B. ureteroileostomy
  B. urinary diversion
bridge
  agar b.
  Albarran reflecting b.
  B. Assurant biliary stent delivery
    system
  colostomy b.
  B. deep surgery forceps
  loop ostomy b.
  mucosal b.
  suture b.
  B. X3 renal stent system
bridging
  b. fibrosis
  b. hepatic necrosis
  mucosal b.
  portal-to-portal b.
  b. therapy
bridle
  control b.
brief
  Ashton b.'s
  Depend fitted b.'s
  Holyoke b.'s
  Kim Care contour b.'s
  B. Male Sexual Function Inventory
    for Urology
  Restore b.'s
  Suretys incontinence b.'s
Brigham sling
bright
  B. disease
  b. light therapy (BLT)
  b. red blood
  b. red blood per rectum (BRBPR)
  b. red vomitus
brim
  pelvic b.
Brinkerhoff
  B. anoscope
  B. rectal speculum
Brinton disease
Bristol
  B. female lower urinary tract
    symptom
  B. nomogram for uroflowmetry
BRM
  basal metabolic rate
  biologic response modifier

broad-based
  b.-b. gait
  b.-b. polyp
broadening
  spectral b.
broad-spectrum
  b.-s. antibiotic
  b.-s. therapy
Brödel line
Broder index
Brodie sign
Broesike fossa
broken stent retrieval device
bromelain, bromelin
bromelin (*var. of* bromelain)
bromfenac
bromide
  cetyldimethylethyl ammonium b.
  clidinium b.
  emepronium b.
  ethidium b.
  hexamethonium b.
  mepenzolate b.
  methantheline b.
  methscopolamine b.
  propantheline b.
  valethamate b.
bromine-75
bromobenzene (B2)
bromocriptine dopaminergic
  medication
5-bromodeoxyuridine (BrDu,
  BUdR)
bromodeoxyuridine (BrDu, BrDU,
  BrdUrd)
  antibody to b.
  b. cell kinetics
bromodiphenhydramine
Bromo Seltzer
brompheniramine
bromsulphalein (BSP)
  b. clearance
bronchi (*pl. of* bronchus)
bronchia (*pl. of* bronchium)
bronchial
  b. carcinoid
  b. obstruction
  b. sound
bronchium, *pl.* **bronchia** (*see also*
  bronchus)
bronchobiliary fistula
Broncho-Cath double-lumen endotracheal
  tube
bronchoesophageal fistula (BEF)
bronchoesophagology
bronchoesophagoscopy
bronchopancreatic fistula
bronchophony
bronchopulmonary foregut malformation

bronchoscope
    Fujinon b.
    Savary b.
bronchospasm
bronchovisceral fistulectomy
bronchus, *pl.* **bronchi** (*see also* **bronchium**)
bronchus-associated lymphoepithelial tissue (BALT)
Bronkosol
Brooke ileostomy
brooklime
broom
    Scotch b.
bropirimine
broth
    cysteine *Brucella* b.
    tryptic soy b.
brown
    B. and Wickham pressure profile method
    b. bowel syndrome
    B. dietary method for colon preparation
    b. pigment gallstone
    b. pigment stone
    b. stool
Brown-Buerger cystoscope
Browne operation
brownian motion
Browning and Parks continence grading system category A, B, C, D
Brown-McHardy
    B.-M. pneumatic dilator
    B.-M. pneumatic mercury bougie dilation
Brown-Mueller
    B.-M. T-bar fastener
    B.-M. T fastener
Broyle
    B. esophagoscope
    B. retrograde cystoscope
B-RTO
    balloon-occluded retrograde transvenous obliteration
Brucella melitensis
brucellosis
Bruel-Kjaer
    B.-K. axial transducer
    B.-K. scanner
    B.-K. 1846 ultrasound system
Bruening esophagoscope
Brugia
    B. lymphatic obstruction
    B. malayi
    B. timori
bruisability
    easy b.

bruit
    abdominal b.
    carotid b.
    femoral b.
    vascular b.
Brunn epithelial nest
Brunner
    B. gland
    B. gland adenoma
    B. gland hamartoma
    B. gland hyperplasia
    B. gland of duodenum
    B. intestinal forceps
    B. ligature set
    B. tissue forceps
brunneroma of duodenum
Brunschwig operation
Brunt score
brush
    Ayre b.
    b. biopsy
    b. border
    b. catheter
    Combo Cath wire-guided cytology b.
    Cragg thrombolytic b.
    b. cytology
    cytology b.
    Cytolong b.
    Endovations disposable cytology b.
    Glassman b.
    Olympus cytology b.
    scraping b.
    sheathed cytology b.
    suction oral b.
brush-border
    b.-b. digestion
    b.-b. disaccharidase specific activity
    b.-b. enzyme activity
    b.-b. hydrolase activity
    b.-b. hydrolysis
    b.-b. marker enzyme
    b.-b. membrane (BBM)
    b.-b. membrane vesicle (BBMV)
brushing
    bile duct b.
    blind esophageal b. (BEB)
    cytologic b.
brushite
Bruton disease
Bruton-type agammaglobulinemia
Bryan-Leishman stain
bryony
    red b.
BS
    bile salt
BSA
    bovine serum albumin
BSA-induced overload proteinuria

BSC
  bile salt concentrate
B-scanner
BSCC
  basaloid squamous cell carcinoma
BSD
  baby soft diet
  bedside drainage
BSD-300 device
BSEP
  bile salt export pump
BSFR
  basal secretory flow rate
    BSFR test
BSGF
  brachiosubclavian bridge graft
    fistula
BSI
  bloodstream infection
BSM
  bile salt metabolism
BSN
  bowel sounds normal
BSNA
  bowel sounds normal and active
BSO
  bile salt output
BSP
  bromsulphalein
    BSP retention
    BSP test
BSQ
  Biliary Symptoms Questionnaire
BSS
  balanced salt solution
  bismuth subsalicylate
BSSL
  bile salt-stimulated lipase
BT
  bladder tumor
BTA
  bladder tumor antigen
    BTA STAT test
    BTA TRAK test
BTG
  beta-thromboglobulin
BTP
  biliary tract pain
BT-PABA
  benzoyl-tyrosyl-paraaminobenzoic acid
    BT-PABA test
B5 tumor marker
BTX
  botulinum toxin
    BTX injection
bubble
  cavitation b.
  collapse of cavitation b.
  Garren-Edwards gastric b.

  Garren gastric b.
  gastric air b.
  GEG b.
  intragastric b.
  intraluminal gas b.
  plasma b.
  b. therapy
bubo
  chancroidal b.
  gonorrheal b.
  indolent b.
  nonvenereal b.
  strumous b.
  venereal b.
bubonocele
buccal
  b. mucosa
  b. mucosal patch graft
  b. mucosal substitution
    urethroplasty
  b. mucosal urethral replacement
  b. smear
buccopharyngeal aponeurosis
bucket-handle incision
Buck fascia
buckling test
buckthorn
Bucladin-S
buclizine
bucrylate sclerosant
bud
  dorsal b.
  B. drainage catheter
  ureteral b.
  ventral b.
Budd
  B. cirrhosis
  B. disease
  B. jaundice
  B. syndrome
Budd-Chiari
  B.-C. disease
  B.-C. syndrome
budesonide capsule
buetschlii
  Iodamoeba b.
Buffaprin caplet
buffer
  barbital-acetate b.
  cacodylate b.
  guanidinium thiocyanate b.
  HEPES b.
  ice-cold sucrose b.
  KHB b.
  Krebs-Ringer bicarbonate b.
  PBS-Tween b.
  Rapid-hyb b.
  b. solution
  b. system

buffered
    b. formalin
    b. saline
Bufferin Arthritis Strength caplet
buffering
    intracellular b.
Bugbee
    B. electrocautery
    B. electrode
Buie
    B. biopsy forceps
    B. fistula probe
    B. fulguration electrode
    B. pile clamp
    B. pile forceps
    B. position
    B. rectal injection cannula
    B. rectal scissors
    B. rectal suction tip
    B. rectal suction tube
    B. sigmoidoscope
Buie-Hirschman anoscope
Buie-Smith retractor
Build Up enteral feeding
bulb
    apex of duodenal b.
    Braasch b.
    b. deformity
    duodenal b.
    genital end b.
    b. of corpus cavernosum
    b. suction
bulbar
    b. artery
    b. colliculus
    b. peptic ulcer
    b. urethra
bulbi (*pl. of* bulbus)
bulbocavernosus
    b. fat pad
    b. reflex (BCR)
bulbocavernous reflex latency measurement
bulbomembranous
    b. stricture
    b. urethra
    b. urethral squamous cell carcinoma
bulboprostatic repair
bulbospongiosus muscle
bulbourethral
    b. artery
    b. carcinoma
    b. gland
    b. stricture
    b. stricture repair
bulbourethralis
    ductus glandulae b.

bulbous
    b. bougie
    b. urethral cuff implantation
bulb-tip
    b.-t. retrograde study
    b.-t. retrograde ureterogram
bulbus, *pl.* **bulbi**
    b. penis
    b. urethrae
bulgaricus
    Lactobacillus b.
bulge
    inguinal b.
    luminal b.
bulging
    anal b.
    b. flank
    b. of perineum
    b. papilla
bulimia nervosa
bulimorexia
bulk
    b. agent
    b. laxative
bulkage
bulking
    b. agent
    b. technique
bulk-producing laxative
bulky
    b. colonic pouch
    b. dressing
    b. malignancy
    b. stool
bulla, *pl.* **bullae**
bullae (*pl. of* bulla)
Bullard intubating laryngoscope
bulldog
    b. clamp
    b. forceps
bullet probe
bullet-tip
    b.-t. catheter
    b.-t. dilator
bullosa
    epidermolysis b. (EB)
    Herlitz junctional epidermolysis b.
bullous
    b. edema
    b. edema vesicae
    b. pemphigoid
bull's-eye
    b.-e. appearance
    b.-e. lesion
bumetanide
Bumex
bumper
    Cloverleaf internal b.
    dome-shaped internal b.

gastrostomy b.
PEG b.
BUN
blood urea nitrogen
bunching
accordion-like b.
b. maneuver
bundle
coherent b.
conjoined fiber b.
fiber b.
fiberoptic b.
IG b.
image guide b.
intermediate filament b.
LG b.
light guide b.
master IG b.
microfilament b.
neovascular b.
b. of His
vasa recta b.
BUN-to-creatinine ratio
BUO
bilateral ureteral obstruction
bupivacaine hydrochloride
buprenorphine narcotic analgesic therapy
bupropion
bur, burr
ultrasonic oscillating b.
Burch
B. colposuspension
B. procedure
B. retropubic colposuspension
B. urethrovesical suspension
Burch-Cooper ligament sling
burden
stone b.
Burdwan fever
burger
barium b.
Bürger-Grütz syndrome
Burhenne
B. steerable catheter
B. stone basket technique
buried
b. bumper syndrome
b. penis
b. suture
b. vaginal island
b. vaginal wall sling
Burkitt lymphoma
burn
genital b.
thermal b.
transmural b.
burned-out
b.-o. mucosa

b.-o. testis cancer
b.-o. tumor
burnet
great b.
burnetii
Coxiella b.
Burnett syndrome
burning
b. drops sign
b. mouth syndrome (BMS)
b. pain
b. sensation
Burnishine disinfectant
Burow vein
burp
burr (*var. of* bur)
b. marigold
burrowing incision
Burrow solution
bursa of Fabricius
bursitis
omental b.
bursoscopy
supragastric b.
burst
oxidative b.
phagocyte respiratory b.
respiratory b.
bursula
Buschke-Löwenstein tumor
Busch umbilical scissors
Buselmeier shunt
buserelin acetate
bush tea
buski
Fasciolopsis b.
Busodium
BuSpar
buspirone hydrochloride
busulfan, busulphan
busulphan (*var. of* busulfan)
butabarbital sodium
Butalan
butalbital
1-butanol
Butibel
Butisol Sodium
butorphanol
butter
b. meal
b. stool
Butterfield cystoscope
butterfly
b. endoluminal gastroplasty procedure
b. hematoma
b.'s in stomach
b. needle
b. rash

butternut
buttock
button
 Bard b.
 b. battery
 b. battery ingestion
 Bentle b.
 Biskra b.
 compression b.
 b. drainage
 b. electrode
 gastrostomy b.
 b. gastrostomy
 Jaboulay b.
 laparoscopic cecostomy b.
 Murphy b.
 b. of duodenum
 Olympus 1-Step B.
 one-step b. (OSB)
 One-Step gastric b.
 B. One-Step gastrostomy device
 OSB 1-step b.
 peritoneal b.
 Surgitek b.
 b. suture
buttonhole
 b. incision
 b. preputial transposition
 b. puncture technique
button-type G tube
buttress
 fascia lata b.
butyl aminobenzoate
butylbromide
 hyoscine b.
butyl-silane extraction column
butyrate
butyricum
 Clostridium b.
Butyrivibrio
butzleri
 Arcobacter b.
BW
 body weight
BXO
 balanitis xerotica obliterans

Byars flap
Byclomine
Byler
 B. disease
 B. syndrome
bypass
 Alden loop gastric b.
 aortic superior mesenteric
  artery b.
 aortorenal b.
 bilioenteric b.
 biliointestinal b. (BIB)
 biliopancreatic b. (BPB)
 bowel b.
 duodenoileal b. (DIB)
 extraanastomotic b.
 extraanatomic b.
 gastric b. (GBP)
 gastroduodenal-to-renal artery b.
 b. graft (BPG)
 Greenville gastric b.
 Griffen Roux-en-Y b.
 Hallberg biliointestinal b.
 hepatic-to-renal artery saphenous
  vein b.
 hepatorenal b.
 ileorenal b.
 intestinal b.
 jejunal b.
 jejunoileal b. (JIB)
 laparoscopic gastric b.
 long-limb surgical b.
 mesenterorenal b.
 partial ileal b. (PIB)
 Payne-DeWind jejunoileal b.
 percutaneous biliary b.
 b. procedure
 Roux-en-Y gastric b.
 Scopinaro pancreaticobiliary b.
 Scott jejunoileal b.
 splenorenal artery b.
 superior mesenterorenal b.
 thoracic aortorenal b.
 venovenous b.
 b. wire
Bywaters syndrome

^{14}C, C-14
carbon-14
^{14}C glucose uptake assay
^{14}C UBT
^{14}C urea breath test
C
C bile
C graft
C loop
C loop of duodenum
C of Hosmer-Lemeshow ratio test
c100
antibody to c100 (anti-c100)
C100-3
C100-3 antigen
C100-3 hepatitis C marker
^{11}C, C-11
carbon-11
C22-3 antigen
C3
C3 convertase
C3, C5 receptor
C3 deposit
C3 immunologic study
seminal plasma C3
C4
leukotriene C_4
C3a
plasma-activated complement 3
C4a
plasma-activated complement 4
C5a
plasma-activated complement 5
CA
carbonic anhydrase
cholic acid
CA cellulose acetate membrane hollow-fiber dialyzer
CA dialyzer
CA 1-18 tumor marker
CA 72-4 tumor marker
CA-125, CA125
cancer antigen 125
CA-19-9
carbohydrate antigen 19-9
CA-19-9 test
Ca2+, Ca^{2+}
calcium ions
inositol 1,4,5-triphosphate Ca2+
CAA
coloanal anastomosis
Ca^{2+}-activated K+
CA-50 antigen

CAB
combined androgen blockade
cable
fiberoptic light c.
internal fiberoptic c.
leakage bypass c.
light c.
Cabot-Nesbit orchiopexy
Cacchi-Ricci
C.-R. disease
C.-R. syndrome
cachectic
c. diarrhea
c. edema
c. fever
c. pallor
cachectin
cachexia
c. aphthosa
Grawitz c.
malignant c.
tumor c.
urinary c.
vascular c.
CaCo2 cell
$CaCO_3$ crystal
cacodylate buffer
cadaver
c. kidney
c. renal preservation
cadaveric
c. intestinal transplant
c. pericardial graft
c. renal transplant
c. renal transplantation
c. segmental graft
cadaveris
Clostridium c.
caddy stool
CA110 dialyzer
cadmium-induced nephrotoxicity
cadmium nephropathy
caecalis
fossa c.
caecum (*var. of* cecum)
cafe
c. coronary
c. coronary syndrome
Cafergot
caffeine
c., alcohol, pepper, spicy foods (CAPS)
c. clearance
c. gut
caffeinism

C

CAG
    cholangiogram
    cholangiography
    chronic atrophic gastritis
cagA
    cytotoxin-associated gene A
        cagA antibody
        cagA gene
        cagA protein
cagA-negative *Helicobacter pylori*
cagA-positive *Helicobacter pylori*
CAGEIN
    catheter-guided endoscopic intubation
cagPAI
    cytotoxin-associated gene pathogenicity
    island
        cagPAI gene
CAH
    chronic active hepatitis
    chronic aggressive hepatitis
    congenital adrenal hyperplasia
CAHP
    cellulose acetate high performance
    CAHP hemodialyzer
CAI
    carbonic anhydrase inhibitor
    Clinical Activity Index
Cajal
    interstitial cells of C. (ICC)
cake kidney
cal
    C. Carb 600 with Vitamin D
    antacid tablet
    C. Carb 600 with Vitamin D
    dietary supplement tablet
    C. Power calorie supplement
calamint
Calan
calbindin
    subserous c.
calbindin-D9k
    vitamin D-dependent c.-D9k
calcaneal ultrasound bone densitometry
calcareous
    c. pancreatitis
    c. renal calculus
Calcibind
Calcidrine syrup
calcific
    c. flocculate
    c. flocculus
    c. pancreatitis
calcification
    carbonate apatite c.
    dystrophic c.
    kidney c.
    laminated c.
    pancreatic c.
    retroperitoneal c.
    rim c.
    scrotal c.
    scrotum c.
    tram-line c.
    ureteral c.
calcified
    c. enterolith
    c. gallstone
    c. zone
calciform cell
calcifying pancreatitis
Calcijex
calcineurin
    c. inhibitor
    c. inhibitor-free immunosuppressive
    regimen
    c. inhibitor toxicity
calcinosis
    c. cutis, Raynaud phenomenon,
    esophageal motility disorder,
    sclerodactyly, and telangiectasia
    (CREST)
    c. cutis, Raynaud phenomenon,
    sclerodactyly, and telangiectasia
    (CRST)
    tumoral c.
calciphylaxis
calcite
calcitonin
    c. gene-related peptide (CGRP)
    serum c.
Cal-Citrate
calcitriol trial
calcium
    c. acetate
    c. ATPase pump
    c. bilirubinate stone
    c. carbonate
    c. carbonate and simethicone
    c. channel (CC)
    c. channel antagonist (CCA)
    c. channel blocker
    c. chloride
    c. concentration
    cytosolic c.
    c. deficiency
    dietary c.
    c. electrolyte
    c. entry blocker
    c. excretion
    exogenous c.
    extracellular c.
    c. gluconate
    c. homeostasis
    c. hydrogen phosphate
    c. infusion test
    intracytoplasmic c.
    c. ionophore
    c. ions (Ca2+, Ca^{2+})

c. metabolism
milk of c.
c. oxalate
c. oxalate calculus
c. oxalate crystallization
c. oxalate dihydrate
c. oxalate dihydrate stone
c. oxalate monohydrate crystal
c. oxalate monohydrate stone
c. oxalate nephrolithiasis
c. oxalate stone former
c. oxalate urolithiasis
c. oxaluria
c. phosphate calculus
c. phosphate homeostasis
c. phosphate nephrocalcinosis
c. phosphate urolithiasis
plasma ionized c.
renal absorption of c.
renal excretion of c.
serum c.
c. supplementation
UFT/leucovorin c.
urinary c.
calcium-activated potassium channel
calcium-binding protein
calcium-calmodulin complex
calcium-creatinine ratio
calcium-free dialysate
calcium-regulated protein
calcium-rich gluten-free diet
calcium-specific binding protein
calcivirus
human enteric c. (HuCV)
calcoaceticus
Acinetobacter c.
calculation
anthropometric c.
c. of renal ammonium excretion
calculi (*pl. of* calculus)
calculosis
calculous
c. anuria
c. cholecystitis
c. cirrhosis
c. formation
c. gallbladder disease
c. pyelitis
calculus, *pl.* **calculi**
alternating calculi
alvine c.
ammonium acid urate c.
apatite c.
asymptomatic c.
biliary c.
bladder c.
blood c.
branched renal c.
branching complex staghorn c.

calcareous renal c.
calcium oxalate c.
calcium phosphate c.
calyceal diverticular c.
carbonate apatite c.
cat's-eye c.
cholesterol c.
combination c.
common duct c.
coral c.
c. culture
cystine c.
decubitus c.
dendritic c.
diagnosing ureteral c.
2,8-dihydroxyadenine c.
encysted c.
fibrin c.
fusible c.
gallbladder c.
gastric c.
gonecystic c.
hemp seed c.
hepatic c.
impacted c.
indigo c.
indinavir c.
infection c.
intestinal c.
intrarenal c.
jackstone c.
lower ureteric c.
male predominance of urinary tract calculi
matrix c.
metabolic c.
midureteral c.
c. migration
mulberry c.
nephritic c.
noncalcareous renal c.
nonstruvite c.
oxalate c.
pancreatic c.
pocketed c.
preputial c.
primary renal c.
prostatic c.
proximal ureteral c.
c. radiography
recurrent urinary c.
renal pelvis c.
salivary c.
secondary renal c.
seminal vesicle c.
silicate c.
small solitary renal c.
solitary lower pole c.
spermatic c.

C

calculus (*continued*)
    spurious c.
    staghorn c.
    stomach c.
    struvite c.
    submucosal c.
    treatment of renal c.
    triamterene c.
    unilateral ureteral c.
    upper urinary tract c.
    urate c.
    ureteral c.
    urethral c.
    uric acid c.
    urinary c.
    urostealith c.
    vesical c.
    vesicoprostatic c.
    Volkmann spoon for pancreatic c.
    weddellite c.
    whewellite c.
    xanthic c.
    xanthine c.
Calcutript
    C. electrohydraulic lithotriptor
    Karl Storz C.
CALD
    chronic active liver disease
caldesmon
Caldwell needle/cannula Quick-Tap paracentesis system
Calglycine
Calgocide disinfectant
caliber
    loop c.
    c. probe
caliber-persistent
    c.-p. artery
    c.-p. artery of stomach
    c.-p. vessel
calibrate
calibration of cardia
calibrator
    c. serum
    Vitros Immunodiagnostic Products HBsAg reagent pack and c.
caliceal (*var. of* calyceal)
    c. diverticulum
calicectasis (*var. of* caliectasis)
calicectomy (*var. of* calicotomy)
calices (*pl. of* calix)
    multiple c.
calicine (*var. of* calycine)
Caliciviridae virus family
Calicivirus gastroenteritis
calicoplasty (*var. of* calioplasty)
calicotomy, calicectomy, caliotomy
Calicylic

caliectasis, pyelocaliectasis, calicectasis
California peppertree
calioplasty, calicoplasty
caliorrhaphy
caliotomy (*var. of* calicotomy)
calipers
    Lange skinfold c.
calix (*var. of* calyx), *pl.* calices
Cal-Lac
Callaway formula
Call-Exner body
Calmette-Guérin
    bacille C.-G. (BCG, bCG)
    C.-G. bacillus
    intravesical bacillus C.-G.
calmodulin
Calmoseptine ointment
Calogen LCT emulsion
caloric
    c. intake
    c. supplement
calorie, calory
    high c.
calorimeter
calory (*var. of* calorie)
Calot
    C. operation
    C. triangle
Calotropis
calpain in acute tubular necrosis
calponin
calprotectin
    c. assay
    fecal c.
calretinin
Caluso PEG gastrostomy tube
calyceal, caliceal
    c. diverticular calculus
    c. drainage
    c. extension
    c. filling time
    c. fistula
    c. fornix
    c. infundibulum
    c. puncture
calyces (*pl. of* calyx)
calycine, calicine
Calymmatobacterium granulomatis
calyx, calix, *pl.* **calyces**
    anomalous c.
    c. clubbing
    c. elongation
    c. enlargement
    extrarenal c.
    kidney c.
    minor c.
    c. obstruction
    c. puncture

CAM
    complementary and alternative
      medicine
Camalox
Cambridge pancreatitis classification
  I–IV
camera
    c. adapter
    Anger scintillation c.
    charge-coupled device
      monochrome c.
    Circon-ACMI MicroDigital-I c.
    endoscopic c.
    field-of-view c.
    Fujinon FG-series endoscopic c.
    gamma scintillation c.
    Gammatone II gamma c.
    instant c.
    Olympus OM-1 reflex c.
    Olympus OM-series endoscopic c.
    Olympus OTV S-series
      miniature c.
    Olympus SCA series
      endoscopic c.
    Pen-F half-frame c.
    Pentax endoscopic c.
    Polaroid c.
    positron c.
    single-lens reflex c.
    still c.
    television c.
Cameron
    C. electrosurgical unit
    C. erosion
    C. lesion
    C. omniangle gastroscope
    C. ulcer
Cameron-Miller
    C.-M. electrocoagulation unit
    C.-M. electrode
    C.-M. monopolar probe
    C.-M. suction-coagulator
Camey
    C. enterocystoplasty
    C. enterocystoplasty urinary
      diversion
    C. I, II detubalarized neobladder
      operation
    C. ileocystoplasty
    C. I orthotopic urinary diversion
    C. neobladder
    C. reservoir
    C. total gastrectomy procedure
    C. urinary pouch
cAMP
    5′-cyclic adenosine monophosphate
    cyclic adenosine monophosphate
      vasopressin-induced cAMP
Campath-1H

Campbell
    C. opening-wedge thoracostomy
      technique
    C. procedure
    C. sound
    C. trocar
camper
    C. angle
    C. chiasm
    C. fascia
    fascia of C.
    C. ligament
    C. plane
Camptosar injection
camptothecin
Campy-BAP culture medium
Campylobacter
    C. cinaedi
    C. coli
    C. doylei
    C. fetus
    C. fetus colitis
    C. fetus enteritis
    C. hyointestinalis
    C. jejuni
    C. lari
    C. pylori
    C. pyloridis gastritis
    C. test
    C. upsaliensis
Campylobacter-like
    C.-l. organism (CLO)
    C.-l. organism test (CLOtest)
Camwrap plastic covering
Canada-Cronkhite syndrome
Canadian
    C. fleabane
    C. Urology Oncology Group
      (CUOG)
canal
    abdominal c.
    Alcock c.
    alimentary c.
    anal c.
    Bernard c.
    epidermoid carcinoma of anal c.
      (ECAC)
    femoral c.
    histologic anal c.
    inguinal c.
    c. of Hering
    c. of Nuck
    c. of Wirsung
    pancreaticobiliary c.
    pecten of anal c.
    pleuroperitoneal c.
    portal c.
    pudendal c.
    pyloric c.

canal (*continued*)
Santorini c.
c. stenosis
ventricular c.
vesicourethral c.
canalicular
c. bile
c. bile plug
c. cholestasia
c. cryptorchidism
canaliculus
apical c.
bile duct c.
biliary c.
c. bilifer
pili torti et c.
pseudobile c.
secretory c.
Canasa suppository
cancelling A's test
cancer
American Joint Committee on C. (AJCC)
American Joint Committee on Cancer/International Union Against C. (AJCC/UICC)
Amsterdam criteria for hereditary nonpolyposis colorectal c.
androgen-independent prostate c. (AIPC)
c. antigen 125 (CA-125, CA125)
antral c.
bile duct c.
bilharzial-related c.
bladder c.
borreliosis classification for advanced gastric c.
Borrmann gastric c.
breast c.
burned-out testis c.
c. cell growth
c. cell heterogeneity
clear cell renal c.
colon c.
colorectal c. (CRC)
columnar cuff c.
cryoablation for prostate c.
de novo liver c.
depressed c.
depressed-type colorectal c.
diagnosis of bladder c.
disseminated c.
c. doubling time
c. drug resistance
duodenal c.
early gastric c. (EGC)
endocrine c.
esophageal c.
esophagogastric junction c.

European Organization for Research and Treatment of C. (EORTC)
exenterative surgery for pelvic c.
extragonadal germ cell c.
extrahepatic bile duct c.
familial colon c.
gastric c.
gastrointestinal c.
GI c.
hereditary nonpolyposis colon c. (HNPCC)
hereditary nonpolyposis colorectal c.
hereditary papillary renal c. (HPRC)
high-grade synchronous colon c.
hypoechoic c.
hypopharyngeal c.
incurable c.
intraepithelial c.
intramucosal c.
Japanese classification of c.
large-bowel c.
liver c.
low-lying rectal c.
lung c.
marker for c.
Matritech NMP22 test for bladder c.
metachronous colon c.
metastatic c.
Mostofi-grade prostate c.
mucin-producing c.
new chemotherapy combinations for advanced bladder c.
nonfixed c.
nonpolyposis colorectal c.
obstructing c.
C. of the Prostate Strategic Urologic Research Endeavor
ovarian c.
pancreatic c. (PC)
pancreaticoduodenal c.
pancreatoduodenal c.
papillary renal c.
polypoid c.
postgastrectomy c.
primary colorectal c. (PCRC)
prostate c. (PCa)
rectal c.
rectosigmoid c.
recurrent colorectal c. (RCRC)
restaging of c.
c. screening
squamous cell c.
staging of c.
stenotic c.
suburothelial infiltrative c.
superficial bladder c.
superficial depressed c.

testicular c.
testis c.
transplanted c.
treatment of bladder c.
Union Internationale Contre le C.
(UICC)
urethral c.
urologic system c.
urothelial c.
Whitmore classification of
prostate c.
cancer-associated
c.-a. sialyl-Lea antigen
transitional cell c.-a. (TCCA)
cancerous erosion
Candela
C. MDA-200 LaserTripter
C. MDL 2000 laser
C. MiniScope
C. pulsed-dye laser
candesartan
luminal c.
Candida
C. *albicans*
C. *esophagitis*
C. *glabrata*
C. *immitis*
C. immunologic study
C. infection
C. *krusei*
C. *neoformans*
C. *peritonitis*
C. symptom
systemic *C.*
C. *tropicalis*
ureteral *C.*
vaginal *C.*
candidal
c. cellulitis
c. cystitis
c. esophagitis
c. infection
c. intertrigo
c. overgrowth
candidemia
candidiasis, candidosis
esophageal c. (EC)
vulvovaginal c. (VVC)
candidosis (*var. of* candidiasis)
candidum
Geotrichum c.
canine sphincter
caninum
Dipylidium c.
canis
Toxocara c.
canister
ATS c.
canker sore

Cannon
C. point
C. ring
cannula, *pl.* **cannulas cannulae**
Buie rectal injection c.
contour ERCP c.
double-lumen irrigation c.
ERCP c.
Flexicath silicone subclavian c.
Fluoro Tip ERCP c.
Franklin-Silverman biopsy c.
Hasson open laparoscopy c.
Intraducer peritoneal c.
Jetco-Spray c.
LaparoSAC single-use obturator and
c.
laparoscopic c.
large-bore c.
Makler c.
Mayo-Ochsner suction trocar c.
Medicut c.
Olympus monopolar c.
perfusion c.
polyethylene c.
portal c.
Ramirez silastic c.
Tandem XL triple-lumen ERCP c.
Teflon ERCP c.
Veress c.
washout c.
c. with preloaded guidewire
cannulae (*pl. of* cannula)
cannulas (*pl. of* cannula)
cannulation, cannulization
bile duct c.
biliary c.
c. catheter
deep c.
duct c.
endoscopic retrograde c.
endoscopic transpapillary c.
ERCP c.
ex vivo c.
freehand c.
c. of biliary tree
postsphincterotomy ERCP c.
retrograde c.
selective ductal c.
stricture c.
transpapillary c.
cannulatome
Cotton c.
cannulization (*var. of* cannulation)
Can-Opt
C.-O. dual-lumen ERCP system
C.-O. stand-alone dual-lumen ERCP
catheter
C-ANP
C-type atrial natriuretic peptide

C22-3 antigen
Cantil
Cantlie line
Cantor tube
Cantwell-Ransley
    C.-R. cavernocavernostomy
    C.-R. epispadias repair
    C.-R. hypospadias repair
      procedure
    C.-R. technique
    C.-R. urethroplasty
CAP
    carcinoma of prostate
    chronic alcoholic pancreatitis
cap
    Assura stoma c.
    Coloplast stoma c.
    continent anal c.
    ConvaTec Active Life stoma c.
    duodenal c. (DC)
    external test c.
    c. method
    phrygian c.
    c. polyposis
    pyloric c.
    stoma c.
    Sur-Fit Natura flange c.
    Sur-Fit stoma c.
    ZE c.
capacitive coupling
capacity
    acid-neutralizing c. (ANC)
    bladder c.
    cystometric bladder c.
    fluid absorptive c.
    functional bladder c.
    galactose elimination c. (GEC)
    gastric c.
    iron-binding c. (IBC)
    maximum bladder c.
    maximum cystometric c.
    peritoneal membrane solute
      transport c.
    PMN oxidative burst c.
    pressure-specific bladder c.
    rectal c.
    total iron-binding c. (TIBC)
    unbound iron-binding c. (UIBC)
capacity-limited kinetics
cap-assisted endoscopic mucosal
  resection
CAPD
    chronic ambulatory peritoneal dialysis
    continuous ambulatory peritoneal
      dialysis
capecitabine
Capener gouge
Cape Town injection sclerotherapy
  technique

cap-fitted
    c.-f. endoscope
    c.-f. gastroscopy
    c.-f. panendoscope
capillarectasia
Capillaria philippinensis
capillariasis
    intestinal c.
capillaritis
    pulmonary c.
capillaropathy
capillary
    bile c.
    c. dilation
    c. endothelial cell
    glomerular c.
    c. hemangioma
    c. hyperfiltration
    c. leak phenomenon
    c. network
    peritubular c.
    c. permeability
    c. refill
    C. System slide holder
    c. wall
capillary-lymphatic invasion
capillata
    Absidia c.
capistration
capita (*pl. of* caput)
capitatum
    Trichosporon c.
capitonnage
caplet
    Buffaprin c.
    Bufferin Arthritis Strength c.
    Renax film-coated c.
    Strovite Advance c.
    Vanquish analgesic c.
Capmul 8210
Capnocytophaga
capnography
capnometry
capotement
Capoten
Capozide
CAPPP
    Captopril Prevention Project
capreomycin (CM)
CAPS
    caffeine, alcohol, pepper, spicy foods
capsaicin
    intravesical c.
CAPS-free diet
capsid
capsid-encoding region
capsula, *pl.* **capsulae**
    c. adiposa renis
    c. fibrosa

c. fibrosa perivascularis hepatis
c. fibrosa renis
c. glomeruli
c. pancreatitis
capsulae (*pl. of* capsula)
capsular
c. artery
c. blood vessel
c. cirrhosis of liver
c. flap pyeloplasty
c. nephritis
c. penetration
c. tear
capsulatum
Histoplasma c.
capsule
acidophilus c.
all-purpose c. (APC)
Bowman c.
budesonide c.
Carey c.
Cenogen-OB c.
Crosby c.
Detrol LA c.
dutasteride c.
c. endoscopy
enteric-coated c.
c. enteroscopy
Entero-Test c.
Entocort EC oral c.
fascial c.
c. flap technique
Gerota c.
Given imaging capsule/
  M2A c.
Glisson c.
hepatic c.
hepatobiliary c.
L-carnitine c.
liver c.
M2A capsule/Given imaging c.
M2A swallowable imaging c.
Max-EPA c.
müllerian c.
mycophenolate mofetil c.
c. of pancreas
Orfadin c.
pH-sensitive radiotelemetry c.
polysaccharide c.
prostatic c.
radioisotope c.
radiotelemetering c.
Rebetol c.
renal c.
ribavirin c.
Sitzmarks radiopaque marker in
  gelatin c.
splenic c.
Synalgos-DC c.

tolterodine tartrate c.
Watson c.
capsule/tablet
Disalcid c./t.
capsulitis
hepatic c.
capsuloma
capsuloplasty
capsulotomy
renal c.
CapSure continence shield
Captiflex polypectomy snare
Captivator polypectomy snare
captivus
penis c.
captopril
c. plasma renin activity test
C. Prevention Project (CAPPP)
c. renogram
c. renography
captopril-DTPA scanning
captopril-enhanced renography
caput, *pl.* **capita**
c. epididymidis
c. gallinaginis
c. medusae
c. pancreatis
Carafate
caraway
carb
carbohydrate
carbachol
carbamazepine hepatotoxicity
carbamoyl phosphate synthetase
  deficiency
carbamylated hemoglobin
carbamylation
carbamylcholine
carbenicillin
carbenoxolone
Carbicarb
carbidopa dopaminergic medication
CarboFlex odor-control dressing
carbohydrate (carb)
c. antigen 19-9 (CA—19-9)
c. antigen 19-9 immunohistochemical
  expression
carbohydrate-free
Ross c.-f. (RCF)
carbohydrate-induced hyperlipidemia
carbohydraturia
carbol fuchsin stain
carbon
c. dioxide (CO_2)
c. dioxide acidosis
c. dioxide insufflator
c. dioxide laser
c. dioxide laser plaque ablation
c. dioxide trapping agent

C

carbon *(continued)*
    c. tetrachloride
    c. tetrachloride-induced liver
      regeneration
    c. tetrachloride nephropathy
carbon-11 (^{11}C, C-11)
carbon-13 urea breath test (^{13}C-UBT)
carbon-14 (^{14}C, C-14)
    c.-14 urea breath test (^{14}C-UBT)
    c.-14 urinary excretion test
carbonate
    aluminum c.
    c. apatite
    c. apatite calcification
    c. apatite calculus
    c. apatite stone
    calcium c.
    dihydroxyaluminum sodium c.
    lanthanum c.
    magnesium c.
carbonic
    c. anhydrase (CA)
    c. anhydrase II
    c. anhydrase inhibitor (CAI)
carbonuria
carboplatin, etoposide, bleomycin (CEB)
carboprost tromethamine
Carbowax
carboxamide
    dimethyltriazenoimidazole c. (DTIC)
    imidazole c.
carboxyamidotriazole
carboxykinase
    phosphoenolpyruvate c. (PEPCK)
carboxylic ester hydrolase (CEH)
carboxyl-terminal amidation
carboxymethylcellulose jelly
carboxypeptidase
    c. B-like enzyme
    porcine c. B
carboxyterminal
    c. noncollagenous domain
    c. PTH
carbuncle
    kidney c.
    renal c.
carbunculoid
carbuterol
Carcassonne perineal ligament
carcinoembryonic antigen (CEA)
carcinogenesis
    chemical c.
    colorectal c.
    oncogene-induced c.
carcinogenicity
carcinogenic nitrosamine
carcinoid
    bronchial c.
    duodenal c.

    c. flush
    gastric c.
    gastroduodenal c.
    hindgut c.
    c. secretory granule
    seminal vesicle c.
    c. syndrome
    testis c.
    c. tumor
carcinoma, *pl.* **carcinomas, carcinomata**
    acinar cell c.
    acinar hepatocellular c.
    adenoid cystic c.
    adenosquamous cell c.
    adrenal cortex c.
    adrenocortical c.
    ameboma mimicking c.
    ampullary c.
    ampullopancreatic c.
    anal epidermoid c.
    anorectal c.
    Astwood-Coller staging system for
      c.
    autolymphocyte-based treatment for
      renal cell c. (ALT-RCC)
    Barrett c.
    basal cell c.
    basaloid squamous cell c. (BSCC)
    Bellini duct c.
    bile duct c.
    biliary c.
    bladder small cell c.
    bladder squamous cell c.
    bladder transitional cell c.
    Borrmann gastric c. type I–IV
    Borrmann scirrhous c.
    bulbomembranous urethral squamous
      cell c.
    bulbourethral c.
    cervical c.
    cholangiocellular c. (CCC)
    cholangitis c.
    clear cell hepatocellular c.
    clear cell nonpapillary c.
    collecting duct c.
    colon c.
    colorectal c. (CRC)
    cortical c.
    cystic renal cell c. (CRCC)
    deleted in colorectal c. (DCC)
    diffuse hepatocellular c.
    downstaging of advanced esophageal
      c.
    Dukes classification of c.
    Edmondson grading system for
      hepatocellular c.
    Edmondson-Steiner histologic grading
      of hepatocellular c. I, II, III, IVa
    embryonal cell c.

embryonal testicular c.
encapsulated renal cell c.
encephaloid gastric c.
endocrine cell c.
endometrial c.
epidermoid c.
esophageal squamous cell c.
excavated gastric c.
c. ex pleomorphic adenoma
fibrolamellar hepatocellular c.
  (FL-HCC)
flat c.
flat-type c.
focal c.
gallbladder c.
gastric c.
genitourinary c.
germ cell c.
hepatocellular c. (HCC)
hereditary nonpolyposis colorectal c.
hilar c.
increased risk of penile c.
c. in situ (CIS)
c. in situ of glans penis
intramucosal c.
invasive c.
islet cell c.
Jass staging for rectal c.
Jewett classification of bladder c.
kidney c.
large-bowel c.
laryngeal c.
linitis plastica c.
liver cell c.
medullary thyroid c.
metastatic prostatic c.
metastatic renal cell c. (MRCC)
microtrabecular hepatocellular c.
monofocal papillary c.
mucin-hypersecreting c.
mucinous c.
mucoepidermoid c.
mutated colorectal c. (MCC)
nodular transitional cell c.
nongerm cell c.
nonseminomatous testicular c.
nonsmall cell lung c.
oat cell c.
obstructing rectosigmoidal c.
c. of prostate (CAP)
oropharyngeal c.
ovarian c.
pancreatic c. (PCA)
pancreatic acinar cell c.
pancreatic islet cell c.
papillary gastric c.
papillary renal cell c.
papillary transitional cell c.
pediatric c.

penile c.
perforated c.
periampullary c.
peritoneal c.
PIVKA-II EIA kit for hepatocellular
  c.
polypoid c.
primary transitional cell c.
prostate gland small cell c.
prostatic urethral transitional cell c.
protuberant c.
rectal linitis plastica colorectal c.
renal cell c. (RCC)
renipelvic transitional cell c.
renomedullary c.
RLP colorectal c.
sarcomatoid squamous cell c.
scirrhous c.
sclerosing hepatic c. (SHC)
secondary metastatic c.
sessile nodular c.
sigmoid colon c.
signet-ring cell c.
signet-ring pattern of gastric c.
splenic flexure c.
sporadic nonfamilial clear cell c.
squamous cell c. (SCC)
stage B, C c.
superficial esophageal c. (SEC)
superficial gastric c.
superficially spreading c.
supraglottic squamous cell c.
testicular c.
TNM classification of c.
TP53-mutated c.
transitional cell c.
transthoracic resection of esophageal
  c.
tubular c.
ulcerating c.
unresectable hepatocellular c.
upper tract transitional cell c.
ureteral c.
urethral c.
urothelial c.
verrucous c.
vulvar c.
yolk sac c.
carcinomas (*pl. of* carcinoma)
carcinomata (*pl. of* carcinoma)
carcinomatosis
peritoneal c.
c. peritonei
carcinosarcoma
bladder c.
gastric c.
kidney c.
polypoid exophytic nonulcerating c.
renal c.

C

card
   Hemoccult II c.
CARD15
   CARD15 gene
   CARD15 polymorphism
cardamom
cardia
   achalasia c.
   calibration of c.
   crescent gastric c.
   gastric c.
   c. intestinal metaplasia (CIM)
   c. of stomach
   patulous c.
cardiac
   c. antrum
   c. beta adrenoreceptor
      hyporesponsiveness
   c. beta receptor
   c. cirrhosis
   c. decompression
   c. glycoside
   c. impression on liver
   c. output
   c. output/cardiac index (CO/CI)
   c. proteinuria
   c. sphincter
   c. stomach
   c. stomach mucosa
   c. sympathovagal tone
cardiac-type
   c.-t. gland
   c.-t. mucosa
cardialgia
cardiectomy
cardinal
   c. ligament
   c. suture
   c. vein
cardinal-sacrouterine ligament
  complex
cardiochalasia
cardiodiosis
cardioesophageal (CE)
   c. junction (CEJ)
   c. mucosal junction
   c. reflex
   c. relaxation
   c. sphincter
cardiofundic gastropathy
cardiohepatic
   c. angle
   c. triangle
cardiohepatomegaly
cardiomegaly
cardiomyopathy
   uremic c.
cardiomyotomy
   Heller c.

cardiopexy
   ligamentum teres c.
cardioplasty
cardiopulmonary
   c. baroreflex
   c. baroreflex dysfunction
   c. baroreflex function
   c. complication
cardiopyloric axis
cardiorespiratory complication
cardiospasm
cardiotomy
cardiotoxicity
   ipecac-induced c.
cardiovascular
   c. complication
   c. disorder
   c. drug hepatotoxicity
   c. mortality
carditis
   gastric c.
Cardizem
CARD15/NOD2 **susceptibility gene**
Cardura
care
   Advanced-RF Natal C.
   cost-effective c.
   Dermacyn wound c.
   c. pathway
   Remedy advanced skin c.
   surgical c.
caretaker gene
Carey capsule
Carey-Coons biliary endoprosthesis
  kit
Ca-Rezz moisture barrier cream
caribi
Carignan syndrome
carina, *pl.* **carinae**
carinae (*pl. of* carina)
carinate abdomen
carinii
   Pneumocystis c.
carious teeth
Carle analytic gas chromatograph
Carlesta
carline thistle
C-arm
   C-a. fluoroscope
   C-a. fluoroscopy
Carmalt
   C. clamp
   C. forceps
   C. hemostat
Carman-Kirklin
   C.-K. meniscus complex
   C.-K. meniscus sign
Carman sign
Carmel clamp

carminative
carmine
    c. blue
    contrast chromoscopy using indigo
      c. (CCIC)
    indigo c.
carmustine (bCNU, BCNU, BiCNU)
Carnett sign
Carney complex
carnitine
Carnitor
carnosinuria
Carnot
    C. function
    C. test
carob
Caroid
Caroli
    C. disease
    C. syndrome
Caroli-Sarles bile duct stricture
  classification
carotene
    serum c.
carotenemia
carotid
    c. artery
    c. bruit
Carpenter syndrome
carphenazine
carrageen, carragheen
carrageenan, carrageenin
carrageenin (*var. of* carrageenan)
carragheen (*var. of* carrageenan)
Carraginate dressing
CarraKlenz skin cleanser
CarraSorb H dressing
Carrel
    C. aortic patch
    C. aortic patch anastomosis
carrier
    Deschamps ligature c.
    Endo-Assist disposable ligature
      c.
    gene c.
    Goldwasser suture c.
    hepatitis c.
    nongene c.
    c. of allele
    Pereyra ligature c.
    Raz double-prong ligature
      c.
    Semb ligature c.
Carr-Locke injection needle
Carson
    C. internal/external endopyelotomy
      stent
    C. Zero Tip balloon dilation
      catheter

cart
    Fujinon videoendoscopy c.
carteolol
Carter-Horsley-Hughes syndrome
Carter-Thomason
    C.-T. port closure device
    C.-T. suture passer
cartilage
    arytenoid c.
cartridge
    Clark hemoperfusion c.
    Dimension RxL PSA Flex
      reagent c.
Cartrol Oral
cartwheel configuration
caruncle
    Morgagni c.
    urethral c.
carvedilol
Cary-Blair medium
Casale
    C. vasectomy
    C. vesicostomy
cascade
    clotting c.
    fibrogenic c.
    intrarenal matrix-degrading
      enzyme c.
    MAP kinase signaling c.
    metastatic c.
    signaling c.
    c. stomach
cascara
    c. sagrada
    c. sagrada and aloe
case
    poor surgical risk c.
    C. Power protein
      supplement
    primary c.
    secondary c.
caseating
    c. granuloma
    c. necrosis
caseation
case-by-case approach
Casec calcium supplement
casei
    Lactobacillus c.
casein refeeding
caseosa
    nephritis c.
caseous nephritis
cashew apple
CAS 200 image cytometer
CaSki cell line
Casodex
Casola cecostomy
Casoni skin test

C

cast
>bacterial c.
>blood c.
>coarse granular c.
>erythrocyte c.
>esophageal c.
>fat c.
>fatty c.
>fine granular c.
>granular c. (GC)
>hematin c.
>hyaline c.
>c. nephropathy
>proteinaceous c.
>red blood cell c.
>c. syndrome
>urinary sediment c.
>white blood cell c.

Castellani paint
Castleman
>C. disease
>C. tumor

castlike tube
castor
>c. oil
>c. oil plant

Castoria
>Fletcher's C.

castrate
castration
>functional c.
>medical c.
>radiologic c.

catabolism
catalase
Catapres
catarrhal
>c. cholangitis
>c. cystitis
>c. dysentery
>c. dyspepsia
>c. gastritis
>c. jaundice
>c. nephritis

catastrophic complication
catatonic trypsinogen DNA screening
catecholamine
>adrenal c.
>c. excess state
>plasma c.
>c. synthetic enzyme
>urinary c.

catecholaminergic
category
>Bosniak lesion c. I-IV
>NIH Classification C. I-IV
>prune-belly syndrome c. I-III

cat-eye syndrome

catgut
>chromic c.

cath
>catheter
>catheterization
>Ash Split Cath

catharsis
cathartic
>c. colitis
>c. colon
>osmotic c.

Cathelin-related antimicrobial peptide (CRAMP)
Cathelin segregator
catheter (cath)
>Ablaser laser delivery c.
>Abscession biliary drainage c.
>Accurate c.
>Achiever balloon dilation c.
>acorn-tipped c.
>Acucise balloon c.
>Acucise endopyelotomy c.
>c. á demeure
>Allis c.
>Amplatz c.
>Angiocath PRN c.
>angiographic endhole c.
>angiography c.
>AngioJet Xpeedior c.
>angioplasty balloon c.
>antibacterial personal c.
>antiseptic-impregnated central venous c.
>Argyle Ingram trocar c.
>Argyle Medicut R c.
>ARROWgard Blue hemodialysis c.
>arteriovenous c.
>aspiration c.
>Atlantic ileostomy c.
>c. bacterial interference
>balloon dilating c.
>Bardex-Foley c.
>Bard gastrostomy c.
>bat-wing c.
>bicoudate c.
>c. bicoudé
>biliary balloon c.
>biliary dilator c.
>Bio-Flex CS c.
>Bio-Flex Tesio c.
>Bitome c.
>blood-contactin c.
>Blue Max balloon c.
>Bozeman-Fritsch c.
>Braasch c.
>brush c.
>BUD drainage c.
>bullet-tip c.
>Burhenne steerable c.

cannulation c.
Can-Opt stand-alone dual-lumen
ERCP c.
Carson Zero Tip balloon dilation
c.
CathLink 20 port system with
Chronoflex c.
central venous c.
Chait Trapdoor cecostomy c.
Chemo-Port c.
Cholangiocath c.
c. cholangiogram
cholangiographic c.
Circle C hemodialysis c.
Clay-Adams c.
coaxial c.
cobra c.
coil c.
Coil-Cath c.
c. coiling sign
colon motility c.
combination biliary brush c.
Comfort Cath I, II c.
Conceptus Soft Seal cervical c.
Conceptus Soft Torque uterine c.
Conceptus VS c.
condom c.
cone-tip c.
conical c.
Conveen female intermittent c.
Conveen olive-tip coudé intermittent
c.
Conveen ultrasecure self-sealing
male external c.
Cook TPN c.
cooled ThermoCath treatment c.
Cope loop nephrostomy c.
Corflo percutaneous access c.
coudé c.
Councill c.
CRE balloon c.
Curity Ultramer Foley c.
Curl Cath c.
DASH ERCP c.
decompression c.
Dentsleeve single multilumen
extrusion c.
de Pezzer c.
Digitrapper c.
dilating c.
dilation c. (DC)
Dormia stone basket c.
Dotter c.
double-J c.
double-lumen balloon c.
double-lumen injection c.
Dover intermittent female c.
Dover red rubber Robinson
intermittent c.

Dover Rob-Nel intermittent c.
Dover 100% silicone Foley c.
Dover Texas c.
Dow-Corning ileal pouch c.
Dowd II prostatic balloon dilation
c.
drainage c.
dual-lumen c.
dual-sensory antimony pH c.
Duo-Coat dual-lumen c.
Duo-Flow c.
DURAglide 3 stone balloon c.
elbowed c.
Eliminator balloon c.
endhole ureteral c.
endoscopic retrograde
cholangiopancreatography c.
EndoSound endoscopic ultrasound c.
epidural c.
ERCP c.
esophageal manometry c.
esophageal motility perfused c.
esophageal perfusion c.
exdwelling ureteral occlusion balloon
c.
exit site of c.
external ureteral c.
Extractor 3-lumen retrieval balloon
c.
female c.
femoral hemodialysis c.
fenestrated c.
fiberoptic c.
Flexima ureteral c.
Flexxicon Blue dialysis c.
Flexxicon II PC internal jugular c.
Fogarty balloon biliary c.
Fogarty irrigation c.
Foley c.
French Cope loop nephrostomy c.
French mushroom-tip c.
French pigtail nephrostomy c.
French Teflon pyeloureteral c.
Gauder Silicon PEG c.
Gazelle balloon dilation c.
Glidex coated Percuflex c.
Glo-tip biliary c.
Gold Probe direct bipolar
hemostasis c.
Gold Probe electrohemostasis c.
Gore-Tex c.
Gouley c.
Graham c.
Greenfield caval c.
Grüntzig balloon c.
c. guide
guiding c.
Hemo-Cath c.
Hemoject injection c.

catheter (*continued*)
    HemoSplit c.
    hooked c.
    Howmedica slit c.
    Hurwitz dialysis c.
    Hydromer grafted c.
    hydrostatic balloon c.
    ILUS c.
    indwelling urinary c.
    injection c.
    intraarterial chemotherapy c.
    intracholedochal manometric c.
    intraductal imaging c.
    intrathecal c.
    intravascular ultrasound c.
    InView male external c.
    c. irrigation
    IVUS c.
    Jackson-Pratt c.
    Jelco c.
    Kaye tamponade balloon c.
    Kendall Foley c.
    Kenguard silicone-coated Foley c.
    kidney internal splint/stent c.
    Kish urethral illuminate c.
    KISS c.
    Konigsberg c.
    Kumpe c.
    Lane gastroenterostomy c.
    large-bore c.
    LeVeen c.
    LifeJet c.
    Lifemed c.
    long-term indwelling c.
    lumen-seeking c.
    Mahurkar c.
    male c.
    Malecot reentry c.
    Malecot suprapubic c.
    Mallinckrodt c.
    manometry c.
    Mark IV Moss decompression feeding c.
    MaxForce TTS biliary balloon dilation c.
    MaxForce TTS high-performance balloon dilation c.
    measuring-mounting c.
    Medicut c.
    Medina ileostomy c.
    Medi-Tech bipolar c.
    Medi-Tech steerable c.
    Memokath c.
    Mentor nonhydrophilic PVC c.
    Mentor straight c.
    metal ball-tip c.
    metallic-tip c.
    Mewissen infusion c.
    microtip sensor c.

microtip transducer c.
Microvasive balloon c.
Millar urodynamic c.
MiniBard c.
Missouri c.
Mistifier spray c.
MM c.
modified aspirating c.
monocrystant antimony pH c.
MS Classique balloon dilation c.
multifiber c.
multilumen manometric c.
mushroom c.
nasobiliary drainage c.
nasocystic c.
nasopancreatic c.
nasovesicular c.
needle-tip c.
Nélaton c.
NeoSoft nephrostomy drainage c.
nephrostomy c.
Niagara temporary dialysis c.
10 o'clock selector c.
olive-tipped c.
Olympus PW-1L wash c.
Olympus PW-5V spray c.
On-Command c.
open-ended ureteral c.
oral suction c.
over-the-wire balloon c.
Passage biliary dilation c.
Passport balloon-on-a-wire dilation c.
PE-MV balloon dilation c.
Percuflex c.
percutaneous femoral vein c.
percutaneous nephrostomy Malecot c.
percutaneous transhepatic biliary drainage c.
percutaneous transhepatic pigtail c.
peritoneal dialysis c. (PDC)
PermCath dual-lumen c.
Pezzer c.
Phantom 5 Plus ST balloon dilation c.
Phillips c.
pigtail c.
Pollack ureteral c.
polyethylene c.
polyurethane nasoenteric c.
polyvinyl chloride c.
polyvinyl manometric c.
Porges c.
Port-A-Cath c.
portal c.
postprostatectomy hemostatic c.
Pourchez XpressO hemodialysis c.
c. probe

c. probe-assisted endoluminal ultrasonography (CP-EUS)
c. probe ultrasound
ProGuide chronic dialysis c.
prostatic c.
PTBD c.
PTHC c.
pulse spray c.
pusher c.
PVC c.
pyeloureteral c.
Quinton c.
Quinton-Mahurkar dual-lumen peritoneal c.
radiopaque ERCP c.
Ranfac cholangiographic c.
Ranfac cholangiography c.
Reddick cystic duct cholangiogram c.
red rubber Robinson c.
Release-NF c.
retrograde occlusion balloon c.
Rigiflex ABD balloon dilation c.
Rigiflex biliary balloon dilation c.
Rigiflex esophageal TTS balloon c.
Rigiflex OTW balloon dilation c.
Rigiflex TTS balloon dilation c.
Ring biliary drainage c.
Robinson c.
ruler c.
Sacks QuickStick c.
Sacks Single-Step c.
SchonCath chronic dialysis c.
Self-Cath hydrogel intermittent urinary c.
self-drainage c.
self-retaining c.
shepherd's hook c.
shepherd's hook-shaped angiographic c.
Siegel-Cohen dilating c.
silastic c.
silicone rubber Dacron cuffed c.
silver c.
SIM 2 c.
Simmons c.
Simplastic c.
single-lumen Broviac silicone c.
SmartCath esophageal balloon c.
Soehendra graduated dilating c.
solid-state esophageal manometry c.
Sonicath endoluminal ultrasound c.
c. sonography
Spectrum silicone Foley c.
spiral-tip c.
Stamey-Malecot c.
Stamey open-tip ureteral c.
standard ERCP c.
stenting c.

Stretta c.
subclavian c.
Suction Buster c.
Supra-Foley c.
SureCath sterile intermittent c.
surgically implanted hemodialysis c. (SIHC)
Surgitek c.
Swan-Ganz pulmonary artery c.
Swan-Ganz thermodilution c.
swan-neck Missouri c.
swan-neck pediatric Coil-Cath c.
SynchroMed infusion system intraspinal c.
synthetic 5-channel water-perfused motility c.
Tandem thin-shaft transureteroscopic balloon dilation c.
tapered-tip hydrophilic-coated push c.
Taut cystic duct c.
Teflon guiding c.
Tenckhoff 2-cuff c.
Tenckhoff peritoneal dialysis c.
Texas-style 2-piece c.
toposcopic c.
Toronto-Western c.
torque c.
Trabucco double balloon c.
Trach-Eze closed suction c.
Tracker c.
transanal c.
transducer c.
translumbar inferior vena cava c.
transurethral c.
Tratner c.
trial without c. (TWOC)
Trilogy low-profile balloon dilation c.
triple-lumen manometry c.
c. tunnel infection
Tyshak c.
Uldall subclavian hemodialysis c.
ureteral occlusion balloon c.
Urocath external c.
urodynamic c.
UroMax II high-pressure balloon c.
Uro-San Plus external c.
van Andel dilating c.
van Sonnenberg gallbladder c.
Vaxcel dialysis c.
Vygon Nutricath S c.
washing c.
water-infusion esophageal manometry c.
water-perfused c.
3-way irrigating c.
whistle-tip ureteral c.
Willscher c.

catheter (*continued*)
    Wilson-Cook fine-needle aspiration c.
    Wilson-Cook Quantum TTC esophageal balloon dilation c.
    winged c.
    Witzel enterostomy c.
    Xpeedior c.
    Z-Med c.
catheter-associated bacteriuria
catheter-based ultrasound probe
catheter-guided endoscopic intubation (CAGEIN)
catheterizable reservoir
catheterization (cath)
    aseptic intermittent c.
    clean intermittent c. (CIC)
    clean intermittent bladder c.
    cystic duct c.
    hepatic vein c.
    in-and-out c.
    intermittent c.
    c. pouch
    c. pouch rupture
    c. reservoir
    retrourethral c.
    Seldinger cystic duct c.
    selective c.
    subclavian vein c.
    c. test
    transhepatic c.
    transnasal bile duct c.
    transpapillary c.
    umbilical vein c.
    ureteral c.
    urethral c.
    urinary c.
catheterize
catheter-related bloodstream infection (CR-BSI, CRBI, CRBSI)
CathLink 20 port system with Chronoflex catheter
Cath-Secure
    C.-S. catheter holder
    C.-S. tape
CathTrack catheter locator system
cation
    cosecreted c.
    c. exchange
    c. exchanger
    c. exchange resin
    c. transport
cationic
    c. colloidal gold (CCG)
    c. dye
cationized ferritin
catnep, catnip
    black c.

catnip (*var. of* catnep)
cat's claw
cat's-eye calculus
Cattell T tube
cauda
    c. epididymis
    c. equina
    c. equina lesion
caudal
    c. block
    c. mesonephros
    c. pancreatic artery
    c. pancreatojejunostomy
    c. pole
    c. regression syndrome
    c. traction
caudate
    c. eminence of liver
    c. lobe
    c. lobe of liver
caustic
    c. acid
    c. alkali
    c. colitis
    c. esophagitis
    c. ingestion
    c. stricture
    c. substance
cauterization
    colon c.
cauterize
cautery
    c. bend
    BICAP II c.
    blind c.
    Bovie c.
    endoscopic laser c.
    c. knife
    looped c.
    c. pencil
    snare c.
cava (*pl. of* cavum)
    inferior vena c. (IVC)
    infrahepatic vena c.
    retrohepatic vena c.
    suprahepatic vena c.
    vena c.
caveola
caveolated cell
caveolin-1
Caverject
CaverMap
    C. procedure
    C. surgical device
cavernitis, cavernositis
    fibrous c.
cavernocavernostomy
    Cantwell-Ransley c.

cavernosal
- c. abscess
- c. alpha blockade
- c. alpha blockade technique
- c. artery
- c. nerve
- c. nerve-sparing radical prostatectomy
- c. systolic pressure
- c. vein

cavernosal-venous shunt
cavernositis (*var. of* cavernitis)
cavernosogram
cavernosography
- dynamic infusion cavernosometry and c.

cavernosometry
- dynamic infusion c.
- gravity c.

cavernosorum
- trabeculae corporum c.
- tunica albuginea corporum c.

cavernospongiosum shunt
cavernostomy
cavernosum
- bulb of corpus c.
- fibrotic corpus c.

cavernosum-dorsal vein shunt
Cavernotome
cavernous
- c. artery blood flow
- c. artery blood flow acceleration
- c. artery dilation
- c. artery disease
- c. artery injury
- c. artery occlusion pressure
- c. autonomic nerve dysfunction
- c. fibrosis
- c. hemangioma
- c. nerve
- c. nerve mapping
- c. transformation of portal vein (CTPV)

cavernovenous leakage
CAVH
- chronic active viral hepatitis
- continuous arteriovenous hemofiltration

CAVH-B
- chronic active viral hepatitis type B

CAVHD
- continuous arteriovenous hemodialysis

CAVHDF
- continuous arteriovenous hemodiafiltration

CAVH-NAB
- chronic active viral hepatitis non-A non-B

caviae
- *Aeromonas c.*

Cavilon
- C. diabetes foot care kit
- C. no-sting barrier film

cavitas peritonealis
cavitating tuberculoma
cavitation
- c. bubble
- c. bubble activity
- pulmonary c.

Cavitron ultrasonic surgical aspirator (CUSA)
cavity
- abdominal c.
- abdominopelvic c.
- Cutinova c.
- intraperitoneal c.
- nephrotomic c.
- peritoneal c.
- retroperitoneal c.
- tension-free closure of abdominal c.

cavoatrial shunt
cavography
- synchronous inferior c.
- synchronous superior c.

cavotomy
CAVU
- continuous arteriovenous ultrafiltration

cavum, pl. cava
- c. pelvis
- c. retzii
- c. vesicouterinum

cayetanensis
- *Cyclospora c.*

CBAVD
- congenital bilateral absence of vas deferens

CBC
- complete blood count

C3b, C4b receptor
CBD
- common bile duct
- CBD 2 choledochoscope
- CBD stone

CBDE
- common bile duct exploration

CBDM
- common bile duct microlithiasis

CBDS
- common bile duct stone

C-beta **gene**
CBH
- chronic benign hepatitis

CBI
- continuous bladder irrigation

^{13}**C-bicarbonate breath test**
CBP
- chronic bacterial prostatitis
- copper-binding protein
- CBP test

^{13}C breath test
CBS
    colloidal bismuth subcitrate
CC
      Adalat CC
CCA
    calcium channel antagonist
CCC
    cholangiocellular carcinoma
    chronic calculous cholecystitis
    cylindrical confronting
      cisterna
cccDNA
    covalently closed circular DNA
CC-chemokine receptor 2
CCD
    charge-coupled device
    cortical collecting duct
      CCD endoscope
      CCD perfusion
CCE
    cholesterol crystal embolization
CCFA
    Crohn and Colitis Foundation of
    America
CCG
    cationic colloidal gold
C-cholylglycine breath excretion test
CCIC
    contrast chromoscopy using indigo
    carmine
CCK
    cholecystokinin
CCK-8, CCK-OP
    cholecystokinin octapeptide
      CCK antagonist
CCK-HIDA
    cholecystokinin dimethyl iminodiacetic
    acid scan
CCK-LI
    cholecystokinin-like immunoreactivity
CCKNOW
    Crohn and Colitis Knowledge
      CCKNOW score
CCK-PZ
    cholecystokinin-pancreozymin
CCL-64 cell
CCL-277 colon cancer cell
CCl4-induced cirrhosis
CCNU
    cyclohexylchloroethylnitrosurea
CCP
    chronic calcifying pancreatitis
    colitis cystica profunda
CCPD
    continuous cycling peritoneal
    dialysis
CCT
    cortical collecting tubule

CCUP
    colpocystourethropexy
C&D
    cystoscopy and dilation
CD
    Clostridium difficile
    cluster of differentiation
    collecting duct
    Crohn disease
    cystic duct
      CD activity index
CD3
    cluster of differentiation 3
      CD3 protein
      CD3 T-cell receptor complex
CD3+
    cluster of differentiation 3+
      CD3+ T cell
CD4
    cluster of differentiation 4
      CD4 lymphocyte count
      CD4 molecule
      CD4 phenotype
      CD4 protein
      CD4 T cell
CD4+
    cluster of differentiation 4+
      autologous HBcAg-specific CD4+
      CD4+ cell
      CD4+ T-cell count
CD8
    cluster of differentiation 8
      CD8 lymphocyte
      CD8 lymphocyte count
      CD8 molecule
      CD8 phenotype
      CD8 protein
CD8+
    cluster of differentiation 8+
      CD8+ cell
      CD8+ T lymphocyte
CD14
    cluster of differentiation 14
      CD14 monoclonal antibody
CD20
    cluster of differentiation 20
      B-cell antigen CD20
CD23
    cluster of differentiation 23
      CD23 enterocyte
CD117
    c-kit protooncogene
CDA
    chenodeoxycholic acid
CDAD
    Clostridium difficile-associated
    diarrhea
CDAI
    Crohn Disease Activity Index

CD25 antigen
CD2-associated protein
CDC
Centers for Disease Control and
Prevention
choledochocholedochostomy
Crohn disease of colon
CDCA
chenodeoxycholic acid
CD4+-CD8+ T-cell ratio
CDC42 protein
CDE
common duct exploration
cystine dimethylester
CDEIS
Crohn Disease Endoscopic Index of
Severity
CDJ
choledochojejunostomy
CDK
cyclin-dependent kinase
cDNA
complementary deoxyribonucleic
acid
complementary DNA
HSP-70 cDNA
cDNA probe
CDNF
ciliary-derived neurotrophic factor
CDNF receptor
CDP
computerized dynamic posturography
CD2-positive cell
CD45RO lymphocyte
CD45RO-positive memory T cell
CDS
commercial dialysis solution
CDY
cystoduodenostomy
CE
cardioesophageal
conjugated estrogen
CEA
carcinoembryonic antigen
CEA test
CE-AD gastric lesion staging by
endoscopy
CEA-Scan
CeaVac
CEB
carboplatin, etoposide, bleomycin
ceca (*pl. of* cecum)
cecal
c. appendage
c. appendix
c. barotrauma
c. bascule
c. botryomycosis
c. colonoscopy

c. cystoplasty
c. dilation
c. diverticulitis
c. diverticulum
c. fissure
c. fold
c. gangrene
c. haustrum
c. hernia
c. homogenate
c. imbrication procedure
c. ligation and puncture
(CLP)
c. mucosal nodule
c. necrosis
c. perforation
c. red patch
c. sacculation
c. serosa
c. ulcer
c. vascular ectasia
c. volvulus
cecectomy
Cecil
C. hypospadias repair procedure
C. operation
C. repair
C. urethral stricture syndrome
C. urethroplasty
cecitis
Ceclor
cecocolic intussusception
cecocolon
cecocolopexy
cecocolostomy
cecocystoplasty
cecofixation
cecoileal reflux
cecoileostomy
cecopexy
cecoplication
cecoproctostomy
cecoptosis
cecorrhaphy
cecosigmoidostomy
cecostomy
blowhole c.
Casola c.
Chait percutaneous c.
ileal Malone c.
Malone c.
percutaneous catheter c.
percutaneous endoscopic c.
tube c.
cecotomy
cecoureterocele
cecum, caecum, *pl.* **ceca**
antimesocolic side of c.
coned c.

cecum (*continued*)
    cone-shaped c.
    conical c.
    watermelon c.
Cedax
CEEA
    curved end-to-end anastomosis
    CEEA stapler
CE-EUS
    contrast-enhanced endoscopic
      ultrasonography
cefaclor
cefadroxil monohydrate
Cefadyl
cefamandole
CE-FAST
    contrast-enhanced fast sequence
cefazolin sodium
cefdinir
cefditoren pivoxil
cefepime
cefixime
cefmenoxime
cefmetazole
Cefobid
cefonicid
cefoperazone
ceforanide
Cefotan
cefotaxime
cefotetan disodium
cefotiam
cefoxitin
cefpirome
cefpodoxime proxetil
cefprozil
cefsulodin
ceftazidime
ceftibuten
Ceftin Oral
ceftizoxime
ceftriaxone
    c. pseudolithiasis
    c. sodium
cefuroxime
CEG
    chronic erosive gastritis
CEGA
    cervical esophagogastric anastomosis
C-EGD
    conventional upper
      esophagogastroduodenoscopy
cEGF
    concentration epidermal growth
      factor
CEH
    carboxylic ester hydrolase
CEJ
    cardioesophageal junction

celandine
    greater c.
    lesser c.
Celebrex
Celestin
    C. dilator bougie
    C. endoprosthesis
    C. esophageal tube
    C. graduated dilator
    C. latex rubber tube
    C. prosthesis
Celestone
celiac
    c. angiogram
    c. angiography
    c. arteriography
    c. axis
    c. axis compression
    c. dimple
    c. disease-specific EMA antibody
    c. flux
    c. lymph node
    c. plexus
    c. plexus block
    c. plexus neurolysis (CPN)
    c. plexus reflex
    c. plexus sectioning
    c. rickets
    c. sprue
    c. sprue disease
    c. syndrome
    c. trunk
    c. tumor
celiacography
celiac-superior mesenteric ganglia
celiacus
    truncus c.
celiagra
celiectomy
celiocentesis
celioenterotomy
celiogastrostomy
celiogastrotomy
celiomesenteric arteriography
celiomyalgia
celiomyomotomy
celioparacentesis
celiopathy
celiorrhaphy
celioscope
celiotomy
    exploratory c.
    c. incision
    vaginal c.
    ventral c.
celitis
cell
    absorptive c.
    acid c.

acinar c.
acinic c.
acinous c.
adelomorphous c.
algoid c.
amine precursor uptake and
  decarboxylation c.
c. analysis system
C. Analysis System 200 image
  cytometer
androgen-presenting c.
aneuploid c.
antigen-presenting c. (APC)
antral D, EC c.
antral gastric c.
argentaffin c.
argyrophilic c.
atypical ductular c.
autologous liver c.
ballooning of c.
Barrett esophagus-associated
  adenocarcinoma c.
basal granular c.
beaker c.
bile duct epithelial c.
biliary epithelial c. (BEC)
binucleate renal tubule
  epithelial c.
bladder mast c.
blast c.
bone marrow-derived B c.
bone marrow stem c.
border c.
CaCo2 c.
calciform c.
capillary endothelial c.
caveolated c.
CCL-64 c.
CCL-277 colon cancer c.
CD2-positive c.
CD45RO-positive memory T c.
CD3+ T c.
CD4 T c.
CD4+ c.
CD8+ c.
central c.
centroacinar c.
chalice c.
chief c.
chromaffin c.
chromogranin A immunoreactive c.
COLO 320 colon cancer c.
colonic epithelial c.
columnar-cuboidal adenocarcinoma c.
connective tissue-type mast c.
  (CTMC)
c. count
crypt c.
cultured rat mesangial c.

c. cycle marker
cytotoxic T c.
D c.
Daudi c.
Davidoff c.
delomorphous c.
dendritic reticular c.
diploid c.
DNA haploid c.
donor dendritic c.
Dukes signet c. A, B, C
dysmorphic red blood c.
dysplastic c.
EC c.
ECL c.
effector c.
endocrine c.
endothelial c.
enteric ganglion c.
enterochromaffin c.
enterochromaffin-like c.
enteroendocrine c.
epithelial endocrine c.
eumorphic red blood c.
F9 c.
fat c.
fat-storing liver c.
fatty liver c. (FLC)
fetal liver-derived B c.
flare c.
flattened epithelial
  microfold c.
flexura hepatica c.
foam c.
gastric pacemaker c.
gastrin c.
gastrin-secreting c.
Gaucher c.
germline stem c.
giant c.
GI pacemaker c.
glitter c.
glomerular contractile c.
glomerular epithelial c.
gluconeogenic-competent human
  proximal tubule c.
goblet c.
graft parenchymal c.
grimelius-positive c.
ground-glass c.
GTL-16 gastric carcinoma c.
haploid c.
HBV-specific T c.
Heidenhain c.
HeLa c.
helper T c.
hemopoietic c.
hepatic stellate c. (HSC)
hepG2 c.

cell (*continued*)

HGF-stimulated renal epithelial c.
histamine-producing mast c.
HLF c.
hobnailed c.
HT-29 c.
human cytotoxic T c.
human intestinal epithelial Coco-2 c.
human umbilical vein endothelial c.
  (HUVEC)
hypochromic red c.
IEC-6 c.
IEL T c.
IgA-producing c.
IgG-producing c.
infiltrating inflammatory c.
infiltrating T c.
intercalated c.
interstitial immunocompetent c.
interstitial mononuclear c.
intestinal absorptive c.
intestinal endocrine c.
intestinal epithelial c. (IEC)
intestinal mucosal mast c. (IMMC)
intraglomerular mesangial c.
IPEC-J2 c.
islet c.
Ito c.
JR-St c.
KATO-III c.
killer T c.
Kulchitsky c.
Kupffer c.
L c.
LAK c.
lamina propria lymphoid c.
Langerhans c.
Langhans c.
LE c.
Leydig c.
LIM 2537 c.
c. line
lipid-laden clear c.
littoral c.
liver-deprived epithelial clonic c.
liver sinusoidal endothelial c.
LLC-PK1-FBPase+ c.
LLC-PK renal tubular c.
lymphocyte target c.
lymphokine-activated killer c.
lymphomononuclear c.
M c.
macula densa c.
mast c.
MDCK epithelial c.
c. membrane
c. membrane epithelial antigen
memory T c.
mesangial c. (MC)

mesenchymal c.
mesenchymal stem c.
microfold c.
MN c.
mucous neck c.
mucus-secreting c.
multinucleated giant c.
murine B16 c.
murine lymphoid c.
murine mesangial c. (MMC)
murine proximal tubule c.
myeloid dendritic c.
myenteric ganglion c.
myointimal c.
natural killer c.
c. necrosis
neuroendocrine c.
NKT c.
nonalpha nonbeta pancreatic
  islet c.
nonantigen-expressing target c.
noncleaved B c.
nonrosetted c.
nuclear factor of activated T c.'s
  (NFAT)
nuclear-tagged c.
oat c.
OKT4 c.
OKT8 c.
OLGC c.
osteoclast-like giant c. (OLGC)
oxyntic c.
P c.
pacemaker c.
packed red blood c.'s (PRBC)
pale c.
pancreatic acinar c.
pancreatic islet c.
Paneth c.
PAP-HT25 c.
paracrine c.
parietal c.
peptic c.
percentage of hypochromic red c.'s
  (%HYPO)
peripheral blood mononuclear c.
  (PBMC)
peripheral T c.
perisinusoidal c.
peritoneal mesothelial c.
peritubular myoid c.
phagocytic stellate c.
phenotypes of mast c.'s
Pick c.
pigment-laden Kupffer c.
pit c.
plasma c.
PLC/PRF5 c.
PMN c.

Pockel c.
polymorphonuclear c.
postreceptor signaling of parietal c.
PP-immunoreactive c.
primed c.
principal c.
proliferating tubular c.
c. proliferation
prostate gland stromal c.
proximal tubular c.
ptyocrinous c.
pulpar c.
purified T c.
Q c.
C. Recovery System (CRS)
rectal epithelial c.
red blood c. (RBC)
renal collecting duct c.
renal proximal tubular c.
renal tubule epithelial c.
renocortical tubule c.
renomedullary interstitial c. (RMIC)
S c.
C. Saver
Schwann c.
schwannian spindle c.
secretory c.
semen round c.
seminiferous tubule Sertoli c.
senescent c.
c. separation technique
serotonin c.
Sertoli c.
Sertoli-Leydig c.
signet-ring c.
silver c.
sinusoidal endothelial c. (SEC)
sinusoidal lining c.
small granule c.
C. Soft semen analyzer
C. Soft system
somatostatin c.
spillage of tumor c.'s
spindle c.
spur c.
squamous c.
stellate c.
stem c.
c. substratum
suppressor T c.
c. surface area
c. surface receptor
SW 480 c.
c. swelling
T84 c.
target c.
T effector c.
tetraploid c.
thymus-derived c.

tolerogenic dendritic c.
transblotting c.
transitional c.
triploid c.
Trypan blue-stained c.
tubular epithelial c.
tumor c.
c. type
undifferentiated c.
unit of packed red blood c.'s
  (UPRBC)
upregulation of monocyte
  chemoattractant protein-1 gene
  cytoplasm of c.'s
ureteral muscle c.
urine glitter c.
vascular permeation of tumor c.
vascular smooth muscle c. (VSMC)
villous-tip c.
villus c.
von Hansemann c.
von Kupffer c.
white blood c. (WBC)
xanthoma c.
XL1-blue c.
zymogenic c.

cell-adhesion molecule
cell-cell
  c.-c. adhesion
  c.-c. contact
  c.-c. interaction
CellCept
cell-mediated
  c.-m. arm
  c.-m. cytotoxicity
  c.-m. hepatic injury
  c.-m. immunity
  c.-m. immunohistological response
  c.-m. mechanism
  c.-m. suppression
cell-only
  Sertoli c.-o. (SCO)
cell-positive margin
cell-surface sialylation
Cell-Track
cellular
  c. atypia
  c. differentiation
  c. electrophysiology
  c. enzyme
  c. immune response
  c. immunity
  c. infiltration
  c. peptide
  c. proliferation
  c. tumor suppressor
cellularis
  balanoposthitis chronica circumscripta
    plasma c.

cellule
cellulitis
    candidal c.
    vaginal cuff c.
cellulosae
    Cysticercus c.
cellulose
    c. acetate
    c. acetate high performance (CAHP)
    c. diacetate membrane
    c. phosphate
cellulose-based membrane
celomic epithelium
celoscope
celoscopy
celotomy
Celsius thermometer
cement
    latex-base skin c.
    Torbot c.
    Wacker Sil-Gel 604 silicone c.
CE-M gastric lesion staging by endoscopy
C-EMR
    cutting endoscopic mucosal resection
CE-24 needle
Cenogen-OB capsule
centaury
center
    anospinal c.
    C.'s for Disease Control and Prevention (CDC)
    freestanding ambulatory surgical c.
    organized germinal c.
    pontine micturition c. (PMC)
    rectovesical c.
    swallowing c.
    The CURE Digestive Diseases Research C.
    vomiting c.
centering balloon
centigrade thermometer
centigray (cGy)
centimeter (cm)
    joules per c. (J/cm)
centipoise
central
    c. adrenergic agent
    c. cell
    c. cystocele
    c. echogenicity
    c. hyaline sclerosis
    c. hyperalimentation
    c. necrosis
    c. nervous system (CNS)
    c. spot
    c. vagal nerve stimulation
    c. venous alimentation
    c. venous catheter

    c. venous pressure (CVP)
    c. venous pressure line
centrifugal pump
centrifugation
    density gradient c.
    Ficoll-Hypaque gradient c.
    Polyprep c.
centrifuge
    Ficoll-Hypaque density gradient c.
centrifuged
centrilobular
    c. acidophilic necrosis
    c. cholestasia
    c. pancreatitis
    c. region of liver
centrizonal necrosis
centroacinar cell
Centrysystem 3 hemodialyzer
Century bicarbonate dialysis control unit
Ceo-Two laxative
cephalad traction
cephalexin
cephalin-cholesterol flocculation test
cephalocyst
cephalosporin
    prophylactic c.
    second-generation c.
    third-generation c.
cephalothin
cephalotrigonal technique
cephapirin sodium
cephradine
Cephulac
Ceplene
CERA
    continuous erythropoiesis receptor activator
Ceralas PDT 633 diode laser system
ceramic element
ceramidase deficiency
ceramide lactoside lipidosis
c-ErbB-2/Neu oncoprotein
cercaria
cercaricidal
cerclage
    McDonald c.
    Shirodkar cervical c.
cerebelloretinal hemangioblastomatosis
cerebral
    c. fluid shunt
    c. hemangioblastoma
    c. palsy
    c. perfusion pressure (CPP)
cerebral-brainstem circuit
cerebral-sacral loop
cerebrohepatorenal syndrome (CHRS)
cerebrooculofacial syndrome
cerebrospinal
    c. fluid (CSF)

cerebrotendinous xanthomatosis
cerebrovascular
    c. complication
    c. disease
Cerespan
Ceretec
cereus
    Bacillus c.
    night-blooming c.
cerevisiae
    Saccharomyces c.
Cerezyme
cerivastatin
ceroid-laden macrophage
cerulein
    exogenous cholecystokinin or c.
ceruloplasmin
    serum c.
cerumen obstruction
cervical
    c. carcinoma
    c. discharge
    c. erosion
    c. esophagogastric anastomosis
    (CEGA)
    c. esophagus
    c. friability
    c. gastroesophagostomy
    c. inflammation
    c. intraepithelial neoplasia
    (CIN)
    c. irregularity
    c. lymphadenopathy
    c. motion tenderness
    c. mucus-sperm interaction
    c. neuroblastoma
    c. polyp
    c. position
    c. spasm
    c. ulcer
    c. wart
cervicitis
    mucopurulent c.
    schistosomal c.
cervicocolpitis
cervicovaginitis
CESD
    cholesterol ester storage
    disease
cesium
cesium-137 wire
CE-SM gastric lesion staging by
  endoscopy
C-1 esterase inhibitor
Cestoda **tapeworm**
cestode, cestoid
cestodiasis
cestoid (*var. of* cestode)
Cetacaine topical anesthetic

cetirizine
CETP
    cholesterol ester transfer protein
Cetuximab
cetyldimethylethyl ammonium
  bromide
Ceylon sore mouth
CF
    cystic fibrosis
    CF epithelium
CF-HM
    CF-HM endoscope
    CF-HM fiberscope
    CF-HM magnifying colonoscope
CF-LB3R colonoscope
C-Flex
    C-F. Amsterdam stent
    C-F. ureteral stent
c-fos
    c-f. induction
    c-f. protooncogene
CFTR
    cystic fibrosis transmembrane
    conductance regulator
    CFTR gene analysis
CFU
    colony-forming unit
CF-UHM colonoscope
CF-UM3 echocolonoscope
CG
    chronic glomerulonephritis
[14]C-glycocholate breath test
C-glycocholic acid breath test
CGM
    coffee-grounds material
cGMP
    5′-cyclic guanosine monophosphate
cGMP-mediated relaxant
CGN
    chronic glomerulonephritis
7C Gold urine test
CGRP
    calcitonin gene-related peptide
c-GVHD
    chronic graft-versus-host disease
CGY
    cystogastrostomy
cGy
    centigray
    cGy radiation measure
CH
    chronic hepatitis
CHA
    common hepatic artery
CH-40 activated charcoal
chaffeensis
    Ehrlichia c.
Chaffin-Pratt drain
Chagas-Cruz disease

Chagas disease
chagasi
    Leishmania donovani c.
chagasic megaesophagus
chain
    alpha-3, -4, -5 c.
    beta c.
    beta-1 c.
    c. cystogram
    c. cystourethrography
    food c.
    gamma light c.
    J c.
    kappa light c.
    monoclonal light c.
    obturator lymphatic c.
    c. suture
    sympathetic c.
chain-of-lakes
    c.-o.-l. deformity
    c.-o.-l. filling defect
    c.-o.-l. sign
chain-terminating inhibitor
chair
    Hausted all-purpose c.
    VESS c.
Chait
    C. percutaneous cecostomy
    C. Trapdoor cecostomy catheter
chalasia, chalasis
chalasis (*var. of* chalasia)
chalaza (*var. of* chalazion)
chalazia (*pl. of* chalazion)
chalazion, chalaza, *pl.* **chalazia**
chalice cell
challenge
    c. diet
    fluid c.
    food c.
    gluten c.
    jejunal gluten c.
    rectal gluten c.
    solid bolus c.
challenging patient population
chamaedrys
    Teucrium c.
chamber
    antropyloroduodenal common c.
     (APDCC)
    deglutitive pharyngeal c.
    hyperbaric oxygen c.
    Makler counting c.
    Microcell c.
    10Pa Amicon c.
    Sigma 34 monoplace
     hyperbaric c.
    Ussing c.
chamomile
    German c.

chancre
    hunterian c.
    Nisbet c.
chancroid
chancroidal bubo
chancrous
change
    blood pressure c.
    degenerative c.
    ductal c.
    enzyme c.
    erosive prepyloric c.
    fibrocystic c.
    fractional weight c.
    large-cell c. (LCC)
    mesangiolytic c.
    mesenchymal c.
    morphologic c.
    morphological c.
    obstructive c.
    orthostatic c.
    pancreatic ductal morphological c.
    phlegmonous c.
    polyneuropathy, organomegaly,
     endocrinopathy, monoclonal protein,
     and skin c.'s (POEMS)
    postsurgical c.
    segmental c.
    sensorium c.
    spatial c.
    trophic c.
    ultrastructural basket-weave c.
channel
    aquaporin water c.
    biopsy c.
    calcium c. (CC)
    calcium-activated potassium c.
    chloride c.
    common c.
    detrusor muscle potassium c.
    epithelial sodium c. (ENaC)
    gastric c.
    ion c.
    ligand-gated c.
    lymph c.
    lymphatic c.
    Malone antegrade continence enema
     c.
    Mitrofanoff catheterizable c.
    pancreatic duct-choledochus c.
    pancreaticobiliary common c.
    potassium c.
    preputial transverse island flap and
     glans c.
    pyloric c.
    Sonotrode c.
    stomalike c.
    stretch-sensitive ion c.
    suction c.

tetrodotoxin-insensitive sodium c.
thin-walled vascular c.
treatment c.
urea c.
voltage-dependent anion c.
voltage-gated c.
water c.
2-channel endoscope
8-channel cross-sectional anal sphincter probe
channelopathy
intestinal c.
sodium c.
chaparral leaf
chaperone
retinoid c.
characteristic
anatomic c.
client-patient c.
performance c.
receiver operating c. (ROC)
characterization
biochemical c.
***c*-Ha-ras gene**
CharcoAid
charcoal
activated c. (AC)
CH-40 activated c.
c. filter
c. hemoperfusion
hemoperfusion with c.
mitomycin adsorbed onto activated c. (M-CH)
C. Plus
c. suspension
CharcoCaps
Charcodote
Aqueous C.
Charcot
C. cirrhosis
C. intermittent fever
C. triad
C. triangle
Charcot-Boettcher crystals and filaments
Chardonna-2
CHARGE
coloboma, heart disease, atresia choanae, retarded growth, genital hypoplasia, and ear abnormalities CHARGE syndrome
charge
urine net c. (UNC)
charge-coupled
c.-c. device (CCD)
c.-c. device endoscope
c.-c. device monochrome camera
Chariker-Jeter wound sealing kit
CHARM trial
Charrière catheter size scale

chasteberry
chaste tree
ChAT
choline acetyltransferase
Chatillon
C. Digital Force gauge
C. dolorimeter
Chauffard point
Chauveau bacterium
Cheatle
C. salt
C. slit
Cheatle-Henry
C.-H. hernia
C.-H. incision
check
Comfort Bath with I-See-Red skin c.
checklist
Hopkins symptom c.
Checklist-90R
Symptom C.-90r
Cheek-Perry syndrome
cheesy
c. necrosis
c. nephritis
Cheetah radiopaque contrast medium
cheilitis, chilitis
granulomatous c.
cheilosis, chilosis
chelate
gadolinium c.
neutral gadolinium c.
chelator
aroylhydrazone c.
Chelidonium majus
Chelsea-Eaton anal speculum
Chemet
chemical
c. anoxia
c. carcinogenesis
c. cholecystitis
c. cystitis
cystogenic c.
c. gastritis
c. gastropathy
c. litholysis
c. peritonitis
c. prostatitis
c. splanchnicectomy
c. urinalysis
chemical-induced esophagitis
chemically defined diet
chemiluminescence, chemoluminescence
enhanced c. (ECL)
luminol-enhanced c.
chemiotaxis (*var. of* chemotaxis)
chemise
bouton en c.

C

chemistry
> phosphoramidite c.

chemo
> chemotherapy

chemoattractant
chemoceptor (*var. of* chemoreceptor)
chemodissolution
chemoembolization
> transarterial c. (TACE)
> transcatheter arterial c. (TACE)

chemoimmunotherapy
chemokine-orchestrated chemotaxis
chemokine receptor
chemoluminescence (*var. of* chemiluminescence)
chemolysis
> intrarenal c.

Chemo-Port catheter
chemoprophylaxis
> long-term low-dose maintenance c.
> traveler's c.

chemoradiation
> neoadjuvant c.
> c. therapy (CRT)

chemoradiotherapy
chemoreceptor, chemoceptor
chemosensitivity
chemosis
chemotactic
> c. factor
> c. peptide

chemotaxis, chemiotaxis
> chemokine-orchestrated c.
> negative c.
> c. of polymorphonuclear leukocyte
> positive c.

chemotherapeutic
> c. agent
> c. agent hepatotoxicity

chemotherapy (chemo)
> adjuvant hepatic arterial infusion c.
> antisarcoma c.
> antiviral c.
> continuous infusion c.
> cytotoxic c.
> c. gonadotoxicity
> hepatic arterial infusion c.
> high-dose c. (HDC)
> intraarterial c.
> intraperitoneal hyperthermic c. (IPHC)
> intrathecal c.
> intravesical c.
> IP c.
> neoadjuvant c.
> c. of primary tumor
> platinum-based consolidation c.
> polyantibiotic c.
> response rate to c.

chemotherapy-induced
> c.-i. nausea
> c.-i. nausea and emesis (CINE)
> c.-i. sterility
> c.-i. vomiting

Chemstrip
> C. bG reagent
> C. LN dipstick

ChemTrak
> C. AccuMeter
> C. AccuMeter screen

Chenix Tablet
chenodeoxycholate
chenodeoxycholic acid (CDA, CDCA)
chenodiol
Cherchevski disease
Cherney incision
cherry
> c. angioma
> c. red spot (CRS)
> c. sponge
> wild c.

Cherry-Crandall method for testing serum lipase
chest
> barrel c.
> flail c.
> c. pain
> c. physiotherapy
> c. tube
> c. tube scar

Chester-Winter urinary stress incontinence repair procedure
chestnut
> Spanish c.

Chevalier
> C. Jackson esophagoscope
> C. Jackson gastroscope

chevron incision
chew-and-spit test
chewing gum diarrhea
CHF
> congenital hepatic fibrosis

CHG
> chlorhexidine gluconate
> CHG Maxi Swabstick

CHI
> creatinine height index

Chiari
> C. disease
> C. malformation

chiasm, chiasma, *pl.* **chiasmata**
> Camper c.

chiasma (*var. of* chiasm)
chiasmata (*pl. of* chiasm)
Chiba
> C. needle
> C. percutaneous cholangiogram

Chibroxin

chicory
chief cell
Chilaiditi
    C. sign
    C. syndrome
child, *pl.* children
    C. class A–C
    C. class A–C patient
    C. classification of hepatic risk
      criteria A–C
    cystinuric c.
    C. esophageal varix classification
    C. hepatic dysfunction classification
    C. intestinal forceps
    C. liver criteria
    C. liver disease classification
    C. operation
    C. pancreatoduodenostomy
childhood
    extraordinary urinary frequency
      syndrome of c.
    papular acrodermatitis of c.
    c. rhabdomyosarcoma
    urolithiasis in c.
    c. visceral myopathy (CVM)
Child-Pugh
    C.-P. class A–C
    C.-P. criteria
    C.-P. liver disease classification
    C.-P. score
children (*pl. of* child)
children's
    c. coma scale
    c. esophagoscope
    C. Hospital intestinal forceps
Childs-Phillips
    C.-P. bowel plication
    C.-P. intestinal plication needle
Child-Turcotte classification (CTC)
Child-Turcotte-Pugh (CTP)
    C.-T.-P. classification
chili-bean pseudopolyp
chilitis (*var. of* cheilitis)
Chilomastix mesnili
chilosis (*var. of* cheilosis)
chimney
    Roux-Y c.
China ink
Chinese
    C. cinnamon
    C. restaurant syndrome (CRS)
chip
    prostatic c.
chiretta
ChiRhoStim
Chiron
    C. RIBA HCV test
    C. RIBA HCV test system second
      generation

chiufa
chlamydia
    C. psittaci
    C. trachomatis
    C. trachomatis infection
    c. urethritis
chloracetic
chloral hydrate
chlorambucil
chloramphenicol
Chlorascrub
chlordiazepoxide
chlorhexidine gluconate (CHG)
chlorhydria
chloride
    adrenalin c.
    ambenonium c.
    c. balance
    benzalkonium c. (BAC)
    benzethonium chloride 0.025%
    benzyl c.
    bethanechol c.
    calcium c.
    c. channel
    choline c.
    c. concentration
    CYT-356 radiolabeled with 111
      indium c.
    c. electrolyte
    endrophonium c.
    mercury c. (HgCl2)
    mivacurium c.
    oxybutynin c.
    polyvinyl c. (PVC)
    potassium c. (KCl)
    c. secretion
    serum c.
    c. shunt
    sodium c.
    strontium-89 c.
    tetramethyl ammonium c. (TEMAC)
    titanous c.
    tridihexethyl c.
    urinary c.
chloride-cation cotransporter (CCC)
chloride-to-phosphate ratio
chloridorrhea
    familial c.
chlorisondamine
chlormadinone acetate
chloroazotemic nephritis
chlorodontia
chloroform toxicity
chlorohydrate
    linsidomine c.
chloroma
    gastric c.
Chloromycetin
chloroplast

C

chloroprocaine
chloroquine-induced damage
chloroquine phosphate
chlorothiazide
chlorotrianisene
chlorozotocin
chlorpheniramine
chlorphenoxamine
chlorpromazine
chlorpromazine-induced cholestasia
chlorprothixene
chlorthalidone
chlorzoxazone toxicity
choana, *pl.* choanae
choanae (*pl. of* choana)
chocolate
    c. agar medium
    c. vine
CHOD-PAP
    cholesterol oxidase phenol
    4-aminoantipyrine peroxidase
    CHOD-PAP cholesterol reagent
Cho/Dyonics 2-portal endoscope
choice
    Medi-Jector C.
Choice2 test
choking
Cholac
cholagogic (*var. of* cholagogue)
cholagogue, cholagogic
cholaneresis
cholangeitis (*var. of* cholangitis)
cholangiectasis
cholangioadenoma
cholangiocarcinoma
    hilar c.
    Klatskin c.
    metastatic c.
    perihilar c.
    peripheral c. (PCC)
    peripheral intrahepatic c.
    type III c.
Cholangiocath catheter
cholangiocatheter
    cystic duct c.
    saline-filled c.
cholangiocellular carcinoma (CCC)
cholangiocholecystocholedochectomy
cholangiodrainage
    endosonography-guided c.
    EUS-guided c.
    percutaneous transhepatic c.
    (PTCD)
cholangiodysplastic pseudocirrhosis
cholangioenterostomy
    intrahepatic c.
cholangiofibroma
cholangiofibromatosis
cholangiogastrostomy

cholangiogram (CAG)
    balloon c.
    catheter c.
    Chiba percutaneous c.
    common duct c.
    contrast selective c.
    cystic duct c.
    endoscopic retrograde c.
    fine-needle percutaneous c.
    fine-needle transhepatic c. (FNTC,
      FNTHC)
    intraoperative c. (IOC)
    intravenous c. (IVC)
    occlusion c.
    operative c.
    percutaneous transhepatic c. (PTC,
      PTHC)
    pernasal c.
    retrograde c.
    serial c.'s
    thin-needle percutaneous c.
    transgastric c.
    transhepatic c. (THC)
    T-tube c. (TTC)
cholangiographic
    c. catheter
    c. finding
cholangiography (CAG)
    balloon occlusion c.
    breath-hold MR c.
    cystic duct c.
    delayed operative c.
    direct percutaneous transhepatic c.
    drip infusion c. (DIC)
    endoscopic retrograde c. (ERC)
    fine-needle transhepatic c. (FNTC)
    intraoperative c. (IOC)
    intravenous c. (IVC)
    magnetic resonance c. (MRC)
    nasobiliary drain c.
    nonbreath-hold MR c.
    operative c.
    percutaneous hepatobiliary c.
    percutaneous transhepatic c. (PTC,
      PTHC)
    postoperative c.
    retrograde c.
    transabdominal c.
    transhepatic c. (TC, THC)
    T-tube c.
cholangiograsper
    Storz c.
cholangiohepatitis
    Oriental c.
    recurrent pyogenic c. (RPC)
cholangiohepatoma
cholangiojejunostomy
    intrahepatic c.
cholangiolar

cholangiole
cholangiolitic
   c. cirrhosis
   c. hepatitis
cholangiolitis
cholangioma
cholangiopancreatography
   endoscopic retrograde c. (ERCP)
   endoscopic ultrasound retrograde c.
   magnetic resonance c. (MRCP)
cholangiopancreatoscopy
   peroral c. (PCPS)
cholangiopathy
   destructive c.
   eosinophilic c.
   Epstein-Barr virus-associated c.
cholangiophytiasis
cholangioscope
   Olympus c.
   prototype c.
cholangioscopic forceps biopsy
cholangioscopy
   intraductal c.
   percutaneous transhepatic c. (PTCS)
   peroral c. (PCS)
cholangiostomy
cholangiotomy
cholangiovenous
   c. communication
   c. reflux
cholangitic
   c. abscess
   c. biliary cirrhosis
cholangitis, cholangeitis
   acute obstructive suppurative c.
    (AOSC)
   acute suppurative c. (ASC)
   ascending c.
   autoimmune c.
   bacterial c.
   biliary c.
   c. carcinoma
   catarrhal c.
   chronic nonsuppurative destructive c.
   destructive c.
   fibrous obliterative c.
   granulomatous c.
   idiopathic autoimmune c.
   intrahepatic sclerosing c.
   c. lenta
   lymphoid c.
   nonsuppurative destructive c.
   obstructive c.
   pleomorphic destructive c.
   postendoscopic c.
   posttransplantation c.
   primary sclerosing c. (PSC)
   progressive suppurative c.
   pyogenic c.

   rejection c.
   sclerosing c.
   secondary sclerosing c.
   septic c.
   small-duct primary sclerosing c.
   suppurative c.
   transient c.
   viral c.
cholanopoiesis
cholanopoietic
cholascos
cholate
cholebilirubin
Cholebrine contrast medium
cholechromopoiesis
cholecyanin
cholecystagogic
cholecystagogue
cholecystalgia
cholecystatony
cholecystectasia
cholecystectomy
   endoscopic laser c.
   laparoscopic c.
   laparoscopic laser c. (LLC)
   minilaparoscope c.
   prophylactic c.
   c. treatment
   3-trocar technique for laparoscopic c.
cholecystendysis
cholecystenteric fistula
cholecystenteroanastomosis
cholecystenterostomy
cholecystenterotomy
cholecystic
cholecystis
cholecystitis
   acalculous c.
   acute c. (AC)
   acute acalculous c.
   calculous c.
   chemical c.
   chronic calculous c. (CCC)
   c. cystica
   c. emphysematosa
   emphysematous c.
   erythromycin-induced c.
   follicular c.
   gangrenous c.
   gaseous c.
   c. glandularis proliferans
   perforated c.
   c. with cholelithiasis
   xanthogranulomatous c.
cholecystobiliary fistula
cholecystocele
cholecystocholangiography
cholecystocholedochal fistula
cholecystocholedocholithiasis

C

cholecystocolonic fistula
cholecystocolostomy
cholecystocolotomy
cholecystoduodenal
    c. band
    c. fistula
    c. ligament
cholecystoduodenocolic
    c. fistula
    c. fold
cholecystoduodenostomy
cholecystoendoprosthesis
    endoscopic retrograde c. (ERCCE)
cholecystoenterostomy
cholecystoenterotomy
cholecystogastric
cholecystogastrostomy
cholecystogram
    oral c. (OCG)
cholecystography
    drip infusion c.
    intravenous c.
    oral c.
    post-fatty meal c.
cholecystoileostomy
cholecystointestinal
cholecystojejunostomy
cholecystokinetic food
cholecystokinin (CCK)
    c. antagonist
    c. cholescintigraphy
    c. dimethyl iminodiacetic acid scan (CCK-HIDA)
    c. octapeptide (CCK-8, CCK-OP)
    c. test
cholecystokinin-like immunoreactivity (CCK-LI)
cholecystokinin-pancreozymin (CCK-PZ)
cholecystolithiasis
cholecystolithotomy
    percutaneous c. (PCCL)
    percutaneous transhepatic c. (PCTCL)
cholecystolithotripsy
cholecystomy (var. of cholecystotomy)
cholecystonephrostomy
cholecystoparesis
    diabetic c.
cholecystopathy
cholecystopexy
cholecystoptosis
cholecystopyelostomy
cholecystorrhaphy
cholecystoscopy
    percutaneous transhepatic c. (PTCC)
cholecystosis
    hyperplastic c.

cholecystostomy
    laparoscopy-guided subhepatic c.
    percutaneous transhepatic c.
cholecystotomy, cholecystomy
    transpapillary endoscopic c. (TEC)
choledochal
    c. basal pressure
    c. cyst grades I, II, III, IV, IVa
    c. region
    c. sphincter
    c. sphincterotomy
choledochectomy
choledochendysis
choledochiarctia
choledochitis
choledochocele
choledochocholedochostomy (CDC)
choledochocolonic fistula
choledochocyst
choledochocystostomy
choledochodochorrhaphy
choledochoduodenal
    c. area
    c. fistula
    c. fistulotomy
    c. junction
    c. junctional stenosis
choledochoduodenostomy
choledochoenteric fistula
choledochoenterostomy
choledochofiberoscopy
    T-tube tract c.
choledochofiberscope
    Olympus translaparoscopic c.
choledochofiberscopic approach
choledochogram
choledochography
choledochohepatostomy
choledochoileostomy
choledochojejunostomy (CDJ)
    end-to-side c.
    loop c.
    retrocolic end-to-side c.
    Roux-en-Y c.
choledocholith
choledocholithiasis
    Glasgow classification of c.
    rendezvous technique for treatment of c.
choledocholithotomy
choledocholithotripsy
choledochopancreatic ductal junction
choledochoplasty
choledochorrhaphy
choledochoscope
    Berci-Shore c.
    CBD 2 c.
    flexible fiberoptic c.

Hopkins rod-lens system for
rigid c.
Machida c.
Olympus c.
choledochoscopic guidance
choledochoscopy
Berci-Shore c.
cystic duct c.
jejunostomy tract c.
operative c.
percutaneous c.
postoperative c.
T-tube tract c.
choledochostomy
choledochotomy
c. incision
longitudinal c.
choledochus
ductus c.
choleglobin
cholehepatic shunt pathway
choleic (*var. of* cholic)
cholelith, chololith
cholelithiasis, chololithiasis
cholecystitis with c.
cholesterol c.
intrahepatic c.
c. prevalence
cholelithic dyspepsia
cholelitholysis
cholelithoptysis
cholelithotomy
cholelithotripsy, cholelithotrity
cholelithotrity (*var. of*
cholelithotripsy)
cholemesis
cholemia
familial c.
Gilbert c.
cholemic nephrosis
cholepathia spastica
choleperitoneum
choleperitonitis
cholepoiesis, cholopoiesis
cholepoietic
choleprasin
cholera
Asiatic c.
bilious c.
c. infantum
c. morbus
c. nostras
pancreatic c.
c. sicca
summer c.
c. toxin
c. toxin-induced diarrhea
Vibrio c. O1
Vibrio c. O139

cholerae
Vibrio c.
choleraesuis
Salmonella c.
choleraic diarrhea
choleresis
choleretic
c. effect
c. enteropathy
cholerheic
choleriform, choleroid
c. enteritis
cholerigenic, cholerigenous
cholerigenous (*var. of* cholerigenic)
cholerine
choleroid (*var. of* choleriform)
cholerrhagia
cholerrhagic
cholescintigram
cholescintigraphy
cholecystokinin c.
hepatobiliary c.
morphine c.
radionuclide c.
Cholestagel
cholestasia, cholestasis
acute drug-induced c.
benign postoperative c.
benign recurrent intrahepatic c.
(BRIC)
bile ductular c.
Bland c.
canalicular c.
centrilobular c.
chlorpromazine-induced c.
contraceptive pill-induced c.
drug-induced c.
estrogen-induced c.
extrahepatic c.
familial c.
hepatocanalicular c.
hepatocellular c.
high-grade c.
intrahepatic c.
methyltestosterone-induced c.
neonatal c.
Norwegian c.
c. patient
pericentral c.
progressive familial intrahepatic c.
(PFIC)
pure c.
recurrent c.
tolbutamide-induced c.
cholestasis (*var. of* cholestasia)
c. of pregnancy
cholestatic
c. hepatosis icterus gravidarum
c. hypersensitivity

C

cholestatic (*continued*)
    c. jaundice
    c. liver disease
    c. reaction
    c. syndrome
    c. viral hepatitis
cholesteatoma
cholesterinosis (*var. of* cholesterolosis)
cholesterol
    c. calculus
    c. cholelithiasis
    c. crystal embolization (CCE)
    dietary c.
    c. embolism
    c. embolus
    c. embolus syndrome
    c. ester
    c. ester storage disease (CESD)
    c. ester transfer protein (CETP)
    high-density lipoprotein c. (HDLC)
    low-density lipoprotein c. (LDLC, LDL-C)
    c. monohydrate crystal
    c. oxidase phenol 4-aminoantipyrine peroxidase (CHOD-PAP)
    c. polyp
    radioactive c.
    c. saturation index (CSI)
    seminal plasma c.
    serum c.
    c. solitaire
    c. stone
    very low density lipoprotein c.
    VLDL c.
cholesterol-cholesteroloxidase-phenol 4-aminophenazone method
cholesterol-containing gallstone
cholesterolosis, cholesterinosis
cholesteryl ester
cholestyramine
    C. Light
    c. therapy
Choletec
choletelin
choletherapy
choleverdin
cholic, choleic
    c. acid (CA)
    c. acid clearance
cholicele
choline
    c. acetyltransferase (ChAT)
    c. chloride
    c. deficiency liver disease
    seminal plasma c.
cholinergic
    c. agonist
    c. innervation

    c. neuron
    c. receptor
    c. syndrome
cholochrome
chologenetic
Cholografin contrast medium
chololith (*var. of* cholelith)
chololithiasis (*var. of* cholelithiasis)
cholopoiesis (*var. of* cholepoiesis)
cholorrhea
choloscopy
Cholybar
cholyl-^{14}C-glycine
chondrocyte
    autologous c.
chondrocyte-alginate gel
chondrodysplasia
    Jansen-type metaphysial c.
Chondrogel
chondrogenic differentiation
chondroitin
chondroitinuria
chondrosarcoma
    bladder c.
Chooz
chorda, *pl.* **chordae**
    c. gubernaculum
    c. penis
    c. spermatica
chordae (*pl. of* chorda)
chordee
    acquired c.
    congenital c.
    c. correction
    fibrous c.
    lateral c.
    residual c.
choreoathetosis
chorioadenoma destruens
choriocarcinoma
    bladder c.
chorioepithelioma
chorionic
chorista
choristoma
choroid plexus cyst (CPC)
Christie gallbladder retractor
Christmas
    C. tree appearance of pancreas
    C. tree sign
Christopher-Williams overtube
chromaffin
    c. cell
    c. tissue
chromaffinoma
chromatofocusing pH range
chromatograph
    Carle analytic gas c.
    QuinTron MicroLyzer 12 c.

chromatography
　column c.
　denaturing high-performance liquid
　　c. (dHPLC)
　gas c.
　gel filtration c.
　high-performance liquid c. (HPLC)
　high-pressure liquid c. (HPLC)
　ion c.
　solid-phase extraction c.
　stool c.
　thin-layer c. (TLC)
　Varian gas c.
chromatopectic, chromopectic,
　chromopexic
chromatopexis, chromopexis
chromic
　c. catgut
　c. catgut suture
　c. gut suture
chromium
　c. deficiency
　c. sesquioxide
51-chromium-labeled
　ethylenediaminetetraacetate (^{51}Cr-EDTA)
chromocystoscopy
chromoendoscope
chromoendoscopy
　acetic acid c.
　crystal violet c.
　high-resolution c.
　Lugol dye spray c.
　magnification c.
　methylene blue c.
　phenol red c.
chromogen
chromogranin
　c. A immunoreactive cell
　serum c. A
　c. stain
chromopectic, chromatopectic,
　chromopexic
chromopexic (*var. of* chromatopectic,
　chromopectic)
chromopexis (*var. of* chromatopexis)
chromophobe
　c. adenoma
　c. cell tumor
chromophobic
chromophore-enhanced laser
　welding
chromoscopy
　gastric c.
chromosomal
　c. abnormality
　c. marker
chromosome
　c. deletion
　human c. 6

　c. insertion
　c. instability
　c. inversion
　c. karyotype
　marker c.
　c. marker
　c. morphology
　Philadelphia c.
　phosphatase and tensin homologue
　　deleted on c. 10
　c. ploidy
　X, Y c.
chromoureteroscopy
chronic
　c. abacterial prostatitis
　c. active gastritis
　c. active hepatitis (CAH)
　c. active liver disease (CALD)
　c. active pouchitis
　c. active viral hepatitis (CAVH)
　c. active viral hepatitis non-A
　　non-B (CAVH-NAB)
　c. active viral hepatitis type B
　　(CAVH-B)
　c. aggressive hepatitis (CAH)
　c. alcoholic cirrhosis
　c. alcoholic pancreatitis (CAP)
　c. alcohol-induced pancreatitis
　c. allograft nephropathy (CAN)
　c. allograft rejection
　c. ambulatory peritoneal dialysis
　　(CAPD)
　c. anoplasty treatment
　c. appendicitis
　c. atrophic duodenitis
　c. atrophic gastritis (CAG)
　c. autoimmune hepatitis
　c. bacterial enteropathy
　c. bacterial prostatitis (CBP)
　c. bacterial pyelonephritis
　c. benign hepatitis (CBH)
　c. calcifying pancreatitis (CCP)
　c. calculous cholecystitis (CCC)
　c. cholestatic liver disease
　c. cicatrizing enteritis
　c. cystic gastritis
　c. diarrhea
　c. diverticulitis
　c. erosion
　c. erosive gastritis (CEG)
　c. fibrosing hepatitis
　c. fibrosing pancreatitis
　c. follicular gastritis
　c. functional constipation
　c. functional gastrointestinal
　　symptom
　c. functional symptomatology
　c. gastrointestinal blood loss
　c. GI blood loss

chronic (*continued*)
  c. glomerular disease
  c. glomerulonephritis (CG, CGN)
  c. graft dysfunction
  c. graft-versus-host disease (c-GVHD)
  c. granulomatous disease
  c. hepatitis (CH)
  c. hepatitis A, B, C, D, E, F
  c. hypokalemic nephropathy
  c. idiopathic constipation
  c. idiopathic intestinal pseudoobstruction (CIIP)
  c. idiopathic jaundice
  c. inflammatory bowel disease (CIBD)
  c. inflammatory cell infiltrate
  c. interstitial gastritis
  c. interstitial hepatitis
  c. intestinal atony
  c. intestinal dysmotility (CID)
  c. intestinal ischemic syndrome
  c. intestinal pseudoobstruction (CIP, CIPO)
  c. intestinal pseudoobstruction syndrome
  c. intravenous supplementation
  c. ischemic colonic lesion caused by phlebosclerosis (CICLP)
  c. lead poisoning
  c. liver disease (CLD)
  C. Liver Disease Questionnaire (CLDQ)
  c. lobular hepatitis (CLH)
  c. low-frequency electrical stimulation
  c. membranous glomerulonephritis (CMGN)
  c. mercury poisoning
  c. metabolic acidosis (CMA)
  c. nonbacterial prostatitis (CNP)
  c. nonimmune gastritis
  c. nonsuppurative destructive cholangitis (CNDC)
  c. obstructive uropathy
  c. pancreatitis (CP)
  c. pancreatitis of Kasugai
  c. parenchymal liver disease
  c. pelvic pain syndrome (CPPS)
  c. peptic esophagitis
  c. periesophagitis
  c. persistent hepatitis (CPH)
  c. persistent hepatitis-chronic active hepatitis (CPH-CAH)
  c. progressive hepatitis
  c. progressive tubulointerstitial disease
  c. prostate pain syndrome (CPPS)
  c. prostatitis-like symptom
  c. prostatitis/pelvic pain syndrome
  c. pyelonephritis (CP, CPN)
  c. radiation-induced proctopathy
  c. radiation proctitis
  c. regurgitation
  c. rejection after renal transplantation
  c. relapsing pancreatitis (CRP)
  c. renal failure (CRF)
  c. renal failure glomerulonephritis
  c. renal insufficiency (CRI)
  c. sacral neuromodulation
  c. sacrospinal nerve stimulation
  c. sclerosing hyaline fibrosis
  c. superficial gastritis (CSG)
  c. transplant rejection
  c. tubular damage
  c. type B hepatitis
  c. ulcer
  c. ulcerative colitis (CUC)
  c. ulcerative proctitis
  c. urate nephropathy
  c. urethral syndrome
  c. urinary retention (CUR)
  c. viral hepatitis

chronica
  enteritis cystica c.
  gastrorrhea continua c.
  ileocolitis ulcerosa c.

chronically inflamed gallbladder

chronic-continuous type

chronicus
  lichen simplex c.

chronobiological parameter

chronotropism

Chronulac

ChronVac DNA vaccine

CHRP
  coagulation and hemostatic resection of prostate

CHRS
  cerebrohepatorenal syndrome

CHUK
  conserved helix-loop-helix ubiquitous kinase

Church deep surgery scissors

Chwalla membrane

chylangioma

chylaqueous

chylectasia

chyle cyst

chyli
  cisterna c.
  receptaculum c.

chylifaction

chylifactive

chyliferous vessel

chylification

chyliform ascites

chylocele
    parasitic c.
chyloderma
chylomediastinum
chylomicron
    c. core
    c. production
    c. retention disease
    c. secretion
chyloperitoneum
chylophoric
chylopoiesis
chylopoietic disease
chylorrhea
chylosa
    diarrhea c.
chylosis
chylosus
    ascites c.
chylothorax
chylous
    c. ascites
    c. ascitic fluid
    c. fistula
    c. leukemia
    c. peritonitis
    c. urine
chyluria
chyme, chymus
    c. discharge
    c. transport
Chymex
chymification
chymobilia
    iatrogenic c.
chymopoiesis
chymorrhea
chymotrypsin
chymus (*var. of* chyme)
CIA
    congenital intestinal
    aganglionosis
Cialis
Ciba-Corning ACS PSA assay
cibalis
    fistula c.
CIBD
    chronic inflammatory bowel
    disease
cibenzoline
cibi
    fastidium c.
CIC
    clean intermittent catheterization
cicatrices (*pl. of* cicatrix)
cicatricial
    c. obliteration
    c. stricture
    c. tissue

cicatrix, *pl.* **cicatrices**
cicatrization
CICLP
    chronic ischemic colonic lesion caused
    by phlebosclerosis
CID
    chronic intestinal dysmotility
Cidecin
Cidex
    C. activated dialdehyde solution
    C. Plus solution
cidofovir
cIEL
    crypt intraepithelial lymphocyte
CIFN
    consensus interferon
    CIFN therapy
cigarette drain
cigar-shaped hyperchromatic nucleus
ciguatera fish poisoning
C-III
    Testred C-III
CIIP
    chronic idiopathic intestinal
    pseudoobstruction
cilastin
ciliary-derived neurotrophic factor (CDNF)
ciliary dysentery
ciliated foregut cyst
ciliate dysentery
Cillium
CIM
    cardia intestinal metaplasia
    cimetidine
cimetidine (CIM)
Cimicifuga heracleifolia
Cimzia
CIN
    cervical intraepithelial neoplasia
cinacalcet
cinaedi
    Campylobacter c.
    Helicobacter c.
CINE
    chemotherapy-induced nausea and
    emesis
cinedefecogram
cinedefecography
cine-esophagogram
cine-esophagoscope
cine-esophagoscopy
cinefluorographic study
cinefluorography
cinefluoroscopic method
cinegastroscopy
cineloop memory function
cineradiographic analysis

cineurography
cinnamic acid
cinnamon
    Chinese c.
Cinobac Pulvules
cinoxacin
cinquefoil
CIP, CIPO
    chronic intestinal pseudoobstruction
ciprofloxacin hydrochloride
Cipro XR
circadian
    c. gastric acidity
    c. periodicity
    c. rhythm
    c. rhythmicity
    c. testosterone pattern
circadian-shaped infusion
Circe device
circinata
    balanitis c.
circinate balanitis
circle
    C. C hemodialysis catheter
    F c.
    c. needle
    c. of death
    Pagenstecher c.
Circon-ACMI
    C.-A. lithotriptor
    C.-A. MicroDigital-I camera
    C.-A. miniscope
    C.-A. MR-6, MR-9 ureteroscope
    C.-A. rigid device
circuit
    cerebral-brainstem c.
    enteric neuronal c.
    enteric secretomotor c.
    extracorporeal cardiopulmonary c.
circuitous
circular
    c. anal dilator
    c. dichroism
    c. folds of Kerckring
    c. muscle
    c. muscle fiber
    c. myotomy
    c. stapled anastomosis
    c. stapler
    c. stapler doughnut
    c. stapling device
    c. suture
    c. tape
    c. vesicomyotomy (CVM)
circulares
    plicae c.
circulating
    c. autoantibody
    c. enzyme

    c. immunocomplex immunologic
      study
    c. tumor-associated antigen
circulation
    arterial c.
    collateral abdominal c.
    cutaneous collateral c.
    enterohepatic c. (EHC)
    hepatic c.
    hyperdynamic c.
    mesenteric c.
    portal c.
    portal-collateral c.
    venous c.
circulatory embarrassment
circumanal
circumcaval ureter
circumcise
circumcised
circumcision
    c. complication
    contraindication to c.
    meatal stenosis after c.
    neonatal c.
    Plastibell c.
    routine neonatal c.
    sleeve-type c.
    trapped penis after c.
circumductive
circumference
    abdominal c.
circumferential
    c. fundoplication
    c. margin
    c. mucosal dissection
    c. transanal sleeve advancement
      flap
circumflex vein
circumintestinal
circumlocution
circumumbilical incision
CIRF
    contrast-induced renal failure
cirrhogenic (*var. of* cirrhogenous)
cirrhogenous, cirrhogenic
cirrhosis
    acholangic biliary c.
    acute juvenile c.
    alcoholic c. (AC)
    atrophic c.
    autoimmune c.
    bacterial c.
    Baumgarten c.
    biliary c.
    Budd c.
    calculous c.
    cardiac c.
    CCl4-induced c.
    Charcot c.

cholangiolitic c.
cholangitic biliary c.
chronic alcoholic c.
compensated c.
congestive c.
CPH-CAH c.
Cruveilhier-Baumgarten c.
cryptogenic c.
decompensated alcoholic c.
decompensated liver c.
drug-induced c.
end-stage c.
fatty c.
focal biliary c.
frank c.
glabrous c.
Glisson c.
Hanot c.
hemochromatotic c.
hepatic c.
hepatitis C antiviral long-term
    treatment to prevent c. (HALT-C)
histologic c.
hypertrophic c.
hypochlorhydric c.
incomplete c.
Indian childhood c.
juvenile c.
Laënnec c.
liver c. (LC)
macronodular c.
Maixner c.
Mayo Clinic system for primary
    biliary c.
micronodular c.
mixed c.
multilobular c.
necrotic c.
nonazotemic c.
nutritional c.
obstructive biliary c.
c. of stomach
periportal c.
pigmentary c.
pipestem c.
portal c.
posthepatitic c.
postnecrotic c.
primary biliary c. (PBC)
progressive familial c.
Roger c.
secondary biliary c.
stasis c.
syndrome of primary biliary c.
Todd c.
toxic c.
type C c.
unilobular c.
vascular c.

cirrhotic
    c. ascites
    c. gastritis
    c. hydrothorax
    c. liver
cirsocele
cirsoid aneurysm
cirsomphalos
CIS
    carcinoma in situ
cisapride
    rectal c.
cisapride-assisted lavage
cisapride-functional dyspepsia trial
CISCA, CisCA
    cisplatin, cyclophosphamide,
    Adriamycin
        CISCA protocol
cis-diaminedichloroplatinum
cisplatin
    bleomycin, etoposide, c. (BEP)
    cisplatin, cyclophosphamide,
        Adriamycin (CISCA, CisCA)
    etoposide, ifosfamide, c.
    methotrexate, c. (MC)
    cisplatin, methotrexate, Velban
        (CMV)
    cisplatin, methotrexate, vinblastine
        (CMV)
    methotrexate, vinblastine,
        Adriamycin, c. (M-VAC)
    methotrexate, vinblastine, epirubicin,
        c. (M-VEC)
    c. nephropathy (CPN)
cisplatin-Lipiodol-Spongel (CLS)
cisterna, *pl.* **cisternae**
    c. chyli
    cylindrical confronting c.
        (CCC)
cisternae (*pl. of* cisterna)
Citra Forte
citrate
    alverine c.
    clomiphene c.
    c. infusion
    lead c.
    magnesium c.
    c. metabolism
    c. of magnesia
    piperazine c.
    potassium c.
    ranitidine bismuth c. (RBC)
    c. replacement fluid
    seminal plasma c.
    sildenafil c.
    sodium c.
    sodium picosulphate and magnesium
        c.
    c. supplementation

C

citrate (*continued*)
   c. synthase
   c. test
   urinary c.
citric
   c. acid
   c. acid bladder mixture
citrinum
   Penicillium c.
Citrobacter
   C. amalonaticus
   C. diversus
   C. freundii
   C. intermedius
Citrocarbonate
Citroma
Citro-Mag
Citro-Nesia
Citrotein liquid feeding
Citrucel Sugar-Free
citrulline
citrullinemia
Civacir
Civiale operation
CIXU
   constant infusion excretory
   urogram
c-jun
   c-j. oncogene
   c-j. protooncogene
c-kit
   c-kit protooncogene (CD117)
CK-MB
   muscle-brain isoenzyme of creatine
   kinase
CKPT
   combined kidney and pancreas
   transplant
CLA
   conjugated linoleic acid
   CLA echoendoscope
^{13}C-labeled cholesteryl octanoate breath test
C-lactose test
Clado ligament
cladribine
Claforan
Clagett-Barrett
   C.-B. esophagogastroscopy
   C.-B. esophagogastrostomy
Clagett esophagogastrostomy
clam
   c. enterocystoplasty
   c. ileocystoplasty
clamp
   Abadie enterostomy c.
   Adson c.
   Allen anastomosis c.
   Allen intestinal c.

Allen-Kocher c.
Allis c.
anastomosis c.
approximator c.
ASSI Microspike approximator c.
atraumatic c.
Babcock c.
Backhaus towel c.
Bainbridge intestinal c.
Baumrucker urinary
  incontinence c.
Beardsley intestinal c.
Best right-angle colon c.
Bihrle dorsal c.
Borge c.
Buie pile c.
bulldog c.
Carmalt c.
Carmel c.
Collins umbilical c.
Cope crushing c.
Cope modification of Martel
  intestinal c.
Crawford c.
Crile appendix c.
Crile hemostatic c.
Cunningham urinary incontinence c.
curved Mayo c.
Daniel colostomy c.
Dardik c.
DeBakey c.
DeMartel appendix c.
DeMartel-Wolfson anastomosis c.
Dennis c.
Dixon-Thomas-Smith c.
Doyen intestinal c.
Earle hemorrhoid c.
Edna towel c.
Fehland intestinal c.
Fogarty c.
Foss anterior resection c.
Foss intestinal c.
Furniss anastomosis c.
Furniss-Clute duodenal c.
Gant c.
Glassman noncrushing gastrointestinal
  c.
Goldblatt c.
Goldstein Microspike approximator
  c.
Gomco umbilical c.
Haberer intestinal c.
Harvey Stone c.
Hayes anterior resection c.
Hayes colon c.
Heaney c.
hemorrhoidal c.
hemostatic c.
Hendren c.

Herrick kidney c.
hilar c.
Hirschmann pile c.
Hunt colostomy c.
Hurwitz esophageal c.
Hurwitz intestinal c.
intestinal c.
Jarvis hemorrhoid c.
Jarvis pile c.
Kane umbilical c.
Kapp-Beck colon c.
Kelly c.
Kelsey pile c.
kidney pedicle c.
Kleinschmidt appendectomy c.
Kocher c.
Kumar Pre-View cholangiography c.
Lane gastroenterostomy c.
Lane intestinal c.
laparoscopic Allis c.
Linnartz intestinal c.
Linton tourniquet c.
Madden intestinal c.
Martel c.
Masters intestinal c.
Masters-Schwartz liver c.
Mayo abdominal c.
Mayo-Robson intestinal c.
McCleery-Miller intestinal c.
McDougal prostatectomy c.
McLean pile c.
Meeker gallbladder c.
metal wing c.
Microspike approximator c.
microvascular c.
Mikulicz c.
Millin T c.
Mixter c.
Mogen c.
Moreno gastroenterostomy c.
mosquito hemostatic c.
Moynihan c.
Myles hemorrhoidal c.
noncrushing bowel c.
Nussbaum intestinal c.
occlusive c.
Ochsner c.
O'Hanlon intestinal c.
Olsen cholangiogram c.
Parker-Kerr intestinal c.
partial-occlusion c.
Payr pyloric c.
Péan c.
pedicle c.
Pemberton sigmoid c.
penile c.
Pennington c.
Petz c.
Phillips rectal c.

Rankin c.
Redo intestinal c.
right-angle c.
Roosevelt c.
rubber-sheathed c.
rubber-shod c.
Satinsky c.
Schwartz c.
Scudder intestinal c.
self-retraction c.
serrefine c.
Shoemaker intestinal c.
Singley intestinal ring c.
slotted nerve c.
Stetten intestinal c.
Stille c.
Stone-Holcombe intestinal c.
Stone intestinal c.
straight mosquito c.
Strelinger colon c.
T c.
tonsil c.
tubing c.
vascular c.
von Petz c.
Wangensteen anastomosis c.
Wirthlin splenorenal c.
Wolfson intestinal c.
Wylie hypogastric c.
Zachary Cope-DeMartel c.
Zeppelin c.
Zipser penile c.

clamping
hyperglycemic c.
clamshell technique
clandestine intake
clapotage, clapotement
clapotement (*var. of* clapotage)
clarithromycin
lansoprazole, amoxicillin, c.
omeprazole, amoxicillin, c. (OAC)
omeprazole, metronidazole, c.
(OMC)
ranitidine bismuth citrate,
amoxicillin, c. (RAC)
c. triple therapy
Clark
C. common duct dilator
C. hemoperfusion cartridge
C. operation
C. sign
Clarke-Reich knot pusher
class
Child class A-C
Child-Pugh class A-C
GR drug c.
c. I, II antigen
c. I, II MHC molecule
Classen-Demling papillotome

classic
    c. achalasia
    c. high-pressure low-flow voiding
    c. triad of Rigler
classical transactivator
classification
    AJCC TNM tumor c.
    Anderson c.
    Ann Arbor Hodgkin disease c.
    Astler-Coller c. A, B1, B2, C1, C2
    Astler-Coller modification of Dukes
      c.
    Banff renal allograft rejection c.
    Bismuth benign bile duct stricture
      c.
    Bismuth c. type I-IV
    Blaivas urinary incontinence c.
    Borrmann gastric cancer c.
    Bosniak renal cystic disease c.
    Cambridge pancreatitis c. I-IV
    Caroli-Sarles bile duct stricture c.
    Child esophageal varix c.
    Child hepatic dysfunction c.
    Child liver disease c.
    Child-Pugh liver disease c.
    Child-Turcotte c. (CTC)
    Child-Turcotte-Pugh c.
    Correa gastritis c.
    Cotton c.
    Couinaud liver anatomy c.
    CTP c.
    Dagradi esophageal variceal c.
    Dubin-Amelar varicocele c.
    Dukes c.
    Forrest c.
    Fredrickson c.
    gastric mucosal pattern c.
    Hald-Bradley c.
    Hetzel-Dent c.
    IGCCCG c.
    International Continence Society
      voiding function c.
    International Germ Cell Cancer
      Collaborative Group c.
    Japanese cancer c.
    Jewett bladder carcinoma c.
    Kasugai pancreatitis c.
    Kelami penile curvature c.
    LA c.
    Lapides c.
    Lauren gastric carcinoma c.
    Los Angeles c.
    Lukes-Collins c.
    Marseille pancreatitis c.
    Marsh c.
    McNeer gastric carcinoma c.
    megaureter c.
    Ming gastric carcinoma c.
    modified Bismuth-Corlette c.

    Mt. Sinai c.
    Musshoff modification of Ann
      Arbor c.
    NIH-CPSI prostatitis c.
    Pugh liver disease c.
    Ranson acute pancreatitis c.
    Rappaport c.
    reflux esophagitis c. I–IV
    Santiani-Stone pancreas head
      gunshot c.
    Siurala gastritis c.
    Solcia gastric dysplasia c.
    Sonnenberg c.
    Stamey c.
    Sumikoshi c.
    Sydney system gastritis c.
    c. system
    TNM c.
    UICC tumor c.
    Visick dysphagia c.
    voiding dysfunction c.
    Whitehead gastritis c.
    WHO gastric carcinoma c.
clathrin-coated pit
claudication
claudin-2-positive zone
claudin-7 intestinal marker
claudin protein
Clave needleless system
clavulanate
clavulanic acid
Clavulin
claw
    cat's c.
    devil's c.
    c. forceps
Clay-Adams catheter
Claybrook sign
clay-colored stool
CLD
    chronic liver disease
      non-B non-C CLD
CLDQ
    Chronic Liver Disease Questionnaire
CLE
    columnar-lined esophagus
      long-segment CLE
      short-segment CLE
clean
    c. intermittent bladder
      catheterization
    c. intermittent catheterization
      (CIC)
clean-catch urine specimen
cleaner
    Endozime AW bacteriostatic
      enzyme c.
cleaning
    diathermic c.

cleanser
- CarraKlenz skin c.
- Rediwash skin c.
- UltraKlenz skin c.

cleansing hypertonic phosphate enema

clean-voided specimen (CVS)

clear
- c. bile
- c. cell adenocarcinoma
- c. cell carcinoma of kidney
- c. cell hepatocellular carcinoma
- c. cell nonpapillary carcinoma
- c. cell renal cancer
- c. cell sarcoma
- c. discharge
- enemas until c.
- c. liquid diet

clearance
- aminopyrine c.
- antipyrine c.
- blood-water c.
- bromsulphalein c.
- caffeine c.
- cholic acid c.
- complete stone c.
- creatinine c. (Crcl)
- ^{51}Cr-labeled albumin c.
- dextran c.
- equivalent residual renal urea c.
- esophageal acid c.
- fractional c.
- hepatic c.
- 24-hour creatinine c.
- hydrogen gas c.
- ICG c.
- I-125 iothalamate c.
- immunoglobulin G c.
- increased peritoneal c.
- indocyanine green c.
- instantaneous c.
- integrated c.
- inulin c.
- in vitro c.
- in vivo c.
- iodoantipyrine c.
- iothalamate c.
- kidney c.
- lithium c. (CLi)
- lowest c.
- luminal acid c.
- mucociliary c.
- osmolar c.
- PAH c.
- paraaminohippurate c.
- plasma c.
- prescribed c.
- renal c.
- retinyl ester c.
- stone c.
- theophylline c.
- urea c.
- whole-blood c.

clearing
- esophageal c.

cleavage
- aspartyl protease-mediated c.
- bacterial c.
- embryonic c.
- c. plane

cleaved extracellular domain

cleft palate

Cleocin

Cleveland
- C. Clinic incontinence score
- C. Clinic technique
- C. Clinic weighted scale of endoscopic procedures

clevudine

CLH
- chronic lobular hepatitis

CLi
- lithium clearance

click
- intermittent c.
- systolic c.

clidinium bromide

client-patient characteristic

clindamycin

Clindex

clinic
- hospital-based c.
- urology c.

clinical
- c. activity
- C. Activity Index (CAI)
- c. determinant
- c. findings
- c. hypergastrinemia
- c. improvement
- c. indication
- c. investigation
- c. monitoring
- C. Outcomes Research Initiative (CORI)
- c. parameter
- c. problem
- c. protocol
- c. rejection
- c. sequela
- c. trial
- c. trial for kidney disease

clinically
- c. insignificant
- c. stable human renal allograft

clinicobiological criteria

clinicopathologic, clinicopathological
- c. staging

C

clinicopathological (*var. of* clinicopathologic)
Clinifeed Iso enteral feeding
Clinitest-negative stool
Clinitest-positive stool
Clinitest stool test
Clinoril
Clinoxide
clip
    absorbable c.
    c. applier
    Heifitz c.
    Hulka c.
    laparoscopic tie c.
    Lapra-Ty c.
    metal c.
    Michel c.
    silver c.
    titanium c.
    towel c.
    von Petz suture c.
    Weck c.
Clipoxide
clipping
    endoluminal c.
    endoscopic c.
    laser c.
Clirans T-series dialyzer
clitoral
    c. index
    c. recession
clitorides (*pl. of* clitoris)
clitoridis
    preputium c.
clitoris, *pl.* **clitorides**
    bifid c.
clitoroplasty
clitorovaginoplasty
CLO
    Campylobacter-like organism
    CLO biopsy
cloaca, *pl.* **cloacae**
    congenital c.
    Enterobacter cloacae
    persistent c.
    c. septation
cloacae (*pl. of* cloaca)
cloacal
    c. anomaly
    c. exstrophy
    c. exstrophy 1-stage repair
    c. exstrophy 2-stage repair
    c. malformation
    c. membrane
    c. plate
    c. remnant
    c. septum
cloacogenic polyp
clodronate

clofazimine
clofibrate
Clomid
clomiphene
    c. citrate
    c. test
clomipramine
clonal
    c. anergy
    c. deletion
    c. dilution
clonality
clonazepam
clone
    gliadin-specific T-cell c.
clonic contraction
clonidine suppression test
cloning
    molecular c.
clonogenic repopulation
clonorchiasis, clonorchiosis
    biliary c.
    hepatic c.
clonorchiosis (*var. of* clonorchiasis)
Clonorchis sinensis
clonus
    left-sided c.
    right-sided c.
Cloquet
    C. hernia
    node of C.
clorazepate dipotassium
clortermine
closed
    c. afferent loop
    c. colon
    c. continuous lavage
    c. drainage
    c. duodenum
    c. efferent loop
    c. esophagus
    c. eyes sign
    c. hemorrhoidectomy
    c. injury
    c. morphology
    c. pylorus
    c. tubule fixation technique
closed-end ostomy pouch
closed-loop intestinal obstruction
closed-suction
    c.-s. drain
    c.-s. drainage system
closing pressure
Clostoban
clostridial nephritis
Clostridium
    C. algidicarnis
    C. botulinum
    C. butyricum

C. *cadaveris*
C. *coccoides*
C. *difficile* (CD)
C. *difficile*-associated diarrhea
 (CDAD)
C. *difficile* enteritis
C. *difficile* enterotoxin
C. *difficile* toxin assay
C. *fallax*
C. *leptum*
C. *perfringens*
C. *ramosum*
C. *tertium*
C. *tetani*
C. *welchii*

closure
Beta-Cap catheter c.
Beta-Cap II c.
bladder neck c. (BNC)
bladder outlet c.
bladder, posterior urethral, abdominal
 wall c.
delayed primary c. (DPC)
exstrophy c.
Graham c.
ileostomy c.
muscularis tunnel c.
primary c.
pyelotomy c.
secondary c.
Smead-Jones c.
stapled c.
Sur-Fit Natura irrigation sleeve tail
 c.
sutureless colostomy c.
Tom Jones c.
Witzel c.
wound c.

clot
adherent c.
c.'s and debris
black c.
blood c.
C. Buster Amplatz thrombectomy
 device
fresh c.
fundic c.
hematuria with c.'s
intraluminal c.
nonadherent c.
overlying c.
sentinel c.

CLOtest
Campylobacter-like organism test
clot-induced urinary tract obstruction
clotrimazole
clotted blood
clotting
c. abnormality

c. cascade
c. factor
c. parameter
c. time

cloud
c. phenomenon
plasma c.

cloudy
c. ascites
c. bile
c. fluid

cloverleaf
c. appearance
c. deformity
c. excision of hemorrhoid
C. internal bumper

cloxacillin-induced cholestatic jaundice
Cloxapen
CLP
cecal ligation and puncture
CLS
cisplatin-Lipiodol-Spongel
club
American Endosonography C. (AEC)
c. moss
clubbed
c. common bile duct
c. finger
c. penis
clubbing
calyx c.
finger c.
c. of fingers and toes
cluster
c. of differentiation (CD)
c. of differentiation 3+ (CD3+)
c. of differentiation 4 (CD4)
c. of differentiation 4+ (CD4+)
c. of differentiation 8 (CD8)
c. of differentiation 8+ (CD8+)
c. of differentiation 14 (CD14)
c. of differentiation 20 (CD20)
c. of differentiation 23 (CD23)
c. of grapelike cysts
clustered
c. jejunal waves
c. waves (CW)
clusterin mRNA
CLVP
contact laser vaporization of
 prostate
clysis
Clysodrast
clyster
cm
centimeter
CMA
chronic metabolic acidosis
cow's milk allergy

c-met
- *c-m.* oncogene
- *c-m.* protein
- *c-m.* receptor

CMG
- cystometrogram
- cystometrography

CMGN
- chronic membranous glomerulonephritis

C-mount adapter

CM1 polyclonal antibody

CMSE
- cow's milk-sensitive enteropathy

CMV
- cisplatin, methotrexate, Velban
- cisplatin, methotrexate, vinblastine
- cytomegalovirus
  - CMV colitis
  - CMV esophagitis
  - CMV inclusion body
  - CMV inclusion cyst
  - CMV infection
  - CMV ulcerative disease

CMV-associated ulceration

CMV-induced esophageal ulceration

CMV-related ulcer

c-myc
- *c-m.* oncogene
- *c-m.* protooncogene

CNDI
- congenital nephrogenic diabetes insipidus

CNNA
- culture-negative neutrocytic ascites

CNP
- chronic nonbacterial prostatitis
- C-type natriuretic peptide

CNS
- central nervous system
- congenital nephrotic syndrome

Co
- coenzyme

CO₂, CO2
- carbon dioxide
  - CO₂ breath test
  - CO₂ electrolyte
  - CO₂ laser
  - CO₂ laser probe

CoA
- coenzyme A

coagulase
- c. waveform
- c. waveform desiccation

coagulase-negative *Staphylococcus*

coagulating
- c. current
- c. electrode
- c. forceps

coagulation
- c. and hemostatic resection of prostate (CHRP)
- argon ion plasma c.
- argon plasma c. (APC)
- BICAP c.
- Bipolar circumactive probe c.
- blood c.
- Bovie c.
- coaptive c.
- disseminated intravascular c. (DIC)
- EHT c.
- electrohydrothermal c.
- endoscopic microwave c.
- free-beam c.
- heater probe c.
- hot biopsy monopolar c.
- infrared c.
- interstitial laser c. (ILC)
- laser c.
- microwave tissue c.
- monopolar c.
- multipolar c.
- c. necrosis
- c. probe
- semen c.
- c. time
- tissue c.

coagulative
- c. laser therapy
- c. necrosis

coagulator
- argon beam c.
- argon plasma c. (APC)
- ERBE Unit argon plasma c.
- infrared c.
- microwave tissue c.
- Redfield infrared c.

Coaguloop resection electrode

coagulopathy
- iatrogenic c.
- c. pancreatitis

coagulum pyelolithotomy

coalesce

coalescence

coalescent ulcer

coalition
- Digestive Disease National C. (DDNC)
- National Prostate Cancer C.

coaptation

coaptive coagulation

coarctation

coarse
- c. granular cast
- c. material
- c. nodularity

coarsely granular kidney

coat
    fibromuscular c.
    hydrated gelatinous c.
    muscular c.
Coat-A-Count Free PSA IRMA test
coated biopsy forceps
coating
    InhibiZone c.
coaxial
    c. catheter
    c. snare
cobalamin deficiency
cobalophilin
cobalt-60
Coban
    C. dressing
    C. 2-layer compression system
    C. tape
Cobas Amplicor HBV monitor test
Cobb collar
cobbler's stitch
cobblestone
    c. appearance
    c. appearance of gastric body
    c. filling defect
    c. mucosa
    c. pattern
    c. pattern of hepatocyte
cobblestonelike monolayer
cobblestoning
    mucosal c.
    c. of colon
    c. of mucosa
    c. sign
Cobe Centrysystem dialyzer 400 HG
COBED tube
^{57}Co B$_{12}$ excretion
cobra catheter
cobra-head
    c.-h. deformity
    c.-h. sign
cocaine
    c. hepatotoxicity
    c. package ingestion
cocarcinogen
cocarcinogenic
    c. FBA
    c. fecal bile acid
coccidia (*pl. of* coccidium)
coccidian
    c. body
    c. *Cyclospora*
    c. sporulation
    unsporulated c.
coccidian-like
coccidioidal

    c. cystitis
    c. endometritis
    c. peritonitis
***Coccidioides immitis* peritonitis**
coccidioidomycosis
coccidiosis
coccidium, *pl.* **coccidia**
coccoides
    Clostridium c.
coccoid form of *Helicobacter pylori*
coccygeal
    c. fistula
    c. pelvis
coccygeus muscle
Cochin China diarrhea
Cochran-Mantel-Haenszel test
Cockcroft-Gault
    C.-G. equation
    C.-G. formula
Cock operation
Cockroft method
cocktail
    GI c.
    lytic c.
CO_2-CO_2 abundance ratio
^{13}C-octanoic acid gastric emptying breath test
coculture system
code
    genetic c.
Coding Systems for a Thesaurus of Adverse Reaction Terms (COSTART)
codominant phenotype
codon
    premature stop c.
coefficient
    glomerular ultrafiltration c.
    inbreeding c.
    mass transfer area c. (MTAC)
    c. of variation
    prostatic pressure c. (PPC)
    sieving c. (SC)
    ultrafiltration c.
coenzyme (Co)
    c. A (CoA)
    hepatic 3-methylglutaryl coenzyme A (HMG-CoA)
coerulea
    Absidia c.
coeundi
    impotentia c.
coexpress
coffee-grounds
    c.-g. emesis
    c.-g. material (CGM)
    c.-g. vomit
    c.-g. vomitus

C

Coffey
    C. ureterointestinal anastomosis
    C. ureterosigmoid transplant
      technique
Cogentin
coglycolide
    polylactide c. (PLG)
cognition
cognitive function
Cohen
    C. antireflux procedure
    C. cross-trigonal reimplantation
    C. cross-trigonal technique
    C. syndrome
    C. test
    C. ureteroneocystostomy
coherent
    c. bundle
    C. 90-K laser
cohosh
    black c.
coil
    c. catheter
    endoanal c.
    endoesophageal MRI c.
    endoprostatic c.
    endorectal-pelvic phased-array c.
    Gianturco c.
    helical c.
    Helmholtz double-surface c.
    intraurethral c.
    interlocking detachable c.'s
    MRCP using HASTE with
      phased-array c.
    pelvic phased-array c.
    secretory c.
    spring-wire c.
    c. stent
    Stylet internal esophageal
      MRI c.
Coil-Cath catheter
coiled
    c. spring appearance
    c. spring sign
coiled-coil motif
coimmunoprecipitate
coincubation
    sperm immunobead c.
coinfection
Colace
**ColActive Ag antimicrobial collagen
  wound dressing**
COL4A3 **gene**
COL4A4 **gene**
COL4A5 **gene**
Colapinto needle
Colaris
    C. genetic susceptibility test
    C. molecular diagnostic test

Colax-C
Colazal
Colazide
colchicine
cold
    c. biopsy forceps
    c. cup biopsy
    c. cup resection
    c. defect
    c. flushing
    c. forceps ablation
    c. ischemia time (CIT)
    c. knife
    c. scissors
    c. snare ablation
    c. snare excision
    C. Spor disinfectant
    c. spot
    c. storage
    c. stress test
cold-knife
    c.-k. endoureterotomy
    c.-k. hook
    c.-k. incision
Cole
    C. duodenal retractor
    C. sign
colectasia
colectomy
    abdominal c.
    blind subtotal c.
    laparoscopic c.
    segmental c.
    subtotal c.
    total abdominal c. (TAC)
    transverse c.
coleoptosis
Colestid
colestipol hydrochloride
Coley toxin
coli
    adenomatous polyposis c. (APC)
    adherent invasive *Escherichia* c.
    attenuated adenomatous
      polyposis c.
    Balantidium c.
    Campylobacter c.
    diffuse adherent *Escherichia* c.
      (DAEC)
    enteroadherent *Escherichia* c.
      (EAEC)
    enteroaggregative *Escherichia* c.
      (EAEC, EaggEC)
    enterohemorrhagic *Escherichia* c.
      (EHEC)
    enteroinvasive *Escherichia* c.
      (EIEC)
    enteropathogenic *Escherichia* c.
      (EPEC)

enterotoxigenic *Escherichia c.*
(ETEC)
Escherichia c. (E. coli)
familial adenomatous polyposis c.
familial polyposis c. (FPC)
flexura lienalis c.
haustra c.
juvenile polyposis c.
labium inferius valvulae c.
labium superius valvulae c.
melanosis c.
nonpathogenic *Escherichia c.*
pneumatosis cystoides c.
(PCC)
polyposis c. (PC)
Shiga toxin-producing *Escherichia c.*
(STEC)
Stx 2-producing *Escherichia c.*
(STEC)
tenia c.

colibacillosis
colic

acute ureteric c.
appendicular c.
c. artery
biliary c.
bilious c.
copper c.
crapulent c.
Devonshire c.
endemic c.
episodic c.
esophageal c.
flatulent c.
gallstone c.
gastric c.
hepatic c.
c. impression
c. impression on liver
infantile c.
intestinal c.
lead c.
mucous c.
multiple recurrent renal c.
c. myoneurosis
c. omentum
painter's c.
pancreatic c.
c. patch
c. patch esophagoplasty
pseudoesophageal c.
pseudomembranous c.
renal c.
saburral c.
c. sacculation
saturnine c.
stercoraceous c.
ureteral c.
uterine c.

vermicular c.
verminous c.
wind c.
worm c.
zinc c.

colica
colicky abdominal pain
colicoplegia
colicystopyelitis
coliform

c. bacillus
c. bacterium
c. urinary infection

colipase
colipase-dependent lipase
coliplication
colipuncture
Colirest
colistimethate
colistin
colitic

c. arthritis
c. mucosa

colitides (*pl. of* colitis)
colitis, *pl.* **colitides**

acute infectious c.
acute self-limited c. (ASLC)
adaptive c.
adenovirus c.
allergic c.
amebic c.
antibiotic-associated c. (AAC)
antibiotic-associated
  pseudomembranous c. (AAPC,
  AAPMC)
bacterial c.
balantidial c.
Balantidium coli c.
Behçet c.
Campylobacter fetus c.
cathartic c.
caustic c.
chronic ulcerative c. (CUC)
CMV c.
collagenous c.
Crohn c.
c. cystica profunda (CCP)
c. cystica superficialis
cytomegalovirus c.
diabetic c.
distal c.
diversion c.
drug-induced c.
eosinophilic c.
familial ulcerative c.
focal c.
fulminant toxic c.
fulminating ulcerative c.
gangrenous ischemic c.

C

colitis (*continued*)
    granulomatous transmural c.
    c. gravis
    hemorrhagic c.
    iatrogenic c.
    idiopathic c.
    indeterminate c. (IC)
    infectious c.
    inflammatory c.
    intractable ulcerative c.
    ischemic c.
    left-sided c.
    lymphocytic c.
    microscopic c.
    milk-sensitive c.
    mucosal ulcerative c. (MUC)
    mucous c.
    myxomembranous c.
    necrotic hemorrhagic c.
    neutropenic c.
    nonantibiotic c.
    nonspecific c.
    pantothenic acid deficiency-induced
      c.
    patchy c.
    c. perineal complication
    peroxynitrite-induced c.
    c. polyposa
    progesterone-associated c.
    pseudomembranous c. (PMC)
    radiation c.
    radiation-induced c.
    regional c.
    Salmonella c.
    segmental ischemic c.
    sexually transmitted c.
    Shigella c.
    single-stripe c. (SSC)
    toxic c.
    Toxoplasma c.
    transmural c. (TMC)
    tuberculous c.
    ulcerative c. (UC)
    uremic c.
    viral c.
    Yersinia enterocolitica c.
colla (*pl. of* collum)
Collaborative Transplant Study (CTS)
collagen
    alpha-2 beta-1 integrin cell-surface
      c.
    bovine dermal c.
    Contigen glutaraldehyde crosslinked
      c.
    degradation of c.
    c. deposition
    glutaraldehyde crosslinked c. (GAX)
    c. injection
    c. maturation

    pressure-injected bovine c.
    c. synthesis
    c. synthesis inhibitor
    c. types I–XIII
    c. vascular disease
collagenase
    interstitial c.
    C. Santyl ointment
collagenofibrotic glomerulopathy
collagenous
    c. colitis
    c. pouchitis
    c. sprue
collapse
    c. of cavitation bubble
    parenchymatous c.
collapsed ileum
collapsing
    c. FSGS
    c. glomerulopathy
collar
    Cobb c.
    polyglycolic acid c.
    preputial c.
    ulcer c.
collar-button
    c.-b. appearance in colon
    c.-b. ulceration
collar-buttonlike ulcer
collateral
    c. abdominal circulation
    vasodilation of portosystemic c.
collecting
    c. duct (CD)
    c. duct carcinoma
    c. system
    c. tube
    c. tubule
    c. venule
collection
    American-type culture c.
    blood c.
    duodenal fluid c.
    encysted intraabdominal c.
    fluid c.
    24-hour urine c.
    pancreatic fluid c. (PFC)
    perinephric fluid c.
    peripancreatic fluid c.
    pus c.
    quantitative stool c.
    semen c.
collector
    Grass force displacement fluid c.
    Misstique female external urinary c.
Colles fascia
colli
    cystitis c.
colliculectomy

colliculi (*pl. of* colliculus)
colliculitis
colliculus, *pl.* colliculi
  bulbar c.
  seminal c.
  c. seminalis
Collidem
collimator
  high-sensitivity c.
Collin
  C. abdominal retractor
  C. intestinal forceps
  C. intestinal retractor
  C. knife
  C. mesher
  C. tissue forceps
  C. tongue forceps
Collin-Duval intestinal thumb forceps
Collings
  C. electrode
  C. electrosurgery knife
Collins
  C. indigo carmine solution
  C. intracellular electrolyte solution
  C. umbilical clamp
colliquative
  c. diarrhea
  c. necrosis
  c. proteinuria
Collis
  C. antireflux operation
  C. gastroplasty
  C. repair
collision block
Collis-Nissen
  C.-N. fundoplication
  C.-N. gastroplasty
colloid
  ^{99m}Tc albumin c.
  ^{99m}Tc sulfur c. (^{99m}Tc SC)
  c. osmotic pressure
  c. shift on liver-spleen scan
  c. solution
  sulfur c. (SC)
  technetium-99m sulfur c. (^{99m}Tc SC)
  technetium-99m tin c.
colloidal
  c. bismuth subcitrate (CBS)
  c. bismuth suspension
  c. oatmeal
  c. thorium
colloid-producing adenocarcinoma
collum, *pl.* colla
  c. glandis penis
  c. vesicae biliaris
  c. vesicae felleae
Colly-Seal wafer-type skin barrier
coloanal anastomosis (CAA)

coloboma, heart disease, atresia choanae, retarded growth, genital hypoplasia, and ear abnormalities (CHARGE)
colobronchial fistula
colocalization
colocalized
ColoCARE fecal occult blood test
colocecostomy
colocentesis
colocholecystic fistula
colocholecystostomy
coloclysis
colocolic intussusception
COLO 320 colon cancer cell
colocolonic
  c. anastomosis
  c. fistula
colocolostomy
colocolponeopoiesis
Colocort
colocutaneous fistula
colocystoplasty
  seromuscular c.
colodyspepsia
coloenteric fistula
coloenteritis
colofixation
cologastrocutaneous fistula
Cologel
colography (*var. of* colonography)
colohepatopexy
coloileal fistula
cololysis
Colombo
colometrometer
colon
  adenomatous polyp of c. (APC)
  aganglionic segment of c.
  anterior band of c.
  antral diverticulum of c. (ADC)
  c. ascendens
  ascending c.
  atonic c.
  c. cancer
  c. cancer resection
  c. cancer screening
  c. carcinoma
  cathartic c.
  c. cauterization
  closed c.
  cobblestoning of c.
  collar-button appearance in c.
  coned-down appearance of c.
  Crohn disease of c. (CDC)
  c. cutoff sign
  c. descendens
  descending c. (DC)
  distal c.
  diverticulum of c.

C

colon (*continued*)
    diverticular disease of c. (DDC)
    endometriosis of c.
    fascia of c.
    foreshortening of c.
    free band of c.
    frenum of valve of c.
    gangrenous c.
    giant c.
    haustra of c.
    hepatic flexure of c.
    hypoganglionosis of c.
    iliac c.
    c. impression
    c. incarceration
    institutional c.
    inverted diverticulum of c.
    irritable c.
    knuckle of c.
    lateral reflection of c.
    c. lavage cytology
    lazy c.
    lead-pipe c.
    left c.
    longitudinal band of c.
    longitudinal fasciculus of c.
    loop of redundant c.
    c. medial reflection
    mesenteric attachment of c.
    mesosigmoid c.
    midsigmoid c.
    c. motility catheter
    pelvic c.
    perforation of c.
    perisigmoid c.
    c. pouch
    c. procedure
    rectosigmoid c.
    right c.
    saccular c.
    sacculation of c.
    c. schistosomiasis
    sigmoid c.
    c. sigmoideum
    c. single-stripe sign
    spastic c.
    spiculation on c.
    spike-burst on electromyogram of c.
    c. splenic flexure
    thrifty c.
    toxic dilation of c.
    c. transit marker study
    transverse c.
    c. transversum
    c. tumor cell lysis
    unstable c.
    c. urinary conduit
    valve of c.
    varix of c.
    volvulus of c.
    watermelon c.
colonalgia
colonic
    c. adenocarcinoma
    c. adenoma
    c. arterial spider
    c. bacterium
    c. biopsy
    c. circular muscle
    c. dilation
    c. distention
    c. diverticulosis
    c. diverticulum
    c. duplication
    c. electromyogram
    c. epithelial cell
    c. epithelial proliferation
    c. explosion
    c. fistula
    c. flora
    c. food
    c. foreign body
    c. gas
    c. hamartoma
    c. hemorrhage
    c. hyperalgesia
    c. ileus
    c. inertia
    c. infiltration
    c. insufflation
    c. interposition
    c. ischemia
    c. J pouch
    c. J-pouch reservoir
    c. lavage
    c. lavage solution
    c. leiomyoma
    c. lesion identification
    c. lipoma
    c. loop
    c. lymphoid nodule
    c. manometry
    c. mass
    c. metaplasia
    c. metastasis
    c. microflora
    c. motility
    c. mucosal line
    c. mucosal pattern
    c. mucosal surface
    c. myenteric plexus
    c. necrosis
    c. neoplasia
    c. nodular lymphoid hyperplasia
    c. obstruction
    c. obstruction technique
    c. orthotopic bladder substitution
    c. patch

c. perforation
c. permeability
c. phenotype
c. pit
c. pitting
c. polyp
c. polyposis
c. polyposis syndrome
c. propulsion
c. prostaglandin
c. pseudoobstruction
c. pseudoobstruction syndrome
c. purge preparation
c. schistosomiasis
c. solitary ulcer syndrome
c. tattoo
c. transabdominal sonography (CTAS)
c. transit study
c. transit test
c. transit time
c. trauma
c. tuberculosis
c. ulcer
c. varix
c. vascular lesion
c. villus
c. volvulus
c. wall
c. Z stent

colonization
gut c.
intestinal c.
jejunal c.
stool c.

Colonlite bowel preparation
colonocyte
colonofiberscope
Olympus CG-P-series c.
colonography, colography
computed tomographic c. (CTC)
CT c.
endoluminal CT c.
magnetic resonance c. (MRC)
colonopathy, colopathy
fibrosing c.
colonorrhagia
colonorrhea
colonoscope, coloscope
ACMI fiberoptic c.
Aeo-O-Scope c.
CF-HM magnifying c.
CF-LB3R c.
CF-UHM c.
double-channel c.
FCS-ML II c.
fiberoptic c.
Fujinon EC-130LT c.
Fujinon EC-200LT c.

Fujinon EC-410MP c.
Fujinon EC-300MS c.
Fujinon FE-100LR c.
Innoflex variable-stiffness c.
Machida FCS-ML II magnifying c.
magnifying c.
Olympus CF-HM-series magnifying c.
Olympus CF-MB/LB c.
Olympus CF-MB-M c.
Olympus CF-MB-series c.
Olympus CF24OZI c.
Olympus CF-PL-series c.
Olympus CF-P20S fiberoptic c.
Olympus CF-1T100L c.
Olympus CF-T-series c.
Olympus CF-TVL-series c.
Olympus CF-UHM-series c.
Olympus CF-UM3 c.
Olympus CF-VL-series c.
Olympus CF-200Z c.
Olympus CV-series c.
Olympus PCF-100 pediatric c.
Olympus PCF-130 pediatric c.
Olympus PCF-series pediatric c.
Olympus SIF-M magnifying c.
PCF-140L pediatric c.
pediatric c.
Pentax FC-series c.
Pentax VSB-P2900 pediatric c.
single-channel c.
small-caliber variable-stiffness c.
standard c.
Toshiba TCE-M-series c.

colonoscopic
c. antegrade contrast enema study
c. appendectomy
c. biopsy
c. decompression
c. diagnosis
c. disimpaction
c. endoluminal ultrasound
c. findings
c. polypectomy
c. removal
c. sclerotherapy
c. study
c. tattoo
c. view of adenoma

colonoscopist
colonoscopy, coloscopy
cecal c.
c. complication
diagnostic c.
emergency c.
high-magnification chromoscopic c.
magnifying c.
pediatric c.
c. screening

C

colonoscopy (*continued*)
    splenic flexure c.
    surveillance c.
    tandem c. (TC)
    c. technique with external
      straightener
    therapeutic c.
    total c.
    upper endoscopy and c.
    urgent c.
    Virtual Vision audiovisual system
      for EGD and c.
colonoscopy-induced hyponatremic
  encephalopathy
colonoscopy-related
    c.-r. emphysema
    c.-r. incarceration
colony count
colony-forming unit (CFU)
colony-stimulating
    c.-s. factor (CSF)
    c.-s. factor-1 (CSF-1)
colopathy (*var. of* colonopathy)
coloperineal fistula
colopexostomy
colopexotomy
colopexy
Coloplast
    C. bag
    C. closed pouch
    C. Conseal plug
    C. drainable pouch
    C. flange minicap
    C. flange pouch
    C. irrigation faceplate
    C. irrigation kit
    C. minipouch
    C. ostomy belt
    C. ostomy irrigation set
    C. skin barrier
    C. skin barrier paste
    C. skin barrier ring
    C. stoma cap
    C. stoma cone
    C. transparent irrigation
      sleeve
coloplasty pouch
coloplication
coloproctectomy
coloproctia
coloproctitis
coloproctology
coloproctostomy
coloptosia (*var. of* coloptosis)
coloptosis, coloptosia
colopuncture
color
    c. Doppler imaging of ureteral jet
      into bladder

    c. Doppler ultrasonography
    c. flow Doppler
    c. flow Doppler imaging
    C. Quad System
    stool c.
    urinalysis c.
    urine c.
color-coded
    c.-c. Doppler sonography
    c.-c. duplex sonography
colorectal
    c. adenocarcinoma
    c. anastomosis (CRA)
    c. biopsy
    c. cancer (CRC)
    c. cancer screening
    c. cancer syndrome
    c. carcinogenesis
    c. carcinoma (CRC)
    c. disease
    c. endoluminal ultrasound
    c. endometriosis
    c. lymphoma
    c. mass
    c. motility
    c. mucosa
    c. neoplasm
    c. physiologic dysfunction
    c. physiologic study
    c. polyp
    c. resection
    c. snare
    c. stricture
    c. surgeon
    c. surgery (CRS)
    c. transition study
    c. trauma
    c. tumor
    c. tumorigenesis
    c. ulcer
    c. variceal bleeding
    c. villous adenoma
ColorectAlert rectal mucus test
colorectal/ovarian (CR/OV)
colorectostomy
colorectum
colorimetric detection
Colormate TLc BiliTest System
colorrhagia
colorrhaphy
colorrhea
coloscope (*var. of* colonoscope)
coloscopy (*var. of* colonoscopy)
ColoScreen
    C. self-test
    C. VPI
Coloshield
colosigmoidostomy
colosigmoid resection

colostomy
    c. bag
    c. bridge
    continent c.
    decompression c.
    descending loop c.
    Devine c.
    diverting loop c.
    divided-stoma c.
    double-barrel c.
    dry c.
    end c.
    end-loop c.
    end-sigmoid c.
    end-to-side ileotransverse c.
    exteriorization c.
    Hartmann c.
    ileoascending c.
    ileosigmoid c.
    ileotransverse c.
    irrigation of c.
    longitudinal c.
    loop transverse c.
    Mikulicz c.
    nonirrigating descending c.
    permanent end c.
    resective c.
    c. rod
    c. shift en masse
    sigmoid-end c.
    sigmoid-loop rod c.
    c. soiling
    takedown of c.
    temporary end c.
    terminal c.
    transverse loop rod c.
    Turnbull c.
    Wangensteen c.
    wet c.
colotomy
    Allingham c.
coloureteral fistula
colouterine fistula
colovaginal fistula
colovenous fistula
colovesical fistula
colpocleisis
    Latzko partial c.
colpocystocele
colpocystotomy
colpocystoureterotomy
colpocystourethropexy (CCUP)
colpogram
colpoperineoplasty
colpopexy
    transvaginal sacrospinous c.
colporectopexy
colporrhaphy
colposuspension

    Burch retropubic c.
    laparoscopic needle c.
    laparoscopic retropubic c.
    retropubic c.
    Stamey c.
colpoureterotomy
column
    anal c.
    butyl-silane extraction c.
    c. chromatography
    C18 Sep-Pack c.
    hemicrypt c.
    c. of Morgagni
    rectal c.
    Sepharose 4B-coupled protein-A c.
    variceal c.
columna, *pl.* **columnae**
    columnae anales
    columnae rectales
    columnae renales
columnae (*pl. of* columna)
columnar
    c. cuff
    c. cuff cancer
    c. epithelium
    c. metaplasia
    c. mucosa
columnar-cuboidal adenocarcinoma cell
columnar-lined esophagus (CLE)
Coly-Mycin M, S
colypeptic
Colyte bowel preparation
coma
    acute hepatic c.
    ammoniagenic c.
    electrolyte imbalance c.
    hepatic c.
comatose
CombiDERM nonadhesive absorbant dressing
Combidex
combination
    c. biliary brush catheter
    c. calculus
    prednisone-colchicine c.
    synergistic c.
combined
    c. androgen blockade (CAB)
    c. antegrade and retrograde dilation
    c. chemoradiation therapy
    c. endoscopic sandwich technique
    c. fat- and carbohydrate-induced hyperlipidemia
    c. hemorrhoids
    c. hiatal hernia
    c. intracavernous injection and stimulation test

C

combined (*continued*)
  c. kidney and pancreas transplant (CKPT)
  c. percutaneous-endoscopic management of perforated esophagus
  c. ureterolysis
comblike redness sign
Combo Cath wire-guided cytology brush
comet sign
Comfeel
  C. Purilon
  C. skin adhesive
  C. skin barrier
Comfort
  C. Bath with I-See-Red skin check
  C. Cath I, II catheter
comfrey
Comhaire grading system
co-mitogen
commensal
  c. bacterium
  c. flora
commercial dialysis solution (CDS)
comminution
  stone c.
Committee
  Joint National C. (JNC)
common
  c. bile duct (CBD)
  c. bile duct compression
  c. bile duct exploration (CBDE)
  c. bile duct microlithiasis (CBDM)
  c. bile duct obstruction
  c. bile duct stent
  c. bile duct stone (CBDS)
  c. bile duct varix
  c. cavity phenomenon
  c. channel
  c. duct (CD)
  c. duct calculus
  c. duct cholangiogram
  c. duct exploration (CDE)
  c. duct sound
  c. hepatic artery (CHA)
  c. hepatic duct
  c. iliac artery
  c. iliac vein
  c. kidney vetch
  c. penile artery
  c. pH electrode
  c. stonecrop
  c. variable immunodeficiency (CVI, CVID)
communicating hydrocele
communication
  anomalous pancreaticobiliary c.
  cholangiovenous c.

horseshoe c.
pseudocyst c.
communis
  arteria hepatica c.
  ductus hepaticus c.
community
  Ashkenazi Jewish c.
comorbid condition
comorbidity
companion
  C. 2
  C. feeding pump
comparison
  c. of depth of tissue injury
  prospective c.
compartment
  infracolic c.
  inframesocolic c.
  posterior pararenal c.
  supracolic c.
Compat enteral feeding pump
compatibility
  in vitro c.
Compazine
Compeed Skinprotector dressing
compendium
  urologic drug c.
compensated
  c. cirrhosis
  c. dysphagia for solid food
compensatory testicular hypertrophy
competent
  c. bowel
  c. ileocecal valve
competitive protein-binding assay
Compleat-B liquid feeding
complement
  c. activation
  c. fixation test
  c. hemolytic activity
  c. level
  plasma-activated c. 3 (C3a)
  plasma-activated c. 4 (C4a)
  plasma-activated c. 5 (C5a)
  prostate gland C3 c.
  c. receptor type 1 (CR1)
  c. regulatory protein
  total hemolytic c.
complementary
  c. and alternative medicine (CAM)
  c. deoxyribonucleic acid (cDNA)
  c. DNA (cDNA)
  c. single-stranded antisense riboprobe
complement-dependent cytotoxicity (CDC)
complement-independent autologous phase
complement-mediated
  c.-m. experimental glomerulonephritis
  c.-m. immune glomerular disease

complete
- c. anatomical recovery
- c. blood count (CBC)
- c. blood count test
- c. bowel obstruction
- c. duplication
- c. hormonal blockage
- c. male epispadias
- c. PEG pull
- c. PEG push
- Pepcid C.
- c. repair of bladder exstrophy
- c. replacement PEG
- c. Savary
- c. stone clearance
- c. stone fragmentation
- c. surgical exploration (CSE)
- c. ureteral stricture
- c. urological imaging

completion gastrectomy

complex
- adenylate cyclase c.
- AIDS-related c. (ARC)
- anisoylated plasminogen-streptokinase activator c.
- c. anorectal fistula
- antimajor histocompatibility c.
- avidin-biotin c. (ABC)
- avidin-biotin-peroxidase c.
- calcium-calmodulin c.
- c. calyceal pattern
- cardinal-sacrouterine ligament c.
- Carman-Kirklin meniscus c.
- Carney c.
- CD3 T-cell receptor c.
- c. class II expression
- dorsal vagal c.
- dorsal vein c. (DVC)
- c. enterocele
- epispadias-exstrophy c.
- exstrophy-epispadias c.
- gastroduodenal artery c.
- Golgi c.
- Heymann nephritis antigenic c. (HNAC)
- histocompatibility c.
- c. hypospadias
- IGFBP-3 c.
- immunostimulating c. (ISCOM)
- inflammatory polyp-fold c. (IPFC)
- interdigestive migrating motor c.
- interdigestive myoelectric c.
- lactase-ceramidase c.
- major histocompatibility c. (MHC)
- membrane-attack c.
- membrane-bound multicomponent enzyme c.
- Meyenburg c.
- migrating motor c. (MMC)

- migrating myoelectric c.
- mitochondrial c.
- muscle-alginate c.
- *Mycobacterium avium* c.
- nephroblastomatosis c. (NBC)
- OEIS c.
- oligohydramnios c.
- oligometric c.
- c. papillary infolding
- penoscrotal transposition c.
- phagocytic respiratory burst oxidase c.
- polysaccharide-iron c. (PIC)
- c. reconstructive surgery
- rectal motor c.
- refined carbohydrate c.
- c. renal procedure
- sling-ring c.
- c. stone
- surface membrane actin cytoskeleton c.
- T-cell antigen receptor/CD3 c.
- thrombin-antithrombin III c.
- tuberous sclerosis c. (TSC)
- urobilin c.
- von Meyenburg c. (VMC)

compliance
- bladder c.
- detrusor c.
- c. of bladder
- rectal c.
- vesical c.

complication
- anastomotic c.
- bacterial c.
- benign pneumatic colonoscopy c.
- bowel preparation c.
- cardiopulmonary c.
- cardiorespiratory c.
- cardiovascular c.
- catastrophic c.
- cerebrovascular c.
- circumcision c.
- colitis perineal c.
- colonoscopy c.
- cystolitholapaxy experienced c.
- endoscopy c.
- extraintestinal c.
- feeding c.
- gastrointestinal c.
- hematologic c.
- infectious c.
- intraoperative c.
- laparoscopy c.
- metabolic c.
- metastatic c.
- neurologic c.
- c. of benign gastric ulcer
- opportunistic c.

complication (*continued*)
    postbiopsy vascular c.
    postoperative c.
    potential c.
    pouch-specific c.
    pulmonary c.
    relatively minimal c.
    renal c.
    sclerotherapy c.
    significant reported c.
    stent-related c.
    urethral reconstruction c.
    vascular access c.

component
    Knodell c.
    lymphoid c.
    secretory c.
    serum amyloid P c.
    shock wave lithotripsy cavitation c.
    suburethral c.
    tachykinin c.

composite prosthesis
composition
    adrenal gland c.
    cystine c.
    stone c.
    urinary c.
    urine c.

compound
    antiobesity c.
    bismuth c.
    c. cyst
    gold c.
    guanidino c.
    nitroso c.
    tetrapyrrol c.

Compound-65 Pulvules
comprehensive review
compressible cavernous body
compression
    abdominal c.
    c. anuria
    c. button
    c. button gastrojejunostomy
    celiac axis c.
    common bile duct c.
    duodenal c.
    esophageal c.
    extramural common bile duct c.
    extrinsic biliary c.
    extrinsic pancreatic c.
    gastric c.
    mechanical variceal c.
    renal venous outflow c.
    spinal cord c.
    c. syndrome
    c. ultrasound (CUS)

compressive base
compressor urethra

compromise
    vascular c.
Compro suppository
computed
    c. tomodensitometry
    c. tomographic angiography (CTA)
    c. tomographic colonography (CTC)
    c. tomography (CT)
    c. tomography arterial portography
    c. tomography during arterial
      portography (CTAP)
    c. tomography enteroclysis
    c. tomography enterography
    c. tomography technology

computer-aided
    c.-a. ambulatory gastrojejunal
      manometry
    c.-a. diagnostic system
**computer-controlled sedation infusion
  system**
computerization
computerized
    c. dynamic posturography (CDP)
    c. electronic endoscopy
    c. image analysis system
    c. phonoenterography
    c. tomographic hepatic angiography
      (CTHA)
    c. tomography (CT)
Compu-void
comutagenic
Comvax
con A/anti-con A perfusion
concealed
    c. hemorrhage
    c. hypospadias
    c. penis
    c. umbilical stoma
    c. vomiting
Concentraid Nasal
concentrate
    bile salt c. (BSC)
    human thrombin c.
    Maalox Therapeutic C.
    therapeutic c. (TC)
concentrated urine
concentration
    albumin plasma c.
    aminothiol c.
    amylase c.
    bile phospholipid c. (BPC)
    blood urea c.
    calcium c.
    chloride c.
    dialysate glucose c.
    endothelin-1 c.
    endothelin-3 c.
    c. epidermal growth factor (cEGF)
    expiratory breath ethanol c.

extrapolated plasma caffeine c.
fasting plasma caffeine c.
fluoroquinolone seminal plasma c.
hepatic iron c. (HIC)
hyaluronic acid c.
hydrogen ion c. (pH)
mean corpuscular hemoglobin c.
  (MCHC)
millimolar c.
minimal inhibitory c. (MIC)
phospholipid-bound choline c.
plasma caffeine c.
plasma-free choline c.
plasma gastrin c.
plasma norepinephrine c.
plasma renin c.
plasma urea c.
predialysis plasma phosphate c.
renal vein renin c. (RVRC)
retinol c.
saturation riboprobe c.
semen sperm c.
serum calcium c.
serum ferritin c.
sodium butyrate c.
spermatozoon c.
subsaturation riboprobe c.
testosterone plasma c.
thyroid hormone serum c.
timed average urea c.
  (TACurea)
total homocysteine plasma c.
total protein c.
urinary c.
urine c.

concentric
c. hyaline inclusion
c. needle
c. needle electrode

concept
evolving c.
exudate-transudate c.
Valsalva leak-point pressure c.

conceptus
c. dose
C. Robust guidewire
C. Soft Seal cervical catheter
C. Soft Torque uterine catheter
C. VS catheter

concern
Rating Form of Inflammatory Bowel
  Disease Patient C.'s (RFIPC)

concomitant
c. antireflux surgery
c. disease
c. hypertension
c. medication effect
c. prolapse

concrement

concretion
bile c.
fecal c.
intestinal c.

concurrent hepatic laceration

concussion
hydraulic abdominal c.

condition
acid-peptic c.
comorbid c.
intersex c.
c. of impaired sodium
  transport
pathologic hypersecretory c.
pathophysiology of c.
physiologic c.
urologic c.

conditioning
c. film
c. film deposition
interceptive c.
semantic c.
c. therapy

condom
c. catheter
c. catheter endoscopic ultrasound
female c.
c. urinal

conductance
potassium c.
selective paracellular c.
urethral electrical c.

conducted current

conduction defect

conductivity
electrical c.

conduit
antirefluxing colonic c.
Bricker ileal c.
colon urinary c.
cutaneous appendiceal c.
ileal urinary c.
jejunal urinary c.
Malone c.
Mitrofanoff c.
nonrefluxing colon c.
sigmoid colon c.
urinary c.
Yang-Monti c.

condyloma, *pl.* **condylomas,**
  condylomata
c. acuminatum
anal c.
flat c.
c. latum
perianal c.
pointed c.

condylomas (*pl. of* condyloma)

condylomata (*pl. of* condyloma)

C

condylomatosis
Condylox
cone
>   c. biopsy
>   Coloplast stoma c.
>   hard sonolucent plastic c.
>   Stone C.
>   vaginal c.

coned cecum
coned-down appearance of colon
cone-shaped cecum
cone-tip catheter
confidence
>   c. interval
>   c. ring

configuration
>   bird-beak c.
>   cartwheel c.
>   golf-hole c.
>   horseshoe c.
>   laparoscopic trocar c.
>   pouch c.
>   rat-tail c.
>   W-pouch c.

confluence
>   high vaginal c.
>   low vaginal c.

confluent hepatic necrosis
confocal
>   c. endomicroscopy
>   c. laser scanning microscopy

conformal radiation therapy
congenital
>   c. adrenal hyperplasia (CAH)
>   c. bifid bladder
>   c. bilateral absence of vas deferens
>   (CBAVD)
>   c. biliary atresia
>   c. biliary cyst
>   c. bladder diverticulum
>   c. chloride diarrhea
>   c. chordee
>   c. cloaca
>   c. curvature
>   c. cystic disease
>   c. cystosis
>   c. diaphragm
>   c. diaphragmatic hernia
>   c. diverticulosis
>   c. double kidney
>   c. duodenal atresia
>   c. enterocele
>   c. enterocyte heparan sulphate
>   deficiency
>   c. epispadias
>   c. esophageal stenosis
>   c. hepatic fibrosis (CHF)
>   c. hydrocele
>   c. hyperbilirubinemia

>   c. hypertrophic pyloric stenosis
>   c. hypoplasia
>   c. intestinal aganglionosis (CIA)
>   c. lactic acidosis
>   c. malrotation of gut
>   c. megacolon
>   c. mesoblastic nephroma
>   c. nephrogenic diabetes insipidus
>   (CNDI)
>   c. nephrosis
>   c. nephrotic syndrome (CNS)
>   c. penile curvature
>   c. penile deviation (CPD)
>   c. polycystic disease (CPD)
>   c. portacaval shunt
>   c. pyloric membrane
>   c. pylorospasm
>   c. renal artery aneurysm
>   c. renal lymphangiectasis
>   c. renal mass
>   c. sodium diarrhea (CSD)
>   c. splenic cyst
>   c. splenomegaly
>   c. ureteral stricture
>   c. ureteropelvic junction
>   obstruction
>   c. urethral stricture
>   c. urethroperineal fistula
>   c. urethrorectal fistula
>   c. urologic abnormality
>   c. uropathy

congenitally altered anatomy
congenitum
>   megacolon c.

congested
>   c. kidney
>   c. mucosa

congestion
>   active c.
>   hepatic c.
>   passive c.
>   renal c.

congestive
>   c. cirrhosis
>   c. hepatomegaly
>   c. hypertensive gastropathy
>   c. splenomegaly

Congo
>   C. red dye
>   C. red stain

congolense
>   *Trypanosoma c.*

congophilic material
congorosa
congruent grade A study
conical
>   c. catheter
>   c. cecum
>   c. centrifuge tube

c. glans
c. trocar
conical-tip electrode
conjoined
c. fiber bundle
c. tendon
conjugate
bilirubin ester c.
bilirubin protein c.
xenobiotic glutathione c.
conjugated
c. bile acid
c. bilirubin
c. estrogen (CE)
c. hyperbilirubinemia
c. linoleic acid (CLA)
conjunctival
c. erythema
c. icterus
ConMed biliary system
connecting tubule
connective
c. tissue
c. tissue disorder
c. tissue-type mast cell
(CTMC)
connector
Luer-Lok c.
T c.
Tuohy-Borst c.
wire-loop c.
Y-port c.
Connell
C. incision
C. stitch
C. suture
connexin 43
conniventes
valvulae c.
Conn syndrome
conorii
Rickettsia c.
Conradi line
Conray 60, 70, 280 contrast material
conscious sedation
Conseal
C. ostomy irrigation set
C. 1-piece continent colostomy
system
consensual reflex
consensus interferon (CIFN)
consequence
metabolic c.
conservation
VP4 protein c.
conservative management
conserved helix-loop-helix ubiquitous kinase (CHUK)

consideration
transplant c.
consistency
doughy c.
consortial approach
consortium
Pediatric Peritoneal Dialysis
Study c.
constant
c. infusion excretory urogram
(CIXU)
Michaelis c.
Constene
constipated
constipation
antepartum c.
atonic c.
chronic functional c.
chronic idiopathic c.
drug-induced c.
functional c.
gastrojejunal c.
geriatric c.
idiopathic c.
intractable c.
outlet obstruction c.
postpartum c.
psychogenic c.
slow-transit c. (STC)
spastic c.
constipation-predominant irritable bowel syndrome
constitutional
c. hepatic dysfunction
c. hyperbilirubinemia
constricting pain
constriction
mesenteric artery c.
c. ring
constrictive pericarditis
construction
Abbe-McIndoe vaginal c.
ileal reservoir c.
Lich ureteral implantation for
neobladder c.
neovagina c.
pelvic ileal reservoir c.
phallic c.
sphincteric c.
U-pouch c.
vaginal c.
constructional apraxia
consult
prompt GI c.
consumption
alcohol c.
EtOH c.
salt c.
whole-cell oxygen c.

C

contact
    c. bleeding
    cell-cell c.
    c. dermatitis
    c. dissolution
    c. laser vaporization
    c. laser vaporization of prostate
      (CLVP)
    c. laxative
    c. lithotripsy
    c. probe
contact-tip laser system
contagiosum
    giant molluscum c.
    molluscum c.
container
    Safe-T-Flex enteral
      feeding c.
contamination
    fecal c.
    c. of food
    c. of water
    postautoclave c.
contemporary urologic
  armamentarium
content
    abdominal c.'s
    bowel c.'s
    brain myoinositol c.
    gastric c.'s
    hepatic malondialdehyde c.
    intestinal c.'s
    luminal c.'s
    mucosal hexosamine c.
    renocortical malondialdehyde c.
    reticulocyte hemoglobin c.
    total glutathione c.
contexture analysis
Contigen
    C. Bard collagen implant
    C. glutaraldehyde crosslinked
      collagen
contiguity
    appendicitis by c.
    spatial c.
contiguous loop
Contimed II pelvic floor muscle
  monitor
continence
    diurnal c.
    fecal c.
    c. nipple
    c. ring
    satisfactory c.
    urinary c.
continence-preserving resection
continent
    c. abdominal wall stoma
    c. anal cap

    c. catheterizable
      appendicovesicostomy using
      Mitrofanoff principle
    c. catheterizable urinary diversion
    c. catheterization reservoir
    c. colostomy
    c. cutaneous appendicocystostomy
    c. cutaneous diversion
    c. cutaneous reservoir
    c. ileal reservoir
    c. ileal reservoir catheterization
      pouch
    c. ileostomy
    c. ileovesicostomy
    c. of stool
    c. supravesical bowel urinary
      diversion
    c. valve
    c. vesicostomy
continuity
    bowel c.
    small-bowel c.
    urinary c.
continuous
    c. ambulatory infusion
    c. ambulatory peritoneal dialysis
      (CAPD)
    c. arteriovenous hemodiafiltration
      (CAVHDF)
    c. arteriovenous hemodialysis
      (CAVHD)
    c. arteriovenous hemofiltration
      (CAVH)
    c. arteriovenous hemofiltration with
      dialysis
    c. arteriovenous ultrafiltration
      (CAVU)
    c. bladder drainage
    c. bladder irrigation (CBI)
    c. catheter drainage
    c. cycler-assisted peritoneal
      dialysis
    c. cycling peritoneal dialysis
      (CCPD)
    c. drip feeding
    c. erythropoiesis receptor activator
      (CERA)
    c. hypothermic pulsatile
      perfusion
    c. incontinence
    c. infusion chemotherapy
    c. murmur
    c. NG suction
    c. prophylaxis
    c. pullthrough technique
    c. renal replacement therapy
      (CRRT)
    c. suction drainage
    c. suture

c. venovenous hemodiafiltration (CVVHDF)
c. venovenous hemodialysis (CVVHD)
c. venovenous hemofiltration (CVVH)

continuous-flow
c.-f. fluorometer
c.-f. resectoscope

continuously perfused probe
ContiRing
contour
c. ERCP cannula
isodose c.
sawtooth irregularity of bowel c.

contraception
contraceptive
c. device
c. pill-induced cholestasia

contractile
c. apparatus
c. ring dysphagia
c. stricture

contractility
normal detrusor c.
ureter c.

contraction
alcohol-induced extracellular volume c.
anal sphincter c.
bladder involuntary c.
clonic c.
crural c.
detrusor c.
fat-induced gallbladder c.
gallbladder c.
giant migrating c. (GMC)
high-amplitude c.
hourglass c.
hunger c.'s
isotonic c.
paradoxical puborectalis c.
peristaltic c.
phase II c.
phasic c.
primary c.
propagated antroduodenal c.
propagation of c.'s
reflex detrusor c.
ringlike c.
secondary c.
sliding filament model of c.
slow phasic c.
sustained detrusor c.
tertiary c.
tonic c.
voluntary sphincter c.

contraction-relaxation cycle
Contractubex gel

contracture
bladder neck c.
postinflammatory c.
severe recurrent bladder neck c.

contradictory result
contraindication
laparoscopy c.
c. to circumcision

Contrajet ERCP contrast delivery system
contralateral
c. reflux
c. testicular biopsy

contrast
c. agent
barium enema with air c.
c. chromoscopy using indigo carmine (CCIC)
Cysto Conray c.
dilute iodinated c.
double c.
dynamic c.
c. enema
c. enhancement
c. esophagography
c. esophagram
c. filling
c. fluid
c. medium
c. selective cholangiogram
Solutrast 300 c.
water-soluble c.

contrast-associated renal failure
contrast-enhanced
c.-e. computed tomography (CECT)
c.-e. endoscopic ultrasonography (CE-EUS)
c.-e. fast sequence (CE-FAST)
c.-e. transabdominal ultrasonography

contrast-induced renal failure (CIRF)
Contreet foam dressing
control
androgen gonadotropin feedback c.
baseline recovered c.
beta-2 microglobulin c.
bleeding c.
c. bridle
electronic pain c.
endoscopic c.
fluoroscopic c.
foot pedal suction c.
gender-matched c.
c. glucose
hemorrhage c.
c. level
neural c.
pain c.
symptom c.

controlled
    c. expansion (CX)
    c. radial expansion (CRE)
controller
    Actis venous flow c.
conus medullaris
ConvaTec
    C. Active Life stoma cap
    C. colostomy pouch
    C. Durahesive Wafer ostomy
    C. Little Ones pediatric ostomy
    product
    C. Sur-Fit Little Ones pouch
    C. Sur-Fit 2-piece pouch
convection
convective transport
Conveen
    C. female intermittent catheter
    C. olive-tip coudé intermittent
    catheter
    C. ultrasecure self-sealing male
    external catheter
conventional
    c. concentric electromyography
    c. cystoscopy
    c. hemodialysis
    c. static scanner
    c. stent
    c. treatment
    c. upper esophagogastroduodenoscopy
    (C-EGD)
Converspaz
convertase
    C3 c.
convexity
convex margin
convolution
    distal c.
Conway Stuart Medical (CSM)
ConXn
COOH-terminal SH2 domain
Cook
    C. biopsy gun
    C. Enforcer
    C. N-Circle tipless stone basket
    C. plastic Luer-Lok adapter
    C. rectal speculum
    C. stent
    C. tissue morcellator
    C. TPN catheter
    C. urologic trocar
Cooke-Apert-Gallais syndrome
coolant
cooled
    c. antenna zone
    c. catheter transurethral microwave
    thermotherapy
    c. catheter TUMT
    c. ThermoCath treatment catheter

cooler
cooling
    external c.
    homogeneous c.
    ice c.
    immersion c.
    nerve c.
    perfusion c.
    surface c.
    transarterial perfusion c.
    urethral c.
    whole body c.
cool-temperature hemodialysis
Cool-tip RF ablation system
Coomassie brilliant blue technique
Coombs test (CT)
Coons/Carey endoprosthesis
Coons guide
Cooper
    C. hernia
    C. herniotome
    C. irritable testis
    C. ligament
    C. ligament hernioplasty
    C. ligament sling
cooperi
    fascia propria c.
coordination
    R-wave c.
copaiba balsam
**Copa Plus ultrasoft foam wound
dressing**
Cope
    C. crushing clamp
    C. loop nephrostomy catheter
    C. loop nephrostomy tube
    C. modification of Martel intestinal
    clamp
    C. sign
    C. viscerotomy anchor
    C. wire
Copegus
copious irrigation
copolymerized substrate
copper
    c. colic
    c. deficiency
    c. deficiency anemia
    c. nephropathy
copper-binding
    c.-b. protein (CBP)
    c.-b. protein test
copracrasia
copremesis
Coprinus **mushroom**
coproantibody
Coprococcus
coprolith
coproma

coproplanesia
coproporphyria
    erythropoietic c. (ECP)
    hereditary c. (HCP)
    variegate c.
coproporphyrin
coprostasis
coracidium
coral calculus
Corbus disease
cord
    Billroth c.
    c. bladder
    genital c.
    gubernacular c.
    hepatic c.
    hepatocytic c.
    c. hydrocele
    inguinal c.
    lipoma of c.
    microsurgical denervation of
      spermatic c.
    nephrogenic c.
    palpable c.
    S c.
    spermatic c.
    c. structure
    tethered spinal c.
    tunic of spermatic c.
    umbilical c.
    vocal c.
Cordis-Hakim shunt
corditis
Cordonnier
    C. technique ureterocolonic
      anastomosis
    C. ureteroileal loop
cordotomy
core
    chylomicron c.
    c. needle biopsy
    c. of tumor
    c. particle
    c. temperature
core-cut system
CoreTherm high-energy device
core-through optical urethrotomy
Corflo
    C. enteral feeding tube
    C. PEG tube
    C. percutaneous access catheter
Corgard
Cori
    C. cycle
    C. disease
CORI
    Clinical Outcomes Research
    Initiative
coriander

coring
    c. out
    uterine c.
coring-out procedure
Corinthian stent
corkscrew
    c. appearance
    c. esophagus
Corlopam
corneae
    Vittaforma c.
corneal
    c. reflex
    c. ulcer
Corneometer MPA5 instrument
corner
    c. suture
    C. tampon
cornerstone immunosuppressant
cornflake esophageal motility test
cornflower
cornstarch-rich diet
cornucopia
    sinusoidal endothelium c.
corona, *pl.* coronae
    c. glandis penis
    c. radiata
coronae (*pl. of* corona)
coronal
    c. adhesion
    c. epispadias
    c. hypospadias
    c. slice
    c. sulcus
coronary
    cafe c.
    c. ligament
    c. sinus
coronavirus
Coronavirus gastroenteritis
Corpak
    C. feeding tube
    C. weighted-tip self-lubricating
    tube
corpora (*pl. of* corpus)
corporal
    c. biopsy
    c. plication procedure
    c. rotation procedure
corporeal
    c. aspiration
    c. fibrosis
    c. reconstruction
    c. sinusoid
    c. venoocclusive dysfunction
corporoplasty
    incisional c.
    modified Essed-Schroeder c.
corporotomy

C

corpus, *pl.* **corpora**
    corpora amylacea
    c. callosum agenesis
    c. cavernosum biopsy
    c. cavernosum dilation
    c. cavernosum muscarinic receptor
    c. cavernosum papaverine injection
    c. cavernosum penile
      electromyography
    c. cavernosum tunica covering
    c. epididymidis
    c. gastricum
    c. gastritis
    Highmore c.
    c. highmori
    c. pancreatis
    c. spongiosum
    c. spongiosum fibrosis
    c. spongiosum hypoplasia
    c. spongiosum penis
    c. ventriculare
    c. ventriculi
    c. vesicae biliaris
    c. vesicae felleae
    c. Wolffi
corpuscle
    Jaworski c.
    juxtamedullary renal c.
    malpighian c.'s
    pacinian c.
    renal c.
Correa gastritis classification
correction
    chordee c.
    Yates c.
Correctol
correlation
    Pearson product c.
    significant c.
    Spearman rank c.
Corrigan pulse
corrosive
    c. esophageal stricture
    c. esophagitis
    c. gastritis
Corson
    C. needle
    C. needle electrosurgical probe
Cortef
Cortenema retention enema
cortex, *pl.* **cortices**
    aberrant suprarenal c.
    adrenal c.
    fetal adrenal c.
    c. glandulae suprarenalis
    kidney c.
    renal c.
    total measured renal c.
Corticaine

cortical
    c. abscess
    c. adenoma
    c. arch
    c. carcinoma
    c. collecting duct (CCD)
    c. collecting tubule (CCT)
    c. interstitial volume fraction
    c. labyrinth
    c. loss
cortices (*pl. of* cortex)
corticoadenoma
    adrenal c.
corticoadrenal
    renal c.
corticomedullary
    c. demarcation
    c. differentiation
    c. junction
corticosteroid
    c. regulation of amiloride-sensitive
      sodium channel subunit
    c. therapy
    c. treatment
corticotropin
corticotropin-releasing hormone (CRH)
Cortifoam
cortisol
    c. hypersecretion
    c. metabolism
    plasma c. (PC)
    urinary c.
cortisone acetate
Cortisporin
Cortone Acetate
Cortrophin-Zinc
Cortrosyn stimulation test
corymbifera
    Absidia c.
    Mucor c.
Corynebacterium
    C. minutissimum
    C. parvum
    C. tenuis
cosecreted cation
cosine curve
cosinor
    c. analysis
    c. rhythmometry
Cosmegen
cosmesis
cost
    c. effectiveness of therapy
    c. of therapy
costal margin
COSTART
    Coding Systems for a Thesaurus of
    Adverse Reaction Terms
    COSTART system

cost-conscious healthcare system
cost-effective care
Costello
    C. laser ablation of prostate
    C. protocol
costive
costiveness
costochondral
    c. junction
    c. tenderness
costocolic fold
costophrenic blunting
costovertebral
    c. angle tenderness (CVAT)
    c. ligament
    c. sulcus
cosyntropin stimulation test
Cotazym-S
cotransporter
    chloride-cation c. (CCC)
    c. mRNA
    NaCl c. (NCC)
    NA+-glucose c.
    Na-KCl c. (NKCC)
    taurine c. (TCT)
Cotrim
cotrimoxazole
cotton
    C. cannulatome
    C. classification
    levan c.
    Oxycel c.
    C. sphincterotome
    c. suture
    c. swab test
    c. tree
Cotton-Huibregtse double-pigtail stent
Cotton-Leung biliary stent
cottonseed oil
cotton-tipped applier
cotton-wool spot (CWS)
coudé catheter
cough stress test
Couinaud liver anatomy classification
Coulter automated autoanalyzer
Coumadin
coumarin
    c. dye laser
    c. flashlamp-pumped pulsed-dye laser
    c. green tunable dye laser lithotripsy
coumestrol
Councill catheter
Councilman
    C. body
    C. lesion
Council-tip tube

count
    Addis c.
    CD4 lymphocyte c.
    CD4+ T-cell c.
    CD8 lymphocyte c.
    cell c.
    colony c.
    complete blood c. (CBC)
    granulocyte c.
    hemolysis, elevated liver enzymes, and low platelet c. (HELLP)
    instrument c.
    lymphocyte c.
    mitosis c.
    needle c.
    c.'s per minute (cpm, CPM)
    peripheral leukocyte c.
    platelet c.
    red blood cell c.
    sponge c.
    too numerous to c. (TNTC)
    white blood cell c.
    whole crypt mitotic c.
counter
    LKB-Wallac scintillation c.
    RackBeta scintillation c.
countercurrent
    c. exchange
    c. mechanism
    c. multiplication
    c. multiplier
    c. multiplier principle
counterirritation
counterstaining
    sequential c.
countertransporter
    sodium-lithium c. (SLC)
coup de sabre
coupling
    capacitive c.
    electromechanical c.
    excitation-contraction c.
    pharmacomechanical c.
    slow-wave c.
    c. stoichiometry
Courtney
    deep postanal space of C.
    C. space
Courvoisier
    C. gallbladder
    C. gastroenterostomy
    C. law
    C. sign
Courvoisier-Terrier syndrome
couvade syndrome
Couvelaire ileourethral anastomosis
CovaClear Ag antimicrobial wound dressing
covalently closed circular DNA (cccDNA)

cover
    Foxy pouch c.
    laparotomy pad c.
    Nu-Hope pouch c.
    pad c.
    Sur-Fit pouch c.
covered
    c. biliary metal stent
    c. self-expanding prosthesis
covering
    Camwrap plastic c.
    corpus cavernosum tunica c.
    Permalume c.
Cowan 1 strain
Cowden
    C. disease
    C. syndrome
Cowdry type A inclusion body
Cowen sign
Cowper
    C. cyst
    C. gland
    C. syringocele
cow's
    c. milk allergy (CMA)
    c. milk protein allergy
    c. milk-sensitive enteropathy
    (CMSE)
cowslip
COX
    cyclooxygenase
    COX enzyme system
    COX mRNA
    COX regression model
COX-1
    cyclooxygenase-1
    COX-1 enzyme
    COX-1 inhibition
COX-2
    cyclooxygenase-2
    COX-2 enzyme
    COX-2 inhibition
    COX-2 inhibitor
    COX-2 selective nonsteroidal
    antiinflammatory drug
Coxiella burnetii
Cox-Mantel test
coxsackievirus infection A, B
CP
    chronic pancreatitis
    chronic pyelonephritis
    CP test
CPA
    cyproterone acetate
CPC
    choroid plexus cyst
CPD
    congenital penile deviation
    congenital polycystic disease

CP-EUS
    catheter probe-assisted endoluminal
    ultrasonography
CPH
    chronic persistent hepatitis
CPH-CAH
    chronic persistent hepatitis-chronic
    active hepatitis
    CPH-CAH cirrhosis
CPK
    creatine phosphokinase
C-plasty
cpm, CPM
    counts per minute
CPN
    celiac plexus neurolysis
    chronic pyelonephritis
    cisplatin nephropathy
    EUS CPN
CPP
    cerebral perfusion pressure
CPPS
    chronic pelvic pain syndrome
    chronic prostate pain syndrome
C1q nephropathy
CR1
    complement receptor type 1
CRA
    colorectal anastomosis
cracker test
cradle
    acoustically transparent c.
Crafoord thoracic scissors
Cragg
    C. Endopro System I stent
    C. thrombolytic brush
cramp
CRAMP
    Cathelin-related antimicrobial
    peptide
crampy abdominal pain
cranberry
    alpine c.
crane-neck deformity
cranesbill
cranial
    c. mesonephros
    c. pole
craniocaudad (*var. of* craniocaudal)
craniocaudal, craniocaudad
Cranley phleborheography
crapulent colic
crapulous diarrhea
crassi
    folliculi lymphatici solitarii
    intestini c.
crater
    ulcer c.
Crawford clamp

CRBI, CR-BSI, CRBSI
    catheter-related bloodstream
      infection
CRC
    colorectal cancer
    colorectal carcinoma
CRCC
    cystic renal cell carcinoma
Crcl
    creatinine clearance
CRE
    controlled radial expansion
      CRE balloon catheter
C-reactive protein (CRP)
cream, creme
      Analpram-HC anorectal c.
      Ca-Rezz moisture barrier c.
      Dermovate c.
      lidocaine-prilocaine c.
      Proctocort c.
      Prudoxin c.
      rectal c.
      Sween 24 superior moisturizing skin
       protectant c.
      Topicort c.
      triamcinolone c.
crease
      inguinal c.
      midline abdominal c.
      skin c.
      torso c.
creatine phosphokinase (CPK)
creatinine
      c. clearance (Crcl)
      c. height index (CHI)
      plasma c.
      pretreatment serum c.
      c. production
      serum c. (SCr)
      c. test
      urinary albumin to c. (UA/C)
creation
      diverting stoma c.
      Politano-Leadbetter tunnel c.
      tunnel c.
creatorrhea
Credé placental removal
 maneuver
^{51}Cr-EDTA
      51-chromium-labeled
      ethylenediaminetetraacetate
      ^{51}Cr-EDTA excretion
creep
      ureter c.
creeping of mesenteric fat
Creevy evacuator
cremaster
      Henle internal c.
      c. muscle

cremasteric
      c. artery
      c. fascia
      c. fiber
      c. muscle
      c. reflex
      c. vessel
creme (*var. of* cream)
Cremer-Ikeda papillotome
cremnocele
crenate margin
Creon 10, 20
crepitus
crescendoing bowel sounds
crescent
      c. fold
      c. gastric cardia
      glomerular c.
      c. snare
crescentic
      c. body
      c. fold disease
      c. glomerulonephritis
      c. nephritis
C-resistance
Crespo operation
cress
      garden c.
crest
      cupula of ampullary c.
      c. factor
      haustral c.
      iliac c.
      jejunal c.
      urethral c.
CREST
      calcinosis cutis, Raynaud phenomenon,
       esophageal motility disorder,
       sclerodactyly, and telangiectasia
      CREST syndrome
Creutzfeldt-Jakob disease
crevicular fluid
CRF
    chronic renal failure
CRH
    corticotropin-releasing hormone
CRI
    chronic renal insufficiency
cricoid
      c. aneurysm
      c. myotomy
cricomyotomy
cricopharyngeal
      c. achalasia
      c. bar
      c. diverticulum
      c. myotomy
      c. spasm
      c. sphincter

C

cricopharyngeus muscle
Crigler-Najjar
    C.-N. disease
    C.-N. jaundice
    C.-N. syndrome type I, II
Crile
    C. angle retractor
    C. appendix clamp
    C. bile duct forceps
    C. gall duct forceps
    C. hemostat
    C. hemostatic clamp
    C. malleable retractor
    C. nerve hook
Crile-Wood needle holder
criminal nerve
crinogenic
crises (*pl. of* crisis)
crisis, *pl.* **crises**
    abdominal c.
    Addison c.
    adrenal c.
    Dietl c.
    gastric c.
    scleroderma renal c.
crista, *pl.* **cristae**
    c. urethralis
    c. urethralis masculinae
    c. urethralis virilis
cristae (*pl. of* crista)
cristate margin
criteria (*pl. of* criterion)
criterion, *pl.* **criteria**
    Amsterdam criteria
    Bosniak criteria
    Child classification of hepatic risk
      criteria A-C
    Child liver criteria
    Child-Pugh criteria
    clinicobiological criteria
    DeMeester criteria
    evidence-based criteria
    Foley criteria
    criteria for grading of clinical
      studies and recommendations
    Forrest criteria
    Ganau criteria
    Harvey and Bradshaw criteria
    histopathologic criteria
    Hogan/Geenen criteria
    King's College ALF criteria
    Lown criteria
    Manning criteria
    manometric criteria
    morphometric criteria
    Munich inclusion criteria
    O'Duffy criteria
    Pugh modification of Child criteria
    Rome criteria I, II

    Ranson criteria
    Savary-Miller criteria
    variceal size inclusion criteria
    well-defined anatomical entry criteria
critical diarrhea
Criticare HN elemental liquid feeding
Crit-Line instrument
Crix belly
Crixivan lithiasis
[51]Cr-labeled
    ^{51}Cr-l. albumin clearance
    ^{51}Cr-l. EDTA
crochet knot
Crohn
    C. and Colitis Foundation of
      America (CCFA)
    C. and Colitis Knowledge
      (CCKNOW)
    C. colitis
    C. disease (CD)
    C. Disease Activity Index (CDAI)
    C. Disease Endoscopic Index of
      Severity (CDEIS)
    C. disease of colon (CDC)
    C. duodenal ulcer
    C. duodenitis
    C. ileitis
    C. ileocolitis
    C. regional enteritis
    C. small intestine
cromakalim
cromoglycate
    disodium c.
    sodium c.
cromolyn sodium
Cronkhite-Canada syndrome
Crosby capsule
Crosby-Kugler capsule for biopsy
cross
    gastrointestinal c.
    Maltese c.
    c. vasovasotomy
crossbar
    c. deformity
    inner c.
    outer c.
    c. symptom of Frankel
crossbridge
    c. cycle
    dephosphorylated myosin c.
    myosin c.
cross-clamped (*var. of* crossclamped)
crossclamped, cross-clamped
Crosseal fibrin sealant
crossed
    c. renal ectopia
    c. testicular ectopia
crossfolding
crosshatch mark

crossmatch
> flow cytometry c. (FCXM)
> T-cell c.

crossmatched blood
crossover vasectomy
cross-phosphorylation
crossreactive group
crossreactivity
> direct c.

cross-section
> c.-s. of collecting duct
> prostate gland c.-s.

cross-sectional
crosstalk
> receptor c.

crosstriagonal repair
cross-trigonal
> c.-t. repair
> c.-t. tunnel

Crotalaria
croton
> C. lechleri
> C. lechleri tree
> c. seed

croupous
> c. cystitis
> c. membrane
> c. nephritis

CR/OV
> colorectal/ovarian
> OncoScint CR/OV

crowding
> variable nuclear c.

crow's-foot pattern
CRP
> chronic relapsing pancreatitis
> C-reactive protein

CRRT
> continuous renal replacement therapy

CRS
> Cell Recovery System
> cherry red spot
> Chinese restaurant syndrome
> colorectal surgery

CRST
> calcinosis cutis, Raynaud phenomenon, sclerodactyly, and telangiectasia
> CRST syndrome

CR326 strain
CRT
> chemoradiation therapy

cruciate incision
cruciferous vegetable
crude
> c. drug
> c. incidence rate
> c. urine

cruentes
> vomitus c.

crunch
> mediastinal c.
> c. stick anastomosis

crura (*pl. of* crus)
crural
> c. banding
> c. contraction
> c. fold
> c. fossa
> c. vein
> c. venous leakage

crus, *pl.* **crura,** *gen.* **cruris**
> c. of diaphragm
> penile c.
> c. penis
> tinea cruris

crush
> c. kidney
> c. syndrome

crusher
crutched
> c. stick-type biliary duct stent
> c. stick-type polyurethane endoprosthesis

Cruveilhier
> C. disease
> C. sign
> C. ulcer

Cruveilhier-Baumgarten
> C.-B. anomaly
> C.-B. cirrhosis
> C.-B. murmur
> C.-B. sign
> C.-B. syndrome

Cruz-Chagas disease
cruzi
> *Trypanosoma c.*

cryaerophilus
> *Arcobacter c.*

cryoablation
> Endocare renal c.
> c. for prostate cancer
> laparoscopic c.
> renal c.
> salvage c.

cryofibrinogenemia
cryogenic ablation
cryoglobulinemia
> essential mixed c.
> mixed essential c.
> type II c.

cryoneedle
> SeedNet Gold ultrathin c.
> c. technology

cryoprecipitate
cryoprecipitated plasma
cryopreservation
> sperm c.
> spermatozoon c.

C

cryoprobe
cryoprostatectomy
cryospray
cryostat
    c. tissue section
    Tissue Tek-II c.
cryosurgery
cryosurgical
    c. ablation
    c. ablation of prostate (CSAP)
cryotherapy
    endoscopic spray c.
CryoVein SG tissue-engineered vascular graft
crypt
    c. abscess
    anal c.
    c. architectural distortion
    c. architecture
    c. atrophy
    c. base
    branched c.
    c. cell
    c. cell apoptosis
    c. defensin
    c. epithelium
    forked c.
    c. hook
    c. hyperplasia
    c. hypertrophy
    ileal c.
    c. intraepithelial lymphocyte (cIEL)
    Lieberkühn c.
    Luschka c.
    Morgagni c.
    mucous c.
    multilocular c.
    c. of Haller
    c. of Littré
Cryptaz
cryptdin
cryptdin-related sequence (CRS)
cryptectomy
cryptitis
    neutrophilic c.
cryptococcal pyelonephritis
cryptococcosis
    adrenal c.
    genital c.
    prostatic c.
    renal c.
Cryptococcus neoformans
cryptogenic
    c. chronic hepatitis
    c. cirrhosis
    c. hypertransaminasemia
    c. liver disease
cryptoglandular

cryptolith
cryptorchidectomy
cryptorchidism, cryptorchism
    abdominal c.
    bilateral c.
    canalicular c.
    ectopic c.
    femoral c.
    inguinal c.
    nonpalpable c.
    pediatric c.
    c. torsion
cryptorchidopexy
cryptorchism (*var. of* cryptorchidism)
cryptosporidial infection
cryptosporidiosis
    biliary c.
Cryptosporidium
    C. muris
    C. oocyst
    C. parvum
    C. species
Cryptosporidium-induced diarrhea
crypt-villus
    c.-v. axis
    c.-v. site
    c.-v. unit
crystal
    c. attachment
    c. binding
    Boettcher c.
    $CaCO_3$ c.
    calcium oxalate monohydrate c.
    cholesterol monohydrate c.
    cystine c.
    c. morphology
    oxalate c.
    phosphate c.
    piezoelectric c.
    quick-dissolving c.
    Reinke c.
    c. retention
    thymol c.
    triple-phosphate c.
    urate c.
    uric acid c.
    urinary c.
    c. violet chromoendoscopy
crystal-cell interaction
crystallization
    c. abnormality
    calcium oxalate c.
crystallography
    optic c.
    x-ray c.
crystalloid
    hypertonic c.
    c. solution
crystalluria

crystalluridrosis
crystal-phospholipid interaction
C&S
>   culture and sensitivity
>> C&S test

CSAP
>   cryosurgical ablation of prostate

CS-5 cryosurgical system
CSD
>   congenital sodium diarrhea

CSE
>   complete surgical exploration

C18 Sep-Pack column
CSF
>   cerebrospinal fluid
>   colony-stimulating factor
>> CSF glucose
>> CSF glutamine
>> CSF glutamine test
>> CSF protein

CSF-1
>   colony-stimulating factor-1

CSG
>   chronic superficial gastritis

CSI
>   cholesterol saturation index

CSM
>   Conway Stuart Medical
>> CSM Stretta system

CT
>   computed tomography
>   computerized tomography
>> CT colonography
>> CT during arterial portography (CTAP)
>> helical CT
>> renal helical CT (RHCT)
>> CT scan
>> CT scan with contrast enhancement
>> spiral CT
>> CT Twin scanner
>> unenhanced helical CT

CTA
>   computed tomographic angiography

CTAP
>   computed tomography during arterial portography
>   CT during arterial portography

CTAS
>   colonic transabdominal sonography

CTC
>   Child-Turcotte classification
>   computed tomographic colonography

Ctenochaetus strigosus
C-terminal propeptide of type I procollagen
CT-guided
>> CT-g. abscess drainage
>> CT-g. celiac plexus neurolysis

>> CT-g. fine-needle aspiration
>> CT-g. liver biopsy
>> CT-g. needle aspiration biopsy
>> CT-g. PEG
>> CT-g. percutaneous endoscopic gastrostomy
>> CT-g. pseudocyst drainage

CTHA
>   computerized tomographic hepatic angiography

CTL
>   cytolytic T lymphocyte
>   cytotoxic T lymphocyte

CTL-mediated lysis
CTMC
>   connective tissue-type mast cell

CTP
>   Child-Turcotte-Pugh
>> CTP classification

CTPV
>   cavernous transformation of portal vein

C-Trak
>> C-T. analyzer
>> C-T. handheld gamma detector
>> C-T. probe
>> C-T. surgical guidance system

^{14}C-triolein breath test
CTS
>   Collaborative Transplant Study

C-type
>> C-t. atrial natriuretic peptide (C-ANP)
>> C-t. natriuretic peptide (CNP)

cube
>   Gelfoam c.

cubilin
cuboidal epithelium
Cub R-200 enteral feeding pump
^{13}C-UBT
>   carbon-13 urea breath test

^{14}C-UBT
>   carbon-14 urea breath test

CUC
>   chronic ulcerative colitis

Cucurbita pepo
cuff
>   c. abscess
>   AS-800 c.
>   bladder c.
>   columnar c.
>   c. electrode
>   laparoscopic extravesical bladder c.
>   rectal muscle c.
>   suprahepatic caval c.
>   vaginal c.

cuffed
>   c. endotracheal tube
>   c. esophageal endoprosthesis

cuffitis
cul-de-sac
c.-d.-s. fluid
c.-d.-s. mass
c.-d.-s. of Douglas
culdocentesis
culdoplasty
McCall c.
culdoscope
culdoscopy
Culp
C. spiral flap pyeloplasty
C. ureteropelvioplasty
Culp-DeWeerd
C.-D. spiral flap pyeloplasty
C.-D. ureteropyeloplasty
culture
aerobic c.
allogenic mixed leukocyte c.
anaerobic c.
c. and sensitivity (C&S)
c. and sensitivity test
bacterial c.
blood c.
calculus c.
fluid c.
glomerular cell c.
hanging-drop c.
keratinocyte serum-free medium c.
c. medium
mixed growth on c.
mixed leukocyte c. (MLC)
c. of biopsy specimen
semiquantitative c.
shell vial c.
stool c.
tissue c.
Transwell cell c.
urine c.
viral c.
cultured rat mesangial cell
Culturelle
culture-negative neutrocytic ascites (CNNA)
cumin
cumuli (*pl. of* cumulus)
cumulative damage hypothesis
cumulus, *pl.* **cumuli**
Cunningham-Cotton sleeve coaxial dilator
Cunninghamella
Cunningham urinary incontinence clamp
CUOG
Canadian Urology Oncology Group
cup
Bard alligator c.
Bard oval c.
c. bladder biopsy

ileostomy c.
stone c.
vaginal fistula c.
cup-and-spill stomach
cupola (*var. of* cupula)
cup-patch ileocystoplasty technique
Cuprimine
cupriuresis
cuprophane membrane
cupula, cupola, *pl.* **cupulae**
gas c.
c. of ampullary crest
cupulae (*pl. of* cupula)
CUR
chronic urinary retention
Curasorb
C. dressing
C. zinc dressing
curative tumor resection
Curcuma longa
curd
alum c.
^{13}C-urea
synthetic ^{13}C-u.
C-urea breath excretion
curet (*var. of* curette)
curette, curet
Spratt c.
C-urinary excretion
Curity
C. irrigation tray
C. Mono-Flo antireflux device
C. Ultramer Foley catheter
Curl Cath catheter
curling
esophageal c.
C. ulcer
Curran syndrome
currant
black c.
c. jelly stool
Currarino triad
current
blended c.
coagulating c.
conducted c.
cutting c.
c. density
electrocoagulating c.
electrosurgical c.
high-frequency electrosurgical c.
membrane c.
Olympus PSD-10 electrosurgical blend c.
pure cutting c.
c. treatment modality
Curschmann disease
curtsy
Vincent c.

curvatura (*var. of* curvature),
  pl. **curvaturae**
  c. gastrica major
  c. gastrica minor
  c. ventriculi major
  c. ventriculi minor
curvature, curvatura
  congenital penile c.
  c. of stomach
  penile c.
curve
  angulus on lesser c.
  anion-cation secretory c.
  cosine c.
  disease-free survival c.
  gallbladder emptying-refilling c.
  Kaplan-Meier c.
  learning c.
  loss of sigmoid c.
  c. of stream
  sigmoid c.
  time-activity c.
  time-concentration c.
  triphasic cystometric c.
curved
  c. bacillus
  c. dissecting forceps
  c. end-to-end anastomosis
    (CEEA)
  c. flank position
  c. hemostat
  c. linear array
  c. linear-array echoendoscope
  c. Maryland forceps
  c. Mayo clamp
  c. Mayo scissors
  c. transjugular needle
curved-array
  c.-a. echoendoscope
  c.-a. transducer
curved-needle surgeon's knot
curvilinear scanning echoendoscope
Curvularia lunata
CUSA
  Cavitron ultrasonic surgical aspirator
  CUSA dissector
Cushing
  C. disease
  C. forceps
  C. medicamentosus syndrome
  C. suture
  C. ulcer
  C. vein retractor
cushingoid facies
Cushing-Rokitansky ulcer
cushion
  air c.
  GasBGon filter seat c.
  hemorrhoidal c.

  partial water bath and water c.
  Positron Plus c.
  c. sign
  tissue c.
  Waffle bariatric seat c.
Custom Ultrasonic automatic reprocessor
cut
  blended c.
  electrosurgical c.
  field c.
  c. surface of liver
  c. waveform
  c. waveform desiccation
cut-and-push method of PEG tube
  removal
cutaneobiliary fistula
cutaneous
  c. advancement flap
  c. appendiceal conduit
  c. collateral circulation
  c. dropsy
  c. EGG
  c. electrical field stimulation
  c. electrogastrogram
  c. hemangioma
  c. horn of penis
  c. hyperesthesia
  c. ileocystostomy
  c. lesion
  c. lichen amyloidosis
  c. loop ureterostomy
  c. metastasis
  c. pyelostomy
  c. recording
  c. reflex
  c. schistosomiasis japonica
  c. T-cell lymphoma
  c. urinary diversion
  c. vesicostomy
cutback
  c. anoplasty
  vaginal c.
cutback-type vaginoplasty
cutdown liver
cuticular flap
Cutinova
  C. cavity
  C. foam
  C. Hydro
  C. Hydro Thin
cutis laxa
cutter
  Endopath endoscopic linear c.
  linear-array staple c.
  linear staple c.
  Nu-Hope hole c.
  Proximate linear c.
  rib c.
  suture c.

C

cutting
    c. current
    c. electrode
    c. endoscopic mucosal resection (C-EMR)
    c. LR needle
    c. wire
CVAT
    costovertebral angle tenderness
CVI, CVID
    common variable immunodeficiency
CVM
    childhood visceral myopathy
    circular vesicomyotomy
CVP
    central venous pressure
CVS
    clean-voided specimen
    cyclic vomiting syndrome
CVVH
    continuous venovenous hemofiltration
CVVHD
    continuous venovenous hemodialysis
CVVHDF
    continuous venovenous hemodiafiltration
CV-1 videoscope
CW
    clustered waves
CWS
    cotton-wool spot
CX
    controlled expansion
    CX Plus prosthesis
CXM prosthesis
C282Y
    C282Y hemochromatosis
    C282Y mutation
cyanate
    urea-derived c.
cyanide
    potassium c.
cyanoacrylate
    c. glue
    c. injection
    N-butyl c.
2-cyanoacrylate
    isobutyl 2-c.
***Cyanobacterium*-like body**
cyanocobalamin
    c. injection
    c. radioactive agent
cyanosis
    enterogenous c.
cyanotic kidney
cybernetic regulation of blood pressure
cyclamate
cyclase
    adenylate c.
    guanylate c.
    guanylyl c.
    ligand-triggered membrane guanylate c.
cycle
    biliary c.
    contraction-relaxation c.
    Cori c.
    crossbridge c.
    cyclin/PCNA during cell c.
    diurnal c.
    gastric c.
    glutathione redox c.
    Krebs c.
    liver-adipose tissue c.
    Schiff biliary c.
    tricarboxylic acid c.
    urea c.
cycler
    Perkin-Elmer thermal c.
cyclic, cyclical
    c. adenosine monophosphate (AMP-c, cAMP)
    c. guanosine monophosphate (cGMP)
    c. proteinuria
    c. urinary disinfectant
    c. vomiting
    c. vomiting syndrome (CVS)
5′-cyclic
    5′-c. adenosine monophosphate (cAMP)
    5′-c. guanosine monophosphate (cGMP)
cyclical (*var. of* cyclic)
cyclin
cyclin-dependent
    c.-d. kinase (CDK)
    c.-d. kinase inhibitor
cycling dialysis
cyclin/PCNA during cell cycle
cyclizine
cyclobenzaprine
cyclocytidine
Cyclogyl
cycloheximide
cyclohexylchloroethylnitrosurea (CCNU)
cyclooxygenase (COX)
    c. inhibition
    c. inhibitor
    c. messenger ribonucleoprotein acid (COX mRNA)
    c. metabolite
    c. mRNA
    c. pathway
cyclooxygenase-1 (COX-1)
cyclooxygenase-2 (COX-2)
    c.-2 inhibitor
    c.-2 selective nonsteroidal antiinflammatory drug
cyclooxygenase-dependent mechanism

cyclopentamine
cyclophosphamide
    escalated methotrexate, vinblastine,
      Adriamycin, cisplatin or c.
      (E-MVAC)
    5-fluorouracil, Adriamycin, c. (FAC)
    cyclophosphamide, Velban,
      actinomycin D, bleomycin, platinum
    vincristine, Adriamycin, c. (VAC)
cycloserine
Cyclospora
    C. cayetanensis
    coccidian *C.*
cyclosporin
    c. A-induced hepatotoxicity
cyclosporine, cyclosporin A
    c. arteriolopathy
    c. for microemulsion
    c. nephrotoxicity
    c. toxicity
    c. tubulopathy
    withdrawal of c.
cyclosporine-induced optic neuropathy
Cyclotrac-SP radioimmunoassay
cycrimine
cylinder
    AMA inflatable c.
    AMS penile prosthesis c.
    banding c.
    Bence Jones c.
    high-pressure inflatable prosthesis c.
    inflated rubber c.
    Mentor Bioflex c.
    suction c.
    Ultrex c.
cylindrical
    c. balloon
    c. confronting cisterna (CCC)
    c. diffuser
    c. mucosal resection
cylindromatosis gene
cylindruria
Cymed Micro Skin 1-piece drainage pouch
CYP
    cyproheptadine
    CYP isoenzyme
CyPat treatment
cypionate
    c. ester
    testosterone c.
cypress spurge
cyproheptadine (CYP)
cyproterone acetate (CPA)
cyst
    adrenal gland c.
    adventitious c.
    air c.
    allantoic c.

    alveolar hydatid c.
    Bartholin c.
    bile duct c.
    biliary c.
    Bowman space c.
    branchiogenous c.
    choledochal c. grades I, II, III, IV, IVa
    choroid plexus c. (CPC)
    chyle c.
    ciliated foregut c.
    cluster of grapelike c.'s
    CMV inclusion c.
    compound c.
    congenital biliary c.
    congenital splenic c.
    Cowper c.
    daughter c.
    dermoid c.
    duplication c.
    Echinococcus liver c.
    endoscopic management of choledochal c.
    Entamoeba coli c.
    enteric c.
    enterogenous c.
    epidermal c.
    epidermoid c.
    epididymal c.
    esophageal duplication c.
    extramucosal c.
    extraparenchymal renal c.
    false c.
    fatty c.
    c. fenestration
    Gartner duct c.
    gas c.
    gastric duplication c.
    glomerular c.
    granddaughter c.
    grapelike c.
    hepatic echinococcal c.
    hydatid c.
    ileal duplication c.
    inclusion c.
    intraluminal c.
    intratesticular c.
    isolated c.
    junctional c.
    kidney c.
    lucent c.
    macroscopic liver c.
    median raphe c.
    mesenteric c.
    mother c.
    müllerian duct c.
    multilocular c.
    multiloculated c.
    neoplastic c.

cyst (*continued*)
    noncommunicating biliary c.
    nonepithelial c.
    nonparasitic splenic c.
    omental c.
    ovarian dermoid c.
    pancreatic c.
    parapelvic c.
    parasitic c.
    paraurethral c.
    parovarian c.
    penile c.
    peripelvic c.
    pilonidal c.
    presacral c.
    prosthetic utricle c.
    c. puncture device
    pyelocalyceal c.
    pyelogenic renal c.
    renal sinus c.
    retention c.
    retrorectal c.
    Rosen c.
    sacrococcygeal pilonidal c.
    scrotal inclusion c.
    scrotum c.
    sebaceous c.
    secondary c.
    seminal vesicle hydatid c.
    simple renal c.
    solitary hepatic c.
    sterile c.
    suburethral epithelial inclusion c.
    tailgut c.
    Tarlov c.
    testicular c.
    tunic c.
    tunica albuginea c.
    unicameral c.
    unilocular ovarian c.
    urachal c.
    urethral c.
    urinary c.
    vitellointestinal c.
cystadenocarcinoma
    biliary c.
    pancreatic mucinous c.
    stage III papillary serous c.
cystadenoma
    biliary c.
    ductal c.
    duct-ectatic mucinous c.
    endoscopic ultrasound-guided ethanol
      lavage of pancreatic c.
    glycogen-rich c.
    hepatic c.
    macrocystic pancreatic c.
    mucinous c.
    ruptured appendiceal c.

Cystagon
cystalgia
cystamine
Cysta-Q
cystathionine gamma lyase
cystatin C
cystatrophia
cysteamine bitartrate
cysteamine-induced duodenal ulcer
cystectasia, cystectasy
cystectasy (*var. of* cystectasia)
cystectomy
    extraperitoneal partial c.
    intraperitoneal partial c.
    palliative c.
    partial c.
    pilonidal c.
    radical c.
    renal c.
    salvage c.
    simple c.
    subtrigonal c.
    supratrigonal c.
    total c.
cysteine
    c. *Brucella* broth
    c. sulfinic acid
cysteinyl leukotriene
cystelcosis
cystendesis
cystenterostome
    diathermic c.
cystenterostomy
    direct c.
    endoscopic c.
cysterethism
cystgastrostomy
cysthypersarcosis
cystic
    c. artery
    c. bile
    c. cystitis
    c. degeneration
    c. dilation
    c. duct (CD)
    c. duct angiogram
    c. duct catheterization
    c. duct cholangiocatheter
    c. duct cholangiogram
    c. duct cholangiography
    c. duct choledochoscopy
    c. duct leakage
    c. duct lumen
    c. duct stenosis
    c. duct stone
    c. echinococcosis
    c. epithelial proliferation
    c. fibrosis (CF)
    c. fibrosis gene probe

c. fibrosis transductance regulator
c. fibrosis transmembrane
   conductance regulator (CFTR)
c. hamartoma
c. liver disease
c. mass
c. nephroma
c. plexus
c. puncture
c. renal cell carcinoma (CRCC)
c. Wilms tumor

cystica
cholecystitis c.
cystitis c.
pyelitis c.
pyeloureteritis c.
ureteritis c.
urethritis c.

cystic-choledochal junction
cysticerci (*pl. of* cysticercus)
cysticercosis
cysticercus, *pl.* **cysticerci**
   C. bovis
   C. cellulosae
   c. disease
cysticohepatic junction
cysticolithectomy
cysticolithotripsy
cysticorrhaphy
cysticotomy
cysticus
ductus c.
polypus c.
cystidoceliotomy (*var. of*
   cystidolaparotomy)
cystidolaparotomy, cystidoceliotomy
cystine
c. calculus
c. composition
c. crystal
c. dimethylester (CDE)
c. metabolism
c. stone
c. supersaturation
c. urolithiasis
cystinosis
neuropathic c.
cystinuria
cystinuric
c. child
c. patient
cystis fellea
Cystistat
cystistaxis, cystostaxis
cystitis
acute hemorrhagic c. (AHC)
allergic c.
amicrobic c.
bacterial c.

candidal c.
catarrhal c.
chemical c.
coccidioidal c.
c. colli
croupous c.
cystic c.
c. cystica
diagnosing interstitial c.
dimethyl sulfate c.
diphtheritic c.
DMSO c.
c. emphysematosa
emphysematous c.
eosinophilic c.
exfoliative c.
follicular c.
c. follicularis
gangrenous c.
glandular c.
c. glandularis
hemorrhagic c.
honeymoon c.
Hunner interstitial c.
incrusted c.
interstitial c.
mechanical c.
nonbacterial c. (NBC)
nonulcerative interstitial c.
panmural c.
papillary c.
radiation c.
recurrent c.
reservoir of underdiagnosed and
   misdiagnosed interstitial c.
c. senilis feminarum
subacute c.
submucous c.
sympathetic c.
uncomplicated c.
viral c.
xanthogranulomatous c.
cystitis-causing strain
cystitome (*var. of* cystotome)
Cysto
C. Conray contrast
C. Flex stent
Urovist C.
Cystocath
cystocele
central c.
grade 4 c.
lateral c.
cystochrome
cystochromoscopy
cystocolostomy
cystocolpoproctography
fluoroscopic c.
cystodiaphanoscopy

C

cystodiathermy
> flexible c.

cystodistention

cystodiverticulum

cystoduodenostomy (CDY)
> endoscopic c.

cystodynia

cystoenterocele

cystoenterostomy

cystoepiplocele

cystoepithelioma

cystofiberscope, cystofibroscope
> Olympus c.

cystofibroma

cystofibroscope (*var. of* cystofiberscope)

cystogastric fistula

cystogastrostomy (CGY)
> endoscopic ultrasound-guided c.
> surgical c.

cystogastrotome

cystogenic chemical

cystogram
> air c.
> chain c.
> excretory c. (XC)
> gravity c.
> micturating c.
> postvoiding c. (PVC)
> retrograde c. (RC)
> static c.
> stress c.
> surveillance c.
> voiding c. (VCG)

cystography
> antegrade c.
> bead-chain c.
> radionuclide c.
> retrograde c.
> suprapubic c.
> triple-voiding c.

cystohepatic triangle

Cysto-Hypaque

cystojejunostomy
> Roux-en-Y c.

cystolateral pancreatojejunostomy

cystolith

cystolithectomy

cystolithiasis

cystolithic

cystolitholapaxy experienced complication

cystolithotomy

cystometer
> Lewis c.

cystometric
> c. biofeedback
> c. bladder capacity

cystometrogram (CMG)
> filling c.

cystometrographic monitoring

cystometrography (CMG)
> voiding c.

cystometry, cystometrography
> filling c.
> gas c.
> multichannel c.
> provoked c.
> saline c.
> screening c.
> simultaneous urethral c.'s
> spontaneous c.
> transballoon c.
> voiding c.
> water c.

cystonephrosis

cystoneuralgia

cystopancreatography

cystopanendoscopy

cystoparalysis

cystopericystectomy

cystoperitoneal shunt

cystopexy

cystophotography

cystophthisis

cystoplasty
> augmentation c.
> autoaugmentation c.
> cecal c.
> flap-valve c.
> Gil-Vernet ileocecal c.
> human lyophilized dura c.
> laparoscopic c.
> nonsecretory sigmoid c.
> sigmoid c.
> urinary tract
> reconstruction-augmentation c.

cystoplegia

cystoproctostomy

cystoprostatectomy
> salvage c.

cystoprostatourethrectomy

cystoprostatovesiculectomy

cystoptosis

cystopyelitis

cystopyelogram

cystopyelography

cystopyelonephritis

cystoradiography

cystorectocele

cystorectostomy

cystoresectoscope
> ALR c.
> anteroposterior c.
> Damon-Julian c.
> Julian c.

cystorrhagia

cystorrhaphy

cystorrhea

cystosarcoma phyllodes
cystoschisis
cystoscope
    Albarran laser c.
    balloon c.
    Braasch direct catheterization c.
    Braasch-Kaplan direct-vision c.
    Brown-Buerger c.
    Broyle retrograde c.
    Butterfield c.
    French c.
    InjecTx c.
    Judd c.
    Kelly c.
    Kidd c.
    Laidley double catheterizing c.
    Lowsley-Peterson c.
    McCarthy-Campbell miniature c.
    McCarthy Foroblique panendoscope
      c.
    McCrea c.
    Miller c.
    Morganstern continuous-flow
      operating c.
    National general purpose c.
    Nesbit c.
    Olympus fiberoptic c.
    Storz c.
    Surgitek graduated c.
    Young c.
cystoscopic
    c. electrohydraulic
      lithotripsy
    c. urography
cystoscopy
    c. and dilation (C&D)
    conventional c.
    fluorescence c.
    percutaneous fetal c.
    steerable c.
    virtual c.
cystose, cystous
cystosis
    congenital c.
cystospasm
Cystospaz
Cystospaz-M
cystospermitis
cystostaxis (*var. of* cystistaxis)
cystostomy
    suprapubic c.
    trocar c.
    c. tube
cystotome, cystitome
    Kelman air c.
    Kelman double-bladed c.
    Kelman knife c.
    Kelman knife-cannula c.
    McIntyre reverse c.

    Mendez ultrasonic c.
    reverse c.
cystotomy
    open c.
    suprapubic c.
cystotrachelotomy
cystoureteritis
cystoureterogram
cystoureterography
cystoureteropyelitis
cystoureteropyelonephritis
cystourethrectomy
    total c.
cystourethritis
cystourethrocele
cystourethrogram (CUG)
    micturating c. (MCU, MCUG)
    micturition c.
    retrograde c.
    voiding c. (VCUG)
cystourethrography
    chain c.
    expression c.
    isotope voiding c. (IVCU)
    micturating c. (MCU)
    radionuclide voiding c.
    voiding c. (VCUG)
cystourethropexy
    autologous fascia lata sling c.
    laparoscopic c.
    Marshall-Marchetti-Krantz c.
    obturator shelf c.
    Pereyra-Raz c.
cystourethroplasty
    Kropp c.
    Leadbetter c.
cystourethroscope
    ACMI c.
    microlens c.
    O'Donoghue c.
    Wappler microlens c.
cystourethroscopy
    dynamic c.
cystous (*var. of* cystose)
Cytadren
cytarabine (Ara-C, ara-C)
Cytocare Prolase II
cytocentrifuge
    c. preparation
    c. set
cytochalasin B
cytochrome
    b558 membrane-bound c.
    c. P450
    c. P450 enzyme system
    c. P450 metabolite
cytochrome-*c* oxidase deficiency
cytodiagnosis
CytoGam

cytogenetic analysis
cytokeratin
    bile duct-type c.
    hepatocyte-type c.
    c. staining
cytokine
    c. antagonist
    antiinflammatory c.
    fibrogenic c.
    fibrosis-promoting c.
    c. gene expression
    GM-CSF c.
    c. profile
    proinflammatory c.
    c. therapy
    c. tumor necrosis factor-alpha
cytologic
    c. biopsy
    c. brushing
    c. diagnosis
    C. software
    c. specimen
cytology
    aspiration biopsy c.
    balloon c.
    biliary brush c.
    brush c.
    c. brush
    colon lavage c.
    endoscopic brush c.
    endoscopic retrograde c.
    endoscopic transesophageal
      fine-needle aspiration c.
    c. examination
    exfoliative c.
    fine-needle aspiration c. (FNAC)
    gastric brush c.
    guided needle aspiration c.
    lavage c.
    needle aspiration c.
    salvage c.
    touch c.
    urine c.
    voiding urine c. (VUC)
    wire-guided c.
Cytolong brush
cytolysis inhibitor
cytolytic
    c. action
    c. therapy
    c. T lymphocyte (CTL)
cytoma
cytomegalovirus (CMV)
    c. colitis
    c. enterocolitis
    c. esophagitis
    c. hepatitis
    c. immune globulin
    c. infection

cytometer
    CAS 200 image c.
    Cell Analysis System 200 image c.
    Dickinson FACS flow c.
    EPICS C-flow c.
    EPICS Elite flow c.
    EPICS V-flow c.
    FACScan flow c.
cytometric
    c. analysis
    c. pattern
cytometry
    deoxyribonucleic acid flow c.
    DNA flow c.
    flow c.
    fluorescence-activated flow c.
    image c.
    static image DNA c.
cytopathologist
cytopenia
cytophilic antibody
cytophotometry
    static c.
cytoplasm
    eosinophilic c.
cytoplasmic
    c. adaptor protein
    c. argyrophilia
    perinuclear antineutrophil c.
      (p-ANC)
    c. staining
    c. urease
cytoprotective prostaglandin
cytoreduction
    ultrasonic c.
cytoreductive
    c. nephrectomy
    c. surgery
Cytosar
Cytoscreen
    C. Human Eotaxin immunoassay
    C. human interferon gamma ELISA
      kit
cytosine
    5-methyl c.
cytoskeletal link
cytoskeleton
    prostate gland c.
cytoskeleton-altering toxin
cytosol
cytosolic
    c. calcium
    c. face
cytospin collection fluid
CytoTAb
Cytotec
cytotoxic
    c. agent
    c. antibody

c. chemotherapy
c. liver disease
c. T cell
c. T-cell response
c. T lymphocyte (CTL)

cytotoxicity
antibody-dependent cell-mediated c. (ADCC)
antibody-dependent cellular c. (ADCC)
Bartel c.
cell-mediated c.
complement-dependent c. (CDC)
lymphocyte c.

cytotoxin
c. assay
c. necrotizing factor

VacA c.
vacuolating toxin gene A c.

cytotoxin-associated
c.-a. gene A (cagA)
c.-a. gene A protein
c.-a. gene pathogenicity island (cagPAI)

Cytoxan
vincristine, actinomycin, bleomycin, cisplatinum, C. (VAB6)

CYT-356 radiolabeled with 111 indium chloride

Czerny
C. rectal speculum
C. suture

Czerny-Kocher-Perthes incision

Czerny-Lembert suture

C

3D

3-dimensional

3D gadolinium-enhanced MR angiography

3D linear endosonography

3D sonography

D

actinomycin C, D

D cell

1,25-dihydroxyvitamin D

hepatitis D

hydroxylated vitamin D

25-hydroxyvitamin D

immunoglobulin D (IgD)

phospholipase D

D3

dihydroxyvitamin D3

1,25-dihydroxyvitamin D3

D_4

leukotriene D_4

da

da Vinci robotic system

da Vinci surgical system

dacarbazine

doxorubicin, bleomycin sulfate, vinblastine, d. (ABVD)

dacliximab

daclizumab

Dacogen

Dacomed

D. Catalyst VCD

D. snap gauge

Dacron

D. interposition graft

D. mesh

D. prosthesis

D. suture

Dacron-impregnated silastic sheet

DAEC

diffuse adherent *Escherichia coli*

DAF

decay-accelerating factor

DAG

diffuse antral gastritis

dimeric acidic glycoprotein

Dagradi esophageal variceal classification

DAH

diffuse alveolar hemorrhage

daidzein

daily

d. hemodialysis

d. intermittent peritoneal dialysis (DIPD)

once d. (OD)

d. protein intake (DPI)

Dairy Ease chewable tablet

daisy

ox-eye d.

white d.

d-ALA

delta-aminolevulinic acid

Dalalone

D. D.P.

D. L.A.

Dale

D. abdominal binder

D. Foley catheter holder

DALM

dysplasia-associated lesion or mass

Dalmane

dalteparin sodium

dam

rubber d.

damage

chloroquine-induced d.

chronic tubular d.

drug-induced esophageal d. (DIED)

flucloxacillin-associated liver d.

gastric mucosal d.

Graham scale for drug-induced gastric d.

histologic d.

hypertensive end-organ d.

indomethacin-induced mucosal d.

ischemic tubular d.

microsomal d.

oropharyngeal d.

parenchymatous d.

probable long-term kidney d.

renal parenchymal d.

renal structural d.

tissue d.

tubular d.

Damon-Julian cystoresectoscope

Danazol

Danbolt-Closs syndrome

Dance sign

dandelion

dandy

d. fever

D. nerve hook

Dane particle

Daniel colostomy clamp

Dansac

D. Karaya Seal 1-piece drainage pouch

D. ostomy irrigation set

D. skin barrier

D. Standard Ileo pouch

dansylcadaverine
Dantec
> D. 12-channel Urocolor Video system
> D. Etude uroflow transducer
> D. Menuet system
> D. rotating disk flowmeter
> D. Urodyn 1000 flowmeter
> D. Urodyn 1000 uroflowmeter

danthron
Dantrium
dantrolene sodium
Danubian endemic familial nephropathy
dapsone
daptomycin for injection
darbepoetin alfa
Darbid
Dardik clamp
D-arginine
> enantiomer D-a.

Daricon PB
Darier disease
darifenacin
dark
> d. adaptation study
> d. burgundy blood
> d. concentrated urine
> spermatogonium d. type A
> d. spot
> d. stool

darting incision
dartoic, dartoid
dartoid (*var. of* dartoic)
dartos
> d. fascia
> d. muscle
> d. pedicle flap
> d. pouch procedure

Darvocet-N 100
Darvon Compound-65 Pulvules
DASH
> dietary approach to stop hypertension
> DASH ERCP catheter
> DASH extraction balloon
> DASH sphincterotome
> DASH system
> DASH tipless extraction basket

Das-1 monoclonal antibody
DAT
> diet as tolerated

data
> long-term followup d.
> multiple testing of d.
> paucity of clinical d.
> perioperative d.
> questionnaire d.
> randomized clinical trial d.

> tolerability d.
> volumetric d.

database
> Medtrax urology d.
> Surveillance, Epidemiology and End Results D. (SEER)

date fever
Daudi cell
daughter
> d. cyst
> d. endoscopic retrograde cholangiopancreatoscopy system
> d. nodule

daunorubicin
DaunoXome
Davidoff cell
David rectal speculum
Davis
> D. interlocking sound
> D. intubated ureterostomy
> D. intubated ureterotomy
> D. loop
> D. spatula
> D. technique

Davol
> D. colon tube
> D. feeding bag
> D. feeding tube
> D. sump drain
> D. tunneler

DAWG
> demucosalized augmentation with gastric segment
> DAWG procedure

daycare diarrhea
daytime incontinence
DAZ **gene**
DBCP
> dibromochloropropane

DBSQ
> Diabetes Bowel Symptom Questionnaire

DBW
> desirable body weight

DC
> descending colon
> duodenal cap
> DC locus allelic specificity

DCBE
> double-contrast barium enema

DCC
> deleted in colorectal carcinoma

DCC **gene**
D-cell density
DCGI
> double-contrast barium examination of upper gastrointestinal tract

DCP
> des-gamma-carboxy prothrombin

3DCRT
    3-dimensional conformal radiation therapy
DCT
    distal convoluted tubule
3DCTP
    3-dimensional CT pancreatography
DCVax-Prostate vaccine
DD
    digestive disease
DD23
    antigen DD23
    DD23 antigen
DDAVP
    deamino-D-arginine-vasopressin
    DDAVP nasal spray
ddC, ddc
    dideoxycytidine
DDC
    diverticular disease of colon
ddI, ddi
    didanosine
D-dimer
DDNC
    Digestive Disease National Coalition
DDS-Acidophilus
DDV
    deep dorsal vein
    DDV ligator
de
    d. novo
    d. novo autoimmune hepatitis
    d. novo liver cancer
    d. novo malignancy
    d. novo needle-knife technique
    d. novo renal disease
    d. Pezzer catheter
    d. Toni-Debré-Fanconi syndrome
    d. Toni-Fanconi-Debré syndrome
DE
    duodenal exclusion
dead
    d. bowel
    d. space
DEAE
    diethylaminoethyl
deafferentation
deafness
    lentigines, electrocardiographic conduction abnormalities, ocular hypertelorism, pulmonary stenosis, abnormal genitalia, retardation of growth, and d. (LEOPARD)
de-air
deaminase
    adenosine d.
    porphobilinogen d. (PBG-D)
deamino-D-arginine-vasopressin (DDAVP)

Dean
    D. stage
    D. stage I, II radiation proctitis
death
    apoptotic cell d.
    circle of d.
    hepatocellular d.
    ischemic tubular cell d.
    liver d.
Deaver
    D. incision
    D. operating scissors
    D. retractor
    window of D.
Deaver-type blade
deazaaminopterin
DeBakey
    D. clamp
    D. forceps
DeBakey-Cooley retractor
Debioclip single-dose delivery system
Debove membrane
DEBRA
    Dystrophic Epidermolysis Bullosa Research Association
debrancher
    d. deficiency
    d. enzyme
    d. glycogen storage disease
Debré-de Toni-Fanconi syndrome
debridement
    endoscopic d.
debris
    clots and d.
    degenerating cellular d.
    purulent d.
    stonelike d.
debrisoquin
debulking
    percutaneous d.
    d. therapy
    tumor d.
DEC
    diethylcarbamazine
Decadron
decanoate
    nandrolone d.
decapacitation factor
Decapeptyl
decapsulation of kidney
decarboxylase
    histidine d. (HDC)
    ornithine d. (ODC)
    uroporphyrinogen d. (UROD)
decarboxylation
    amine precursor uptake and d. (APUD)
decay-accelerating factor (DAF)
decerebrate posturing

D

Decholin
decidualis
    periappendicitis d.
Declomycin
decompensated
    d. alcoholic cirrhosis
    d. liver cirrhosis
    d. neobladder
decompensation
    bladder d.
    detrusor muscle d.
decompression
    abdominal d.
    balloon d.
    biliary d.
    bladder d.
    cardiac d.
    d. catheter
    colonoscopic d.
    d. colostomy
    ductal d.
    endoscopic biliary d.
    gastric d.
    hydrostatic d.
    intestinal d.
    long intestinal tube d.
    nasogastric d.
    operative d.
    palliative d.
    PEG-assisted d.
    percutaneous transhepatic d.
    pericardial d.
    portal d.
    surgical d.
    transduodenal endoscopic d.
    d. tube
    tube d.
    variceal d.
decongestant
decontamination
    selective gut d.
    selective intestinal d. (SID)
decorin
    proteoglycan d.
decorticate posturing
decortication
    renal cyst d.
decreased
    d. peristalsis
    d. postprandial-to-fasting power
    ratio
decrescendo
decubitus
    d. calculus
    lateral d.
    d. position
    d. ulcer
dedifferentiate
deep

    d. abdominal ring
    d. artery
    d. breathing
    d. cannulation
    d. cervical fascia
    d. dorsal vein (DDV)
    d. interloop abscess
    d. jaundice
    d. muscular plexus
    d. pain
    d. perineal space
    d. postanal anorectal space
    d. postanal space of Courtney
    d. trigone
deepithelialization, deepithelization
deepithelialized flap
deepithelization (*var. of*
    deepithelialization)
deep-seated fungal infection
defecate
    urge to d.
defecating proctogram
defecation
    balloon d.
    disordered d.
    fragmentary d.
    infrequent d.
    obstructive d.
    painful d.
    d. syncope
defecatory
    d. difficulty
    d. dyschezia
    d. straining
    d. urgency
defecogram
defecography
    FECOM artificial stool for d.
defecometry
defect
    acidemia d.
    acidification d.
    acinar d.
    acquired neutrophil chemotaxis d.
    amorphous filling d.
    bony d.
    chain-of-lakes filling d.
    cobblestone filling d.
    cold d.
    conduction d.
    fascial d.
    fetal alcohol syndrome ureter d.
    filling d.
    frondlike filling d.
    hernial d.
    hot d.
    inherited d.
    interventricular d.
    intraluminal filling d.

intrapelvic filling d.
isolation d.
lobulated filling d.
mesenteric d.
plaquelike linear d.
polypoid filling d.
portal perfusion d.
renal concentrating d.
tailing d.
uterine lateral fusion d.

defensin
crypt d.

deferens
ampulla of vas d.
congenital bilateral absence of vas
d. (CBAVD)
ductus d.
ectopic vas d.
vas d.

deferentectomy
deferential artery
deferentis
ampulla ductus d.
diverticula ampullae ductus d.

deferentitis
deferoxamine mesylate infusion test
defervescence
deficiency
acquired lactose d.
adenine phosphoribosyltransferase d.
(APRT)
adult lactase d.
aldosterone d.
alpha-1-antitrypsin d.
17-alpha-hydroxylase d.
amylo-1,6-glucosidase d.
androgen d.
antithrombin III d.
APRT d.
arginase d.
11-beta-hydroxylase d.
3-beta hydroxysteroid dehydrogenase
d.
bile salt d.
biotin d.
brancher d.
calcium d.
carbamoyl phosphate
synthetase d.
ceramidase d.
chromium d.
cobalamin d.
congenital enterocyte heparan
sulphate d.
copper d.
cytochrome-*c* oxidase d.
debrancher d.
20,22-desmolase d.
dietary d.

disaccharidase d.
enteropeptidase d.
essential fatty acid d. (EFAD)
estrogen d.
familial high-density
lipoprotein d.
folate d.
follicle-stimulating hormone d.
fructose aldolase d.
fructose diphosphatase d.
fumarylacetoacetate hydrolase d.
glucose-6-phosphatase d.
glucuronyl transferase d.
gonadotropin-releasing hormone d.
growth hormone d.
hepatic phosphorylase d.
hypoxanthine-guanine
phosphoribosyltransferase d.
IgA d.
immune d.
intestinal lactase d.
intrinsic sphincter d. (ISD)
iron d.
lactase d.
long-chain acyl-CoA dehydrogenase
d.
magnesium d.
medium-chain acyl-CoA
dehydrogenase d.
niacin d.
nutritional d.
ornithine carbamoyl transferase d.
pancreatic lipase d.
PiZZ alpha-1-antitrypsin d.
potassium d.
protein C, S d.
pyridoxal 5′-phosphate d.
riboflavin d.
S-adenosylmethionine d.
sodium d.
sucrose-isomaltase d. (SID)
testosterone d.
thiamine d.
triglyceride enzyme d.
UDPGT d.
uridine diphosphate
glucuronosyltransferase d.
vaginal estrogen d.
vitamin A, D d.
zinc d.

deficiens
ejaculatio d.

deficit
lateralizing sensory d.
neurologic d.

defined-formula diet
deflated lumen technique
deflazacort
defloration pyelitis

Deflux
  D. injectable gel
  D. injectable implant
  D. system implant
deformability
  hepatic d.
deformans
  peritonitis d.
deformity
  Akerlund d.
  bell-clapper d.
  bulb d.
  chain-of-lakes d.
  cloverleaf d.
  cobra-head d.
  crane-neck d.
  crossbar d.
  duodenal bulb d.
  gross d.
  hourglass d.
  keyhole d.
  limb d.
  nasal d.
  penile d.
  phrygian cap d.
  swan-neck d.
  trefoil d.
  ureterocele cobra-head d.
  Whitehead d.
  Z-type d.
defunctionalization
defunctionalized bladder
defunctioning efficiency
Defyne urethral assist device
degassed water
degenerating cellular debris
degeneration
  acidophilic d.
  acute hepatocellular d.
  alcoholic foamy d.
  Armanni-Ehrlich d.
  ballooning d.
  cystic d.
  feathery d.
  fistulous d.
  hepatocerebral d.
  hepatolenticular d.
degenerative
  d. change
  d. nephritis
degloving
  penile shaft d.
deglutible
deglutition
  d. disorder
  d. mechanism
  d. reflex
deglutitive
  d. inhibition

  d. pharyngeal chamber
deglutitory
Degos
  D. disease
  D. syndrome
degradation
  gastric mucosal d.
  haptocorrin d.
  d. of collagen
  proteolytic d.
degradative enzyme
degranulation
  mast cell d.
degree
  d. of hyperreflexia
  d. of objectivity
dehisced
dehiscence
  abdominal incision d.
  Killian d.
  d. of cystic stump
  staple line d.
  suture line d.
  wound d.
dehydrated ethanol
dehydration
  absolute d.
  d. fever
  hyperosmotic nonketotic d.
dehydrocholaneresis
dehydroemetine
dehydroepiandrosterone (DHA)
  d. sulfate (DHAS)
dehydrogenase
  alcohol d. (ADH)
  aldehyde d. (ALDH)
  alpha ketoacid d.
  benzaldehyde d.
  beta hydroxyacyl-coenzyme A d.
  3-beta hydroxysteroid d.
  branched-chain alpha ketoacid d.
  glutamate d. (GLDH)
  glyceraldehyde phosphate d. (GAPD)
  glyceraldehyde-3-phosphate d.
    (GAPDH, G3PDH)
  inosine monophosphate d. (IMPDH)
  ketoglutarate d. (KGDH)
  lactate d. (LDH)
  lactic acid d. (LAD, LDH)
  long-chain 3-hydroxyacyl coenzyme
    A d. (LCHAD)
  medium-chain acyl-CoA d.
    (MCAD)
  pyruvate d. (PDH)
  sorbitol d. (SDH)
  succinate d.
  xanthine d. (XDH)
deionized formamide
Deisting technique

dejecta
dejection
Dejerine-Sottas syndrome
Delatestryl
delavirdine
delay
    excretory d.
    gastric emptying d.
    outlet d.
delayed
    d. anastomosis
    d. blush
    d. capillary refill
    d. colonic transit
    d. cutaneous hypersensitivity
    (DCH)
    d. gallbladder emptying
    d. graft function
    d. hyperacute transplant rejection
    d. liquid gastric emptying
    d. nephrogram
    d. operative cholangiography
    d. primary closure (DPC)
    d. primary intention
    d. primary intention healing
    d. upstroke
    d. ureteral anastomotic stenosis
    d. vesicoureteral reflux
delayed-release tablet
delayed-type hypersensitivity (DTH)
del Castillo syndrome
deleted
    d. in colon carcinoma gene
    d. in colorectal carcinoma
    (DCC)
deletion
    d. and mutation detection
    enhancement gel
    chromosome d.
    clonal d.
    d. mutation
    d. polymorphism
    somatic allelic d.
Delflex peritoneal dialysis solution
delivery
    energy d.
    PlasmaKinetic radiofrequency energy
    d.
    vectorial d.
delomorphous cell
Delorme
    D. operation for rectal prolapse
    D. rectal prolapse repair
    D. rectal prolapse repair procedure
    D. transrectal excision
delta
    d. agent hepatitis
    d. antigen
    d. bilirubin

    d. hepatitis superinfection
    d.'s per mil
    d. virus
delta-aminolevulinic acid (d-ALA)
Delta-Cortef
delta-5-pregnenolone
Deltasone
Deltatrac metabolic monitor
delusional
Demadex
demand
    increased clinical d.
demarcate
demarcation
    corticomedullary d.
DeMartel
    D. appendix clamp
    D. appendix forceps
DeMartel-Wolfson
    D.-W. anastomosis clamp
    D.-W. clamp holder
demasculinization
demeclocycline-induced ascites
DeMeester
    D. acid score
    D. criteria
dementia
    dialysis d.
    HIV-associated d.
Demerol
demethylchlortetracycline
demeure
    catheter á d.
Deming operation
Demling-Classen sphincterotome
demonstrated hypertensive rate
demucosalized augmentation with gastric
    segment (DAWG)
denaturation
denaturing high-performance liquid
    chromatography (dHPLC)
Denck esophagoscope
dendritic
    d. calculus
    d. cell therapy
    d. reticular cell
dendriticum
    Diphyllobothrium d.
denervated sphincter of Oddi
denervation
    bladder d.
    detrusor d.
    partial bladder d.
    peripheral bladder d.
    sinoaortic d. (SAD)
dengue
    hemorrhagic d.
    d. hemorrhagic fever
    d. hemorrhagic fever infection

D

dengue (*continued*)
 d. shock syndrome
 d. virus
Denhardt solution
Denis
 D. Browne abdominal retractor
 D. Browne operation
 D. Browne pouch
 D. Browne urethroplasty technique
Dennis
 D. clamp
 D. colorectal tube
 D. intestinal forceps
 D. intestinal tube
Dennis-Brooke ileostomy
Dennis-Varco pancreatoduodenostomy
Denonvilliers fascia
densa
 lamina d.
 macula d.
 nascent macula d.
dense
 d. adhesion
 d. polyposis
densitometer
 Hoefer laser d.
 Hologic d.
densitometer/absorptiometer
 QDR 1000 d.
densitometric unit
densitometry
 calcaneal ultrasound bone d.
 double x-ray d.
density
 current d.
 D-cell d.
 electrosurgical current d.
 fat d.
 filtration slit-length d.
 gastrin mRNA:G-cell d.
 d. gradient centrifugation
 grain d.
 intramural microvessel d.
 lumbar spine bone mineral d.
 prostate-specific antigen d.
  (PSAD)
 radiopaque d.
 rectal telangiectasia d.
 slit pore length d.
Dent
 D. disease
 D. supplement
dentate
 d. line
 d. margin
denticulatum
 pentastomum d.
Dentsleeve
 D. device

 D. extruded silastic perfused manometric assembly
 D. pneumohydraulic perfusion system
 D. single multilumen extrusion catheter
 D. sleeve sensor
denuded mucosa
denutrition
Denver
 D. peritoneovenous shunt
 D. pleuroperitoneal shunt
Denys-Drash syndrome
deodorized tincture of opium (DTO)
deoxycholate
 sodium d.
deoxycholic acid
deoxycorticosterone
deoxycytidine
 fluoromethylene d.
deoxydoxorubicin
deoxyepinephrine
5′-deoxy-5-fluorouridine (5′-DFUR)
1-deoxy-galactonojirimicin (DGJ)
deoxyribonucleic
 d. acid (DNA)
 d. acid flow cytometry
 d. acid synthesizer
deoxyspergualin (DSG)
15-deoxyspergualin
DePage-Janeway gastrostomy
Depakene
deparaffinization
Depen
dependent rubor
Depend fitted briefs
dephosphorylated myosin crossbridge
depleted lysate
depletion
 mucus d.
 nephropathy of potassium d.
 plasma volume d.
 potassium d.
 protein d.
 syndrome of chloride d.
deployment
 stent d.
depMedalone
depolarization
Depo-Predate
Depo-Provera
deposit
 C3 d.
 electron-dense mesangial d.
 fatty d.
 hemosiderin d.
 liver d.
 mesangial d.

peritoneal d.
seminal vesicle amyloid d.
subendothelial d.
subepithelial d.
deposition
collagen d.
conditioning film d.
heavy-chain d.
incrustation d.
ion beam-assisted d.
matrix d.
microdroplet fat d.
perisinusoidal fibrin d.
Depostat
depot
d. injection
Lupron D.
Sandostatin LAR D.
Trelstar D.
Depo-Testosterone
depressed
d. adenoma
d. cancer
d. tumor
depressed-type colorectal cancer
depression
pterygoid d.
respiratory d.
spermatogenesis d.
d. surface
deprivation
androgen d.
neoadjuvant hormonal d.
depsipeptide
deranged hemostatic mechanism
derangement
metabolic d.
derivative
atropine d.
ergot d.
fibrate d.
hematoporphyrin d. (HpD)
isoxazole d.
Photofrin d.
Photoscan-3 hematoporphyrin d.
photosensitizing hemoporphyrin d.
pivalate d.
purified protein d. (PPD)
sialylated d.
sphingolipid d.
derma
Dermacyn wound care
Dermaginate dressing
Dermagran-B
dermal
d. island-flap anoplasty
d. suture
Dermalene suture
Dermalon suture

dermatan sulfate
dermatitidis
Blastomyces d.
dermatitis
allergic d.
d. artefacta
atopic d.
contact d.
factitial d.
d. herpetiformis (DH)
irritant d.
perineal d.
seborrheic d.
Toxicodendron d.
dermatofibroma (DF)
dermatologic tumor
dermatolymphatic invasion
dermatomyositis
paraneoplastic d.
dermatopathic enteropathy
dermatophyte infection
dermatoses (*pl. of* dermatosis)
dermatosis, *pl.* **dermatoses**
acute febrile neutrophilic d.
neutrophilic d.
d. of hemodialysis
reactive inflammatory
vascular d.
dermoid cyst
Dermovate cream
DeRoyal Surgical grab bag
DES
diethylstilbestrol
diffuse esophageal spasm
desaturation
arterial oxygen d.
oxygen d.
descendens
colon d.
descending
d. colon (DC)
d. diaphragm
d. duodenum
d. inhibitory reflex
d. loop colostomy
d. perineum syndrome
d. urography
descensus
d. aberrans testis
bladder d.
d. paradoxus testis
rectal d.
renal d.
d. uteri
d. ventriculi
descent
open renal d.
pelvic floor d.
perineal d.

D

descent (*continued*)
 testicular d.
 total d.
 vaginal d.
Deschamps ligature carrier
DESD
 detrusor external sphincter
 dyssynergia
deserpidine
Desferal Mesylate challenge for
 hemochromatosis
desferrioxamine
des-gamma-carboxy
 d.-g.-c. prothrombin (DCP)
 d.-g.-c. prothrombin level
desiccation
 blend waveform d.
 coagulase waveform d.
 cut waveform d.
 electrosurgical d.
desipramine hydrochloride
desirable body weight (DBW)
Desjardins
 D. gallbladder forceps
 D. gallbladder probe
 D. gallbladder scoop
 D. gall duct probe
 D. gallstone forceps
 D. gallstone probe
 D. gallstone scoop
 D. point
Desmarres paracentesis knife
Desmet/Scheurer staging system
desmin
desmoid tumor
desmolase
20,22-desmolase deficiency
desmoplastic
 d. reaction
 d. response
desmopressin (DDAVP)
 d. acetate
 d. response
desmosomal junction
desmosome
desoximetasone, desoxymethasone
desoxymethasone (*var. of*
 desoximetasone)
desquamated epithelium
desquamation
 tubular cell d.
dessusception
destruction
 fibroproliferative d.
 long-term graft d.
 d. of laminin
destructive
 d. cholangiopathy
 d. cholangitis

destruens
 chorioadenoma d.
Desyrel
detachable miniloop ligation
detachment
 mucosal d.
 transvesical laparoscopic d.
detachment-induced apoptosis
Detachol adhesive remover
detail
 outstanding anatomical d.
detailed stepwise approach
detection
 antiliver microsomal antibody d.
 breath isotope bacterial urease d.
 colorimetric d.
 fluorescent d.
 gastroenteropathy d.
 hepatitis B DNA d.
 hepatitis C virus RNA d.
 immunohistochemical d.
 d. of malignancy
 radioactive d.
 d. rate
 RIGScan CR49 test for colorectal
 cancer d.
detector
 C-Trak handheld gamma d.
 Early D.
deterioration
 marked d.
 d. of graft function
 renal d.
determinant
 antigenic d.
 clinical d.
 MAb IOT2-recognizing monomorphic
 DR d.
determination
 IHA d.
 indirect hemagglutination d.
detorsion
Detrol
 D. LA
 D. LA capsule
detrusodetrusor facilitative reflex
detrusor
 acontractile d.
 d. acontractility
 d. activity index
 d. areflexia
 d. compliance
 d. contraction
 d. contraction strength
 d. denervation
 d. external sphincter dyssynergia
 (DESD)
 d. hyperactivity
 d. hyperreflexia

hypocontractile d.
d. hypocontractility
d. instability
d. muscle decompensation
d. muscle flap
d. muscle inhibition
d. muscle instability
d. muscle leak-point pressure
d. muscle myosin
d. muscle overactivity
d. muscle potassium channel
d. muscle pressure-flow micturition study
d. muscle protrusion junction
d. muscle stability
d. muscle trabeculation
d. muscle underactivity
d. myectomy
d. recovery
d. urethral dyssynergia
d. urinae
detrusorectomy
detrusorrhaphy
detrusosphincteric inhibitory reflex
detrusourethral inhibitory reflex
detubularization principle
detubularized
d. right colon reservoir
d. small bowel
detumescence
deuterium oxide
devascularization
paraesophagogastric d.
Sugiura paraesophagogastric d.
devastated urethra
devazepide
developer
Hemoccult Sensa d.
developing high-grade dysplasia
development
dynamic d.
embryologic d.
deviation
axis d.
congenital penile d. (CPD)
tongue d.
tracheal d.
uvular d.
device
Accutorr oscillometric d.
ACMI ulcer measuring d.
Acucise balloon cutting d.
AcuSnare polypectomy d.
AcuTrainer handheld electronic d.
angled delivery d.
Arena hemodialysis d.
Argon Beamer 2 d.
Assura AC closure d.
Assura EasiClose d.

autostapling d.
band-ligator d.
BAS-300 transurethral thermotherapy d.
BetaSorb d.
BiliChek breath analyzer d.
bioartificial liver support d.
BladderManager portable ultrasonic d.
broken stent retrieval d.
BSD-300 d.
Button One-Step gastrostomy d.
Carter-Thomason port closure d.
CaverMap surgical d.
charge-coupled d. (CCD)
Circe d.
Circon-ACMI rigid d.
circular stapling d.
Clot Buster Amplatz thrombectomy d.
contraceptive d.
CoreTherm high-energy d.
Curity Mono-Flo antireflux d.
cyst puncture d.
Defyne urethral assist d.
Dentsleeve d.
Digiflator digital inflation d.
Digitrapper MK III ambulatory d.
Dilamezinsert d.
DomeTip CleverCut d.
DomeTip Ultratome XL d.
double-headed P190 stapling d.
Eagle Claw VII d.
EEA stapling d.
endoscopically deliverable tissue-transfixing d.
endoscopic hemoclip d.
endoscopic mucosal resection with ligating d.
endoscopic transilluminator d.
ErecAid vacuum erection d.
Erlangen magnetic colostomy d.
EsophyX endoluminal fundoplication d.
external urethral barrier d.
extracorporeal bioartificial liver d.
extracorporeal liver assist d. (ELAD)
fingerstick d.
flexible delivery d.
flexible endoscopic suturing d.
flexible Olympus GF-EUM3 d.
Flexible Sew-Right d.
Flexible Ti-Knot d.
fog reduction/elimination d. (FRED)
gastroesophageal antireflux d. (GARD)
Gastro-Port II feeding d.
GIA autosuture d.

device (*continued*)

Gore Viatorr ePTFE d.
Gould polygraph gastric motility measuring d.
head-mounted d.
hemoclipping application d.
Hepatix d.
HX-5/6-1 endoscopic clipping d.
implantable penile venous compression d.
indwelling stomal d.
infection prevention d.
Insuflon insulin delivery d.
InterStim d.
IntraSonix TULIP laser d.
Isobar barostat distention d.
KeraPac d.
ligation d.
linear-array stapling d.
linear stapling d.
Macroplastique implantation d.
Makler insemination d.
Makler sperm-counting d.
Menuet Compact urodynamic testing d.
Microgyn II urinary incontinence d.
Microvasive Gold probe bipolar electrocautery d.
miniature ultrasound suction d.
Mission vacuum constriction d.
Mission vacuum erection d.
multiband ligating d.
multiclip d.
Multifire Endo GIA stapling d.
Nachlas-Linton esophagogastric balloon tamponade d.
needlescope d.
Nottingham KeyMed introducing d.
NovolinPen d.
Ntrap d.
Olympus clip-fixing d.
Olympus LUS-1 rigid d.
Olympus LUS-2 ultrasonic energy rigid d.
Olympus UES-series snare cautery d.
OraSure salivary collection d.
OSB gastrostomy d.
pneumatic compression d. (PCD)
PortSaver PercLoop d.
Pos-T-Vac vacuum erection d.
Procon incontinence d.
Prometheus d.
prophylactic d.
Prostathermer d.
Prostatron transurethral thermotherapy d.

ProTack tacking d.
Puritan DM Stick wound measuring d.
pyxigraphic d.
Q-Maxx side-firing laser d.
Quantum inflation d. (QID)
Relia-Flow d.
reposable d.
Resolution Clip d.
Richard Wolf ultrasonic energy rigid d.
Rigiflator handheld inflation/deflation d.
RigiScan d.
ring-type rigidity measuring d.
robotic automated assist d.
Roticulator stapling d.
Sepet artificial liver support d.
shape-locking d.
silicone pressure sensor d.
Soehendra stent retrieval d.
SofPulse noninvasive pulsed electromagnetic therapy d.
SofTouch vacuum erection d.
Sonoblate ablation d.
Sony Promavica still capture d.
Stone Cone nitinol stone retrieval d.
SuturTek fascia closure d.
Swiss Lithoclast Master d.
Synergist vacuum erection d.
targeted cryoablation d.
TA stapling d.
Techstar percutaneous closure d.
temporary endoprosthetic d.
testicular hypothermia d.
TherMatrx hyperthermia d.
TherMatrx TMx-2000 d.
Thermex-II transurethral prostate heating d.
thread-locking d.
TissueLink Floating Ball radiofrequency d.
transparent elastic band ligating d.
TriClip endoscopic clipping d.
Trimedyne Optilase 1000 d.
Turapy d.
Uri-Drain male incontinence d.
UV-Flash ultraviolet germicidal exchange d.
vacuum constriction d. (VCD)
vacuum entrapment d.
vacuum erection d. (VED)
vacuum extraction d.
vacuum tumescence d.
variceal pressure measuring d.
Visiport d.
VTU-1 vacuum erection d.
Wallstent delivery d.

Wedge electrosurgical resection d.
wire-guided metal spiral retrieval d.
Wolf Piezolith 2300 lithotripsy d.
device-related urinary tract infection
2-devices-in-1-channel method
devil's claw
Devine
D. colostomy
D. exclusion
D. hypospadias repair
Devine-Devine procedure
Devine-Horton flip-flap for hypospadias repair
devitalization
devolvulization
endoscopic d.
Devonshire colic
Dew sign
DEXA
dual-energy x-ray absorptiometry
DEXA absorption
dexamethasone
d. sodium phosphate
d. suppression test
vincristine, Adriamycin, d. (VAD, VDD)
dexamethasone-encapsulated erythrocyte
Dexatrim
dexbrompheniramine
Dexedrine
dexfenfluramine
dexloxiglumide (DEX)
Dexol 300
Dexon
D. polyglycolic acid mesh
D. suture
dexpanthenol
dexter
ductus hepaticus d.
ductus lobi caudati d.
dextofisopam
dextra
arteria colica d.
arteria gastrica d.
arteria gastroomentalis d.
flexura coli d.
dextran
d. 40, 70, 75
d. clearance
iron d.
d. sieving
d. sodium sulfate (DSS)
dextrin
dextrinase
alpha d.
dextrinizing time
dextrinosis
limit d.
dextroamphetamine

dextrogastria
dextropropoxyphene
dextrose
DFT
Doppler flow test
5'-DFUR
5'-deoxy-5-fluorouridine
d-galactosamine
DGER
duodenal gastroesophageal reflux
duodenogastroesophageal reflux
DGHAL
Doppler-guided hemorrhoidal artery ligation
DGJ
1-deoxy-galactonojirimicin
DGR
duodenogastric reflux
DH
dermatitis herpetiformis
diaphragmatic hernia
DHA
dehydroepiandrosterone
DHAD
mitoxantrone
DHA-paclitaxel
Taxoprexin DHA-p.
DHAS
dehydroepiandrosterone sulfate
DHD
donor hepatic duct
DHFK
Dow hollow-fiber kidney
DHP
dihydropyridine
DHPG
dihydroxypropoxymethyl guanine
dHPLC
denaturing high-performance liquid chromatography
DHSI
Digestive Health Status Instrument
DiaBeta
diabetes
alimentary d.
D. Bowel Symptom Questionnaire (DBSQ)
fibrocalculous pancreatic d. (FCPD)
gestational d.
d. home screening test
d. insipidus (DI)
insulin-dependent d.
d. mellitus (DM)
pancreatic d.
diabetic
d. autonomic neuropathy
d. cholecystoparesis
d. colitis
d. diarrhea

diabetic (*continued*)
    d. diet
    d. enteropathy
    d. gastroparesis
    d. gastropathy
    d. impotence
    insulin-treated d.
    d. ketoacidosis (DKA)
    d. microangiopathy
    d. nephropathy
    d. patient
    Resource D.
    d. urine
diabetica
    balanitis d.
diabeticorum
    gastroparesis d.
DiabetiSweet
DiabetiTrim
Diabinese
diabrosis
DiaCan fistula needle
diacetate
    2′,7′-dichlorofluoresin d.
diachorema
diachoresis
Diacol
diacylglycerol
Diacyte DNA ploidy analysis
Diagnex
    D. Blue test
    D. Blue test for gastric
      acid
diagnoses (*pl. of* diagnosis)
diagnosing
    d. interstitial cystitis
    d. ureteral calculus
diagnosis, *pl.* **diagnoses**
    colonoscopic d.
    cytologic d.
    differential d.
    endoscopic ultrasonographic d.
    endoscopic ultrasound d.
    enteroscopy d.
    histologic d.
    missed d.
    needle biopsy d.
    noninvasive d.
    d. of bacterial prostatitis
    d. of bladder cancer
    d. of testicular tumor
    pancreatic tumor d.
    pathologic d.
    photodynamic d.
    prenatal d.
    scintigraphic d.
    serologic d.
    ultrasonic d.
    wastebasket d.

diagnostic
    d. angiography
    d. aspiration
    d. colonoscopy
    d. duodenoscope
    d. fiberoptic stomatoscopy
    d. imaging evaluation
    d. laparoscope
    d. laparoscopy
    d. paracentesis
    d. surgery
    d. technique
    d. upper endoscopy
    d. uroradiology
    d. yield
diagram
    schematic d.
diagraph
Dialose
Dialume
Dialyflex dialysis fluid
dialysance
dialysate
    bicarbonate d.
    calcium-free d.
    ethanol and phosphate-enriched d.
    d. glucose concentration
    high-calcium d.
    low-calcium d.
    peritoneal d.
dialysate-to-plasma ratio
dialysis
    d. access infection
    d. access surgery
    d. adequacy
    albumin d.
    automated peritoneal d. (APD)
    chronic ambulatory peritoneal d.
      (CAPD)
    continuous ambulatory peritoneal d.
      (CAPD)
    continuous arteriovenous
      hemofiltration with d.
    continuous cycler-assisted peritoneal
      d.
    continuous cycling peritoneal d.
      (CCPD)
    cycling d.
    daily intermittent peritoneal d.
      (DIPD)
    d. dementia
    d. disequilibrium syndrome
    d. equilibrium syndrome
    d. encephalopathy syndrome
    extended daily d. (EDD)
    extracorporeal d.
    high-efficiency d.
    high-flux d.
    home d.

d. modality
nightly intermittent peritoneal d. (NIPD)
d. osteomalacia
D. Outcomes Quality Initiative (DOQI)
peritoneal d. (PD)
profiled d.
renal d.
short daily d.
d. shunt
single-pass albumin d. (SPAD)
slow low-efficiency d. (SLED)
sustained low-efficiency d. (SLED)
terminal anuria vesical d.
d. to plasma
dialysis-associated hypotension
dialysis-related ascites
dialytic
d. treatment
d. ultrafiltration
dialyzer
AN69 membrane d.
Asahi d.
CA110 d.
CA cellulose acetate membrane hollow-fiber d.
Clirans T-series d.
double d.
Fresenius AG d.
Gambro d.
high-flux d.
hollow-fiber d.
d. membrane
parallel plate d.
polysulfone d.
Renaflo hollow-fiber d.
Renalin d.
Renatron d.
Terumo d.
diameter
distal bile duct d.
inner d.
lower infundibular d.
luminal d.
maximum d.
outer d.
renal artery d.
unequal calf d.
diaminedichloroplatinum
diamine oxidase (DAO, DO)
diaminobenzidine
3′,3-diaminobenzidine tetrahydrochloride
diamond
d. flap
D. stent
D. tube
diamond-jaw needle holder
diamorphine

Dianeal K-141
diaphoresis
diaphoretic
diaphragm
accessory d.
congenital d.
crus of d.
descending d.
d. disease
duodenal d.
endoscopic ablation of antral d.
leaf of d.
mucosal ileal d.
pelvic d.
prepyloric antral d.
slit d.
urogenital d.
diaphragmatic
d. abscess
d. breathing
d. hernia (DH)
d. hernia trauma
d. hiatus
d. hump
d. injury
d. muscle
d. pinch
d. pinchcock
d. surface of liver
diaphragmatocele
diaphragmlike
d. stenosis
d. stricture
diarrhea
acute infectious d.
Aeromonas d.
alcoholic d.
d. and vomiting (D&V)
antibiotic-associated d. (AAD)
antibiotic-induced d.
anxiety-related d.
bacterial toxigenic d.
beta-lactam-associated d.
bile acid d. type 1, 2
bile salt d.
bilious d.
bloody d.
Brainerd d.
cachectic d.
chewing gum d.
choleraic d.
cholera toxin-induced d.
chronic d.
d. chylosa
Clostridium difficile-associated d. (CDAD)
Cochin China d.
colliquative d.
congenital chloride d.

D

diarrhea (*continued*)
    congenital sodium d. (CSD)
    crapulous d.
    critical d.
    Cryptosporidium-induced d.
    daycare d.
    diabetic d.
    Dientamoeba d.
    dysenteric d.
    elixir d.
    endemic d.
    enteral d.
    enterotoxin d.
    explosive d.
    factitious d.
    familial chloride d.
    fatty acid d.
    fermentative d.
    flagellate d.
    fructose d.
    functional d.
    gastrogenic d.
    gastrogenous d.
    gluten-sensitive d.
    hemorrhagic d.
    Hill d.
    ileostomy d.
    infantile d.
    infectious nosocomial d.
    infectious viral d.
    inflammatory d.
    intermittent d.
    intractable d.
    irritative d.
    lactose-associated d.
    lienteric d.
    liquid d.
    magnesium-induced d.
    malabsorptive d.
    maldigestive d.
    mechanical d.
    morning d.
    mucous d.
    nausea, vomiting, d. (NVD)
    neurogenic secretory d.
    nocturnal d.
    osmotic d.
    d. pancreatica
    pancreatogenous d.
    paradoxical d.
    parenteral d.
    postvagotomy d. (PVD)
    putrefactive d.
    raw milk-associated d.
    rotavirus d.
    rotavirus-associated d.
    runner's d.
    secretory d.
    serous d.
    severe secretory d.
    sodium anion d.
    sorbitol d.
    stercoraceous d.
    d. stool
    summer d.
    toddler's d.
    toxic d.
    toxigenic d.
    traveler's d.
    tropical d.
    tubercular d.
    unrelenting d.
    viral d.
    virulent d.
    watery d.
    white d.
diarrheagenic (*var. of* diarrheogenic)
diarrheal, diarrheic, diarrhetic
diarrhea-predominant irritable bowel syndrome (IBS-D)
diarrheic (*var. of* diarrheal)
diarrheogenic, diarrheagenic
diarrhetic (*var. of* diarrheal)
diary
    voiding d.
DiaScreen 10 reagent strip
Diasonics
    D. DRF ultrasound unit
    D. Therasonic lithotriptor
Diasorb
diastase
    d. digestion
    pancreatic d.
    d. predigestion
diastasis
    palpable rib d.
    pubic d.
    rectus d.
    d. rectus abdominis
    wide pubic d.
Diastate AcuDiet
diastatic serosal tear
Diastat vascular access graft
diastematomyelia
diathermal snare
diathermic
    d. cleaning
    d. cystenterostome
    d. fistulotomy
    d. loop
    d. loop biopsy
    d. precut needle
    d. puncture
    d. resection
diathermocoagulation
diathermy
    BICAP bipolar d.

d. hemorrhoidectomy
d. mark
d. scissors
d. technique
d. wire
diatheses (*pl. of* diathesis)
diathesis, *pl.* **diatheses**
diatrizoate
    meglumine d.
    postdilation meglumine d.
    d. sodium enema
    sodium methylglucamine d.
diatrizoic acid
diazepam emulsified injection
diaziquone (AZQ)
diazoxide
DIB
    duodenoileal bypass
dibasic
    d. aminoacidopathy
    d. amino acid residue
Dibent injection
Dibenzyline
dibromochloropropane (DBCP)
dibucaine
DIC
    disseminated intravascular coagulation
    drip infusion cholangiography
    DIC parameter
dichlorofluorescein
2′,7′-dichlorofluoresin diacetate
dichotomization
dichroism
    circular d.
Dickinson
    Becton D. (BD)
    D. FACS flow cytometer
Dickson osteotomy
diclofenac
    d. analgesic therapy
    d. sodium
dicloxacillin
dicyclomine
Di-Dak-Sol dressing
didanosine (ddI, ddi)
didelphys
    uterus d.
dideoxycytidine (ddC, ddc)
Didrex
Didronel
didymalgia
didymitis
DIED
    drug-induced esophageal damage
dientamoeba
    D. diarrhea
    D. fragilis
diet
    absolute d.

acid-ash d. (AAD)
ADA d.
advance to regular d.
alkaline-ash d.
Andresen d.
ape d.
d. as tolerated (DAT)
Atkins d.
baby soft d. (BSD)
balanced d.
basal d.
basic d.
bland d.
blenderized d.
blood-type d.
BRAT d.
BRATT d.
calcium-rich gluten-free d.
CAPS-free d.
challenge d.
chemically defined d.
clear liquid d.
cornstarch-rich d.
defined-formula d.
diabetic d.
disease-specific d.
Ebstein d.
elemental d.
elimination d.
exclusion d.
fasting d.
fen-phen d.
fiber-deficient d.
fractionated d.
fructose-free d.
full liquid d.
galactose-free d.
gastric d.
Giordano-Giovannetti d.
gluten-free d. (GFD)
gluten-rich d.
grapefruit d.
high-bulk low-fat d.
high-calorie d.
high-carbohydrate d.
high-fat d.
high-fiber d. (HFD)
high-protein d.
high-roughage d.
high-starch d.
hypercaloric d.
hyperprotidic d.
immune-enhancing d.
K d.
K+2 d.
lactose-free d.
liquid d.
liver d.
low available carbohydrate d.

D

diet (*continued*)
    low-calorie d.
    low-fat d.
    low-fiber d. (LFD)
    low-lactose d.
    low-oxalate d.
    low-residue d.
    low-roughage d.
    low-sodium d.
    low-tyrosine, low-phenylalanine d.
    Meulengracht d.
    milk d.
    modified liver d.
    Moro-Heisler d.
    Paleolithic d.
    phen-fen d.
    Portagen d.
    progressive d.
    reducing d.
    regular d.
    rice-fruit d.
    Schmidt d.
    semielemental d. (SED)
    Sippy d.
    smooth d.
    soft bland d.
    steroid-dependent d.
    steroid-refractory d.
    d. therapy
    Travasorb Hepatic D.
    Travasorb Renal D.
    vegetarian d.
    very low calorie d. (VLCD)
    Weight Watchers d.
    Western d.
dietary
    d. approach to stop hypertension
      (DASH)
    d. calcium
    d. cholesterol
    d. deficiency
    d. energy intake
    d. fat
    d. fiber
    d. gluten
    d. habit
    d. L-arginine supplementation
    d. nitrite
    d. oxalate
    d. phosphate
    d. phosphorus
    d. potassium
    d. protein
    d. protein intolerance
    d. protein restriction
    d. purine
    d. sodium
dietetic regimen
dietetics

diethylaminoethyl (DEAE)
diethylcarbamazine (DEC)
diethylenetriamine
    d. pentaacetic acid (DTPA)
    d. pentaacetic acid renal scan
    d. pentaacetic acid renography
diethylenetriamine-pentaacetic
  acid-galactosyl-human serum albumin
diethylpropion
diethylstilbestrol (DES)
dieting plateau
dietitian
Dietl crisis
Dieulafoy
    D. anomaly
    D. cirsoid aneurysm
    D. disease
    D. gastric erosion
    D. gastric lesion
    D. theory
    D. triad
    D. ulcer
    D. vascular malformation
difference
    potential d. (PD)
    substantial regional d.
    transmembrane electrical
      potential d.
    transmucosal potential d. (TMPD)
differential
    d. diagnosis
    d. loading
    d. neuroaxial blockade
    d. renal function test
    d. ureteral catheterization test
    WBC d.
    white blood count d.
differentiated teratoma
differentiation
    cellular d.
    chondrogenic d.
    cluster of d. (CD)
    cluster of d. 3+ (CD3+)
    cluster of d. 3 (CD3)
    cluster of d. 4+ (CD4+)
    cluster of d. 4 (CD4)
    cluster of d. 8+ (CD8+)
    cluster of d. 8 (CD8)
    cluster of d. 14 (CD14)
    cluster of d. 20 (CD20)
    cluster of d. 23 (CD23)
    corticomedullary d.
    endothelial cell d.
    genital d.
    gonadal d.
    impaired cell d.
    osteogenic d.
    rhabdomyoblastic d.
    sexual d.

DiffGAM
difficile
    Clostridium d. (CD)
difficult nephrectomy
difficulty
    defecatory d.
Diff-Quik stain
diffractometry
    x-ray d.
Diffu-K
diffuse
    d. adherent *Escherichia coli*
      (DAEC)
    d. alveolar hemorrhage (DAH)
    d. alveolar hemorrhage syndrome
    d. angiodysplasia
    d. angiokeratoma
    d. antral gastritis (DAG)
    d. diabetic glomerulosclerosis
    d. esophageal spasm (DES)
    d. hepatocellular carcinoma
    d. hyperplastic polyposis
    d. irregular narrowing of pancreatic
      duct
    d. liver disease
    d. lobular fibrosis
    d. malignant mesothelioma (DMM)
    d. mesangial proliferation
    d. mesangial sclerosis (DMS)
    d. metastasis
    d. mucosal polyposis
    d. nodular hyperplasia (DNH)
    d. pain
    d. pancreatitis
    d. patchy nephrogram
    d. proliferative glomerulonephritis
      (DPGN)
    d. redness
    d. suppurative nephritis
    d. tenderness
    d. varioliform gastritis
    d. vasculitis of polyarteritis nodosa
      type
diffusely tender abdomen
diffuser
    cylindrical d.
diffusion
    disk d.
    interstitial d.
    pericapillary d.
    transcapillary d.
diffusive transport
diffusum
    angiokeratoma corporis d.
Diflucan
diflunisal
difluoromethylornithine
DIF-test
    direct immunofluorescence test

digastric
    d. anterior muscle
    d. impression
    d. posterior muscle
    d. triangle
Di-Gel
DiGeorge anomaly
Digepepsin
digestant
digestion
    brush-border d.
    diastase d.
    duodenal d.
    proteolytic d.
    RNAse d.
    solid food d.
digestive
    d. apparatus
    d. disease (DD)
    D. Disease National Coalition
      (DDNC)
    d. enzyme
    d. fever
    d. gastrosuccorrhea
    d. glycosuria
    D. Health Status Instrument
      (DHSI)
    D. Health Status Instrument survey
    d. system
    d. tract
    d. tube
digestive-respiratory
    d.-r. fistula (DRF)
    d.-r. fistula stent
digestorius
    apparatus d.
    tubus d.
Digibar 190
Digiflator digital inflation device
digit
    sausage d.
digital
    d. manipulation of pubic hair
    d. rectal evacuation
    d. rectal examination (DRE)
    d. stream segment
    d. venous subtraction angiography
      (DVSA)
digitalis
digitally guided biopsy
digitonin
Digitrapper
    D. catheter
    D. Gold MK III solid-state data
      logger
    D. Mark II pH monitoring system
    D. MK III
    D. MK III ambulatory device
    D. MK III portable digital recorder

D

diglycoaldehyde
Dignity incontinence pants
digoxin
dihydrate
    calcium oxalate d.
    octahedral-shaped d.
dihydrochloride
    histamine d.
    nolatrexed d.
dihydroergotoxine
dihydropyridine (DHP)
dihydrotestosterone (DHT)
    d. gel
    d. synthesis
2,8-dihydroxyadenine calculus
dihydroxyadenine urolithiasis
dihydroxyaluminum
    d. aminoacetate
    d. sodium carbonate
dihydroxyeicosatrienoic acid
dihydroxyphenylalanine
  (DOPA)
dihydroxypropoxymethyl guanine
  (DHPG)
dihydroxy salt
1,25-dihydroxyvitamin
    1,25-d. D
    1,25-d. D3 (1,25(OH)2 D3)
dihydroxyvitamin D3
diiodohydroxyquin
diisopropyliminodiacetic
    d. acid (DISDA, DISIDA)
    d. acid enterogastroesophageal reflux
    study
Dilamezinsert (DMI)
    D. device
    D. penile prosthesis
    D. urologic instrument
Dilantin
dilatation (*var. of* dilation)
dilatator (*var. of* dilator)
dilated
    d. bile duct
    d. gallbladder
    d. loop of bowel
    d. pupil
    d. vein
dilating
    d. catheter
    d. catheter-gastrostomy tube
    assembly
    d. set
dilation, dilatation
    achalasia balloon d.
    anal d.
    aneurysmal d.
    balloon d.
    biliary d.
    bowel d.

Brown-McHardy pneumatic mercury
  bougie d.
capillary d.
d. catheter
cavernous artery d.
cecal d.
colonic d.
combined antegrade and
  retrograde d.
corpus cavernosum d.
cystic d.
cystoscopy and d. (C&D)
ductal d.
Eder-Puestow d.
endoscopic balloon d. (EBD)
endoscopic balloon sphincter d.
  (EBSD)
endoscopic papillary balloon d.
  (EPBD)
esophageal d.
extrahepatic biliary cystic d.
gastric d.
Grüntzig balloon d.
hepatic web d.
hydrostatic balloon d.
inadequate d.
intrahepatic biliary cystic d.
intrahepatic ductal d.
ITS balloon d.
Lord d.
Maloney d.
mechanical ureteral d.
medical d.
mucosal vascular d.
d. of esophagus
d. of hemorrhoid
d. of stomach
percutaneous balloon d.
periportal sinusoidal d.
peroral esophageal d.
pneumatic bag esophageal d.
pneumatic balloon catheter d.
pneumostatic d.
prostate gland transurethral
  balloon d.
pyloric d.
d. range
rectal d.
Rigiflex pneumatic d.
submucosal vascular d.
d. therapy
through-the-scope balloon d.
tract d.
transurethral balloon d.
TTS balloon d.
upper tract d.
urethral d.
Uromat d.
Wirsung d.

dilator, dilatator
  achalasia d.
  Achiever balloon d.
  American Endoscopy d.
  Amplatz fascial d.
  anal d.
  Backhaus d.
  Bakes common duct d.
  balloon d.
  Barnes common duct d.
  biliary balloon d.
  bougie d.
  Brown-McHardy pneumatic d.
  bullet-tip d.
  Celestin graduated d.
  circular anal d.
  Clark common duct d.
  Cunningham-Cotton sleeve coaxial d.
  Dotter d.
  Eder-Puestow metal olive d.
  Einhorn d.
  Eliminator PET biliary balloon d.
  ERCP d.
  esophageal balloon d.
  Ferris biliary duct d.
  fluoroscopy-guided balloon d.
  French d.
  Garrett d.
  Grüntzig d.
  Hegar rectal d.
  high-diameter d.
  Hurst bullet-tip d.
  Hurst mercury-filled d.
  Hurst-Tucker pneumatic d.
  hydrostatic d.
  InScope optical d.
  KeyMed advanced d.
  Kollmann d.
  Kron bile duct d.
  Kron gall duct d.
  Maloney-Hurst d.
  Maloney mercury-filled
    esophageal d.
  Maloney tapered-tip d.
  mercury-filled d.
  mercury-weighted d.
  metal olive d.
  Microvasive CRE esophageal d.
  Microvasive Rigiflex balloon d.
  modified polyethylene d.
  Mosher d.
  Murphy common duct d.
  Nottingham One-Step tapered d.
  Nottingham ureteral d.
  Olbert balloon d.
  olive-tipped plastic d.
  Optilume prostate balloon d.
  over-the-endoscope Witzel d.
  d. placement

  d. placement failure
  Plummer d.
  pneumatic balloon d.
  polyethylene balloon d.
  polyvinyl d.
  probe d.
  prostate balloon d.
  Quantum TTC balloon d.
  Ramstedt pyloric stenosis d.
  rectal d.
  Rider-Moeller d.
  Rigiflex achalasia d.
  Rigiflex TTS balloon d.
  Russell peel-away sheath d.
  Savary-Gilliard over-the-wire d.
  Savary tapered thermoplastic d.
  Sippy esophageal d.
  Soehendra catheter d.
  Starck d.
  Stucker bile duct d.
  tapered-tip d.
  through-the-scope d.
  TTS d.
  Tucker spindle-shaped d.
  vessel d.
  Walther d.
  Witzel pneumatic d.
Dilaudid
dilaurate
  fluorescein d. (FDL)
dildo, dildoe
dildoe (*var. of* dildo)
dilemma of distal ureter
dilevalol
dilinoleoylphosphatidylcholine (DLPC)
Dilomine
diltiazem therapy
dilute iodinated contrast
dilution
  agar d.
  clonal d.
  serial d.
dilutional hyponatremia
dimenhydrinate
dimension
  D. Free prostate-specific antigen
    Flex reagent cartridge test
  D. RxL PSA Flex reagent
    cartridge
2-dimensional flow cytometric analysis
3-dimensional (3D)
  3-d. conformal radiation therapy
    (3DCRT)
  3-d. CT pancreatography (3DCTP)
  3-d. endoscopic ultrasonography
  3-d. linear endoscopic ultrasound
  3-d. linear endosonography
  3-d. optical coherence tomography
  3-d. pelvicaliceal endocast

D

dimercaptosuccinic
    d. acid (DMSA)
    d. acid renal scan
    d. acid scintigraphy
dimeric
    d. acidic glycoprotein (DAG)
    d. IgA
dimerization
dimethyl
    d. iminodiacetic acid scan
    d. sulfate cystitis
    d. sulfoxide (DMSO)
dimethylester
    cystine d. (CDE)
1,2-dimethylhydrazine
dimethyl-4-phenylpiperazinium (DMPP)
dimethylpolysiloxane (DMPS)
dimethyltriazenoimidazole carboxamide (DTIC)
diminished
    d. bowel sounds
    d. branching abnormality
    d. gag reflex
diminuta
    Hymenolepis d.
diminutive
    d. adenomatous polyp
    d. colonic polyp
    d. hyperplastic polyp
dimorphic
dimple
    celiac d.
dimpling
    focal d.
    postanal d.
    skin d.
Dinamap Plus monitor
dinitrate
    d. and mononitrate ester
    isosorbide d.
dinitrochlorobenzene (DNCB)
Dinitrophenol
dinner
    d. pad
    test d.
Dinophysis
    D. acuminata
    D. fortii
dinucleotide
    flavin adenine d.
    nicotinamide adenine d. (NADH)
Diocto-C, -K
diode
    interstitial d.
    d. laser
Diodrast
Dioeze
Diogenes syndrome

Diomed laser
Dionex 2000 system
Diosuccin
dioxide
    carbon d. (CO_2)
    thorium d.
DiPAS-positive granule
DIPD
    daily intermittent peritoneal dialysis
Dipentum
dipeptidase
    N-acetylated alpha-linked d.
dipeptide
diphallia (*var. of* diphallus)
diphallus, diphallia
diphemanil methylsulfate
Diphenatol
diphenhydramine
diphenoxylate
diphenylthiazole
diphosphatase
    adenosine d. (ADPase)
diphosphate (DP, D.P.)
    adenosine d. (ADP)
    d. buffer solution
5′-diphosphate
    uridine 5′.-d. (UDP)
diphosphonate
    methylene d. (MPD)
    ^{99m}Tc-labeled stannous methylene d.
diphtheria
diphtheritic
    d. cystitis
    d. enteritis
diphyllobothriasis
Diphyllobothrium
    D. alascence
    D. dendriticum
    D. latum
    D. latum infection
    D. nihonkaiense
    D. nihonkaiense infection
    D. pacificum
    D. parvum
    D. taenioides
    D. ursi
dipivoxil
diploid
    d. cell
    d. tumor
diploidy
dipole
dipotassium
    clorazepate d.
dipropionate (DP, D.P.)
    beclomethasone d. (BDP)
Diprospan
dipslide
    Uricult d.

dipstick
    Chemstrip LN d.
    d. protein
    urinalysis d.
    urine d.
Dipylidium caninum
dipyridamole
direct
    d. bilirubin
    d. cautery puncture
    d. crossreactivity
    d. cystenterostomy
    d. extension
    d. fragmentation technique
    d. immunobead test
    d. immunofluorescence test
    (DIF-test)
    d. inguinal hernia
    d. laryngoscopy
    d. manipulation
    d. nerve stimulation graciloplasty
    d. percutaneous endoscopic
    jejunostomy (DPEJ)
    d. percutaneous jejunostomy (DPJ)
    d. percutaneous jejunostomy tube
    d. percutaneous transhepatic
    cholangiography
    d. repeat
    d. secretin endoscopic pancreatic
    function test
    d. tubular toxicity
    d. vesicoureteral scintigraphy (DVS)
    d. vision
direct-beam coupler for TURP
direct-current
    d.-c. electrocoagulation
    d.-c. electrotherapy trial
direction
    isoperistaltic d.
director
    grooved d.
    D. guidewire system
    Larry rectal d.
    probe and groove d.
direct-reading bilirubinometer
direct-vision
    d.-v. internal urethrotomy
    (DVIU)
    d.-v. liver biopsy
Direx Tripter X-1 lithotriptor
dirithromycin
Disa
    D. electromyography
    D. needle electrode
    D. 5500 urograph
disaccharidase
    d. assay
    d. deficiency
    d. enzyme activity

disaccharide
    d. intolerance
    d. lactose
    nonabsorbable d.
    d. tripeptide
disaggregation
Disalcid capsule/tablet
disappearing phenomenon
disassembly
    penile d.
    technique of penile d.
disc (*var. of* disk)
discharge
    anal d.
    bloody d.
    cervical d.
    chyme d.
    clear d.
    nasal d.
    nipple d.
    purulent d.
    urethral d.
    vaginal d.
discoid
    d. lupus erythematosus
    d. rash
discoloration
discomfort
    epigastric d.
    postligation d.
    posttreatment d.
    preexisting d.
disconnection
    ureteroendoscopic d.
discontinuation
    transient d.
discontinuity
    pelvic d.
discrete
    d. bleeding source
    d. mass
    d. narrowing
    d. nodule
    d. organ enlargement
discriminant function
discriminator
    EMI APED amplifier d.
    gamma camera d.
DISDA
    diisopropyliminodiacetic acid
disease
    acalculous gallbladder d.
    acid-peptic d.
    acquired cystic kidney d. (ACKD)
    acquired renal cystic d.
    (ARCD)
    actinomycotic esophageal d.
    acute abdominal vascular d.
    acute graft-versus-host d.

D

disease (*continued*)

acute idiopathic inflammatory bowel d.
acute on chronic liver d. (AOCLD)
acute polycystic d.
Addison d.
adrenal d.
adult celiac d. (ACD)
adult familial hyaline membrane d.
adult polycystic kidney d. (APCD, APKD)
adult polycystic liver d. (APLD)
adynamic bone d. (ABD)
African-American Study of Kidney D.
Ajmalin liver d.
Albarran d.
alcoholic liver d. (ALD)
alpha-1-antitrypsin d. (AATD)
alpha-1-antitrypsin deficiency d.
alpha chain d.
alpha heavy-chain d.
Alstrom d.
alveolar hydatid d.
American Association for the Study of Liver D.'s (AASLD)
American Foundation for Urologic D.'s (AFUD)
amyloidosis-associated kidney d.
Andersen d.
anorectal d.
anti-GBM d.
antiglomerular basement membrane d.
aplastic bone d.
arteriosclerotic renal artery d. (ASO-RAD)
atheroembolic renal d. (AERD)
atherosclerotic renovascular d.
atypical distribution of d.
atypical gallbladder d.
autoimmune thyroid d. (ATD)
autosomal-dominant polycystic kidney d. (ADPKD)
autosomal-dominant polycystic kidney d. 1 (ADPKD1)
autosomal-dominant polycystic kidney d. 2 (ADPKD2)
autosomally recessive inherited d.
autosomal-recessive polycystic kidney d. (ARPKD)
Banti d.
Barrett d.
Bassen-Kornzweig d.
Behçet d.
benign anorectal d. (BAD)
Berger d.
Besnier-Boeck-Schaumann d.
Biermer d.

big liver and spleen d. (BLSD)
biliary tract d.
black liver d.
bleeding acid-peptic d.
Blount d.
bone d.
Botkin d.
Bouchard d.
Bourneville d.
bowel d.
Bowen d.
Bradley d.
brancher glycogen storage d.
branch renal artery d.
Bright d.
Brinton d.
Bruton d.
Budd d.
Budd-Chiari d.
Byler d.
Cacchi-Ricci d.
calculous gallbladder d.
Caroli d.
Castleman d.
cavernous artery d.
celiac sprue d.
cerebrovascular d.
Chagas d.
Chagas-Cruz d.
Cherchevski d.
Chiari d.
cholestatic liver d.
cholesterol ester storage d. (CESD)
choline deficiency liver d.
chronic active liver d. (CALD)
chronic cholestatic liver d.
chronic glomerular d.
chronic graft-versus-host d. (c-GVHD)
chronic granulomatous d.
chronic inflammatory bowel d. (CIBD)
chronic liver d. (CLD)
chronic parenchymal liver d.
chronic progressive tubulointerstitial d.
chylomicron retention d.
chylopoietic d.
clinical trial for kidney d.
CMV ulcerative d.
collagen vascular d.
colorectal d.
complement-mediated immune glomerular d.
concomitant d.
congenital cystic d.
congenital polycystic d. (CPD)
Corbus d.
Cori d.

Cowden d.
crescentic fold d.
Creutzfeldt-Jakob d.
Crigler-Najjar d.
Crohn d. (CD)
Cruveilhier d.
Cruz-Chagas d.
cryptogenic liver d.
Curschmann d.
Cushing d.
cysticercus d.
cystic liver d.
cytotoxic liver d.
Darier d.
debrancher glycogen storage d.
Degos d.
de novo renal d.
Dent d.
diaphragm d.
Dieulafoy d.
diffuse liver d.
digestive d. (DD)
diverticular d.
drug-related liver d.
Dubin-Sprinz d.
Ducrey d.
duodenal ulcer d.
Durand-Nicholas-Favre d.
early-onset graft-versus-host d.
Ebstein d.
echinococcal cyst d.
endoscopy-negative reflux d. (ENRD)
end-stage liver d. (ESLD)
end-stage renal d. (ESRD)
Epstein d.
estrogen-induced liver d.
extensive pelvic d.
extraabdominal d.
extracapsular d.
extraintestinal d.
extramammary Paget d. (EMPD)
Fabry d.
familial Crohn d.
fatty liver d.
Fenwick d.
fibroobliterative d.
fibropolycystic liver d.
fistulizing Crohn d.
fistulous Crohn d.
Forbes d.
Fournier d.
fulminant Crohn d.
functional bowel d.
gamma heavy-chain d.
Gamna d.
gastric mucosal d.
gastritis-associated peptic ulcer d.
gastroduodenal Crohn d.
gastroesophageal reflux d. (GERD)

Gaucher d.
Gee d.
Gee-Herter d.
Gee-Herter-Heubner d.
Gee-Thaysen d.
Gierke d.
Gilbert d.
glomerular basement membrane d.
glomerulocystic kidney d.
glycogen storage d.
Goldstein d.
gonococcal perihepatis pelvic
  inflammatory d.
Goodpasture d.
Gordon d.
G protein d.
graft-versus-host d. (GVHD)
granulomatous bowel d.
Graves d.
Grey Turner d.
Gross d.
H d.
Hailey-Hailey d.
halothane-induced d.
Hanot d.
Harley d.
Hartnup d.
HBsAg-negative anti-HCV-negative
  chronic liver d.
heavy-chain deposition d.
Hebra d.
hemorrhage in inflammatory
  bowel d.
hepatic cystic d.
hepatic Hodgkin d.
hepatic metastatic d.
hepatic venoocclusive d.
hepatic venous web d.
hepatitis C virus-associated
  venoocclusive d.
hepatobiliary fibropolycystic d.
hepatobiliary tract d.
hepatocellular d.
hepatolenticular d.
herring-worm d.
Hers d.
Herter d.
Herter-Heubner d.
Heubner-Herter d.
Hirschsprung d.
Hodgkin d.
homologous protein overload d.
hookworm d.
Hutinel d.
hydatid cyst d.
hyperacute graft-versus-host d.
hypertensive autosomal-dominant
  polycystic kidney d.
hypoplastic glomerulocystic d.

D

disease (*continued*)

idiopathic inflammatory bowel d.
  (IIBD)
ileocolic Crohn d.
immunodeficiency d.
immunoproliferative small intestinal
  d. (IPSID)
inactive Crohn d.
infantile celiac d.
infantile polycystic d. (IPCD)
infiltrative d.
inflammatory bowel d. (IBD)
intramural atheromatous d.
iron overload d.
iron storage d.
ischemic bowel d. (IBD)
Johne d.
juvenile nephronophthisis-medullary
  cystic d.
Kashin-Beck d.
Katayama d.
Kennedy d.
Keshan d.
kidney glomerulocystic d.
Kimmelstiel-Wilson d.
Kimura d.
Kinnier Wilson d.
Klebs d.
Klemperer d.
Kohlmeier-Degos d.
Kyasanur Forest d.
Kyrle d.
Lafora d.
Lane d.
Larrey-Weil d.
Leigh d.
Leiner d.
Leyden d.
Lhermitte-Duclos d.
Liddle d.
light-chain deposition d. (LCDD)
Lignac d.
Lignac-Fanconi d.
liver hydatid d.
Löwe d.
luminal Crohn d.
lung d.
Lyell d.
Lyme d.
lysosomal storage d. (LSD)
Mackenzie d.
macrovascular d.
Madelung d.
malabsorption d.
malignant biliary obstructive d.
Manson d.
maple syrup urine d. (MSUD)
Marchiafava-Micheli d.
Marie-Strümpell d.

Marion d.
medullary cystic d.
Ménétrier d.
Ménière d.
Menkes d.
mesenteric inflammatory
  venoocclusive d. (MIVOD)
mesenteric vascular d.
metabolic liver d.
metabolic stone d.
metastatic Crohn d. (MCD)
microvillus inclusion d.
Milroy d.
minimal-change d.
Model for End-Stage Liver D.
  (MELD)
modification of diet in renal d.
  (MDRD)
mucosal lesion of acid peptic d.
multicystic kidney d. (MCKD)
Munk d.
muscle layer d.
mycobacterial d.
myeloproliferative d.
National Institute of Diabetes,
  Digestive and Kidney D. (NIDDK)
neoplastic d.
neurogenic bladder d.
neurohumoral d.
Niemann-Pick d.
nil d.
Nisbet d.
non-A–G chronic liver d.
nonalcoholic fatty liver d. (NAFLD)
non-B non-C chronic liver d.
  (NBNC CLD)
noncalculous d.
noncommunicating polycystic d.
nondiabetic proteinuric renal d.
nonerosive gastroesophageal
  reflux d.
nonerosive reflux d. (NERD)
nonobstructive hepatic
  parenchymal d.
nonorgan-confined d.
oasthouse urine d.
obstructive gastroduodenal
  Crohn d.
Ohara d.
oral d.
organic neurologic d.
Ormond d.
Osler-Weber-Rendu d.
ovarian d.
Paget extramammary d.
Paget perianal d.
panacinar d.
pancreatic d.
pancreaticobiliary d.

parasitic liver d.
parathyroid d.
parenchymatous liver d.
Parkinson d.
paroxysmal motor d.
Payr d.
pediatric endstage liver d. (PELD)
pediatric stone d.
pelvic inflammatory d. (PID)
peptic reflux d.
peptic ulcer d. (PUD)
perforated ulcer d.
perianal Crohn d.
perineal Crohn d.
Peyronie d.
pilonidal sinus d.
polycystic kidney d. (PCKD)
polycystic liver d. (PCLD, PLD)
Pompe d.
post jejunoileal bypass hepatic d.
Potter d.
predominant hyperparathyroid bone
  d. (PHBD)
preeclamptic liver d.
preexisting d.
primary glomerular d.
primary sclerosing cholangitis
  inflammatory bowel d. (PSC-IBD)
protozoan d.
pseudoalcoholic liver d.
pseudo-Whipple d.
radiation-induced d.
Rayer d.
recessive polycystic kidney d.
rectal d.
recurrent episodes of *Clostridium*
  difficile d.
reflux d.
Refsum d.
Reichmann d.
Reiter d.
renal arterial occlusive d.
renal bone d.
renal cystic d.
renal fibromuscular d.
renal hydatid d.
Rendu-Osler-Weber d.
renovascular d.
rheumatic d.
Rokitansky d.
Rossbach d.
Ruysch d.
Saunders d.
Schilder d.
Schindler d.
schistosomal liver d.
Schönlein-Henoch d.
Schultz d.
scleroderma bowel d.

segmental colitis associated with
  diverticular d.
sexually related intestinal d.
sexually transmitted d. (STD)
sickle cell d.
sigmoid d.
Simple Endoscopic Score for Crohn
  D. (SES-CD)
skeletal muscle d.
skin d.
small-intestinal Crohn d.
space-occupying d.
Spencer d.
steely-hair d.
Steinert d.
steroid-dependent Crohn d.
steroid-refractory Crohn d.
Still d.
Stokvis d.
stone d.
Strachan d.
stress-related mucosal d. (SRMD)
Stühmer d.
subacute liver d.
subserous d.
suprahilar d.
systemic mast cell d.
Tangier d.
terminal ileal d.
testicular Hodgkin d.
Thaysen d.
thin basement membrane d.
thin glomerular basement
  membrane d.
thromboembolic d.
thyroid d.
Tis d.
transfusion-related chronic liver d.
transmittable d.
tubulointerstitial d.
tufting d.
tunnel d.
unilocular hydatid d.
upper tract d.
uremic medullary cystic d.
urinary tract d.
urologic d.
valvular heart d.
van Bogaert d.
van Buren d.
van den Bergh d.
vascular d.
venereal d. (VD)
venoocclusive liver d.
venous outflow obstructive d.
venous web d.
Vienna classification of Crohn d.
von Gierke d.
von Hippel-Lindau d.

D

disease (*continued*)
    von Recklinghausen d.
    von Rokitansky d.
    von Willebrand d.
    Wassilieff d.
    Weber-Christian d.
    Weil d.
    Werdnig-Hoffman d.
    Westphal-Strümpell d.
    Whipple d.
    Wilkie d.
    Wilson d.
    Wolman d.
    X-linked chronic granulomatous d.
    (X-CGD)
diseased organileal pouch-anal anastomosis
disease-free survival curve
disease-specific diet
dish
    Side-Fire reflecting d.
disialosyl Lea
DISIDA
    diisopropyliminodiacetic acid
    DISIDA enterogastroesophageal
      reflux study
    ^{99m}Tc DISIDA
    DISIDA scan
disimpaction
    colonoscopic d.
disinfectant
    Abocide d.
    Actril d.
    Asepti-steryl d.
    Burnishine d.
    Calgocide d.
    Cold Spor d.
    cyclic urinary d.
    Endospore d.
    Enzol d.
    Metricide d.
    Omnicide d.
    ProCide d.
    Sporacidin d.
    Vespore d.
    Wavicide d.
disinfection
    high-level d.
disintegration
    endoscopic stone d.
DisIntek reagent strip
disjoined pyeloplasty
disk, disc
    anal d.
    bilaminar embryonic d.
    d. diffusion
    d. kidney
    laser d.
    d. margin

    Marlen double-faced adhesive d.
    Molnar d.
dislodgement
    electrode d.
dislodger
    stone d.
dismembered
    d. anastomosis
    d. pyeloplasty
    d. reimplanted appendicocystostomy
dismutase
    superoxide d. (SD)
disobliteration
disodium
    balsalazide d.
    cefotetan d.
    d. cromoglycate
    d. edetate
Disolan
Disonate
disopyramide phosphate (DP)
disorder
    absence of comorbid d.'s
    acid-base d.
    acid-related d. (ARD)
    acid secretory d.
    anorexia nervosa and associated d.'s
    (ANAD)
    appetite d.
    autoimmune connective tissue d.
    autosomal-dominant d.
    binge-eating d. (BED)
    blood coagulation d.
    cardiovascular d.
    connective tissue d.
    deglutition d.
    esophageal motility d. (EMD)
    esophageal motor d.
    evacuation d.
    fat storage d.
    feeding d.
    functional bowel d. (FBD)
    functional esophageal d. (FED)
    functional gastrointestinal d.
    (FGID)
    gastric motility d.
    Hartnup d.
    humoral immunodeficiency d.
    International Foundation for
      Functional Gastrointestinal D.'s
    intestinal motility d.
    iron overload d.
    lower motor neuron bladder d.
    lymphoproliferative d.
    metabolic d.
    minor cognitive motor d. (MCMD)
    mixed connective tissue d.
    motility d.
    myeloproliferative d.

National Association of Anorexia
  Nervosa and Associated D.'s
neurodegenerative d.
neurogenic d.
neurologic d.
nonspecific esophageal motility d.
  (NEMD)
papulosquamous d.
pelvic floor d.
posttransplant lymphoproliferative d.
  (PTLD)
psychological d.
psychophysiologic d.
psychosomatic d.
pulmonary d.
rectal evacuatory d. (RED)
seizure d.
spastic motor d.
umbilical d.
urachal d.
vasomotor d.
vesiculobullous d.
wound healing d.

disordered
  d. acrosome reaction of
    spermatozoon
  d. defecation
  d. motility

Di-Sosul
dispar
  Entamoeba d.

Di-Spaz
Dispenstirs
displacement
  bowel d.
  fiber lock d.
  fish-hook d.
  gallbladder d.
  tumor d.

disposable
  d. forceps
  d. pudendal nerve electrode
  d. trocar

disposable-sheath
  d.-s. flexible gastroscope
  d.-s. flexible sigmoidoscope

disrupted peristalsis
disruption
  pancreatic duct d.

disruptor
  endocrine d.

Disse
  space of D.

dissecting
  d. abdominal aneurysm
  d. balloon
  d. renal artery aneurysm

dissection
  aortic d.

autonomic nerve-preserving
  3-space d.
blunt and sharp d.
circumferential mucosal d.
dorsal artery d.
electrosurgical d.
en bloc d.
endoscopic submucosal d. (ESD)
extended obturator node and
  iliopsoas node d.
extraperitoneal endoscopic pelvic
  lymph node d. (EEPLND)
3-field d.
flap d.
iliac fossa d.
intersphincteric rectal d.
intracapsular d.
intramural air d.
laparoscopic pelvic lymph node d.
  (LPLND)
laparoscopic retroperitoneal lymph
  node d.
lateral node d.
limited obturator node d.
lymph node d. (LND)
d. margin
meticulous d.
minilaparotomy pelvic lymph
  node d.
nerve-sparing lymph node d.
node d.
partial zonal d. (PZD)
pelvic lymph node d. (PLND)
per anum intersphincteric rectal d.
plane of d.
rectal d.
renal hilar d.
retroperitoneal lymph node d.
  (RLND)
d. scissors
scissors d.
sharp d.
3-space d.
spontaneous d.
submucosal d.
suprahilar lymph node d.
ultrasonic d.
ureteral d.
water-jet d.

dissector
  Beaver d.
  CUSA d.
  Kittner d.
  McDonald stone d.
  Mixter d.
  peanut d.
  Spacemaker balloon d.
  sponge d.
  ultrasonic aspirator and d.

D

disseminated
    d. cancer
    d. CMV infection
    d. histoplasmosis
    d. intravascular coagulation
      (DIC)
    d. lupus erythematosus (DLE)
    d. metastasis
    d. peritoneal adenomucinosis
    d. strongyloidiasis
dissemination
    metastatic d.
dissimilatory sulfate reduction
dissociated medium
dissolution
    contact d.
    MTBE gallstone d.
    d. of gallstone
distal
    d. bile duct
    d. bile duct diameter
    d. blind stomach
    d. colitis
    d. colon
    d. convoluted tubule (DCT)
    d. convolution
    d. duodenum
    d. esophageal ring
    d. esophageal stenosis
    d. esophageal stricture
    d. esophagus
    d. gastrectomy
    d. ileitis
    d. intestine
    d. neoplasia
    d. nephron segment
    d. pancreatectomy
    d. pouch leak
    d. renal tubular acidosis (dRTA)
    d. renal tubular necrosis
    d. shave section
    d. splenorenal shunt (DSRS)
    d. tubular acting agent
    d. tubule
    d. ureter
    d. ureteral anatomy
    d. ureterectomy
    d. venous plexus
distance
    peritoneal-anal d.
distant
    d. abscess
    d. metastasis
    d. pH probe location
distasonis
    Bacteroides d.
distended
    d. abdomen
    d. bladder

distensae
    striae d.
distensibility
distension (*var. of* distention)
distention, distension
    abdominal d.
    colonic d.
    esophageal balloon d.
    gaseous d.
    gastric d.
    intestinal d.
    intraesophageal balloon d. (IEBD)
    intraluminal d.
    isobaric gastric d.
    postprandial d.
    rectal d.
    d. ulcer
    visible abdominal d.
distomatosis (*var. of* distomiasis)
distomiasis, distomatosis
    intestinal d.
distorted crypt architecture
distortion
    crypt architectural d.
distress
    epigastric d.
    functional bowel d. (FBD)
    mild d.
    moderate d.
    respiratory d.
distribution
    folate d.
    geographic d.
    hit-skip d.
    intrarenal d.
    liver d.
    node d.
    d. ratio (DR)
    d. ratio 2 (DR2)
    d. ratio 3 (DR3)
    d. ratio 4 (DR4)
    d. ratio 5 (DR5)
    d. ratio 7 (DR7)
    vasoactive intestinal peptide d.
    volume of d.
disturbance
    acid-base d.
    gait d.
    phytoestrogen-induced menstrual
      cycle d.
disulfide crosslinked fibril
disulfiram
disulfiram-like effect
dithiothreitol (DTT)
Ditropan XL
Dittel
    D. operation
    D. sound
Diucardin

Diupres
diuresis
> alcohol d.
> osmotic d.
> postobstructive d.
> solute d.
> tubular d.
> water d.

diuretic
> high-ceiling d.
> hydragogue d.
> kaliuretic d.
> loop d.
> d. nuclear renography
> osmotic d.
> potassium-sparing d.
> refrigerant d.
> d. renal quantitative camera study
> d. renal scintigraphy
> thiazide d.

diuretic-induced hypokalemia
diuria
Diurigen
diurnal
> d. continence
> d. cycle
> d. enuresis
> d. incontinence
> d. urine osmolality
> d. variation

Diutensen-R
diutinum
> erythema elevatum d.

divalent
> d. metal transporter 1 (DMT1)
> d. mineral

diversion
> acidosis after urinary intestinal d.
> biliopancreatic d.
> Bricker urinary d.
> Camey enterocystoplasty urinary d.
> Camey I orthotopic urinary d.
> d. colitis
> continent catheterizable urinary d.
> continent cutaneous d.
> continent supravesical bowel urinary d.
> cutaneous urinary d.
> double-T pouch urinary d.
> Duke pouch cutaneous urinary d.
> external biliary d.
> fecal d.
> Gil-Vernet ileocecal cystoplasty urinary d.
> Gil-Vernet orthotopic urinary d.
> Hammock technique urinary d.
> hemi-Kock urinary d.
> heterotopic d.

> ileal conduit urinary d.
> ileal neobladder urinary d.
> ileocecal cutaneous d.
> ileocolic pouch urinary d.
> Indiana continent reservoir urinary d.
> initial proximal d.
> jejunal cutaneous urinary d.
> Kock pouch cutaneous urinary d.
> Leadbetter ileal loop d.
> Le Bag urinary d.
> LeDuc technique urinary d.
> Mainz pouch cutaneous urinary d.
> Mainz pouch I continent urinary d.
> orthotopic urinary d.
> palliative urinary d.
> partial external biliary d.
> primary urinary d.
> d. proctitis
> rectal bladder urinary d.
> split-nipple technique urinary d.
> stone in urinary d.
> Studer reservoir urinary d.
> subcutaneous urinary d.
> supravesical urinary d.
> tunneled technique urinary d.
> urinary intestinal d.
> Wallace technique urinary d.

diversionary ileostomy
diversus
> *Citrobacter d.*

diverticula (*pl. of* diverticulum)
diverticular
> d. abscess
> d. bleeding
> d. disease
> d. disease of colon (DDC)
> d. hemorrhage
> d. phlegmon

diverticulectomy
> bladder d.
> endocavitary bladder d.
> extravesical/intravesical d.
> Harrington esophageal d.
> pharyngoesophageal d.
> urethral d.
> vesical d.

diverticulitis
> acute d.
> cecal d.
> chronic d.
> duodenal d.
> d. evaluation
> Meckel d.
> perforating d.
> sigmoid d.

diverticulogram
diverticuloma
diverticulopexy

D

diverticuloscope
soft d.
diverticulosis
acquired d.
bleeding d.
colonic d.
congenital d.
esophageal intramural d.
gastric d.
giant d.
jejunal d.
diverticulostomy
endoscopic stapling d.
diverticulotomy
endoscopic clip-and-cut d.
diverticulum, *pl.* **diverticula**
diverticula ampullae ductus
deferentis
angioarchitecture of arterial supply
of d.
biliary d.
bladder congenital d.
bleeding d.
caliceal d.
cecal d.
colonic d.
congenital bladder d.
cricopharyngeal d.
Dohlman endoscopic repair of
Zenker d.
duodenal d.
epiphrenic d.
esophageal d.
false d.
fluid-filled d.
d. fulguration
Ganser d.
giant colonic d. (GCD)
Graser d.
Heister d.
hepatic d.
Hutch d.
hypopharyngeal d.
d. ilei verum
inflamed d.
intestinal d.
intraluminal duodenal d.
(IDD)
intramural d.
inverted sigmoid d.
juxtapapillary duodenal d.
Kirchner d.
Kommerell d.
long-neck d.
Meckel d.
midesophageal d.
mucosal d.
noncommunicating d.
d. of Akerlund

d. of colon
d. of Nuck
pancreatic d.
perforated d.
periampullary duodenal d.
peripapillary d.
Pertik d.
pharyngeal d.
pharyngoesophageal d.
pressure d.
Rokitansky d.
ruptured sigmoid d.
sigmoid d.
solitary d.
supradiaphragmatic d.
thin-walled d.
traction d.
unroofing of d.
urachal d.
ureteral d.
urethral d.
vesical d.
vesicourachal d.
volvulated Meckel d.
Zenker d.
diverting
d. loop colostomy
d. loop ileostomy
d. stoma
d. stoma creation
divided
d. appendix
d. pancreas
divided-stoma colostomy
division
urethral plate d.
divisum
incomplete pancreas d. (IPD)
pancreas d. (PD)
Dixon-Thomas-Smith clamp
Dizac
DJJ
duodenojejunal junction
DKA
diabetic ketoacidosis
DLE
disseminated lupus erythematosus
DLG5 **gene variant**
DLPC
dilinoleoylphosphatidylcholine
DMEM
Dulbecco modified Eagle medium
DMI
Dilamezinsert
DMI urologic instrument
DMPP
dimethyl-4-phenylpiperazinium
DMPS
dimethylpolysiloxane

DMS
diffuse mesangial sclerosis
DMSA
dimercaptosuccinic acid
^{99m}Tc DMSA
DMSA scan
DMSA scintigraphy
DMSO
dimethyl sulfoxide
DMSO cystitis
DMT1
divalent metal transporter 1
DNA
deoxyribonucleic acid
DNA aneuploidy
DNA array
branched-chain DNA
complementary DNA (cDNA)
covalently closed circular DNA
(cccDNA)
fecal DNA (F-DNA)
DNA flow cytometry
genomic DNA
DNA haploid cell
HBV genomic DNA
hepatitis B-like DNA
DNA hypomethylation
DNA immunization
DNA labeling kit
DNA laddering
DNA microarray technology
DNA ploidy analysis
DNA ploidy pattern
DNA polymerase
DNA polymorphism
DNA proliferation
DNA sequencing system
single-parameter DNA
DNA stemline
DNA synthesis
DNCB
dinitrochlorobenzene
DNCB immunologic study
DNH
diffuse nodular hyperplasia
Dobbhoff
D. biofeedback monitor
D. bipolar coagulation probe
D. enteral feeding bag
D. gastrectomy feeding tube
D. gastric decompression tube
D. PEG tube
dobutamine
docetaxel
dock
D. test meal
water d.
Docucal-P
docusate sodium

dodecadactylitis
dodecadactylon
dog-ear of anastomosis
Dogiel type I, II morphology
dog rose
dogwood
Asiatic d.
DO2 haplotype
Dohlman
D. endoscopic repair of Zenker
diverticulum
D. esophagoscope
dolasetron
dolichocolon with pseudoobstruction
**DoLi S extracorporeal shock wave
lithotriptor**
Dolobid
dolorimeter
Chatillon d.
dolorosa
nephritis d.
dolphin grasping forceps
dolphin-type atraumatic forceps
domain
alternative cell attachment d.
carboxyterminal noncollagenous d.
cleaved extracellular d.
COOH-terminal SH2 d.
effector d.
Kringle d.
membrane-spanning d. (MSD)
NH2-terminal SH2 d.
nucleotide-binding d. (NBD)
SH2-binding d.
src-homology 2 d.
trefoil d.
dome
gallbladder d.
d. of bladder
d. of liver
trabeculation of bladder d.
Domeboro solution
dome-shaped internal bumper
DomeTip
D. Autotome
D. CleverCut device
D. Ultratome XL device
dome-tip electrode
domiciliary urinary tract infection
dominant inheritance model
Domino transplant
domperidone
domperidone-functional dyspepsia trial
donation
live renal d.
organ d.
Donnagel
Donnagel-PG
Donnamar

D

Donna-Sed
Donnatal No. 2
Donnazyme
donor
    d. age-dependent effect
    antigen-matched d.
    artificial insemination d. (AID)
    d. dendritic cell
    d. hematopoietic cell
      microchimerism
    d. hepatectomy
    d. hepatic duct (DHD)
    kidney d.
    d. kidney
    living d.
    living adult-to-adult d.
    living related d. (LRD)
    living unrelated d. (LURD)
    marginal kidney d.
    d. nephrectomy
    nitric oxide d.
    d. of nitric oxide
    related living d. (RLD)
    sulfhydryl d.
donor/recipient race matching
donor-specific
    d.-s. alloantibody
    d.-s. transfusion (DST)
donor-type microchimerism
Donovan body
donovani
    Leishmania donovani d.
donovanosis
Donphen
donut (*var. of* doughnut)
doom
    triangle of d.
DOPA
    dihydroxyphenylalanine
dopamine
    d. agonist
    d. antagonist
    d. beta-hydroxylase
dopaminergic
    d. agonist
    d. medication
Dopar
dopexamine
Doppler
    D. assistance
    color flow D.
    D. color flow imaging
    D. effect
    endoscopic color D.
    D. flow test (DFT)
    D. operation
    penile D.
    D. perfusion index (DPI)
    D. probe

    pulsed D.
    D. QAD1
    D. Quantum color flow system
    D. sonography of SMA
    D. ultrasonography
    D. ultrasonography/angiography
    D. ultrasound
    D. ultrasound intestinal blood flow
      measurement
Doppler-guided hemorrhoidal artery
  ligation (DGHAL)
DOQI
    Dialysis Outcomes Quality Initiative
Dor fundoplication
Dormia
    D. noose
    D. stone basket
    D. stone basket catheter
Dornier
    D. compact lithotriptor
    D. electrohydraulic lithotriptor
    D. extracorporeal shock wave
      lithotripsy
    D. gallstone lithotriptor
    D. MFL lithotriptor
    D. MFL 5000 urological
      workstation
    D. MPL 9000 electrohydraulic
      lithotriptor ultrasound focusing
      system
    D. MPL gallstone lithotripsy
    D. MPL lithotriptor
    D. Urotract cystoscopy table
dorsal
    d. artery dissection
    d. bud
    d. curve plication
    d. lithotomy
    d. lithotomy position
    d. lumbotomy
    d. lumbotomy incision
    d. mesogastrium
    d. nerve conduction velocity
    d. nerve of penis
    d. pancreatic artery
    d. pancreatic duct
    d. penile artery
    d. point
    d. rhizotomy
    d. root ganglion
    d. slit
    d. tunical tuck
    d. vagal complex
    d. vein
    d. vein complex (DVC)
    d. vein patch graft
dorsalis
    arteria pancreatica d.
    tabes d.

dorsocranial
dorsosacral position
dorsum
    d. of penis
    d. of testis
dosage
    radiation d.
    sclerosant d.
dose
    arthritic d. (A/D)
    breakthrough d.
    conceptus d.
    d. response
dose-optimized therapy (DOT)
dosepak
    Hytrin D.
dosimeter
    single-channel in vivo
      light d.
Dostent
DOT
    dose-optimized therapy
    TherMatrx DOT
dot-blot hybridization
dot-plotted probe
Dotter
    D. catheter
    D. dilator
Doubilet
    D. sphincterotome
    D. sphincterotomy
double
    d. accessory channel therapeutic
      endoscope
    d. bladder
    d. bubble duodenal sign
    d. contrast
    d. dialyzer
    d. duct sign
    d. enterostomy
    d. gallbladder
    d. gracilis wrap
    d. halo sign
    d. incontinence
    d. intussusception
    d. J-shaped reservoir
    d. penis
    d. pyloroplasty
    d. pylorus
    d. reverse alpha-sigmoid
      loop
    d. stapling technique (DST)
    d. strength (DS)
    d. tracking of barium
    d. uterus
    d. x-ray densitometry
double-antibody sandwich system
double-balloon
    d.-b. endoscopy system

    d.-b. method of enteroscopy
    d.-b. technique
double-barrel
    d.-b. colostomy
    d.-b. ileostomy
    d.-b. reservoir
double-bite biopsy
double-blind randomized study
double-chamber hemodiafiltration
double-channel
    d.-c. colonoscope
    d.-c. endoscope
    d.-c. esophagram
    d.-c. fistulotome
    d.-c. sphincterotome
    d.-c. videoendoscope
double-contrast
    d.-c. barium enema (DCBE)
    d.-c. barium enema examination
    d.-c. barium examination of upper
      gastrointestinal tract (DCGI)
    d.-c. barium meal
    d.-c. esophagram
    d.-c. radiography
    d.-c. roentgenography
double-cuff urinary sphincter
double-dose IV Timentin
double-endoscope method
double-faced island flap for hypospadias
repair
double-folded cup-patch ileocystoplasty
technique
double-headed
    d.-h. P190 stapler
    d.-h. P190 stapling device
double-head spermatozoon
double-J
    d.-J catheter
    d.-J indwelling catheter stent
    d.-J silicone stent
    d.-J Surgitek catheter stent
    d.-J ureteral stent
double-loop
    d.-l. pouch
    d.-l. tourniquet
double-lumen
    d.-l. balloon catheter
    d.-l. endoprosthesis
    d.-l. gastric laryngeal mask airway
    d.-l. injection catheter
    d.-l. irrigation cannula
    d.-l. tapered-tip papillotome
    d.-l. tube
double-peaked wave
double-pigtail
    d.-p. endoprosthesis
    d.-p. prosthesis
    d.-p. stent
double-puncture laparoscopy

D

double-spoon forceps
double-stapled
    d.-s. ileal pouch-anal anastomosis
    d.-s. ileal reservoir
double-staple technique
DoubleStent
    D. biliary endoprosthesis
    D. biliary endoprosthesis stent
double-tail spermatozoon
double-T pouch urinary diversion
double-wing shape
doubling time
doubly ligated
doughnut, donut
    circular stapler d.
    d. lesion
    stapler d.
doughnut-shaped balloon
doughy
    d. abdomen
    d. consistency
Douglas
    D. abscess
    cul-de-sac of D.
    D. fold
    line of D.
    D. pouch
    D. rectal snare
    rectouterine pouch of D.
    semicircular line of D.
doula
Dover
    D. intermittent female catheter
    D. red rubber Robinson intermittent
    catheter
    D. Rob-Nel intermittent catheter
    D. 100% silicone Foley catheter
    D. Texas catheter
Dow-Corning ileal pouch catheter
Dowd II prostatic balloon dilation
  catheter
Dow hollow-fiber kidney (DHFK)
down
    D. syndrome
    tacked d.
downhill esophageal varix
downregulation after furosemide
  treatment
downscatter
downstage
downstaging
    hormonal d.
    d. of advanced esophageal
    carcinoma
downstream
    d. signaling protein
    d. signal transduction
downward retraction
doxacurium

doxazosin
    d. gastrointestinal therapy system
    d. mesylate
doxepin
doxercalciferol injection
Doxinate
doxorubicin
    doxorubicin, bleomycin sulfate,
      vinblastine (ABV)
    doxorubicin, bleomycin sulfate,
      vinblastine, dacarbazine (ABVD)
doxycycline-metronidazole-bismuth
  subcitrate triple therapy
doxycycline monohydrate
Doyen
    D. abdominal retractor
    D. abdominal scissors
    D. gallbladder forceps
    D. intestinal clamp
    D. intestinal forceps
    D. operation
    D. raspatory
    D. rib elevator
doylei
    Campylobacter d.
DP, D.P.
    diphosphate
    dipropionate
    disopyramide phosphate
    Dalalone D.P.
DPC
    delayed primary closure
DPEG
    dual percutaneous endoscopic
    gastrostomy
DPEJ
    direct percutaneous endoscopic
    jejunostomy
D-penicillamine
DPGN
    diffuse proliferative glomerulonephritis
DPI
    daily protein intake
    Doppler perfusion index
DPJ
    direct percutaneous jejunostomy
    DPJ tube
DP-1 lithotriptor
D-P urea ratio
DQ2 haplotype
DR
    distribution ratio
DR1 HLA-DRB tissue type
DR2
    distribution ratio 2
      DR2 1501 HLA-DRB tissue type
      DR2 1502 HLA-DRB tissue type
      DR2 1601 HLA-DRB tissue type
      DR2 1602 HLA-DRB tissue type

DR3
  distribution ratio 3
    DR3 HLA-DRB tissue type
DR4
  distribution ratio 4
    DR4 HLA-DRB tissue type
DR5
  distribution ratio 5
    heterozygous DR5
DR7
  distribution ratio 7
    DR7 haplotype
    DR7 HLA-DRB tissue type
DR9
  distribution ratio 9
    DR9 HLA-DRB tissue type
drag
  solvent d.
dragon pyelogram
dragon's blood
drain
  Blair silicone d.
  Chaffin-Pratt d.
  cigarette d.
  closed-suction d.
  Davol sump d.
  ERCP nasobiliary d.
  fluted J-Vac d.
  Hemovac Suction standard d.
  Hollister irrigator d.
  Jackson-Pratt d.
  J-Vac d.
  Mikulicz d.
  nasobiliary d. (NBD)
  nasocystic d.
  Nélaton rubber tube d.
  Penrose sump d.
  perineal d.
  Pezzer d.
  Quad-Lumen d.
  Redivac suction d.
  Redon d.
  Relia-Vac d.
  Snyder d.
  stab-wound d.
  suction d.
  sump d.
  surgical d.
  T d.
  Teflon nasobiliary d.
  transnasal pancreaticobiliary d.
  transpapillary d.
  T-tube d.
  van Sonnenberg sump d.
  d. volume
  Wangensteen d.
  2-wing Malecot d.
  4-wing Malecot d.
drainable ostomy pouch

drainage
  antegrade ureteral d.
  bedside d. (BSD)
  biliary d.
  button d.
  calyceal d.
  d. catheter
  closed d.
  continuous bladder d.
  continuous catheter d.
  continuous suction d.
  CT-guided abscess d.
  CT-guided pseudocyst d.
  duodenal d.
  endoscopic biliary d.
  endoscopic nasobiliary catheter d.
  endoscopic pancreatic d.
  endoscopic retrograde biliary d.
    (ERBD)
  endoscopic transgastric d.
  endoscopic transpapillary cyst d.
    (ETCD)
  endoscopic transpapillary
    nasopancreatic d.
  external d.
  gravity-dependent d.
  guided percutaneous d.
  incision and d. (I&D)
  internal biliary d.
  J-Vac closed wound d.
  lymphocele internal d.
  lymphocele percutaneous d.
  nasobiliary d.
  nasogastric d.
  nasopancreatic d.
  open d.
  pancreaticoduodenal venous d.
  passive chest d.
  percutaneous abscess d.
  percutaneous antegrade biliary d.
  percutaneous biliary d. (PBD)
  percutaneous transhepatic d. (PTD)
  percutaneous transhepatic biliary d.
    (PTBD)
  postoperative irrigation-suction d.
  Pyridium test of vaginal d.
  sanguineous d.
  serosanguineous d.
  suction d.
  suprapubic d.
  tidal d.
  transduodenal d.
  transgastric d.
  transhepatic biliary d.
  transluminal pseudocyst d.
  transmural d. (TMD)
  transpapillary d.
  T-tube d.
  d. tube

D

drainage *(continued)*
    Wangensteen d.
    wound d.
drainage-resistant pseudocyst
draining sinus
drain-trap stomach
Drake uroflowmeter
Drake-Willock
    D.-W. delivery system
    D.-W. peritoneal dialysis system
Dramamine
Drapanas shunt
drape
    barrier d.
    fenestrated d.
    Lingeman 3-in-1 procedure d.
    Lingeman TUR d.
    O'Connor d.
    surgical d.
Drash syndrome
DRB **gene**
DRE
    digital rectal examination
Dreiling
    D. tube
    D. tube pancreatic function
    test
Dremel Moto-Tool
dressing
    Acticoat composite d.
    Acticoat foam d.
    Adaptic d.
    adhesive d.
    Algidex Ag Silver d.
    Amerigel d.
    anorectal d.
    antiseptic d.
    Aquacel Ag d.
    Arglaes powder d.
    Askina Derm film d.
    Biatain foam d.
    bioocclusive d.
    bolus d.
    bulky d.
    CarboFlex odor-control d.
    Carraginate d.
    CarraSorb H d.
    Coban d.
    ColActive Ag antimicrobial collagen
      wound d.
    CombiDERM nonadhesive
      absorbant d.
    Compeed Skinprotector d.
    Contreet foam d.
    Copa Plus ultrasoft foam
      wound d.
    CovaClear Ag antimicrobial
      wound d.
    Curasorb zinc d.

Dermaginate d.
Di-Dak-Sol d.
dry sterile d.
Elastoplast d.
Flexzan topical wound d.
d. forceps
gauze d.
Gentleheal d.
Hyalofill-F biopolymeric d.
Hydrocol II d.
hydrocolloid island d.
Hydrofera blue bacteriostatic foam
  wound d.
hydrofiber d.
Hydrovase wound d.
Integra bilayer wound d.
Kalginate d.
Kaltostat d.
Kling d.
Lyofoam d.
Maxorb d.
Melgisorb d.
Mepilex Border Lite d.
Mepilex Transfer d.
Montgomery strap d.
nanocrystalline silver-containing d.
nonadhesive d.
occlusive collodion d.
Op-Site d.
Optifoam d.
pressure d.
QuadraFoam d.
SaliCept freeze-dried d.
Signa Dress hydrocolloid d.
sterile d.
Tegaderm absorbent clear
  acrylic d.
Tegaderm foam adhesive d.
Telfa d.
Tielle Plus hydropolymer d.
tie-over d.
VAC GranuFoam silver d.
wound contact d.
DRF
  digestive-respiratory fistula
dribble
    postmicturition d.
    postvoid d.
dribbling
    urinary d.
drilling tract
drink
    Boost nutritional energy d.
    HeartBar orange d.
drinking
    d. habit
    psychogenic water d.
    voluntarily stopping eating and d.
    (VSED)

drip

alkaline milk d.
d. infusion cholangiography (DIC)
d. infusion cholecystography
intragastric d.
intravenous d.
Murphy d.
postnasal d.

driver

automatic needle d.
Heaney needle d.
laparoscopic needle d.
long vascular needle d.
needle d.
Szabo-Berci needle d.

dromedary hump
dronabinol
drooling
droop

flank d.

drooping lily sign
droperidol
dropped bladder
dropsical

d. nephritis
d. nephropathy

dropsy

abdominal d.
cutaneous d.
nutritional d.
peritoneal d.

Drosophila melanogaster
dRTA

distal renal tubular acidosis

drug

aminobisphosphonate gastrotoxic d.
anorectic d.
antagonistic d.
anticholinergic d.
antiemetic d.
antilipemic d.
antimotility d.
antimuscarinic d.
antimycobacterial d.
antisecretory d.
antispasmodic d.
aquaretic d.
d. carrier system
COX-2 selective nonsteroidal
   antiinflammatory d.
crude d.
cyclooxygenase-2 selective
   nonsteroidal antiinflammatory d.
d. hepatotoxicity
H2 receptor-blocking d.
hydrocholeretic d.
immunoregulatory d.
immunosuppressive d.
d. intoxication

lipid-lowering d.
d. metabolism
mucosal protective d.
neurolytic d.
neuropsychotropic d.
nitric oxide-releasing nonsteroidal
   antiinflammatory d.'s (NO-NSAIDs)
nonnephrotoxic d.
nonsteroidal antiinflammatory d.
   (NSAID)
parasympatholytic d.
parasympathomimetic d.
portal hypotensive d.
prokinetic d.
psychotropic d.
d. reaction
recreational d.
d. resistance
second-line d.
serotonergic d.
d. therapy
vasoactive d.

drug-induced

d.-i. acute hepatic injury
d.-i. acute pancreatitis
d.-i. acute tubular necrosis
d.-i. cholestasia
d.-i. cirrhosis
d.-i. colitis
d.-i. constipation
d.-i. erection
d.-i. esophageal damage (DIED)
d.-i. esophagitis
d.-i. gastritis
d.-i. hepatitis
d.-i. pain
d.-i. priapism
d.-i. renal failure
d.-i. steatosis
d.-i. ulcer

3-drug regimen
drug-related liver disease
Drummond

artery of D.
marginal artery of D.

DRw8 HLA-DRB tissue type
DRw10 HLA-DRB tissue type
DRw11 HLA-DRB tissue type
DRw12 HLA-DRB tissue type
DRw13 HLA-DRB tissue type
DRw14 HLA-DRB tissue type
dry

d. colostomy
d. ejaculation
d. heaves
d. mucous membranes
d. skin
d. sterile dressing
d. swallow

D

dry (*continued*)
    d. swallow on esophageal
       manometry
    d. vomiting
    d. weight (DW)
DS
    double strength
       Bactrim DS
       Septra DS
       Sulfatrim DS
       trimethoprim-sulfamethoxazole
         DS
DSG
    deoxyspergualin
D4S231 marker
D4S414 marker
D16S84 marker
D16S283 marker
D16S291 marker
DSRS
    distal splenorenal shunt
DSS
    dextran sodium sulfate
DST
    donor-specific transfusion
    double stapling technique
    duodenal secretin test
DTH
    delayed-type hypersensitivity
DTIC
    dimethyltriazenoimidazole carboxamide
DTPA
    diethylenetriamine pentaacetic acid
       indium-111 DTPA
       DTPA renal scan
       DTPA renography
DTT
    dithiothreitol
Dua antireflux stent
dual
    d. percutaneous endoscopic
       gastrostomy (DPEG)
    d. percutaneous gastrostomy tube
dual-axis confocal microscope
dual-endoscope technique
dual-energy
    d.-e. CT scan
    d.-e. x-ray absorptiometry (DEXA,
       DXA)
    d.-e. x-ray absorption
dual-lumen
    d.-l. catheter
    d.-l. papillotome
DualMesh hernia repair
dual-phase helical computed tomography
dual-photon absorptiometry
dual-plane catheter-based ultrasound
dual-port system
dual-pulse lithotriptor

dual-sensory antimony pH catheter
Dubin-Amelar varicocele classification
Dubin-Johnson
    D.-J. pigment
    D.-J. syndrome
Dubin-Sprinz
    D.-S. disease
    D.-S. syndrome
Dubowitz syndrome
Duchenne-type muscular dystrophy
duck-bill forceps
Duckett
    D. meatal advancement
    D. tubularized neourethra procedure
Ducrey disease
ducreyi
    Haemophilus d.
duct
    absence of diluted d.
    accessory pancreatic d.
    anomalous junction of
      pancreaticobiliary d.'s (AJPBD)
    anomalous pancreaticobiliary d.
     (APBD)
    arborization of d.'s
    beaded hepatic d.
    Bellini d.
    Bernard d.
    bifurcation of common bile d.
    bile d.
    biliary d.
    branched pancreatic d.
    d. cannulation
    clubbed common bile d.
    collecting d. (CD)
    common bile d. (CBD)
    common hepatic d.
    cortical collecting d. (CCD)
    cross-section of collecting d.
    cystic d. (CD)
    diffuse irregular narrowing of
     pancreatic d.
    dilated bile d.
    distal bile d.
    donor hepatic d. (DHD)
    dorsal pancreatic d.
    ductal d.
    ejaculatory d.
    epididymis lymphatic d.
    excretory d.
    extrahepatic bile d.
    fusiform widening of d.
    gall d.
    Gartner d.
    genu of pancreatic d.
    hepatic d.
    horseshoe anomaly of pancreatic
     d.
    impacted cystic d.

infected bile d.
infundibulum of bile d.
inner medullary collecting d.
   (IMCD)
interlobular bile d.
intrahepatic bile d.
intrapancreatic bile d.
irregular d.
left hepatic d.
Leydig d.
d. lumen
Luschka d.
main pancreatic d. (MPD)
medullary collecting d.
mesonephric d.
middle extrahepatic bile d.
Müllerian d.
narrow-caliber d.
nontransected pancreatic d.
normal-caliber d.
d. of Santorini
d. of Wirsung
d. of Wolff
outer medullary collecting d.
pancreatic d.
papillomatosis of intrahepatic bile d.
perilobular d.
peripheral bile d.
preampullary portion of bile d.
prepapillary bile d.
proximal bile d.
Rathke d.
right hepatic d.
serpiginous microcystic d.
Skene d.
spiral fold of cystic d.
Stensen d.
subvesical d.
tapered common bile d.
tear d.
terminal bile d.
terminal inner medullary collecting
   d.
thoracic d.
upstream pancreatic d.
vitelline d.
vitellointestinal d. (VID)
Wharton d.
wolffian d.

ductal
d. adenocarcinoma of prostate
d. change
d. cystadenoma
d. decompression
d. dilation
d. duct
d. epithelial hyperplasia
d. epithelium
d. hypertension

d. obstruction
d. stricture
d. system
d. system perforation
duct-ectatic
d.-e. mucinous cystadenoma
d.-e. tumor
ductogram
pancreatic d.
ductography
peroral retrograde pancreaticobiliary
   d.
postsphincterotomy d.
ductopenia
idiopathic adulthood d.
mild idiopathic adulthood biliary d.
   (MIAD)
ductopenic rejection
ductular structure
ductule
biliary d.'s
inferior aberrant d.
superior aberrant d.
ductuli (*pl. of* ductulus)
ductulus, *pl.* **ductuli**
d. aberrans superior
ductuli aberrantes
ductuli biliferi
ductuli efferentes
ductuli interlobulares
ductuli prostatici
ductus, *pl.* **ductus**
d. biliaris
d. biliferi
d. choledochus
d. cysticus
d. deferens
d. ejaculatorius
d. epididymidis
d. excretorius vesiculae seminalis
d. glandulae bulbourethralis
d. hepaticus communis
d. hepaticus dexter
d. hepaticus sinister
d. lobi caudati dexter
d. lobi caudati sinister
d. mesonephricus
d. muelleri
d. pancreaticus
d. pancreaticus accessorius
d. paraurethrales urethrae femininae
d. prostatici
d. Wolffi
Duette
D. double-lumen ERCP instrument
D. multiband variceal ligator
Duffield deep surgery scissors
Dufourmentel pilonidal cyst and sinus
   closure technique

D

DUG
    dynamic urinary graciloplasty
Duhamel
    D. laparoscopic pullthrough
      anastomosis
    D. operation
    D. pullthrough procedure
Duke
    D. pouch
    D. pouch cutaneous urinary
      diversion
Dukes
    D. B-1
    D. classification
    D. classification of carcinoma
    D. signet cell A, B, C
    D. stage
    D. staging system
**Dulbecco modified Eagle medium
(DMEM)**
Dul45 cell line
Dulcolax bowel preparation
dull
    d. pain
    d. to percussion abdomen
dullness, dulness
    hepatic d.
    liver d.
    shifting d.
    splenic d.
    d. to percussion
    tympanitic d.
dulness (*var. of* dullness)
dumbbell-shaped
    d.-s. calyceal extension
    d.-s. shadow
Dumdum fever
dumerili
    Seriola d.
Dumon-Gilliard
    D.-G. endoprosthesis system
    D.-G. prosthesis introducer
    D.-G. prosthesis pushing tube
dumping
    late d.
    d. stomach
    d. syndrome
dump kidney
**Dunnigan-type familial partial
lipodystrophy**
Duo-Coat dual-lumen catheter
duocrinin
duodenal
    d. acidification
    d. adenocarcinoma
    d. adenoma
    d. ampulla
    d. antrum
    d. atresia

d. biopsy
d. bleeding
d. brake
d. bulb
d. bulb deformity
d. cancer
d. cap (DC)
d. carcinoid
d. C loop
d. cluster unit
d. compression
d. diaphragm
d. digestion
d. diverticulitis
d. diverticulum
d. drainage
d. effect
d. electrical stimulation
d. endoscopic polypectomy
d. erosion
d. exclusion (DE)
d. fistula
d. fluid collection
d. fold
d. foreign body
d. fossa
d. gastrinoma
d. gastroesophageal reflux (DGER)
d. hemangiomatosis
d. hematoma
d. histoplasmosis
d. impression
d. impression on liver
d. injury
d. juice
d. leiomyoma
d. lesion
d. lumen
d. lymphoma
d. lymphonodular hyperplasia
d. mass
d. metastasis
d. mucosa
d. neurofibroma
d. obstruction
d. orifice
d. papilla
d. polyp
d. polyposis
d. pressure wave
d. secretin test (DST)
d. seromyectomy
d. smear
d. stenosis
d. stump
d. sweep
d. switch
d. telangiectasia
d. terminus

d. trauma
d. tube
d. tuberculosis
d. tumor
d. ulcer
d. ulceration
d. ulcer disease
d. ulceroinflammatory ulcer
d. ulcer perforation (DUP)
d. varix
d. villus
d. wall hamartoma
d. web
duodenale
    Ancylostoma d.
duodenalis
    Giardia d.
duodenectomy
duodenitis
chronic atrophic d.
Crohn d.
erosive d.
duodenobiliary
d. pressure gradient
d. reflux
duodenocaval fistula
duodenocholangeitis
duodenocholecystostomy
duodenocholedochotomy
duodenocolic fistula
duodenocystostomy
duodenoduodenostomy
duodenoenterocutaneous fistula
duodenoenterostomy
duodenogastric reflux (DGR)
duodenogastroesophageal reflux (DGER)
duodenogastroscopy
retrograde d. (RDG)
duodenogastrostomy
end-to-side d.
duodenogram
duodenography
barium contrast hypotonic d.
hypotonic d.
duodenohepatic
duodenoileal bypass (DIB)
duodenoileostomy
duodenojejunal
d. angle
d. flexure
d. fold
d. fossa
d. hernia
d. junction (DJJ)
d. recess
d. sphincter
duodenojejunalis
flexura d.

duodenojejunostomy
suprapapillary Roux-en-Y d.
duodenolysis
duodenomesocolic fold
duodenopancreatic reflux
duodenorrhaphy
duodenoscope
diagnostic d.
endoscopic ultrasound d.
Fujinon DUO-XT d.
Fujinon ED7-XT d.
Fujinon ED-200XU d.
Fujinon ED-310XU d.
Fujinon ED-410XU d.
Fujinon EVD-XT d.
Fujinon FD-100XU d.
JF-200 d.
JF-IT20 d.
large-channel therapeutic d.
master d.
Olympus EW-series fiberoptic d.
Olympus JF1T10 fiberoptic d.
Olympus PJF-series pediatric d.
Olympus TJF-10, -100, -200 d.
Pentax d.
side-viewing fiberoptic d.
standard d.
therapeutic side-viewing d.
TJF-100, -130 large-channel d.
duodenostomy
Witzel d.
duodenotomy
transverse d.
duodenovideoscope
small-caliber d.
duodenum
Brunner gland of d.
brunneroma of d.
button of d.
C loop of d.
closed d.
d. deformed by scarring
descending d.
distal d.
gastric metaplasia of d.
mucous crypt of d.
obstruction d.
scarified d.
ulcer d.
duodenum-preserving pancreatic head resection
Duodopa
Duo-Flow catheter
Duosol
Duotab
Symax D.
Duo-Tube feeding tube
DUP
duodenal ulcer perforation

Dupan-2 tumor marker
Duphalac
Duplay operation
duplex
    d. collecting system
    d. Doppler endosonography
    d. ileum
    d. sonography
duplicated gallbladder
duplicate uterus
duplication
    alimentary tract d.
    d. anomaly
    biliary tree d.
    bladder d.
    colonic d.
    complete d.
    d. cyst
    gastric cystic d.
    incomplete d.
    renal d.
    tubular colonic d.
    urethra d.
Dupuytren
    D. suture
    D. tourniquet
durable healing
Duracep biopsy forceps
DURAglide 3 stone balloon catheter
Dura-II positionable penile prosthesis
Duralone
dural patch reconstruction
Duramorph
Durand-Nicholas-Favre disease
Duraphase inflatable penile prosthesis
Durasphere injectable bulking agent
duration
    esophageal body contraction d.
    mean treatment d.
    phasic wave d.
    d. time
Duricef
Durrani dorsal vein complex ligation
  needle
duskiness
    stomal d.
dusky stoma
dutasteride capsule
Duval
    D. distal pancreatojejunostomy
    D. pancreaticojejunostomy procedure
Duverney foramen
Duvoid
D&V
    diarrhea and vomiting
DVC
    dorsal vein complex
DVIU
    direct-vision internal urethrotomy

DVS
    direct vesicoureteral scintigraphy
DVSA
    digital venous subtraction
     angiography
DW
    dry weight
dwarf kidney
dwell period
DXA
    dual-energy x-ray absorptiometry
D-xylose
    D-x. absorption test
    D-x. malabsorption
dyad
    mother-infant d.
dyadic relationship
Dyazide
Dyclone
dye
    Alcian blue d.
    basic d.
    cationic d.
    Congo red d.
    Evans blue d.
    HpD d.
    indigo carmine d.
    indocyanine green d.
    iodine d.
    Kiton red d.
    d. laser
    metachromatic d.
    methylene blue d.
    orthochromatic d.
    radiopaque d.
    rapid emptying of d.
    rhodamine 6G d.
    d. scattering method
    d. sham intrarenal lesion
    d. spraying
dye-exclusion test
dye-injection endoscopic retrograde
  pancreatography
Dynabac
DynaCirc
Dynaflex
    D. penile implant
    D. penile prosthesis
Dynalink biliary self-expanding stent
  system
dynamic
    d. closure pressure
    d. contrast
    d. cystourethroscopy
    d. development
    d. fluorescein angiography
    d. fluorescence videoendoscopy
    d. ileus
    d. infusion cavernosometry

d. infusion cavernosometry and cavernosography
d. proctography
d. urethral profile study
d. urinary graciloplasty (DUG)
dynamoscopy
dynograph
dynorphin
dyphylline
Dyrenium
dysarthric
dysautonomia
    familial d.
    Riley-Day syndrome of familial d.
dysbiosis
dyschezia
    defecatory d.
dyscinesia (*var. of* dyskinesia)
dyscoordinate hyoid movement
dysenteriae
    Shigella d.
dysenteric
    d. algid malaria
    d. arthritis
    d. diarrhea
dysentery
    amebic d.
    d. antitoxin
    bacillary d.
    d. bacillus
    balantidial d.
    bilharzial d.
    catarrhal d.
    ciliary d.
    ciliate d.
    epidemic d.
    flagellate d.
    Flexner d.
    fulminant d.
    fulminating d.
    giardiasis d.
    helminthic d.
    institutional d.
    Japanese d.
    malarial d.
    malignant d.
    protozoan d.
    schistosomal d.
    scorbutic d.
    Shiga d.
    Shigella d.
    Sonne d.
    spirillar d.
    spirochetal d.
    sporadic d.
    viral d.
dysesthesia
dysfunction
    anal sphincter d.

anorectal sensorimotor d.
autonomic d.
balanced voiding d.
bladder neck d.
Bradley classification of voiding d.
brain-gut d.
cardiopulmonary baroreflex d.
cavernous autonomic nerve d.
chronic graft d.
colorectal physiologic d.
constitutional hepatic d.
corporeal venoocclusive d.
ejaculatory d.
erectile d. (ED)
esophageal body motor d.
evidence-based review of sphincter of Oddi d.
gastric d.
geriatric voiding d.
hereditary spastic paraplegia voiding d.
hindgut d.
International Continence Society classification of voiding d.
intracorporeal therapy of erectile d.
intraurethral therapy of erectile d.
intrinsic sphincter d. (ISD)
Lapides classification of voiding d.
late graft d.
lower urinary tract d. (LUTD)
low-pressure low-flow voiding d.
mechanoreceptor d.
multiple-organ system d. (MOSD)
neurogenic erectile d.
neuroimmune d.
neuropathic voiding d.
neutrophil d.
nondiabetic neurogenic erectile d.
nonneurogenic voiding d.
oral therapy of erectile d.
outlet d.
pancreatic exocrine d.
pediatric voiding d.
pelvic floor d.
platelet d.
postgastrectomy d.
postparacentesis circulatory d. (PCD)
posttransplant renal d.
progressive renal d.
psychogenic erectile d.
psychological d.
puborectalis d.
reflex voiding d.
sensory voiding d.
sphincter d.
sphincter of Oddi d. (SOD)
transfer d.
traumatic corporeal venoocclusive d.
tubular cell d.

D

dysfunction (*continued*)
 urodynamic d.
 venoocclusive d.
 visceral d.
dysfunctional
 d. bleeding
 d. voiding
dysgenesia (*var. of* dysgenesis)
dysgenesis, dysgenesia
 anorectal d.
 gonadal d.
 mixed gonadal d.
dysgenetic
 d. fibrous band
 d. gonad
dysgenitalism
dysgerminoma
dysgeusia
dyskeratosis follicularis
dyskinesia, dyskinesis, dyscinesia
 bile duct d.
 biliary d.
 primary ciliary d.
dyskinesis (*var. of* dyskinesia)
dyskinetic
 d. cilia syndrome
 d. puborectalis
dyslipidemia
dyslipidosis
dysmetabolic syndrome
dysmorphic
 d. erythrocyte
 d. red blood cell
 d. vessel
dysmorphy
 extrarenal d.
dysmotility
 chronic intestinal d. (CID)
 d. dyspepsia
 esophageal d.
 gallbladder d.
dysmotility-like dyspepsia
dysnatremia
dysorexia
dyspareunia
dyspepsia
 acid d.
 adhesion d.
 appendicular d.
 appendix d.
 atonic d.
 biliary d.
 catarrhal d.
 cholelithic d.
 dysmotility d.
 dysmotility-like d.
 fermentative d.
 flatulent d.
 functional d.

 gastric d.
 gastroduodenal d.
 mononuclear d.
 nervous d.
 nonorganic d.
 nonulcer d. (NUD)
 Optimal Regimen Cures
  Helicobacter-Induced D.
  (ORCHID)
 postcholecystectomy flatulent d.
 Quality of Life in Reflux and D.
  (QOLRD)
 reflex d.
 reflux d.
 refluxlike d.
 ulcer d.
 ulcerlike d.
dyspeptic
 d. symptom
 d. urine
dyspeptica
 angina d.
dysperistalsis
dysphagia, dysphagy
 d. after antireflux surgery
 d. aortica
 Atkinson scoring system for d.
 contractile ring d.
 esophageal d.
 d. inflammatoria
 liquid food d.
 d. lusoria
 malignant d.
 d. nervosa
 neurogenic d.
 onset of d.
 oropharyngeal d.
 d. paralytica
 postvagotomy d.
 preesophageal d.
 progressive d.
 sideropenic d.
 soft food d.
 solid food d.
 d. spastica
 transfer d.
 vallecular d.
 d. valsalviana
dysphagic
dysphagy (*var. of* dysphagia)
dysphasia
 polyostotic fibrous d.
dysphonia
dysphoria
dysplasia
 acrocephalopolydactylous d.
 anal squamous d.
 anal transitional zone d.
 arteriohepatic d. (AHD)

Barrett d.
bladder d.
developing high-grade d.
epithelial d.
fibromuscular d. (FMD)
fibrous d.
flat d.
genital d.
high-grade d. (HGD)
kidney d.
liver cell d.
low-grade d. (LGD)
lung d.
malignant d.
mucosal d.
multicystic renal d.
neuroectodermal d.
nonulcer d.
panostotic fibrous d.
polypoid d.
renal segmental renal d.
urothelial d.
vesicourethral reflux and renal d.
dysplasia-associated lesion or mass (DALM)
dysplasia-to-carcinoma sequence
dysplastic
d. cell
d. focus
d. kidney
d. mucosa
dyspnea
Dysport
dysraphic malformation
dysreflexia
autonomic d.
dysregulated immune response
dysrhythmia
ESWL-related d.
gastric electrical d.
glucagon-evoked gastric d.
dysspermatogenic sterility
dyssynergia, dyssynergy

biliary d.
detrusor external sphincter d. (DESD)
detrusor urethral d.
pelvic floor d.
rectoanal d.
rectosphincteric d.
vesical external sphincter d.
vesicosphincteric d.
dyssynergy (*var. of* dyssynergia)
dystonia
dystonic phenomenon
dystopia
d. transversa externa testis
d. transversa interna testis
dystopic kidney
dystrophia (*var. of* dystrophy)
dystrophic
d. calcification
D. Epidermolysis Bullosa Research Association (DEBRA)
d. penis
dystrophica
epidermolysis bullosa d.
dystrophy, dystrophia
adiposogenital d.
asphyxiating thoracic d. (ATD)
Duchenne-type muscular d.
hyperplastic d.
Jeune asphyxiating thoracic d.
muscular d.
myotonic muscular d.
oculocerebrorenal d.
oculopharyngeal muscular d.
Steinert myotonic d.
dystrypsia
dysuresia
dysuria, dysury
psychic d.
dysuria-pyuria syndrome
dysuric
dysury (*var. of* dysuria)
dyszoospermia

D

E

E rosetted
E sign
E test

E1

E1, E2, E6 protein
prostaglandin E1 (PGE1)

E2

prostaglandin E2 (PGE2)

eAb seroconversion

EABV

effective arterial blood volume

Eadie-Hofstee

E.-H. plot
E.-H. transformation

EAEC

enteroadherent *Escherichia coli*
enteroaggregative *Escherichia coli*

EAGER

exertion-associated gastroesophageal
reflux

Eagle

E. Claw VII device
E. minimal essential medium
(EMEM)

Eagle-Barrett syndrome

EAP

etoposide, Adriamycin, Platinol

ear

bladder e.
elephant e.

Earle

E. hemorrhoid clamp
E. medium
E. rectal probe
E. sign
E. solution

early

E. Detector
e. dumping syndrome
e. gastric cancer (EGC)
e. growth response factor-alpha
e. preimplantation cell screening
(EPICS)
e. satiety
e. signs of dilutional hyponatremia
e. virologic response (EVR)

early-onset graft-versus-host disease

earth

e. eating
E. Radiation Budget Experiment
(ERBE)

Easi-Lav lavage

easily reducible hernia

EasiVac evacuator

Easprin

EAST1

enteroaggregative *Escherichia coli*
heat-stable enterotoxin 1

**Eastern Cooperative Oncology Group
(ECOG)**

Eastman cystic duct forceps

EasyBand adjustable gastric band

easy bruisability

EATCL

enteropathy-associated T-cell lymphoma

eater

liver e.

eating

earth e.

EAUS

endoanal ultrasound

EB

epidermolysis bullosa
Epstein-Barr

EBA

extrahepatic biliary atresia

E-Base

**Ebbehoj penile straightening-reinforcing
procedure**

EBCT

electron-beam computerized
tomography

EBD

endoscopic balloon dilation

EBL

endoscopic band ligation
estimated blood loss

Ebola hemorrhagic fever

E1b protein

ebrotidine

EBS

estrogen binding site

EBSD

endoscopic balloon sphincter dilation

Ebstein

E. diet
E. disease
E. lesion

EBV

Epstein-Barr virus

EC

enteric-coated
esophageal candidiasis
EC cell
Entocort EC
thymic EC

ECA

enterobacterial common antigen

Ecabet Sodium

E

ECAC
    epidermoid carcinoma of anal canal
E-cadherin
ECF
    extracellular fluid
ECFV
    extracellular fluid volume
ECGF
    endothelial cell growth factor
Echinacea purpurea
echinococcal
    e. cyst disease
    e. liver abscess
echinococciasis (*var. of* echinococcosis)
echinococcosis, echinococciasis
    alveolar e.
    biliary e.
    cystic e.
    hepatic e.
    hepatic-alveolar e.
    renal e.
Echinococcus
    E. granulosus
    life cycle of *E.*
    E. liver cyst
    E. multilocularis
echinostomiasis
echo
    gradient e.
    magnetization prepared-rapid
        gradient e. (MP-RAGE)
    e. pattern
    e. sign
echocolonoscope
    CF-UM3 e.
    Olympus CF-UM3 flexible e.
echo-Doppler
echoduodenoscope
echoduodenoscopy
echoendoscope
    CLA e.
    curved-array e.
    curved linear-array e.
    curvilinear scanning e.
    electronic radial-array e.
    linear-array e.
    linear-oriented radial
        scanning e.
    oblique viewing e.
    Olympus CF-UM-series e.
    Olympus EUM-20 e.
    Olympus GF-UC30P e.
    Olympus GF-UCT30P linear-array
        e.
    Olympus GF-UM29 radial
        scanner e.
    Olympus GF-UM30P e.
    Olympus GIF20 e.
    Olympus GIF-EUM2 e.

    Olympus GIF-series e.
    Olympus GIF-1T10 e.
    Olympus JF-UM20 e.
    Olympus UM-20 radial e.
    Olympus VU-M2 e.
    Olympus XIF-UM3 e.
    Pentax FG-36-UX linear-array e.
    radial-sector scanning e.
echoendoscopy
echogastroscope
echogenic
    e. cardiac focus
    e. duct margin
    e. liver
echogenicity
    central e.
echographic
echolucent
echomorphologic
echo-poor
    e.-p. layer
    e.-p. lesion
echoprobe
    Olympus catheter e.
echo-rich
**EchoSeed radioactive iodine-125
  brachytherapy seed**
echotexture
EchoTip Ultra endoscopic needle
ECHO virus infection
ECI automatic reprocessor
Eck fistula
Eckhout vertical gastroplasty
ECL
    enhanced chemiluminescence
    enterochromaffin-like
        ECL cell
        ECL cell hyperplasia
        E. hypertrophy and hyperplasia
        ECL Western blot
ECLoma
    enterochromaffin-like gastric carcinoid
        tumor
ECLP
    extracorporeal liver perfusion
ECM
    esophagocardiomyotomy
    extracellular matrix
    extracolonic malignancy
ECOG
    Eastern Cooperative Oncology
        Group
        ECOG performance status scale
E. coli
    Escherichia coli
ecology
    microbial e.
Econolith lithotriptor
Ecotrin

ECP
  erythropoietic coproporphyria
ECPL
  endocavitary pelvic lymphadenectomy
ectacolia
ectasia, ectasis
  antral vascular e.
  Boley vascular e.
  cecal vascular e.
  gastric antral vascular e.
    (GAVE)
  gastric vascular e. (GVE)
  mucinous ductal e. (MDE)
  precaliceal canalicular e.
  tortuous venous e.
  vascular e.
  venous e.
ectasis (*var. of* ectasia)
ectatic
  e. vascular lesion
  e. vessel
ecthyma gangrenosum
ectocolon
ectoderm
ectodermal
ectoperitoneal
ectoperitonitis
ectopia, ectopy
  acquired gastric e.
  crossed renal e.
  crossed testicular e.
  gastric mucosal e.
  intraabdominal transverse
    testicular e.
  renal e.
  transverse testicular e.
  ureteral e.
  e. vesicae
ectopic
  e. adrenal rest
  e. anus
  e. cryptorchidism
  e. gastric mucosa
  e. gestation
  e. kidney
  e. pancreas
  e. pheochromocytoma
  e. schistosomiasis
  e. scrotum
  e. sigmoid pregnancy
  e. testis
  e. ureter
  e. ureterocele
  e. varix
  e. vas deferens
ectopy (*var. of* ectopia)
ectoscopy
ECU
  extracorporeal ultrafiltration

ECV
  esophageal collateral vein
ED
  erectile dysfunction
ED1
  monoclonal antibody ED1
EDA+
  extradomain A positive
EDAP lithotriptor
EDD
  extended daily dialysis
Edebohls
  E. operation
  E. position
edema
  acute idiopathic scrotal e.
  alimentary e.
  angioneurotic e.
  antral e.
  bullous e.
  cachectic e.
  focal e.
  idiopathic e.
  laryngeal e.
  nephritic e.
  nephrotic e.
  pedal e.
  penile e.
  perianal e.
  pericholecystic e.
  peripheral extremity e.
  pitting e.
  pulmonary e.
  sacral e.
edematous
  e. gallbladder
  e. hyperemic mucosa
  e. pancreatitis
  e. tag
edentulous
Eder-Bernstein gastroscope
Eder-Chamberlin gastroscope
Eder gastroscope
Eder-Hufford
  E.-H. gastroscope
  E.-H. rigid esophagoscope
Eder-Palmer
  E.-P. semiflexible fiberoptic
    endoscope
  E.-P. semiflexible gastroscope
Eder-Puestow
  E.-P. bougie
  E.-P. dilation
  E.-P. dilator shaft
  E.-P. guidewire
  E.-P. metal olive dilator
  E.-P. olive
edetate
  disodium e.

E

Edex
edge
- e. enhancement
- heaped-up e.
- hepatic e.
- ligament reflecting e.
- liver e.
- Poupart ligament shelving e.
- ulcer with heaped-up e.

EdGr
- Edmondson grading
- EdGr system

edible vaccine
Edlich gastric lavage tube
Edmondson
- E. grading (EdGr)
- E. grading system
- E. grading system for hepatocellular carcinoma

Edmondson-Steiner histologic grading of hepatocellular carcinoma I, II, III, IVa
Edmonston-Zogreb (EZ)
Edna towel clamp
EDP
- endoscopic digital pancreatography

EDRF
- endothelium-derived relaxing factor

edrophonium
- e. provocation
- e. test

ED-Spaz
EDTA
- ethylenediaminetetraacetic acid
- ^{51}Cr-labeled EDTA

Edwardsiella tarda
Edwards syndrome
EEA
- end-to-end anastomosis
  - EEA stapler gun
  - EEA stapling device
  - EEA stapling of varix

EEG
- electroencephalography

EEGF
- esophageal epidermal growth factor

EEJ
- electroejaculation

e10 electrosurgery system
EEPLND
- extraperitoneal endoscopic pelvic lymph node dissection

EES
- expandable esophageal stent

EFA
- essential fatty acid

EFAD
- essential fatty acid deficiency

efavirenz

effacement
- villous e.

effect
- analgesic e.
- antinociceptive e.
- antiproliferative e.
- antiproteinuric e.
- banana peel e.
- blooming e.
- Bohr e.
- choleretic e.
- concomitant medication e.
- disulfiram-like e.
- donor age-dependent e.
- Doppler e.
- duodenal e.
- esophageal e.
- first-pass e.
- gastric e.
- gender e.
- gene-inductive e.
- Haldane e.
- halo e.
- hypothermic e.
- inhibitory e.
- intracellular flush e.
- irradiation e.
- J-curve e.
- kaliuretic e.
- kidney shock wave e.
- local alcohol instillation e.
- long-term renal functional e.
- membrane e.
- metabolic e.
- mitogenic e.
- mutagenic e.
- normothermic e.
- octreotide e.
- e. of inhibition
- physiologic trophic e.
- pinchcock e.
- placebo e.
- preservation time e.
- proapoptotic e.
- prokinetic e.
- sieving e.
- snowstorm e.
- soar-crash e.
- systemic e.
- tubulotoxic e.

effective
- e. arterial blood volume (EABV)
- e. dose-equivalent radiation
- e. lithotriptor
- e. renal plasma flow (ERPF)

effector
- e. cell
- e. domain

locally acting paracrine e.
e. response
EFFERdose
Zantac E.
efferent
e. glomerular arteriole
e. limb
e. loop
e. loop syndrome
e. renal sympathetic nerve activity (ERSNA)
efferentes
ductuli e.
Effer-Syllium
efficacious noninvasive anesthesia-independent first-line method
efficacy
e. of neuromodulation
poor long-term e.
efficiency
defunctioning e.
effluent
anal e.
ileal e.
ileostomy e.
peritoneal dialysis e. (PDE)
transverse colostomy e.
efflux
effort rupture of esophagus
effusion fluid
E2F protein
EFTR
endoscopic full-thickness resection
EFV
extracellular fluid volume
EGBT
esophagogastric balloon tamponade
EGC
early gastric cancer
EGD
esophagogastroduodenoscopy
EGE
eosinophilic gastroenteritis
egesta
EGF
epidermal growth factor
intragastric EGF
luminal EGF
subcutaneous EGF
EGFR
epidermal growth factor receptor
EGG
electrogastrogram
electrogastrography
cutaneous EGG
egg
e. yolk-cobalamin absorption test (EYCAT)

eggerthii
Bacteroides e.
EGM
extraglomerular mesangium
EGS 100 electrogalvanic stimulator
EGT
endoscopic gastrin test
EGTA
esophageal gastric tube airway
ethyleneglycoltetraacetic acid
Egyptian splenomegaly
EHBDA
extrahepatic bile duct atresia
EHC
enterohepatic circulation
EHEC
enterohemorrhagic *Escherichia coli*
EHL
electrohydraulic lithotripsy
endoscopic hemorrhoid ligation
EHL probe
Ehlers-Danlos syndrome
EHM
extrahepatic metastasis
EHPVO
extrahepatic portal vein obstruction
Ehrlich
E. abdominoplasty
E. diazo reaction
E. reagent
Ehrlichia chaffeensis
Ehrmann alcohol test meal
EHT
electrohydrothermal
EHT coagulation
EHT electrode
EIA
enzyme immunoassay
HCV EIA II
Helicobacter pylori stool antigen EIA
EIA kit
EIA-2
second-generation enzyme immunoassay
eicosanoid synthesis
eicosapentaenoic acid (EPA)
EIEC
enteroinvasive *Escherichia coli*
Einhorn
E. dilator
E. string test
EIP
ethanol injection therapy of prostate
EIS
endoscopic injection sclerotherapy
Eisenberger technique
Eitest MONO P-II test

E

ejaculatio
  e. deficiens
  e. praecox
  e. retardata
ejaculation
  antegrade e.
  dry e.
  electrostimulation-induced e.
  e. failure
  premature e.
  retrograde e.
ejaculatorius
  ductus e.
ejaculatory
  e. duct
  e. duct obstruction
  e. duct reflux
  e. duct transurethral resection
  e. duct ultrasonography
  e. dysfunction
  e. impotence
ejaculum
ejecta
ejection
ekiri
eKru
  equivalent residual renal urea
  clearance
Ektachem slide test
ELAD
  extracorporeal liver assist device
ELAM-1
  endothelial leukocyte adhesion
  molecule-1
  ligand for ELAM-1
Elastalloy
  E. esophageal endoprosthesis
  E. esophageal stent
elastase
  neutrophil e.
  serum e. 1
elastic
  e. band ligation
  e. bougie
  e. ligature
  e. O ring
  e. scattering spectroscopy
  e. silicone membrane
elastica interna
elasticum
  pseudoxanthoma e.
elastin stain
elastolysis
  generalized e.
Elastoplast dressing
elastosis perforans serpiginosa
Elavil
ELBF
  estimated liver blood flow

ELBNS
  extraperitoneal laparoscopic bladder
  neck suspension
elbowed
  e. bougie
  e. catheter
Elecsys
  E. anti-HBs immunoassay
  E. 1010, 2010 immunoanalyzer
  E. PreciControl anti-HBs
elective resection
electric
  e. tissue morcellator
  e. zone
electrical
  e. blocking
  e. conductivity
  e. waveform
electroblotting
electrocautery
  bipolar e.
  blended e.
  Bovie e.
  Bugbee e.
  e. knife
  light e.
  monopolar e.
  multipolar e.
  needle-knife e. (NKE)
  Neomed e.
  e. pencil
  e. resection
electrocholecystectomy
electrocholecystocausis
electrocoagulating
  e. biopsy forceps
  e. current
electrocoagulation
  bipolar e. (BPEC)
  direct-current e.
  endoscopic e.
  Gold Probe e.
  monopolar e.
  multipolar e. (MPEC)
  e. necrosis
  snare e.
  transendoscopic e.
electrocystography
electrode
  abdominal patch e.
  ACMI monopolar e.
  antimony monocrystalline e.
  antimony pH e.
  ASSI laparoscopic e.
  ball e.
  bayonet-tip e.
  bipolar glass e.
  Bugbee e.
  Buie fulguration e.

button e.
Cameron-Miller e.
coagulating e.
Coaguloop resection e.
Collings e.
common pH e.
concentric needle e.
conical-tip e.
cuff e.
cutting e.
Disa needle e.
e. dislodgement
disposable pudendal nerve e.
dome-tip e.
EHT e.
e. electrolyte
Eppendorf needle e.
flat spatula e.
foramen e.
glass pH e.
Greenwald Control Tip
  cystoscopic e.
Gyrus bipolar e.
hook-tip laparoscopic e.
indifferent e.
intraluminal reference e.
ion-specific e.
e. jelly
J-hook-tip laparoscopic e.
knife e.
loop-tipped e.
McCarthy e.
Medtronic thin flexible antimony e.
Microelectrode MI-506 small-caliber
  pH e.
Microglass pH e.
midgastric e.
e. migration
modified thermal nitinol e.
needle e.
needle-tip laparoscopic e.
Neil-Moore e.
pencil-tipped e.
e. placement
e. probe
3-quarter circle e.
renal sympathetic nerve activity
  recording e.
reusable laparoscopic e.
right-angle e.
rollerball e.
Smith e.
spatula-tip laparoscopic e.
spoon-tip laparoscopic e.
St. Mark pudendal e.
surface e.
unipolar glass e.
VaporTrode e.
wire e.

electrodiathermy
electroejaculation (EEJ)
  rectal probe e.
electroejaculator
  G&S e.
electroencephalography
  (EEG)
electroendosmosis
electroevaporation
electrofulguration
electrogalvanic
  e. stimulation (EGS)
  e. stimulator
electrogastrogram (EGG)
  cutaneous e.
electrogastrograph
electrogastrography (EGG)
electrohemostasis
electrohydraulic
  e. generator
  e. lithotripsy (EHL)
  e. lithotripsy probe
  e. lithotriptor
  percutaneous transhepatic
    choledochoscopic e.
  e. shock wave lithotripsy
    (ESWL)
electrohydrothermal (EHT)
  e. coagulation
electroimmunodiffusion assay
electroincision
electrolyte, *pl.* **electrolytes**
  e. abnormality
  e. balance
  bicarbonate e.
  calcium e.
  chloride e.
  CO_2 e.
  electrode e.
  e. excretion
  e. flush solution
  e. imbalance coma
  e. lavage solution
  e. loss
  potassium e.
  e. preparation
  sodium e.
  stool e.
electrolyte-polyethylene glycol lavage
  solution
electrolytes (*pl. of* electrolyte)
electromagnetic
  e. flowmeter
  e. flow transducer
  e. force (E, EMF)
  e. lithotriptor
electromechanical
  e. coupling
  e. impactor (EMI)

E

electromicroscopy
electromyogram (EMG)
    colonic e.
electromyography
    conventional concentric e.
    corpus cavernosum penile e.
    Disa e.
    intraanal e.
    needle electrode e.
    noninvasive intraanal e.
    e. of penile corpus cavernosum
       muscle
    pelvic floor e.
    rhabdosphincter e.
    single-fiber needle e.
    surface pelvic floor e.
    ureteral e.
    video pressure flow e.
electron
    e. immunoperoxidase observation
    e. microscopy
electron-beam computerized tomography
  (EBCT)
electron-dense mesangial deposit
electronic
    e. barostat
    e. pain control
    e. radial-array echoendoscope
    e. radial-array endoscope
electron-microscopic evidence
electrophoresis
    agarose gel e.
    horizontal e.
    e. immunoblot analysis
    immunofixation e. (IFE)
    polyacrylamide gel e. (PAGE)
    pulsed-field gel e. (PFGE)
    serum protein e. (SPEP)
    sodium dodecyl
       sulfate-polyacrylamide gel e.
       (SDS-PAGE)
    urine protein e. (UPEP)
electrophoretic
    e. mobility
    e. mobility shift assay
electrophysiology
    cellular e.
    GI e.
    e. of gastric musculature
electropneumatic endoscopic
  lithotriptor
electroresection
electrosensitivity
    mucosal e. (MES)
electrostimulation
electrostimulation-induced ejaculation
electrosurgery
    EUS probe-guided e.
    microprocessor-controlled e.

electrosurgical
    e. current
    e. current density
    e. curved scissors
    e. cut
    e. cutting knife
    e. desiccation
    e. dissection
    e. fulguration
    e. generator
    e. monopolar spatula probe
    e. needle
    e. snare
    e. snare polypectomy
    e. spatula
    e. unit
electrotherapy
electrovaporization
    prostate gland e.
    transurethral e.
Elema-Siemens AB pressure transducer
element
    acute-phase response e. (APRE)
    androgen receptor e.
    ceramic e.
    estrogen response e. (ERE)
    glucocorticoid response e.
    hepatic subcellular e.
    interferon-stimulated regulatory e.
       (ISRE)
    thyroid hormone response e.
       (TRE)
elemental
    e. diet
    e. phosphate
elephant ear
elephantiasis
    genital e.
    e. scroti
elevated WBC
elevation
    mucosal e.
elevator
    Alexander e.
    Doyen rib e.
    Ellik kidney stone e.
    Freer e.
    Stille e.
eleventh
    e. rib flank incision
    e. rib transperitoneal incision
ELF
    etoposide, leucovorin, 5-fluorouracil
       ELF chemotherapy protocol
ELG
    endoluminal gastroplication
Elgiloy stent
Eligard sustained-release subcu
  injection

elimination
>e. diet
>pyelography by e.
>spontaneous partial e.
>stool e.

eliminator
>E. balloon catheter
>E. biliary stent
>Fecal Odor E.
>E. nasobiliary catheter set
>E. pancreatic stent
>E. PET biliary balloon dilator
>E. stone extraction basket

ELISA
>enzyme-linked immunosorbent assay
>first-generation ELISA
>gliadin ELISA
>Heprofile ELISA
>ELISA Kit Alfa-gliatest
>sensitive and specific ELISA
>TG ELISA
>tissue transglutaminase ELISA (TG ELISA)
>ELISA titer

ELISA-I
>enzyme-linked immunosorbent assay I
>ELISA-I test

ELISA-II
>enzyme-linked immunosorbent assay II
>ELISA-II test

ELISA-III
>enzyme-linked immunosorbent assay III
>ELISA-III test

ELISA-like assay
elixir
>e. diarrhea
>Hemocyte-F e.
>Susano e.

Ellik
>E. evacuator
>E. kidney stone basket
>E. kidney stone elevator

Elliot position
Elliott gallbladder forceps
ellipsoid method
elliptical incision
Ellis type 1, 2 glomerulonephritis
EL2-LS2 flexible videolaparoscope
Ellsner gastroscope
elm bark
Elmiron
Elmiskop 101 electron microscope
Elocalcitol
elongated pseudostratified nucleus
elongation
>calyx e.

Eloxatin
ELP
>enterocolic lymphocytic phlebitis

Elspar
ELT
>endoscopic laser therapy

eltor
>*Vibrio choleraE* biotype *e.*

eluate
>acetonitrile e.

elucidation
EluHair
ELUS
>endoluminal rectal ultrasonography

elusive
>e. polyp
>e. ulcer

eluted antibody
elutriation
>T-cell depletion by e.

El-Zimaity triple stain
EMA
>endomysial antibody
>antibody to EMA
>IgA EMA

emaciation
EMAG
>environmental metaplastic atrophic gastritis

emasculation
EMB
>eosin-methylene blue
>EMB agar

embarrassment
>circulatory e.
>respiratory e.

embolectomy
>renal artery e.

emboli (*pl. of* embolus)
embolic
>e. agent
>e. nephritis

embolism
>air e.
>bile pulmonary e.
>cholesterol e.
>hemodialysis air e.
>mesenteric arterial e.
>postoperative cholesterol e.
>pulmonary bile e.
>renal artery e.

embolization
>angiographic variceal e.
>arterial e.
>arteriographic e.
>bilateral pudendal artery e.
>cholesterol crystal e. (CCE)
>Gelfoam e.
>hyperselective e.
>iliac artery e.
>e. of aneurysm
>percutaneous transhepatic liver biopsy with tract e.

E

embolization (*continued*)
    portal e.
    renal artery cholesterol e.
    splenic arterial e.
    superselective transcatheter e.
    transarterial catheter e.
      (TACE)
    transcatheter hepatic arterial e.
    transcatheter splenic arterial e.
      (TSAE)
    transcatheter variceal e.
    transhepatic e. (THE)
    varicocele e.
embolotherapy
    transcatheter e.
embolus, *pl.* **emboli**
    cholesterol e.
    metallic e.
    pulmonary e.
    renal cholesterol e.
    talc e.
embryoid body
embryologic development
embryology
embryoma of kidney
embryonal
    e. adenoma
    e. adenomyosarcoma
    e. adenosarcoma
    e. cell carcinoma
    e. nephroma
    e. testicular carcinoma
    e. transitory bladder
    e. tumor
embryonic cleavage
Emcyt
EMD
    esophageal motility disorder
EMEM
    Eagle minimal essential
    medium
emepronium bromide
Emerge biomaterial
emergency
    e. appendectomy
    e. colonoscopy
    e. laparotomy
emergent appendectomy
emerging profile
emesis
    bilious e.
    chemotherapy-induced nausea and e.
      (CINE)
    coffee-grounds e.
emetatrophia
Emete-Con
emetic reflex
emetine

emetocathartic
emetogenic injury
Emetrol
EMF
    electromagnetic force
      EMF oral liquid
EMG
    electromyogram
      MyoTrac EMG
      sphincter EMG
EMI
    electromechanical impactor
      EMI APED amplifier
      discriminator
emissary vein of penis
emission
    gamma e.
    nocturnal e.
Emitasol nasal therapy
Emitrip
emitter
    light e.
EMLA
    eutectic. mixture of local anesthetics
      EMLA anesthetic
Emmett needle
emollient laxative
Emory score
EMPD
    extramammary Paget disease
emperipolesis
emphysema
    alpha-1-antitrypsin disease-
      related e.
    colonoscopy-related e.
    endoscopy-related e.
    intestinal e.
    panacinar e.
    panlobular e.
    subcutaneous e.
    unilateral periorbital e.
emphysematosa
    cholecystitis e.
    cystitis e.
emphysematous
    e. cholecystitis
    e. cystitis
    e. gastritis
    e. pyelonephritis
empty
    e. intestine
    e. sella syndrome
emptying
    bladder e.
    delayed gallbladder e.
    delayed liquid gastric e.
    e. delta volume
    gastric e.

liquid e.
neorectal e.
rapid gastric e.
rectal e.
Roux limb e.
solid e.
T-1/2 time of gastric e.

empyema
e. of gallbladder
spontaneous bacterial e.

empyocele

EMR
endoscopic magnetic resonance
endoscopic mucosal resection

EMRC
endoscopic mucosal resection, cap
method

EMRL
endoscopic mucosal resection with
ligation

EMRT
endoscopic mucosal resection, tube
method

EMS
esophageal manometric sequence

emtricitabine

emulsion
Biafine wound dressing e.
Calogen LCT e.
intralipid fat e.
intravenous lipid e.
lipid e.
Panafil SE spray e.
papain, urea, chlorophyllin copper
complex sodium spray e.
e. proteinuria

Emulsoil bowel preparation

E-MVAC
escalated methotrexate, vinblastine,
Adriamycin, cisplatin or
cyclophosphamide

E-Mycin

en
e. bloc dissection
e. bloc distal pancreatectomy
e. bloc endoscopic resection
e. bloc kidney transplantation
e. bloc technique
e. bloc ureter
e. bloc vein resection
e. coup de sabre
e. face
e. face view

ENA
extracted nuclear antigen
ENA screen

ENaC
epithelial sodium channel

enalapril
enalaprilat
enalkiren
enamel pellicle formation
ENANB
enterically transmitted non-A non-B
ENANB hepatitis

enanthate
e. ester
testosterone e.

enantiomer D-arginine

encapsulated
e. carcinoid tumor
e. plasmodium
e. renal cell carcinoma

encapsulation
peritoneal e.
tumor e.

Encare tube-feeding formula

encasement
pancreatic duct e.
ureteral e.

encelialgia

enceliitis (*var. of* encelitis)

encelitis, enceliitis

Encephalitozoon intestinale

encephaloid gastric carcinoma

encephalomyocarditis virus

encephalomyopathy
mitochondrial neurogastrointestinal e.
(MNGIE)

encephalopathia (*var. of* encephalopathy)

encephalopathy, encephalopathia
bilirubin e.
colonoscopy-induced hyponatremic e.
hepatic e. (HE)
myoclonic e.
portosystemic e. (PSE)
postshunt e.
Rue hepatic e.
subclinical hepatic e. (SHE)
uremic e.
Wernicke e.

encircle

encirclement
anal e.

encoding virulence

encopresis

encroachment
scrotal e.

encrustation
biofilm-related e.

encystation

encysted
e. bladder
e. calculus
e. hydrocele
e. intraabdominal collection

E

end

advanced glycation e. (AGE)
e. colostomy
esophageal Z stent with fully
  coated flange e.'s
e. ileostomy
e. stoma

endarterectomy

e. knife
renal e.
transaortic e.

end-cutaneous ureterostomy

endeavor

Cancer of the Prostate Strategic
  Urologic Research E.

endemic

e. colic
e. deep mycosis
e. diarrhea
e. hematuria
e. nonbacterial infantile
  gastroenteritis

end-end stapler

Endep

**end-expiratory intragastric
pressure**

end-filling pressure

endfire transrectal probe

endhole ureteral catheter

end-labeling

nick e.-l.

endloop

e. colostomy
e. ileocolostomy
e. ileostomy
e. stoma

endo

E. Catch bag
E. GIA suture stapler
E. hernia stapler
E. pants

endoabdominal fascia

endoanal

e. coil
e. fast spin-echo T2-weighted MR
  image
e. magnetic resonance imaging
e. mucosectomy
e. probe
e. ultrasound (EAUS)
e. ultrasound scan

EndoAnchor

endoappendicitis

Endo-Assist

E.-A. disposable atraumatic grasping
  forceps
E.-A. disposable hemostat
E.-A. disposable ligature carrier

E.-A. disposable needle holder
E.-A. reusable knot pusher

endoauscultation

Endo-Avitene

E.-A. MCH
E.-A. microfibrillar collagen
  hemostat

Endo-Babcock stapler

endobag

endobiliary ascariasis

endoblade

LaserSonics E.

endobrachyesophagus

endobronchial

e. fistula
e. stent

Endocam

endocamera

Polaroid e.

Endocare renal cryoablation

endocast

3-dimensional pelvicaliceal e.

endocavitary

e. bladder diverticulectomy
e. pelvic lymphadenectomy
  (ECPL)
e. radiation

endocholedochal

EndoCinch suturing system

Endoclip applier

EndoCoil

E. biliary stent
E. esophageal stent

endocolitis

endocrine

e. cancer
e. cell
e. cell carcinoma
e. disruptor
e. mimic
e. screening
e. system
e. therapy

endocrinopathy

Endocut

endocutter

Long 45 e.

endocystitis

endocytosis

fluid-phase e.

endocytotic vesicle

endodermal, endodermic

endodermic (*var. of* endodermal)

**Endo-Dop transendoscopic Doppler
catheter probe system**

Endodynamics suction polyp trap

endoenteritis

endoesophageal MRI coil

endoesophagitis
endogastric
endogastritis
Endo-Gauge
endogenic (*var. of* endogenous)
endogenous, endogenic
    e. biotin
    e. lipophilic antioxidant
    e. mutation
    e. obesity
    e. opioid
    e. peroxidase
    e. peroxidase activity
    e. pyrogen
    e. renal antigen
endograsper
endoherniorrhaphy
Endolav
    E. lavage pump
    Meditron EL-100 E.
endoligature
Endoloop
    E. ligation
    E. suture
EndoLumina bougie
endoluminal
    e. clipping
    e. CT colonography
    e. endoscopy
    e. gastroplasty
    e. gastroplication
    e. rectal ultrasonography
      (ELUS)
    e. ultrasonography-guided fine-needle
      aspiration biopsy
    e. ureteral ultrasound
Endomark India ink
EndoMate grab bag
endometrial carcinoma
endometrioid
endometrioma
    ovarian e.
endometriosis
    colorectal e.
    e. of colon
    e. vesicae
endometritis
    coccidioidal e.
endometrium
endomicroscopy
    confocal e.
endomorph
endomorphic
endomorphy
endomysial
    e. antibody (EMA)
    e. antibody test
    e. IgA

endomysium
    e. antibody
    e. antigen
EndoNet
    Pentax E.
endonuclease
    restriction e.
Endopath
    E. EMS hernia stapler
    E. endoscopic linear cutter
    E. Optiview laparoscopic obturator
endopeptidase
    neutral e.
    pancreatic e.
    prolyl e.
endoperitoneal
endoperitonitis
endoperoxide
    prostaglandin G2 e. (PGG2
      endoperoxide)
    prostaglandin H2 e. (PGH2
      endoperoxide)
endophlebitis hepatica obliterans
endophotography
endophytic
endoplasmic
    e. reticulum
    e. reticulum-bound polysome
Endo-P-Probe
endoprobe
    rotating e.
endoprostatic coil
endoprosthesis
    biliary e.
    Celestin e.
    Coons/Carey e.
    crutched stick-type polyurethane e.
    cuffed esophageal e.
    double-lumen e.
    double-pigtail e.
    DoubleStent biliary e.
    Elastalloy esophageal e.
    endoscopic biliary e.
    esophageal e.
    exchange of e.
    expandable biliary e.
    expandable metal mesh e.
    IntraStent DoubleStrut biliary e.
    KeyMed Atkinson e.
    large-bore biliary e.
    Medoc-Celestin e.
    pancreatic e.
    peroral e.
    pigtail e.
    3/4-pigtail plastic e.
    plastic e.
    polyethylene e.
    Proctor-Livingston e.

E

endoprosthesis (*continued*)

    self-expandable stainless steel braided e.
    straight e.
    Titan e.
    transpapillary endoscopic e.
    UroLume e.
    Viabil biliary e.
    Wallstent e.
    Wilson-Cook e.

endopyeloplasty

    percutaneous e.

endopyelotomy

    Acucise e.
    antegrade e.
    e. failure
    e. incision
    retrograde e.
    e. stent
    ureteroscopic e.

endopyeloureterotomy

    percutaneous e.

endoradiosonde

endorectal

    e. advancement flap
    e. coil magnetic resonance imaging
    e. ileal pouch
    e. ileal pullthrough
    e. probe
    e. pullthrough procedure
    e. surface coil MRI
    e. ultrasound (ERUS)

endorectal-pelvic phased-array coil

endosac

endoscissors

    rotating e.

endoscope

    AccuSharp e.
    ACMI e.
    activated capsule e.
    battery-powered e.
    cap-fitted e.
    CCD e.
    CF-HM e.
    2-channel e.
    charge-coupled device e.
    Cho/Dyonics 2-portal e.
    double accessory channel therapeutic e.
    double-channel e.
    Eder-Palmer semiflexible fiberoptic e.
    electronic radial-array e.
    end-viewing e.
    EVIS 140 Q-series e.
    EVIS 140 S wide-screen e.
    FCS 2-channel ultrahigh-magnification e.

    FG-series 2-channel e.
    FGS-ML-series 2-channel e.
    FGS-series 2-channel e.
    FGS-SML-series 2-channel e.
    fiberoptic e.
    flexible fiberoptic e.
    forward-viewing e.
    Fujinon EG-FP-series e.
    Fujinon EVE-series e.
    Fujinon EVG-CT e.
    Fujinon EVG-F-series e.
    Fujinon EVG-FP-series e.
    Fujinon FP-series e.
    GIF N30 fiberoptic pediatric e.
    GIF-Q240 upper digestive tract e.
    GIF XP20 e.
    GIF XQ10 upper e.
    Hirschowitz e.
    e. impaction
    intraductal e.
    JFB III e.
    JF-20 side-viewing fiberoptic e.
    J-shaped e.
    Karl Storz e.
    Kussmaul e.
    large-channel e.
    lateral-viewing e.
    looping of e.
    LoPresti fiberoptic e.
    magnifying e.
    Messerklinger e.
    mother-daughter e.
    Navigator flexible e.
    near-infrared electronic e.
    nonferromagnetic MR e.
    oblique viewing e.
    Olympus Aloka GF-EU-series e.
    Olympus CF 2301 e.
    Olympus CF-UM20 ultrasonic e.
    Olympus CF-UM20 ultrasound e.
    Olympus CF-200Z e.
    Olympus CV-series e.
    Olympus DES-series e.
    Olympus EUM-20 e.
    Olympus EUS-series e.
    Olympus EVIS Q-series e.
    Olympus GF-UM30P e.
    Olympus GF-UM20 radial scanning e.
    Olympus GF-UM3 ultrasonic e.
    Olympus GF-UM20 ultrasound e.
    Olympus GIF-D2 e.
    Olympus GIF-HM-series e.
    Olympus GIF-J-series e.
    Olympus GIF-P e.
    Olympus GIF-Q200 e.
    Olympus GIF-2T10 e.
    Olympus GIF-2T200 e.
    Olympus GIF-T-series e.

Olympus GIF-XP-series e.
Olympus GIF-XQ240 e.
Olympus GIF-XV-series e.
Olympus high-definition e.
Olympus JF1T e.
Olympus JF-T-series e.
Olympus JF-TV-series e.
Olympus JF-V-series e.
Olympus PJF e.
Olympus PJF-series pediatric e.
Olympus P-series e.
Olympus SIF-SW fiberoptic e.
Olympus SIF-100 video push e.
Olympus 2T100 e.
Olympus TJF-100 e.
Olympus UM-series e.
Olympus V-series e.
Olympus XCF-XK-series e.
Olympus XGF-UCT30 e.
Olympus XP-series e.
Olympus Zoom e.
pediatric e.
Pentax EG-2901, -2940, -3800 e.
Pentax ESI-2000 fiberoptic e.
Pentax FG-38X e.
Pentax VSB-2000 fiberoptic e.
PillCam ESO capsule e.
rigid e.
semiflexible e.
semirigid e.
side-viewing e.
Simpson e.
Surgenomic e.
therapeutic e.
transcutaneous sonogram e.
UGI e.
ultrasonic e.
ultrasound e.
ultrathin e.
upper GI e.
variable-stiffness e.
Visicath e.
Weerda e.
wireless capsule e.
endoscope-body position relationship
endoscopic
　e. ablation of antral diaphragm
　e. access
　e. adrenalectomy
　e. alligator forceps
　e. ampullectomy
　e. atrophic gastritis
　e. balloon dilation (EBD)
　e. balloon sphincter dilation (EBSD)
　e. band ligation (EBL)
　e. band ligation of varix
　e. band ligator
　e. BICAP probe
　e. biliary decompression

e. biliary drainage
e. biliary endoprosthesis
e. biliary sphincterotomy
e. biliary stent
e. biliary stent placement
e. biopsy forceps
e. biopsy site
e. botulinum toxin injection
e. brush cytology (EBC)
e. camera
e. clip-and-cut diverticulotomy
e. clipping
e. color Doppler
e. color Doppler assessment
e. color Doppler ultrasonography
e. control
e. cystenterostomy
e. cystoduodenostomy
e. data acquisition
e. debridement
e. detachable miniloop ligation
e. devolvulization
e. digital pancreatography (EDP)
e. diverticulotomy
e. Doppler optical coherence tomography
e. Doppler probe
e. Doppler ultrasound-guided injection therapy
e. electrocoagulation
e. electrohydraulic lithotripsy
e. enterogastric reflux gastritis
e. enucleation
e. epinephrine injection
e. erythematous/exudative gastritis
e. esophageal mucosal resection tube technique
e. esophagitis
e. esophagogastric variceal ligation
e. examination
e. extraction of pancreatic duct stone
e. findings
e. fine-needle puncture
e. fistulotomy
e. flowprobe
e. fulguration
e. full-thickness resection (EFTR)
e. gastrin test (EGT)
e. gastroenteric anastomosis with magnets
e. gastrostomy tube
e. grasping forceps
e. guidance
e. heater probe thermocoagulation
e. heat probe
e. hemoclip device
e. hemoclipping
e. hemoclip therapy

E

endoscopic (*continued*)

e. hemorrhagic gastritis
e. hemorrhoid ligation (EHL)
e. hemostasis
e. hemostatic therapy
e. Ho:YAG lithotripsy
e. incision
e. India ink injection
e. injection sclerosis
e. injection sclerotherapy (EIS)
e. injection therapy
e. intervention
e. jejunostomy
e. large-balloon sphincteroplasty
e. laser cautery
e. laser cholecystectomy
e. laser recanalization
e. laser therapy (ELT)
e. light source
e. magnet-assisted nonsurgical technique
e. magnetic extractor
e. magnetic resonance (EMR)
e. magnetic resonance scanning
e. management
e. management of choledochal cyst
e. manipulator
e. manometry
e. membranectomy
e. metallic stent lithotripsy
e. microwave
e. microwave coagulation
e. monitoring
e. mucosal resection (EMR)
e. mucosal resection, cap method (EMRC)
e. mucosal resection, tube method (EMRT)
e. mucosal resection with ligating device
e. mucosal resection with ligation (EMRL)
e. nasobiliary catheter drainage
e. oblique aspiration mucosectomy
e. optical coherence tomography
e. optical urethrotomy
e. pancreatic drainage
e. pancreatic duct sphincterotomy
e. pancreatic stenting (EPS)
e. pancreatic therapy
e. papillary balloon dilation (EPBD)
e. papillotomy
e. papillotomy and stenting
e. patchiness
e. photography
e. pulsed-dye laser
e. pulsed-dye laser lithotripsy
e. pyloromyotomy
e. 4-quadrant tattoo

e. raised erosive gastritis
e. reflectance
e. reflectance spectrophotometry
e. removal of fragment
e. rendezvous technique
e. resection of antral web
e. retroflexion
e. retrograde biliary drainage (ERBD)
e. retrograde biliary stenting
e. retrograde cannulation
e. retrograde cholangiogram
e. retrograde cholangiography (ERC)
e. retrograde cholangiopancreatography (ERCP)
e. retrograde cholangiopancreatography catheter
e. retrograde cholecystoendoprosthesis (ERCCE)
e. retrograde cytology
e. retrograde ileography
e. retrograde pancreatography (ERP)
e. retrograde parenchymography (ERP)
e. retrograde parenchymography of pancreas (ERPP)
e. retrograde sclerotherapy
e. rugal hyperplastic gastritis
e. scissors
e. sessile polypectomy
e. sewing machine
e. sewing machine technology
e. sigmoidopexy
e. small-bowel biopsy
e. snare
e. snare ampullectomy
e. snare resection
e. sphincterectomy
e. sphincter of Oddi manometry
e. sphincterotomy (ES)
e. sphincterotomy-induced duodenal perforation
e. sphincterotomy-induced pancreatitis
e. spray cryotherapy
e. stapling diverticulostomy
e. stent exchange
e. stigma
e. stigmata of hemorrhage
e. stone disintegration
e. stone manipulation
e. stone removal
e. stricturotomy
e. strip biopsy
e. submucosal dissection (ESD)
e. surveillance
e. suture-cutting forceps
e. system

e. thermal ablation
e. thermodisinfector
e. transbronchial real-time ultrasound-guided biopsy
e. transesophageal fine-needle aspiration
e. transesophageal fine-needle aspiration cytology
e. transgastric distal pancreatectomy (ETDP)
e. transgastric drainage
e. transgastric lymphadenectomy
e. transilluminator device
e. transpancreatic ampullary septotomy
e. transpapillary biopsy
e. transpapillary cannulation
e. transpapillary catheterization of gallbladder (ETCG)
e. transpapillary cyst drainage (ETCD)
e. transpapillary drainage of pancreatic abscess
e. transpapillary nasopancreatic drainage
e. treatment
e. ultrasonographic diagnosis
e. ultrasonographic imaging
e. ultrasonography (EUS)
e. ultrasound (EUS)
e. ultrasound-assisted band ligation
e. ultrasound diagnosis
e. ultrasound duodenoscope
e. ultrasound evaluation
e. ultrasound-guided alcohol ablation
e. ultrasound-guided celiac plexus block
e. ultrasound-guided celiac plexus neurolysis
e. ultrasound-guided cystogastrostomy
e. ultrasound-guided ethanol lavage of pancreatic cystadenoma
e. ultrasound-guided fine-needle aspiration (EUS-FNA)
e. ultrasound-guided fine-needle injection
e. ultrasound-guided pancreatic gastrostomy
e. ultrasound probe
e. ultrasound retrograde cholangiopancreatography
e. variceal band ligation
e. variceal ligation (EVL)
e. variceal sclerotherapy
e. video autofluorescence imaging
e. video information system (EVIS)
e. washing pipe
e. Waterpik

endoscopically
e. deliverable tissue-transfixing device
e. guided segmental gut lavage
e. normal patient
endoscopic-controlled lithotripsy
endoscopist
endoscopy
acetic acid-enhanced magnifying e.
advanced therapeutic e.
American Society for Gastrointestinal E. (ASGE)
5-aminolevulinic acid-induced fluorescence e.
anal e.
autofluorescence e.
capsule e.
CE-AD gastric lesion staging by e.
CE-M gastric lesion staging by e.
CE-SM gastric lesion staging by e.
e. complication
computerized electronic e.
diagnostic upper e.
endoluminal e.
enhanced magnification e.
Erlanger active stimulator for interventional e.
fiberoptic e.
flexible e.
fluorescein electronic e.
fluorescence e.
fluorescent electronic e.
gastrointestinal e.
high-altitude e.
high-definition e.
high-magnification e.
high-resolution e.
infrared e.
intestinal e.
intraoperative biliary e.
light-induced fluorescence e. (LIFE)
magnification e.
open-access e. (OAE)
outpatient e.
pancreaticobiliary e.
pediatric e.
peripartum e.
peroral e.
PillCam ESO capsule e.
postsurgical e.
primary diagnostic e.
e. procedure
rapid alternating recorder exchange in capsule e.
rapid exchange technique for therapeutic e.
screening e.
string-capsule e.
e. suite

E

endoscopy (*continued*)
    surveillance e.
    TEM transanal e.
    therapeutic pancreaticobiliary e.
    therapeutic upper e.
    transcolonic e.
    transesophageal e.
    transmural e.
    transnasal e.
    UGI e.
    ultrahigh-magnification e.
    ultrathin e.
    upper alimentary e.
    upper gastrointestinal e. (UGIE)
    videocapsule e.
    virtual e.
    white light e.
    wireless capsule e. (WCE)
    e. with iodine staining
endoscopy-negative reflux disease (ENRD)
endoscopy-related emphysema
Endoshears
EndoSheath
    Vision System E.
endosnare
endosonographer
endosonographically targeted injection
endosonographic staging
endosonography
    anal e. (AES)
    anorectal e.
    3-dimensional linear e.
    3D linear e.
    duplex Doppler e.
    high-frequency e.
    e. instrument
    rectal e.
endosonography-guided
    e.-g. celiac plexus neurolysis (EUS-CPN)
    e.-g. cholangiodrainage
    e.-g. drainage of pancreatic pseudocyst
EndoSound
    E. endoscopic ultrasound catheter
    E. ultrasound probe
Endospore disinfectant
Endostapler
Endostat II bipolar/monopolar electrosurgical generator
endostethoscope
ENDOstim
EndoTAG 1
Endotek machine
endothelia (*pl. of* endothelium)
endothelial
    e. cell
    e. cell differentiation

    e. cell growth factor (ECGF)
    e. leukocyte adhesion molecule-1 (ELAM-1)
    e. tube
endothelial-dependent relaxation
endothelialis
    hepatic e.
endothelin (ET)
    e. A (EtA)
    e. antagonist
    e. A receptor
    e. B (EtB)
    renal e.
    selective e. A
endothelin-1 (ET-1)
    e.-1 concentration
endothelin-3 (ET-3)
    e.-3 concentration
endothelioma
endotheliosis
    glomerular e.
endothelium, *pl.* **endothelia**
    gastrointestinal e.
    sinusoidal e.
endothelium-dependent
    e.-d. fibrinolysis
    e.-d. vasodilation
endothelium-derived
    e.-d. nitric oxide (EDNO)
    e.-d. relaxing factor (EDRF)
    e.-d. relaxing hormone
EndoTherapy
Endotorque
    Greenen E.
endotoxemia
    systemic e.
endotoxin
    e. antibody
    bacterial e.
endotracheal
    e. intubation
    e. tube (ET, ETT)
    e. tube placement
Endo-Tube nasojejunal feeding tube
endoureteral ultrasound sonography
endoureterotomy
    cold-knife e.
endourologic
    e. biopsy
    e. cold-knife incision
    e. failure
    e. management
endourological
    e. procedure
    e. training
endourology
    reconstructive e.
    therapeutic e.

endovascular
    e. stent grafting
    e. stenting
    e. treatment
Endovations disposable cytology brush
endovenous
Endozime
    E. AW bacteriostatic enzyme
     cleaner
    E. sponge
end-plate (*var. of* endplate)
endplate, end-plate
    motor e.
endpoint dilution titer
Endrate
endrophonium chloride
end-sigmoid colostomy
end-stage
    e.-s. cirrhosis
    e.-s. liver disease (ESLD)
    e.-s. renal disease (ESRD)
    e.-s. renal failure (ESRF)
end-to-end
    e.-t.-e. anastomosis (EEA)
    e.-t.-e. anastomotic repair
    e.-t.-e. branch reanastomosis
    e.-t.-e. enterostomy
end-to-side
    e.-t.-s. anastomosis (ESA)
    e.-t.-s. arteriotomy
    e.-t.-s. choledochojejunostomy
    e.-t.-s. duodenogastrostomy
    e.-t.-s. ileotransverse colostomy
    e.-t.-s. portacaval shunt
    e.-t.-s. reimplantation
    e.-t.-s. vasoepididymostomy technique
Enduron
Enduronyl
end-viewing
    e.-v. endoscope
    e.-v. gastroscope
Enecat CT concentrated rectal
** suspension**
enema
    air-contrast barium e. (ACBE)
    5-aminosalicylic acid e.
    analeptic e.
    antegrade colonic e. (ACE)
    antegrade continence e. (ACE)
    5-ASA e.
    barium e. (BE)
    blind e.
    cleansing hypertonic phosphate e.
    contrast e.
    Cortenema retention e.
    diatrizoate sodium e.
    double-contrast barium e. (DCBE)
    flatus e.
    Fleet Babylax e.

    flocculation on barium e.
    full-column barium e.
    Gastrografin e.
    glycerin e.
    high e.
    hydrocortisone e.
    hydrogen peroxide e.
    Hypaque e.
    Kayexalate e.
    lactulose e.
    Malone antegrade colonic e.
    Malone antegrade continence e.
     (MACE)
    Malone antegrade continence e.
    meglumine diatrizoate e.
    mesalamine e.
    methylene blue e.
    nuclear e.
    NuLYTELY e.
    nutrient e.
    oil retention e.
    pancreatic e.
    phosphate e.
    Phospho-soda e.
    povidone-iodine e.
    prednisolone e.
    puddling on barium e.
    retention e.
    retrograde flow on barium e.
    Rowasa e.
    saline cleansing e.
    single-contrast barium e. (SCBE)
    small bowel e.
    soapsuds e. (SSE)
    sorbitol e.
    steroid foam e.
    sucralfate retention e.
    sulfasalazine e.
    tap water e.
    theophylline olamine e.
    tranexamic acid e.
    turpentine e.
    e.'s until clear
    water-soluble contrast e.
enemator
energy
    apparent digestive e. (ADE)
    e. delivery
    interstitial photon radiation e.
    mean e.
Enfamil
    E. LIPIL formula
    E. Low Iron liquid
    E. with iron formula
enflurane
Enforcer
    Cook E.
Engerix-B
    HBV E.-B

E

engineering
> bladder tissue e.
> fetal tissue e.
> genital tissue e.

English plantain

engorgement
> liver e.
> venous e.

engraftment

enhanced
> e. chemiluminescence (ECL)
> e. chemiluminescence Western blot
> e. magnification endoscopy
> e. reverse transcriptase polymerase chain reaction assay
> e. technical feasibility
> e. virulence
> e. visualization

enhancement
> abnormal bowel wall e.
> contrast e.
> CT scan with contrast e.
> edge e.
> hybrid rapid acquisition with relaxation e. (HRARE)

enlarged
> e. prostate
> e. uterus

enlargement (enl)
> benign prostatic e. (BPE)
> bladder e.
> calyx e.
> discrete organ e.
> ovarian e.
> parotid gland e.
> penile e.
> salivary gland e.
> tonsillar e.
> tube e.
> uterine e.

enolase
> neuron-specific e. (NSE)

Enovil

enoxacin

enoxaparin
> e. sodium
> e. sodium injection

ENRD
> endoscopy-negative reflux disease

Enrich
> E. feeding
> E. protein and calorie supplement

ENS
> enteric nervous system

ensheathing trocar

ensnarement

Ensure
> E. HIN tube-feeding formula
> E. Plus

> E. Plus formula
> E. Plus liquid feeding
> E. pudding

EN-tabs
> Azulfidine EN-t.

entactin

entamebiasis

entamebic abscess

Entamoeba
> *E. coli* cyst
> *E. dispar*
> *E. histolytica*
> *E. histolytica* abscess

entecavir

enteradenitis

EnteraFlo feeding tube

enteral
> e. absorption
> e. alimentation
> e. diarrhea
> e. feeding
> e. nutrition

enteralgia, enterdynia

EnteraLite Infinity feeding pump

enterdynia (*var. of* enteralgia)

enterectasis

enterectomy

enterelcosis

enteric
> e. adenovirus
> e. cyst
> e. excitatory motor neuron
> e. fever
> e. fistula
> e. ganglion
> e. ganglion cell
> e. hormone
> e. hyperoxaluria
> e. immunogen
> e. infection
> e. inhibitory motor neuron
> e. interneuron
> e. nervous system (ENS)
> e. neuronal circuit
> e. neuronal reflex
> e. oxaluria
> e. pathogen
> e. secretomotor circuit
> e. vasodilator neuron

enterically
> e. transmitted non-A non-B (ENANB)
> e. transmitted non-A non-B hepatitis (ET-NANBH)

enteric-coated (EC)
> e.-c. aspirin
> e.-c. capsule
> e.-c. pancreatic enzyme

entericus
> liquor e.
> succus e.

enteritidis
> *Salmonella* e.

enteritis
> e. anaphylactica
> *Campylobacter fetus* e.
> choleriform e.
> chronic cicatrizing e.
> *Clostridium difficile* e.
> Crohn regional e.
> e. cystica chronica
> diphtheritic e.
> eosinophilic e.
> granulomatous e.
> e. gravis
> hemorrhagic e.
> idiopathic diffuse ulcerative
>   nongranulomatous e.
> leishmanial e.
> mucomembranous e.
> mucous e.
> myxomembranous e.
> e. necroticans
> pellicular e.
> phlegmonous e.
> e. polyposa
> protozoan e.
> pseudomembranous e.
> radiation e.
> regional e.
> segmental e.
> *Streptococcus* e.
> tuberculous e.
> ulcerative e.
> viral e.
> *Yersinia* e.

enteroadherent *Escherichia coli* **(EAEC)**
enteroaggregative
> e. *Escherichia coli* (EAEC,
>   EaggEC)
> e. *Escherichia coli* heat-stable
>   enterotoxin 1 (EAST1)

enteroanastomosis
enteroanthelone
enteroapocleisis
Enterobacter
> *E. aerogenes*
> *E. cloacae*
> *E. hafniae*
> *E. liquefaciens*

Enterobacteriaceae
enterobacterial common antigen (ECA)
enterobiliary
Enterobius vermicularis
enterocele
> complex e.
> congenital e.
> iatrogenic e.
> partial e.
> e. pulsion
> rectocele, cystocele, e.
> e. sac
> secondary e.
> simple e.
> e. traction

enterocele-like central hernia
enterocentesis
enteroceptive
enterocholecystostomy
enterocholecystotomy
enterochromaffin cell
enterochromaffin-like (ECL)
> e.-l. cell
> e.-l. gastric carcinoid tumor
>   (ECLoma)

enterocleisis
> omental e.

enteroclysis
> computed tomography e.
> multidetector spiral computed
>   tomography e.
> small-bowel e.
> e. tube

enterococcal sepsis
enterococci (*pl. of* enterococcus)
enterococcus, *pl.* **enterococci**
> *E. faecalis*
> vancomycin-resistant e. (VRE)

enterocolectomy
enterocolic
> e. fistula
> e. lymphocytic phlebitis (ELP)

enterocolitica
> *Yersinia* e.

enterocolitis
> *Aeromonas*-associated e.
> antibiotic e.
> antibiotic-induced e.
> bacterial e.
> cytomegalovirus e.
> gangrenous ischemic e.
> granulomatous e.
> hemorrhagic e.
> Hirschsprung-associated e. (HAEC)
> necrotizing e. (NEC)
> nontuberculous
>   mycobacteria-associated e.
> pericrypt eosinophilic e.
> pseudomembranous e.
> radiation e.
> regional e.
> *Salmonella typhimurium* e.

enterocolostomy
enterocutaneous
> e. fistula
> e. intubation

E

255

enterocyst, enterocystoma
enterocystocele
enterocystoma (*var. of* enterocyst)
enterocystoplasty
    augmentation e.
    Camey e.
    clam e.
    Mainz e.
    sigmoid e.
enterocyte
    e. apoptosis
    CD23 e.
    intestinal e.
    small-intestinal e.
Enterocytozoon bieneusi
enterodiol
enterodynia
enteroendocrine cell
enteroenteral fistula
enteroenteric
    e. anastomosis
    e. fistula
enteroenterostomy
    Braun e.
    2-layer e.
    Parker-Kerr closed method of
    end-to-end e.
enterogastric reflex
enterogastritis
enterogastrone
enterogenous
    e. cyanosis
    e. cyst
enteroglucagon
enterogram
enterograph
enterography
    computed tomography e.
enterohemorrhagic *Escherichia coli*
  (EHEC)
enterohepatic
    e. circulation (EHC)
    e. recirculation
enterohepatitis
enterohepatocele
enteroidea
enteroinsular axis
enterointestinal
enteroinvasive *Escherichia coli* (EIEC)
enterokinase
enterokinesis
enterokinetic
enterolactone
enterolith
    calcified e.
enterolithiasis
enterolithotomy
enterology
enterolysis

enteromegalia (*var. of* enteromegaly)
enteromegaly, enteromegalia
enteromenia
enteromesenteric occlusion
enterometer
enteromycodermitis
enteromycosis
enteromyiasis
enteronitis
    polytropous e.
Enteron Pharmaceuticals, Inc.
enteroparesis
enteropathic
    e. organism
    e. reactive arthritis
enteropathica
    acrodermatitis e.
enteropathogen
enteropathogenic *Escherichia coli*
  (EPEC)
enteropathy
    allergic e.
    bile salt-losing e.
    choleretic e.
    chronic bacterial e.
    cow's milk-sensitive e. (CMSE)
    dermatopathic e.
    diabetic e.
    food-sensitive e.
    gluten e.
    gluten-sensitive e. (GSE)
    HIV-1 e.
    idiopathic e.
    protein-losing e.
    radiation e.
    soya-induced e.
enteropathy-associated T-cell lymphoma
  (EATCL)
enteropeptidase deficiency
enteroperitoneal abscess
enteropexy
enteroplasty
enteroplegia
Enteroport feeding pump
enteroproctia
enteroptosia (*var. of* enteroptosis)
enteroptosis, enteroptosia
enterorrhagia
enterorrhaphy
enterorrhea
enterorrhexis
enteroscope
    magnifying e.
    Olympus SIF-10 e.
    Olympus SIF-Q240 e.
    Olympus SIF-100 video push e.
    Pentax VSB-P-series e.
    push e.
    Sonde e.

temporary e.
tube e.
variable-stiffness e.
video push e.

enteroscopy
antegrade double-balloon e.
capsule e.
e. diagnosis
double-balloon method of e.
intraoperative e. (IOE)
pull e.
push e.
push-and-pull e.
push-type e.
Roux-en-Y limb e.
small-bowel e. (SBE)
Sonde e.
total peroral intraoperative e.
transgastrostomic e. (TGE)
videocapsule e.
video small-bowel e.
virtual e.

enterosepsis
enterosorption
enterospasm
enterostasis
enterostaxis
enterostenosis
enterostomal
e. therapy (ET)
e. therapy nurse

enterostomy
double e.
end-to-end e.
gun-barrel e.
tube e.
Witzel e.

Entero-Test capsule
enterotome
enterotomy
antimesenteric e.
inadvertent e.
e. incision
longitudinal e.

enterotoxemia
enterotoxication
enterotoxigenic *Escherichia coli* **(ETEC)**
enterotoxin
Clostridium difficile e.
e. diarrhea
enteroaggregative *Escherichia coli*
heat-stable e. 1 (EAST1)
heat-labile e.
heat-stable e.

enterotoxism
enterotropic
enterourethral fistula
enterourethrostomy
enterourinary fistula

enterovaginal fistula
enterovenous
enterovesical fistula
enterovesical/urethral fistulae
enterovirus
enterozoon
Enterprise hospital bed
Enterra
E. gastrointestinal pacemaker
E. Therapy
E. Therapy implantable
neurostimulation system

Enteryx
E. GERD procedure kit
E. implant
E. implantation
E. injectable polymer
intentional injection of E.
E. procedure
E. technology for GERD

enthesis
enthetic
entocele
Entocort
E. EC
E. EC oral capsule

entoderm
Entolase
Entralife HN tube-feeding formula
entrapment
e. of bowel
e. sac

Entri-Pak
E.-P. enteral feeding bag
E.-P. tube-feeding formula

EntriStar
E. feeding tube
E. polyurethane PEG tube

Entrition
E. Entri-Pak feeding
E. tube-feeding formula

EntroEase
E. Dry powder for oral suspension
E. oral radiopaque contrast medium
suspension

entry site
enucleation
endoscopic e.

enucleator
Young e.

Enulose
enuresis
adult-onset nocturnal e.
e. alarm
e. alarm technique
diurnal e.
learned e.
monosymptomatic nocturnal e.
(MNE)

E

enuresis (*continued*)
    nocturnal e.
    psychologic e.
    sleep e.
enuretic absence
envelope 2 antigen (anti-E2)
environment
    acidic e.
    bactericidal stomach e.
environmental metaplastic atrophic gastritis (EMAG)
enzimoimmunoassay MEIA Abbott
Enzol disinfectant
Enzygnost anti-HIV 1+2 test
enzymatic, enzymic
    e. fat necrosis
    e. protein
    e. spectrophotometric analysis
enzyme
    angiotensin-converting e. (ACE)
    AP marker e.
    brancher e.
    brush-border marker e.
    carboxypeptidase B-like e.
    catecholamine synthetic e.
    cellular e.
    e. change
    circulating e.
    COX-1 e.
    COX-2 e.
    debrancher e.
    degradative e.
    digestive e.
    enteric-coated pancreatic e.
    gluconeogenesis-associated e.
    glycolytic e.
    glycosaminoglycan-degrading e.
    HK e.
    e. immunoassay (EIA)
    e. immunoassay E-1023
    immunoreactive trypsin e.
    insulin-degrading e. (IDE)
    Ku-Zyme HP pancreatic e.
    lactase e.
    LDH e.
    lipase e.
    lipolytic e.
    liver e.
    lysosomal e.
    NAG lysosomal marker e.
    pancreatic isoamylase e.
    plasma e.
    proteinase e.
    proteolytic e.
    e. replacement therapy
    restriction e.
    SDH e.
    zinc-requiring e.
enzyme-conjugated anti-IgA antibody

enzyme-linked
    e.-l. immunosorbent assay (ELISA)
    e.-l. immunosorbent assay I (ELISA-I)
    e.-l. immunosorbent assay II (ELISA-II)
    e.-l. immunosorbent assay III (ELISA-III)
enzymic (*var. of* enzymatic)
enzymology
Enzymun test
EOA
    esophageal obturator airway
EORTC
    European Organization for Research and Treatment of Cancer
eosin
    hematoxylin and e. (H&E)
    e. stain
eosin-methylene
    e.-m. blue (EMB)
    e.-m. blue agar
eosinophil (E, EO, eos, EOS, eosin), eosinophile
    e. cationic protein
    e. protein X (EPX)
eosinophile (*var. of* eosinophil)
eosinophilia
eosinophilic
    e. ascites
    e. ballooning
    e. cholangiopathy
    e. colitis
    e. cystitis
    e. cytoplasm
    e. enteritis
    e. esophagitis
    e. gastritis
    e. gastroenteritis (EGE)
    e. gastroenteritis syndrome
    e. gastroenteropathy
    e. granuloma
    e. ileal perforation
    e. major basic protein
eosinophiluria
Eovist
EPA
    eicosapentaenoic acid
EPBD
    endoscopic papillary balloon dilation
EPEC
    enteropathogenic *Escherichia coli*
EP2-EP3 protein
ephedrine sulfate
EPI
    exocrine pancreatic insufficiency
epicardia
epicardial

epicritic pain
EPICS
    early preimplantation cell screening
        EPICS C-flow cytometer
        EPICS Elite flow cytometer
        EPICS flow cytometer
        EPICS V-flow cytometer
epicystitis
epicystotomy
epidemic
    e. dysentery
    e. gangrenous proctitis
    e. hemorrhagic fever
    e. hepatitis
    e. hypochlorhydria
    e. nausea
    e. nephritis
    e. nephropathy
    e. nonbacterial gastroenteritis
    e. vomiting
epidemica
    nephropathia e.
epidemiologic, epidemiological
epidemiological (*var. of* epidemiologic)
epidemiology
epidermal, epidermatic
    e. cyst
    e. growth factor (EGF)
    e. growth factor receptor
    (EGFR)
    e. stria
epidermatic (*var. of* epidermal)
epidermidis
    Staphylococcus e.
epidermoid
    e. carcinoma
    e. carcinoma of anal canal
    (ECAC)
    e. cyst
epidermolysis
    e. bullosa (EB)
    e. bullosa acquisita
    e. bullosa dystrophica
Epidermophyton floccosum
epididymal
    e. abscess
    e. cyst
    e. infection
    e. sarcoidosis
    e. sperm aspiration (ESA)
    e. sperm procurement technique
    e. tubule
    e. tunic
epididymectomy
epididymides (*pl. of* epididymis)
epididymis, *pl.* **epididymides**
    appendix epididymidis
    body of e.
    caput epididymidis

    cauda e.
    corpus epididymidis
    ductus epididymidis
    e. epithelium
    e. filariasis
    e. lymphatic duct
    e. marsupialization
    e. micropuncture
    microsurgical extraction of sperm
      from e. (MASE)
    e. obstruction
    e. percutaneous puncture
    e. secretion
epididymitis
    acute e.
    mumps e.
    spermatogenic e.
epididymodeferentectomy
epididymodeferential
epididymography
epididymoorchitis
    pediatric cryptococcal e.
epididymoplasty
epididymotomy
epididymovasectomy
epididymovasostomy
    microsurgical e. (MSEV)
epididymovesiculography
epidural
    e. catheter
    e. space
epifluorescence microscopy
epigastralgia
epigastric
    e. angle
    e. artery
    e. discomfort
    e. distress
    e. fold
    e. fossa
    e. hernia
    e. incision
    e. pain
    e. puncture
    e. reflex
    e. spot
    e. zone
epigastrica
    plica e.
epigastrium
    palpation in e.
epigastrocele
epigastrography
    impedance e.
epigenetic
epiglottis
    omega-shaped e.
epiillumination
EpiLeukin

E

Epimorph
epinephrectomy
epinephrine
epinephritis
epinephroma
epinephros
epiphenomenon
epiphrenic diverticulum
epiplocele
epiploectomy
epiploenterocele
epiploic
    e. abscess
    e. appendage
    e. appendix
    e. foramen
epiploicum
    foramen e.
epiploitis
epiploon
    great e.
    lesser e.
epiplopexy
epiploplasty
epiplorrhaphy
epipodophyllotoxin
epirubicin
episcleritis, episclerotitis
episclerotitis (*var. of* episcleritis)
episiotomy scar
episode
    mitochondrial encephalomyopathy,
      lactic acidosis and strokelike e.'s
      (MELAS)
    multiple acute rejection e.'s
    e. of pouchitis
    reduced rejection e.
    subsequent rejection e.
    urinary incontinence e.
episodic
    e. colic
    e. vomiting
epispadiac, epispadial
    e. opening
    e. orifice
epispadial (*var. of* epispadiac)
epispadias
    balanitic e.
    complete male e.
    congenital e.
    coronal e.
    female e.
    incontinent e.
    male e.
    penile e.
    penopubic e.
    e. repair
    subsymphysial e.
epispadias-exstrophy complex

epistaxis
    Gull renal e.
    renal e.
epitaxial nucleation
epithelia (*pl. of* epithelium)
epithelial
    e. cell
    e. dysplasia
    e. endocrine cell
    e. growth factor
    e. inclusion body
    e. membrane antigen
    e. regenerative process
    e. restitution and renewal
    e. sodium channel (ENaC)
    e. tumor
epitheliitis
epithelioid
    e. granuloma
    e. leiomyoma
epithelium, *pl.* **epithelia**
    adenomatous e.
    airway e.
    Barrett e.
    bladder e.
    celomic e.
    CF e.
    columnar e.
    crypt e.
    cuboidal e.
    desquamated e.
    ductal e.
    epididymis e.
    flattening of ileal e.
    follicle-associated e.
    gastric foveolar e.
    gastric-type surface e.
    germinal e.
    heterotopic cylindric ciliated e.
    hyperplastic foveolar e.
    metaplastic e.
    nonkeratinizing squamous e.
    nontumorous e.
    oviduct e.
    parietal e.
    proliferation of gastric e.
    renal tubular e.
    seminiferous tubule e.
    short-segment Barrett e.
    specialized columnar e. (SCE)
    squamous e.
    surface e.
    transitional e.
    tumorous e.
    villous e.
epithelium-lined tubule
epitope
    antibody to GOR e.
    B-cell e.

Goodpasture e.
HLA class II-restricted T-cell e.
immunodominant T-cell e.
Lewis Y carbohydrate e.
nephritogenic e.
T-cell e.
epitrochlear
epityphlitis
epityphlon
Epivir-HBV
EPL
extracorporeal piezoelectric lithotripsy
Piezolith EPL
EPO, Epo
erythropoietin
glycosylation of EPO
Epodyl
epoetin
e. alfa
e. beta
Epogen
Epon 812 resin
epoöphoron
epoprostenol sodium
epoxyeicosatrienoic acid (EET)
EPP
erythropoietic protoporphyria
Eppendorf
E. needle electrode
E. tube
Epping jaundice
EPS
endoscopic pancreatic stenting
EPS-21
PerryMeter anal electromyographic
sensor EPS-21
epsilon aminocaproic acid (EACA)
EPSP
excitatory postsynaptic potential
Epstein
E. disease
E. nephrosis
E. syndrome
Epstein-Barr (EB)
E.-B. virus (EBV)
E.-B. virus-associated
cholangiopathy
E.-B. virus infection
EPX
eosinophil protein X
Equagesic
Equalactin
equal fluid balance
Equalizer bead technology
equation
Cockcroft-Gault e.
Harris-Benedict energy
requirement e.
Henderson-Hasselbalch e.

Nernst e.
Portsmouth predictor e.
Equilet
equilibrium
acid-base e.
Gibbs-Donnan e.
solute e.
equina
cauda e.
equivalent
meconium ileus e. (MIE)
e. residual renal urea clearance
(eKru)
equivocal
equol
ER
estrogen receptor
extended release
ER alpha
ER beta
ERA
estrogen receptor assay
eradication therapy
ERBD
endoscopic retrograde biliary
drainage
ERBE
Earth Radiation Budget Experiment
ERBE electrical coagulation
instrument
ERBE electrical cutting instrument
ERBE electrocautery unit
ERBE Unit argon plasma
coagulator
Erbitux
erbium:YAG laser
Erbotom F2 electrocoagulation unit
ERC
endoscopic retrograde cholangiography
ERCCE
endoscopic retrograde
cholecystoendoprosthesis
ERCP
endoscopic retrograde
cholangiopancreatography
ERCP balloon extractor
ERCP cannula
ERCP cannulation
ERCP catheter
ERCP conventional prosthesis
ERCP dilator
ERCP guidewire
ERCP manometry
ERCP nasobiliary drain
ERCP sphincterotome
ERCP-guided biopsy
ERCP-induced splenic rupture
ERE
estrogen response element

E

ErecAid
    E. vacuum erection device
    E. vacuum system
erectile
    e. dysfunction (ED)
    e. potency
    e. sinusoid
erection
    artificial e.
    drug-induced e.
    e. hemodynamics
    intraoperative penile e.
    Medicated Urethral System for E.
      (MUSE)
    medication-associated e.
    nocturnal e.
    nonbuckling e.
    penile e. (PE)
    pharmacologically induced e.
    psychogenic e.
    reflex e.
    reflexogenic e.
    vacuum constriction e.
ERF
    esophagorespiratory fistula
Ergamisol
ergonovine test
ergot
    e. alkaloid
    e. derivative
ergotamine
erigendi
    impotentia e.
erigentes
    nervi e.
Erlangen
    E. magnetic colostomy device
    E. papillotome
    E. pull-type precut papillotomy
    E. pull-type sphincterotomy
**Erlanger active stimulator for
  interventional endoscopy**
erlotinib
eroded polyp
erosion
    aphthous e.
    bladder e.
    Cameron e.
    cancerous e.
    cervical e.
    chronic e.
    Dieulafoy gastric e.
    duodenal e.
    gastric antral e.
    gastric mucosal e.
    gravity-induced e.
    idiopathic chronic e.
    implant e.

    limiting plate e.
    linear e.
    linear-array e.
    mucosal e.
    salt-and-pepper duodenal e.
    small-bowel e.
    stress e.
erosive
    e. duodenitis
    e. esophagitis
    e. gastritis
    e. gastropathy
    e. prepyloric change
erosive-hemorrhagic gastritis
erotic vomiting
ERP
    endoscopic retrograde pancreatography
    endoscopic retrograde
    parenchymography
ERPF
    effective renal plasma flow
ERPP
    endoscopic retrograde
    parenchymography of pancreas
ERSNA
    efferent renal sympathetic nerve
      activity
ERT
    estrogen replacement therapy
ertapenem sodium
eructation
    nervous e.
ERUS
    endorectal ultrasound
**ERxin multicomponent penile
  injection**
Eryc
eryngo
EryPed
erysipelas
Ery-Tab
erythema
    conjunctival e.
    e. elevatum diutinum
    joint e.
    e. multiforme
    necrolytic migratory e.
    e. nodosum
    palmar e.
    e. toxicum
    urethromeatal e.
erythematosus
    discoid lupus e.
    disseminated lupus e. (DLE)
    lupus e. (LE)
    procainamide-induced systemic lupus
      e.
    systemic lupus e. (SLE)

erythematous
  e. gastropathy
  e. streak
erythrasma
Erythrocin
erythrocyte
  e. aggregation
  e. cast
  dexamethasone-encapsulated e.
  dysmorphic e.
  eumorphic e.
  e. lysis assay
  neuraminidase-treated sheep e.
  e. sedimentation rate (ESR)
  e. sedimentation rate test
  e. sickling
erythrocytosis
  absolute e.
  stress e.
erythrocyturia
erythroid
  e. colony formation
    (ECF)
  e. hypoplasia
erythromycin
  e. base
  e. estolate hepatotoxicity
  e. ethylsuccinate
  e. gluceptate
  e. lactobionate
erythromycin-induced cholecystitis
erythroplasia
  Queyrat e.
  Zoon e.
erythropoiesis
  ineffective e.
erythropoietic
  e. coproporphyria (ECP)
  e. protoporphyria (EPP)
erythropoietin (EPO, Epo)
  human recombinant e.
  e. hyporesponsiveness
  recombinant human e. (rh-EPO)
  e. therapy
ES
  endoscopic sphincterotomy
ESA
  end-to-side anastomosis
  epididymal sperm aspiration
Esbach method
escalated methotrexate, vinblastine, Adriamycin, cisplatin or cyclophosphamide (E-MVAC)
Escape nitinol stone basket retrieval basket
Escherichia
  E. coli (E. coli)
  E. faecalis

escutcheon
  female e.
  male e.
Esdifan
E-selectin expression
Esidrix
ESI fiberoptic sigmoidoscope
Esimil
ESLD
  end-stage liver disease
esmolol
esogastritis
esomeprazole magnesium
EsophaCoil
  E. prosthesis
  E. self-expanding esophageal stent
esophagalgia
esophageal
  e. A, B ring
  e. achalasia
  e. acid clearance
  e. acid infusion test
  e. acid sensitivity
  e. adenocarcinoma
  e. atresia
  e. balloon dilator
  e. balloon distention
  e. balloon tamponade
  e. banding
  e. banding technique
  e. band ligation
  e. biopsy
  e. biopsy specimen
  e. body contraction amplitude
  e. body contraction duration
  e. body motor dysfunction
  e. bougienage
  e. cancer
  e. candidiasis (EC)
  e. cast
  e. clearing
  e. colic
  e. collateral vein (ECV)
  e. compression
  e. condyloma acuminatum
  e. condyloma virus
  e. contractile ring
  e. curling
  e. dilation
  e. dilation treatment
  e. diverticulum
  e. duplication cyst
  e. dysmotility
  e. dysphagia
  e. ectopic sebaceous gland
  e. effect
  e. endoprosthesis
  e. epidermal growth factor (EEGF)

E

esophageal (*continued*)
    e. extirpation
    e. fistula
    e. foreign body
    e. function test
    e. fungal infection
    e. gastric tube airway (EGTA)
    e. globus
    e. globus sensation
    e. groove
    e. hyperkeratosis
    e. hyperkinesis
    e. hypomotility
    e. impression
    e. inlet
    e. intramural diverticulosis
    e. intramural hematoma
    e. intramural pseudodiverticulosis
    e. intubation
    e. I stent
    e. leiomyoma
    e. Lewy body
    e. lumen
    e. malignancy
    e. manometric sequence (EMS)
    e. manometry
    e. manometry catheter
    e. mass
    e. motility
    e. motility disorder (EMD)
    e. motility perfused catheter
    e. motor disorder
    e. mucosa
    e. mucosal gland
    e. mucosal ring
    e. muscular ring
    e. myotomy
    e. obstruction
    e. obturator airway (EOA)
    e. osteophyte
    e. paralysis
    e. perforation
    e. perfusate
    e. perfusion catheter
    e. peristalsis
    e. peristaltic pressure
    e. pH monitoring
    e. photodynamic therapy
    e. plexus
    e. polyp
    e. prosthesis
    e. reflux
    e. resection
    e. rupture
    e. scleroderma
    e. shunt
    e. single balloon
    e. sling procedure
    e. sound

    e. spasm
    e. sphincter
    e. sphincter relaxation
    e. squamous cell carcinoma
    e. squamous papilloma
    e. stenosis
    e. stethoscope
    e. Strecker stent
    e. stricture
    e. tear
    e. transection
    e. transit scan
    e. transit time
    e. trauma
    e. tube
    e. tuberculosis
    e. tumor
    e. ulcer
    e. ulceration
    e. valve
    e. variceal bleeding
    e. variceal hemorrhage (EVH)
    e. variceal sclerosant
    e. variceal sclerosis
    e. variceal sclerotherapy (EVS)
    e. varix
    e. wall
    e. wall thickness
    e. web
    e. Z stent with anchors
    e. Z stent with Dua antireflux stent
    e. Z stent with Dua antireflux valve
    e. Z stent with fully coated flange ends

esophagectasia, esophagectasis
esophagectasis (*var. of* esophagectasia)
esophagectomy
    Ivor Lewis 2-stage subtotal e.
    transhiatal blunt e.
    transhiatal radical e.
    transhiatal simple e.
    transthoracic e.
    e. with thoracotomy
esophagi (*pl. of* esophagus)
esophagism
    hiatal e.
esophagismus
esophagitis
    acid-pepsin reflux e.
    acid-peptic e.
    acute corrosive e.
    acute necrotizing e.
    alkaline reflux e.
    allergic eosinophilic e.
    aspergillosis e.
    bacterial e.
    Barrett e.

Candida esophagitis
candidal e.
caustic e.
chemical-induced e.
chronic peptic e.
CMV e.
corrosive e.
cytomegalovirus e.
e. dissecans superficialis
drug-induced e.
endoscopic e.
eosinophilic e.
erosive e.
herpes simplex e.
herpetic e.
herpetiform e.
histologic e.
infectious e.
Leishmania e.
Los Angeles classification grade A,
  B, C, D e.
Monilia e.
monilial e.
mucormycosis e.
nonerosive e.
nonreflux e.
nonspecific e.
peptic e.
pill e.
pill-induced e.
polycystic chronic e.
radiation e.
reflux e.
refractory e.
retention e.
Savary-Gilliard e. grade I, II
Savary-Miller grade I-III
  erosive e.
Savary-Miller grade I-III reflux e.
severe erosive e.
severe reflux e.
stasis e.
streptococcal e.
tetracycline-induced spongiotic
  e.
thrush e.
tuberculous infectious e.
ulcerative reflux e.
esophagobronchial fistula
esophagocardial malignancy
esophagocardiomyotomy (ECM)
esophagocardioplasty
esophagocele
esophagocolic anastomosis
esophagocologastrostomy
esophagocoloplasty
esophagoduodenoscopy
  ultrathin e. (UT-EGD)
esophagoduodenostomy

esophagodynia
esophagoenterostomy
esophagoesophagostomy
esophagofiberscope
esophagofundopexy
esophagogastrectomy (EG)
  Ivor Lewis e.
  thoracoabdominal e.
esophagogastric
  e. balloon tamponade (EGBT)
  e. fat pad
  e. intubation
  e. junction
  e. junction cancer
  e. pH-metry
  e. variceal bleeding
  e. varix
esophagogastroanastomosis
esophagogastroduodenoscopy (EGD)
  conventional upper e. (C-EGD)
  pediatric e.
  small-caliber e.
esophagogastromyotomy
esophagogastropexy
  intercostal pedicle e.
esophagogastroplasty
  Grondahl-Finney e.
esophagogastroscopy
  Abbott e.
  Clagett-Barrett e.
  intrathoracic e.
  Johnson e.
  Thal e.
  Woodward e.
esophagogastrostomy
  Abbott e.
  Barrett-Clagett e.
  Clagett e.
  Clagett-Barrett e.
  intrathoracic e.
  Johnson e.
  Thal e.
  Woodward e.
esophagogram (*var. of* esophagram)
esophagography
  contrast e.
esophagojejunal anastomosis
esophagojejunoplasty
esophagojejunostomy
  loop e.
  Roux-en-Y e.
esophagolaryngectomy
esophagology
esophagomalacia
esophagomediastinal fistula
esophagometer
esophagomycosis
esophagomyotomy
  Heller e.

E

esophagopharynx
esophagoplasty
    colic patch e.
esophagopleural fistula
esophagoplication
esophagoprobe
    Olympus ultrasonic e.
esophagoproximal
  gastrectomy
esophagoptosia (*var. of*
  esophagoptosis)
esophagoptosis, esophagoptosia
esophagopulmonary fistula
esophagorespiratory fistula
  (ERF)
esophagosalivary reflex
esophagosalivation
esophagoscope
    ACMI fiberoptic e.
    ballooning e.
    Blom-Singer e.
    Boros e.
    Broyle e.
    Bruening e.
    Chevalier Jackson e.
    children's e.
    Denck e.
    Dohlman e.
    Eder-Hufford rigid e.
    fiberoptic e.
    Foregger rigid e.
    Foroblique fiberoptic e.
    full-lumen e.
    Haslinger e.
    Holinger e.
    infant e.
    Jackson e.
    Jesberg e.
    J-scope e.
    large-bore rigid e.
    LoPresti fiberoptic e.
    Moersch e.
    Mosher e.
    Moure e.
    Negus rigid e.
    Olympus EF-series e.
    optic e.
    oval open e.
    Roberts folding e.
    Roberts oval e.
    Sam Roberts e.
    Schindler e.
    Storz e.
    Tesberg e.
    Tucker e.
    Universal e.
    Yankauer e.
esophagoscopy
    flexible e.

    prospective blind study of
      diagnostic e.
    rigid e.
esophagospasm
esophagostenosis
esophagostoma
esophagostomy
esophagotome
esophagotomy
esophagotracheal fistula
esophagram, esophagogram
    barium e.
    contrast e.
    double-channel e.
    double-contrast e.
    solid-column e.
    tube e.
esophagus, *pl.* **esophagi**
    abdominal part of e.
    achalasia-like e.
    aperistaltic e.
    A ring of e.
    atonic e.
    Barrett e. (BE)
    black e.
    B ring of e.
    cervical e.
    closed e.
    columnar-lined e. (CLE)
    combined percutaneous-endoscopic
      management of perforated e.
    corkscrew e.
    dilation of e.
    distal e.
    effort rupture of e.
    external coat of e.
    feline e.
    Heller-Belsey correction of achalasia
      of e.
    Heller-Nissen correction of achalasia
      of e.
    hypersensitive e.
    long-segment Barrett e. (LSBE)
    nutcracker e.
    pneumatic bag dilation of e.
    primary malignant melanoma of e.
      (PMME)
    pseudosarcoma of e.
    pseudowatermelon e.
    ringed e.
    scleroderma of e.
    short-segment Barrett e. (SSBE)
    spastic e.
    strictured e.
    thoracic e.
    tortuous e.
    variceal sclerotherapy in e.
EsophyX endoluminal fundoplication
device

esorubicin
ESPGHAN
European Society of Pediatric Gastroenterology, Hepatology, and Nutrition
esprolol plus Viagra
ESR
erythrocyte sedimentation rate
ESR immunologic study
ESRD
end-stage renal disease
ESRF
end-stage renal failure
Essed
E. plication method
E. surgical procedure
essential
e. amino acid
e. fatty acid (EFA)
e. fatty acid deficiency (EFAD)
e. hematuria
e. mixed cryoglobulinemia
estazolam
Esteem
E. advanced vacuum therapy for impotence
E. synergy ostomy system
ester
cholesterol e.
cholesteryl e.
cypionate e.
dinitrate and mononitrate e.
enanthate e.
injectable e.
esterase
leukocyte e.
e. stain
urinary leukocyte e.
esterification
esterified fecal acid
esthesioneuroblastoma
estimate
significant parameter e.
ultrasonography e.
estimated
e. blood loss (EBL)
e. liver blood flow (ELBF)
estimation
Kaplan-Meier e.
Estracyt
estradiol-releasing silicone vaginal ring
estradiol transdermal patch
estramustine
e. phosphate
e. phosphate sodium
estramustine-binding protein
Estring estradiol vaginal ring
estrogen
e. binding site (EBS)

conjugated e. (CE)
e. deficiency
e. receptor (ER)
e. receptor alpha (ER alpha)
e. receptor assay (ERA)
e. receptor beta (ER beta)
e. replacement therapy (ERT)
e. response element (ERE)
e. testicular secretion
estrogen-induced
e.-i. cholestasia
e.-i. liver disease
estrone
oleyl e.
Estroven
ESWL
electrohydraulic shock wave lithotripsy
Modulith device for ESWL
ESWL-related dysrhythmia
ET
endothelin
endotracheal tube
ET-1
endothelin-1
ET-3
endothelin-3
EtA
endothelin A
EtA antagonist
EtA receptor
etanercept
EtB
endothelin B
EtB antagonist
EtB receptor
ETCD
endoscopic transpapillary cyst drainage
ETCG
endoscopic transpapillary catheterization of gallbladder
ETEC
enterotoxigenic Escherichia coli
ethacrynic acid
ethambutol
Ethamolin
ethanol (EtOH)
e. abuse
e. and phosphate-enriched dialysate
dehydrated e.
GFPM of e.
hydrolyzed in e.
e. injection
e. injection therapy
e. injection therapy of prostate (EIP)
e. sclerotherapy
ethanolamine oleate sclerosant
ethanol-enriched dialysate
ethanol-induced tumor necrosis (ETN)
ethanolism

E

ethanol-specific impairment
Ethaquin
ethaverine
ethchlorvynol
ether
    methyl-*tert*-butyl e. (MTBE)
    tert-butyl e.
    trimethylsilyl e.
Ethezyme debriding ointment
Ethibond suture
Ethicon
    E. CDH29 stapler
    E. TLH30 stapler
    E. trocar
ethidium
    e. bromide
    e. bromide staining
Ethiflex suture
Ethilon suture
ethinylestradiol
ethiofos
ethionamide
ethmoid
ethoglucid
ethopropazine
ethosuximide
Ethox feeding tube
ethoxysclerol
Ethril
ethyl alcohol (EtOH)
ethylcellulose
ethylchlorformate polymerized antigen
ethylene
    e. glycol
    e. oxide (ETO)
ethylenediamine
    theophylline e.
ethylenediaminetetraacetate
    51-chromium-labeled e. (^{51}Cr-EDTA)
ethylenediaminetetraacetic acid (EDTA)
ethyleneglycoltetraacetic acid (EGTA)
ethylene-vinyl alcohol
ethylsuccinate
    erythromycin e.
5-ethynyluracil
Ethyol
etidronate
etiology
etiopathogenesis
ETN
    ethanol-induced tumor necrosis
ET-NANBH
    enterically transmitted non-A non-B
    hepatitis
ETO
    ethylene oxide
      ETO gas
      ETO sterilization

etodolac
EtOH
    ethanol
    ethyl alcohol
      EtOH consumption
etomidate
etoposide (VP-16)
    e., Adriamycin, Platinol (EAP)
    e., ifosfamide, cisplatin
    e. injection
    e., leucovorin, 5-fluorouracil
      (ELF)
    platinum, e. (PE)
etoricoxib
ETT
    endotracheal tube
eubacterial strain
Eubacterium
    E. lentum
    E. limosum
    E. rectale
eucalyptus
Eucestoda
euchlorhydria
eucholia
euglycemic hyperinsulinism
Eulexin plus LHRH-A chemotherapy/radiation therapy protocol
eumorphic
    e. erythrocyte
    e. red blood cell
eupancreatism
eupepsia, eupepsy
eupepsy (*var. of* eupepsia)
eupeptic
euperistalsis
Euphorbia resinifera
Euro-Collins
    E.-C. fluid
    E.-C. solution
European
    E. 5-finger grass
    E. goldenrod
    E. mistletoe
    E. Organization for Research and
      Treatment of Cancer (EORTC)
    E. peony
    E. primary sclerosing cholangitis
      patient
    E. retrospective study
    E. Society of Pediatric
      Gastroenterology, Hepatology, and
      Nutrition (ESPGHAN)
Eurotransplant kidney allocation
EUS
    endoscopic ultrasonography
    endoscopic ultrasound
      EUS CPN

evaluation of pancreatic cystic
lesions with EUS
EUS probe-guided electrosurgery
**EUS-AD gastric lesion staging by
endoscopic ultrasonography**
EUS-CPN
endosonography-guided celiac plexus
neurolysis
EUS-FNA
endoscopic ultrasound-guided
fine-needle aspiration
EUS-guided
EUS-g. celiac plexus neurolysis
EUS-g. cholangiodrainage
EUS-g. fine-needle aspiration
EUS-g. FNA
EUS-g. Tru-Cut needle biopsy
**EUS-M gastric lesion staging by
endoscopic ultrasonography**
EUSN-1 EchoTip needle
**EUS-SM gastric lesion staging by
endoscopic ultrasonography**
eutectic
e. mixture
e. mixture of local anesthetics
(EMLA)
Eutonyl
euvolemic hyponatremia
Evac-Q-Kwik bowel preparation
evacuation
digital rectal e.
e. disorder
hemobilia e.
ileal reservoir e.
e. pouchography
e. proctography
rectal e.
stool e.
evacuator
Creevy e.
EasiVac e.
Ellik e.
McCarthy e.
Toomey e.
Urovac bladder e.
Evac-U-Gen
Evac-U-Lax
evagination
Evalose
evaluation
Acute Physiology and Chronic
Health E. (APACHE)
adolescent urologic e.
diagnostic imaging e.
diverticulitis e.
endoscopic ultrasound e.
followup e.
genomic e.
geriatric incontinence e.

Heart Outcomes Prevention E.
(HOPE)
manometric e.
medical e.
metabolic e.
e. of pancreatic cystic lesions with
EUS
e. of symptomatic hydronephrosis
percutaneous nerve e. (PNE)
peripheral nerve e. (PNE)
postoperative e.
presurgical medical e.
pretransplant e.
prospective e.
risk e.
serum metabolic e.
sexual e.
status e.
urinary tract 4-glass e.
urodynamic e.
videourodynamic e.
evanescent
Evans
E. blue
E. blue dye
EVE Fujinon videocolonoscope
event
thromboembolic e.
eventration
Everett pile forceps
Everett-TeLinde operation
**ever-expanding armamentarium of
therapeutic modalities**
everolimus pharmacokinetics
eversion
e. normal
e. operation
e. orchiopexy
vaginal e.
everted umbilicus
everting suture
evidence
electron-microscopic e.
e. of inflammation
solid e.
evidence-based
e.-b. criteria
e.-b. dietary/fluid modification
e.-b. position statement
e.-b. review of sphincter of Oddi
dysfunction
eviration
EVIS
endoscopic video information system
EVIS EXERA video system
Olympus EVIS 140
Olympus EVIS Q-200V
EVIS 140 Q-series endoscope
EVIS 140 S wide-screen endoscope

E

evisceration
  pelvic e.
  total abdominal e. (TAE)
EVL
  endoscopic variceal ligation
evoked potential
evolving concept
EVR
  early virologic response
EVS
  esophageal variceal sclerotherapy
Ewald
  E. breakfast
  E. gastroscope
  E. node
  E. test meal
  E. tube
Ewing sarcoma
ex
  e. vivo
  e. vivo bench surgery with renal
    transplantation
  e. vivo cannulation
  e. vivo liver-directed gene
    therapy
  e. vivo perfusion
exacerbation of pain
exam (*var. of* examination)
examination, exam
  abdominal tomodensitometric e.
  adolescent genitourinary e.
  anorectal e.
  arterioportographical e.
  bidigital rectal e.
  bladder e.
  cytology e.
  digital rectal e. (DRE)
  double-contrast barium enema e.
  endoscopic e.
  fistula in ano endoscopic e.
  followup e.
  merthiolate fresh stool e.
  microscopic urine e.
  motor e.
  nonrehydrated guaiac e.
  parasite e.
  peroral pneumocolon e.
  physical e.
  prostate gland color flow Doppler
    e.
  radial e.
  rectal e.
  reflux small-bowel e.
  retrograde small-bowel e.
  tomodensitometric e.
exanthematicus
  ichthyismus e.
exanthesis arthrosia
excavated gastric carcinoma

excavatio
  e. rectouterina
  e. rectovesicalis
  e. vesicouterina
excavation
  ischiorectal e.
  rectoischiadic e.
Excel disposable biopsy forceps
excess
  base e.
  e. mucus
  severe aldosterone e.
excessive
  e. bleeding
  e. straining
exchange
  anion e.
  cation e.
  countercurrent e.
  endoscopic stent e.
  extensive plasma e.
  guidewire e.
  e. of endoprosthesis
  plasma e.
  rapid e. (RX)
  short-dwell hypertonic e.
  sodium e.
  stent e.
  wire-guided balloon-assisted
    endoscopic biliary stent e.
exchanger
  cation e.
  heat e.
  thymocyte NA+/H+ e.
excision
  abdominoperineal e.
  adrenal gland laparoscopic e.
  Allingham rectum e.
  bladder e.
  cold snare e.
  Delorme transrectal e.
  full-thickness local e.
  Gibson e.
  laparoscopic abdominoperineal e.
  laser hemorrhoid e.
  mesorectal e.
  plaque e.
  pouch e.
  sinus e.
  total mesorectal e. (TME)
  transanal e.
  urachal cyst e.
excitation-contraction coupling
excitatory
  e. junction potential (EJP)
  e. postsynaptic potential (EPSP)
excitotoxic food poisoning
exclusion
  Devine e.

e. diet
duodenal e. (DE)
subtotal gastric e.
excoriation
excrement
excrementitious
excrescence
polypoid e.
excreta
excrete
excretion
basal renal e.
biliary e.
calcium e.
calculation of renal ammonium e.
^{57}Co B_{12} e.
^{51}Cr-EDTA e.
C-urea breath e.
C-urinary e.
electrolyte e.
fecal fat e. (FFE)
glucose e.
24-hour fecal fat e.
net acid e. (NAE)
pulmonary methane e.
e. pyelography
quantified protein e.
renal acid e.
renal ammonium e.
renal phosphate e.
renal sodium e.
renal urate e.
urinary chloride e.
urinary glycosaminoglycan e.
urinary kallikrein e.
urinary oxalate e.
urinary protein e.
urinary sodium e. (UNaV)
urinary urea nitrogen e.
(UUN)
waste nitrogen e.
water e.
whole-kidney fractional e.
excretor
methane e.
non-CH4 e.
excretory
e. azoospermia
e. cystogram (XC)
e. delay
e. duct
e. function
e. urogram (XU)
e. urography (EU, EXU)
excursion
respiratory e.
excystation
exdwelling ureteral occlusion balloon catheter

exendin
exenteration
anterior pelvic e.
pelvic e.
posterior pelvic e.
supralevator pelvic e.
total pelvic e.
exenterative surgery for pelvic cancer
exenteritis
exercise
Kegel pelvic muscle e.
pelvic floor e. (PFE)
pelvic floor muscle e. (PFME)
vaginal cone for pelvic floor e.
exercise-associated acute renal failure
exercise-induced hematuria
exeresis
palliative e.
exertional rhabdomyolysis
exertion-associated gastroesophageal reflux (EAGER)
exertion-induced pain
exfoliative
e. cystitis
e. cytology
e. gastritis
exisulind
exit
e. site
e. site infection
e. site of catheter
Ex-Lax
Exna
exocolitis
exocrine
e. function
e. pancreas
e. pancreatic hypoplasia
e. pancreatic insufficiency (EPI)
exocytosis
granulocyte e.
exoenzyme-S
exogastric
exogastritis
exogenous
e. androgen
e. calcium
e. cholecystokinin or cerulein
e. hyperglyceridemia
e. IGF-1
e. obesity
e. PGE2
exomphalos
exon 1–5
exopeptidase
pancreatic e.
exophytic
e. adenocarcinoma
e. lesion

E

exophytic (*continued*)
  e. mass
  e. wart
exotoxin
  Pseudomonas exotoxin A
expandable
  e. biliary endoprosthesis
  e. esophageal stent (EES)
  e. intrahepatic portacaval shunt
  stent
  e. metallic stent
  e. metal mesh endoprosthesis
  e. olive
expander
  intraperitoneal tissue e.
  rectal e.
expanding retroperitoneal hematoma
expansile abdominal mass
expansion
  controlled e. (CX)
  controlled radial e. (CRE)
  intravascular volume e.
  mesangial matrix e.
  plasma volume e.
  sudden e.
  volume e.
expenditure
  resting energy e. (REE)
experience
  initial clinical e.
  personal e.
experiment
  Earth Radiation Budget E.
  (ERBE)
  Nussbaum e.
experimental
  e. background
  e. glomerulonephritis
  e. maneuver
expiratory breath ethanol concentration
explant
exploration
  common bile duct e. (CBDE)
  common duct e. (CDE)
  complete surgical e. (CSE)
  laparoscopically guided transcystic e.
  laparoscopic transcystic duct e.
  prior negative inguinal e.
  renal e.
  repeat e.
  transcystic duct/common bile duct e.
  (TCD/CBDE)
exploratory
  e. celiotomy
  e. laparotomy
explosion
  colonic e.
explosive
  e. diarrhea

  e. doubling time
  e. vomiting
exponential rate
exposure
  occupational toxin e.
  postural quantitative analysis of acid
  e.
  radiation e.
  tobacco dose e.
  toxin e.
expression
  breast cancer-associated protein pS2
  e.
  carbohydrate antigen 19-9
  immunohistochemical e.
  complex class II e.
  e. cystourethrography
  cytokine gene e.
  E-selectin e.
  fibronectin e.
  e. of hemin receptor
  p53 e.
  phenotypic e.
  renal tissue kallikrein e.
  tissue-specific gene e.
expulsion
  rectal balloon e.
exquisite
  e. pain
  e. tenderness
exquisitely tender abdomen
exsanguinating hemorrhage
exsanguination
exsiccation fever
exstrophic bladder plate
exstrophy
  bladder e.
  cloacal e.
  e. closure
  complete repair of bladder e.
  vesical e.
exstrophy-epispadias complex
extended
  e. criteria donor graft
  e. daily dialysis (EDD)
  e. left subcostal incision
  e. obturator node and iliopsoas
  node dissection
  e. pelvic lymphadenectomy
  e. pyelolithotomy
  e. pyelotomy
  e. release (ER, XL, XR)
  e. right hepatectomy
extensibility
  penile e.
extension
  calyceal e.
  direct e.
  dumbbell-shaped calyceal e.

extraprostatic e.
e. fiber
full e.
superficial e.

extensive
e. fibrosis
e. pelvic disease
e. plasma exchange

exteriorization colostomy
exteriorize
externa
fascia spermatica e.
lamina rara e. (LRE)
muscularis e.

external
e. abdominal ring
e. anal sphincter (EAS)
e. anal sphincter muscle
e. anorectal mucosal prolapse
e. biliary diversion
e. biliary fistula
e. biliary lavage
e. coat of esophagus
e. cooling
e. cooling appliance
e. drainage
e. hemorrhoid
e. iliac artery
e. inguinal ring
e. ligament
e. oblique
e. oblique aponeurosis
e. oblique fascia
e. oblique muscle
e. pressure transducer
e. proctotomy
e. receiving
e. recording
e. rectal sphincter
e. rotation
e. shock wave lithotripsy
e. skin tag
e. spermatic fascia
e. spermatic vein
e. sphincter ani profundus muscle
e. sphincterotomy
e. stimulus
e. straightener
e. striated urethral sphincter
e. swelling
e. test cap
e. trauma
e. ureteral catheter
e. urethral barrier device
e. urethrotomy
e. vacuum therapy

external-beam
e.-b. irradiation
e.-b. radiation therapy (EBRT)

externally releasable knot
externi
urethritis orificii e.

extirpation
esophageal e.
surgical e.

extra
e. heart sound
E. Stiff Amplatz wire

extraabdominal disease
extraanastomotic bypass
extraanatomical renal revascularization technique
extraanatomic bypass
extracapillary crescent formation
extracapsular
e. disease
e. tumor

extracellular
e. calcium
e. fluid (ECF)
e. fluid volume (ECFV, EFV)
e. hyperosmolarity
e. lipid
e. matrix (ECM)
e. matrix molecule
e. potassium
e. signal-regulated protein kinase (ERK)
e. superoxide

extracellulary
extracolonic malignancy (ECM)
extracorporeal
e. anastomosis
e. bioartificial liver device
e. cardiopulmonary circuit
e. dialysis
e. liver assist device (ELAD)
e. liver perfusion (ECLP)
e. liver support
e. partial nephrectomy
e. piezoelectric lithotripsy (EPL)
e. piezoelectric lithotriptor
e. piezoelectric shock wave lithotripsy
e. renal preservation
e. repair
e. shock
e. shock wave
e. shock wave lithotriptor
e. surgery
e. ultrafiltration (ECU)
e. whole-organ perfusion

extract
lipidosterol e.
Mycobacterium phlei cellular e.
numerous plant e.'s
pollen e.
pygeum e.

E

extract (*continued*)
    Serenoa repens e.
    E. specimen bag
extracted
    e. ductal sperm
    e. nuclear antigen (ENA)
extraction
    e. balloon
    e. balloon technique
    basket e.
    bolus e.
    foreign body e.
    harpoon e.
    microdissection testicular sperm e.
    e. of bile duct stone
    e. of pancreatic stone
    stone e.
    testicular sperm e. (TESE)
    ultrasound basket e.
extractor
    Applied Biosystems nucleic acid e.
    endoscopic magnetic e.
    ERCP balloon e.
    Glassman stone e.
    E. 3-lumen retrieval balloon catheter
    NCompass multiwire nitinol stone e.
    Soehendra stent e.
    E. XL triple-lumen retrieval balloon
extradomain A positive (EDA+)
extradural electrical stimulation
extraesophageal symptom
extraglandular endocrine cell proliferation
extraglomerular mesangium (EGM)
extragonadal
    e. germ cell cancer
    e. germ cell neoplasm
extrahepatic
    e. bile duct
    e. bile duct atresia (EHBDA)
    e. bile duct cancer
    e. bile duct obstruction
    e. biliary atresia (EBA)
    e. biliary cystic dilation
    e. biliary obstruction
    e. biliary stricture
    e. cholestasia
    e. manifestation
    e. metastasis (EHM)
    e. portal vein
    e. portal vein obstruction (EHPVO)
    e. portal venous hypertension
    e. shunt
extraintestinal
    e. complication
    e. disease
extralymphatic metastasis
extramammary Paget disease (EMPD)

extramedullary
    e. hemopoiesis
    e. plasmacytoma
extramucosal
    e. cyst
    e. mass
extramural
    e. common bile duct compression
    e. lesion
    e. pseudocyst
Extraneal 7.5% peritoneal dialysis solution
extraordinary urinary frequency syndrome of childhood
extrapancreatic
    e. nerve plexus
    e. pseudocyst
extraparenchymal renal cyst
extraperitoneal
    e. bladder rupture
    e. endoscopic pelvic lymph node dissection (EEPLND)
    e. excision of lower 1/3 of ureter
    e. fascia
    e. hand-assisted laparoscopy
    e. laparoscopic bladder neck suspension (ELBNS)
    e. laparoscopic nephrectomy
    e. partial cystectomy
    e. supracostal live-donor nephrectomy
    e. tissue
    totally e. (TEP)
extrapolated plasma caffeine concentration
extraprostatic extension (EPE)
extraprostatitis
extrapudendal pelvic nerve
extrapulmonary *Pneumocystis carinii* **infection**
extrapyramidal function assessment
extrarenal
    e. antigen
    e. azotemia
    e. calyx
    e. dysmorphy
    e. mass
    e. renal pelvis
    e. uremia
    e. vasculitis
extrasphincteric
    e. anal fistula
    e. approach
extraurethral incontinence
extravaginal torsion
extravasated
    e. bile
    e. iodinated contrast material

extravasation
  e. of contrast medium
  peripelvic e.
  pyelosinus e.
  red blood cell e.
  urinary e.
  urine e.
extravascular space
extraversion
  urinary e.
extravesical
  e. anastomosis
  e. bladder cuff technique
  e. pathology
  e. reimplantation
  e. seromuscular tunnel
  e. ureteral reimplantation technique
  e. ureterolysis
extravesical/intravesical diverticulectomy
extravisceral aneurysm
extremitas (*var. of* extremity)
extremitates
extremity, extremitas
  anterior e.
  inferior e.
  posterior e.
  superior e.
  e. weakness
extrinsic
  e. biliary compression
  e. mass
  e. pancreatic compression
  e. ureteral obstruction
  e. ureteropelvic junction obstruction

extrude
extruding mucus
extubate
extussusception
EXU
  excretory urography
exuberant granulation tissue
exudate
  fibrinopurulent e.
  mucopurulent e.
  pharyngeal e.
  whitish e.
exudate-transudate concept
exudative
  e. ascites
  e. nephritis
  e. peritonitis
Exuderm odor shield
exulceratio simplex
EYCAT
  egg yolk-cobalamin absorption test
eye
  bull's e.
eyelet
EZ
  Edmonston-Zogreb
    EZ Detect colorectal screening test
    kit
    EZ vascular linear stapler
Ez-HBT
  Ez-*Helicobacter* blood test
Ez-*Helicobacter* blood test (Ez-HBT)
EZH2 protein
E-Z Paque

E

F

F circle
F value

F-18, ^{18}F

fluorine-18

Faber

F. anemia
F. syndrome

fabianii

Hansenula f.

FABP

fatty acid-binding protein

Fabricius

bursa of F.

Fabry disease

FAC

5-fluorouracil, Adriamycin,
cyclophosphamide

face

cytosolic f.
en f.
linear-array streaks en f.
linear streaks en f.
stable f.

faceplate

Coloplast irrigation f.
Marlen Neoprene All-Flexible f.
Sur-Fit Natura irrigation adapter f.
Torbot f.
United Surgical Hypalon f.

faceted gallstone

facies (F)

f. abdominalis
cushingoid f.
f. diaphragmatica hepatis
moon f.
Potter f.

facile working knowledge

faciodigital syndrome

FACS

fluorescence-activated cell sorter

FACScan

fluorescence-activated cell sorter scan
FACScan flow cytometer

F-actin filament

factitial

f. dermatitis
f. proctitis

factitious diarrhea

Factive

factor

acidic fibroblast growth f.
acid inhibitory f.
adverse prognostic f.
alcoholic prognostic f.

analysis of virulence f.
angiogenic f.
atrial natriuretic f. (ANF)
autocrine motility f. (AMF)
bacterial virulence f.
basic fibroblast growth f. (bFGF)
basic fibroblastic growth f.
f. beta-1
f. beta-2
f. beta-3
beta fibroblastic growth f.
beta-HCG autocrine motility f.
binary f.
bladder cancer angiogenic f.
brain-derived neurotrophic f. (BDNF)
chemotactic f.
ciliary-derived neurotrophic f.
(CDNF)
clotting f.
colony-stimulating f. (CSF)
concentration epidermal growth f.
(cEGF)
crest f.
cytotoxin necrotizing f.
decapacitation f.
decay-accelerating f. (DAF)
endothelial cell growth f. (ECGF)
endothelium-derived relaxing f.
(EDRF)
epidermal growth f. (EGF)
epithelial growth f.
esophageal epidermal growth f.
(EEGF)
fibroblast-derived f.
fibroblast growth f. (FGF)
gastric inhibitor f.
glial cell line-derived neurotrophic f.
(GDNF)
glial-derived neurotrophic f. (GDNF)
glycosylation-inhibiting f. (GIF)
glycyrrhetinic acidlike f. (GALF)
granulocyte colony-stimulating f.
(G-CSF)
granulocyte-macrophage
colony-stimulating f. (GM-CSF)
growth f.
guanine nucleotide-releasing f.
(GNRF)
f. H
heat-labile f. (HLF)
hematopoietic growth f. (HGF)
heparin-binding epidermal growth f.
(HB-EGF)
hepatocyte growth f. (HGF)
hepatocyte nuclear f. 1 (HNF1)

F

factor (*continued*)
    histamine-releasing f. (HRF)
    host f.
    human epidermal growth f. (h-EGF)
    human growth f. (HGF)
    important risk f.
    independent positive predictive f.
    independent risk f.
    insulinlike growth f. (IGF)
    intrinsic f.
    keratinocyte growth f. (KGF)
    Kruppel-like f. 6 (KLF6)
    Kruppel-like f. 11
    luminal CCK-releasing f.
    luteinizing hormone
      follicle-stimulating
      hormone-releasing f.
    macrophage colony-stimulating f.
      (M-CSF)
    maternal age as risk f.
    migration inhibition f. (MIF)
    mineralocorticoid-independent f.
    müllerian inhibiting f.
    negative anatomical f.
    nerve growth f. (NGF)
    neurohumoral f.
    new differentiation f. (NDF)
    nonimmune f.
    nuclear roundness f.
    osteoclast-activating f.
    oxidase cytosolic f.
    paracrine f.
    pathogenetic f.
    patient f.
    platelet f. 4
    platelet-activating f. (PAF)
    platelet-derived growth f. (PDGF)
    P-Mod-S f.
    polypeptide growth f.
    prognostic f.
    progression f.
    prostatic antibacterial f.
    psychological f.
    review f.
    salivary epidermal growth f. (sEGF)
    scatter f.
    serum blocking f.
    serum inducible f. A (SIF-1)
    somatotropin release-inhibiting f.
      (SRIF)
    sperm motility-inhibiting f.
    sperm survival f.
    testis-determining f.
    thrombotic risk f.
    transcription f.
    transfer f.
    transforming growth f. (TGF)
    trefoil f.
    tumor necrosis f. (TNF)

    urethral resistance f. (URA)
    vascular endothelial growth f.
      (VEGF)
    vascular permeability f. (VPF)
    f. VIII antigen
    virulence f.
    von Willebrand f.
    washout f.
    well-known virulence f.
    Wyanoids Relief F.
    f. Xa
    f. XIa
    f. XIIa

factor-1
    colony-stimulating f.-1 (CSF-1)
    heparin-binding growth f.-1
      (HBGF-1)
    insulinlike growth f.-1 (IGF-1)
    salivary epidermal growth f.-1

factor-2
    insulinlike growth f.-2 (IGF-2)

factor-alpha
    cytokine tumor necrosis f.-a.
    early growth response f.-a.

factor-1R
    insulinlike growth f.-1R (IGF-1R)

Fader Tip ureteral stent

faecalis
    Enterococcus f.
    Escherichia f.
    Streptococcus f.

FAG
    fundic atrophic gastritis

Fahrenheit thermometer

failed
    f. adaptation
    f. antireflux surgery
    f. nipple valve
    f. recovery of potency
    f. transplant

failure
    acute hepatic f.
    acute intrinsic renal f.
    acute liver f. (ALF)
    acute on chronic liver f.
    acute renal f. (ARF)
    anatomic fundoplication f.
    anemia of chronic renal f.
    bile secretory f.
    chronic renal f. (CRF)
    contrast-associated renal f. (CIRF)
    contrast-induced renal f.
    dilator placement f.
    drug-induced renal f.
    ejaculation f.
    endopyelotomy f.
    endourologic f.
    end-stage renal f. (ESRF)
    exercise-associated acute renal f.

fulminant hepatic f. (FHF)
fulminant hepatocellular f.
fulminant liver f.
hyperacute liver f. (HALF)
intubation f.
irradiation f.
kidney f.
late-onset hepatic f.
liver f.
multiorgan system f. (MOF)
multiple-organ f. (MOF)
multiple-organ system f. (MOSF)
multiple-system organ f. (MSOF)
multisystem organ f. (MSOF)
nephrotoxic acute renal f.
nonoliguric acute renal f.
oliguric renal f.
paracetamol acute liver f.
parenchymatous acute renal f.
postischemic acute renal f.
pouch f.
radiocontrast-induced acute renal f.
renal f.
respiratory f.
shock wave lithotripsy f.
sling f.
subacute liver f. (SALF)
subfulminant liver f.
surgical f.
f. to thrive
treatment f.
vascular access f.

Fairley
F. bladder washout localization
technique
F. bladder washout test

falciform
f. body
f. ligament

falciparum
f. fever
f. malaria
Plasmodium f.

Falk appendectomy spoon
fallax
Clostridium f.

fallopian
f. arch
f. tube

Fallot tetralogy
F2-alpha
prostaglandin F2-a. (PGF2-alpha)

false
f. aneurysm
f. channel formation
f. colonic obstruction
f. cyst
f. diverticulum
f. membrane

f. negative
f. positive
f. schisandra
f. tympanites

false-negative rate in high-risk patient
false-positive scintiscan
FAM
5-fluorouracil, Adriamycin, mitomycin
C

famciclovir
FAMe
fluorouracil, Adriamycin, methyl-CCNU

familial
f. adenomatous polyposis (FAP)
f. adenomatous polyposis coli
f. aggregation
f. amyloid polyneuropathy (FAP)
f. atypical multiple-mole melanoma
(FAMMM)
f. atypical multiple-mole melanoma
syndrome
f. benign hematuria
f. chloride diarrhea
f. chloridorrhea
f. cholemia
f. cholestasia
f. chronic idiopathic jaundice
f. chylomicronemia syndrome
f. colon cancer
f. colonic varix
f. colorectal polyposis
f. combined hyperlipidemia
f. Crohn disease
f. dysautonomia
f. fat-induced hyperlipidemia
f. gastrointestinal polyposis
f. hamartomatous polyposis
f. hepatitis
f. high-density lipoprotein deficiency
f. hyperaldosteronism
f. hyperbetalipoproteinemia and
hyperprebetalipoproteinemia
f. hypercholesteremic xanthomatosis
f. hypercholesterolemia
f. hypercholesterolemia with
hyperlipidemia
f. hyperchylomicronemia
f. hyperchylomicronemia with
hyperprebetalipoproteinemia
f. hyperlipoproteinemia type II
f. hypertriglyceridemia
f. hypocalciuric hypercalcemia
(FHH)
f. hypocalciuric hypocalcemia
f. intestinal neurofibromatosis
f. intestinal polyposis
f. intestinal pseudoobstruction
f. juvenile nephronophthisis
f. juvenile polyposis (FJP)

F

familial (*continued*)
  f. lipoprotein lipase inhibitor
  f. Mediterranean fever (FMF)
  f. microvillus atrophy
  f. nephritis
  f. nephrosis
  f. nonhemolytic jaundice
  f. pancreatitis
  f. paroxysmal polyserositis (FPP)
  f. pheochromocytoma
  f. polyposis coli (FPC)
  f. polyposis syndrome
  f. predisposition
  f. pseudohyperkalemia
  f. recurrent polyserositis
  f. ulcerative colitis
  f. unconjugated hyperbilirubinemia
  f. visceral myopathy (FVM)
  f. visceral neuropathy (FVN)

family
  Caliciviridae virus f.
  inter-alpha inhibitor f.
  secretin-glucagon-vasoactive intestinal
    peptide f.
  S100 super f.
  tachykinin-bombesin f.
  trefoil factor f. 1–3

FAMMM
  familial atypical multiple-mole
  melanoma
  FAMMM syndrome

famotidine
  f. maintenance treatment
  f. pharmacokinetics

FAMTX
  fluorouracil, Adriamycin, methotrexate
  with leucovorin rescue

FANA
  fluorescent antinuclear antibody

Fanconi-de Toni-Debré syndrome
Fanconi syndrome
fan elevator retractor
fanolesomab
fan-shaped biopsy technique
Fansidar
fan-type laparoscopic retractor
FAP
  familial adenomatous polyposis
  familial amyloid polyneuropathy
  5-fluorouracil, Adriamycin, Platinol

Farabeuf retractor
farmer's lung
farnesoid
  f. X receptor
  f. X receptor agonist

Fas
  F. gene
  F. immunostaining
  soluble F.

fascia, *pl.* **fasciae, fascias**
  anal f.
  anterior rectus f.
  anterior renal f.
  autologous rectus f.
  Buck f.
  Camper f.
  Colles f.
  cremasteric f.
  dartos f.
  deep cervical f.
  Denonvilliers f.
  f. diaphragmatis pelvis inferior
  f. diaphragmatis pelvis superior
  endoabdominal f.
  external oblique f.
  external spermatic f.
  extraperitoneal f.
  fusion f.
  Gerota f.
  inferior f.
  internal abdominal f.
  internal oblique f.
  internal spermatic f.
  investing f.
  ischiorectal f.
  kidney Gerota f.
  f. lata
  f. lata buttress
  f. lata suburethral sling
  lateral oblique f.
  levator f.
  lumbodorsal f.
  lumbosacral f.
  f. of Camper
  f. of colon
  f. of urogenital trigone
  paraconal f.
  pelvic f.
  f. pelvis
  f. pelvis visceralis
  f. penis profunda
  f. penis superficialis
  perineal f.
  perirenal f.
  posterior renal f.
  prevertebral f.
  f. propria cooperi
  prostatic f.
  psoas f.
  pubocervical f.
  pubovesicocervical f.
  rectal f.
  rectosacral f.
  rectovesical f.
  rectus f.
  renal f.
  f. renalis
  rim of f.

Scarpa f.
spermatic f.
f. spermatica externa
f. spermatica interna
subperitoneal f.
subserous f.
superficial f.
transversalis f.
umbilicovesical f.
vesicopelvic f.
Waldeyer f.

fasciae (*pl. of* fascia)
fascial

f. capsule
f. defect
f. layer
f. sling approach
f. stranding

fascias (*pl. of* fascia)
fasciculata

zona f.

fasciculated bladder
fasciculation
fasciitis, fascitis

necrotizing f.

fasciocutaneous flap
Fasciola

F. gigantica
F. hepatica
F. hepatica infestation

fascioliasis

biliary f.
hepatic f.

Fascioloides magna
fasciolopsiasis
Fasciolopsis buski
fascitis (*var. of* fasciitis)
fashion

Heineke-Mikulicz f.
helical f.
LeDuc f.
retrograde f.

fast

f. cholinergic input
f. spin-echo acquisition MRI

fasted-to-fed pattern
fastener

Brown-Mueller T f.
Brown-Mueller T-bar f.
ROC XS suture f.
T f.

fastidium cibi
fasting

f. C-peptide level
f. diet
intermediate f.
f. motor pattern
partial f.

f. plasma caffeine concentration
f. serum gastrin
f. serum gastrin level
total f.

FastPack system
Fastrac

F. gastric access port
F. hydrophilic coated guidewire

FasTracker 325 coaxial microcatheter
fast-twitch striated muscle fiber
fat

abdominal f.
autologous f.
f. cast
f. cell
creeping of mesenteric f.
f. density
dietary f.
fecal f.
herniated preperitoneal f.
f. indigestion
f. infiltration
ischiorectal f.
macrovesicular f.
microvesicular f.
f. pad
paratesticular f.
pericolic f.
perinephric f.
peripelvic f.
perirectal f.
perirenal f.
perivesical f.
preperitoneal f.
properitoneal f.
protruding f.
f. quantitation
retroperitoneal f.
serosal creeping f.
f. storage disorder
subcutaneous f.
submucosal f.
f. wrapping

fat-free supper (FFS)
fatigue

structural f.
suture f.

fat-induced gallbladder contraction
fat-soluble

f.-s. bilirubin
f.-s. vitamin

fat-storing liver cell
fat-suppressed spin-echo (FSSE)
fatty

f. acid
f. acid-binding protein (FABP)
f. acid diarrhea
f. acid-free bovine serum albumin
f. acyl CoA oxidase (FACO)

F

fatty (*continued*)
    f. ascites
    f. cast
    f. cirrhosis
    f. cyst
    f. deposit
    f. food
    f. food intolerance
    f. infiltration of liver
    f. kidney
    f. liver
    f. liver and kidney syndrome (FLKS)
    f. liver cell (FLC)
    f. liver disease
    f. liver hepatitis
    f. liver of pregnancy
    f. meal
    f. meal sonogram (FMS)
    f. metamorphosis
    f. necrosis
    f. omental apron
    f. stool
    f. tissue

favorable outcome

favored gait

FBA
    fecal bile acid
        cocarcinogenic FBA

FBD
    functional bowel disorder
    functional bowel distress

FBDSI
    Functional Bowel Disorder Severity
    Index

FBI
    foodborne illness

FB-25K jumbo biopsy forceps

5-FC
    5-fluorocytosine

***FCC-COCA1* gene**

F9 cell

FCIS
    Flint colon injury scale

FCPD
    fibrocalculous pancreatic diabetes

FCS
    fluorescence correlation spectroscopy
        FCS 2-channel
            ultrahigh-magnification endoscope

FCS-ML
    fluorescence correlation spectroscopy
    magnifying light
        FCS-ML II colonoscope
        FCS-ML II fiberscope
        FCS-ML II gastroscope

FCXM
    flow cytometry crossmatch

FDI
    frequency-duration index

FDL
    fluorescein dilaurate
        FDL test

F-DNA
    fecal DNA

FDP
    fibrin/fibrinogen degradation product
    fibrinogen degradation product

Fe
    iron
        Slow Fe

feasibility
    enhanced technical f.

feathery degeneration

feature
    manometric f.
    pathognomonic f.
    unique esophageal f.

febrile
    f. agglutinin
    f. morbidity
    f. pleomorphic anemia
    f. proteinuria
    f. urine

fecal
    f. abscess
    f. alpha-1-antitrypsin test
    f. analysis
    f. bile acid (FBA)
    f. calprotectin
    f. concretion
    f. contamination
    f. contamination of food
    f. contamination of water
    f. continence
    f. diversion
    f. DNA (F-DNA)
    f. DNA testing
    f. fat
    f. fat excretion (FFE)
    f. fat test
    f. fistula
    f. flora
    f. fluid
    f. frequency
    f. homogenate
    f. impaction
    f. incontinence
    f. lactoferrin
    f. leukocyte
    f. leukocyte count test
    f. marker
    f. material
    f. microbiota
    f. obstruction
    f. occult blood test (FOBT)
    f. occult blood testing
    F. Odor Eliminator
    f. paradoxical puborectalis spasm

f. peritonitis
f. PMN-elastase
f. reservoir
f. residue
f. seepage
f. soiling
f. spillage
f. stasis
f. tagging
f. transmission
f. tumor
f. urobilinogen
f. vomiting
fecalith
fecaloid
fecaloma, scatoma
fecal-oral
f.-o. route
f.-o. transmission
fecaluria
Fecatest
feces
impacted f.
inspissated f.
retained f.
Fechtner syndrome
FECOM artificial stool for defecography
feculence
feculent vomitus
fecundity
FED
functional esophageal disorder
fed
f. motor pattern
f. response
Federici sign
fedotozine
feedback
tubuloglomerular f. (TGF)
feeding
Amin-Aid powdered f.
bolus f.
Build Up enteral f.
Citrotein liquid f.
Clinifeed Iso enteral f.
Compleat-B liquid f.
f. complication
continuous drip f.
Criticare HN elemental liquid f.
f. disorder
Enrich f.
Ensure Plus liquid f.
enteral f.
Entrition Entri-Pak f.
Finkelstein f.
Flexical enteral f.
forced f.
forcible f.

Fortison enteral f.
gastric f.
gastrostomy f.
f. gastrostomy
f. gastrostomy tube
gavage f.
half-strength f.
Hepatic-Aid powdered f.
HN f.
hyperosmotic f.
intermittent drip f.
intravenous f.
Isocal HCN liquid f.
Isotein HN f.
isotonic f.
jejunostomy elemental diet f.
jejunostomy tube f.
lactose-free f.
Lonalac f.
low-residue f.
Magnacal liquid f.
Meritene liquid f.
modified sham f.
nasal f.
nasoenteric f.
nasojejunal f.
Osmolite HN enteral f.
parenteral f.
Portagen f.
postoperative regimen for oral early
f. (PROEF)
Precision Isotein HN powdered f.
Precision Isotonic powdered f.
Precision LR powdered f.
Renu enteral f.
Resource enteral f.
semielemental enteral f.
sham f.
Stresstein liquid f.
Sustacal HC liquid f.
Sustagen liquid f.
thermic effect of f. (TEF)
transitional f.
transpyloric f.
TraumaCal enteral f.
Traum-Aid HBC enteral f.
Travasorb HN powdered f.
Travasorb MCT liquid f.
Travasorb STD liquid f.
tube f.
f. tube placement
f. vessel
Vital HN f.
Vitaneed f.
Vivonex HN powdered f.
Vivonex TEN f.
Feen-a-Mint
FEFEK
fractional excretion of potassium

F

Fehland intestinal clamp
Feldene
FELI
    fractional excretion of lithium
Felig insulin pump
feline esophagus
felineus
    Opisthorchis f.
felis
    Helicobacter f.
fellea
    cystis f.
    vesica f.
felleae
    collum vesicae f.
    corpus vesicae f.
    fundus vesicae f.
felodipine
Felty syndrome
female
    f. catheter
    f. condom
    f. epispadias
    f. escutcheon
    f. hypospadias
    f. pelvis
    f. perineum
    f. urethral syndrome
feminae
    hydrocele f.
    ostium urethrae externum f.
    tunica spongiosa urethrae f.
feminarum
    cystitis senilis f.
Femina vaginal weight
feminina
    ductus paraurethrales urethrae
      femininae
    urethra f.
feminizing
    f. genitoplasty
    f. surgery
femoral
    f. artery (FA)
    f. bruit
    f. canal
    f. cryptorchidism
    f. hemodialysis catheter
    f. hernia
    f. ligament
    f. nerve
    f. testis
    f. triangle
FemSoft insert
fenbufen
fencing reflex
fenestrated
    f. catheter
    f. cup biopsy forceps

    f. drape
    f. ellipsoid spiked open-span biopsy
      forceps
    f. spiked open-span jumbo biopsy
      forceps
fenestration
    cyst f.
fenfluramine
Fenger
    F. gallbladder probe
    F. nondismembered pyeloplasty
fennelliae
    Helicobacter f.
fenofibrate
fenoldopam
fenoprofen
fen-phen diet
fentanyl
fenugreek
Fenwick disease
Fenwick-Hunner ulcer
Feosol
Ferguson
    F. abdominal scissors
    F. anal retractor
    F. anoscope
    F. gallstone scoop
    F. hemorrhoidectomy
    F. needle
    F. technique
    F. tenaculum forceps
Ferguson-Moon rectal retractor
Feridex IV
fermentation
fermentative
    f. diarrhea
    f. dyspepsia
Ferrein
    F. tube
    F. tubule
ferric hyaluronate gel
ferricytochrome-C
Ferris
    F. biliary duct dilator
    F. common duct scoop
ferritin
    anionic f.
    cationized f.
    serum f.
ferrofluid
ferromagnetic tamponade
ferroportin
    f. 1 (fp1)
    basolateral transporter f. 1
ferrous
    f. salt poisoning
    f. sulfate
fertile eunuch syndrome
fertility status

fertilization
    in vitro f. (IVF)
FertilMARQ home diagnostic screening test kit
ferumoxides injectable solution
ferumoxsil
Ferumoxtran-10
FerX-Ella antireflux stent
Festalan
Festal II
fetal
    f. adrenal cortex
    f. adrenal gland hemorrhage
    f. alcohol syndrome ureter defect
    f. arginine vasopressin
    f. bladder aspiration
    f. liver-derived B cell
    f. macrosomia
    f. sulfoglycoprotein antigen (FSA)
    f. tissue engineering
fetalis
    nonimmune hydrops f. (NIHF)
fetid
fetoprotein
    alpha f. (AFP)
    anti-alpha f.
    beta f.
    fucosylation index of alpha f.
    gamma f.
    ^{99m}Tc-labeled anti-alpha f.
fetor hepaticus
fetus
    Campylobacter f.
Feulgen
    F. reaction
    F. staining
fever
    Aden f.
    Assam f.
    beaver f.
    bilious remittent f.
    bouquet f.
    breakbone f.
    Burdwan f.
    cachectic f.
    Charcot intermittent f.
    dandy f.
    date f.
    dehydration f.
    dengue hemorrhagic f.
    digestive f.
    Dumdum f.
    Ebola hemorrhagic f.
    enteric f.
    epidemic hemorrhagic f.
    exsiccation f.
    falciparum f.
    familial Mediterranean f. (FMF)
    filarial f.

    food f.
    hemorrhagic f.
    hepatic intermittent f.
    inanition f.
    intermittent hepatic f.
    Katayama f.
    Kinkiang f.
    Korean hemorrhagic f.
    Lassa hemorrhagic f.
    low-grade f.
    Manchurian hemorrhagic f.
    Mediterranean f.
    polka f.
    Q f.
    solar f.
    spiking f.
    thirst f.
    typhoid f.
    urticarial f.
    viral hemorrhagic f.
    Yangtze Valley f.
fexofenadine
F&F
    filiform and follower
FFE
    fecal fat excretion
^{18}F-fluorodeoxyglucose
F-18 fluorodeoxyglucose positron emission tomography
F2 focal point
FFP
    fresh frozen plasma
FFS
    fat-free supper
FGF
    fibroblast growth factor
FGID
    functional gastrointestinal disorder
FG-series 2-channel endoscope
FGS-ML II gastroscope
FGS-ML-series 2-channel endoscope
FGS-series 2-channel endoscope
FGS-SML-series 2-channel endoscope
FG-32UA
    Pentax F.-32UA
    Pentax/Hitachi F.-32UA
FHF
    fulminant hepatic failure
FHH
    familial hypocalciuric hypercalcemia
FHVP
    free hepatic venous pressure
fialuridine
fiber, fibra, fibre
    afferent nerve f.
    autonomic nerve f.
    f. bundle
    f. bundle volume
    circular muscle f.

F

fiber (*continued*)
  cremasteric f.
  dietary f.
  extension f.
  fast-twitch striated muscle f.
  GBM collagen f.
  hypogastric f.
  Indigo diffuse f.
  intrapelvic somatic f.
  f. lock displacement
  oblique gastric f.
  optic f.
  oxidative-glycolytic f.
  pain f.
  PediaSure with F.
  psyllium husk f.
  ragged red f.
  sacral afferent f.
  slow-twitch striated muscle f.
  SLT 7 laser f.
  splanchnic afferent f.
  Trimedyne Flex MAX f.
  UltraLine f.
  Urolase neodymium:YAG laser f.
  viscoelastic collagen f.
Fiberall
fibercolonoscope
  Olympus CF-20 f.
FiberCon
fiber-deficient diet
fiberduodenoscope
fiberendoscope
fibergastroscope
  fluorescence f.
fiberoptic
  f. bundle
  f. catheter
  f. colonoscope
  f. endoscope
  f. endoscopy
  f. esophagoscope
  f. gastroscope
  f. injection sclerotherapy
  f. instrument technology
  f. light cable
  f. panendoscopy
  f. sensor
  f. sigmoidoscope
  f. sigmoidoscopy
fiberoptics
fiberscope
  CF-HM f.
  FCS-ML II f.
  gastrointestinal f.
  GIF-HM f.
  Hirschowitz gastroduodenal f.
  Olympus Aloka EU-MI ultrasound
    gastrointestinal f.
  Olympus GF-EU1 gastrointestinal f.

  Olympus GIF-Q30 f.
  Olympus OES f.
  Olympus XK-series oblique-viewing
    flexible f.
  pediatric f.
  Pentax f.
  side-viewing f.
  ultrasound gastrointestinal f.
Fibersure
fibra (*var. of* fiber), *pl.* fibrae
fibrae obliquae tunicae muscularis
fibrate derivative
fibre (*var. of* fiber)
fibril
  disulfide crosslinked f.
  twisted beta-pleated sheet f.
fibrillary glomerulonephritis
fibrin
  f. calculus
  f. glue
  f. injection
  f. score
  f. seal
  f. sealant
  f. split product (FSP)
  f. sponge
  f. spraying
  f. strand
  f. tissue adhesive
**fibrin/fibrinogen degradation product
  (FDP)**
**fibrinogen degradation product
  (FDP)**
fibrinoid necrosis
fibrinolysis
  accelerated f.
  endothelium-dependent f.
fibrinolytic activity
fibrinopeptide-A
fibrinopurulent exudate
fibroadenoma
fibroadenomatosis
  biliary f.
fibroadipose tissue
fibroblast
  f. ECM adhesion assay
  f. growth factor (FGF)
  HE9 f.
  human synovial f.
  interstitial f.
  perivascular f.
  f. PMN adhesion assay
  quiescent human f.
  3T3 murine f.
fibroblast-derived factor
fibroblastic polyp
fibrocalculous pancreatic diabetes (FCPD)
fibrocollagenous tissue
fibrocongestive splenomegaly

fibrocystic
  f. change
  f. disease of pancreas
fibrodysplastic
fibroelastic
  f. connective tissue stroma
  f. tissue
fibroelastosis
fibrofatty
  f. adventitia
  f. infiltration of pancreas
fibrogenesis
fibrogenic
  f. cascade
  f. cytokine
fibroid
  f. induration
  f. polyp
  uterine f.
fibrolamellar
  f. hepatocarcinoma
  f. hepatocellular carcinoma
  (FL-HCC)
  f. hepatoma
fibrolipomatous nephritis
fibroma
  kidney f.
  f. of testis
  ovarian f.
  renal f.
  testicular f.
  ungual f.
fibromatogenic
fibromatoid
fibromatosis
  aggressive f.
  mesenteric f.
  penile f.
fibromatous
fibromectomy
fibromuscular
  f. coat
  f. dysplasia (FMD)
  f. hyperplasia
fibromyalgia
  f. syndrome
fibromyoma
fibromyxoma
fibronectin
  f. expression
  f. monoclonal antibody
  plasma f.
  urinary f.
fibronectin-binding protein
fibroobliterative disease
fibroplasia
  adventitial f.
  intimal f.
  medial f.

perimedial f.
string-of-beads appearance of renal
  medial f.
subadventitial f.
fibroplastica
  gastritis granulomatosa f.
fibropolycystic liver disease
fibroproliferative destruction
fibropurulent perisplenitis
fibrosa, *pl.* **fibrosae**
  appendix f.
  capsula f.
  tunica f.
fibrosae (*pl. of* fibrosa)
fibrosarcoma
  kidney f.
fibrosing
  f. cholestatic hepatitis (FCH)
  f. cholestatic hepatitis B
  f. colonopathy
  f. piecemeal necrosis
fibrosis
  acholangic biliary f.
  alcoholic f.
  anal f.
  arachnoid f.
  biliary f.
  bridging f.
  cavernous f.
  chronic sclerosing hyaline f.
  congenital hepatic f. (CHF)
  corporeal f.
  corpus spongiosum f.
  cystic f. (CF)
  diffuse lobular f.
  extensive f.
  hepatic f.
  idiopathic retroperitoneal f. (IRF)
  interlobular f.
  interstitial f.
  intralobular f.
  liver f.
  mixed intralobular f.
  noncirrhotic portal f. (NCPF)
  pancreatic f.
  paravariceal f.
  penile f.
  pericentral f.
  periductal f.
  perilobular f.
  perinephritic f.
  peripancreatic f.
  periportal f.
  periportal-perisinusoidal f.
  perisinusoidal f.
  periureteral f.
  perivenular f.
  portal-to-portal f.
  portal tract f.

F

fibrosis (*continued*)
    postoperative retroperitoneal f.
    progressive perivenular alcoholic f.
    (PPAF)
    retroperitoneal f.
    f. score
    secondary biliary f.
    segmental bile duct f.
    sinusoidal f.
    stripe interstitial f.
    transmural f.
    tubulointerstitial f.
    vesical f.
fibrosis-promoting cytokine
fibrostenosing
FibroTest
fibrotic corpus cavernosum
fibrous, fibrosa
    f. adhesion
    f. appendage of liver
    f. capsule of liver
    f. cavernitis
    f. chordee
    f. dysplasia
    f. histiocytoma
    f. nephritis
    f. obliterative cholangitis
    f. septum
    f. sheath
    f. stroma
    f. tissue
    f. tunic
    f. tunic of liver
fibrovascular polyp
Fick principle
Ficoll-Hypaque
    F.-H. density gradient centrifuge
    F.-H. gradient centrifugation
    F.-H. gradient sedimentation
field
    f. cut
    high-power f. (hpf)
2-field lymphadenectomy
3-field
    3-f. dissection
    3-f. lymphadenectomy
field-of-view camera
Fiessinger-Leroy-Reiter syndrome
figure-of-8 suture
filament
    actin f.
    Charcot-Boettcher crystals
    and f.'s
    F-actin f.
filamentous morphology
filarial
    f. abscess
    f. fever
    f. funiculoepididymitis

    f. hydrocele
    f. lymphedema
    f. orchitis
filariasis
    amicrofilaremic f.
    epididymis f.
    late-period f.
    occult f.
    prepatent-period f.
filiform
    f. and follower (F&F)
    f. bougie
    f. polyp
    f. polyposis
    f. stricture
    f. tip
filling
    bladder f.
    contrast f.
    f. cystometrogram
    f. cystometry
    f. defect
    gallbladder f.
    muscle f.
    rectal f.
film
    Bard protective barrier f.
    Cavilon no-sting barrier f.
    conditioning f.
    high abdominal plain f.
    organic conditioning f.
    plain f.
    postevacuation f.
    soft x-ray f.
filmy adhesion
filter
    Amicon f.
    Baermann stool f.
    Baxter f.
    charcoal f.
    fluorescence excitation f.
    Fresenius f.
    Gambro f.
    Gene Screen nylon membrane f.
    Greenfield f.
    Hospal Biospal f.
    interference barrier f.
    Millex-GS pore-size f.
    Millex-GV f.
    Millipore f.
    nitrocellulose f.
    Percoll f.
    Renal System f.
    suprarenal Greenfield f.
    Sur-Fit auto-lock closed-end pouch
    with f.
    Sur-Fit Natura opaque closed-end
    pouch with f.
    Zeta probe nylon f.

filtered
    f. fraction
    f. glucose
filtering
    high-pass f.
filtrate
    Folin f.
filtration
    f. barrier
    f. fraction
    glomerular f.
    kidney magnesium f.
    f. slit-length density
    f. slit membrane
    f. slit pore
    spontaneous ascites f.
fimbria, *pl.* **fimbriae**
fimbriae (*pl. of* fimbria)
final
    f. motor neuron
    f. position
finasteride
finding
    anatomic f.
    cholangiographic f.
    clinical f's
    colonoscopic f's
    endoscopic f's
    focal f.
    intraoperative f's
    manometric f.
    physical examination f.
    preliminary f.
    relevant gastroduodenal f.
    RNA-based f's
    roentgen f.
    sensory f.
    spinal f.
    ultrasonographic f.
    unexplained f.
fine
    f. gastric mucosal pattern
    f. granular cast
    f. needle
    f. reticular pattern
    f. tissue forceps
finely
    f. fatty foamy liver
    f. granular kidney
fine-needle
    f.-n. aspiration (FNA)
    f.-n. aspiration biopsy (FNAB)
    f.-n. aspiration cytology (FNAC)
    f.-n. capillary biopsy
    f.-n. percutaneous cholangiogram
    f.-n. transhepatic cholangiogram (FNTC)

    f.-n. transhepatic cholangiography (FNTC)
    f.-n. vasography
fine-toothed forceps
finger
    clubbed f.
    f. clubbing
    f. fracture technique
    f. ring
    zinc f.
fingerbreadth
2-finger grip
3-finger grip
fingerlike
    f. epithelial process
    f. villus
fingerprick latex agglutination test
fingerprinting
    peptide mass f.
fingerstick device
fingertip lesion
Finkelstein feeding
Finney
    F. Flexirod penile prosthesis
    F. gastroenterostomy
    F. operation
    F. pyloroplasty
    F. stricturoplasty
Finochietto retractor
Fioricet
Fiorinal
Firlit-Kluge stent
First-Choice drainable pouch
first-degree relative
first-generation ELISA
first-line treatment
first-order kinetics
first-pass
    f.-p. effect
    f.-p. metabolism (FPM)
first-set phenomenon
first variceal bleeding
Fischer test meal
FISH
    fluorescence in situ hybridization
fish
    f. bone ingestion
    f. oil
    f. oil supplementation
    f. tapeworm
Fishberg method
Fisher
    F. Accumet pH meter
    F. capillary system
    F. exact probability test
    F. 2-tailed exact test
fish-hook displacement
Fishman-Doubilet test

F

fishmouth
>f. anastomosis
>f. incision

fish-scale gallbladder

fissura *pl.* **fissurae**
>f. ligamenti teretis
>f. ligamenti venosi

fissurae (*pl. of* fissura)

fissural

fissure
>Allingham f.
>anal f.
>anterior f.
>cecal f.
>f. in ano
>longitudinal f.
>f. of ligamentum teres
>f. of ligamentum venosum
>f. of round ligament
>portal f.
>posterior f.
>transverse f.
>umbilical f.

fissurectomy

fissured tongue

fissurelike ulceration

fist fornication

fistula, *pl.* **fistulae, fistulas**
>abdominal f.
>airway-arterial f.
>anal f.
>anorectal f.
>anovaginal f.
>antecubital arteriovenous f.
>anterior f.
>aortoduodenal f. (ADF)
>aortoenteric f.
>aortoesophageal f.
>aortogastric f.
>aortograft duodenal f.
>aortosigmoid f.
>arterial-enteric f.
>arterioportal f.
>arteriovenous f. (AVF)
>AV f.
>benign duodenocolic f.
>benign gastrocolic-pancreatic f.
>biliary f.
>biliary-bronchial f.
>biliary-cutaneous f.
>bilioduodenal f.
>bilioenteric f.
>biliopancreatic f.
>f. bimucosa
>bladder f.
>blind f.
>Blom-Singer tracheoesophageal f.
>brachioaxillary bridge graft f. (BAGF)

>brachiosubclavian bridge graft f. (BSGF)
>Brescia-Cimino f.
>bronchobiliary f.
>bronchoesophageal f. (BEF)
>bronchopancreatic f.
>calyceal f.
>cholecystenteric f.
>cholecystobiliary f.
>cholecystocholedochal f.
>cholecystocolonic f.
>cholecystoduodenal f.
>cholecystoduodenocolic f.
>choledochocolonic f.
>choledochoduodenal f.
>choledochoenteric f.
>chylous f.
>f. cibalis
>coccygeal f.
>colobronchial f.
>colocholecystic f.
>colocolonic f.
>colocutaneous f.
>coloenteric f.
>cologastrocutaneous f.
>coloileal f.
>colonic f.
>coloperineal f.
>coloureteral f.
>colouterine f.
>colovaginal f.
>colovenous f.
>colovesical f.
>complex anorectal f.
>congenital urethroperineal f.
>congenital urethrorectal f.
>cutaneobiliary f.
>cystogastric f.
>digestive-respiratory f. (DRF)
>duodenal f.
>duodenocaval f.
>duodenocolic f.
>duodenoenterocutaneous f.
>Eck f.
>endobronchial f.
>enteric f.
>enterocolic f.
>enterocutaneous f.
>enteroenteral f.
>enteroenteric f.
>enterourethral f.
>enterourinary f.
>enterovaginal f.
>enterovesical f.
>enterovesical/urethral fistulae
>esophageal f.
>esophagobronchial f.
>esophagomediastinal f.
>esophagopleural f.

esophagopulmonary f.
esophagorespiratory f. (ERF)
esophagotracheal f.
external biliary f.
extrasphincteric anal f.
fecal f.
forearm graft arteriovenous f.
f. formation
gastric f.
gastrocolic f.
gastrocutaneous f.
gastroduodenal f.
gastroenteric f.
gastrointestinal f.
gastrojejunocolic f.
genitourinary f.
graft-enteric f.
hepatic f.
hepaticopulmonary f.
hepatopleural f.
horseshoe f.
H-type f.
iatrogenic prostatourethral-rectal f.
iatrogenic rectourethral f.
ileosigmoid f.
ileovesical f.
f. in ano
f. in ano endoscopic examination
intersphincteric anal f.
intestinal f.
intrahepatic AV f.
intrahepatic spontaneous
  arterioportal f.
ischiorectal f.
jejunocolic f.
kidney arteriovenous f.
low intersphincteric anal f.
malignant esophagopericardial f.
Mann-Bollman f.
mesenteric arteriovenous f.
mucous f.
pancreatic cutaneous f.
pancreaticopleural f.
pancreatic-portal vein f.
pararectal f.
parietal f.
pelvirectal f.
perianal f.
perianal and enterourethral fistulae
perineal urinary f.
perirectal f.
pleurobiliary f.
postbiopsy f.
postoperative pleurobiliary f.
posttraumatic pancreatic-cutaneous f.
pouch f.
primary arteriovenous f.
f. probe
prostatourethral f.

prostatourethral-rectal f.
pseudocystobiliary f.
psuedocystolonic f.
radiation-induced vesicovaginal f.
radiocephalic f.
rectal f.
rectolabial f.
rectoneovaginal f.
rectourethral f.
rectourinary f.
rectovaginal f.
rectovesical f.
rectovestibular f.
rectovulvar f.
renal arteriovenous f.
renogastric f.
residual rectoperineal f.
respiratory-esophageal f.
retroperitoneal f.
seton treatment of high anal f.
sigmoidovesical f.
spermatic f.
splanchnic AV f.
splenic AV f.
splenobronchial f.
stercoraceous f.
suprapapillary f.
suprasphincteric f.
sylvian f.
thigh graft arteriovenous f.
Thiry f.
Thiry-Vella f. (TVF)
thoracic f.
tracheoesophageal f. (TEF)
f. tract
transsphincteric anal f.
ulcerogenic f.
umbilical f.
urachal f.
ureterocolic f.
ureterocutaneous f.
ureterouterine f.
ureterovaginal f.
urethral f.
urethrocavernous f.
urethrocutaneous f.
urethrorectal f.
urethrovaginal f.
urinary umbilical f.
urogenital f.
vaginal f.
vasocutaneous f.
Vella f.
vesical f.
vesicocolic f.
vesicocutaneous f.
vesicoenteric f.
vesicointestinal f.
vesicorectal f.

F

fistula (*continued*)
    vesicosalpingovaginal f.
    vesicoumbilical f.
    vesicouterine f.
    vesicovaginal f. (VVF)
    vesicovaginorectal f.
    vulvorectal f.
fistulae (*pl. of* fistula)
fistulas (*pl. of* fistula)
fistulation, fistulization
    spreading f.
fistulectomy
    bronchovisceral f.
fistulization (*var. of* fistulation)
fistulizing Crohn disease
fistuloenterostomy
fistulogram
fistulography
fistulotome
    double-channel f.
    needle-knife f.
fistulotomy
    choledochoduodenal f.
    diathermic f.
    endoscopic f.
    laying-open f.
    needle-knife f. (NKF)
    Parks method of anal f.
    Parks staged f.
    primary f.
fistulous
    f. Crohn disease
    f. degeneration
    f. orifice
    f. tract
FITC
    fluorescein isothiocyanate
Fite stain
Fitz
    F. law
    F. syndrome
Fitz-Hugh and Curtis syndrome
FIV-ASA
    mesalamine
    FIV-ASA suppository
Fix and Perm permeabilizing kit
fixation
    f. anomaly
    iliococcygeus f.
    intestinal f.
    pubic f.
    sacrospinalis ligament vaginal f.
    sacrospinous ligament vaginal f.
    scrotal f.
    superior passive f.
    tissue f.
fixative
    Saccomanno f.
    Zamboni f.

fixed
    f. and dynamic urethral compression
      treatment
    f. drain pipe urethra
    f. drug reaction
    f. ring retractor
    f. segment of bowel
FJP
    familial juvenile polyposis
FK-13K-1 jumbo biopsy forceps
flabby abdomen
flaccid penis
flagella (*pl. of* flagellum)
flagellate
    f. diarrhea
    f. dysentery
flagellin
flagellum, *pl.* **flagella**
    polar sheathed f.
Flagyl
flail chest
flame photometry
flammeus
    nevus f.
flange
    Assura pediatric skin barrier f.
flank
    f. approach
    f. approach adrenalectomy
    bulging f.
    f. droop
    f. incision
    f. mass
    f. nephrectomy
    f. pain
    f. position
    f. roll positioning
    f. surgery
flanking sequence
FLAP
    fluorouracil, leucovorin rescue,
      Adriamycin, Platinol
flap
    abdominal fasciocutaneous f.
    advancement of rectal f.
    advancement sleeve f.
    axial f.
    Bakamjian f.
    Boari bladder f.
    Boari-Ockerblad ureteral f.
    Byars f.
    circumferential transanal sleeve
      advancement f.
    cutaneous advancement f.
    cuticular f.
    dartos pedicle f.
    deepithelialized f.
    detrusor muscle f.
    diamond f.

f. dissection
endorectal advancement f.
fasciocutaneous f.
forearm f.
foreskin f.
Fortunoff f.
gracilis muscle f.
House sliding advancement f.
ischemia or sloughing of f.
island groin f.
island pedicle f.
latissimus dorsi free f.
liver f.
Martius labial fat pad f.
Mathieu island onlay f.
microvascular f.
musculocutaneous f.
myocutaneous f.
Ockerblad-Boari ureteral f.
omental pedicle f.
onlay island f.
paraexstrophy skin f.
parameatal-based f.
pedicle island f.
pedicle muscle f.
penile island f.
random f.
rectus abdominis
  musculocutaneous f.
rectus femoris f.
renal capsular f.
Scardino vertical pyeloplasty f.
surgical f.
f. technique
tensor fascia lata f.
tubed groin f.
tubularized cecal f.
upper arm f.
U-shaped skin f.
vaginal f.
f. valve
vastus lateralis muscle f.
ventrum penis f.
flapping tremor sign
flap-valve
    f.-v. antireflux procedure
    f.-v. cystoplasty
    f.-v. mechanism
    f.-v. principle
flare
    f. cell
    pancreatic f.
flare-up
flashlamp pumped-dye laser
**flash pulmonary edema with
anuria**
flat
    f. adenoma
    f. carcinoma

f. condyloma
f. depressed lesion
f. dysplasia
f. elevated lesion
f. hyperplasia
f. plate of abdomen
f. polycyclic ulceration
f. rectal adenocarcinoma
f. spatula electrode
f. ulcer
flattened
    f. duodenal fold
    f. epithelial microfold cell
flattening
    histogram f.
    f. of ileal epithelium
flat-type carcinoma
flatulence
flatulent
    f. colic
    f. dyspepsia
Flatulex
flatus
    f. enema
    f. incontinence
Flavimonas
flavin, flavine
    f. adenine dinucleotide
    f. mononucleotide
flavine (*var. of* flavin)
flavivirus
Flavobacterium meningosepticum
flavonol
flavoxate hydrochloride
flavus
    Aspergillus f.
flax
    mountain f.
FLC
   fatty liver cell
fleabane
    Canadian f.
flea-bitten kidney
flecainide
Fleet
    F. Accu-Prep
    F. Babylax enema
    F. Bisacodyl
    F. bowel preparation
    F. enema mineral oil
    F. flavored castor oil
    F. Phospho-soda
    F. Phospho-soda buffered saline
      laxative
fleroxacin
Fletcher's Castoria
flex knife
flexed
Flexeril

F

flexible
> f. aspiration needle
> f. bronchoscopy simulator
> f. cystodiathermy
> f. delivery device
> f. dental suction
> f. endoscopic overtube
> f. endoscopic suturing device
> f. endoscopy
> f. esophagoscopy
> f. fiberoptic choledochoscope
> f. fiberoptic endoscope
> f. forward-viewing panendoscope
> f. gastroscope
> f. laparoscopy
> f. nephroscope
> f. nephroscopy
> f. Olympus GF-EUM3 device
> f. scope
> F. Sew-Right device
> f. sigmoidoscope
> f. sigmoidoscopy
> F. Ti-Knot device
> f. ureteropyeloscopy
> f. ureterorenoscopy
> f. ureteroscope
> f. videolaparoscope

flexible-tip guidewire
Flexical enteral feeding
Flexicath silicone subclavian cannula
Flexi-Flate
> F.-F. I, II penile prosthesis
> F.-F. penile implant

Flexiflo
> F. Companion enteral feeding pump
> F. II enteral feeding pump
> F. Inverta-PEG gastrostomy kit
> F. Inverta-PEG tube
> F. Lap J laparoscopic jejunostomy kit
> F. over-the-guidewire gastrostomy kit
> F. stoma-creator tube
> F. Stomate low-profile gastrostomy tube
> F. Top-Fill enteral nutrition system
> F. tungsten weighted feeding tube
> F. Versa-PEG tube

Flexima
> F. biliary stent
> F. ureteral catheter

Flexirod penile prosthesis
Flexi-Seal FMS fecal diversion and containment system
Flexi-Stent
> Freeman pancreatic F.-S.

Flexner dysentery
flexneri
> *Shigella f.*

FlexSure
> F. anti-*H. pylori* IgG antibody
> F. HP test
> F. in-office rapid serology test kit
> F. OBT
> F. whole-blood test

flexura, *pl.* **flexurae**
> f. coli dextra
> f. coli sinistra
> f. duodeni inferior
> f. duodeni superior
> f. duodenojejunalis
> f. hepatica cell
> f. lienalis coli
> f. perinealis recti
> f. sacralis recti

flexurae (*pl. of* flexura)
flexural rigidity
flexure
> anorectal f.
> colon splenic f.
> duodenojejunal f.
> hepatic f.
> left colonic f.
> perineal f.
> right colonic f.
> sigmoid f.
> splenic f.

Flexxicon
> F. Blue dialysis catheter
> F. II PC internal jugular catheter

Flexxus endoscopic biliary stent
Flexzan topical wound dressing
FLH
> focal lymphoid hyperplasia

FL-HCC
> fibrolamellar hepatocellular carcinoma

Flint colon injury scale (FCIS)
flip-flap
> Mathieu-Horton-Devine f.-f.
> f.-f. procedure
> f.-f. technique

flipped T wave
FLKS
> fatty liver and kidney syndrome

floating
> f. gallbladder
> f. gallstone
> f. stent
> f. stool
> f. table

Flocare 500 feeding pump
floccosum
> *Epidermophyton f.*

flocculate
> calcific f.

flocculation on barium enema
flocculi (*pl. of* flocculus)

flocculus, *pl.* **flocculi**
    calcific f.
Flo-Gard pump
Flolan
Flomax
Flomaxtra XL
Flood syndrome
floor
    inguinal f.
    f. of inguinal region
    pelvic f.
FloPoint test
floppy
    f. Nissen fundic wrap
    f. Nissen fundoplication
floppy-tipped guidewire
flora
    bacterial f.
    colonic f.
    commensal f.
    fecal f.
    GI tract f.
    gut f.
    intestinal f.
    normal f.
    protective probiotic f.
    proximal human colonic f.
Flora-Q
Florastor Kids
florid
    f. bile duct lesion
    f. polyposis
Florida
    F. pouch urinary reservoir
    F. Prostate Cancer Network
    F. urinary pouch
Floropryl
flosulide
flow
    azygos blood f.
    bile f.
    blood f.
    cavernous artery blood f.
    f. cytometric analysis
    f. cytometric study
    f. cytometry
    f. cytometry analysis
    f. cytometry crossmatch (FCXM)
    effective renal plasma f.
    estimated liver blood f. (ELBF)
    forearm blood f.
    gastric mucosal blood f. (GMBF)
    hepatic blood f.
    hepatofugal f.
    hepatopetal f.
    high-velocity f.
    light f.
    f. microsphere fluorescent
      immunoassay technique

    mucosal blood f.
    nephron plasma f.
    noninvasive assessment of urinary f.
    obstruction of bile f.
    outer cortical blood f.
    pancreatic blood f.
    peak f.
    plasma f.
    f. rate
    renal blood f. (RBL)
    renal plasma f. (RPF)
    splanchnic blood f.
    splenic venous blood f.
    tubular fluid f.
    turbulent f.
    urinary f.
    f. volume
flower
    pasque f.
    passion f.
flowmeter
    Dantec rotating disk f.
    Dantec Urodyn 1000 f.
    electromagnetic f.
    laser Doppler f.
    Life-Tech f.
    Transonics laser-Doppler f.
flowprobe
    endoscopic f.
Flow-Thru feeding tube
Floxin
floxuridine (FUDR, FUdR)
flucloxacillin
flucloxacillin-associated liver damage
flucloxacillin-induced delayed cholestatic
  hepatitis
fluconazole
fluctuance
fluctuant mass
fluctuation
    GB vol+ f.
    spontaneous f.
flucytosine
fludarabine phosphate
Fluhrer rectal probe
fluid
    f. absorptive capacity
    f. analysis
    ascitic tumor f. (ATF)
    BiCart dialysis f.
    bile-stained f.
    bile-tinged f.
    bloody peritoneal f.
    cerebrospinal f. (CSF)
    f. challenge
    chylous ascitic f.
    citrate replacement f.
    cloudy f.
    f. collection

F

fluid (*continued*)
    contrast f.
    crevicular f.
    cul-de-sac f.
    f. culture
    cytospin collection f.
    Dialyflex dialysis f.
    effusion f.
    Euro-Collins f.
    extracellular f. (ECF)
    fecal f.
    follicular f. (FF)
    forward motility protein of
      epididymal f.
    free f.
    f. intake postoperatively
    intracellular f. (ICF)
    intraglandular f.
    irrigating f.
    IV f.
    LDH level of ascitic f.
    LKB Optiphase 2 scintillation f.
    f. loss
    malodorous f.
    milky f.
    motor oil peritoneal f.
    Niflex PEG-based lavage f.
    nonmalodorous f.
    oviductal f.
    peripancreatic f.
    peritoneal f.
    peritubular f.
    f. phase marker
    primary infection of ascitic f.
    prune juice peritoneal f.
    renal tubular f.
    f. replacement therapy
    f. restriction
    f. resuscitation
    sanguineous f.
    seminal f.
    f. sequestration
    serosanguineous f.
    f. shift
    straw-colored f.
    synovial f.
    testicular interstitial f. (TIF)
    f. transport
    turbid peritoneal f.
    University of Wisconsin
      preservation f.
    f. wave
fluid-air interface
fluid-debris level
fluid-filled
    f.-f. balloon
    f.-f. diverticulum
    f.-f. sac
    f.-f. small bowel

fluidity
    hepatocellular basolateral plasma
      membrane f.
**fluidjet technology-assisted mucosal
    resection**
fluid-phase
    f.-p. endocytosis
    f.-p. pinocytosis
fluid:ultrafiltrate
    tubular f:u. (TF/UF)
fluke
    giant intestinal f.
    liver f.
flulike syndrome
flumazenil
flumecinol
flunarizine
flunisolide
fluocinolone
fluorescein
    f. dilaurate (FDL)
    f. dilaurate test
    f. electronic endoscopy
    f. isothiocyanate (FITC)
    f. isothiocyanate conjugated
      antibody
    f. isothiocyanate-labeled monoclonal
      antibody
    linear f.
    linear-array f.
    scattered f.
    sodium f. (NaF)
    f. string test
    superficial f.
fluoresceinuria
fluorescence
    f. angiography
    f. correlation spectroscopy (FCS)
    f. correlation spectroscopy
      magnifying light (FCS-ML)
    f. cystoscopy
    f. endoscopy
    f. excitation filter
    f. fibergastroscope
    f. in situ hybridization (FISH)
    f. intensity
    pericentral pyridine nucleotide f.
    periportal pyridine nucleotide f.
fluorescence-activated
    f.-a. cell sorter (FACS)
    f.-a. cell sorter scan (FACScan)
    f.-a. flow cytometry
fluorescent
    f. antinuclear antibody (FANA)
    f. detection
    f. electronic endoscopy
    f. gene scanning
    f. image analysis
    f. light intensity (FLI)

f. treponemal antibody absorption (FTA-ABS)

f. treponemal antibody absorption test

fluoride

phenyl-methane-sulfonyl f.

fluorine-18 (F-18, ^{18}F)

5-fluorocytosine (5-FC)

18-fluorodeoxyglucose positron emission tomography

fluorodeoxyuridine (FUdR, FUDR)

fluorodopan

fluorometer

continuous-flow f.

fluorometholone

fluoromethylene deoxycytidine

FluoroPlus Roadmapper

fluoropyrimidine

fluoroquinolone

f. seminal plasma concentration

f. therapy

fluoroscope

C-arm f.

fluoroscopic

f. control

f. cystocolpoproctography

f. guidance

f. monitoring

fluoroscopy

C-arm f.

oblique f.

pulse f.

fluoroscopy-guided balloon dilator

Fluoro Tip ERCP cannula

Fluorotome double-lumen sphincterotome

5-fluorouracil (5-FU)

5-f., Adriamycin, cyclophosphamide (FAC)

5-f., Adriamycin, mitomycin C (FAM)

5-f., Adriamycin, Platinol (FAP)

etoposide, leucovorin, 5-f. (ELF)

5-f., mitomycin C radiation (FUMIR)

fluorouracil

fluorouracil, Adriamycin, methotrexate with leucovorin rescue (FAMTX)

fluorouracil, Adriamycin, methyl-CCNU (FAMe)

fluorouracil, leucovorin rescue, Adriamycin, Platinol (FLAP)

methotrexate, Oncovin, f. (MOF)

fluorourodynamics

fluoxetine hydrochloride

fluoxymesterone

FLUP

front-loading ultrasound probe

fluphenazine

flurbiprofen

flush

carcinoid f.

saline f.

f. stoma

flushing

cold f.

f. syndrome

flush-tank sign

flutamide therapy

fluted J-Vac drain

fluvastatin

fluvialis

Vibrio f.

fluvoxamine

flux

bilious f.

celiac f.

lumen-to-bath sodium f.

paracellular f.

proton f.

sodium f.

FMD

fibromuscular dysplasia

FMF

familial Mediterranean fever

fMLP

N-formyl-methionyl-leucyl-phenylalanine

fMLP chemoattractant receptor

fMLP-stimulated O_2

fMRI, f-MRI

functional magnetic resonance imaging

FMS

fatty meal sonogram

FNA

fine-needle aspiration

EUS-guided FNA

FNAB

fine-needle aspiration biopsy

FNAC

fine-needle aspiration cytology

FNH

focal nodular hyperplasia

FNTC, FNTHC

fine-needle transhepatic cholangiogram

fine-needle transhepatic cholangiography

foal adhesion kinase

foam

f. cell

Cutinova f.

hydrocortisone f.

foamy

f. liver

f. stool

Fobi pouch

FOBT

fecal occult blood test

FOBT positive

F

focal
- f. accumulation of tracer
- f. bacterial nephritis
- f. biliary cirrhosis
- f. carcinoma
- f. colitis
- f. collagen synthesis
- f. colonic mucosal ulcer
- f. dimpling
- f. edema
- f. fatty infiltration
- f. fatty infiltration of liver
- f. finding
- f. hepatocellular necrosis
- f. ileus
- f. lymphoid hyperplasia (FLH)
- f. necrotizing glomerulonephritis
- f. nodular hyperplasia (FNH)
- f. nonfatty infiltration of liver
- f. pancreatitis
- f. proliferative glomerulonephritis
- f. sclerosis
- f. segmental glomerulosclerosis (FSGS)
- f. stricture
- f. tenderness
- f. tumor

foci (*pl. of* focus)

focus, *pl.* **foci**
- aberrant crypt f.
- dysplastic f.
- echogenic cardiac f.
- f. of tumor
- tumor f.

focused shock wave

Foerster
- F. abdominal ring retractor
- F. sponge forceps

foetida
- asa f.

Fogarty
- F. balloon
- F. balloon biliary catheter
- F. biliary probe
- F. clamp
- F. irrigation catheter

fog reduction/elimination device (FRED)

folate
- f. anemia
- f. deficiency
- f. distribution
- f. malabsorption
- polyglutamate f.
- red blood cell f.
- serum f.

fold
- aryepiglottic f.
- cecal f.
- cholecystoduodenocolic f.
- costocolic f.
- crescent f.
- crural f.
- Douglas f.
- duodenal f.
- duodenojejunal f.
- duodenomesocolic f.
- epigastric f.
- flattened duodenal f.
- gastric f.
- gastropancreatic f.
- giant gastric f.
- gluteal f.
- haustral f.
- Heister f.
- Hensing f.
- hepatopancreatic f.
- ileocolic f.
- inferior duodenal f.
- inguinal f.
- interhaustral f.
- Jonnesco f.
- Kerckring f.
- left pancreaticogastric f.
- middle rectal f.
- mucosal f.
- Nélaton f.
- palatopharyngeal f.
- paraduodenal f.
- parietocolic f.
- f. pattern
- rectal f.
- rugal f.
- semilunar-shaped f.
- sentinel f.
- sigmoid f.
- spiral f.
- superior duodenal f.
- Treves f.
- triradiate cecal f.
- vascular cecal f.
- vertical f.

folded fundus

Foley
- F. catheter
- F. criteria
- nitrofurazone F.
- F. operation
- F. V-V pyeloplasty
- F. Y-plasty
- F. Y-plasty pyeloplasty
- F. Y-type ureteropyeloplasty
- F. Y-V plasty
- F. Y-V pyeloplasty
- F. Y-V ureteropyeloplasty

Folgard

foliaceus
- pemphigus f.

foliate papillae

folic
    f. acid
    f. acid malabsorption
Folin
    F. filtrate
    F. gravimetric method
    F. phenol reagent
Folin-Benedict-Myers method
Folin-Denis method
folinic acid
follicle
    ileal f.
    Lieberkühn f.
    lymphoid f.
    mucosal lymphoid f.
follicle-associated epithelium
follicle-stimulating
    f.-s. hormone (FSH)
    f.-s. hormone deficiency
    f.-s. hormone inhibin regulation
    f.-s. hormone secretion
follicular
    f. atresia
    f. cholecystitis
    f. cystitis
    f. fluid
    f. gastritis
    f. lymphoid hyperplasia
follicularis
    cystitis f.
    dyskeratosis f.
    keratosis f.
folliculi (*pl. of* folliculus)
folliculitis
folliculus, *pl.* **folliculi**
    f. lymphatica
    folliculi lymphatici aggregati
    folliculi lymphatici gastrici
    folliculi lymphatici recti
    folliculi lymphatici solitarii
    folliculi lymphatici solitarii intestini
      crassi
    folliculi lymphatici solitarii intestini
      tenuis
    folliculi lymphatici splenici
follitropin alfa for injection
Follmann balanitis
follower
    filiform and f. (F&F)
following bougie
followthrough
    small-bowel f. (SBFT)
follow-up (*var. of* followup)
followup, follow-up
    f. evaluation
    f. examination
    median f.
fomepizole
Fontana-Masson stain

food
    f. allergen
    f. allergy
    f. ball
    bland f.
    f. bolus
    f. bolus impaction
    f. bolus obstruction
    caffeine, alcohol, pepper, spicy f.'s
      (CAPS)
    f. chain
    f. challenge
    cholecystokinetic f.
    colonic f.
    compensated dysphagia for solid f.
    contamination of f.
    fatty f.
    fecal contamination of f.
    f. fever
    gas-producing f.
    Lactobacillus plantarum-fermented f.
    medical f.
    methionine-rich f.
    NutraPrep f.
    f. particle
    f. poisoning
    f. protein-induced enterocolitis
      syndrome (FPIES)
    f. residue
    sieving of solid f.
    solid f.
    f. supplement
foodborne illness (FBI)
FoodSCAN food allergy test
food-sensitive enteropathy
fool's parsley
foot
    f. pedal suction control
    f. process
foramen
    Duverney f.
    f. electrode
    epiploic f.
    f. epiploicum
    greater sciatic f.
    f. of Bochdalek
    f. of Bochdalek hernia
    f. of Morgagni
    f. of Winslow
    omental f.
    f. omentale
    pleuroperitoneal f.
Forbes disease
force
    electromagnetic f. (E, EMF)
    isometric f.
forced
    f. alimentation
    f. feeding

F

forceps

ACMI Martin endoscopy f.
Adair-Allis f.
Adson-Brown tissue f.
Adson tissue f.
Allen intestinal f.
alligator jaws Olympus grasping f.
alligator-type grasping f.
Allis f.
angled dissecting f.
3-armed basket f.
atraumatic locking/grasping f.
Babcock intestinal f.
Backhaus towel f.
Bainbridge intestinal f.
Ballenger f.
Bard Precisor direct bite f.
Barrett intestinal f.
Barrett-Murphy intestinal thumb f.
basket f.
basket-type crushing f.
bayonet-type f.
Beardsley intestinal f.
Beasley-Babcock f.
Beck aorta f.
Beebe hemostatic f.
Behrend cystic duct f.
Best gallstone f.
Bevan gallbladder f.
Billroth f.
biopsy f.
bipolar coagulating f.
bite biopsy f.
Blake gallstone f.
Blalock pulmonary artery f.
Blanchard hemorrhoid f.
bowel f.
Bozeman f.
Bridge deep surgery f.
Brunner intestinal f.
Brunner tissue f.
Buie biopsy f.
Buie pile f.
bulldog f.
Carmalt f.
Child intestinal f.
Children's Hospital intestinal f.
claw f.
coagulating f.
coated biopsy f.
cold biopsy f.
Collin-Duval intestinal thumb f.
Collin intestinal f.
Collin tissue f.
Collin tongue f.
Crile bile duct f.
Crile gall duct f.
curved dissecting f.
curved Maryland f.

Cushing f.
DeBakey f.
DeMartel appendix f.
Dennis intestinal f.
Desjardins gallbladder f.
Desjardins gallstone f.
disposable f.
dolphin grasping f.
dolphin-type atraumatic f.
double-spoon f.
Doyen gallbladder f.
Doyen intestinal f.
dressing f.
duck-bill f.
Duracep biopsy f.
Eastman cystic duct f.
electrocoagulating biopsy f.
Elliott gallbladder f.
Endo-Assist disposable atraumatic
  grasping f.
endoscopic alligator f.
endoscopic biopsy f.
endoscopic grasping f.
endoscopic suture-cutting f.
Everett pile f.
Excel disposable biopsy f.
FB-25K jumbo biopsy f.
fenestrated cup biopsy f.
fenestrated ellipsoid spiked
  open-span biopsy f.
fenestrated spiked open-span jumbo
  biopsy f.
Ferguson tenaculum f.
fine tissue f.
fine-toothed f.
FK-13K-1 jumbo biopsy f.
Foerster sponge f.
foreign body retrieving f.
Foss intestinal clamp f.
Fujinon biopsy f.
gallstone f.
Gavin-Miller intestinal f.
Gemini gall duct f.
Gerald f.
Gilbert cystic duct f.
Glassman-Allis intestinal f.
Glenn diverticulum f.
Gold deep surgery f.
grasping f.
grasp tripod f.
Gray cystic duct f.
Green cystic duct f.
Haberer intestinal f.
Halsted f.
Hamilton deep surgery f.
Harrington f.
Hasson bullet-tip f.
Hasson needle-nose f.
Hasson ring f.

Hasson spike-tooth f.
Healy intestinal f.
high-frequency hemostatic f.
hook f.
hot biopsy f.
hot flexible f.
Jarvis hemorrhoid f.
jeweler's f.
Johns Hopkins gallbladder f.
Judd-Allis intestinal f.
Judd-DeMartel gallbladder f.
Julian splenorenal f.
jumbo biopsy f.
Keen Edge disposable biopsy f.
Kelly f.
Kelly-Murphy f.
Kent deep surgery f.
Kleppinger f.
Kocher f.
Koerte gallstone f.
Lahey-Babcock f.
Lahey gall duct f.
Lalonde hook f.
lancet-shaped biopsy f.
Lane intestinal f.
Laplace f.
Lawrence deep surgery f.
Leonard deep surgery f.
Lillie intestinal f.
Lockwood-Allis intestinal f.
long-jaw disposable f.
loop-type snare f.
loop-type stone-crushing f.
Lovelace f.
Lower gall duct f.
Luer hemorrhoid f.
Maxum reusable f.
Mayo-Blake gallstone f.
Mayo-Péan f.
Mayo-Robson intestinal f.
Mazzariello-Caprini f.
McGill f.
McGivney hemorrhoid f.
McNealey-Glassman-Mixter f.
Medicon-Jackson rectal f.
Michigan intestinal f.
Microvasive disposable
  alligator-shaped f.
Microvasive radial-jaw large-capacity
  biopsy f.
Mikulicz peritoneal f.
Miller rectal f.
Millin f.
Mill-Rose RiteBite biopsy f.
Mixter gallstone f.
mosquito f.
Moynihan artery f.
Moynihan gall duct f.
Muir hemorrhoid f.

Multibite biopsy f.
Nelson f.
Nissen gall duct f.
no-scalpel vasectomy fixator ring
  clamp f.
Nussbaum intestinal f.
Ochsner f.
O'Hara f.
Olympus alligator-jaw endoscopic f.
Olympus basket-type endoscopic f.
Olympus endotherapy disposable
  biopsy f.
Olympus FB-20C endoscopic f.
Olympus FB-25K endoscopic f.
Olympus FB-24U biopsy f.
Olympus FG-12U wide-mouth f.
Olympus FK-13-1 biopsy f.
Olympus FS-K-series endoscopic
  suture-cutting f.
Olympus grasping rat-tooth f.
Olympus hot biopsy f.
Olympus magnetic extractor f.
Olympus minisnare f.
Olympus pelican-type endoscopic f.
Olympus rat-tooth endoscopic f.
Olympus reusable oval-cup f.
Olympus rubber-tip endoscopic f.
Olympus shark-tooth endoscopic f.
Olympus tripod-type endoscopic f.
Olympus W-shaped endoscopic f.
Ombrédanne f.
Orr gall duct f.
packing f.
Payr pyloric f.
Péan f.
pelican biopsy f.
Pennington f.
Percy intestinal f.
perforating f.
pinch f.
Porter duodenal f.
Positrap 3-prong nonretracting
  grasping f.
Potts f.
Potts-Smith f.
Precisor Direct Bite biopsy f.
Precisor disposable biopsy f.
3-pronged grasping f.
Quire mechanical finger f.
Radial Jaw hot biopsy f.
Radial Jaw III Max Capacity 1589
  biopsy f.
Radial Jaw III Max Capacity needle
  biopsy f.
Radial Jaw III single-use biopsy f.
Rampley sponge-holding f.
Randall stone f.
Ratliff-Blake gallstone f.
Ratliff-Mayo f.

F

forceps (*continued*)
  rat-tooth Olympus FG 8L grasping
    f.
  Reich-Nechtow f.
  f. removal
  ring f.
  RiteBite biopsy f.
  Robbers f.
  Robson intestinal f.
  Rochester-Carmalt f.
  Rochester gallstone f.
  Rochester-Mixter f.
  Rochester-Ochsner f.
  Rochester-Péan f.
  Rudd Clinic hemorrhoidal f.
  Russian tissue f.
  Schindler peritoneal f.
  Schnidt gall duct f.
  Schnidt thoracic f.
  Schoenberg intestinal f.
  Scudder intestinal f.
  Seitzinger tripolar cutting f.
  Semken tissue f.
  Shark disposable biopsy f.
  shark-tooth f.
  Singley intestinal f.
  smooth tissue f.
  SOLOS endoscopy clip-applying f.
  spiral gallstone f.
  sponge f.
  sponge-holding f.
  spoon f.
  Steinmann intestinal f.
  Stille-Barraya intestinal f.
  Stille gallstone f.
  stone-grasping f.
  stone-holding basket f.
  straight Maryland f.
  SureBite biopsy f.
  Therma Jaw disposable hot biopsy
    f.
  Therma Jaw hot urologic f.
  Thorek gallbladder f.
  Thorek-Mixter gallbladder f.
  tissue f.
  tonsil f.
  toothed tissue f.
  traumatic grasping f.
  tripod grasping f.
  Troutman rectus f.
  Turner-Warwick stone f.
  Turrell-Wittner rectal f.
  Varco gallbladder f.
  Westphal gall duct f.
  Williams intestinal f.
  W-shaped f.
  Yeoman rectal biopsy f.
  Yeoman-Wittner rectal f.
  Young intestinal f.

forcible feeding
Forder retractor
Fordyce
  angiokeratoma of F.
  F. granule
  F. spot
forearm
  f. blood flow
  f. flap
  f. graft arteriovenous fistula
Foregger rigid esophagoscope
foregut
foreign
  f. body
  f. body appendicitis
  f. body extraction
  f. body ingestion
  f. body management
  f. body reaction
  f. body removal
  f. body retrieving forceps
  f. body sensation
  f. body trauma
  f. object
foreshortening of colon
foreskin
  f. flap
  f. manual retraction
  f. restoration
Forest I, II lesion
forestomach
forgotten stent
fork
  stimulation f.
forked crypt
form
  band f.
  trophozoite f.
  wax-matrix slow-release f.
  WBC immature f.'s
Formad kidney
formaldehyde
  gelatin, resorcinol, f.
  f. solution
formalin
  buffered f.
  intravesical f.
formalin-fixed tissue
formamide
  deionized f.
formate
formation
  abscess f.
  adhesion f.
  bacterial biofilm f.
  beta-pleated sheet f.
  bile acid-independent bile f.
    (BAIBF)
  biofilm f.

bone f.
branching tubule f.
calculous f.
enamel pellicle f.
erythroid colony f.
extra-capillary crescent f.
false channel f.
fistula f.
gallstone f.
germinal center f.
Gothic arch f.
idiopathic calcium renal stone f.
indicator of reactive oxygen
  species f.
kerion f.
median bar f.
micelle f.
nurse cell f.
physicochemical basis of gallstone f.
prostanoid f.
prosthesis-related seroma f.
pseudoaneurysm f.
recurrent calcium stone f.
renal stone f.
scar tissue f.
stercoraceous f.
stone granuloma f.
struvite crystal f.
ultimate fistula f.
formatio reticularis
forme
  f. fruste
  f. tardive
formed stool
former
  calcium oxalate stone f.
  pouch f.
  stone f.
formigenes
  Oxalobacter f.
formin
formononetin
formula, *pl.* **formulas, formulae**
  Advance f.
  Attain tube-feeding f.
  Callaway f.
  Cockcroft-Gault f.
  F. EM oral suspension
  Encare tube-feeding f.
  Enfamil LIPIL f.
  Enfamil with iron f.
  Ensure HIN tube-feeding f.
  Ensure Plus f.
  Entralife HN tube-feeding f.
  Entri-Pak tube-feeding f.
  Entrition tube-feeding f.
  heartburn relief f. (HRF)
  hydrolyzed whey f.
  Isomil SF f.

I-Soyalac f.
Jevity tube-feeding f.
Lofenalac f.
Lonalac f.
Natural stool f.
Nursoy f.
Nutramigen f.
Portagen f.
predigested protein f.
Pregestimil f.
ProSobee liquid f.
RCF f.
Reabilan HN tube-feeding f.
Similac PM 60/40 low-iron f.
SMA f.
Soyalac f.
soy-based f.
F. 2 tube-feeding formula
Van Slyke f.
Vitaneed tube-feeding f.
formulae (*pl. of* formula)
formulas (*pl. of* formula)
Formulex
formyl peptide receptor
fornication
  fist f.
fornices (*pl. of* fornix)
fornix, *pl.* fornices
  calyceal f.
  gastric f.
Foroblique
  F. fiberoptic esophagoscope
  F. lens
  F. optic laparoscope
  F. resectoscope
Forrest
  F. classification
  F. classification of gastroduodenal
    ulcer
  F. criteria
Forssell sinus
FortaPerm surgical sling
Fortaz
Forte
  Citra F.
  Pamine F.
  Robinul F.
fortii
  Dinophysis f.
Fortison enteral feeding
fortuitum
  Mycobacterium f.
Fortuna syringe
Fortunoff flap
Forvia
forward
  f. motility protein of epididymal
    fluid
  f. optic laparoscope

F

forward-viewing
    f.-v. endoscope
    f.-v. position
    f.-v. telescope
    f.-v. videocolonoscope
foscarnet
    f. therapy
    f. treatment
fosfomycin tromethamine
fosinopril
Fosrenol
Foss
    F. anterior resection clamp
    F. bifid gallbladder retractor
    F. biliary duct retractor
    F. intestinal clamp
    F. intestinal clamp forceps
fossa, *pl.* **fossae**
    Biesiadecki f.
    Broesike f.
    f. caecalis
    crural f.
    duodenal f.
    duodenojejunal f.
    epigastric f.
    Gruber-Landzert f.
    Hartmann f.
    hypochondriac f.
    iliac f.
    inferior digital f.
    intrabulbar f.
    ischiorectal f.
    Jonnesco f.
    Landzert f.
    lateral f.
    f. navicularis urethrae
    f. of male urethra
    f. of Morgagni
    f. ovalis
    paravesical f.
    piriform f.
    prostatic f.
    rectal f.
    retrocolic f.
    f. subinguinalis
    subsigmoid f.
    Treitz f.
    f. vesicae biliaris
fossae (*pl. of* fossa)
fotemustine
Fothergill sign
Fouchet test
Fougera Vitamin A+D ointment
foul-smelling
    f.-s. odor
    f.-s. stool
foundation
    American Digestive Health F. (ADHF)
    American Liver F. (ALF)
    Gastro-Intestinal Research F.
    National Kidney F. (NKF)
    National Pancreas F.
    The Magic F.
Fourier
    F. transform analysis
    F. transform infrared spectroscopy
Fournier
    F. disease
    F. gangrene
    F. sign
    syphiloma of F.
fovea
    Morgagni f.
foveola, *pl.* **foveolae**
    gastric f.
    f. gastrica
foveolae (*pl. of* foveola)
foveola-gland ratio
foveolar
    f. gastric mucosa
    f. hyperplasia
foveolate
Fowler position
Fowler-Stephens
    F.-S. laparoscopic orchiopexy
    F.-S. spermatic vessel division procedure
    F.-S. spermatic vessel ligation maneuver
    F.-S. test
Foxy pouch cover
fp1
    ferroportin 1
FPC
    familial polyposis coli
FPIES
    food protein-induced enterocolitis syndrome
FPM
    first-pass metabolism
FPP
    familial paroxysmal polyserositis
fPSA
    free PSA
fraction
    alpha-gliadin f.
    anionic IgG 4 f.
    cortical interstitial volume f.
    filtered f.
    filtration f.
    gallbladder ejection f. (GBEF)
    globulin f.
    mesangial volume f.
    micronized flavonidic f.
    nonnuclear f.
    non-T-cell f.
    nuclear f.
    packing f.

plasma protein f.
recombination f.

fractional
f. clearance
f. excretion of lithium (FELI)
f. excretion of potassium (FEFEK)
f. excretion of sodium (FENa)
f. percentage of inspired oxygen (FIO$_2$)
f. proximal reabsorption
f. weight change

fractionated
f. diet
f. plasma separation and absorption (FPSA)
f. voiding

fractionation of bilirubin

fracture
pelvis f.
penis f.
trabecular bone f.

fragilis
Bacteroides f.
Dientamoeba f.

fragment
anucleate f.
autotransplantation of splenic f.
endoscopic removal of f.
N-terminal f.
nuclear f.
residual f.

fragmentary defecation

fragmentation
complete stone f.
laser-induced f.
stone f.
ultrasonic f.

Fragmin

Fraley
F. sign
F. syndrome

frame
nitinol mesh-covered f.
polyprotein open reading f. (PORF)
Stryker f.

frameshift

Framingham risk-factor approach

Francis test

Franco operation

frank
f. blood
f. blood in stool
f. cirrhosis
F. operation
f. pus

Frankel
crossbar symptom of F.

Frankfeldt rectal snare

Franklin-Silverman biopsy cannula

Franseen needle

Franz abdominal retractor

Fraser syndrome

Frazier
F. suction tip
F. suction tube

FreAmine amino acid solution

FRED
fog reduction/elimination device

FREDDY
frequency-doubled double pulse
FREDDY Nd:YAG laser

Frederick-Miller tube

frederiksenii
Yersinia f.

Fredet-Ramstedt
F.-R. operation
F.-R. pyloromyotomy

Fredrickson classification

free
f. acetate
f. air
f. band of colon
f. fatty acid
f. fecal bile acid
f. fluid
f. hepatic venous pressure (FHVP)
f. jejunal graft
f. prostate-specific antigen
f. PSA (fPSA)
f. radical
f. radical scavenger
f. reflux
f. resection
f. ribosome
f. subphrenic gas
symptom f.
f. testosterone
f. thyroxine (FT4)
f. tie

free-beam
f.-b. coagulation
f.-b. laser system

Freedom
F. Clear long-seal male external catheter line
F. Clear LS male external catheter line
F. Clear sport-sheath male external catheter line
F. Clear SS male external catheter line

free-floating testis

free-GEPA graft

freehand
f. biopsy
f. cannulation

freeing up of adhesions

Freeman pancreatic Flexi-Stent

F

Freer elevator
freestanding ambulatory surgical center
free-to-total
  f.-t.-t. prostate-specific antigen
    (FTPSA)
  f.-t.-t. PSA
  f.-t.-t. PSA ratio
freezing
  gastric f.
Freiburg biopsy set
fremitus
frena (*pl. of* frenum)
frenal
French
  F. bougie
  F. Cope loop nephrostomy catheter
  F. cystoscope
  F. dilator
  F. double-J ureteral stent
  F. introducer set
  F. mushroom-tip catheter
  F. Pharmacovigilance system
  F. pigtail nephrostomy catheter
  F. scale
  F. Swan-Ganz balloon
  F. tarragon
  F. Teflon pyeloureteral catheter
  F. T tube
French-eye needle
frenectomy
frenoplasty
Frenta
  F. Mat feeding pump
  F. System II feeding pump
frenula (*pl. of* frenulum)
frenulum, *pl.* **frenula**
  f. of duodenal papilla
  f. of ileocolic valve
  f. preputii penis
  f. valvae ileocecalis
frenum, *pl.* **frena**
  f. of Morgagni
  f. of valve of colon
frequency
  fecal f.
  f. of stool
  operating f.
  pulse repetition f. (PRF)
  urinary f.
frequency-doubled
  f.-d. double pulse (FREDDY)
  f.-d. double pulse ND:YAG laser
frequency-duration index (FDI)
frequency-urgency-pain syndrome
frequent
  f. hemodialysis
  f. joint manifestation
Fresenius
  F. AG dialyzer

F. filter
F. hemodialysis machine
F. volumetric dialysate balancing
  system
fresh
  f. clot
  f. frozen plasma (FFP)
Freter theory
Freund adjuvant
freundii
  Citrobacter f.
Frey
  F. gastric pit
  F. hair
Freyer operation
friability
  cervical f.
friable mucosa
friction-fit adapter
friction knot
Friderichsen-Waterhouse syndrome
Friedländer bacillus
Friedman perineal retractor
Frimberger-Karpiel 12 o'clock
  papillotome
fringe tree
Fritsch retractor
Froehlich (*var. of* Fröhlich)
frogleg position
frog-spawnlike mucosa
Fröhlich, Froehlich
  F. syndrome
frondlike filling defect
frontal tenderness
front-loading ultrasound probe
  (FLUP)
Frostberg reversed-3 sign
frothy
frozen section
fructose
  f. aldolase
  f. aldolase deficiency
  f. diarrhea
  f. diphosphatase deficiency
  f. intolerance
  seminal plasma f.
fructose-1,6-bisphosphatase
fructose-free diet
fruity odor
fruste
  forme f.
Frykman-Goldberg
  F.-G. operation for rectal prolapse
  F.-G. procedure
FSA
  fetal sulfoglycoprotein antigen
FSGS
  focal segmental glomerulosclerosis
  collapsing FSGS

FSH
follicle-stimulating hormone
FSP
fibrin split product
F60S polysulfone
FSSE
fat-suppressed spin-echo
FT4
free thyroxine
FTA-ABS
fluorescent treponemal antibody
absorption
fluorescent treponemal antibody
absorption test
FTA-ABS test
FTPSA
free-to-total prostate-specific antigen
5-FU
5-fluorouracil
fucosidosis
fucosylation index of alpha fetoprotein
fucosyltransferase gene
FUDR, FUdR
floxuridine
fluorodeoxyuridine
fugax
proctalgia f.
Fujinon
F. biopsy forceps
F. bronchoscope
F. CEG-FP-series videoelectroscope
F. DUO-XT duodenoscope
F. EC7-CM2 videocolonoscope
F. EC-130LT colonoscope
F. EC-200LT colonoscope
F. EC-410MP colonoscope
F. EC-300MS colonoscope
F. ED7-XT duodenoscope
F. ED7-XU2 videoduodenoscope
F. ED-200XU duodenoscope
F. ED-310XU duodenoscope
F. ED-410XU duodenoscope
F. EG-310D gastroscope
F. EG-200FP gastroscope
F. EG-FP-series endoscope
F. EG-410HR gastroscope
F. ES-200ER sigmoidoscope
F. EVC-M videocolonoscope
F. EVD-XL videoduodenoscope
F. EVD-XT duodenoscope
F. EVE-series endoscope
F. EVG-CT endoscope
F. EVG-FP-series endoscope
F. EVG-F-series endoscope
F. FD-100XU duodenoscope
F. FE-100LR colonoscope
F. FG-series endoscopic camera
F. FP-series endoscope

F. FS-100ER sigmoidoscope
F. GF-100PE gastroscope
F. PRO-PC flexible fiberoptic
sigmoidoscope
F. 400-series super image
videogastroscope
F. SIG-E2 fiberoptic
sigmoidoscope
F. SIG-EK-series flexible fiberoptic
sigmoidoscope
F. SIG-E-series flexible fiberoptic
sigmoidoscope
F. SIG-ET-series flexible fiberoptic
sigmoidoscope
F. SP-501 sonoprobe system
F. UGI-FP-series videoendoscope
F. videoendoscopy cart
F. videoendoscopy system
F. 310XU videoduodenoscope
FUL
functional urethral length
fulguration
direct f.
diverticulum f.
electrosurgical f.
endoscopic f.
indirect f.
full
f. extension
f. liquid diet
f. liquids
f. Monti procedure
f. Monti technique
full-bladder technique
full-column barium enema
Fuller
F. operation
F. rectal shield
full-length viral genome
full-lumen esophagoscope
fullness
abdominal f.
adnexal f.
postprandial f.
pyloric f.
full-surface micromesh teeth
full-thickness
f.-t. biopsy
f.-t. graft
f.-t. local excision
fulminant
f. Crohn disease
f. dysentery
f. hepatic failure (FHF)
f. hepatitis A–E
f. hepatocellular failure
f. liver failure
f. toxic colitis
f. viral hepatitis (FVH)

F

fulminating
  f. appendicitis
  f. dysentery
  f. pancreatitis
  f. ulcerative colitis
fumagillin
fumarylacetoacetate hydrolase deficiency
fumigatus
  Aspergillus f.
FUMIR
  5-fluorouracil, mitomycin C radiation
fumitory
function
  anal sphincter f.
  bladder neck sphincteric f.
  bladder storage f.
  bowel f.
  cardiopulmonary baroreflex f.
  Carnot f.
  cineloop memory f.
  cognitive f.
  delayed graft f.
  deterioration of graft f.
  discriminant f.
  excretory f.
  exocrine f.
  gallbladder f.
  gastrin cell f.
  graft f.
  impaired colonic motor f.
  International Index of Erectile F.
    (IIEF)
  kidney f.
  Leydig cell secretory f.
  Maddrey discriminant f.
  native kidney f.
  neoanal f.
  organ f.
  P450 f.
  pharyngoesophageal f.
  preoperative f.
  proximal tubule f.
  PTEN suppressor gene f.
  puborectalis muscle f.
  pudendal nerve f.
  rectoanal f.
  rectosigmoid f.
  renal f.
  Sertoli cell secretory f.
  sexual f.
  sieving f.
  sphincter f.
  splenic f.
  split renal f.
functional
  f. bladder capacity
  f. bleeding
  f. bowel disease
  f. bowel disorder (FBD)

F. Bowel Disorder Severity Index
  (FBDSI)
  f. bowel distress (FBD)
  f. bowel syndrome
  f. castration
  f. constipation
  f. cystic duct obstruction
  f. diarrhea
  f. disorder of stomach
  f. dyspepsia
  f. esophageal disorder (FED)
  f. gastrointestinal disorder (FGID)
  f. hepatic volume
  f. impotence
  f. incontinence
  f. magnetic resonance imaging
    (fMRI, f-MRI)
  f. pain
  f. plasminogen
  f. profile length
  f. reconstruction
  f. trauma
  f. urethral length (FUL)
Fund
  American Kidney F.
fundal
  f. gastritis
  f. plication
  f. pouch
  f. varix
fundectomy
fundi (*pl. of* fundus)
fundic
  f. atrophic gastritis (FAG)
  f. biopsy
  f. clot
  f. gland atrophy
  f. gland gastritis
  f. gland heterotopia
  f. gland polyp
  f. mucosa
  f. plexus
  f. varix
fundic-antral junction
fundiform ligament
fundoplasty
  Gomez f.
  Thal f.
fundoplication
  anatomically correct f.
  Belsey Mark IV f.
  Belsey partial f.
  Belsey 2/3 wrap f.
  circumferential f.
  Collis-Nissen f.
  Dor f.
  floppy Nissen f.
  Hill esophageal f.
  intrathoracic Nissen f.

laparoscopic Nissen and Toupet f.
Nissen laparoscopic f.
partial f.
Rossetti modification of Nissen f.
slipped Nissen f.
supraphysiologic f.
Toupet partial posterior f.
fundopyloric mucosal border
fundus, *pl.* **fundi**
bald gastric f.
folded f.
gallbladder f.
gastric f.
f. gastricus
f. of stomach
f. rotation gastroplasty
f. ventricularis
f. ventriculi
f. vesicae biliaris
f. vesicae felleae
f. vesicae urinariae
fundusectomy
fungal
f. ball
f. bezoar
f. infection
f. liver abscess
f. peritonitis
f. pyelonephritis
f. spore
fungating growth
fungemia
fungi (*pl. of* fungus)
Fungi-Fluor
F.-F. chitin stain
F.-F. procedure
fungiform papilla
Fungizone
fungoides
mycosis f.
fungosa
gastrosia f.
funguria
fungus, *pl.* **fungi**
ovoid f.
f. testis
funicular
f. hydrocele
f. inguinal hernia
f. stump
funiculi (*pl. of* funiculus)
funiculitis
funiculoepididymitis
filarial f.
funiculopexy

funiculus, *pl.* **funiculi**
hepatic f.
f. spermaticus
funis
funisitis
funnel
stent f.
funnel-neck prostate
Furacin
Furadantin
fura-2 pentapotassium salt
furazolidone
Furlow
F. cylinder inserter
F. introducer
**Furlow-Fisher modification of Virag 1
erectile failure microsurgical operation**
Furniss
F. anastomosis clamp
F. ureterointestinal anastomosis
Furniss-Clute duodenal clamp
furnissii
Vibrio f.
furor medicus
furosemide washout renogram
Furoxone
furrier suture
furrow
Liebermeister f.
furuncle
furunculosis
Fusarium solani
fused kidney
fusible calculus
fusiform
f. renal artery aneurysm
f. widening of duct
fusion
f. fascia
splenogonadal f.
tissue f.
urethrohymenal f.
viral membrane f.
Fusobacterium
Futura resectoscope sheath
**future role of target of rapamycin
inhibitors in renal transplantation**
FVH
fulminant viral hepatitis
FVM
familial visceral myopathy
FVN
familial visceral neuropathy
Fx1A antibody
fyn protein

F

G
G protein
G protein disease
G syndrome
G tube

G1
immunoglobulin G1 (IgG1)

G4
immunoglobulin G4 (IgG4)

G2a
immunoglobulin G2a (IgG2a)

GABA
gamma-aminobutyric acid

gabapentin
gabexate mesylate
Gabriel proctoscope
gadolinium
g. chelate
g. EOB-DTPA (Gd-EOB-DTPA)
g. EOB-DTPA contrast agent

gadolinium-enhancement magnetic resonance
Gadolite oral suspension
GAG
glycosaminoglycan

gag
Millard mouth g.
mouth g.
g. reflex
g. response

GAGUA
glycosaminoglycan uronate

gain
interdialytic weight g. (IDWG)
symptomatic fluid g.
weight g.

galactitol
Galacto-Light assay
galactoma
galactopexy
galactose
beta g.
g. elimination capacity (GEC)

galactose-free diet
galactosemia
Indiana variant g.
Rennes variant g.

galactose-1 — phosphate uridyltransferase
galactosidase
beta g.

galactosyltransferase isoenzyme II
galacturia
galanga (*var. of* galangal)
galangal, galanga
lesser g.

galanin antiserum
Galant reflex
Galeati gland
galeni
porus g.

galenic preparation
GALF
glycyrrhetinic acidlike factor

gall
g. duct
g. duct spoon

gallamine
gallbladder (GB)
adenomyoma of g.
g. adenomyomatosis
g. bag positioner
g. bed
bilobed g.
g. calculus
g. carcinoma
chronically inflamed g.
g. contraction
Courvoisier g.
dilated g.
g. displacement
g. dome
double g.
duplicated g.
g. dysmotility
edematous g.
g. ejection fraction (GBEF)
g. ejection rate (GBER)
g. emptying-refilling curve
empyema of g.
endoscopic transpapillary
   catheterization of g. (ETCG)
g. filling
fish-scale g.
floating g.
g. function
g. function test
g. fundus
gangrene of g.
hourglass constriction of g.
g. hydrops
g. ileus
inflamed g.
infundibulum of g.
g. lift
mobile g.
mucocele of g.
multiseptate g.
nonfunctioning g.
nonvisualization of g.
notch of g.

G

gallbladder (*continued*)
    palpable g.
    perforation of g.
    porcelain g.
    robin's egg-blue g.
    g. scan
    g. scoop
    g. series (GBS)
    g. sludge
    g. stasis
    stasis g.
    g. stone
    strawberry g.
    thick-walled g.
    thin-walled g.
    g. torsion
    torsion of g.
    g. trauma
    trauma of g.
    g. trocar
    g. varix
    g. volume
    g. wall
    g. wall abscess
    wandering g.
Gallie transplant
gallinaginis
    caput g.
gallium
    g. imaging
    g. nitrate
    g. scan
gallium-67
gallop rhythm
Galloway-Mowat syndrome
gallows-type retractor
gallstone
    asymptomatic g.
    bilirubin pigment g.
    black pigment g.
    brown pigment g.
    calcified g.
    cholesterol-containing g.
    g. colic
    dissolution of g.
    faceted g.
    floating g.
    g. forceps
    g. formation
    g. ileus
    g. incidence
    innocent g.
    intragastric g.
    g. migration
    mixed cholesterol g.
    mulberry g.
    g. pancreatitis
    g. pattern
    pigmented g.

    g. probe
    radiolucent g.
    retained g.
    silent g.
    g. solubilizing agent
    symptomatic g.
    unextractable g.
Gal 4 protein
GALT
    gastrointestinal-associated lymphoid
      tissue
    gut-associated lymphoepithelial tissue
    gut-associated lymphoid tissue
galvanic probe
Gambee
    G. anastomosis
    G. stitch
    G. suture
Gambian sleeping sickness
Gambro
    G. dialyzer
    G. filter
    G. Lundia Minor artificial kidney
    G. machine
gamete
    g. intrafallopian transfer (GIFT)
    g. micromanipulation
gametic
gametocidal
gametocide
gametocyst
gamma
    basal interferon g.
    g. camera discriminator
    g. emission
    g. fetoprotein
    g. globulin (GG)
    g. globulin therapy
    g. glutamyltransferase (GGT)
    g. glutamyltransferase level
    g. glutamyl transpeptidase (GGTP)
    g. heavy-chain disease
    HLA class II-restricted interferon g.
    g. interferon
    interferon g. (IFN-G)
    g. light chain
    g. lyase
    nucleocapsid antigen-stimulated
      interferon g.
    g. scintillation camera
    g. seminoprotein
    g. split-sling wrap
    g. transverse colon loop
gamma-aminobutyric
    g.-a. acid (GABA)
    g.-a. acid accumulation
    g.-a. acidergic neuron
gammaglobulin
    antithymocyte g. (ATGAM)

gamma-glutamyltransferase
  serum g.-g. (SGGT)
Gammatone II gamma camera
gammopathy
  monoclonal g.
Gamna
  G. disease
  G. nodule
Ganau criteria
ganciclovir
Gandy-Gamna nodule
ganglia (*pl. of* ganglion)
ganglial
ganglion, *pl.* **ganglia, ganglions**
  basal ganglia
  celiac-superior mesenteric ganglia
  g. cell loss
  dorsal root g.
  enteric g.
  intramural g.
  nodose g.
  subserous g.
  Troisier g.
ganglionated plexus
ganglioneuroblastoma
ganglioneuroma
  adrenal cortex g.
ganglioneuromatosis
ganglion-free muscle strip
ganglions (*pl. of* ganglion)
ganglioside
  GM3 g.
gangraenosa
  balanitis g.
gangrene
  cecal g.
  Fournier g.
  gas g.
  ischemic penile g.
  g. of gallbladder
gangrenosum
  ecthyma g.
  pyoderma g.
gangrenous
  g. appendicitis
  g. appendix
  g. balanitis
  g. bowel
  g. cholecystitis
  g. colon
  g. cystitis
  g. ischemic colitis
  g. ischemic enterocolitis
  g. necrosis
GAN-19 needle
Gans
  incisura dextra of G.
Ganser diverticulum
Gant clamp

Gantrisin
gantry
GAP
  glans approximation procedure
  GTPase-activating protein
  GAP test
gap
  anion g.
  glottic g.
  g. junction
  osmolarity g.
  stool osmotic g.
  underwater spark g.
  urinary anion g.
GAPD, GAPDH
  glyceraldehyde phosphate
    dehydrogenase
  glyceraldehyde-3-phosphate
    dehydrogenase
Garamycin
GARD
  gastroesophageal antireflux device
garden
  g. cress
  G. prognostic system
Gardner-Diamond syndrome
Gardnerella vaginalis
Gardner syndrome
gargle
  viscous Xylocaine g.
garlic
  bear's g.
Garren
  G. balloon
  G. gastric bubble
Garren-Edwards
  G.-E. balloon
  G.-E. gastric (GEG)
  G.-E. gastric bubble
Garrett dilator
Gartner
  G. duct
  G. duct cyst
gas
  g. abscess
  arterial blood g. (ABG)
  bowel g.
  g. chromatography
  g. chromatography/mass spectroscopy
    (GC/MS)
  colonic g.
  g. cupula
  g. cyst
  g. cystometry
  g. density line
  ETO g.
  free subphrenic g.
  g. gangrene
  hydrogen g.

G

gas (*continued*)
    g. isotope ratio mass spectrometry
    g. metabolism
    g. pattern
    g. sterilization
    g. thermometer
GaSampler collection system
GasBGon filter seat cushion
gas-bloat syndrome
gaseous
    g. cholecystitis
    g. distention
    g. pericholecystitis
gas-forming
    g.-f. liver abscess
    g.-f. organism in bowel wall
    g.-f. pyogenic liver infection
gasket
    United Surgical Seal-Tite g.
gasless
    g. laparoscopic approach
    g. laparoscopy
GASP
    gastric augment and single-pedicle
    GASP tube
gas-producing food
gasserian syndrome
Gasser syndrome
gassiness
gassy
gaster
gastradenitis, gastroadenitis
gastralgia
gastrectasia (*var. of* gastrectasis)
gastrectasis, gastrectasia
gastrectomized patient
gastrectomy
    antecolic g.
    Billroth I, II g.
    completion g.
    distal g.
    esophagoproximal g.
    high subtotal g.
    Horsley g.
    partial g.
    physiologic g.
    Pólya g.
    proximal g.
    subtotal g.
    total g.
gastric, gastricus
    g. accommodation test
    g. achlorhydria
    g. acid
    g. acidity
    g. acidity reduction
    g. acid pump inhibitor
    g. acid rebound
    g. acid secretion

    g. actinomycosis
    g. adenocarcinoma
    g. adenoma
    g. adenopapillomatosis
    g. air bubble
    g. analysis
    g. aneurysm
    g. angiodysplasia
    g. angioma
    g. angiomyolipoma
    g. anisakiasis
    g. anoxia
    g. antral erosion
    g. antral sessile polyp
    g. antral vascular ectasia (GAVE)
    g. antrum
    g. arteriography
    g. arteriovenous malformation
    g. artery
    g. aspirate
    g. aspiration
    g. aspiration tube
    g. atony
    g. atresia
    g. augment and single-pedicle (GASP)
    g. augment and single-pedicle tube
    g. bacterial overgrowth (GBO)
    g. balloon
    g. balloon implantation
    g. barostat
    g. bezoar
    g. bladder
    g. bladder replacement
    g. bleeding time (GBT)
    g. brush cytology
    g. bypass (GBP)
    g. bypass surgery (GBS)
    g. calculus
    g. cancer
    g. capacity
    g. carcinoid
    g. carcinoid tumor
    g. carcinoma
    g. carcinosarcoma
    g. cardia
    g. carditis
    g. cell kinetics
    g. channel
    g. chloroma
    g. chromoscopy
    g. coin removal
    g. colic
    g. compression
    g. contents
    g. crisis
    g. cycle
    g. cystic duplication
    g. decompression

g. diet
g. dilation
g. distention
g. diverticulosis
g. duplication cyst
g. dysfunction
g. dyspepsia
g. effect
g. electrical dysrhythmia
g. electrical stimulation
g. emptying
g. emptying breath test (GEBT)
g. emptying delay
g. emptying half-time (GET1/2)
g. emptying scan
g. emptying scintigraphy
g. emptying time (GET)
g. epithelial cell infiltration
g. epithelial cell replication
g. feeding
g. first-pass metabolism (GFPM)
g. fistula
g. fold
g. foreign body
g. fornix
g. foveola
g. foveolar epithelium
g. freezing
g. function test
g. fundus
g. fundus wrap
Garren-Edwards g. (GEG)
g. gland
g. hemorrhage
g. heterotopia
g. hyperacidity
g. hyperemia
g. hyperplastic polyp
g. hypersecretion
g. hypochlorhydria
g. hypomotility
g. hypothermia
g. hypothermia machine
g. ileus
g. impression
g. impression on liver
g. indigestion
g. inflammatory fibroid polyp
g. inhibitor factor
g. inhibitory peptide (GIP)
g. inhibitory polypeptide (GIP)
g. insufficiency
g. intestinal metaplasia
g. juice
g. juice ammonia assay
g. Kaposi sarcoma
g. laryngeal mask airway (GLMA)
g. lavage
g. lavage tube

g. leiomyoma
g. leiomyosarcoma
g. lesion
g. lipoma
g. luminal pH
g. lymphoma
g. malaria
g. mass
g. mechanosensory threshold
g. metaplasia of duodenum
g. microenvironment
g. motility disorder
g. mucormycosis
g. mucosal atrophy
g. mucosal barrier (GMB)
g. mucosal blood flow (GMBF)
g. mucosal damage
g. mucosal degradation
g. mucosal disease
g. mucosal ectopia
g. mucosal ectopia in rectum
(GMER)
g. mucosal erosion
g. mucosal injury
g. mucosal laminin receptor
g. mucosal pattern classification
g. mucosal prolapse
g. mucus
g. muscularis mucosa
g. mycosis
g. myoelectrical activity
g. neobladder
g. neobladder procedure
g. neurasthenia
g. neurectomy
g. notch
g. omentum
g. outlet
g. outlet obstruction (GOO)
g. outline
g. oxyntic cell receptor
g. pacemaker cell
g. pacemaker region
g. parietography
g. partition
g. peptide TFF1, TFF2
g. perforation
g. petechia
g. pH monitor
g. pigment
g. pit
g. pitting
g. plasma
g. plasmacytoma
g. plexus
g. pneumocystosis
g. polypectomy
g. polyposis
g. pool

G

315

gastric (*continued*)
g. pouch
g. pseudolymphoma
g. red spot
g. remnant
g. resection
g. residuum
g. retention
g. rupture
g. sclerosis
g. secretory test
g. sedative
g. serosa
g. stapling
g. stasis
g. stump
g. syphilis
g. tear
g. teratoma
g. tetany
g. tone
g. transit time
g. transposition
g. trauma
g. tuberculosis
g. ulcer
g. ulceration
g. urease activity
g. variceal ligation
g. varix
g. varix bleeding
g. vascular ectasia (GVE)
g. vein
g. venacaval shunt
g. vertigo
g. volume
g. volvulus
g. window
g. xanthoma
g. xanthomatosis
gastrica
achylia g.
adenasthenia g.
area g.
foveola g.
myasthenia g.
myxorrhea g.
ruga g.
gastrici
folliculi lymphatici g.
gastric-type surface epithelium
gastricum
corpus g.
gastricus (*var. of* gastric)
fundus g.
liquor g.
status g.
succus g.
Gastrimmune

gastrin
antral g.
basic g.
g. cell
g. cell function
g. cell hyperfunction
fasting serum g.
g. gene
g. mRNA
g. mRNA:G-cell density
g. mRNA level
g. mRNA species
g. receptor
G. RIA kit II
serum g.
g. stain
g. stimulation test
gastrin-17
gastrinoma
duodenal g.
g. triangle
gastrin-releasing
g.-r. peptide (GRP)
g.-r. peptide/bombesin
gastrin-secreting
g.-s. cell
g.-s. nonbeta islet cell tumor
gastritis
active chronic g.
acute erosive g. (AEG)
acute hemorrhagic g.
alcoholic hemorrhagic g.
alkaline reflux g. (ARG)
antral g.
antral atrophic g. (AAG)
antral-predominant g.
aspirin-induced g.
atrophic g.
autoimmune metaplastic atrophic g. (AMAG)
bile reflux g.
bleeding g.
Campylobacter pyloridis g.
catarrhal g.
chemical g.
chronic active g.
chronic atrophic g. (CAG)
chronic cystic g.
chronic erosive g. (CEG)
chronic follicular g.
chronic interstitial g.
chronic nonimmune g.
chronic superficial g. (CSG)
cirrhotic g.
corpus g.
corrosive g.
g. cystica polyposa
g. cystic profunda
diffuse antral g. (DAG)

diffuse varioliform g.
drug-induced g.
emphysematous g.
endoscopic atrophic g.
endoscopic enterogastric reflux g.
endoscopic erythematous/exudative g.
endoscopic hemorrhagic g.
endoscopic raised erosive g.
endoscopic rugal hyperplastic g.
environmental metaplastic atrophic g.
  (EMAG)
eosinophilic g.
erosive g.
erosive-hemorrhagic g.
exfoliative g.
follicular g.
fundal g.
fundic atrophic g. (FAG)
fundic gland g.
giant hypertrophic g.
g. granulomatosa fibroplastica
granulomatous g.
Helicobacter pylori-induced g.
hemorrhagic g.
histologic chronic active g.
hyperpeptic g.
hypertrophic lymphocytic g.
  (HLG)
idiopathic chronic erosive g.
interstitial g.
isolated granulomatous g.
lymphocytic g. (LG)
metaplastic atrophic g.
multifocal atrophic g. (MAG)
mycotic g.
nonautoimmune fundic atrophic g.
nonerosive nonspecific g.
nonspecific erosive g.
oxyntic mucosal g.
phlegmonous g.
polypous g.
postgastrectomy g.
postoperative g.
proliferative hypertrophic g.
pseudomembranous g.
purulent g.
radiation g.
reflux bile g.
severe g.
specific g.
stress g.
superficial g.
suppurative g.
Sydney classification of g.
syphilitic g.
toxic g.
tuberculous g.
type A, B antral g.
ulcerative g.

uremic g.
varioliform g.
g. varioliformis
verrucous g.
viral g.
zonal g.
**gastritis-associated peptic ulcer
  disease**
gastroadenitis (*var. of* gastradenitis)
gastroadynamic
gastroalbumorrhea
gastroanastomosis
gastroatonia
gastroblennorrhea
gastrocamera
  Olympus GTF-A g.
gastrocardiac syndrome
Gastroccult test
gastrocele
gastrochronorrhea
gastrocolic
  g. fistula
  g. ligament
  g. omentum
  g. reflex
gastrocolitis
gastrocolostomy
gastrocutaneous
  g. fistula
  g. fistula tract
gastrocystoplasty
gastrodiaphanoscopy
gastrodiaphany
gastroduodenal
  g. angiodysplasia
  g. artery (GDA)
  g. artery complex
  g. carcinoid
  g. Crohn disease
  g. double ulcer
  g. dyspepsia
  g. fistula
  g. hypertrophy
  g. lumen
  g. misperfusion
  g. mucosa
  g. mucosal injury
  g. mucosal protection
  g. outflow obstruction (GOO)
gastroduodenal-to-renal
  g.-t.-r. artery bypass
  g.-t.-r. artery bypass graft
gastroduodenectomy
gastroduodenitis
  neutrophilic g.
gastroduodenoenterostomy
gastroduodenopancreatectomy
gastroduodenoscopy
  Billroth g.

G

gastroduodenostomy
    Billroth I g.
    Jaboulay g.
gastrodynia
gastroenteralgia
gastroenteric fistula
gastroenteritis
    acute g. (AGE)
    acute infectious nonbacterial g.
    astrovirus g.
    Calicivirus g.
    Coronavirus g.
    endemic nonbacterial
      infantile g.
    eosinophilic g. (EGE)
    epidemic nonbacterial g.
    infantile g.
    infectious g.
    nonbacterial g.
    Norwalk g.
    rotavirus g.
    viral g. (VGE)
    winter g.
gastroenteroanastomosis
gastroenterocolitis
gastroenterocolostomy
gastroenterologic
gastroenterologist
gastroenterology (GE)
    American College of G.
      (ACG)
gastroenteropancreatic (GEP)
    g. tumor
gastroenteropathy
    g. detection
    eosinophilic g.
    protein-losing g.
gastroenteroplasty
gastroenteroptosis
gastroenterostomy (GE)
    Balfour g.
    Billroth g. type I, II
    Braun-Jaboulay g.
    Courvoisier g.
    Finney g.
    Heineke-Mikulicz g.
    Hill esophageal g.
    Hofmeister g.
    percutaneous g. (PGE)
    Pólya g.
    Roux-en-Y g.
    Schoemaker g.
    truncal vagotomy and g.
gastroenterotomy
gastroepiploic
    g. arcade
    g. artery (GEA, GEPA)
    g. artery graft (GEA graft)
    g. blood vessel

gastroesophageal (GE)
    g. antireflux device (GARD)
    g. flap valve
    g. hernia
    g. incompetence
    g. junction (GEJ)
    g. reflux (GER)
    g. reflux disease (GERD)
    g. reflux scan
    g. scintigraphy
    g. scintiscan
    g. sphincter
    g. variceal plexus
    g. varix type 1, 2
gastroesophagitis
gastroesophagostomy
    cervical g.
gastrogastrostomy
gastrogavage
gastrogenic diarrhea
gastrogenous diarrhea
Gastrografin
    G. contrast medium
    G. enema
    G. GI series
    G. swallow
GastrograpH
    G. ambulatory pH monitoring
    system
    G. Mark III pH analyzer
gastrohepatic
    g. bare area
    g. ligament
    g. omentum
gastrohydrorrhea
gastroileac, gastroileal
    g. augmentation
    g. reflex
gastroileal (*var. of* gastroileac)
gastroileitis
gastroileostomy
gastrointestinal (GI)
    g. absorption
    g. allergy
    g. assistant (GIA)
    g. autonomic nerve tumor
    g. biota
    g. bleed
    g. bleeding (GIB)
    g. blood loss test
    g. cancer
    g. cancer-associated antigen (GICA)
    g. complication
    g. cross
    g. endoscopy
    g. endothelium
    g. eosinophilic granuloma
    g. fiberscope
    g. fistula

g. fungal ball
g. hamartomatous polyp
g. histoplasmosis
g. immunodeficiency syndrome
g. intubation
g. Kaposi sarcoma
g. lavage
g. lesion
g. lipoma
g. motility
g. myenteric plexus
g. needle
g. neuroendocrinology
g. neurofibroma
g. peptide hormone
g. polyposis (GIP)
g. reflux
g. regularity peptide
g. smooth muscle
g. stoma
g. stromal tumor (GIST)
G. Symptom Rating Scale (GSRS)
g. system (GIS)
g. telangiectasia
g. therapeutic system (GITS)
g. tract (GIT)
g. tract hemorrhage
g. transit
G. Tumor Study Group (GITSG, GTSG)
upper g. (UGI)
gastrointestinal-associated lymphoid tissue (GALT)
gastrointestinalis
mycetism g.
pseudoleukemia g.
Gastro-Intestinal Research Foundation
gastrojejunal
g. constipation
g. loop obstruction syndrome
gastrojejunocolic fistula
gastrojejunostomy
antecolic long-loop isoperistaltic g.
Billroth g. type I, II
compression button g.
Hofmeister-Shoemaker g.
loop g.
percutaneous endoscopic g. (PEG-J)
gastrokinesograph
gastrokinetic agent
gastrolavage
gastrolienal ligament
gastrolith
gastrolithiasis
gastrologist
gastrology
gastrolysis
Gastrolyte oral solution

gastromalacia
GastroMark
gastromegaly
gastromotor insufficiency
gastromycosis
gastromyotomy
gastromyxorrhea
gastronesteostomy
gastropancreatic
g. fold
g. ligament
g. reflex
gastropancreatitis
GastroPanel assay kit
gastroparalysis
gastroparesis
diabetic g.
g. diabeticorum
idiopathic g.
nondiabetic g.
postvagotomy g.
transient g.
gastroparietal
gastropathic
gastropathy
aphthous g.
benign hyperplastic g.
cardiofundic g.
chemical g.
congestive hypertensive g.
diabetic g.
erosive g.
erythematous g.
hemorrhagic g.
hypertensive g.
hypertrophic hypersecretory g. (HHG)
idiopathic hypertrophic g.
nonsteroidal antiinflammatory drug g.
NSAID g.
papulous g.
portal hypertensive g. (PHG)
prolapse g.
protein-losing g.
varioliform g.
gastroperiodynia
gastroperitonitis
gastropexy
Boerema anterior g.
Hill posterior g.
Horsley g.
gastrophotography
gastrophrenic ligament
gastrophthisis
gastroplasty
Collis g.
Collis-Nissen g.
Eckhout vertical g.

G

gastroplasty (*continued*)
endoluminal g.
fundus rotation g.
Gomez horizontal g.
greater curvature banded g.
horizontal g.
Laws g.
Mason vertical banded g.
silastic ring vertical g.
silicone elastomer ring vertical g.
(SRVG)
Stamm g.
tubular vertical g.
unbanded g.
vertical banded g. (VBG)
vertical ring g. (VRG)
vertical silastic ring g.
gastroplegia
gastroplication
endoluminal g. (ELG)
Gastro-Port II feeding device
gastroprokinetic
gastroprotection
adaptive g.
gastroprotective
gastroptosia (*var. of* gastroptosis)
gastroptosis, gastroptosia
gastropylorectomy
gastropyloric
**Gastroreflex ambulatory pH
monitor/recorder**
gastrorenal shunt
gastrorrhagia
gastrorrhaphy
gastrorrhea continua chronica
gastrorrhexis
gastroschisis
silastic silo reduction of g.
gastroscope
ACMI g.
Benedict g.
Bernstein g.
Cameron omniangle g.
Chevalier Jackson g.
disposable-sheath flexible g.
Eder g.
Eder-Bernstein g.
Eder-Chamberlin g.
Eder-Hufford g.
Eder-Palmer semiflexible g.
Ellsner g.
end-viewing g.
Ewald g.
FCS-ML II g.
FGS-ML II g.
fiberoptic g.
flexible g.
Fujinon EG-310D g.
Fujinon EG-200FP g.

Fujinon EG-410HR g.
Fujinon GF-100PE g.
Herman-Taylor g.
Hirschowitz g.
Housset-Debray g.
Janeway g.
Jenning-Streifeneder g.
Kelling g.
Krentz g.
Mancke flex-rigid g.
Mikulicz g.
Olympus GFT g.
Olympus GIF-K-series g.
Olympus GIFxP10 g.
Olympus GIF-XQ30 flexible g.
Olympus 2T-2000 twin-channel
therapeutic g.
Olympus XQ230 g.
pediatric g.
Pentax EUP-EC124
ultrasound g.
peroral g.
Q200 g.
Schindler semiflexible g.
Sielaff g.
Taylor g.
Tomenius g.
Universal g.
Wolf-Henning g.
Wolf-Knittlingen g.
Wolf-Schindler semiflexible g.
gastroscopic
gastroscopy
cap-fitted g.
high-magnification g.
infrared transillumination g.
Gastrosed
gastrosia fungosa
gastrosis
**GastroSoft data reduction and
prognostic software package**
gastrospasm
Gastrospirillum hominis
gastrosplenic
g. ligament
g. omentum
gastrostaxis
gastrostenosis
gastrostogavage
gastrostolavage
gastrostomy
Beck g.
Beck-Jianu g.
g. bumper
g. button
button g.
CT-guided percutaneous endoscopic
g.
DePage-Janeway g.

dual percutaneous endoscopic g.
  (DPEG)
endoscopic ultrasound-guided
  pancreatic g.
g. feeding
feeding g.
Glassman g.
Janeway g.
jejunal tube through percutaneous
  endoscopic g. (JETPEG)
Kader g.
Martin g.
Olympus g.
percutaneous g.
percutaneous endoscopic g.
  (PEG)
plug g.
Russell percutaneous endoscopic g.
g. scarring
Ssabanejew-Frank g.
Stamm g.
Surgitek One-Step percutaneous
  endoscopic g.
g. tube (G-tube)
g. tube migration
ultrasound-assisted percutaneous
  endoscopic g.
venting percutaneous g.
  (VPG)
Witzel g.
gastrosuccorrhea
  digestive g.
  g. mucosa
gastrotome
gastrotomy
gastrotonometer
gastrotonometry
gastrotoxic
gastrotoxin
gastrotropic
Gastrovist contrast medium
gastroxia
Gastrozepine
Gas-X
gate
  sampling g.
gatekeeper
  g. gene
  G. reflux repair system
Gates
  method of G.
gatifloxacin
Gatta prognostic system
Gaucher
  G. cell
  G. disease
  G. splenomegaly
Gauderer-Ponsky PEG operation
Gauder Silicon PEG catheter

Gau gastric balloon
gauge
  Chatillon Digital Force g.
  Dacomed snap g.
  intraabdominal pressure g.
  LeVeen inflator with pressure g.
  g. of instrument
  snap g.
  Statham P23 strain g.
Gaur balloon distention technique
Gautier ureteroscope
gauze
  g. dressing
  iodoform g.
  g. pack
  g. sponge
  Surgicel g.
  Vaseline g.
  Xeroform g.
gavage
  g. bag
  g. feeding
Gavard muscle
GAVE
  gastric antral vascular ectasia
  GAVE syndrome
Gavin-Miller intestinal forceps
Gaviscon, Gaviscon-2
gay bowel syndrome
Gaymar water-circulating blanket
Gazayerli
  G. endoscopic retractor
  G. knot pusher
Gazelle balloon dilation catheter
GB
  gallbladder
  Guillain-Barré
  GB virus C/hepatitis G virus
  RNA
  GB vol+ fluctuation
GBEF
  gallbladder ejection fraction
GBER
  gallbladder ejection rate
GBM
  glomerular basement membrane
  GBM collagen fiber
  perimesangial GBM
  GBM polyanion
GBO
  gastric bacterial overgrowth
GBP
  gastric bypass
GBS
  gallbladder series
  gastric bypass surgery
  Guillain-Barré syndrome
GBT
  gastric bleeding time

G

GBV-C/HGV
  Guillain-Barré virus C/hepatitis G
  virus
    GBV-C/HGV RNA
GCD
  giant colonic diverticulum
G-cell
    G-c. gastrin release
    G-c. hyperplasia
GC/MS
  gas chromatography/mass spectroscopy
G-CSF
  granulocyte colony-stimulating
  factor
GCW
  glomerular capillary wall
GDA
  gastroduodenal artery
    GDA aneurysm
G:D-cell ratio
Gd-EOB-DTPA
  gadolinium EOB-DTPA
GDNF
  glial cell line-derived neurotrophic
  factor
  glial-derived neurotrophic factor
GDSS
  Glasgow Dyspepsia Severity
  Score
GE
  gastroenterology
  gastroesophageal
    GE junction
    GE reflux
    GE RT 3200 Advantage II
GEA
  gastroepiploic artery
    GEA graft
GEBT
  gastric emptying breath test
Gee disease
Gee-Herter disease
Gee-Herter-Heubner
    G.-H.-H. disease
    G.-H.-H. syndrome
Geenan Endotorque guidewire
Gee-Thaysen disease
GEG
  Garren-Edwards gastric
    GEG bubble
GEJ
  gastroesophageal junction
gel
    agar g.
    agarose g.
    Betadine g.
    chondrocyte-alginate g.
    Contractubex g.
    Deflux injectable g.

deletion and mutation detection
  enhancement g.
dihydrotestosterone g.
ferric hyaluronate g.
g. filtration chromatography
Ile-Sorb absorbent g.
IntraDose g.
Iodosorb g.
Optase wound care g.
oxybutynin ATD g.
percutaneous testosterone g.
polyacrylamide g.
Sephacryl S-300 HR g.
Simaal G. 2
viscoelastic g.
Gelamal
gelatin
  gelatin, resorcinol, formaldehyde
    (GRF)
  g. sponge
  g. sponge packing
gelatinous
  g. ascites
  g. nodule
gelatin-subbed slide
gelcap
  Anemagen OB g.'s
Gelclair
GELdose
  Zantac G.
Gelfoam
  G. cube
  G. embolization
  G. particle transarterial embolization
    treatment
Gellhorn pessary
Gelpi self-retaining retractor
gelsolin
  recombinant human g.
Gelusil, Gelusil-II, Gelusil-M
  open-label G.
Gelusil-II (*var. of* Gelusil)
Gelusil-M (*var. of* Gelusil)
Gély suture
gemcitabine HCl
Gemella
gemfibrozil
gemifloxacin
Gemini
  G. gall duct forceps
  G. paired-wire helical basket
Gemzar
Genasense
genavense
  Mycobacterium g.
gender
  g. effect
  g. reassignment
gender-matched control

gene

 g. A
 ABCB4 g.
 adenomatous polyposis coli g.
 ADPKD1 g.
 alpha g.
 angiotensin-converting enzyme g.
 APC tumor suppressor g.
 APOB g.
 apolipoprotein B g.
 ATP7A g.
 break cluster homology g.
 cagA g.
 cagPAI g.
 CARD15 g.
 CARD15/NOD2 susceptibility g.
 caretaker g.
 g. carrier
 C-beta g.
 c-Ha-ras g.
 G. Clean II kit
 COL4A3 g.
 COL4A4 g.
 COL4A5 g.
 cylindromatosis g.
 cytotoxin-associated gene A (cagA, CagA)
 DAZ g.
 DCC g.
 deleted in colon carcinoma g.
 DRB g.
 Fas g.
 FCC-COCA1 g.
 fucosyltransferase g.
 gastrin g.
 gatekeeper g.
 HDA-DR3 g.
 HFE g.
 HLA class II g.
 HLA-DQw2 g.
 HLA-DR3 g.
 hMLH1 g.
 human kidney chloride channel g.
 immunogenic g.
 integrase g.
 interferon-stimulated g.
 Jagged 1 g.
 KAL1 g.
 kallikreinlike g.
 Kirsten-ras g.
 KLF6 g.
 Klotho g.
 K-ras g.
 Kruppel-like factor 6 g.
 g. linkage
 LMP g.
 MCC g.
 MCH g.
 MDM2 g.

 MDR1 g.
 Menkes disease g.
 metastasis g.
 MLH1 g.
 MSH2 g.
 MTS1 g.
 MTS2 g.
 MUC-1 g.
 multidrug-resistance g.
 MutL g.
 MutS g.
 NM23 g.
 NOD2 g.
 OB g.
 p15 g.
 p16 g.
 p18 g.
 p53 g.
 PAX2 g.
 PAX8 g.
 phospholipid export pump g.
 P15/INK4B g.
 PKD1, PKD2 g.
 P27Kip1 g.
 polymorphic g.
 prodynorphin g.
 proenkephalin g.
 proopiomelanocortin g.
 P21/WAF1 g.
 Ras effector RASSF2 tumor-suppressor g.
 Rb g.
 G. Screen nylon membrane filter
 serine threonine kinase g. 11
 SRY g.
 STK11 g.
 suppressor g.
 TAP g.
 TAP2 peptide transporter g.
 TGF-beta-1 g.
 g. therapy
 TNF-alpha g.
 TP40 g.
 TP53 g.
 g. transfer therapy
 tuberous sclerosis g. TS1
 tuberous sclerosis g. TS2
 tumor suppressor g.
 uromodulin g.
 vacuolating toxin g. A (VacA)
 V-alpha g.
 V-beta g.
 VHL g.
 von Hippel-Lindau g.
 WTI g.

gene-blotting study
gene-inductive effect
gene-linkage analysis

G

general
- G. Electric Signa scanner
- g. endotracheal anesthesia (GETA)
- g. peptic ulcer
- g. practice urologist

generalized
- g. abdominal tenderness
- g. distal renal tubular acidosis
- g. elastolysis
- g. glycogenosis
- g. peritonitis

generation
- anti-HCV antibody third g.
- Chiron RIBA HCV test system second g.
- interdialytic urea g.
- Ortho HCV ELISA test system second g.

generator
- banana plug dipolar g.
- electrohydraulic g.
- electrosurgical g.
- Endostat II bipolar/monopolar electrosurgical g.
- implantable pulse g. (IPG)
- isolated g.
- Itrel pulse g.
- Medstone STS shock wave g.
- microexplosive g.
- Northgate SD-100 EHL g.
- piezoelectric g.
- spark-gap shock wave g.
- Symmetry endobipolar g.
- Valleylab II g.
- Valleylab SSE-2L g.

genetic
- g. aberration
- g. alteration
- g. code
- g. hemochromatosis
- g. heterogeneity
- g. marker
- g. predisposition
- g. susceptibility

Genetics Systems microplate reader spectrophotometer
geniohyoid muscle
genistein
genital
- g. burn
- g. cord
- g. cryptococcosis
- g. differentiation
- g. dysplasia
- g. elephantiasis
- g. end bulb
- g. human papillomavirus
- g. mesonephros
- g. rash
- g. reconstruction
- g. scabies
- g. swelling
- g. tissue engineering
- g. tract
- g. tuberculosis
- g. ulcer
- g. wart

genitalia
- adolescent g.
- ambiguous external g.
- anomalous g.

genitocerebral evoked potential study
genitocrural
genitofemoral nerve
genitography
- retrograde g.

genitoinfectious
genitomesenteric band
genitoplasty
- feminizing g.
- masculinizing g.

genitourinary (GU)
- g. carcinoma
- g. fistula
- g. neoplasm
- g. prolapse
- g. region
- g. surgeon
- g. tract
- g. tuberculosis

genodermatosis
genome
- full-length viral g.
- retroviral g.

genome/ml
genomewide screen
genomic
- g. deoxyribonucleic acid
- g. DNA
- g. DNA probe
- g. evaluation
- g. imprinting
- g. instability
- g. sequence
- g. site

genotoxic
genotype
- ADPKD1 g.
- ADPKD2 g.
- HCV g. 1b
- hepatitis C virus g.
- g. II
- g. III
- g. III 2a
- g. V 3

Genta
- G. method
- G. stain

Gentafair
Gentamar
gentamicin sulfate
gentian
 g. violet
 yellow g.
gentle
 G. Nature
 G. Touch colostomy appliance
Gentleheal dressing
genuine
 g. cystine stone
 g. stress incontinence (GSI)
 g. stress urinary incontinence
  (GSUI)
genu of pancreatic duct
Geocillin
geographic
 g. distribution
 g. tongue
 g. variance
Geopen
geophagia, geophagism, geophagy
geophagism (*var. of* geophagia)
geophagy (*var. of* geophagia)
geotrichosis
Geotrichum candidum
GEP
 gastroenteropancreatic
GEPA
 gastroepiploic artery
GER
 gastroesophageal reflux
Gerald forceps
GERD
 gastroesophageal reflux disease
 Enteryx technology for GERD
 Los Angeles classification of GERD
 RS associated with GERD
GERDcheck ambulatory esophageal pH
monitoring system
GERDyzer tool
Gerhardt
 G. table
 G. test
geriatric
 g. constipation
 g. incontinence
 g. incontinence evaluation
 g. urinary tract infection
 g. urology
 g. voiding dysfunction
geriatrics
Geridium
Geriplex-FS
Gerlach valve
germ
 g. cell carcinoma
 g. cell hypoplasia

 g. cell neoplasm
 g. cell tumor
 g. layer
German
 G. chamomile
 G. sarsaparilla
germander
 water g.
germicide
 liquid chemical g. (LCG)
germinal
 g. center formation
 g. epithelium
germinomatous
germline
 g. mutation
 g. stem cell
Gerota
 G. capsule
 G. fascia
gestation
 ectopic g.
gestational
 g. diabetes
 g. thyrotoxicosis
 g. trophoblastic tumor
GET
 gastric emptying time
GET1/2
 gastric emptying half-time
GFD
 gluten-free diet
GFPM
 gastric first-pass metabolism
 GFPM of ethanol
GFR
 glomerular filtration rate
 single-nephron GFR
GFS Mark II inflatable penile
prosthesis
GF-UM2, -UM3, -UM20 radial-sector
scan transducer
GFX Genomic blood DNA purification
kit
GG
 gamma globulin
 Lactobacillus GG
GGT
 gamma glutamyltransferase
 GGT test
GGTP
 gamma glutamyl transpeptidase
GGTP liver function test
GGU
 giant gastric ulcer
Ghedini-Weinberg serologic test
GHP
 growth hormone promoter
 ^{99m}Tc GHP

G

ghrelin
GI
> gastrointestinal
> Gingival Index
> > GI bleed
> > GI bleeding
> > GI bleeding of obscure origin
> > GI bleeding scan
> > GI cancer
> > GI cocktail
> > GI electrophysiology
> > Imagent GI
> > GI pacemaker cell
> > GI tract
> > GI tract flora

GIA
> gastrointestinal assistant
> > GIA autosuture apparatus
> > GIA autosuture device
> > GIA instrument
> > GIA stapler

Gianotti-Crosti syndrome
giant
> g. anorectal condyloma
> acuminatum
> g. cell
> g. cell adenocarcinoma
> g. cell hepatitis
> g. cell transformation
> g. colon
> g. colonic diverticulum (GCD)
> g. diverticulosis
> g. fibrous mesothelioma
> g. gastric fold
> g. gastric polyp
> g. gastric ulcer (GGU)
> g. hypertrophic gastritis
> g. hypertrophy of gastric mucosa
> g. intestinal fluke
> g. migrating contraction (GMC)
> g. milkweed
> g. mitochondria
> g. molluscum contagiosum
> g. nonpancreatic pseudocyst
> g. peptic ulcer

Gianturco
> G. coil
> G. expandable self-expanding
> metallic biliary prosthesis
> G. expandable self-expanding
> metallic biliary stent
> G. metal urethral stent
> G. Z stent

Gianturco-Rosch
> G.-R. biliary Z stent
> G.-R. self-expandable Z stent

Gianturco-Roubin flexible coil stent
Giardia
> *G. duodenalis*

> *G. intestinalis*
> *G. lamblia*

giardiasis dysentery
giardin
GIB
> gastrointestinal bleeding

Gibbon
> G. hernia
> G. hydrocele
> G. indwelling ureteral stent

Gibbs-Donnan equilibrium
Gibson
> G. excision
> G. incision

Gibson-Balfour abdominal retractor
GICA
> gastrointestinal cancer-associated antigen

Giemsa
> G. method
> G. stain

Giemsa-stained section
Gierke disease
GIF
> glycosylation-inhibiting factor
> > G.IF N30 fiberoptic pediatric
> > endoscope
> > GIF XP20 endoscope
> > GIF XQ10 upper endoscope

GIF-HM fiberscope
GIF-Q240 upper digestive tract endoscope
GIFT
> gamete intrafallopian transfer

GIF1T130
> Olympus large-channel endoscope
> GIF1T130

gigantica
> *Fasciola g.*

Gigasept
Gilbert
> G. cholemia
> G. cystic duct forceps
> G. disease
> G. sign
> G. syndrome

Gilbert-Behçet syndrome
Gilbert-Dreyfus syndrome
Gilchrist
> G. ileocecal bladder
> G. urinary diversion procedure

Gill renal tourniquet
Gilman-Abrams gastric tube
Gil-Vernet
> G.-V. anti-vesicoureteral reflux technique
> G.-V. dorsal lumbotomy incision
> G.-V. extended pyelolithotomy
> G.-V. ileocecal cystoplasty
> G.-V. ileocecal cystoplasty urinary
> diversion
> G.-V. ileocecocystoplasty procedure

G.-V. operation
G.-V. orthotopic urinary diversion
G.-V. position
G.-V. retractor

ginger root

gingival

G. Index (GI)
g. papilloma

gingivostomatitis

herpetic g.

ginkgo

ginseng

Giordano-Giovannetti diet

Giordano sphincter

GIP

gastric inhibitory peptide
gastric inhibitory polypeptide
gastrointestinal polyposis
glucose-dependent insulinotropic peptide

GIP/MEDI-Globe needle

Giraldes

organ of G.

girdle

Neptune g.
shoulder g.

Gironcoli hernia

girth

abdominal g.

GIS

gastrointestinal system

GIST

gastrointestinal stromal tumor

GIT

gastrointestinal tract

Gitelman syndrome

GITS

gastrointestinal therapeutic system

GITSG

Gastrointestinal Tumor Study Group

Gittes

G. bladder neck suspension
G. genitourinary technique
G. needle
G. urethral suspension procedure
G. urethrocystopexy

Gittes-Loughlin

G.-L. bladder neck suspension
G.-L. needle bladder suspension
procedure

Given

G. diagnostic imaging system
G. imaging capsule/M2A capsule
G. Imaging Ltd.
G. M2A endoscopic videocapsule
G. videocapsule system

glabella reflex

glabrata

Candida g.
Torulopsis g.

glabrous cirrhosis

Glahn test

gland

accessory adrenal g.
accessory parotid g.
accessory sex g.
accessory thyroid g.
acid g.
adrenal g.
Albarran g.
anal intramuscular g.
Bartholin g.
biliary g.
Brunner g.
bulbourethral g.
cardiac-type g.
Cowper g.
esophageal ectopic
sebaceous g.
esophageal mucosal g.
Galeati g.
gastric g.
hilum of suprarenal g.
Home g.
Lieberkühn g.
Littré g.
Luschka cystic g.
medulla of suprarenal g.
metaplastic gastric fundic g.
middle g.
misplaced g.
mucous g.
mucus-secreting g.
oxyntic g.
paraurethral g.
periductal g.
periurethral g.
preputial g.
pyloric g.
Skene g.
suprarenal g.
trapped prostate g.
urethral g.
vestibular g.
von Ebner g.

glandula, *pl.* **glandulae**

glandulae (*pl. of* glandula)

glandular

g. cystitis
g. metaplasia
g. structure

glandularis

cystitis g.
pyelitis g.
ureteritis g.
urethritis g.

glandule

glandulectomy

glandulopexy

G

glandulous
glans
> g. approximation procedure (GAP)
> conical g.
> g. hyperemia
> g. penis
> g. penis papilla
> septum glandis

glans-cavernosal shunt
glansplasty
> meatal advancement and g.
> (MAGPI)

glanular hypospadias
glanuloplasty
Glasgow
> G. alcoholic hepatitis score
> G. classification of
> choledocholithiasis
> G. criteria for severity of
> pancreatitis
> G. Dyspepsia Severity Score
> (GDSS)

glass
> g. penile prosthesis
> g. pH electrode

Glasser gastrostomy tube
Glassman
> G. basket
> G. brush
> G. gastrostomy
> G. noncrushing gastrointestinal
> clamp
> G. stone extractor

Glassman-Allis intestinal forceps
4-glass test
Glaxo stain
Gleason
> G. cancer grade
> G. grading system
> G. score

gleet
gleety
Gleevec, Glivec
Glenn
> G. diverticulum forceps
> G. technique

Glenn-Anderson
> G.-A. advancement
> G.-A. technique
> G.-A. ureteroneocystostomy

gliadin
> g. ELISA
> g. IgA
> wheat g.

gliadin-specific T-cell clone
glial cell line-derived neurotrophic factor
(GDNF)
glial-derived neurotrophic factor (GDNF)
glibenclamide

glibornuride
gliclazide
glidewire
> angle-tip g.
> G. Gold surgical guidewire
> Terumo g.

Glidex coated Percuflex catheter
glimepiride
glioblastoma multiforme
glioma-polyposis syndrome
gliopathy
glipizide
glischruria
Glisson
> G. capsule
> G. cirrhosis
> G. sphincter

glissonitis
glitter cell
Glivec (*var. of* Gleevec)
GLMA
> gastric laryngeal mask airway

global sclerosis
globi (*pl. of* globus)
globoside
globular
> g. albuminuria
> g. hyalin
> g. proteinuria

globulin
> alpha-1 g.
> alpha-1 antitrypsin g.
> antilymphocyte g. (ATGAM)
> antithymocyte g. (ATG, ATGAM)
> Bence Jones g.
> cytomegalovirus immune g.
> g. fraction
> gamma g. (GG)
> hepatitis B hyperimmune g.
> human hepatitis B immune g.
> immune serum g.
> lymphocyte immune g. (LIG)
> Minnesota antilymphocyte g.
> prophylactic gamma g.
> sex hormone-binding g. (SHBG)
> testosterone-binding g.
> testosterone-estrogen-binding g.
> tetanus g.
> thyroxine-binding g.

globulinuria
globus, *pl.* **globi**
> esophageal g.
> g. hystericus
> g. major
> g. minor
> g. sensation

glomerular, glomerulose
> g. accumulation
> g. arteriole

g. basement membrane (GBM)
g. basement membrane disease
g. capillary
g. capillary healing
g. capillary hypertension
g. capillary pressure
g. capillary wall (GCW)
g. cell culture
g. cell proliferation
g. contractile cell
g. crescent
g. cyst
g. endothelial myxovirus-like microtubular inclusion
g. endotheliosis
g. epithelial cell
g. epithelial cell toxin puromycin aminonucleoside
g. extracellular matrix
g. fibronectin mRNA
g. filtration
g. filtration rate (GFR)
g. hematuria
g. hypercellularity
g. hyperfiltration
g. hypertrophy
g. injury
g. ischemia
g. macrophage infiltration
g. mesangium
g. metabolism
g. microvascular thrombosis
g. morphology
g. necrosis
g. neutrophil infiltration
g. podocyte
g. proteinuria
g. sclerosis
g. tip lesion (GTL)
g. tuft
g. ultrafiltrate
g. ultrafiltration
g. ultrafiltration coefficient
glomerulation
glomeruli (*pl. of* glomerulus)
glomerulitis
glomerulocapillary
glomerulocapsular nephritis
glomerulocystic kidney disease
glomerulonephritides (*pl. of* glomerulonephritis)
glomerulonephritis (GN), *pl.*
  glomerulonephritides
    acute g. (AGN)
    acute mesangial proliferative g.
    acute poststreptococcal g. (APSGN)
    anti-GBM g.
    antiglomerular basement membrane g.

antithymocyte antibody-induced g.
biopsy-verified chronic g.
chronic g. (CG, CGN)
chronic membranous g. (CMGN)
chronic renal failure g.
complement-mediated experimental g.
crescentic g.
diffuse proliferative g. (DPGN)
Ellis type 1, 2 g.
experimental g.
fibrillary g.
focal necrotizing g.
focal proliferative g.
idiopathic crescentic g.
idiopathic membranous g.
idiopathic rapidly progressive g. (IRPGN)
IgA g.
immune complex g. (ICGN, IC-GN)
immunotactoid g.
membranous g. (MGN)
mesangiocapillary g.
mesangioproliferative g. (MPGN)
membranoproliferative g. type I, II (MPGN)
necrotizing crescentic g. (NCGN)
pauciimmune antineutrophil cytoplasmic antibody-associated g.
pauciimmune crescentic g.
postinfectious g. (PIGN)
postinfective g.
poststreptococcal g. (PSGN)
poststreptococcal acute g.
proliferative g. (PGN)
rapidly progressive g. (RPGN)
recurrent focal sclerosing g.
tropical mesangiocapillary g.
type I mesangiocapillary g.
glomerulopathy
  Adriamycin g.
  amyloidlike g.
  collagenofibrotic g.
  collapsing g.
  immunotactoid g. (ITGP)
  inflammatory g.
  lipoprotein g.
  nonamyloid g.
  proteinuric g.
  toxic g.
glomerulosa
  zona g.
glomerulosclerosis
  diffuse diabetic g.
  focal segmental g. (FSGS)
  segmental g.
glomerulose (*var. of* glomerular)
glomerulotubular balance

glomerulus, *pl.* **glomeruli**
    afferent vessel of g.
    amyloidotic g.
    atubular g.
    capsula glomeruli
    human g.
    kidney g.
    malpighian g.
    obsolescent g.
    pooled glomeruli
    renal g.
    Ruysch g.
    vas afferens g.
    vas efferens g.
glomus tumor
glory
    morning g.
glossitis
    Rider-Moeller g.
glossodynia
Glo-tip biliary catheter
glottic
    g. gap
    g. spasm
glove
    SensiCare synthetic powder-free
      surgical g.
    Tactyl 1 g.
GLPT
    glutamate pyruvate transaminase
glucagon
    g. precipitation
    g. stain
glucagon-evoked gastric dysrhythmia
glucagonoma syndrome
gluceptate
    erythromycin g.
glucoamylase
    maltase g.
glucocerebrosidase
glucocorticoid
    g. kinase
    g. response element
    g. treatment
glucocorticoid-induced
    g.-i. hypercalcemia
    g.-i. hypercalcemic
      nephrolithiasis
gluconate
    calcium g.
    chlorhexidine g. (CHG)
    iron g.
    quinidine g.
gluconeogenesis
gluconeogenesis-associated enzyme
gluconeogenic-competent human proximal tubule cell
gluconeogenic pathway
glucoreceptor

glucose
    G. Analyzer II test
    control g.
    CSF g.
    g. excretion
    filtered g.
    g. intolerance
    luminal g.
    g. test
    g. tolerance
    g. transport
    g. transporter
    g. uptake
    urinary g.
glucose-dependent insulinotropic peptide (GIP)
glucose-galactose malabsorption
glucose-6-phosphatase deficiency
glucose-6-phosphate isomerase
glucosuria
    renal g.
Glucotrol
glucuronate
    trimetrexate g.
glucuronidase
glucuronidation
glucuronide, glucuronoside
glucuronoside (*var. of* glucuronide)
glucuronosyltransferase
    uridine diphosphate g. (UDPGT)
glucuronyl
    g. transferase
    g. transferase deficiency
glue
    cyanoacrylate g.
    fibrin g.
    hemostatic surgical g.
    tissue g.
glutamate
    g. dehydrogenase (GLDH)
    g. pyruvate transaminase (GLPT)
glutamic
    g. acid
    g. acid hydrochloride
glutamic-oxaloacetic transaminase (GOT)
glutamic-pyruvic transaminase (GPT)
glutaminase
    mitochondrial phosphate-dependent g.
    phosphate-dependent g.
    phosphate-independent g.
glutamine
    g. aminotransferase pathway
    CSF g.
    g. nitrogen
    g. test
glutamylcysteine synthetase heavy subunit (GCS-HS)
glutamyltransferase
    gamma g. (GGT)

glutamyl transpeptidase (GTP)
glutaral
glutaraldehyde
> activated alkaline g.
> g. alarm
> g. crosslinked collagen
> g. crosslinked collagen injection

glutaraldehyde-induced proctitis
glutathione (GSH)
> g. metabolism
> g. peroxidase
> g. redox cycle
> g. S-transferase M1
> g. transferase

gluteal
> g. artery
> g. fold
> g. nerve

gluten
> g. challenge
> dietary g.
> g. enteropathy
> g. sensitivity
> g. solution
> wheat g.

gluten-dependent population
gluten-free diet (GFD)
gluten-rich diet
gluten-sensitive
> g.-s. diarrhea
> g.-s. enteropathy (GSE)

gluteus
> g. maximus
> g. maximus transposition

glyburide
glycated albumin
glyceraldehyde phosphate dehydrogenase (GAPD, GAPDH)
glyceraldehyde-3-phosphate dehydrogenase (GAPDH, G3PDH)
glycerin (*var. of* glycerol)
> g. enema
> g. suppository

glycerol, glycerin
Glycerol-T
glycero-monooctanoin
> alpha-1 g.-m.

glycerylphosphorylcholine
> alpha g.

glyceryl trinitrate
glycine
glycocalyx
> podocyte g.

glycochenodeoxycholate
glycogen
> g. inclusion
> g. nephrosis
> g. phosphorylase
> g. storage disease

glycogenic acanthosis
glycogenosis
> brancher deficiency g.
> generalized g.
> hepatophosphorylase deficiency g.
> hepatorenal g.
> type III g.

glycogen-rich cystadenoma
glycol
> ethylene g.
> polyethylene g. (PEG)
> polyethylene g. 600

glycolate
glycolipid
> mucin-type g.

glycolysis
> aerobic g.
> anaerobic g.

glycolytic
> g. enzyme
> g. inhibition

2-glycoprotein
> seminal plasma Zn-alpha 2-g.

glycoprotein
> g. accumulation
> acidic epididymal g.
> alpha-1 acid g.
> B2 g, I
> dimeric acidic g. (DAG)
> heterodimeric g.
> microfil-associated g. (MAGP)
> N-linked g.
> TAG-72 g.
> viral g.

glycoprotein-2
> sulfated g.-2 (SGP-2)

glycoprotein-producing tumor
glycopyrrolate test
glycosaminoglycan (GAG)
> g. heparin
> g. layer
> g. uronate (GAGUA)

glycosaminoglycan-degrading enzyme
glycosidase
glycoside
> anthracene g.
> cardiac g.

glycosphingolipid
glycosuria
> alimentary g.
> digestive g.

glycosylated phosphoprotein
glycosylation
> nonenzymic g.
> g. of EPO
> g. process

glycosylation-inhibiting factor (GIF)
glycosyltransferase
glycyl prolinuria

G

glycyltryptophan test
glycyrrhetinic acidlike factor (GALF)
glycyrrhiza
    syrup of g.
Glynazan
glyoxylate
glypican
Glypressin
GMB
    gastric mucosal barrier
GMBF
    gastric mucosal blood flow
GMC
    giant migrating contraction
GM-CSF
    granulocyte-macrophage
     colony-stimulating factor
      GM-CSF cytokine
Gmelin test
GMER
    gastric mucosal ectopia in rectum
GM3 ganglioside
GMP
    guanosine monophosphate
    guanosine 5'-monophosphate
GN
    glomerulonephritis
gnawing pain
GNRF
    guanine nucleotide-releasing factor
GnRH
    gonadotropin-releasing hormone
goblet
    g. cell
    g. cell hyperplasia
    g. cell metaplasia
Goelet retractor
goiter
    nontoxic g.
gold
    cationic colloidal g. (CCG)
    g. compound
    G. deep surgery forceps
    g. nephropathy
    G. Probe
    G. Probe direct bipolar hemostasis
     catheter
    G. Probe electrocoagulation
    G. Probe electrohemostasis catheter
    g. salt
    g. seed implant
    g. seed implantation technique
Goldberg Anorectic Attitude scale
Goldblatt
    G. clamp
    G. hypertension
    G. kidney
    G. phenomenon
Goldenhar syndrome

goldenrod
    European g.
goldenseal
Goldman classification of operative risk
Goldschmiedt technique
Goldstein
    G. disease
    G. hematemesis
    G. Microspike approximator clamp
    G. Microspike approximator clamp
     for vasoepididymostomy
    G. Microspike approximator clamp
     for vasovasostomy
Goldston syndrome
Goldwasser suture carrier
golf-hole configuration
Golgi
    G. apparatus
    G. complex
    G. vesicle
Goligher
    G. extraperitoneal ileostomy
    G. modification
    G. retractor
GoLYTELY
    G. bowel preparation
    G. solution
Gomco
    G. suction
    G. suction tube
    G. umbilical clamp
Gomez
    G. fundoplasty
    G. horizontal gastroplasty
    G. horizontal gastroplasty with
     reinforced stoma
gompertzian tumor kinetics
gonad
    dysgenetic g.
    intersex g.
    streak g.
    vanishing g.
gonadal
    g. artery
    g. differentiation
    g. dysgenesis
    g. ligament
    g. vein
    g. vein valve
    g. vessel
gonadectomize
gonadectomy
gonadial
gonadoblastoma
gonadoliberin
gonadopathy
gonadotherapy
gonadotoxic

gonadotoxicity
    chemotherapy g.
gonadotroph
gonadotrophin (*var. of* gonadotropin)
gonadotropic hormone
gonadotropin, gonadotrophin
    human chorionic g. (HCG, hCG)
    human menopausal g. (HMG)
gonadotropin-releasing
    g.-r. hormone (GnRH, hMG)
    g.-r. hormone deficiency
    g.-r. hormone pulsatile secretion
    g.-r. hormone test
gonaduct
Gonal-f
gonangiectomy
gondii
    Toxoplasma g.
gonecyst, gonecystis
gonecystic calculus
gonecystis (*var. of* gonecyst)
gonecystitis
gonecystolith
gonecystopyosis
gonococcal
    g. perihepatis pelvic inflammatory
      disease
    g. proctitis
    g. urethritis (GU)
gonococcus
gonocyte
    seminiferous tubule g.
gononephrotome
gonophore, gonophorus
gonophorus (*var. of* gonophore)
gonorrhea
    rectal g.
gonorrheal
    g. bubo
    g. proctitis
    g. urethritis
gonorrhoeae
    Neisseria g.
GOO
    gastric outlet obstruction
    gastroduodenal outflow obstruction
good
    g. performance unit
    g. voiding
Goodpasture
    G. disease
    G. epitope
    G. reactivity
    G. syndrome
Goodsall rule
Goodwin
    G. cup-patch principle
    G. orthotopic ileal neobladder
      technique

    G. sound
    G. technique ureterocolonic
      anastomosis
Goodwin-Hohenfellner ureteric
  reimplantation technique
Goodwin-Scott plastic reconstruction of
  prepuce technique
Gopalan syndrome
GOR
    antibody to GOR (anti-GOR)
Gordon
    G. disease
    G. syndrome
gordonae
    Mycobacterium g.
Gore-Tex (GTX)
    G.-T. Acuseal cardiovascular patch
    G.-T. catheter
    G.-T. graft
    G.-T. sling reinforcement
    G.-T. soft tissue patch
    G.-T. strip
Gore Viatorr ePTFE device
gorge
gorget
    probe g.
    Teale g.
Gorlin basal cell nevus syndrome
Gorlin-Chaudhry-Moss syndrome
goserelin acetate
Gosset appendectomy retractor
GOT
    glutamic-oxaloacetic transaminase
Gothic arch formation
Gott
    G. shunt
    G. tube
Gottron sign
gotu kola
gouge
    Capener g.
Gould
    G. inverted mattress suture
    G. polygraph gastric motility
      measuring device
    G. pressure monitor
    G. pressure transducer
Goulding procedure
Gouley catheter
gout
gouty
    g. kidney
    g. proteinuria
    g. urethritis
    g. urine
Gowers
    G. attack
    G. sign
    G. syndrome

G

Goyrand hernia
G3PDH
    glyceraldehyde-3-phosphate
     dehydrogenase
GPT
    glutamic-pyruvic transaminase
Grabstald Memorial staging system
gracilis
    g. muscle
    g. muscle flap
    g. musculocutaneous unit
    g. myocutaneous neovagina
    g. neosphincter
graciloplasty
    direct nerve stimulation g.
    dynamic urinary g. (DUG)
    intramuscular perineural stimulation
     g.
    stimulated g.
grade
    g. 4 cystocele
    Gleason cancer g.
    hemorrhoid g.
    Hetzel-Dent esophagitis g.
    high g. (HG)
    Matts g. 1–4
    M.D. Anderson g.
    mucosal PMN g.
    Roenigk g.
    Savary-Miller II g.
    tumor g.
graded
    g. alcohol
    g. esophageal balloon distention test
gradient
    A-a g.
    acinar g.
    albumin g.
    biliary-duodenal pressure g.
    duodenobiliary pressure g.
    g. echo
    hepatic venous pressure g. (HVPG)
    serum-ascites albumin g. (SAAG)
    transcapillary hydrostatic pressure g.
    transmural hydrostatic pressure g.
    transtubular potassium g. (TTKG)
grading
    Edmondson g. (EdGr)
    histologic g.
    tumor g.
graft
    aortoenteric g.
    aortohepatic arterial g.
    aortorenal bypass g.
    g. atherosclerosis
    autogenous tunica vaginalis g.
    g. bed
    biologic collagen-based
     tissue-matrix g.

    bladder mucosal g.
    bovine g.
    branched vascular g.
    buccal mucosal patch g.
    bypass g.
    C g.
    cadaveric pericardial g.
    cadaveric segmental g.
    CryoVein SG tissue-engineered
     vascular g.
    Dacron interposition g.
    Diastat vascular access g.
    dorsal vein patch g.
    extended criteria donor g.
    free-GEPA g.
    free jejunal g.
    full-thickness g.
    g. function
    gastroduodenal-to-renal artery bypass
     g.
    gastroepiploic artery g.
     (GEA graft)
    Gore-Tex g.
    hepatic-to-renal artery saphenous
     vein bypass g.
    hepatorenal bypass g.
    HLA-identical kidney g.
    Horton-Devine dermal g.
    iliac-to-renal artery bypass g.
    Impra g.
    Intering vascular g.
    interposition Dacron g.
    live-donor segmental g.
    lobe g.
    loop forearm g.
    g. loss
    Marlex g.
    Martius g.
    meshed g.
    mucosal g.
    omental pedicle flap g.
    g. parenchymal cell
    patch g.
    pedicle g.
    pedicled omental g.
    g. placement
    portacaval H g.
    postauricular Wolfe g.
    prosthetic arterial g.
    quality of kidney g.
    reduced-size g.
    renal artery g.
    segmental liver g.
    seromuscular intestinal patch g.
    skin g.
    g. spatulation
    splenorenal bypass g.
    split-thickness skin g.
    g. substitute

superior mesenteric to renal artery
  saphenous vein bypass g.
sural nerve g.
Surgisis Gold hernia repair g.
g. survival
synthetic vascular g.
Thiersch g.
Thiersch-Duplay tube g.
tube g.
tubed free skin g.
vascular access g.
Vectra hemodialysis access g.
V-Y sliding skin g.
Y-V sliding skin g.
graft-enteric fistula
grafting
  endovascular stent g.
graft-versus-host disease (GVHD)
Graham
  G. catheter
  G. closure
  G. closure with omental pouch
  G. deep surgery scissors
  G. plication
  G. scale for drug-induced gastric
   damage
  G. test
grain density
Gram
  G. stain
  G. stain of stool
  G. stain of stool test
gram-negative
  g.-n. bacterium
  g.-n. rod
  g.-n. sepsis
gram-positive
  g.-p. bacterium
  g.-p. organism
  g.-p. sepsis
gram-stain morphology
granddaughter cyst
granisetron
granny knot
Grant gallbladder retractor
granular
  g. cast
  g. cell myoblastoma
  g. cell tumor
  g. induration
  g. kidney
granularity
granulation
  healing by g.
granule
  acidophilic PAS-positive g.
  acrosomal g.
  Birbeck g.
  carcinoid secretory g.

DiPAS-positive g.
Fordyce g.
hemosiderin g.
Kretz g.
mucin g.
perichromatin g.
Weibel-Palade g.
zymogen g.
granulocyte
  g. colony-stimulating factor
   (GCSF)
  g. count
  g. exocytosis
granulocyte-macrophage colony-stimulating factor (GM-CSF)
granulocytic
  g. sarcoma
  g. sarcoma of stomach
granulocytopenia
granuloma, *pl.* **granulomata**
  amebic g.
  barium g.
  caseating g.
  eosinophilic g.
  epithelioid g.
  gastrointestinal eosinophilic g.
  hepatic g.
  g. inguinale
  noncaseating tuberclelike g.
  nonnecrotizing g.
  plasma cell g.
  portal zone g.
  pulmonary g.
  pyogenic g.
  g. pyogenicum
  sperm g.
  stone g.
  suture g.
  umbilical g.
granulomata (*pl. of* granuloma)
granulomatis
  Calymmatobacterium g.
granulomatosa
  Miescher cheilitis g.
granulomatosis
  lipophagic intestinal g.
  Wegener g.
granulomatous
  g. bowel disease
  g. cheilitis
  g. cholangitis
  g. enteritis
  g. enterocolitis
  g. gastritis
  g. hepatitis
  g. ileitis
  g. peritonitis
  g. prostatitis
  g. transmural colitis

G

granulosa
appendicitis g.
g. cell tumor
urethritis g.
granulosa-theca cell tumor
granulosus
Echinococcus g.
granzyme
g. B
g. B ELISPOT assay
grapefruit diet
grapelike cyst
Graser diverticulum
grasp
g. biopsy
palmar g.
plantar g.
g. tripod forceps
grasper
Allis tooth g.
atraumatic g.
bowel g.
laparoscopic g.
Polaris g.
polyp g.
3-pronged g.
4-pronged polyp g.
traumatic locking g.
tripod g.
umbilical port g.
grasping
g. forceps
g. instrument
grass
G. force displacement fluid collector
G. SIU5A stimulation isolation unit
G. S9 stimulator
Grassi
nerve of G.
Graves
G. disease
G. technique
gravidarum
cholestatic hepatosis icterus g.
hyperemesis g.
icterus g.
nephritis g.
gravid uterus
gravimetric
g. technique
g. weighing
gravis
colitis g.
enteritis g.
icterus g.
myasthenia g.
gravity
g. cavernosometry
g. cystogram

urinalysis specific g.
g. urinary incontinence
urinary specific g.
urine specific g.
gravity-dependent drainage
gravity-induced erosion
Grawitz
G. cachexia
G. tumor
gray (Gy), grey
G. cystic duct forceps
g. scale
gray-scale
g.-s. imaging
g.-s. sonography
g.-s. ultrasonography
g.-s. ultrasound
great
g. burnet
g. epiploon
g. lacuna
g. pancreatic artery
greater
g. bindweed
g. celandine
g. curvature banded gastroplasty
g. curvature of stomach
g. curvature ulcer
g. curve position
g. omentum
g. peritoneal sac
g. sciatic foramen
greedy bowel
green
G. cystic duct forceps
g. fluorescent protein
g. hellebore
indocyanine g. (ICG)
g. Mersilene suture
g. sputum
g. stool
g. tea
Greene
G. renal implant stent set
G. retractor
Greenen
G. Endotorque
G. pancreatic stent
Greenfield
G. caval catheter
G. filter
Greenville gastric bypass
Greenwald
G. Control Tip cystoscopic electrode
G. needle
G. Roth Grip-Tip suture guide
G. sound
Greer EZ Access drainage pouch

Gregoir-Lich ureteroneocystostomy procedure
Greishaber self-retaining retractor
grey (*var. of* gray)
    G. Turner disease
    G. Turner sign
    G. Turner sign of retroperitoneal hemorrhage
Grice suture needle
gridiron incision
Griess test
Griffen Roux-en-Y bypass
Griffith point
Grimelius
    G. silver stain
    G. staining
    G. technique
grimelius-positive cell
grip
    2-finger g.
    3-finger g.
    hand g. (HG)
    hook g.
    power g.
    precision g.
grippe
Grip-Tip suture guide
griseofulvin
grit-free solution
gritty tumor
gRNA
    guide RNA
GRNVAC1 vaccine
Grocco sign
Grocott methenamine silver stain
groin incision
gromwell
    purple g.
Grondahl-Finney esophagogastroplasty
groove
    anal intersphincteric g.
    esophageal g.
    innominate g.
    intersphincteric g.
    Liebermeister g.
    oval-form colonic g.
    g. pancreatitis
    paracolic g.
    radial g.
    spindle colonic g.
grooved director
grooving
gross
    g. deformity
    G. disease
    g. hematuria
    G. test
ground-glass
    g.-g. appearance

    g.-g. cell
    g.-g. hepatocyte
groundsel
group
    ABH blood g.
    ABO blood g.
    antibiotic g.
    Astra/Merck G.
    Benelux Multicentre Trial Study G.
    g. B streptococcus (GBS)
    Canadian Urology Oncology G. (CUOG)
    crossreactive g.
    g. C rotavirus
    Eastern Cooperative Oncology G. (ECOG)
    Gastrointestinal Tumor Study G. (GITSG, GTSG)
    hydroxyl g.
    International Germ Cell Cancer Collaborative G. (IGCCCG)
    Laparoscopic Colorectal Surgery G.
    Leuprolide Depot Neoadjuvant Prostate Cancer Study G.
    Lewis blood g.
    nadolol g.
    National Prostatic Cancer Treatment G. (NPCTG)
    National Wilms Tumor Study G. (NWTSG)
    Permixon g.
    phytyl g.
    population-based control g.
    radical resection g.
growth
    cancer cell g.
    g. factor
    g. factor beta
    g. factor isoform
    fungating g.
    g. hormone deficiency
    g. hormone promoter (GHP)
    g. hormone secretagogue receptor (GHSR)
    g. of coagulase-negative *Staphylococcus*
    g. regulation
    somatic g.
GRP
    gastrin-releasing peptide
Gruber-Landzert fossa
Grüntzig
    G. balloon
    G. balloon catheter
    G. balloon dilation
    G. dilator
Grynfeltt
    G. hernia
    G. triangle

G

GSA
  guanidinosuccinic acid
  ^{99m}Tc GSA
  technetium GSA
GSE
  gluten-sensitive enteropathy
G&S electroejaculator
GSH
  glutathione
  GSH prodrug
GSI
  genuine stress incontinence
GSRS
  Gastrointestinal Symptom Rating
  Scale
GSUI
  genuine stress urinary incontinence
GTL
  glomerular tip lesion
GTL-16 gastric carcinoma cell
GTP
  glutamyl transpeptidase
  guanosine triphosphate
GTPase-activating protein (GAP)
GTP-dependent signaling protein
GTP-regulatory protein
GTSG
  Gastrointestinal Tumor Study
  Group
G-tube
  gastrostomy tube
GTX
  Gore-Tex
GU
  genitourinary
guaiac
  bicolor g.
  g. gum
  g. test
guaiac-impregnated slide
guaiac-negative stool
guaiac-positive stool
guanabenz
guanadrel
guanethidine
  parenteral g.
guanfacine
guanidine thiocyanate
guanidinium thiocyanate buffer
guanidino compound
guanidinosuccinic acid (GSA)
Guanilib
guanine
  dihydroxypropoxymethyl g.
  (DHPG)
  g. nucleotide
  g. nucleotide-regulatory protein
  g. nucleotide-releasing factor
  (GNRF)

guanoclor
guanosine
  g. monophosphate (GMP)
  g. 5′-monophosphate (GMP)
  g. monophosphate pathway
  g. triphosphate (GTP)
guanoxan
guanylate cyclase
guanylyl cyclase
guarana
guard
  Protection Plus male g.
Guardian overtube
guarding
  abdominal g.
  involuntary g.
  muscle g.
  g. reflex
  g. sign
  voluntary g.
guard-ring tocodynamometer
Guardus overtube
guar gum
gubernacular
  g. cord
  g. vein
gubernaculum
  chorda g.
Guenzberg test
Guérin
  valve of G.
guidance
  choledochoscopic g.
  endoscopic g.
  fluoroscopic g.
guide
  catheter g.
  Coons g.
  Greenwald Roth Grip-Tip suture g.
  Grip-Tip suture g.
  image g. (IG)
  J-wire g.
  light g. (LG)
  Lunderquist-Ring torque g.
  master image g.
  g. RNA (gRNA)
  Roth Grip-Tip suture g.
  ShapeLock endoscopic g.
  shape-locking g.
  soft-tipped wire g.
  suture g.
  TFE-coated wire g.
  Tracer Hybrid wire g.
guided
  g. fine-needle pass
  g. needle aspiration cytology
  g. percutaneous drainage
  g. transcutaneous biopsy
guide-eye instrument

guideline
Appropriate Use of Gastrointestinal
Endoscopy g.'s
string g.
guidewire, guide wire
Amplatz Super Stiff g.
g. and minisnare technique
Bard Director g.
Bentson floppy-tipped g.
Bentson-type Glidewire g.
cannula with preloaded g.
Conceptus Robust g.
Eder-Puestow g.
ERCP g.
g. exchange
FasTrac hydrophilic coated g.
flexible-tip g.
floppy-tipped g.
Geenan Endotorque g.
Glidewire Gold surgical g.
hydrophilic-coated g.
hydrophilic polymer-coated steerable
g.
Hydro Plus coated g.
Jagwire g.
Lumina g.
Lunderquist g.
Microvasive angled hydrophilic g.
Microvasive Geenen Endotorque g.
Microvasive Glidewire g.
nonconductive g.
olive over g.
g. passage
Pathfinder exchange g.
Placer g.
slipper-tipped g.
g. sphincterotomy
Teflon-coated g.
Terumo hydrophilic g.
Terumo/Meditech g.
Terumo-Radiofocus hydrophilic
polymer-coated g.
Wilson-Cook Protector g.
Wilson-Cook THSF-series g.
Wilson-Cook Tracer g.
Zebra exchange g.
guidewire/basket lasso
guiding catheter
Guillain-Barré (GB)
G.-B. syndrome (GBS)
Guillian-Barré virus C/hepatitis G
virus (GBV-C/HGV)
guillotine
g. incision
g. needle biopsy
gullet
Gull renal epistaxis
gum
g. arabic

guaiac g.
guar g.
Karaya g.
gumma, *pl.* **gummata, gummas**
gummas (*pl. of* gumma)
gummata (*pl. of* gumma)
gummatous necrosis
gummosa
periarteritis g.
gun
Bard Biopty g.
biopsy g.
Biopty g.
Cook biopsy g.
EEA stapler g.
introducer g.
Mentor g.
modified caulking g.
Moss T-anchor introducer g.
spring-loaded biopsy g.
gun-barrel enterostomy
gunpowder lesion
gurgle
gurgling bowel sounds
Gussenbauer suture
gustatory
g. hyperesthesia
g. hypesthesia
g. sweating
gustatory-salivary reflex
gut
artificial g.
g. barrier integrity
caffeine g.
g. colonization
congenital malrotation of g.
g. flora
g. hormone
nervous g.
plain g.
g. rest
gut-associated
g.-a. lymphoepithelial tissue
(GALT)
g.-a. lymphoid tissue (GALT)
gut-hormone profile
gut-liver axis
gutter
lateral g.
left g.
paracolic g.
right g.
guttered T tube
Guyon
G. sign
G. sound
GVAX pancreatic cancer vaccine
GVE
gastric vascular ectasia

G

GVHD
   graft-versus-host disease
Gy
   gray
Gymnodinium breve
gynandroblastoma
Gynecare TVT support system
gynecologic laparoscopy

gynecomastia, gynecomasty
gynecomastia-aspermatogenesis
   syndrome
gynecomasty (*var. of* gynecomastia)
Gyromitra
Gyrus
   G. bipolar electrode
   G. endourology system

H
factor H
Preparation H
prostaglandin H
H2
histamine-2
H2 blocker
H2 breath test
H2 receptor
H2 receptor-blocker
H2 receptor-blocking drug
HAA
hepatitis-associated antigen
HAART
highly active antiretroviral therapy
Haberer
H. abdominal spatula
H. intestinal clamp
H. intestinal forceps
vena marginalis epididymis of H.
Haber-Weiss reaction
habit
bowel h.
dietary h.
drinking h.
habitus
body h.
marfanoid h.
Hadefield-Clarke syndrome
Hadera continent reservoir
Hadju-Cheney acroosteolysis syndrome
HAE
hereditary angioedema
HAEC
Hirschsprung-associated enterocolitis
haeckelii
Psorospermium h.
haematobium
Schistosoma h.
haemoglobin (*var. of* hemoglobin)
haemolyticus
Haemophilus h.
Haemophilus
H. *ducreyi*
H. *haemolyticus*
H. *influenzae*
haemorrhagica
achylia gastrica h.
haemostasis (*var. of* hemostasis)
Hafnia alvei
hafniae
Enterobacter h.
Hagedorn
neutral, protamine H. (NPH)
Hagner operation

HAI
hepatic arterial infusion
histologic activity index
Hailey-Hailey disease
hair
h. ball
digital manipulation of pubic h.
Frey h.
hairline
pubic h.
hairy
h. leukoplakia
h. tongue
HAL
hand-assisted laparoscopy
Halban culdoplasty procedure
Halcion
Haldane effect
Haldane-Priestly tube
Hald-Bradley classification
Haldol
Hale
H. colloidal iron stain
H. colloidal iron technique
Haley's M-O
HALF
hyperacute liver failure
half-body irradiation
half-Fourier acquisition single-shot turbo spin-echo (HASTE)
half-hitch knot
half-life
HalfLytely
half-normal saline
half-strength feeding
half-time
gastric emptying h.-t. (GET1/2)
haliphagia
halitosis
Hallberg biliointestinal bypass
Halle point
Haller
crypt of H.
HALNU
hand-assisted laparoscopic nephroureterectomy
halo effect
haloperidol
halothane hepatotoxicity
halothane-induced
h.-i. disease
h.-i. hepatitis
HALS
hand-assisted laparoscopic surgery

H

341

Halsted
    H. anastomosis
    H. forceps
    H. hemostat
    H. hernioplasty
    H. inguinal herniorrhaphy
    H. interrupted mattress suture
    H. interrupted quilt suture
    H. method
    H. operation
Halsted-Bassini
    H.-B. hernia repair
    H.-B. herniorrhaphy
HALT-C
    hepatitis C antiviral long-term
    treatment to prevent cirrhosis
    HALT-C study
Haltran
Ham
    H. F12 medium
    H. test
hamartoma
    ampullary h.
    angiomatous lymphoid h.
    Brunner gland h.
    colonic h.
    cystic h.
    duodenal wall h.
    mesenchymal h.
    pancreatic h.
    Peutz-Jeghers h.
    renal h.
hamartomatous
    h. gastric polyp
    h. lesion
    h. polyposis
Hamilton deep surgery forceps
Hamilton-Thorn motility analyzer
hammock
    omental h.
    H. technique
    H. technique urinary
      diversion
Hampton
    H. line
    H. sign
hand
    h. grip
    h. temperature
hand-assisted
    h.-a. laparoscopic donor nephrectomy
    h.-a. laparoscopic nephroureterectomy
      (HALNU)
    h.-a. laparoscopic partial
      nephrectomy
    h.-a. laparoscopic sigmoidectomy
    h.-a. laparoscopic surgery (HALS)
    h.-a. laparoscopy (HAL)
1-handed knot

handheld retractor
Handi-Cath catheter kit
handling
    renal tubular sodium h.
    tubular sodium h.
HandPort system
handsewn anastomosis
Hanger test
hanging-drop culture
hanging panniculus
Hank
    H. balanced salt solution
      (HBSS)
    H. buffer solution
Hanley
    H. method
    H. rectal bladder procedure
Hanot
    H. cirrhosis
    H. disease
    H. syndrome
Hanot-Chauffard syndrome
Hanot-Rössle syndrome
Hansel stain
Hansenula fabianii
H2-antagonist therapy
Hantavirus
HAP
    hepatic arterial-dominant phase
    high-amplitude peristalsis
    HAP image
hapatotoxic range
HA-PI
    hepatic arterial pulsatility index
haploid cell
haplotype
    DO2 h.
    DQ2 h.
    DR7 h.
    histocompatibility h.
    HLA-DQ2 h.
    HLA-DR17 h.
haptocorrin degradation
haptoglobin
    serum h.
Hara classification of gallbladder inflammation
hard
    h. adhesion
    h. sonolucent plastic cone
    h. stool
harderoporphyria
harderoporphyrinogen
Harley disease
harmonic
    h. scalpel
    h. scalpel coagulating shears
Harnal
haronga

harpoon extraction
Harrington
    H. Deaver retractor
    H. esophageal diverticulectomy
    H. forceps
    H. splanchnic retractor
Harrington-Mayo scissors
Harris
    H. band
    H. hematoxylin
    H. segregator
    H. tube
    H. tube suction
Harris-Benedict energy requirement equation
Harrison spot test
hartford
    Salmonella h.
Hartmann
    H. closure of rectum
    H. colostomy
    H. fossa
    H. operation
    H. point
    H. pouch
    H. reconstruction technique
    H. resection of intestine procedure
    H. solution
Hartnup
    H. disease
    H. disorder
    H. syndrome
Harvard pump
harvest
harvester
    Arandel cell h.
    Brandel cell h.
harvesting en bloc
Harvey
    H. and Bradshaw criteria
    H. Stone clamp
Harvey-Bradshaw index
Hashimoto
    H. struma
    H. thyroiditis
Hashizume endoscopic ligator kit
Hashmat shunt
Hashmat-Waterhouse shunt
Haslinger esophagoscope
Hasson
    H. bullet-tip forceps
    H. method
    H. needle-nose forceps
    H. open laparoscopy cannula
    H. ring forceps
    H. spike-tooth forceps
    H. technique
    H. trocar

HASTE
    half-Fourier acquisition single-shot turbo spin-echo
    HASTE sequence
HAstV
    human *Astrovirus*
HAT
    hepatic artery thrombosis
hatching
    blastocyst h.
    h. test
H+-ATPase
    vacuolar H+-ATPase
Haudek sign
Hauri penile revascularization technique
Hausted all-purpose chair
haustra (*pl. of* haustrum)
haustral
    h. blunting
    h. crest
    h. fold
    h. indentation
    h. marking
    h. pattern
    h. pouch
haustration
haustrum, *pl.* **haustra**
    cecal h.
    haustra coli
    haustra of colon
Hautmann ileal neobladder
HAV
    hepatitis A virus
Havrix
Hawaii
    H. agent
    H. virus
Hawes-Pallister-Landor syndrome
Hayem
    H. icterus
    H. jaundice
Hayes
    H. anterior resection clamp
    H. colon clamp
Hayflick phenomenon
Hay test
hazel
    witch h.
HB
    histamine blocker
    Recombivax HB
    Tagamet HB
HBAg
    hepatitis B antigen
HBC
    hepatitis C virus
HBcAb
    hepatitis B core antibody

H

HBcAg
> hepatitis B core antigen
>> HBcAg immunostaining
>> recombinant HBcAg
>> (rHBcAg)

HBe
> hepatitis Be
>> HBe antibody

HB$_e$Ab
> hepatitis B early antibody

HBeAb
> hepatitis Be antibody
> hepatitis B early antibody
>> HBeAb antibody

HBeAg
> hepatitis B early antigen
>> HBeAg immunologic study
>> HBeAg positive
>> purified HBeAg

HB-EGF
> heparin-binding epidermal growth
> factor

HBGF-1
> heparin-binding growth factor-1

HBIg
> hepatitis B immunoglobulin

HBO
> hyperbaric oxygen

HBsAb
> antibody to hepatitis B surface
> antigen
> hepatitis B surface antibody

HBsAg
> hepatitis B surface antigen
>> HBsAg immunologic study
>> HBsAg subtype

**HBsAg-negative anti-HCV-negative
chronic liver disease**

HBSS
> Hank balanced salt solution

HBV
> hepatitis B virus
>> HBV Engerix-B
>> HBV genomic DNA
>> HBV virion

HBV-associated DNA polymerase

HBV-specific T cell

HBVV
> hepatitis B virus vaccine

HC, HC-1
> hydrocortisone
>> AnaMantle HC
>> Anusol HC, HC-1

HCA
> hepatocellular adenoma

HCC
> hepatocellular carcinoma

hCG, HCG
> human chorionic gonadotropin

HCl
> hydrochloric acid
> hydrochloride
>> alfuzosin HCl
>> alosetron HCl
>> alprostadil/prazosin HCl
>> atrasentan HCl
>> benazepril HCl
>> gemcitabine HCl
>> liposomal daunorubicin HCl
>> lomefloxacin HCl
>> 1% pramoxine HCl
>> sibutramine HCl
>> sulamserod HCl
>> tamsulosin HCl
>> Tris HCl
>> Vancocin HCl
>> vardenafil HCl

HCN
> high calorie and nitrogen
>> Isocal HCN

HCO3, HCO
> bicarbonate
>> luminal HCO3
>> peritubular HCO3
>> HCO3 reabsorption

HCP
> hereditary coproporphyria

HCS
> hematocystic spot

HCTZ
> hydrochlorothiazide

HCV
> hepatitis C virus
>> HCV antibody
>> HCV DupliType test
>> HCV ELISA test
>> HCV genotype 1b
>> HCV protein
>> HCV QuantaSure Plus
>> HCV QuantaSure Plus
>> test

HDA-DR3 gene

HDAg
> hepatitis D antigen

HDL
> high-density lipoprotein
>> HDL cholesterol

H63D mutation

HDV
> hepatitis D virus

H&E
> hematoxylin and eosin
>> H&E stain

HE
> hepatic encephalopathy

head
>> Medusa h.
>> h. of pancreas

pancreatic h.
h. symptom
headlamp
Keeler Magnalite h.
head-mounted device
healed
h. ulcer
h. yellow atrophy
healing
h. by first intention
h. by granulation
h. by primary intention
h. by secondary intention
h. by second intention
delayed primary intention h.
durable h.
glomerular capillary h.
h. per primam intentionem
h. per secundam intentionem
wound h.
health
National Institutes of H. (NIH)
h. outcome
Healy intestinal forceps
Heaney
H. clamp
H. needle driver
H. retractor
heaped-up edge
heart
H. Outcomes Prevention Evaluation (HOPE)
h. rate monitoring
h. transplant
h. transplantation
Wistar-Kyoto h.
HeartBar orange drink
heartbeating simulator
heartburn
nocturnal h.
h. of pregnancy
h. relief formula (HRF)
spontaneous h.
symptom of chronic h.
heart-kidney transplant
Heartsease
heat
h. exchanger
h. probe
h. probe thermocoagulation
h. shock protein (HSP)
h. shock protein-70 (HSP-70)
h. therapy
heater
h. probe (HP)
h. probe coagulation
h. probe therapy
h. probe thermocoagulation
telescope h.

heather
heating
preferential h.
heat-labile
h.-l. enterotoxin
h.-l. factor (HLF)
h.-l. toxin
heat-stable enterotoxin
heat-sterilized by autoclave
heaven
tree of h.
heaves
dry h.
heavy-chain
h.-c. deposition
h.-c. deposition disease
heavy silk suture
Hebra disease
Hectorol injection
hedge-hyssop
hedrocele
heel tap test
HE9 fibroblast
Hegar
H. intrarectal bougie
H. rectal dilator
h-EGF, hEGF
human epidermal growth factor
Heibronn technique
heidelberg
Salmonella h.
Heidenhain
H. cell
H. pouch
Heifitz clip
heilmannii
Helicobacter h.
Heimlich maneuver
Heineke-Mikulicz
H.-M. fashion
H.-M. gastroenterostomy
H.-M. incision
H.-M. operation
H.-M. principle
H.-M. pyloroplasty
H.-M. stricturoplasty
Heiss
H. flexible endoscopic scissors
H. loop
Heister
H. diverticulum
H. fold
spiral valve of H.
H. valve
Heitz-Boyer procedure
HeLa cell
helical
H. basket
h. coil

H

helical (*continued*)
    h. computed tomography
      (HCT)
    h. CT
    h. fashion
helical-ridged ureteral stent
Helicide
helicine artery
Helicobacter
    H. bilis
    H. cinaedi
    H. felis
    H. fennelliae
    H. heilmannii
    H. hepaticus
    H. pylori (HP)
    H. pylori breath excretion test
    H. pylori cagA strain
    H. pylori-induced gastritis
    H. pylori-like organism (HPLO)
    H. pylori stool antigen (HpSA)
    H. pylori stool antigen EIA
    H. pylori stool assay
Helicobacter-**induced gastric injury**
Helicoblot 2.1 test
Helicosol
Helidac therapy
heliotrope sign
Heliotropium
Helisal
    H. rapid blood diagnostic kit
    H. rapid blood test
helium insufflation
helium-neon laser
Helivax vaccine
helix-loop-helix protein
helix-turn-helix protein
hellebore
    black h.
    green h.
    white h.
Heller
    H. cardiomyotomy
    H. esophagomyotomy
    H. myotomy
    H. operation
Heller-Belsey correction of achalasia of esophagus
Heller-Dor procedure
Heller-Nelson syndrome
Heller-Nissen correction of achalasia of esophagus
HELLP
    hemolysis, elevated liver enzymes, and
    low platelet count
      HELLP syndrome
Helmholtz double-surface coil
helminthemesis
helminthiasis, helminthism

helminthic (*var. of* helmintic)
    h. dysentery
    h. pseudotumor
helminthism (*var. of* helminthiasis)
helmintic, helminthic
    h. abscess
    h. appendicitis
    h. infection
    h. pseudotumor
Helmstein balloon
helper T cell
Helvetius ligament
Hemaccel
hemacytometer (*var. of* hemocytometer)
hemagglutination
    indirect h. (IHA)
hemangioblastoma
    cerebral h.
    spinal h.
hemangioblastomatosis
    cerebelloretinal h.
    von Hippel-Lindau cerebellar h.
hemangioendothelial sarcoma
hemangioepithelioma
hemangioma, *pl.* **hemangiomata**
    capillary h.
    cavernous h.
    cutaneous h.
    hepatic h.
    h. laser treatment
    polypoid colorectal cavernous h.
    renal h.
    scrotal h.
    strawberry h.
    urethral h.
    vascular h.
hemangiomata (*pl. of* hemangioma)
hemangiomatosis
    duodenal h.
    splenic capillary h.
hemangiopericytoma
hemangiosarcoma
Hemaseel APR kit fibrin sealant
hematemesis
    Goldstein h.
Hematest test
hemathorax (*var. of* hemothorax)
hematin cast
hematobilia (*var. of* hemobilia)
hematocele
hematochezia
    severe h.
hematochyluria
hematocolpos
hematocrit
    hemoglobin and h. (H&H)
    multivariate analysis of h.
hematocystic spot (HCS)
hematocystis

hematocyturia
hematogenic, hematogenous
    h. metastasis
    h. micrometastasis
    h. proteinuria
    h. pyelitis
    h. pyelonephritis
    h. spread of infection
hematogenous (*var. of* hematogenic)
hematologic
    h. abnormality
    h. complication
    h. stain
    h. study
hematoma
    butterfly h.
    duodenal h.
    esophageal intramural h.
    expanding retroperitoneal h.
    intrahepatic h.
    intramural duodenal h. (IDH)
    kidney h.
    mesenteric h.
    parenchymatous h.
    perianal h.
    perinephric h.
    perirenal h.
    pulsatile h.
    rectus abdominis h.
    rectus sheath h. (RSH)
    renal h.
    retroperitoneal h.
    scrotal h.
    septal h.
    subcapsular h.
    warfarin-associated subcapsular h.
    wound h.
hematometrocolpos
hematomphalocele
hematonephrosis
hematopathology
hematopoiesis (*var. of* hemopoiesis)
hematopoietic (*var. of* hemopoietic)
    h. growth factor (HGF)
hematoporphyrin
    h. derivative (HPD, HpD)
    h. derivative therapy
hematospermatocele
hematospermia
hematotympanum (*var. of* hemotympanum)
hematoxylin
    h. and eosin (H&E)
    h. and eosin stain (H&E stain)
    Harris h.
hematuresis
hematuria
    adolescent stress h.
    angioneurotic h.
    anticoagulant-induced h.

    benign familial h.
    endemic h.
    essential h.
    exercise-induced h.
    familial benign h.
    glomerular h.
    gross h.
    idiopathic h.
    initial h.
    macroscopic h.
    microscopic h.
    nonglomerular h.
    painful h.
    painless h.
    renal h.
    stress h.
    terminal h.
    total h.
    urethral h.
    vesical h.
    h. with clots
hematuria-dysuria syndrome
HemaWipe test
heme
    h. pigment-induced acute tubular necrosis
    h. test
heme-albumin
    intravenous h.-a.
heme-negative stool
heme-porphyrin assay
heme-positive
    h.-p. NG aspirate
    h.-p. stool
HemeSelect
hemiacidrin irrigation
hemianopia, hemianopsia
hemianopsia (*var. of* hemianopia)
hemiballism (*var. of* hemiballismus)
hemiballismus, hemiballism
hemiblock
    anterior h.
hemibody irradiation
hemicolectomy
    laparoscopic-assisted h.
hemicolon
hemicrypt column
hemifundoplication
    Toupet h.
hemigastrectomy and vagotomy (H&V)
hemihepatectomy
hemihypertrophy
hemi-Kock
    h.-K. neobladder
    h.-K. pouch
    h.-K. procedure
    h.-K. system
    urethral h.-K.
    h.-K. urinary diversion

H

heminephrectomy
heminephroureterectomy
hemiorchiectomy
hemiparesis
hemipelvectomy
    Jaboulay-Doyen-Winkleman h.
hemiplegia
hemipylorectomy
hemipyonephrosis
hemiscrotectomy
hemiscrotum
hemispheria (*pl. of* hemispherium)
hemispherium, *pl.* **hemispheria**
    h. bulbi urethrae
hemi-T
    h.-T augmentation
    h.-T augmentation procedure
hemizona assay
hemobilia, hematobilia
Hemo-Cath catheter
Hemoccult
    H. ICT fecal occult
     test
    H. II
    H. II card
    H. II test
    H. Sensa
    H. Sensa developer
    H. Sensa slide
    H. Sensa test
hemocholecyst
hemochromatosis
    African h.
    C282Y h.
    Desferal Mesylate challenge
     for h.
    genetic h.
    hereditary human leukocyte
     antigen-linked h.
    idiopathic h.
    non-HFE h.
    perinatal h.
    precirrhotic h.
hemochromatotic cirrhosis
hemoclip
    Hx-5LR-1 h.
hemoclipping
    h. application device
    endoscopic h.
hemoconcentration
hemoculture
hemocyanin
    keyhole limpet h. (KLH)
Hemocyte-F
    H.-F elixir
    H.-F tablet
Hemocyte Plus tablet
hemocytometer, hemacytometer
hemodiadsorption system

hemodiafiltration
    continuous arteriovenous h.
     (CAVHDF)
    continuous venovenous h.
     (CVVHDF)
    double-chamber h.
    online h.
hemodialysis
    h. air embolism
    continuous arteriovenous h.
     (CAVHD)
    continuous venovenous h. (CVVHD)
    conventional h.
    cool-temperature h.
    daily h.
    dermatosis of h.
    frequent h.
    intermittent h. (IHD)
    nocturnal h. (NHD)
    h. patient
    h. population
    sequential ultrafiltration h.
    simplified nocturnal home h.
     (SNHHD)
    single-pass h.
    sorbent h.
    standard h.
    h. vascular access
    venovenous continuous h.
hemodialysis-associated
    h.-a. anemia
    h.-a. ascites
hemodialyzer
    Altra-Flux h.
    Altra Nova h.
    Altrex h.
    Baxter h.
    CAHP h.
    Centrysystem 3 h.
    ultrafiltration h.
hemoductal pancreatitis
hemodynamics
    erection h.
    hepatic arterial h.
    intraglomerular h.
    intrarenal h.
    renal h.
hemofilter
hemofiltration
    arteriovenous h.
    continuous arteriovenous h. (CAVH)
    continuous venovenous h. (CVVH)
    simultaneous hemodialysis and h.
    h. therapy (HFT)
    venovenous h.
hemoflagellate parasite
hemoglobin, haemoglobin
    h. and hematocrit (H&H)
    carbamylated h.

h. content index (IHb)
mean corpuscular h. (MCH)
mucosal blood h.
hemoglobinemia
paroxysmal nocturnal h.
hemoglobinopathy
sickle h.
hemoglobinuria
intermittent h.
paroxysmal nocturnal h. (PNH)
Hemoject
H. injection catheter
H. needle
hemolysin
hemolysis
hemolysis, elevated liver enzymes,
and low platelet count (HELLP)
sulfasalazine-induced oxidative h.
hemolytic
h. anemia
h. jaundice
h. splenomegaly
h. streptococcus
hemolytic-uremic syndrome (HUS)
hemonephrosis
hemoperfusion
albumin-coated resin h.
charcoal h.
hepatic venous isolation by direct
h. (HVI-DHP)
h. with charcoal
hemopericardium
hemoperitoneum
Hemophan membrane
hemophilia
renal h.
hemophiliac
hemopoiesis, hematopoiesis
extramedullary h.
hepatic extramedullary h.
hemopoietic, hematopoietic
h. cell
h. cell transplantation
h. lineage
hemoptysis
hemopyelectasia (*var. of* hemopyelectasis)
hemopyelectasis, hemopyelectasia
HemoQuant
H. assay
H. fecal blood test
hemorrhage
acute nonvariceal upper
gastrointestinal h.
adrenal h.
bland pulmonary h.
colonic h.
concealed h.
h. control
diffuse alveolar h. (DAH)

diverticular h.
endoscopic stigmata of h.
esophageal variceal h. (EVH)
exsanguinating h.
fetal adrenal gland h.
gastric h.
gastrointestinal tract h.
Grey Turner sign of retroperitoneal
h.
hepatic h.
h. in inflammatory bowel disease
internal h.
intestinal h.
intraabdominal h.
intramural intestinal h.
intraperitoneal h.
kidney h.
lower gastrointestinal h.
neonatal adrenal gland h.
nonvariceal upper GI h.
pancreatitis-related h.
postgastrectomy h.
postpolypectomy h.
refractory variceal h.
renal cyst h.
retroperitoneal h. (RPH)
stigmata of recent h. (SRH)
stress ulcer h.
subcapsular h.
subepithelial h.
submucosal gastric h.
torrential h.
upper GI h. (UGIH)
variceal h.
hemorrhagic
h. ascites
h. colitis
h. cystitis
h. dengue
h. diarrhea
h. enteritis
h. enterocolitis
h. fever
h. fever with renal syndrome
h. gastritis
h. gastropathy
h. hypotension
h. necrotizing pancreatitis
h. nephritis
h. nephrosonephritis
h. radiation injury
h. speck
h. telangiectasia
hemorrhoid
bleeding h.
cloverleaf excision of h.
combined h.'s
dilation of h.
external h.

H

hemorrhoid (*continued*)
    h. grade
    internal h.
    ligation of h.
    Lord dilation of h.
    mixed h.'s
    mucocutaneous h.
    necrotic h.
    prolapsed internal h.
    prolapsing fourth-degree h.
    h. reduction
    rubber band ligation of h.
    strangulated h.
    thrombosed internal and external h.'s
hemorrhoidal
    h. banding
    h. clamp
    h. cushion
    h. plexus
    h. prolapse
    h. sclerotherapy
    h. tag
    h. zone
hemorrhoidectomy
    ambulatory h.
    closed h.
    diathermy h.
    Ferguson h.
    laser h.
    Longo h.
    Lord method of h.
    Milligan-Morgan h.
    modified Whitehead h.
    open h.
    radical h.
    semiopen h.
    stapled h.
    sutured h.
HemoSelect test
hemosiderin
    h. deposit
    h. granule
hemosiderin-laden macrophage
hemosiderosis
hemospermia
    h. spuria
    h. vera
HemoSplit catheter
hemostasia (*var. of* hemostasis)
hemostasis, hemostasia
    endoscopic h.
hemostat
    Carmalt h.
    Crile h.
    curved h.
    Endo-Assist disposable h.
    Endo-Avitene microfibrillar collagen h.
    Halsted h.
    Kelly h.
    Kocher h.
    microfibrillar collagen h. (MCH)
    Mixter h.
    mosquito h.
    Ochsner h.
    Rochester-Péan h.
    Westphal h.
hemostatic
    h. agent
    h. bond strength
    h. clamp
    h. surgical glue
    h. suture
    h. therapy
hemosuccus pancreaticus
HemoTherapies liver dialysis unit
hemothorax, hemathorax
hemotympanum, hematotympanum
Hemovac Suction standard drain
hemp
    Indian h.
    h. seed calculus
Henderson-Hasselbalch equation
Hendren
    H. clamp
    H. technique
Henke triangle
Henle
    H. ampulla
    H. band
    H. internal cremaster
    internal cremaster of H.
    H. loop
    loop of H.
    H. sphincter
    thick ascending limb of H.
    H. tubule
henna
Henning sign
Henoch-Schönlein purpura (HSP)
Henry approach
henselae
    Bartonella h.
Hensing fold
hep G2 cell line
Hepa
    Amino Mel H.
Hepadnaviridae
hepadnavirus
HepaGam B
Hepahydrin
Hepaplastin test
hepar
    h. lobatum
heparan sulfate proteoglycan (HSPG)
heparin
    h. bolus
    glycosaminoglycan h.

intravesical h.
low molecular weight h. (LMWH)

heparinase

heparin-binding
h.-b. epidermal growth factor
(HB-EGF)
h.-b. growth factor-1 (HBGF-1)

heparin-induced
h.-i. lipolysis
h.-i. thrombocytopenia (HIT)

heparinization
regional h.

heparinized saline

hepaRV cell line

hepatalgia

HepatAmine amino acid solution

HepatAssist liver support system

hepatectomy
donor h.
extended right h.
partial h.
recipient h.
triple-lobe h.

hepatic
h. abnormality
h. abscess
h. adenoma
h. adhesion
h. allograft
h. amebiasis
h. amyloidosis
h. angiomatosis
h. angiosarcoma
h. architecture
h. arterial-dominant phase (HAP)
h. arterial hemodynamics
h. arterial infusion (HAI)
h. arterial infusion chemotherapy
h. arterial pulsatility index (HA-PI)
h. arterial vascular resistance
h. arteriogram
h. arteriography
h. artery
h. artery aneurysm
h. artery infusion pump
h. artery ligation
h. artery thrombosis (HAT)
h. bed
h. bifurcation
h. blood flow
h. blood pool scan
h. calculus
h. candidal infection
h. capsule
h. capsulitis
h. circulation
h. cirrhosis
h. clearance
h. clonorchiasis

h. colic
h. coma
h. congestion
h. copper overload
h. cord
h. cystadenoma
h. cystic disease
h. deformability
h. diverticulum
h. duct
h. duct stone
h. dullness
h. echinococcal cyst
h. echinococcosis
h. edge
h. encephalopathy (HE)
h. endothelialis
h. extramedullary hemopoiesis
h. fascioliasis
h. fibrosis
h. fistula
h. flexure
h. flexure of colon
h. funiculus
h. funiculus of Rauber
h. glycogen store
h. granuloma
h. hemangioma
h. hemorrhage
h. hilar region
h. hilum
h. Hodgkin disease
h. hydrothorax
h. hypoxia
h. insufficiency
h. intermittent fever
h. iron concentration (HIC)
h. iron index (HII)
h. lectin
h. leiomyosarcoma
h. ligament
h. lipase
h. lobectomy
h. malignancy
h. malondialdehyde content
h. mass lesion
h. metabolism
h. metastatic disease
h. 3-methylglutaryl coenzyme A
(HMG-CoA)
h. osteodystrophy
h. outflow tract
h. parenchyma
h. peliosis
h. perfusion index (HPI)
h. phosphorylase deficiency
h. porphyria
h. resection
h. rudiment

H

hepatic (*continued*)
    h. rupture
    h. sarcoidosis
    h. schistosomiasis
    h. sclerosis
    h. segmentectomy
    h. sinusoid
    h. span
    h. steatosis
    h. stellate cell
    h. stimulatory substance (HSS)
    h. subcellular element
    h. subsegmentectomy
    h. telangiectasia
    h. toxemia
    h. trauma
    h. triad
    h. triglyceride lipase (HTGL)
    h. tumor
    h. tumor index (HTI)
    h. uptake
    h. urea
    h. uroporphyrinogen decarboxylase activity
    h. vein
    h. vein catheterization
    h. vein injury
    h. vein occlusion
    h. vein thrombosis
    h. vein wedge pressure
    h. venogram
    h. venography
    h. venoocclusive disease
    h. venous isolation by direct hemoperfusion (HVI-DHP)
    h. venous outflow
    h. venous outflow obstruction (HVOO)
    h. venous pressure
    h. venous pressure gradient (HVPG)
    h. venous pressure gradient reduction
    h. venous web disease
    h. venule
    h. web
    h. web dilation
hepatica
    Fasciola h.
Hepatic-Aid powdered feeding
hepatic-alveolar echinococcosis
hepaticocholedochostomy
hepaticocystic junction
hepaticodochotomy
hepaticoduodenostomy, hepatoduodenostomy
hepaticoenterostomy, hepatocholangioenterostomy

hepaticogastrostomy
hepaticojejunal anastomosis
hepaticojejunostomy, hepatojejunostomy
    Roux-en-Y h.
hepaticoliasis
hepaticolithotomy
hepaticolithotripsy
hepaticopulmonary fistula
hepaticostomy
hepaticotomy
hepatic-to-renal
    h.-t.-r. artery saphenous vein bypass
    h.-t.-r. artery saphenous vein bypass graft
hepaticus
    fetor h.
    Helicobacter h.
    peliosis h.
hepatis
    area nuda h.
    capsula fibrosa perivascularis h.
    facies diaphragmatica h.
    impressio esophagealis h.
    incisura vesicae felleae h.
    ligamentum teres h.
    peliosis h.
    pons h.
    ponticulus h.
    porta h.
hepatitic
hepatitides (*pl. of* hepatitis)
hepatitis, *pl.* **hepatitides**
    h. A
    active chronic h.
    acute h.
    acute alcoholic h. (AAH)
    acute lobular h.
    acute mononucleosis-like h.
    acute parenchymatous h.
    acute self-limited h.
    acute viral h. (AVH)
    h. A inactivated hepatitis B recombinant vaccine
    alcoholic h.
    amebic h.
    anesthetic h.
    anicteric viral h.
    autoimmune h. (AIH)
    h. A virus (HAV)
    h. A virus antigen reduction assay
    h. A virus radioimmunoassay
    h. B
    h. B antigen (HBAg)
    h. B core antibody (HBcAb)
    h. B core antigen (HBcAg)
    h. B DNA detection
    h. Be antibody (HBeAb)
    h. Be antigen
    h. B early antibody (HBeAb)

h. B early antigen (HBeAg)
h. B hyperimmune globulin
h. B immunoglobulin (HBIG, HBIg)
h. B-like DNA
h. B-like DNA virus
bloodborne non-A non-B h.
h. B surface antibody (HBsAb)
h. B surface antigen (HBsAg)
h. B surface antigen subdeterminant
h. B virus (HBV)
h. B virus-encoded antigen
h. B virus vaccine (HBVV)
h. C
h. C antiviral long-term treatment to prevent cirrhosis (HALT-C)
h. carrier
cholangiolitic h.
cholestatic viral h.
chronic h. (CH)
chronic h. A, B, C, D, E, F
chronic active h. (CAH)
chronic active viral h. (CAVH)
chronic active viral h. type B (CAVH-B)
chronic aggressive h. (CAH)
chronic autoimmune h.
chronic benign h. (CBH)
chronic fibrosing h.
chronic interstitial h.
chronic lobular h. (CLH)
chronic persistent h. (CPH)
chronic persistent hepatitis-chronic active h. (CPH-CAH)
chronic progressive h.
chronic type B h.
chronic viral h.
cryptogenic chronic h.
h. C viremia
h. C virus (HCV)
h. C virus-associated venoocclusive disease
h. C virus DupliType test
h. C virus enzyme immunoassay
h. C virus genotype
h. C virus RNA
h. C virus RNA detection
cytomegalovirus h.
h. D
h. D antigen (HDAg)
delta agent h.
h. delta virus
de novo autoimmune h.
drug-induced h.
h. D superinfection
h. D virus (HDV)
h. E
ENANB h.
enterically transmitted non-A non-B h. (ET-NANBH)

epidemic h.
h. E virus (HEV)
h. E virus antigen (HEVAg)
h. F
familial h.
fatty liver h.
fibrosing cholestatic h.
fibrosing cholestatic h. B
flucloxacillin-induced delayed cholestatic h.
H. Foundation International
fulminant h. A–E
fulminant viral h. (FVH)
giant cell h.
granulomatous h.
h. G virus (HGV)
halothane-induced h.
herpetic h.
hyperglobulinemic h.
idiopathic autoimmune chronic h.
inapparent h.
h. infection A–E
infectious h.
interface h.
intrahepatic h.
ischemic h.
isoniazid-induced h.
lobular h.
long incubation h.
lupoid h.
malarial h.
MS-1, -2 h.
murine h.
NANB h.
neonatal h.
newborn h.
non-A–E h.
non-A–G fulminant h.
non-A non-B h.
non-A non-B non-C h.
non-A non-B posttransfusion h.
nonspecific reactive h.
normal carrier h.
occult h.
Ortho HCV 2.0 ELISA test system for h. C
oxacillin-associated anicteric h.
persistent chronic h.
persistent viral h. (PVH)
persistent viral h. type B (PVH-B)
plasma cell h. (PCH)
posttransfusion h.
quiescent h.
h. serologic marker
serum h.
short incubation h.
spontaneous reactivation of h.
subacute h.
subclinical h.

H

hepatitis (*continued*)
 superimposed alcoholic h.
 syphilitic h.
 terbutaline h.
 toxic h.
 transfusion h.
 transfusion-associated h.
 h. type 1
 type 1, 2 autoimmune h.
 vaccine-preventable h. (VPH)
 viral h.
 viral h. type A, B
 virus A, B h.
hepatitis-associated antigen (HAA)
Hepatix device
hepatization
hepatobiliary
 h. capsule
 h. cholescintigraphy
 h. fibropolycystic disease
 h. malignancy
 h. manifestation
 h. sarcoidosis
 h. scan
 h. scintigraphy
 h. tract disease
 h. tree
hepatoblastoma
hepatocanalicular
 h. cholestasia
 h. jaundice
hepatocarcinogenesis
hepatocarcinogenic
hepatocarcinoma
 fibrolamellar h.
hepatocele
hepatocellular
 h. adenoma (HCA)
 h. adnexa
 h. atypia
 h. ballooning
 h. basolateral plasma membrane
  fluidity
 h. carcinoma (HCC)
 h. cholestasia
 h. death
 h. disease
 h. injury
 h. jaundice
 h. necrosis
 h. protein
hepatocerebral degeneration
hepatocholangeitis
hepatocholangiocarcinoma
hepatocholangiocystoduodenostomy
hepatocholangioduodenostomy
hepatocholangioenterostomy (*var. of*
 hepaticoenterostomy)
hepatocholangiogastrostomy

hepatocholangiojejunostomy
hepatocholangiostomy
hepatocholangitis
hepatocirrhosis
hepatocolic ligament
hepatocystic
Hepatocystis
hepatocystocolic ligament
hepatocyte
 allogenic h.
 ballooned h.
 ballooning degeneration of h.
 cobblestone pattern of h.
 ground-glass h.
 h. growth factor (HPG, HGF)
 lipid-laden h.
 h. lysosome
 h. necrosis
 h. nuclear factor 1 (HNF1)
 periportal h.
 polygonal h.
 porcine h.
 h. proliferation inhibitor (HPI)
 h. protein synthesis
 pseudoductular transformation of h.
 h. transplantation
hepatocyte-type cytokeratin
hepatocytic cord
hepatoduodenal
 h. ligament
 h. reflection
hepatoduodenal-peritoneal reflection
hepatoduodenostomy (*var. of*
 hepaticoduodenostomy)
hepatodynia
hepatodysentery
hepatoenterostomy
hepatofugal
 h. arterioportal shunt
 h. flow
 h. portosystemic venous shunt
hepatogastric ligament
hepatogastroduodenal ligament
hepatogastroenterology
hepatogenic, hepatogenous
 h. jaundice
hepatogenous (*var. of* hepatogenic)
hepatography
hepatohemia
hepatoid adenocarcinoma
hepatoiminodiacetic acid (HIDA)
hepatojejunostomy (*var. of*
 hepaticojejunostomy)
hepatojugular reflux
hepatolenticular
 h. degeneration
 h. disease
hepatolith
hepatolithectomy

hepatolithiasis
hepatologist
hepatology
hepatoma
 fibrolamellar h.
hepatomegalia (*var. of* hepatomegaly)
hepatomegaly, hepatomegalia
 congestive h.
hepatomphalocele, hepatomphalos
hepatomphalos (*var. of* hepatomphalocele)
hepatonephoric syndrome
hepatonephric (*var. of* hepatorenal)
hepatonephromegaly
hepatopancreatica
 ampulla h.
hepatopancreatic fold
hepatopancreatoduodenectomy
hepatopathic
hepatopathy
 radiation h.
hepatopetal flow
hepatopexy
hepatophosphorylase deficiency glycogenosis
hepatophrenic ligament
hepatopleural fistula
hepatoportal sclerosis
hepatoportoenterostomy
 Kasai-type h.
hepatoptosis
hepatopulmonary syndrome (HPS)
hepatorenal, hepatonephric
 h. angle
 h. bypass
 h. bypass graft
 h. glycogenosis
 h. ligament
 h. space of Morison
 h. syndrome (HRS)
hepatorrhagia
hepatorrhaphy
hepatorrhea
hepatorrhexis
hepatoscopy
hepatosplenic T-cell lymphoma
hepatosplenomegaly (HSM)
hepatosplenopathy
hepatostomy
hepatotherapy
hepatotomy
hepatotoxemia
hepatotoxic
hepatotoxicity
 acetaminophen h.
 Amanita mushroom h.
 anesthetic h.
 anticonvulsant agent h.
 antidepressant drug h.
 antidiabetic agent h.

 antineoplastic drug h.
 antipsychotic drug h.
 antithyroid drug h.
 carbamazepine h.
 cardiovascular drug h.
 chemotherapeutic agent h.
 cocaine h.
 cyclosporin A-induced h.
 drug h.
 erythromycin estolate h.
 halothane h.
 hydrazide h.
 nitrofurantoin h.
 2-nitropropane h.
 phenylbutazone h.
 potentiation of drug h.
 valproic acid h.
 yellow phosphorus h.
hepatotoxin
hepatoumbilical ligament
Hep-B-Gammagee
HepBzyme
hepcidin mRNA
HEPES
 N-2-hydroxyethyl-piperazine-*N*-2-ethane-sulfonic acid
 HEPES buffer
 HEPES solution
HepeX-5
hepG2 cell
Heprofile ELISA
Hepsera
heptacarboxyl
heptahelical receptor protein
Heptalac
Heptavax-B
Heptazyme
Heptimax hepatitis C viral load test
heracleifolia
 Cimicifuga h.
herald
 h. bleed
 h. patch
herb
 Mercury h.
 h. Robert
Herbgels
 BioFit H.
Herculink
 H. Plus biliary stent
 RX H. 14
hereditary
 h. aceruloplasminemia
 h. angioedema (HAE)
 h. coproporphyria (HCP)
 h. flat adenoma syndrome (HFAS)
 h. fructose intolerance (HFI)
 h. hemorrhagic telangiectasia (HHT)

H

hereditary (*continued*)
    h. human leukocyte antigen-linked hemochromatosis
    h. internal anal sphincter myopathy
    h. nephritis
    h. nonpolyposis colon cancer (HNPCC)
    h. nonpolyposis colorectal cancer (HNPCC)
    h. nonpolyposis colorectal cancer syndrome
    h. nonpolyposis colorectal carcinoma
    h. osteoonychodysplasia
    h. pancreatitis
    h. papillary renal cancer (HPRC)
    h. prostate cancer 1 locus (HPC-1)
    h. spastic paraplegia voiding dysfunction
    h. tyrosinemia
Hering
    canal of H.
Herlitz junctional epidermolysis bullosa
Hermansky-Pudlak syndrome
Herman-Taylor gastroscope
hermaphrodism (*var. of* hermaphroditism)
hermaphroditism, hermaphrodism
hermetically
HER-2/neu oncogene
hernia, *pl.* **herniae**
    abdominal wall h.
    acquired h.
    antevesical h.
    axial hiatal h.
    Barth h.
    Béclard h.
    bladder h.
    Bochdalek h.
    cecal h.
    Cheatle-Henry h.
    Cloquet h.
    combined hiatal h.
    congenital diaphragmatic h.
    Cooper h.
    diaphragmatic h. (DH)
    direct inguinal h.
    duodenojejunal h.
    easily reducible h.
    enterocele-like central h.
    epigastric h.
    femoral h.
    foramen of Bochdalek h.
    funicular inguinal h.
    gastroesophageal h.
    Gibbon h.
    Gironcoli h.
    Goyrand h.
    Grynfeltt h.
    Hesselbach h.

Hey h.
hiatal h.
hiatus h.
Holthouse h.
h. hydrocele
incarcerated intrathoracic h.
h. incarceration
incisional h.
incomplete h.
indirect inguinal h.
inguinal h.
inguinofemoral h.
inguinoscrotal h.
inguinosuperficial h.
interstitial h.
intraepiploic h.
intrailiac h.
irreducible h.
h. knife
Krönlein h.
Larrey h.
lateral ventral h.
Laugier h.
Lesgaft h.
levator ani h.
Littré h.
Madden repair of incisional h.
Maydl h.
mesenteric h.
mesentericoparietal h.
mesocolic h.
metachronous contralateral herniae
Morgagni h.
multiorgan h.
obturator h.
occult levator ani h.
pantaloon h.
paracolostomy h.
paraduodenal h.
paraesophageal diaphragmatic h.
paraesophageal hiatal h.
paraesophageal h. type I, II
parahiatal h.
paraileostomal h.
parapubic h.
parastomal h.
parietal h.
h. pouch
properitoneal h.
reducible h.
h. repair
retrograde h.
retroperitoneal h.
retrosternal h.
Richter h.
Rieux h.
right inguinal h.
Rokitansky h.
rolling hiatal h.

h. sac
sciatic h.
scrotal h.
sliding esophageal hiatal h.
spigelian h.
h. stapler
strangulated h.
traumatic diaphragmatic h.
Treitz h.
umbilical h.
ureteral h.
h. uteri inguinale
Velpeau h.
ventral h.
vesicle h.
voluminous hiatus h.
w h.
herniae (*pl. of* hernia)
hernial defect
herniated preperitoneal fat
herniation
paracolostomy h.
ureteroneocystostomy h.
hernioenterotomy
herniolaparotomy
hernioplasty
Cooper ligament h.
Halsted h.
Lichtenstein open tension-free
mesh h.
mesh-plug h.
open mesh-plug h.
herniorrhaphy
Anson-McVay femoral h.
Bassini inguinal h.
Halsted-Bassini h.
Halsted inguinal h.
Hill hiatus h.
Lichtenstein h.
Macewen h.
Madden incisional h.
McVay h.
pants-over-vest h.
Ponka h.
Shouldice inguinal h.
ventral h.
vest-over-pants h.
herniotome
Cooper h.
herniotomy
herpangina
herpes
anorectal h.
h. labialis
h. pharyngitis
h. progenitalis
h. simplex
h. simplex esophagitis
h. simplex infection

h. simplex virus (HSV)
h. simplex virus-thymidine kinase
(HSV-tk)
h. zoster
h. zoster virus
Herpesviridae
herpesvirus, herpes virus
human h. 6 (HHV-6)
Kaposi sarcoma-associated h. (KSHV)
h. simplex (HVS)
herpetic
h. esophagitis
h. gingivostomatitis
h. hepatitis
h. stomatitis
h. ulcer
herpetiform esophagitis
herpetiformis
dermatitis h. (DH)
Herrick kidney clamp
herring worm
herring-worm disease
Hers disease
Herter
H. disease
H. infantilism
Herter-Heubner disease
Herzberg test
hesitancy
urinary h.
Hesselbach
H. hernia
H. ligament
H. triangle
Hess operation
20-HETE
20-hydroxyeicosatetraenoic acid
HETE
hydroxyeicosatetraenoic acid
HETE acid
heterochromatin
heteroconjugate
antilymphocyte h.
heterodimer
heterodimeric
h. glycoprotein
h. protein
heteroduplex analysis
heterogeneity, heterogenicity
cancer cell h.
genetic h.
intratumoral h.
heterogeneous
h. pseudocyst
h. texture
heterogenicity (*var. of* heterogeneity)
heterologous
h. anti-GBM antibody
h. liver perfusion

H

heterotopia, heterotopy
    fundic gland h.
    gastric h.
heterotopic
    h. cylindric ciliated
      epithelium
    h. diversion
    h. gastric mucosa
    h. pancreas
heterotopic-aberrant pancreas
heterotopy (*var. of* heterotopia)
heterotrimer
heterotrimeric G protein
heterozygosis (*var. of* heterozygosity)
heterozygosity, heterozygosis
    loss of h.
heterozygote
heterozygous
    h. DR5
    h. ornithine transcarbamylase
      (HOTC)
Hetzel-Dent
    H.-D. classification
    H.-D. esophagitis grade
    H.-D. scale
Heubner-Herter disease
HEV
    hepatitis E virus
**Hewlett-Packard IVUS imaging
system**
Hexabrix
Hexadrol Phosphate
hexagon snare
hexamethonium bromide
hexapeptide inhibitor
hexobarbital
hexocyclium
hexokinase (HK)
Hexvix
Hey
    H. hernia
    H. ligament
Heyde syndrome
Heyer-Schulte
    H.-S. Small-Carrion sizing
      set
    H.-S. stent
Heymann
    H. antibody
    H. nephritis
    H. nephritis antigenic complex
      (HNAC)
    H. nephrosis
HFE **gene**
HFI
    hereditary fructose
      intolerance
HFT
    hemofiltration therapy

HFUPS
    high-frequency ultrasound probe
      sonography
HG
    high grade
      Cobe Centrysystem dialyzer 400 HG
HGD
    high-grade dysplasia
HGF
    hematopoietic growth factor
    hepatocyte growth factor
    human growth factor
      recombinant HGF
HGF-stimulated renal epithelial cell
HGPRT
    hypoxanthine-guanine
      phosphoribosyltransferase
      HGPRT deficiency
HGV
    hepatitis G virus
H&H
    hemoglobin and hematocrit
HHG
    hypertrophic hypersecretory gastropathy
H3 histone
HHM
    humoral hypercalcemia of malignancy
HHT
    hereditary hemorrhagic telangiectasia
HHV-6
    human herpesvirus 6
5-HIAA
    5-hydroxyindoleacetic acid
HIAA
    hydroxyindoleacetic acid
hiatal
    h. esophagism
    h. hernia
hiatus
    aortic h.
    diaphragmatic h.
    h. hernia
    patulous h.
    vaginal h.
    vena cava h.
Hibiclens
Hibidil solution
hibiscus
Hibistat
Hibond N+ nylon membrane
HIC
    hepatic iron concentration
hiccough (*var. of* hiccup)
hiccup, hiccough
HIDA
    hepatoiminodiacetic acid
HIDA
    ^{99m}Tc HIDA
    HIDA scan

hidden antigen
hidradenitis suppurativa
hiemis
>hyperemesis h.

Higgins India ink
high
>h. abdominal plain film
>h. anion gap metabolic acidosis
>h. calorie
>h. calorie and nitrogen (HCN)
>h. cutaneous loop ureterostomy
>h. enema
>h. failure rate
>h. false-positive rate
>h. fundal lesion
>h. grade (HG)
>h. intermuscular abscess
>h. intraluminal pressure
>h. ligation
>h. ligation of hernia sac
>h. lithotomy
>h. mallow
>h. neurological lesion
>h. nitrogen (HN)
>h. rectal washout
>h. resting anal pressure
>h. small-bowel obstruction
>h. subtotal gastrectomy
>h. testis
>h. transection
>h. transection of inferior mesenteric artery
>h. vaginal confluence

high-affinity
>h.-a. low-capacity system
>h.-a. receptor
>h.-a. sodium-dependent phosphate transport system

high-altitude endoscopy
high-amplitude
>h.-a. contraction
>h.-a. peristalsis (HAP)

high-bulk low-fat diet
high-calcium dialysate
high-calorie diet
high-carbohydrate diet
high-ceiling diuretic
high-compliance latex balloon
high-definition endoscopy
high-density
>h.-d. endocavity probe
>h.-d. lipoprotein (HDL)
>h.-d. lipoprotein cholesterol

high-diameter dilator
high-dose
>h.-d. chemotherapy (HDC)
>h.-d. consensus interferon
>h.-d. intravenous urography
>h.-d. IVU
>h.-d. pulse steroid

high-echoic area
high-efficiency dialysis
high-ending vagina
high-energy
>h.-e. amplitude
>h.-e. modification
>h.-e. protocol
>h.-e. transurethral microwave thermotherapy (HE-TUMT)
>h.-e. TUMT

higher
>h. host susceptibility
>h. incidence of rejection

high-fat diet
high-fiber diet (HFD)
high-flow priapism
high-flux
>h.-f. dialysis
>h.-f. dialysis membrane
>h.-f. dialyzer
>h.-f. polysulfone
>h.-f. polysulfone membrane

high-frequency
>h.-f. electrosurgical current
>h.-f. endosonography
>h.-f. hemostatic forceps
>h.-f. intraluminal ultrasound
>h.-f. miniprobe
>h.-f. probe ultrasonography
>h.-f. ultrasound probe sonography (HFUPS)

high-grade
>h.-g. cholestasia
>h.-g. dysplasia (HGD)
>h.-g. hydronephrosis
>h.-g. obstruction
>h.-g. prostatic intraepithelial neoplasia (HGPIN)
>h.-g. synchronous colon cancer
>h.-g. tumor

high-intensity
>h.-i. focused ultrasonography
>h.-i. focused ultrasound

high-level disinfection (HLD)
highlight
>human genome h.

high-loop cutaneous ureterostomy
highly
>h. active antiretroviral therapy (HAART)
>h. selective vagotomy (HSV)

high-lying side
high-magnification
>h.-m. chromoscopic colonoscopy
>h.-m. endoscopy
>h.-m. gastroscopy

H

359

Highmore
- H. body
- H. corpus

highmori
- corpus h.

high-pass filtering
high-performance liquid chromatography (HPLC)
high-pitched bowel sounds
high-power
- h.-p. field (hpf)
- h.-p. photomicrograph

high-pressure
- h.-p. antireflux barrier
- h.-p. arterial baroreceptor
- h.-p. inflatable prosthesis cylinder
- h.-p. liquid chromatography (HPLC)
- h.-p. zone

high-protein diet
high-resolution
- h.-r. chromoendoscopy
- h.-r. endoluminal sonography (HRES)
- h.-r. endoscopy
- h.-r. real-time scanner
- h.-r. ultrasonography

high-riding bladder
high-roughage diet
high-sensitivity collimator
high-speed electrical tissue morcellator
high-starch diet
high-throughput screening assay
high-velocity flow
HII
- hepatic iron index

hila (*pl. of* hilum)
hilar
- h. bile duct stenting
- h. carcinoma
- h. cholangiocarcinoma
- h. clamp
- h. mass
- h. plate
- h. retractor
- h. structure scar tissue

hill
- H. antireflux operation
- H. diarrhea
- H. esophageal antireflux repair
- H. esophageal fundoplication
- H. esophageal gastroenterostomy
- H. hiatus hernia repair
- H. hiatus herniorrhaphy
- H. median arcuate repair
- H. posterior gastropexy
- H. rectal retractor

Hill-Ferguson rectal retractor
Hilton white line
hilum, *pl.* **hila**

hepatic h.
liver h.
h. of suprarenal gland
renal h.
h. renale
splenic h.
h. stimulation

hindgut
- h. carcinoid
- h. dysfunction
- h. pattern

hind kidney
Hind-SITE 20/20 system
Hinkle-James rectal speculum
Hinman
- H. reflux
- H. stress incontinence procedure
- H. syndrome

Hinman-Allen syndrome
Hippel-Lindau
- H.-L. syndrome
- von H.-L. (VHL)

hippocratic succussion
Hippuran clearance technique
hippurate
- methenamine h.

hippuric acid
Hiprex
hirschfeldii
- *Salmonella h.*

Hirschmann
- H. anoscope
- H. pile clamp
- H. speculum

Hirschowitz
- H. endoscope
- H. gastroduodenal fiberscope
- H. gastroscope

Hirschsprung-associated enterocolitis (HAEC)
Hirschsprung disease
Hirshberg Foundation for Pancreatic Cancer Research
hirsute papilloma of penis
hirsuties (*var. of* hirsutism)
hirsutism, hirsuties
- adrenal h.

hirsutoid papilloma
His
- angle of H.
- bundle of H.

Hismanal
Histalog stimulation test
histamine
- h. antagonist
- h. blocker (HB)
- h. dihydrochloride
- h. fish poisoning
- h. test

histamine-2 (H2)
    h.-2 receptor antagonist (H2RA)
histamine-fast
histamine-producing mast cell
histamine-releasing factor (HRF)
histamine-resistant achlorhydria
histaminergic type 2 receptor
histatin
histidine
    h. decarboxylase (HDC)
    h. residue
histiocyte, histocyte
    pigmented h.
histiocytic lymphoma
histiocytoma
    fibrous h.
    kidney malignant fibrous h.
histiocytosis, histocytosis
    Langerhans cell h.
    malignant h.
Histoacryl injection
histochemical pattern
histochemical-ultrastructural analysis
histochemistry
histocompatibility
    h. antigen
    h. complex
    h. haplotype
    h. testing
histocyte (*var. of* histiocyte)
histocytochemical technique
histocytosis (*var. of* histiocytosis)
Histofine
    H. SAB kit
    H. SAB-PO kit
histogram flattening
histologic, histological
    h. activity index (HAI)
    h. anal canal
    h. chronic active gastritis
    h. cirrhosis
    h. damage
    h. diagnosis
    h. esophagitis
    h. grading
    h. patchiness
    h. sign
histological (*var. of* histologic)
histology
    bladder h.
histolytica
    Entamoeba h.
histometry
histomorphometric
histone
    H3 h.

histopathologic
    h. criteria
    h. nature of tumor
histopathology
    renal h.
Histoplasma capsulatum
histoplasmosis
    disseminated h.
    duodenal h.
    gastrointestinal h.
    intestinal h.
    mediastinal h.
    recurrent colonic h.
history
    positive family h.
    psychosexual h.
    significant clinical h.
histrelin implant
histrionic personality
His-Wiz device endoscopic plicator
HIT
    heparin-induced thrombocytopenia
Hitachi
    H. analyzer
    H. 737 autoanalyzer
    H. F-2000 fluorescence spectrophotometer
hitch
    psoas h.
hit-skip distribution
HIV
    human immunodeficiency virus
    HIV infection
    HIV P24 antigen
HIVAN
    human immunodeficiency virus-associated nephropathy
HIV-associated dementia
Hi-Vegi-Lip
HIV-1 enteropathy
hives
HK
    hexokinase
    HK enzyme
hK3
    human glandular kallikrein 3
H+/K+-ATPase
    H.-A. acid pump inhibitor
    H.-A. enzyme system
HK-ATPase proton pump
HLA
    human leukocyte antigen
    HLA class II gene
    HLA class II phenotype
    HLA class II restricted
    HLA class II-restricted interferon gamma
    HLA class II-restricted T-cell epitope

H

HLA (*continued*)
    HLA mismatch
    solubilized HLA
    HLA typing
    HLA typing immunologic study
HLA-A, -B, -B8
HLA-DP allele
HLA-DQ2
    HLA-DQ2 haplotype
    HLA-DQ2 marker
    HLA-DQ2 molecule
HLA-DQ8 marker
HLA-DQ typing
HLA-DQw2 **gene**
HLA-DR
    human leukocyte antigen-D related
    HLA-DR antigen
    HLA-DR DNA typing
    HLA-DR matching
HLA-DR+
HLA-DR4
HLA-DR3 **gene**
HLA-DR17 haplotype
HLA-DR2 subtyping
HLA-identical
    H.-i. kidney graft
    H.-i. sibling
HLA-matched kidney
HLF
    heat-labile factor
    HLF cell
HLG
    hypertrophic lymphocytic gastritis
^{1}H magnetic resonance spectroscopy
HMB-45, HMB, HMB45
    homatropine methylbromide
    H.-4. monoclonal antibody
    H.-4. monoclonal antibody marker
    HMB — 45 staining
HM-CAP serological test
hMG, HMG
    human menopausal gonadotropin
HMG-CoA
    hepatic 3-methylglutaryl coenzyme A
    HMG-CoA reductase
    HMG-CoA reductase inhibitor
hMLH1 **gene**
HM4 lithotriptor
HM175 strain
HN
    high nitrogen
    hypertensive nephrosclerosis
    HN feeding
HNAC
    Heymann nephritis antigenic
      complex
HNF1
    hepatocyte nuclear factor 1
H-600 normothermic irrigation

HNPCC
    hereditary nonpolyposis colon cancer
hoarhound (*var. of* horehound)
hobnailed cell
hobnail liver
Hochenegg operation
hockey stick incision
Hodge intestinal decompression tube
Hodgkin disease
Hodgson
    H. technique of modified Lich
      procedure
    H. XX procedure
hoe
    Joe h.
Hoefer laser densitometer
Hoehn and Yahr stage
Hoesch test
Hoffmann-Steinberg gastric reservoir
Hofmeister
    H. anastomosis
    H. gastrectomy procedure
    H. gastroenterostomy
    H. operation
    H. technique
Hofmeister-Pólya anastomosis
Hofmeister-Shoemaker gastrojejunostomy
Hogan/Geenen criteria
Hoguet hernial sac conversion maneuver
H_2O_2-induced injury
HoLAP
    holmium laser ablation of prostate
holder
    Adson needle h.
    Bihrle dorsal clamp-T-C needle h.
    Bookler swivel-ball laparoscope h.
    Bovie h.
    Capillary System slide h.
    Cath-Secure catheter h.
    Crile-Wood needle h.
    Dale Foley catheter h.
    DeMartel-Wolfson clamp h.
    diamond-jaw needle h.
    Endo-Assist disposable needle h.
    Jacobson needle h.
    Kilner needle h.
    Lloyd-Davis knee and leg h.
    Mason needle h.
    Mayo-Hegar needle h.
    microneedle h.
    microvascular needle h.
    needle h.
    Sarot needle h.
    Stratte needle h.
    T-C needle h.
    Young needle h.
holdup
    bolus h.
Holinger esophagoscope

Hollander test
Hollande solution
Hollenhorst plaque
hollisae
    Vibrio h.
Hollister
    H. convex insert
    H. First Choice pouch
    H. Guardian F skin barrier
    H. Holligard pouch
    H. irrigator drain
    H. Karaya 5 ostomy pouch
    H. Karaya Seal pouch
    H. Premium paste
    H. Premium pouch
    H. urostomy bag
hollow-fiber dialyzer
hollow viscus
holmium
    h. laser
    h. laser ablation of prostate
      (HoLAP)
    h. laser resection of prostate
      (HoLRP)
holmium:YAG laser
holmium:yttrium-aluminum-garnet
  (Ho:YAG)
holodiastolic
Hologic densitometer
holosystolic
HoLRP
    holmium laser resection of prostate
Holter
    H. pediatric pump
    H. valve
    vesicovaginal H.
Holthouse hernia
Holt-Oram syndrome
Holyoke
    H. brief
    H. pants
homatropine methylbromide (HMB-45,
  HMB, HMB45)
home
    h. automated telemanagement (HAT)
    H. Care Simplimatt Plus zoned
      foam mattress
    h. dialysis
    H. gland
    H. lobe
    h. parenteral nutrition (HPN)
    h. screening test
    h. uroflowmetry
homeostasis
    calcium phosphate h.
    sodium h.
homeostatic therapy
Homer Wright rosette
HomeSelect test

homing
    lymphoblast h.
hominis
    Blastocystis h.
    Gastrospirillum h.
    Mycoplasma h.
    Trichomonas h.
homocladic anastomosis
homocysteine
    h. level
    plasma h.
    protein-bound h.
    total h.
homocystinuria
homodimer
homodimerization
    ligand-dependent receptor h.
homogenate
    cecal h.
    fecal h.
    mucosal h.
    sphincter of Oddi h.
homogeneity
    assumption of h.
homogeneous
    h. ablation
    h. cooling
    h. nucleation
    h. radioimmunoassay
    h. texture
homogenous
homologous
    h. protein overload disease
    h. serum jaundice
homosexual rectal trauma
homotransplant (*var. of*
  homotransplantation)
homotransplantation, homotransplant
    renal h.
homovanillic acid (HVA)
homozygote
homozygous sickle cell anemia
honeycomb
    h. mucosa
    h. pattern
honeymoon cystitis
hood
    latex h.
hooded prepuce
hook
    Adson dissecting h.
    Barr fistula h.
    cold-knife h.
    Crile nerve h.
    crypt h.
    Dandy nerve h.
    h. forceps
    h. grip
    Joseph h.

H

hook (*continued*)
    h. knife
    Neivert polyp h.
    nerve h.
    Pratt crypt h.
    Pratt rectal h.
    Pucci-Seed h.
    Rosser crypt h.
    h. scissors
    Shambaugh fistula h.
    Stewart crypt h.
    Whitaker h.
hooked catheter
hooklet
    hydatid h.
hook-tip laparoscopic electrode
hookworm disease
Hooper deep surgery scissors
HOPE
    Heart Outcomes Prevention Evaluation
    HOPE study
Hopkins
    H. II rod lens
    H. rod-lens system for rigid
    choledochoscope
    H. symptom checklist
    H. telescope
hordein
hordeolum
horehound, hoarhound
Horizon prostatic stent
horizontal
    h. electrophoresis
    h. folds of rectum
    h. gastroplasty
    h. mattress suture
    h. transmission
hormonal
    h. downstaging
    h. therapy
hormone
    adrenocorticotropic h. (ACTH)
    h. antagonist
    antidiuretic h. (ADH)
    corticotropin-releasing h. (CRH)
    endothelium-derived relaxing h.
    enteric h.
    follicle-stimulating h. (FSH)
    gastrointestinal peptide h.
    gonadotropin-releasing h. (GnRH)
    gut h.
    human menopausal h.
    international unit of male h.
    luteinizing h. (LH)
    luteinizing hormone
    follicle-stimulating h. (LH-FSH)
    luteinizing hormone-releasing h.
    (LHRH)
    parathyroid h. (PTH)

    peptide h.
    plasma parathyroid h.
    h. receptor
    recombinant growth h.
    secosteroid h.
    syndrome of inappropriate secretion
    of antidiuretic h. (SIADH)
    thyroid h.
    thyrotropin-releasing h.
hormone-secreting tumor syndrome
hormone-stimulated cAMP synthesis
horn
    anterior h.
    H. sign
Horner syndrome
horseradish peroxidase-conjugated
  antirabbit IgG
horseshoe
    h. abscess
    h. anomaly of pancreatic duct
    h. communication
    h. configuration
    h. fistula
    h. kidney
    h. track
Horsley
    H. anastomosis
    H. gastrectomy
    H. gastropexy
    H. pyloroplasty
    H. suture
hortobezoar
Horton-Devine
    H.-D. dermal graft
    H.-D. flip-flap hypospadias repair
    H.-D. hypospadias flip-flap procedure
    H.-D. operation
hose-pipe appearance of terminal ileum
Hospal Biospal filter
hospital-based clinic
host
    h. factor
    immunocompetent h.
    immunocompromised h.
    h. side
    h. tyrosine phosphorylation
hostility score
hot
    h. appendix
    h. biopsy
    h. biopsy forceps
    h. biopsy monopolar coagulation
    h. biopsy technique
    h. defect
    h. flexible forceps
    h. spot
    h. squeeze
    h. wire balloon
Hounsfield unit (HU)

24-hour
> 2.-h. ambulatory esophageal pH monitoring
> 2.-h. ambulatory gastric pH monitor
> 2.-h. ambulatory manometry study
> 2.-h. ambulatory pH-metry
> 2.-h. ambulatory pH test
> 2.-h. creatinine clearance
> 2.-h. esophageal pH probe
> 2.-h. fecal fat excretion
> 2.-h. gastric acidity test
> 2.-h. home pH-metry
> 2.-h. intraesophageal pH study
> 2.-h. spectrophotometric bilirubin monitoring
> 2.-h. urine collection

hour
72-hour fecal fat test
hourglass
> h. constriction of gallbladder
> h. contraction
> h. deformity
> h. narrowing
> h. stomach
> h. stricture

12-hour home pad test
hourly scratching activity (HSA)
1-hour office pad test
House
> H. advancement anoplasty
> H. sliding advancement flap

houseleek
Housset-Debray gastroscope
Houston
> H. muscle
> H. valve
> valve of H.

Howard test
Howel-Evans syndrome
Howell
> H. needle
> H. Rotatable BII papillotome

Howell-Jolly body
Howmedica slit catheter
Howship-Romberg sign
Ho:YAG
> holmium:yttrium-aluminum-garnet

HP
> heater probe
> *Helicobacter pylori*
> hyperplastic polyp
> HP Chek screening system
> Ku-Zyme HP
> HP thermocoagulation

HPA
> hypothalamic-pituitary-adrenal
> hypothalamic-pituitary axis

HPC-1
> hereditary prostate cancer 1 locus

HPC-2 standard needle knife
HpD
> hematoporphyrin derivative
> HpD dye
> low-dose HpD

hpf
> high-power field

Hpfast rapid urease test
HPI
> hepatic perfusion index
> hepatocyte proliferation inhibitor

HPLC
> high-performance liquid chromatography
> high-pressure liquid chromatography
> HPLC fluorescence assay

HPLO
> *Helicobacter pylori*-like organism

HPN
> home parenteral nutrition

HP-NAP
> neutrophil-activating protein of *Helicobacter pylori*

HP7754 pneumohydraulic capillary infusion system
HPRC
> hereditary papillary renal cancer
> HPRC syndrome

HPS
> hepatopulmonary syndrome
> hypertrophic pyloric stenosis

HpSA
> *Helicobacter pylori* stool antigen
> Premier Platinum HpSA
> HpSA test

Hp-test
> Jatrox HP-t.

HPV
> human papillomavirus

H2RA
> histamine-2 receptor antagonist
> H2-receptor antagonist
> H2-r. antagonist therapy

H-related protein
HRES
> high-resolution endoluminal sonography

HRF
> heartburn relief formula
> histamine-releasing factor
> Maalox HRF

HRS
> hepatorenal syndrome

HSE
> hypertonic saline-epinephrine
> HSE solution

H-shaped
> H-s. ileal pouch-anal anastomosis
> H-s. tilt tag

HSM
> hepatosplenomegaly

H

HSP
    heat shock protein
    Henoch-Schönlein purpura
HSP-70
    heat shock protein-70
        HSP-70 cDNA
        HSP-70 messenger ribonucleoprotein
        acid level
        HSP-70 mRNA
HSPG
    heparan sulfate proteoglycan
HSS
    hepatic stimulatory substance
HSV
    herpes simplex virus
    highly selective vagotomy
HSV-tk
    herpes simplex virus-thymidine
    kinase
5-HT, 5HT
    5-hydroxytryptamine
5-HT4 agonist
HT-29 cell
HTGL
    hepatic triglyceride lipase
5-HT₃, 5-HT₄ antagonist
3H-thymidine
        3H-thymidine uptake
H-thymidine
HTI
    hepatic tumor index
HTLV-1
    human T-cell leukemia virus type I
    antibody to HTLV-1 (anti-HTLV-I)
HTLV-I-associated myelopathy
5HTM3 receptor antagonist
HTP
    hydroxytryptophan
    Bio-Gel HTP
5-HT3 receptor
5-HT test
H-type fistula
HU
    Hounsfield unit
    hydroxyurea
Huan
        Jin Bu H.
HuCV
    human enteric calcivirus
Hueter maneuver
Huggins operation
Huibregtse biliary stent
Huibregtse-Katon papillotome
Hulka clip
human
        h. adenovirus 12
        h. apo A-I DNA probe
        h. *Astrovirus* (HAstV)
        h. betaretrovirus (HBRV)

        h. case report
        h. chorionic gonadotropin (HCG,
        hCG)
        h. chromosome 6
        h. cytochrome P-450 enzyme system
        h. cytotoxic T cell
        h. enteric calcivirus (HuCV)
        h. epidermal growth factor (hEGF,
        h-EGF)
        h. fibronectin cDNA probe
        h. gastrin probe
        h. genome highlight
        h. glandular kallikrein 3 (hK3)
        h. glomerulus
        h. growth factor (HGF)
        h. gut bacterium
        h. hepatitis B immune globulin
        h. herpesvirus 6 (HHV-6)
        h. immunodeficiency virus (HIV)
        h. immunodeficiency virus-associated
        nephropathy (HIVAN)
        h. insulin
        h. intestinal epithelial Coco-2 cell
        h. kidney chloride channel gene
        h. leukocyte antigen (HLA)
        h. leukocyte antigen-D related
        (HLA-DR)
        h. leukocyte antigen renal allograft
        h. lymphoblastoid interferon (L-IFN)
        h. lymphocyte chromosomal
        aberration test
        h. lyophilized dura cystoplasty
        h. menopausal gonadotropin (HMG,
        hMG)
        h. menopausal hormone
        h. motilin receptor
        h. papillomavirus (HPV)
        h. PDGF receptor
        h. proximal tubule
        h. recombinant erythropoietin
        h. recombinant TGF
        h. serum albumin
        h. serum I-FABP
        h. serum jaundice
        h. synovial fibroblast
        h. T-cell leukemia virus type I
        (HTLV-1)
        h. T-cell lymphotrophic virus type
        I, II
        h. thrombin concentrate
        h. umbilical vein endothelial cell
        (HUVEC)
**humanized anti-CD3 monoclonal
    antibody**
Humicade
Humira
humoral
        h. antibody response
        h. arm

h. hypercalcemia of malignancy (HHM)
h. immunity
h. immunodeficiency disorder
hump
diaphragmatic h.
dromedary h.
hunger
h. contractions
h. pain
hungry bone syndrome
Hunner
H. interstitial cystitis
H. stricture
H. ulcer
Hunt
H. colostomy clamp
H. test
hunterian chancre
Hunter line
Hunt-Lawrence pouch
Hunt-Limo-Basto gastric reservoir
Hurst
H. bougienage
H. bullet-tip dilator
H. mercury bougie
H. mercury-filled dilator
Hurst-Tucker pneumatic dilator
Hurst-type bougie
Hurwitz
H. dialysis catheter
H. esophageal clamp
H. intestinal clamp
HUS
hemolytic-uremic syndrome
husband
artificial insemination h. (AIH)
Huschke ligament
husk
ispaghula h.
Hutch diverticulum
Hutinel disease
HUVEC
human umbilical vein endothelial cell
H&V
hemigastrectomy and vagotomy
HVA
homovanillic acid
HVI-DHP
hepatic venous isolation by direct hemoperfusion
HVOO
hepatic venous outflow obstruction
HVPG
hepatic venous pressure gradient
HVS
herpesvirus simplex
HX-5/6-1 endoscopic clipping device

Hx-5LR-1 hemoclip
Hyalgan
hyalin
alcoholic h.
globular h.
Mallory h.
hyaline, hyaloid
h. arteriolar nephrosclerosis
h. cast
hyalinized stroma
hyalinosis
arteriolar h.
Hyalofill-F biopolymeric dressing
hyaloid (*var. of* hyaline)
hyaluronan
polysaccharide h.
hyaluronate
sodium h.
hyaluronic
h. acid
h. acid concentration
hyaluronidase activity
hybrid
H. Capture system
h. metallic stent
h. rapid acquisition with relaxation enhancement
hybridization
dot-blot h.
fluorescence in situ h. (FISH)
in situ h.
nucleic acid h.
quantitative liquid h.
reverse dot h.
sequence-sequence oligonucleotide h.
Southern blot h.
hybridoma-derived monoclonal antibody
Hybritech
H. method
H. PSA scan
H. Tandem prostate-pecific antigen assay
H. Tandem PSA ratio test
H. Tandem-R assay kit
H. Tandem-R PSA assay
Hy-Cal calorie supplement
Hycamtin
hycanthone mesylate
hydatid
h. cyst
h. cyst disease
h. cyst intrahepatic rupture
h. hooklet
h. mole
Morgagni h.
h. resonance
h. sand
hydatidiform mole, hydatid mole
hydatidocele

H

hydatidosis
    renal h.
hydatidosus
    polypus h.
hydatiduria
Hydeltrasol
Hydeltra-T.B.A.
Hydergine
Hyde shunt
Hydra
    H. Vision Es urologic imaging system
    H. Vision IV urology system
    H. Vision Plus DR urologic imaging system
hydraeroperitoneum
hydragogue diuretic
hydralazine
HydraLife oral rehydration therapy
hydramnion (*var. of* hydramnios)
hydramnios, hydramnion
    acute h.
hydrargyria, hydrargyrism
hydrargyrism (*var. of* hydrargyria)
hydrate
    chloral h.
hydrated
    h. gelatinous coat
    h. pyelogram
hydration
    intravenous h.
HydraTrend urine test strip
hydraulic
    h. abdominal concussion
    h. capillary infusion system
    h. hinge penile prosthesis
hydrazide hepatotoxicity
hydrazine sulfate
Hydrea
hydremic
    h. ascites
    h. nephritis
hydrepigastrium
hydrindantin
hydro
    Cutinova H.
    H. Plus coated guidewire
    H. Plus stent
hydroappendix
hydrobilirubin
hydrobromide
hydrocalycosis
hydrocele
    abdominoscrotal h.
    communicating h.
    congenital h.
    cord h.
    encysted h.
    h. feminae

    filarial h.
    funicular h.
    Gibbon h.
    hernia h.
    Maunoir h.
    meconium h.
    noncommunicating h.
    Nuck h.
    postoperative h.
    h. repair
    simple h.
    h. wall
hydrocelectomy
    h. bottle procedure
    h. dartos pouch procedure
    h. plication technique
    h. scleral therapy
hydrochloric
    h. acid (HCl,)
    h. acid secretion
    h. acid test
hydrochloride (HCl)
    alosetron h.
    amiloride h.
    amitriptyline h.
    bethanechol h.
    bupivacaine h.
    buspirone h.
    ciprofloxacin h.
    colestipol h.
    desipramine h.
    flavoxate h.
    fluoxetine h.
    glutamic acid h.
    hydroxyzine h.
    imipramine h.
    irinotecan h.
    lomefloxacin h.
    meperidine h.
    midazolam h.
    naloxone h.
    nefazodone h.
    oxyphencyclimine h.
    papaverine h.
    phenazopyridine h.
    phenoxybenzamine h.
    1% pramoxine h.
    prazosin h.
    procaine h.
    propoxyphene h.
    pseudoephedrine h.
    quinine urea h.
    ranitidine h.
    sevelamer h.
    tetracycline h.
    thioridazine h.
    tocainide h.
    tolazoline h.
    trospium h.

vancomycin h.
yohimbine h.
hydrochlorothiazide (HCTZ)
h. and reserpine
h. and spironolactone
h. and triamterene
hydrocholecystis
hydrocholeretic drug
Hydrocil Instant
hydrocirsocele
hydrocodone
Hydrocol II dressing
hydrocolloid island dressing
hydrocolpos
hydrocortisone (HC, HC-1)
1% h.
h. acetate
h. acetate rectal aerosol
h. enema
h. foam
Hydrocortone Acetate
hydrodilation
hydrodistention
bladder h.
HydroDIURIL
Hydrofera blue bacteriostatic foam wound dressing
hydrofiber dressing
Hydroflex
H. penile implant
H. penile prosthesis
H. sphincter
hydroflumethiazide
hydrogel
Maxgel h.
hydrogen
h. adenosine triphosphatase
h. breath test
h. gas
h. gas clearance
h. gas clearance technique
h. ion
h. ion concentration (pH)
h. ion production
h. peroxide
h. peroxide enema
h. peroxide ultrasound
hydrography
MR h.
hydrohematonephrosis
hydrohepatosis
hydrolase
carboxylic ester h. (CEH)
lactase-phlorizin h. (LPH)
hydrolysis
brush-border h.
intragastric h.
urea h.
hydrolyze

hydrolyzed
h. in ethanol
h. whey formula
Hydromer-coated polyurethane stent
Hydromer grafted catheter
hydrometrocolpos
hydromorphone
Hydromox
hydronephrosis
bilateral h.
evaluation of symptomatic h.
high-grade h.
h. in utero
prenatal fetal h.
significant h.
hydronephrotic
hydroosmotic action of vascopressin
hydropancreatosis
Hydro-Par
hydroperinephrosis
hydroperitoneum, hydroperitonia
hydroperitonia (*var. of* hydroperitoneum)
hydroperoxide
lipid h.
hydrophila
Aeromonas h.
hydrophilic
h. polymer-coated steerable guidewire
h. wire
hydrophilic-coated guidewire
hydrophilicity
hydrophobic binding region
hydrophone
needle h.
hydropic nephrosis
hydropigenous nephritis
hydropneumoperitoneum
hydropneumothorax
Hydropres-25
hydrops
h. abdominis
gallbladder h.
nonimmune h.
hydropyonephrosis
hydrorachis
hydrosarcocele
hydroscheocele
Hydro-Serp
Hydroserpine
hydrostatic
h. balloon
h. balloon catheter
h. balloon dilation
h. decompression
h. dilator
h. pressure
h. pressure therapy
h. ultrafiltration

H

hydrothorax
    cirrhotic h.
    hepatic h.
Hydro-T Tabs
hydroureter
hydroureteronephrosis
hydroureterosis
Hydrovase wound dressing
Hydroxacen
hydroxide
    aluminum h.
    ammonium h.
    magnesium h.
    potassium h. (KOH)
hydroxyapatite, hydroxylapatite
6-hydroxybenzoate
hydroxychloroquine
18-hydroxycorticosterone
18-hydroxycortisol
20-hydroxyeicosatetraenoic acid (20-HETE)
hydroxyeicosatetraenoic acid (HETE)
5-hydroxyindoleacetic acid (5-HIAA)
hydroxyindoleacetic acid (HIAA)
hydroxyl
    h. group
    h. radical
    h. radical scavenger
hydroxylamine
hydroxylapatite (*var. of* hydroxyapatite)
hydroxylase
    alpha h.
    beta h.
    dopamine beta h.
    tryptophan h. 1
hydroxylated vitamin D
3-hydroxy-3-methylglutaric aciduria
hydroxypropyl methylcellulose (HPMC)
hydroxyquinoline
hydroxysteroid
    3-beta h.
hydroxystilbamidine
5-hydroxytryptamine (5-HT)
hydroxytryptophan (HTP)
hydroxyurea (HU)
25-hydroxyvitamin
    25-h. D
    25—h. D3
    25-h. D level
hydroxyzine hydrochloride
hygiene
    h. hypothesis
    perianal h.
hygroscopicus
    Streptomyces h.
Hygroton
hymen
    imperforate h.

hymenal band
hymenolepiasis
Hymenolepis
    H. diminuta
    H. nana
hymenotomy
hyodeoxycholate
hyodysenteriae
    Serpulina h.
hyointestinalis
    Campylobacter h.
hyoscine butylbromide
hyoscyamine
    sublingual h.
    h. sulfate
    h. sulfate orally disintegrating tablet
Hyosophen
hypanakinesia, hypanakinesis
hypanakinesis (*var. of* hypanakinesia)
Hypaque
    H. contrast medium
    H. enema
    H. swallow
hypazoturic nephropathy
hyperabduction
hyperabsorption
hyperacid
hyperacidity
    gastric h.
hyperactive
    h. bowel sounds
    h. rectosigmoid junction
hyperactivity
    detrusor h.
hyperacute
    h. graft-versus-host disease
    h. liver failure (HALF)
    h. rejection
hyperadiposis, hyperadiposity
hyperadiposity (*var. of* hyperadiposis)
hyperaldosteronism
    familial h.
    primary h.
    secondary h.
hyperalgesia, hyperalgia
    colonic h.
    selective jejunal h.
    visceral h.
hyperalgia (*var. of* hyperalgesia)
hyperalimentation
    central h.
    intravenous h. (IVH)
    parenteral h.
    peripheral h.
hyperalimentosis
hyperalkalinity
hyperaminoaciduria
hyperammonemia (*var. of* ammonemia)

hyperammonemic syndrome
hyperamylasemia
hyperanacinesia (*var. of* hyperanakinesia)
hyperanakinesia, hyperanakinesis,
  hyperanacinesia
hyperanakinesis (*var. of* hyperanakinesia)
hyperandrogenism
hyperbaric
    h. oxygen (HBO)
    h. oxygen chamber
    h. oxygen therapy
    h. oxygen toxicity
hyperbetalipoproteinemia
hyperbilirubinemia
    congenital h.
    conjugated h.
    constitutional h.
    familial unconjugated h.
    idiopathic unconjugated h.
    neonatal conjugated h.
    unconjugated h.
hypercalcemia
    familial hypocalciuric h. (FHH)
    glucocorticoid-induced h.
    iatrogenic h.
    h. of malignancy
hypercalcemic
    h. nephrolithiasis
    h. nephropathy
hypercalcinuria (*var. of* hypercalciuria)
hypercalciuria, hypercalcinuria,
  hypercalcuria
    absorptive h.
    idiopathic h.
    renal h.
    resorptive h.
hypercalcuria (*var. of* hypercalciuria)
hypercaloric diet
hypercarbia
hypercatabolic
hypercatharsis
hypercathartic
hypercellularity
    glomerular h.
    interstitial h.
    mesangial h.
hyperchloremia
hyperchloremic metabolic acidosis
hyperchlorhydria, hyperhydrochloria
hypercholecystokininemia
hypercholesteremia (*var. of*
  hypercholesterolemia)
hypercholesterinemia (*var. of*
  hypercholesterolemia)
hypercholesterolemia, hypercholesteremia,
  hypercholesterinemia
    familial h.
hypercholesterolemic cadaveric renal
  transplant

hypercholesterolia
hypercholia
hyperchromatic nucleus
hyperchylia
hyperchylomicronemia
    familial h.
hypercinesia (*var. of* hyperkinesis)
hypercinesis (*var. of* hyperkinesis)
hypercoagulability
hypercoagulable state
hypercontinence
hypercontinent
hypercontractile external sphincter
  response
hyperdense
hyperdibasic aminoaciduria
hyperdiploidy
hyperdistention
hyperdiuresis
hyperdopaminemia
hyperdynamic
    h. circulation
    h. ileus
    h. precordium
    h. syndrome
hypereccrisia
hypereccritic
hyperechoic
    h. shadowing
    h. spot
    h. stranding
hyperemesis
    h. gravidarum
    h. hiemis
hyperemetic
hyperemia
    gastric h.
    glans h.
    postprandial portal h.
    reactive h.
    splanchnic h.
hyperemic
    h. border zone
    h. mucosa
hypereosinophilia syndrome
hyperesthesia
    cutaneous h.
    gustatory h.
hyperesthetic
hyperferremia
hyperferritinemia
hyperfibrinogenemia
hyperfiltration
    capillary h.
    glomerular h.
    h. injury
    renal h.
    h. theory
hyperfractionated radiation therapy

H

hyperfunction
adrenal cortex h.
antral gastrin cell h.
gastrin cell h.
hyperganglionosis
hypergastrinemia
clinical h.
h. with acid hypersecretion
hypergenitalism
hyperglobulinemic hepatitis
hyperglycemia
hyperglycemic clamping
hyperglyceridemia
exogenous h.
hyperglycogenolysis
hypergonadotropic hypogonadism
HyperHep
hyperhepatia
hyperhidrosis
hyperhomocysteinemia
hyperhydrochloria (*var. of*
hyperchlorhydria)
hypericin
intravascular instillation of h.
hyperinfection
hyperingestion
hyperinsulinemia (*var. of* hyperinsulinism)
hyperinsulinism, hyperinsulinemia
alimentary h.
euglycemic h.
hyperkalemia, hyperkaliemia
hyperkaliemia (*var. of* hyperkalemia)
hyperkaluria
hyperkeratosis
esophageal h.
h. palmaris et plantaris
hyperkinesia (*var. of* hyperkinesis)
hyperkinesis, hyperkinesia, hypercinesis,
hypercinesia
esophageal h.
paroxysmal anal h.
hyperleydigism
hyperlipemia (*var. of* hyperlipidemia)
hyperlipidemia, hyperlipemia
carbohydrate-induced h.
combined fat- and
carbohydrate-induced h.
familial combined h.
familial fat-induced h.
familial hypercholesterolemia
with h.
idiopathic h.
mixed h.
hyperlipoproteinemia
acquired h.
familial h. type II
hyperlithic
hyperlithuria
hypermagnesemia

hypermetabolic state
hypermethylation
promotor h.
hypermobile kidney
hypermobility
bladder neck h.
urethral h.
hypermotility
hypernatremia
hypervolemic h.
hypovolemic h.
hypernephritis
hypernephroid
hypernephroma
hypernephronia
hypernutrition
hyperorchidism
hyperorexia
hyperosmolar
h. liquid
h. perfusate
hyperosmolarity
extracellular h.
hyperosmotic
h. feeding
h. laxative
h. nonketotic dehydration
h. urine
hyperoxaluria
absorptive h.
acquired h.
enteric h.
idiopathic h.
mild h.
primary h. type I, II (PH-I, -II)
hyperoxaluric stone
hyperpancreatism
hyperparathyroidism (HPT)
primary h. (PrHPT)
secondary h. (sHPT)
tertiary h. (tHPT)
hyperpepsia
hyperpepsinia
hyperpeptic gastritis
hyperperfusion
hyperperistalsis
hyperphagia
weight loss with h.
hyperphagic
hyperphosphatemia
hyperpigmentation
reticulated poikilodermatous h.
hyperpipecolatemia
hyperplasia
adenomatous h.
adrenal zona glomerulosa h.
antral G-cell h.
atypical adenomatous h. (AAH)
benign prostatic h. (BPH)

biliary epithelial h.
bilobar h.
Brunner gland h.
colonic nodular lymphoid h.
congenital adrenal h. (CAH)
crypt h.
diffuse nodular h. (DNH)
ductal epithelial h.
duodenal lymphonodular h.
ECL cell h.
ECL hypertrophy and h.
fibromuscular h.
flat h.
focal lymphoid h. (FLH)
focal nodular h. (FNH)
follicular lymphoid h.
foveolar h.
G-cell h.
goblet cell h.
incomplete basal cell h.
insulin h.
intimal h.
islet cell h.
lymphonodular h.
median lobe h.
mesonephric h.
mesothelial h.
musculomucoid intimal h.
myointimal h.
neointimal h.
nodular lymphoid h. (NLH)
nodular regenerative h. (NRH)
nonantral endocrine cell h.
papillary h.
parathyroid h.
polypoid gastric rugal h.
polypoid lymphoid h.
polypoid lymphomatous h.
postatrophic h.
prostate gland benign h.
prostatic h.
Rokitansky-Aschoff sinus h.
scrotal h.
symptomatic benign prostatic h.
trilobar h.

hyperplasiogenic polyp
hyperplastic
h. adenomatous polyp
h. arteriolar nephrosclerosis
h. cholecystosis
h. dystrophy
h. epithelial gastric polyp
h. foveolar epithelium
h. gastric polyp
h. nodule
h. obesity
h. polyp (HP)
h. polyposis
hyperplasticity

hyperpolarization
membrane h.
hyperprebetalipoproteinemia
familial hyperbetalipoproteinemia and
h.
familial hyperchylomicronemia with
h.
hyperprochoresis
hyperprolactinemia
hyperproliferation
hyperproteinemia
hyperproteosis
hyperprotidic diet
hyperpyrexia
hyperreflexia
autonomic h.
degree of h.
detrusor h.
neurogenic h.
pathogenesis of h.
hyperreflexic
h. bladder
h. motor urge incontinence
hyperreninemia
hyperreninemic
hyperresonance
hyperresonant abdomen
hyperresponsiveness
hyperrugosity
hypersalivation
hypersecreting tumor
hypersecretion
acid h.
cortisol h.
gastric h.
hypergastrinemia with acid h.
salivary h.
hypersecretion-obstruction hypothesis
hyperselective embolization
hypersensitive esophagus
hypersensitivity
h. angiitis
antiepileptic drug h.
cholestatic h.
delayed cutaneous h.
delayed-type h. (DTH)
paraaminosalicylate h.
phenindione h.
h. reaction
visceral h.
hyperspectral imaging
hypersplenism
hypersthenuria
hyperstimulation
hypersuprarenalism
hypertension
accelerated h.
African-American Study of Kidney
Disease and H. (AASK)

H

hypertension (*continued*)
    allograft-mediated h.
    angiotensin-dependent h.
    concomitant h.
    dietary approach to stop h.
      (DASH)
    ductal h.
    extrahepatic portal venous h.
    glomerular capillary h.
    Goldblatt h.
    idiopathic portal h. (IPH)
    impact of donor h.
    intraglomerular h.
    intrahepatic portal h.
    isolated systolic h. (ISH)
    JNC VI classification of h.
    lithotripsy-induced h.
    noncirrhotic portal h.
    pancreatic ductal h.
    portal h. (PHTN)
    portopulmonary h.
    presinusoidal intrahepatic portal h.
    refractory h.
    renal h.
    renin-mediated renovascular h.
    renovascular h. (RVH)
    h. resistance axis
    salt-sensitive h.
    secondary h.
    sinistral portal h.
    splenoportal h.
    systemic h.
hypertensive
    h. autosomal-dominant polycystic
      kidney disease
    h. end-organ damage
    h. gastropathy
    h. lower esophageal sphincter
    h. lower esophageal sphincter
      syndrome
    h. nephrosclerosis (HN)
    h. renal injury
hypertestosteronism
hyperthermia
    malignant h.
    microwave h.
    transrectal prostatic h. (TPH)
hyperthyroidism
hyperthyroxinemia
hypertonia, hypertonicity, hypertonus
    anal canal h.
hypertonic
    h. bladder
    h. crystalloid
    h. infusion
    h. saline
    h. saline-epinephrine (HSE)
    h. saline-epinephrine solution
hypertonicity (*var. of* hypertonia)

hypertonus (*var. of* hypertonia)
hypertransaminasemia
    cryptogenic h.
hypertrichosis lanuginosa acquisita
hypertriglyceridemia
    familial h.
hypertrophic
    h. cirrhosis
    h. hypersecretory gastropathy
      (HHG)
    h. lymphocytic gastritis (HLG)
    h. obesity
    h. pyloric stenosis (HPS)
    h. pylorus
hypertrophy
    benign prostatic h. (BPH)
    Billroth h.
    bilobar h.
    compensatory testicular h.
    crypt h.
    gastroduodenal h.
    glomerular h.
    muscle h.
    h. of column of Bertin
    prostatic h.
    renal h.
    renovascular h.
    rugal h.
    symptomatic benign prostatic h.
    trilobar h.
hypertyrosinemia
hyperuricemia
hyperuricuria
hypervariable
    h. deoxyribonucleic acid
    h. region 1
hypervolemia
hypervolemic hypernatremia
hypes
    hypesthesia
hypesthesia (hypes), hypoesthesia
    gustatory h.
hyphema
hyphemia (*var. of* hypovolemia)
Hypnovel
hypoacidity
    luminal h.
hypoactive bowel sounds
hypoactivity
hypoadiponectinemia
hypoalbuminemia
hypoalbuminemic patient
hypoaldosteronism
    hyporeninemic h.
    isolated h.
hypoalimentation
hypoandrogenism
hypobetalipoproteinemia
hypobicarbonatemia

hypocalcemia
    asymptomatic h.
    familial hypocalciuric h.
hypochloremia
hypochloremic-hypokalemic metabolic alkalosis
hypochlorhydria
    epidemic h.
    gastric h.
hypochlorhydric cirrhosis
hypochloruric nephropathy
hypocholia
hypochondria (*pl. of* hypochondrium)
hypochondriac
    h. fossa
    h. region
hypochondriacal patient
hypochondriasis
hypochondrium, *pl.* **hypochondria**
hypochromic
    h. microcytic anemia
    h. red cell
hypochylia
hypocitraturia
hypocomplementemia
hypocontractile detrusor
hypocontractility
    detrusor h.
hypocupremia
hypocystotomy
hypodiaphragmatic
hypodiploidy
hypodipsia
hypoeccrisis
hypoeccritic
hypoechoic
    h. cancer
    h. lesion
    h. periphery
    h. ringed layer
    h. thickening
hypoesthesia
hypoestrogenic urethritis
hypoestrogenism
hypofibrinogenemia
hypofunction
hypogammaglobinemia (*var. of* hypogammaglobulinemia)
hypogammaglobulinemia, hypogammaglobinemia
hypogammaglobulinemic
hypoganglionosis of colon
hypogastric
    h. artery
    h. artery aneurysm
    h. fiber
    h. nerve
    h. node
    h. papillary zone
    h. plexus
    h. region
    h. vessel
hypogastrium
hypogastrocele
hypogastroschisis
hypogenetic nephritis
hypogenitalism
hypogeusia
hypoglycemia
    alcohol-induced h.
    postprandial h.
hypoglycin
    acetyl coenzyme h. A
hypogonadal state
hypogonadism
    hypergonadotropic h.
hypohepatia
hypohydrochloria
hypokalemia, hypopotassemia
    diuretic-induced h.
hypokalemic
    h. metabolic alkalosis
    h. nephropathy
    h. nephrosis
    h. renal tubular acidosis
hypokaluria
hypolactasia
    adult h.
hypoleydigism
hypomagnesemia
hypomagnesuria
hypometabolic
hypometabolism
hypomethylation
    DNA h.
hypomotility
    esophageal h.
    gastric h.
hypomyxia
hyponatremia
    dilutional h.
    early signs of dilutional h.
    euvolemic h.
    thiazide-induced h.
hypoorchidism
hypoosmotic urine
hypopancreatism
hypopancreorrhea
hypoparathyroidism
hypopepsia
hypopepsinia
hypoperfusion
    renal h.
hypoperistalsis syndrome
hypoperistaltic
hypopharyngeal
    h. cancer
    h. diverticulum

H

hypopharynx
hypophosphatasia
hypophosphatemia
    X-linked h.
hypophosphatemic rickets
hypophosphaturia
hypophrenic
hypophysectomy
hypoplasia
    bile duct h.
    bladder h.
    congenital h.
    corpus spongiosum h.
    erythroid h.
    exocrine pancreatic h.
    germ cell h.
    intrahepatic biliary duct h.
    oligonephronic h.
    prostate gland h.
    thymic h.
    unilateral renal h.
hypoplastic
    h. blind-ending spermatic
      vessel
    h. glomerulocystic disease
    h. kidney
hypoposia
hypopotassemia (*var. of* hypokalemia)
hypoproteinemia
hypoproteinosis
hypoprothrombinemia
hyporeninemic hypoaldosteronism
hyporesponsiveness
    cardiac beta adrenoreceptor h.
    erythropoietin h.
hyposensitivity
    rectal h.
hypospadiac
hypospadias
    anterior h.
    balanic h.
    complex h.
    concealed h.
    coronal h.
    female h.
    glanular h.
    middle h.
    penile h.
    penoscrotal h.
    perineal h.
    posterior h.
    pseudovaginal perineoscrotal h.
      (PPSH)
    scrotal h.
    subcoronal h.
hypospermatogenesis
hyposplenism
hypostasis
hypostatic

hyposthenuria
    renal h.
hyposuprarenalism
hypotension
    dialysis-associated h.
    hemorrhagic h.
    intradialytic h. (IDH)
    systemic h.
hypotestosteronism
hypothalamic-pituitary-adrenal
  (HPA)
hypothalamic-pituitary axis (HPA)
hypothalamic-pituitary-testicular-penile
  axis
hypothalamic suppression
hypothalamus
hypothermia
    gastric h.
    intraoperative kidney h.
    renal h.
hypothermic
    h. effect
    h. pulsatile perfusion
    h. storage
hypothesis
    affinity-avidity h.
    cumulative damage h.
    hygiene h.
    hypersecretion-obstruction h.
    iron shuttle h.
    Keller h.
hypothromboplastinemia (HTP)
hypothyroidism
hypotonia, hypotonus, hypotony
    rectal h.
hypotonic
    h. bladder
    h. duodenography
hypotonus (*var. of* hypotonia)
hypotony (*var. of* hypotonia)
hypouremia
hypouresis
hypouricemia
hypouricuria
hypourocrinia
hypoventilation
    benzodiazepine-induced h.
    sedation-induced h.
hypovolemia, hyphemia
    intertropical h.
    nephrosis with h.
    nephrosis without h.
    watery diarrhea, hypokalemia, and
      h. (WDHH)
hypovolemic
    h. anemia
    h. hypernatremia
    h. shock
    h. variance

hypoxanthine-guanine
> h.-g. phosphoribosyltransferase
> (HGPRT)
> h.-g. phosphoribosyltransferase
> deficiency

hypoxemia

hypoxia
> hepatic h.
> pericentral h.

hypoxia-induced rhabdomyolysis

Hypoxis rooperi

Hyrtl sphincter

hysterectomy (hys)

hysterical vomiting

hystericus
> globus h.

hysterocele

hysterocystopexy

hysterosacropexy
> Ivalon sponge h.
> polyvinyl alcohol
> sponge h.

hysterosalpingectomy
> laparoscopic h.

hysteroscopy

Hy-Tape

Hytrin Dosepak

Hyzine-50

H

I-125, ^{125}I
   iodine-125
      ^{125}I albumin
      I-125 iothalamate clearance
I-131, ^{131}I
   iodine-131
      ^{131}I paraaminohippuric acid
I-alpha-hydroxyvitamin D3
IAS
   internal anal sphincter
   intraabdominal sepsis
iatrogenic
   i. chymobilia
   i. coagulopathy
   i. colitis
   i. enterocele
   i. hypercalcemia
   i. hypercalcemic nephrolithiasis
   i. immunodeficiency syndrome
   i. intraoperative ureteral injury
   i. malabsorption
   i. pancreatic trauma
   i. pneumothorax
   i. prostatourethral-rectal fistula
   i. rectourethral fistula
   i. tumor perforation
   i. urolithiasis
IB
   ibuprofen
IBB
   intestinal brush border
IBC
   iron-binding capacity
IBD
   inflammatory bowel disease
IBDQ
   Inflammatory Bowel Disease
      Questionnaire
ibotenic acid
IBS
   inflammatory bowel syndrome
   irritable bowel syndrome
IBS-D
   irritable bowel syndrome
      diarrhea-predominant
IBStat
ibuprofen (IB)
IBW
   ideal body weight
ICA
   islet cell antibody
      ICA test
ICAM-1
   intercellular adhesion
    molecule-1

ICC
   interstitial cells of Cajal
ICDB
   Interstitial Cystitis Data Base
ice
   i. cooling
   i. slush
ice-cold sucrose buffer
iced
   i. intestine
   i. lactated Ringer solution
   i. saline
   i. saline lavage
Iceland moss
IceSeeds
ice-water
   i.-w. swallow
   i.-w. test
ICG
   indocyanine green
      ICG clearance
      ICG dye
      ICG test
ICGN, IC-GN
   immune complex glomerulonephritis
iChem urine chemistry analyzer
ichthyismus exanthematicus
ICIT
   intracavernosal injection therapy
**icodextrin 7.5% peritoneal dialysis
solution**
ICP
   intrahepatic cholestasis of pregnancy
**ICR strain-derived glomerular nephritis
(ICGN)**
ICS
   International Continence Society
ICSI
   intracytoplasmic sperm injection
ICT
   isolated cortical tubule
ictal
icteric
   i. necrosis
   i. sclerae
   i. skin
icterogenic
icterohepatitis
icteroid
icterus
   benign familial i.
   conjunctival i.
   i. gravidarum
   i. gravis
   Hayem i.

icterus (*continued*)
    i. melas
    i. neonatorum
    i. praecox
    scleral i.
ictometer
ictus
I&D
    incision and drainage
idarubicin
IDD
    intraluminal duodenal diverticulum
IDDM
    insulin-dependent diabetes mellitus
IDE
    insulin-degrading enzyme
ideal
    i. body weight (IBW)
    i. patient profile
identifiable intrascrotal lesion
identification
    colonic lesion i.
    lesion i.
IDH
    intradialytic hypotension
    intramural duodenal hematoma
idiopathic
    i. achalasia
    i. adulthood ductopenia
    i. ammonemia
    i. ascites
    i. autoimmune cholangitis
    i. autoimmune chronic hepatitis
    i. bile acid malabsorption
    i. calcium renal stone formation
    i. chronic erosion
    i. chronic erosive gastritis
    i. colitis
    i. constipation
    i. crescentic glomerulonephritis
    i. diffuse ulcerative nongranulomatous enteritis
    i. edema
    i. enteropathy
    i. esophageal ulcer (IEU)
    i. fibrosing pancreatitis
    i. fibrous retroperitonitis
    i. gastric acid secretion
    i. gastroparesis
    i. hematuria
    i. hemochromatosis
    i. hypercalciuria
    i. hypereosinophilic syndrome (IHES)
    i. hyperlipidemia
    i. hyperoxaluria
    i. hypertrophic gastropathy
    i. hypertrophic pyloric stenosis

    i. hypocomplementemic interstitial nephritis
    i. infertility
    i. inflammatory bowel disease (IIBD)
    i. intestinal pseudoobstruction
    i. megacolon
    i. megarectum
    i. membranous glomerulonephritis
    i. myointimal hyperplasia of mesenteric vein
    i. nephralgia
    i. nephrotic syndrome
    i. nonfamilial visceral neuropathy
    i. obstruction
    i. portal hypertension (IPH)
    i. proctitis
    i. proctocolitis
    i. rapidly progressive glomerulonephritis (IRPGN)
    i. recurrent pancreatitis (IRP)
    i. retroperitoneal fibrosis (IRF)
    i. steatorrhea
    i. thrombocytopenic purpura
    i. unconjugated hyperbilirubinemia
    i. varix
    i. volvulus
idiotype-antiidiotype interaction
idioventricular
IDL
    intermediate density lipoprotein
IDPN
    intradialytic parenteral nutrition
idremcinal
IDST
    intraductal secretin test
IDUS
    intraductal ultrasonography
    intraductal ultrasound
IDWG
    interdialytic weight gain
IEBD
    intraesophageal balloon distention
IEC
    intestinal epithelial cell
IEC-6 cell
IEHL
    intracorporeal electrohydraulic lithotripsy
IEL
    intraepithelial leukocyte
    intraepithelial lymphocyte
        IEL T cell
IEM
    ineffective esophageal motility
IEU
    idiopathic esophageal ulcer

I-FABP
intestinal fatty acid-binding protein
human serum I-FABP
IFE
immunofixation electrophoresis
Ifex, Taxol, Platinol (ITP)
IFN
interferon
IFN alfa
IFN alfa-2b therapy
IFN alfa therapy
IFNa, IFN-alpha
interferon alfa
IFNa-2a
interferon alfa-2a
IFN-G
interferon gamma
IFN-gamma
IFOBT
immunologic fecal occult blood
test
IFP
inflammatory fibroid
polyp
IG
image guide
intragastric
IG bundle
Ig
immunoglobulin
IgA
immunoglobulin A
IgA antigliadin
IgA deficiency
dimeric IgA
IgA EMA
endomysial IgA
gliadin IgA
IgA glomerulonephritis
IgA immunologic study
jejunal IgA
IgA kappa-chain myeloma
IgA nephropathy
IgA neuropathy
IgA polymerization
secretory IgA (sIgA)
IgA tTG
IgA tTG assay
IgA1
immunoglobulin A1
IgA2
immunoglobulin A2
IgA-producing cell
IGCCCG
International Germ Cell Cancer
Collaborative Group
IGCCCG classification
IgD
immunoglobulin D

IgE
immunoglobulin E
IgE titer
IGF
insulinlike growth
factor
IGF-1
insulinlike growth factor-1
exogenous IGF-1
IGF-2
insulinlike growth factor-2
IGF-binding protein-1 mRNA
IGFBP-1
insulinlike growth factor-binding
protein-1
IGFBP-3
insulinlike growth factor-binding
protein-3
IGFBP-3 complex
IGF-1R
insulinlike growth factor-1R
IFG-1R mRNA
IFG-1R RNA
IgG
immunoglobulin G
IgG AGA
IgG alpha gliadin antibody
IgG anti-HAV-positive
horseradish peroxidase-conjugated
antirabbit IgG
IgG immunologic study
polyclonal IgG
IgG reticulin antibody
IgG serology
IgG1
immunoglobulin G1
IgG4
immunoglobulin G4
IgG2a
immunoglobulin G2a
IgG2a antibody
IgG-producing cell
IgG4
immunoglobulin G4
IgG4 titer
Iglesias
I. fiberoptic resectoscope
I. method of aspiration
IgM
immunoglobulin M
IgM antigliadin
IgM anti-HAV
IgM anti-HAV antibody
IgM anti-HBc antibody
anti-Helicobacter pylori
IgM
IgM immunologic study
monoclonal IgM
IgM nephropathy

IgM-HA
 IgM-hepatitis A
  IgM-HA antibody
IgM-hepatitis
  I.-h. A (IgM-HA)
  I.-h. E virus (IgM-HEV)
IgM-HEV
 IgM-hepatitis E virus
  IgM-HEV antibody titer
IGS
 implantable gastric stimulation
IGV
 isolated gastric varix
  IGV type 1, 2
IHA
 indirect hemagglutination
 intrahepatic atresia
  IHA determination
IHb
 hemoglobin content index
IHD
 intermittent hemodialysis
IHES
 idiopathic hypereosinophilic syndrome
IHPS
 infantile hypertrophic pyloric stenosis
IIBD
 idiopathic inflammatory bowel
  disease
IIEF
 International Index of Erectile
  Function
IIF
 indirect immunofluorescence
I1307K allele
IK allele
IkBa protein
IL
 interleukin
  IL 750 AA spectrophotometer
IL-1
 interleukin-1
IL-2
 interleukin-2
IL-6
 interleukin-6
IL-8
 interleukin-8
IL-10
 interleukin-10
  recombinant I.-10
ILA
 inferolateral angle
  ILA surgical stapler
ILC
 interstitial laser coagulation
ILDL
 intermediate low density lipoprotein
ileac

ileal
 i. artery
 i. artery stent
 i. atresia
 i. biopsy
 i. bladder
 i. blood vessel
 i. brake
 i. conduit urinary diversion
 i. crypt
 i. duplication cyst
 i. effluent
 i. follicle
 i. ileoscopy
 i. inflow tract
 i. interposition
 i. intestinal antireflux valve
 i. J pouch
 i. loop
 i. loopography
 i. low-pressure bladder substitute
 pouch
 i. low-pressure reservoir
 i. Malone cecostomy
 i. neobladder
 i. neobladder urinary diversion
 i. neobladder urinary pouch
 i. nipple valve
 i. orthotopic bladder substitute
 i. outflow tract
 i. papilla
 i. patch ureteroplasty
 i. pouch-anal anastomosis (IPAA)
 i. pouch-distal rectal anastomosis
 i. pullthrough
 i. reflux
 i. resection
 i. reservoir construction
 i. reservoir evacuation
 i. segment
 i. sleeve
 i. S pouch
 i. spout
 i. stasis
 i. ureter
 i. ureteral substitution
 i. urinary conduit
 i. varix
 i. W pouch
ileales
 arteriae i.
ilealis
 papilla i.
ileectomy
ileitis
 backwash i.
 Crohn i.
 distal i.
 granulomatous i.

I

Meckel i.
obstructive dysfunctional i.
pouch i.
prestomal i.
regional i.
terminal i.
ileoanal
  i. anastomosis
  i. endorectal pullthrough
  i. pouch
  i. pullthrough procedure
  i. reservoir
ileoascending colostomy
ileocecal
  i. bladder
  i. continent urinary reservoir
  i. cutaneous diversion
  i. fat pad
  i. insufficiency
  i. intestinal antireflux valve
  i. intussusception
  i. junction
  i. papilla
  i. pouch
  i. region
  i. resection
  i. segment
  i. segment transposition
  i. sphincter
  i. syndrome
  i. tuberculosis
  i. ureterocolostomy
  i. valve lipohyperplasia
ileocecale
  ostium i.
ileocecalis
  frenulum valvae i.
  plica i.
  valva i.
ileocecocystoplasty bladder augmentation
ileocecostomy
ileocolectomy
ileocolic, ileocolonic
  i. anastomosis
  i. artery
  i. bladder
  i. Crohn disease
  i. fold
  i. intussusception
  i. neobladder
  i. plexus
  i. pouch
  i. pouch urinary diversion
  i. resection
  i. transit
  i. vessel
ileocolica
  arteria i.

ileocolitis
  Crohn i.
  transmural i.
  tuberculous i.
  i. ulcerosa chronica
ileocolonic (*var. of* ileocolic)
ileocolonoscopy
ileocolostomy
  endloop i.
  LeDuc-Camey i.
ileocolotomy
ileoconduit
ileocystoplasty
  Camey i.
  clam i.
  LeDuc-Camey i.
ileocystostomy
  cutaneous i.
ileoentectropy
ileogastric reflex
ileogastrostomy
ileogram
ileography
  endoscopic retrograde i.
ileoileal intussusception
ileoileostomy
ileojejunitis
ileopexy
ileoproctostomy (IP)
ileorectal anastomosis (IRA)
ileorectostomy
ileorenal bypass
ileorrhaphy
ileoscopy
  ileal i.
ileosigmoid
  i. anastomosis
  i. colostomy
  i. fistula
  i. knot
ileosigmoidostomy
ileostogram
ileostomate
ileostomy
  i. bag
  Bishop-Koop i.
  blowhole i.
  Brooke i.
  i. closure
  continent i.
  i. cup
  Dennis-Brooke i.
  i. diarrhea
  diversionary i.
  diverting loop i.
  double-barrel i.
  i. effluent
  end i.
  endloop i.

ileostomy (*continued*)
Goligher extraperitoneal i.
incontinent i.
J-loop i.
Kock continent i.
Kock reservoir i.
loop end i.
mucosal i.
permanent loop i.
pouched i.
i. rod
split i.
i. stoma
temporary loop i.
terminal i.
Turnbull end-loop i.
ileotomy
ileotransverse
i. colon anastomosis
i. colostomy
ileotransversostomy
ileovesical
i. anastomosis
i. fistula
ileovesicostomy
continent i.
incontinent i.
laparoscopy-assisted ileocystoplasty
and i.
Monti-Yang i.
transverse retubularized i.
Yang-Monti i.
Ile-Sorb absorbent gel
ileum
antimesenteric border of distal i.
collapsed i.
duplex i.
hose-pipe appearance of
terminal i.
neoterminal i.
i. nipple
terminal i.
ileus
adhesive i.
adynamic i.
colonic i.
dynamic i.
focal i.
gallbladder i.
gallstone i.
gastric i.
hyperdynamic i.
mechanical i.
meconium i.
occlusive i.
paralytic i.
i. paralyticus
postoperative i.
spastic i.

i. subparta
terminal i.
verminous i.
iLEX skin protectant paste
ilia (*pl. of* ilium)
iliac
i. artery
i. artery aneurysm
i. artery embolization
i. bend
i. colon
i. crest
i. fossa
i. fossa dissection
i. roll
i. spine
i. vein
iliac-to-renal artery bypass graft
iliacus muscle
iliococcygeus
i. fixation
i. muscle
iliocolotomy
iliohypogastric nerve
ilioinguinal
i. nerve
i. ring
iliopectineal line
iliopsoas
i. ring
i. sign
i. test
^{131}**I-lipiodol isotope**
ilium, *pl.* **ilia**
ILL
intracorporeal laser lithotripsy
illness
foodborne i. (FBI)
severe morbid i.
illuminated St. Mark retractor
illumination system
ilodecakin
Ilopan
iloprost
Ilosone
Ilotycin
Ilozyme
IL-2, -3, -4, -6, -8 receptor
ILS
intraluminal stapler
ILUS
intraluminal ultrasound
ILUS catheter
IM
intramuscular
Rocephin IM
image
i. analysis
axial i.

B-mode ultrasound i.
i. cytometry
endoanal fast spin-echo T2-weighted
  MR i.
i. guide (IG)
i. guide bundle
HAP i.
longitudinal i.
point-counting i.
probe i.
i. processing
sagittal i.
spin-echo T1-weighted MR i.
thumbnail i.
transverse i.
T1-weighted i. (T1WI)
T2-weighted i. (T2WI)
image-guided therapy
Imagent GI
image-processing unit
imager
Tesla Signa MR i.
imaging
anorectal i.
autofluorescence and
  reflectance i.
biomarker-based i.
bladder i.
i. bladder support
B-mode i.
color flow Doppler i.
complete urological i.
Doppler color flow i.
endoanal magnetic resonance i.
endorectal coil magnetic
  resonance i.
endoscopic ultrasonographic i.
endoscopic video autofluorescence i.
functional magnetic resonance i.
  (fMRI)
gallium i.
gray-scale i.
hyperspectral i.
internet-based digital i.
LaparoScan laparoscopic
  ultrasonic i.
magnetic endoscopic i.
magnetic resonance i.
  (MRI)
i. method
mucosal i.
narrow-band i.
nuclear hepatobiliary i.
parathyroid i.
photodynamic i.
planar i.
radiolabeled i.
radionuclide renal i.
renal helical CT i.

RHCT i.
sonoelasticity i.
technetium i.
i. technology
thallium i.
thermal i.
transcutaneous ultrasound i.
uniplanar i.
imaging-guided minimally invasive
  procedure
imapatumumab
imatinib mesylate
imbalance
acid-base i.
imbedded microtransducer
imbricate, imbricated
imbricated (*var. of* imbricate)
IMCD
inner medullary collecting duct
IMED 430 enteral feeding pump
Imerslund syndrome
imidazole
i. aminoaciduria
i. carboxamide
imidoacetic acid radioactive agent
imiglucerase
iminodiacetic acid (IDA)
iminoglycinuria
imipenem
imipenem-cilastatin
imipramine hydrochloride
imiquimod
immature teratoma
IMMC
intestinal mucosal mast cell
intravesical mitomycin C
immediate blush
immersion
i. cooling
water i.
immitis
Candida i.
immoCare fecal occult blood test
immortelle
immotile cilia syndrome
ImmTher
Immu-4
Immudia-HemSp
ImmuFact® IMP321
Immulite
I. 2000 anti-HBc IgM analyzer
I. 2000 free PSA assay
I. 2000 HBsAg immunoanalyzer
I. HBsAg immunoassay analyzer
I. 2000 third-generation PSA assay
immune
i. complex glomerulonephritis
  (ICGN, IC-GN)
i. deficiency

immune (*continued*)
    i. electron microscopy
    i. rabbit antibody
    i. response
    i. serum
    i. serum globulin
    i. signaling
    i. suppression
    i. system
immune-enhancing diet
immune-mediated
    i.-m. infertility
    i.-m. interstitial nephritis
    i.-m. reaction
immunity
    acquired i.
    adaptive i.
    cell-mediated i.
    cellular i.
    humoral i.
    immunologic i.
    innate i.
    natural i.
    nonimmunologic i.
immunization
    DNA i.
    parenteral i.
immunoadsorption
immunoanalyzer
    Elecsys 1010, 2010 i.
    Immulite 2000 HBsAg i.
immunoassay
    Abbott TDx monoclonal fluorescence polarization i.
    Advia Centaur HAV IgM i.
    Advia Centaur HBc Total i.
    Cytoscreen Human Eotaxin i.
    Elecsys anti-HBs i.
    enzyme i. (EIA)
    hepatitis C virus enzyme i.
    Magic Lite chemiluminometric i.
    microparticle enzyme i. (MEIA)
    rapid enzyme i.
    RIVA HCV 2.0 Strip i.
    second-generation enzyme i. (EIA-2)
    TDx fluorescence polarization i.
immunobead
    i. assay
    i. reacting antigen
immunobiology
immunoblot test
ImmunoCard
    I. serum antibody test
    I. STAT!
    I. STAT! Rotavirus test
immunocompetency
immunocompetent host

immunocompromised host
immunocyte
immunocytochemical stain
immunocytochemistry
    vacuolar-type proton pump i.
immunocytology
ImmunoCyt test
immunodeficiency
    acquired i.
    common variable i. (CVID)
    i. disease
    severe combined i. (SCID)
immunodepression
immunodiffusion
    radial i.
    i. test
immunodominant T-cell epitope
immunoelectrophoresis
immunoenhancing
immunofixation electrophoresis (IFE)
immunofluorescence
    indirect i. (IIF)
    i. microscopy
    negative i.
immunofluorescent antibody test
immunogen
    enteric i.
immunogenic gene
immunoglobulin (Ig)
    i. A (IgA)
    i. A1 (IgA1)
    i. A2 (IgA2)
    i. A endomysial antibody
    i. A nephropathy
    anti-gp330 i. G
    i. A transglutaminase antibody (IgA tTG)
    biliary i.
    i. D (IgD)
    i. E (IgE)
    i. G (IgG)
    i. G1 (IgG1)
    i. G4 (IgG4)
    i. G2a (IgG2a)
    i. G2a antibody
    i. G antigliadin antibody (IgG AGA)
    i. G clearance
    i. G4 staining
    hepatitis B i. (HBIg)
    intravenous i. (IVIg)
    i. M (IgM)
    i. neuropathy
    secretory i. A
    i. superfamily adhesion molecule
immunohistochemical
    i. detection
    i. method

i. stain
i. staining
immunohistochemistry
p53 i.
immunohistology
Immuno I complex PSA test
immunologic, immunological
i. abnormality
i. fecal occult blood test
(IFOBT)
i. immunity
i. rapid urease test
immunological (*var. of* immunologic)
immunology
intestinal i.
immunomodulator
immunomodulatory
i. action
i. gene therapy
immunonephelometry
immunoneutralization
immunoperoxidase
light and electron i.
i. stain
i. staining
i. staining technique
immunophenotypical profiling of patient
immunopositivity
immunoprecipitation
**immunoproliferative small intestinal
disease (IPSID)**
immunoradiometric assay (IRMA)
immunoreactive
i. methionine-enkephalin (IRME)
i. trypsin enzyme
i. trypsinogen (IRT)
immunoreactivity
cholecystokinin-like i. (CCK-LI)
PYY-like i.
vasoactive intestinal polypeptide i.
(VIP-IR)
immunoregulator
immunoregulatory drug
immunoscintigraphy
^{111}In-CYT-103 i.
immunosorbent
immunostain
immunostaining
Fas i.
HBcAg i.
in situ i.
i. of transversely sectioned tubule
i. technique
immunostimulating complex (ISCOM)
immunosuppressant
antiproliferative i.
cornerstone i.
immunosuppressed patient

immunosuppression
posttransplant i.
immunosuppressive
i. agent
i. drug
i. regimen
i. therapy
immunosurveillance
immunotactoid
i. glomerulonephritis
i. glomerulopathy (ITGP)
immunotherapy
adoptive i.
BCG i.
intravesical i.
Pacis BCG bladder cancer i.
specific i.
immunotyping
Imodium
I. A-D
I. Advanced
IMP321
ImmuFact® IMP321
impact
I. lithotriptor system
I. nutritional supplement
i. of donor hypertension
i. of microwave antenna on
treatment outcome
impacted
i. ampullary stone
i. calculus
i. cystic duct
i. feces
i. stool
i. ureteral stone
impaction
acute esophageal food i. (AEFI)
endoscope i.
fecal i.
food bolus i.
meat i.
rectal i.
stone and basket i.
impactor
electromechanical i. (EMI)
stone i.
impaired
i. cell differentiation
i. colonic motor function
i. gastric absorption
i. lecithin synthesis
i. regeneration syndrome (IRS)
i. urinary concentrating ability
impairment
anabolic steroid spermatogenesis i.
ethanol-specific i.
memory i.

impar
impassable ureter
impedance
    i. epigastrography
    intraluminal electrical i.
    i. planimetry
    i. plethysmography (IPG)
    rectal i.
impedancometry
    intraluminal electrical i.
    multiple intraluminal i.'s
imperforate
    i. anus
    i. hymen
implant
    Alpha I penile i.
    BrachySeed Pd-103 i.
    Contigen Bard collagen i.
    Deflux injectable i.
    Deflux system i.
    Dynaflex penile i.
    Enteryx i.
    i. erosion
    Flexi-Flate penile i.
    gold seed i.
    histrelin i.
    Hydroflex penile i.
    iridium 192 wire i.
    islet cell i.
    Jonas i.
    leuprolide acetate i.
    Lifecath peritoneal i.
    Macroplastique i.
    malleable i.
    palladium-103 seed i.
    penile i.
    PTQ i.
    Rapid Strand i.
    i. reabsorption
    retropubic i.
    Septopal i.
    Surgitek Flexi-Flate II penile i.
    Tegress endoscopic urethral i.
    testicular i.
    transperineal seed i.
    Zoladex i.
implantable
    i. gastric stimulation (IGS)
    i. gastric stimulation system
    i. neuromodulation system
    i. penile venous compression device
    i. pulse generator (IPG)
implantation
    artificial genitourinary sphincter i.
    artificial urinary sphincter i.
    bulbous urethral cuff i.
    Enteryx i.
    gastric balloon i.
    intracavitary i.

    i. metastasis
    metastatic i.
    i. of prosthetic material
    penile prosthesis i.
    percutaneous transperineal seed i.
    radioactive seed i.
    real-time 3D biplanar transperineal
      prostate i.
    second-cuff i.
    ureter i.
    ureterointestinal i.
important risk factor
impotence, impotency
    arteriogenic i.
    diabetic i.
    ejaculatory i.
    Esteem advanced vacuum therapy
      for i.
    functional i.
    organic i.
    orgastic i.
    paretic i.
    psychic i.
    psychogenic i.
    secondary i.
    symptomatic i.
    vasculogenic i.
    venogenic i.
    venous leak i.
impotency (*var. of* impotence)
impotentia
    i. coeundi
    i. erigendi
Impra graft
impressio (*var. of* impression), (*pl.*
  impressiones)
    i. esophagealis hepatis
impression, impressio
    colic i.
    colon i.
    digastric i.
    duodenal i.
    esophageal i.
    gastric i.
    liver i.
    renal i.
    suprarenal i.
impressiones
Impress Softpatch
imprinting
    genomic i.
improved
    i. graft survival
    i. visualization
improvement
    clinical i.
    subjective i.
IMPT
    intensity-modulated proton therapy

IMRT
  intensity-modulated radiation therapy
Imuran
IMx
  isobutyl-methyl-xanthine
    IMx Hg assay
    IMx PSA system
¹¹¹In, In-111
  indium-111
    In-111 pentetreotide
In
  indium
in
    i. situ
    i. situ end labeling (ISEL)
    i. situ hybridization
    i. situ immunostaining
    i. utero programming
    i. vitro
    i. vitro clearance
    i. vitro compatibility
    i. vitro fertilization (IVF)
    i. vitro incubation
    i. vitro model
    i. vitro synergism
    i. vivo
    i. vivo clearance
    i. vivo microscopy
    i. vivo veritas
inactivated pepsin (IP)
inactivation
    oncogene i.
inactive
    i. Crohn disease
    i. schistosomiasis
inactivity
    physical i.
inadequate
    i. bowel preparation
    i. dilation
inadvertent enterotomy
in-and-out catheterization
inanimate simulator
inanition fever
inapparent hepatitis
Inapsine
inborn error of metabolism
inbreeding coefficient
Inc.
  Incorporated
    Enteron Pharmaceuticals, Inc.
    Kidney Urology Foundation of
      America, Inc.
    Pediatric Crohn's and Colitis
      Association, Inc.
    Vision Sciences Inc. (VSI)
incarcerated
    i. bowel
    i. intrathoracic hernia

    i. omentum
    i. prolapse
    i. snare
incarceration
    colon i.
    colonoscopy-related i.
    hernia i.
    penile i.
    string method for treatment of
      penile i.
    i. symptom
InCare PRES 9300 system
incidence
    angle of i.
    gallstone i.
    i. of acute rejection
    i. of bacteremia
incidental
    i. adenoma
    i. appendectomy
    i. splenectomy
incidentaloma
    adrenal gland i.
incipient
    i. nephropathy
    i. proteinuria
Incise pouch
incision
    Amussat i.
    i. and drainage (I&D)
    anterolateral thoracotomy i.
    apron skin i.
    Battle i.
    Battle-Jalaguier-Kammerer i.
    Bevan abdominal i.
    bilateral subcostal i.'s
    bilateral transabdominal i.'s
    bucket-handle i.
    burrowing i.
    buttonhole i.
    celiotomy i.
    Cheatle-Henry i.
    Cherney i.
    chevron i.
    choledochotomy i.
    circumumbilical i.
    cold-knife i.
    Connell i.
    cruciate i.
    Czerny-Kocher-Perthes i.
    darting i.
    Deaver i.
    dorsal lumbotomy i.
    eleventh rib flank i.
    eleventh rib transperitoneal i.
    elliptical i.
    endopyelotomy i.
    endoscopic i.
    endourologic cold-knife i.

incision (*continued*)
    enterotomy i.
    epigastric i.
    extended left subcostal i.
    fishmouth i.
    flank i.
    Gibson i.
    Gil-Vernet dorsal
      lumbotomy i.
    gridiron i.
    groin i.
    guillotine i.
    Heineke-Mikulicz i.
    hockey stick i.
    infraumbilical i.
    inguinal i.
    inverted-U abdominal i.
    Joel-Cohen i.
    Kammerer-Battle i.
    Kehr i.
    Kocher i.
    LaRoque herniorrhaphy i.
    less morbid lower abdominal
      transverse i.
    i. line
    lower abdominal transverse i.
    low transverse i.
    lumbodorsal i.
    lumbotomy i.
    Mallard i.
    McBurney i.
    median i.
    midabdominal transverse i.
    midline lower
      abdominal i.
    midline upper abdominal i.
    minilaparotomy i.
    mini-Pfannenstiel i.
    modified Gibson i.
    muscle-cutting i.
    muscle-splitting i.
    oblique i.
    omega-shaped i.
    paramedian i.
    pararectus i.
    perineal i.
    Pfannenstiel i.
    plaque i.
    posterior transthoracic i.
    precut i.
    pyelotomy i.
    4-quadrant i.
    radial i.
    relaxing i.
    Rockey-Davis i.
    Salmon backcut i.
    Sanders i.
    Schuchardt relaxing i.
    smiling i.

    stab i.
    steri-stripped i.
    subcostal flank i.
    subcostal transperitoneal i.
    supracostal i.
    surgical i.
    teardrop i.
    thoracoabdominal i.
    transperitoneal anterior subcostal i.
      (TASI)
    transpubic i.
    transurethral i. (TUI)
    transverse semilunar skin i.
    Turner-Warwick i.
    unilateral subcostal i.
    vertical midline i.
    Wangensteen i.
    xiphoid-to-pubis midline
      abdominal i.
    xiphoid-to-umbilicus i.
    Y-shaped i.

incisional
    i. biopsy
    i. corporoplasty
    i. hernia

incisor

incisura, incisure, *pl.* **incisurae**
    i. angularis
    i. dextra of Gans
    i. vesicae felleae hepatis

incisurae (*pl. of* incisura)

incisure (*var. of* incisura)

inclusion
    i. body
    concentric hyaline i.
    i. cyst
    glomerular endothelial myxovirus-like
      microtubular i.
    glycogen i.
    intracytoplasmic tuboreticular i.
    tubuloreticular i. (TRI)

incompatible
    ABO i.

incompetence, incompetency
    gastroesophageal i.
    LES i.
    neurogenic sphincteric i.

incompetency (*var. of* incompetence)

incompetent
    i. ileocecal valve
    i. sphincter

incomplete
    i. basal cell hyperplasia
    i. cirrhosis
    i. duplication
    i. hernia
    i. pancreas divisum (IPD)
    i. passage
    i. polypectomy

i. rectal prolapse
i. relaxation
i. voiding
inconspicuous penis
incontinence, incontinentia
adolescent i.
anal i.
anatomic stress i.
anterior fecal i.
bladder i.
Blaivas classification of urinary i.
bowel i.
continuous i.
daytime i.
diurnal i.
double i.
extraurethral i.
fecal i.
flatus i.
functional i.
genuine stress i. (GSI)
genuine stress urinary i. (GSUI)
geriatric i.
gravity urinary i.
hyperreflexic motor urge i.
ischemic fecal i.
mixed i.
mixed urinary i. (MUI)
Miyazaki-Bonney test for stress i.
neurogenic refractory urge i.
nocturnal i.
overflow fecal i.
pad test for urinary i.
paradoxical i.
paralytic i.
passive i.
postprostatectomy i.
posttraumatic i.
postvoid i.
rectal i.
recurrent stress i.
reflex i.
refractory motor urge i.
i. related
Resident Assessment Protocol for i.
i. score
secondary i.
sphincteric i.
stool i.
stress i. type 0, I, II, III
stress urinary i. (SUI)
i. surgery
Teflon paste injection for i.
transdermal oxybutynin for urinary
   i.
unconscious i.
urge i.
urgency i.
urge urinary i. (UUI)

urinary exertional i.
urinary stress i.
incontinent
i. epispadias
i. ileostomy
i. ileovesicostomy
incontinentia (*var. of* incontinence)
i. alvi
i. urinae
incoordination
pharyngeal-UES i.
Incorporated (Inc.)
increased
i. bladder permeability
i. clinical demand
i. in proportion
i. peritoneal clearance
i. risk of penile carcinoma
incretin
incrustation
i. analysis
i. deposition
i. of biomaterial
i. of stent
stent i.
incrusted
i. cystitis
i. pyelitis
i. ureteral stent
incubation
in vitro i.
incurable cancer
Incystene
^{111}In-CYT-103 immunoscintigraphy
indapamide
indentation
haustral i.
independent
i. positive predictive factor
i. predictor
i. risk factor
Inderal
Indermil adhesive
indeterminate colitis (IC)
index, *pl.* **indices**
American Urological Association
   symptom i.
apoptotic i.
AUA symptom i.
biliary saturation i.
body mass i. (BMI)
Bouchard i.
BPH impact i. (BII)
brachial pressure i.
Broder i.
cardiac output/cardiac i. (CO/CI)
CD activity i.
cholesterol saturation i. (CSI)
Clinical Activity I. (CAI)

i. carmine stain
i. carmine-stained normal saline
I. diffuse fiber
I. LaserOptic treatment system
I. Optima laser
I. Optima laser system
indinavir calculus
indinavir-induced nephrolithiasis
indirect
i. bilirubin
i. hemagglutination (IHA)
i. hemagglutination determination
i. hernia sac
i. immunofluorescence (IIF)
i. immunofluorescence assay
i. immunolocalization technique
i. inguinal hernia
indispensable diagnostic modality
indium (In)
i. 64-labeled white blood cell scan
i. leukocyte scan
i. pentetreotide
indium-111 (^{111}In, In-111)
i.-111 DTPA
i.-111 murine anti-CEA monoclonal antibody
i.-111 pentetreotide
^{111}indium-labeled autologous leukocyte test
indium-labeled leukocyte scan
individual
intermediate cystinuric i.
i. parameter
individualization
Indocin
indocyanine
i. green (ICG)
i. green clearance
i. green dye
indolalkylamine alkaloid
indole
indolent
i. bubo
i. radiation-induced rectal ulcer
indomethacin (IM, IMT, IND, INDO)
indomethacin-induced mucosal damage
indoramin
indoxyl
indoxyluria
induced nitric oxide synthase (iNOS)
inducer
interferon i.
induction
c-fos i.
indurated appendix
induration
bowel wall i.
fibroid i.
granular i.

indurative nephritis
industrial toxin
indwelling
i. stomal device
i. ureteral stent
i. urinary catheter
ineffective
i. colonic propulsion
i. erythropoiesis
i. esophageal motility (IEM)
inertia
colonic i.
inevitable postoperative pain
infancy
melanotic neuroectodermal tumor of i. (MNTI)
infant
i. esophagoscope
i. reflex
infantile
i. celiac disease
i. colic
i. diarrhea
i. food protein-induced enterocolitis syndrome
i. gastroenteritis
i. hypertrophic pyloric stenosis (IHPS)
i. leishmaniasis
i. nephrotic syndrome
i. pellagra
i. polycystic disease (IPCD)
infantilism
Herter i.
sexual i.
infantis
Bifidobacterium i.
Salmonella i.
infantum
cholera i.
Leishmania i.
Leishmania donovani i.
infarct, infarction
bile i.
bilirubin i.
Brewer i.
small-bowel i.
uric acid i.
Zahn i.
infarcted bowel
infarction, infarct
acute nonocclusive bowel i.
intestinal i.
mesenteric i.
myocardial i. (MI)
nonocclusive intestinal i.
occlusive i.
omental i.
segmental ileal i.

infarction (*continued*)
 segmental testicular i.
 small-intestinal i.
 total i.
infected
 i. bile duct
 i. pancreatic necrosis (IPN)
 i. pseudocyst
 i. tract
infection
 active systemic bacterial i.
 adenovirus i.
 i. after renal transplantation
 antifungal esophageal i.
 antifungal-resistant opportunistic i.
 Aspergillus i.
 asymptomatic urinary tract i.
  (AUTI)
 bacterial i.
 biomaterial-associated i.
 bladder *Candida* i.
 bloodstream i. (BSI)
 i. calculus
 Candida i.
 candidal i.
 catheter-related bloodstream i.
  (CR-BSI, CRBI, CRBSI)
 catheter tunnel i.
 Chlamydia trachomatis i.
 CMV i.
 coliform urinary i.
 coxsackievirus i. A, B
 cryptosporidial i.
 cytomegalovirus i.
 deep-seated fungal i.
 dengue hemorrhagic fever i.
 dermatophyte i.
 device-related urinary tract i.
 dialysis access i.
 Diphyllobothrium latum i.
 Diphyllobothrium nihonkaiense i.
 disseminated CMV i.
 domiciliary urinary tract i.
 echovirus i.
 enteric i.
 epididymal i.
 Epstein-Barr virus i.
 esophageal fungal i.
 exit site i.
 extrapulmonary *Pneumocystis carinii*
  i.
 fungal i.
 gas-forming pyogenic liver i.
 geriatric urinary tract i.
 helmintic i.
 hematogenic spread of i.
 hepatic candidal i.
 hepatitis i. A-E
 herpes simplex i.

HIV i.
intestinal i.
intraabdominal i.
isolated urinary tract i.
liver cyst i.
metasynchronous bacterial urinary
 tract i.
monilial i.
multiple hepatitis virus i.'s
Mycobacterium i.
necrotizing i.
nematode i.
nosocomial fungal i.
nosocomial urinary tract i.
Okadaella gastrococcus i.
opportunistic i.
parasitic i.
pediatric urinary tract i.
perianal i.
perineal i.
peristomal i.
peritoneal fungal i.
pneumococcal i.
polymicrobial i.
Polyomavirus i.
postsplenectomy i.
preventing urinary tract i.
i. prevention device
recurrent urinary tract i.
renal allograft i.
renal cyst i.
retroperitoneal i.
retrovirus i.
rotavirus i.
seminal vesicle i.
i. stone
strongyloid i.
synchronous urinary tract i.
torulopsis i.
tunnel i.
uncomplicated urinary tract i. (UUTI)
unresolved urinary tract i.
urinary tract i. (UTI)
varicella-zoster i.
Vibrio fetus i.
viral i.
whipworm i.
wound i.
infection-related interstitial nephritis
infectious
 i. avian nephrosis
 i. colitis
 i. complication
 i. esophagitis
 i. gastroenteritis
 i. hepatitis
 i. jaundice
 i. mononucleosis heterophil antibody
 i. nosocomial diarrhea

i. pancreatic necrosis
i. splenomegaly
i. viral diarrhea
infective
i. jaundice
i. splenomegaly
INFeD
Infergen
inferior
i. aberrant ductule
i. adrenal vein
i. anal nerve
i. anal plexus
arteria epigastrica i.
arteria mesenterica i.
arteria pancreatica i.
arteria rectalis i.
i. digital fossa
i. duodenal fold
i. extremity
i. fascia
fascia diaphragmatis pelvis i.
flexura duodeni i.
i. hemorrhoidal artery
i. hypogastric plexus
i. mesenteric artery
i. mesenteric vein
i. pancreatic artery
i. pancreaticoduodenal artery
i. phrenic artery
plica duodenalis i.
i. pole
i. rectal nerve
i. rectal vein
i. vena cava (IVC)
i. vena cava thrombosis
inferiores
arteriae pancreaticoduodenales i.
inferolateral angle (ILA)
inferomedial
infertility
i. androgyny
idiopathic i.
immune-mediated i.
tubal i.
infestation
Ascaris i.
biliary i.
Fasciola hepatica i.
parasitic i.
infiltrate
chronic inflammatory cell i.
lobular inflammatory i.
lobular mononuclear cell i.
MN i.
mononuclear histiocytic portal i.
PMN i.
polymorphonuclear inflammatory i.
sparse inflammatory i.

infiltrating
i. adenocarcinoma
i. inflammatory cell
i. T cell
infiltration
bacterial mucosal i.
cellular i.
colonic i.
fat i.
focal fatty i.
gastric epithelial cell i.
glomerular macrophage i.
glomerular neutrophil i.
lymphohistiocytic i.
massive malignant i.
neutrophilic i.
panmucosal inflammatory cell i.
perirectal fat i.
plasma cell portal i.
portal plasma cell i.
serosal i.
tumor i.
infiltrative
i. disease
i. lymphoma
inflamed
i. appendix
i. diverticulum
i. gallbladder
i. mucosa
inflammation
cervical i.
evidence of i.
Hara classification of gallbladder i.
interstitial i.
intralobular i.
kidney i.
i. marker
microbiliary i.
parenchymatous i.
periportal i.
portal eosinophilic i.
portal tract i.
refractory pouch i.
transmural i.
traumatic i.
tubulointerstitial i.
vaginal i.
inflammatoria
dysphagia i.
inflammatory
i. bowel disease (IBD)
I. Bowel Disease Questionnaire (IBDQ)
i. bowel syndrome (IBS)
i. colitis
i. diarrhea
i. fibroid polyp (IFP)
i. glomerulopathy

inflammatory (*continued*)
    i. myofibroblastic tumor (IMT)
    i. pancreatitis
    i. polyp-fold complex (IPFC)
    i. prostatic mass (IPM)
    i. pseudotumor
    i. reaction
    i. renal mass
    i. response
inflatable penile prosthesis (IPP)
inflated rubber cylinder
inflator
    LeVeen i.
InflatoRing
infliximab IV infusion
influenzae
    Haemophilus i.
influenza virus
influx
    Rb i.
infold
infolding
    complex papillary i.
Informatics
    American College of Medical I.
    (ACMI)
infracolic compartment
infradiaphragmatic radiotherapy
infragastric pancreatoscopy
infrahepatic vena cava
inframammary region
inframesocolic compartment
infraorbital
infrared
    i. coagulation
    i. coagulator
    i. endoscopy
    i. photocoagulation
    i. spectroscopy
    i. transillumination gastroscopy
    i. videoendoscope
infrarenal template procedure
infraumbilical
    i. incision
    i. mound
infravesical prostatic obstruction
infrequent
    i. defecation
    i. voider-lazy bladder syndrome
Infumorph
infundibular
    i. neck
    i. stenosis
    i. width
infundibuliform
infundibulopelvic
    i. angle
    i. ligament
    i. stenosis

infundibuloplasty
infundibulum
    calyceal i.
    lower i.
    i. of bile duct
    i. of gallbladder
    single midline calyceal i.
Infusaid
    I. chemotherapy implantable pump
    I. hepatic pump
infuser, infusor
    UROS i.
infusion
    acid i.
    atropine i.
    Avastin IV i.
    BabyBIG powder for IV i.
    bladder i.
    circadian-shaped i.
    citrate i.
    continuous ambulatory i.
    hepatic arterial i. (HAI)
    hypertonic i.
    infliximab IV i.
    Infuvite Pediatric IV i.
    insulin/glucagon i.
    intraarterial vasopressin i.
    intraduodenal lipid i.
    intravariceal i.
    intravenous urea i.
    intravenous vasopressin i.
    lipid i.
    monooctanoin i.
    multiple vitamins for i.
    i. nephrotomography
    Normosol-M IV i.
    pentagastrin i.
    Protonix IV powder for i.
    i. pump (IP)
    i. pyelography
    Remicade IV i.
    saline i.
    solvent i.
    total dose i.
    transcatheter arterial i.
    vasopressin i.
infusor (*var. of* infuser)
Infuvite Pediatric IV infusion
ingested
    i. foreign body
    i. foreign object
ingestion
    acid i.
    alkali i.
    battery i.
    button battery i.
    caustic i.
    cocaine package i.
    fish bone i.

I

foreign body i.
lye i.
mercuric oxide battery i.
razor blade i.
safety pin i.
Ingold M3, M4 glass electrode pH monitor
ingrowth
  mesodermal i.
  i. of tumor
inguinal
  i. adenopathy
  i. bulge
  i. canal
  i. cord
  i. crease
  i. crease compound nevus
  i. cryptorchidism
  i. floor
  i. fold
  i. hernia
  i. incision
  i. laparoscopy
  i. ligament
  i. ligament of Blumberg
  i. lymphadenectomy
  i. lymphadenopathy
  i. lymph node
  i. orchiectomy
  i. orchiopexy
  i. reservoir inserter
  i. ring
  i. sphincter
  i. triangle
  i. varicocelectomy
inguinale
  granuloma i.
  hernia uteri i.
inguinoabdominal
inguinocrural
inguinofemoral hernia
inguinoperitoneal
inguinoscrotal hernia
inguinosuperficial hernia
inhalation aerosol
inhaler
  Allis i.
  Vanceril i.
inherent to linkage
inheritance
  kallikrein i.
inherited defect
inhibin
  beta i.
inhibition
  alcohol dehydrogenase i.
  5-alpha-reductase i.
  antisense DNA i.
  i. assay

bladder i.
COX-1 i.
COX-2 i.
cyclooxygenase i.
deglutitive i.
detrusor muscle i.
effect of i.
glycolytic i.
laminin receptor i.
lipoxygenase i.
micturition reflex i.
presynaptic i.
renin i.
secretory leukocyte proteinase i. (SLPI)
spinobulbospinal micturition reflex i.
inhibitor
  ACE i.
  alkaline protease i. (API)
  alpha-glucosidase i.
  5-alpha-reductase i.
  angiotensin-converting enzyme i. (ACEI)
  aromatase i.
  ATPase i.
  azasteroid i.
  BILN 2061 protease i.
  Bowman Birk protease i.
  calcineurin i.
  carbonic anhydrase i. (CAI)
  C-1 esterase i.
  chain-terminating i.
  collagen synthesis i.
  COX-2 i.
  cyclin-dependent kinase i.
  cyclooxygenase i.
  cyclooxygenase-2 i.
  cytolysis i.
  familial lipoprotein lipase i.
  gastric acid pump i.
  hepatocyte proliferation i. (HPI)
  hexapeptide i.
  H+/K+-ATPase acid pump i.
  HMG-CoA reductase i.
  inter-alpha-trypsin i.
  5-lipoxygenase i.
  lipoxygenase i.
  metalloproteinase i.
  monoamine oxidase i. (MAOI)
  nitric oxide synthase i.
  nonnucleoside reverse transcription i. (NNRTI)
  pancreatic secretory trypsin i. (PSTI)
  PDE5 i.
  phosphodiesterase i. (PDE-I)
  plasminogen activator i. (PAI)
  plasminogen activator i. type 1, 2 (PAI-1, -2)

inhibitor (*continued*)
- protease i.
- proteinase i.
- proton pump i. (PPI)
- purine synthesis i.
- rapamycin i.
- rectoanal i.
- RNAse i.
- sertraline serotonin reuptake i.
- serum alpha$_1$-protease i.
- topoisomerase I i.
- trypsin i.
- tumor-derived angiogenic i.
- urinary trypsin i. (UTI)
- VX950 protease i.
- wheat amylase i.

inhibitory
- i. effect
- i. intestinointestinal reflex
- i. postsynaptic potential (IPSP)
- i. syndrome

InhibiZone coating
inhomogeneity of parenchyma
inhomogeneous hyperechoic mass
initial
- i. broad-spectrum therapy
- i. clinical experience
- i. hematuria
- i. in-plan record
- i. proximal diversion
- i. treatment

initiation
- micturition reflex manual i.
- voiding i.

initiative
- Clinical Outcomes Research I. (CORI)
- Dialysis Outcomes Quality I. (DOQI)
- Kidney Disease Outcomes Quality I. (K/DOQI)
- National Kidney Foundation-Data Outcomes Quality I. (NKF-DOQI)

InjecAid system
injectable
- i. ester
- Macroplastique i.

injection
- adrenalin i.
- Albunex i.
- Antizol for i.
- BayGam IM i.
- BCG live intravesical i.
- Benzacot i.
- biopolymer i.
- botulinum toxin i.
- Bovie GAX collagen i.
- BTX i.
- Camptosar i.
- i. catheter
- collagen i.
- corpus cavernosum papaverine i.
- cyanoacrylate i.
- cyanocobalamin i.
- daptomycin for i.
- depot i.
- diazepam emulsified i.
- Dibent i.
- doxercalciferol i.
- Eligard sustained-release subcu i.
- endoscopic botulinum toxin i.
- endoscopic epinephrine i.
- endoscopic India ink i.
- endoscopic ultrasound-guided fine-needle i.
- endosonographically targeted i.
- enoxaparin sodium i.
- ERxin multicomponent penile i.
- ethanol i.
- etoposide i.
- fibrin i.
- follitropin alfa for i.
- glutaraldehyde crosslinked collagen i.
- i. gold probe
- Hectorol i.
- Histoacryl i.
- intracytoplasmic sperm i. (ICSI)
- intralesional steroid i.
- intraperitoneal i.
- intrasphincteric botulinum toxin i.
- intravariceal i.
- iopamidol i.
- iron sucrose i.
- lipiodol i.
- local depot i.
- meropenem for i.
- moxisylyte i.
- ^{99m}Tc DISIDA contrast i.
- mycophenolate mofetil intravenous for i.
- N-butyl-2-cyanoacrylate i.
- 2-octyl cyanoacrylate i.
- papaverine i.
- paravariceal i.
- PEG-interferon alfa-2b powder for i.
- PEG-Intron powder for i.
- percutaneous ethanol i. (PEI)
- periurethral collagen i.
- PGE$_1$ i.
- Plenaxis powder for IM i.
- polidocanol i.
- Polytef i.
- polytetrafluoroethylene paste i.
- polytetrafluoroethylene periurethral i.
- Renovist i.
- sclerosant i.
- i. sclerosis
- i. sclerotherapy

sham i.
i. site
sodium hyaluronate i.
sodium morrhuate i.
sodium tetradecyl i.
somatropin i.
submucosal saline i.
submucosal Teflon i.
subureteric Teflon i. (STING)
synthetic porcine secretin for i.
tangential colonic submucosal i.
technetium-99m Exametazime i.
i. therapy
Tisseel fibrin sealant i.
transduodenal i.
Twinrix IM i.
zoledronic acid for i.
Zometa for i.
Zorbtive powder for subcu i.

injector
Olympus i.
Teflon i.
Virag i.

InjecTx cystoscope
injured allograft
injury
acid i.
Ajmalin liver i.
alcohol-induced gastric i.
alkaline i.
antecedent pancreatic i.
bile salt i.
bladder i.
blast i.
blunt testicular i.
bowel i.
cavernous artery i.
cell-mediated hepatic i.
closed i.
comparison of depth of tissue i.
diaphragmatic i.
drug-induced acute hepatic i.
duodenal i.
emetogenic i.
gastric mucosal i.
gastroduodenal mucosal i.
glomerular i.
Helicobacter-induced gastric i.
hemorrhagic radiation i.
hepatic vein i.
hepatocellular i.
H_2O_2-induced i.
hyperfiltration i.
hypertensive renal i.
iatrogenic intraoperative ureteral i.
intestinal radiation i.
ischemia-reperfusion i.
juxtahepatic venous i.
liver transplantation preservation i.

major deceleration i.
medication-induced i.
microangiopathic renal i.
mitochondrial i.
mucosal i.
NSAID-induced gastric i.
NSAID-induced intestinal i.
obstetric i.
open i.
oxidant i.
oxidative cell i.
pancreatic i.
paraquat-induced upper
  gastrointestinal i.
pill-induced esophageal i.
pinch i.
PMN-mediated endothelial
  cell i.
radiation i.
rectal i.
renovascular i.
reperfusion i.
scrotum avulsion i.
spinal cord i. (SCI)
splenic i.
straddle i.
stress-related mucosal i.
treatment of nonspecific
  inflammatory i.
tubular epithelial cell i.
tubular morphologic i.
tubulointerstitial i.
ureteral i.
urethra blowout i.
vascular i.

ink
autoclaved India i.
China i.
Endomark India i.
Higgins India i.
India i.
Koh-I-Noor Universal India i.
osmolarity of i.
Pelikan brand India i.
solution-diluted India i.

inlay
Turner-Warwick i.

Inlay-Tabs
Ursinus I.-T.

inlet
esophageal i.
i. patch
i. patch mucosa
i. port
i. pouch (IP)
thoracic i.

[111]In-leukocyte technique
inline blood gas monitor
innate immunity

inner
- i. crossbar
- i. diameter
- i. medulla
- i. medullary collecting duct (IMCD)

innervation
- adrenal gland i.
- afferent i.
- bladder i.
- cholinergic i.
- intrinsic excitatory i.
- kidney i.
- pelvis i.
- prostate gland i.
- rectal i.
- seminal vesicle i.
- serosal afferent i.
- striated muscle i.

innocens
- *Serpulina i.*

innocent gallstone

innocuous

Innoflex variable-stiffness colonoscope

Innohep

Inno-LiPA assay

innominate
- i. bone
- i. groove

Innova home incontinence therapy system

inoculated medium

inoculum size

inorganic iodine

inosine monophosphate dehydrogenase (IMPDH)

inositol
- i. lipid
- i. ring
- i. triphosphate (IP3)
- i. 1,4,5-triphosphate
- i. 1,4,5-triphosphate Ca2+

input
- fast cholinergic i.
- nociceptive sensory i.

InScope optical dilator

insemination
- intrauterine i. (IUI)
- subzonal i. (SUZI)

insensible loss of water

insert
- FemSoft i.
- Hollister convex i.
- Nu-Hope convex i.
- Reliance urinary control i.
- Sur-Fit Natura disposable convex i.
- United Surgical convex i.
- urinary control urethral i.

inserter
- Furlow cylinder i.
- inguinal reservoir i.

insertion
- biliary endoprosthesis i.
- chromosome i.
- jejunal tube i.
- J-tube i.
- i. mutation
- PEG i.
- Sengstaken-Blakemore tube i.
- subclavian catheter i.
- i. tube

InSIGHT
- I. manometry
- I. manometry system

insignificant
- clinically i.

insipidus
- congenital nephrogenic diabetes i. (CNDI)
- diabetes i.
- nephrogenic diabetes i. (NDI)
- neurogenic diabetes i.

insorption

inspiration

inspiratory

inspissated
- i. bile
- i. bile syndrome
- i. feces
- i. sump syndrome

instability
- bladder postcystourethropexy i.
- chromosome i.
- detrusor i. (DI)
- detrusor muscle i.
- genomic i.
- microsatellite i. (MSI)

instant
- i. camera
- Hydrocil I.
- i. photography

instantaneous clearance

InStent EsophaCoil stent

instillation
- intravesical i.
- i. therapy

Institute-1640
- Roswell Park Memorial I.-1640 (RPMI-1640)

instituted GI bleeding management program

institutional
- i. colon
- i. dysentery

institutionalized patient

instrument
- Accurate Surgical and Scientific I.'s (ASSI)
- automated anastomotic i.
- Bard Biopty i.
- Bard BladderScan bladder volume i.
- biopsy i.
- BIP biopsy i.
- Corneometer MPA5 i.
- i. count
- Crit-Line i.
- Digestive Health Status I. (DHSI)
- Dilamezinsert urologic i.
- DMI urologic i.
- Duette double-lumen ERCP i.
- endosonography i.
- ERBE electrical coagulation i.
- ERBE electrical cutting i.
- gauge of i.
- GIA i.
- grasping i.
- guide-eye i.
- mechanical radial scanning i.
- oblique forward-viewing i.
- quality-of-life i.
- Quinton suction biopsy i.
- Radiometer 85 i.
- Roboprep G i.
- Sharpoint cutting i.
- slotted i.
- small-diameter endosonographic i.
- spring-loaded-type biopsy i.
- standardized i.
- Tewameter MPA5 i.

instrumentation
- biliary i.
- Karl Storz i.
- Microvasive i.
- retrograde i.

instrument-track seeding

insufficiency
- acute renal i. (ARI)
- adrenal i.
- angiotensin-converting enzyme inhibition in progressive renal i. (AIPRI)
- chronic renal i. (CRI)
- exocrine pancreatic i. (EPI)
- gastric i.
- gastromotor i.
- hepatic i.
- ileocecal i.
- pancreatic exocrine i.
- primary adrenal i.
- progressive renal i.
- pyloric i.
- renal i.
- underlying chronic renal i.
- vascular i.
- velopharyngeal i. (VPI)

insufflation
- air i.
- colonic i.
- helium i.
- i. of stomach

insufflator
- carbon dioxide i.
- nitrous oxide i.
- PROTOCO$_2$L i.

Insuflon insulin delivery device
insular structure
insulated
- i. curved scissors
- i. straight scissors

insulated-tip electrosurgical knife
insulation-tipped electrosurgical knife
insulin
- human i.
- i. hyperplasia
- Lente i.
- NPH i.
- protamine zinc i.
- i. reaction
- i. receptor-related receptor
- i. resistance
- i. resistance syndrome
- Semilente i.
- i. sensitivity index
- i. stain
- Ultralente i.

insulin-degrading enzyme (IDE)
insulin-dependent
- i.-d. diabetes
- i.-d. diabetes mellitus (IDDM)

insulin/glucagon
- i./g. infusion
- putative hepatotrophic factors i./g.

insulinlike
- i. growth factor (IGF)
- i. growth factor-1 (IGF-1)
- i. growth factor-2 (IGF-2)
- i. growth factor-binding protein-1 (IGFBP-1)
- i. growth factor-binding protein-3 (IGFBP-3)
- i. growth factor-1R (IGF-1R)

insulinoma
insulinopenia
insulin-transferrin-sodium selenite
insulin-treated diabetic
insult
- ischemic i.

InSure
- I. brush sampling
- I. immunochemical fecal occult blood test

intact
> i. hormone assay
> i. PTH

intake
> i. and output (I&O)
> caloric i.
> clandestine i.
> daily protein i. (DPI)
> dietary energy i.

Intal

Integra bilayer wound dressing

integrase gene

integrated
> i. assessment
> i. automatic stone-tissue detection system
> i. clearance

integrating spherical power meter

integration
> Advanced Systems I. (ASI)

integrin
> alpha-3 beta-1 i.
> alpha-5 beta-1 i.
> B1, B2 i.
> beta-1 chain i.
> i. mediated
> membrane-spanning i.

integrity
> gut barrier i.
> mucosal i.

integument

intensified radiographic imaging system (IRIS)

intensity
> fluorescence i.
> fluorescent light i. (FLI)
> light fluorescent i.

intensity-modulated
> i.-m. proton therapy (IMPT)
> i.-m. radiation therapy (IMRT)

intention
> delayed primary i.
> healing by first i.
> healing by primary i.
> healing by second i.
> healing by secondary i.

intentional injection of Enteryx

intentionem
> healing per primam i.
> healing per secundam i.

IntePro polypropylene mesh

interaction
> bacterial host i.
> cell-cell i.
> cervical mucus-sperm i.
> crystal-cell i.
> crystal-phospholipid i.
> idiotype-antiidiotype i.
> protein-crystal i.

> shock wave-gas bubble i.
> vasoactive peptide-cytokine i.

interactive video technology

inter-alpha inhibitor family

inter-alpha-trypsin inhibitor (ITI)

intercalated cell

intercalatum
> *Schistosoma i.*

intercapillary nephrosclerosis

Interceed absorbable adhesion barrier

intercellular
> i. adhesion molecule-1 (ICAM-1)
> i. space

Intercept
> I. esophagus microcoil
> I. prostate microcoil
> I. urethra microcoil

interceptive conditioning

Interceptor M3 triple-channel solid-state monitor

intercolonoscopy

interconversion

intercostal
> i. pedicle esophagogastropexy
> i. scan
> i. space

intercourse
> receptive anal i.

interdialytic
> i. urea generation
> i. weight gain (IDWG)

interdigestive
> i. antroduodenal motility
> i. migrating motor complex
> i. myoelectric complex

interdigitate

interdigitating teeth

interface
> fluid-air i.
> i. hepatitis

interference
> bacterial i.
> i. barrier filter
> catheter bacterial i.
> ribonucleic acid i.

interferential electrical stimulation

interferon (IFN)
> i. alfa (IFNa)
> alfa i.
> i. alfa-2a (IFNa-2a)
> i. alfa 2-beta
> i. alfa-2b therapy
> i. alfacon-1
> i. alfa-n1
> i. alfa-n3
> i. alfa therapy
> alpha-2a i.
> beta i.
> i. beta (IFN beta)

consensus i. (CIFN)
gamma i.
i. gamma (IFN-G)
i. gamma stimulation
high-dose consensus i.
human lymphoblastoid i. (L-IFN)
i. inducer
low-dose i.
pegylated i.
recombinant human alfa i.
i. sensitivity determining region
i. treatment
type I i.
interferon-stimulated
i.-s. gene (ISG)
i.-s. regulatory element (ISRE)
interfoveolar muscle
Intergel
I. adhesion prevention solution
I. irrigating solution
interhaustral
i. fold
i. septum
interiliacus
plexus i.
Intering vascular graft
interlabial
i. rhabdomyosarcoma
i. sarcoma botryoid
interleukin (IL)
interleukin-1 (IL-1)
i.-1 receptor antagonist
interleukin-1b urinary marker
interleukin-2 (IL-2)
i.-2 receptor-blocking agent
recombinant i.-2 (rIL-2)
serum i.-2
interleukin-6 (IL-6)
serum i.-6
interleukin-8 (IL-8)
serum i.-8
interleukin-10 (IL-10)
interlobar
i. renal artery
i. vein
interlobular
i. bile duct
i. fibrosis
interlobulares
ductuli i.
interlocking
i. detachable coils
i. ligature
interloop abscess
intermedia
Yersinia i.
intermediate
i. biomarker
i. cystinuric individual

i. density lipoprotein (IDL)
i. fasting
i. filament bundle
i. junction
i. low density lipoprotein (ILDL)
i. mesenteric lymph node
i. polyposis
i. space
thiol i.
intermedius
Citrobacter i.
intermesenteric abscess
intermicrovillar area
intermittent
i. calcitriol therapy
i. catheterization
i. click
i. diarrhea
i. drip feeding
i. hemodialysis (IHD)
i. hemoglobinuria
i. hepatic fever
i. hormone therapy
i. obstruction
i. pain
i. positive-pressure breathing (IPPB)
i. proteinuria
i. pulse
i. self-catheterization (ISC)
i. self-obturation
i. suctioning
interna
elastica i.
fascia spermatica i.
lamina rara i. (LRI)
internal
i. abdominal fascia
i. abdominal ring
i. absorption
i. anal sphincter (IAS)
i. biliary drainage
i. biliary lavage
i. biliary stent
i. cremaster of Henle
i. fiberoptic cable
i. hemorrhage
i. hemorrhoid
i. iliac artery
i. iliac vein
i. inguinal ring
i. oblique
i. oblique fascia
i. oblique muscle
I. Ostomy Association (IOA)
i. procidentia
i. proctotomy
i. pudendal artery
i. pudendal vein
i. rectal sphincter

internal (*continued*)
    i. ribosome entry site
    i. rotation
    i. septation
    i. spermatic fascia
    i. spermatic vessel
    i. sphincterotomy
    i. urethrotomy
international
    i. androgen unit
    I. Association for Enterostomal
      Therapy
    I. Autoimmune Hepatitis Group
      score
    I. Biomedical microcapillary infusion
      system
    I. Continence Society (ICS)
    I. Continence Society classification
      of voiding dysfunction
    I. Continence Society voiding
      function classification
    I. Foundation for Functional
      Gastrointestinal Disorders
    I. Germ Cell Cancer Collaborative
      Group (IGCCCG)
    I. Germ Cell Cancer Collaborative
      Group classification
    Hepatitis Foundation I.
    I. Index of Erectile Function (IIEF)
    I. Prognostic Index score
    I. Prostate Symptom Score (IPSS)
    i. unit of male hormone
    i. units per liter (IU/L)
internet-based digital imaging
interneuron
    enteric i.
internist tumor
internodal strand
internum
    ostium urethrae i.
interobserver reliability
interosseous
interpersonal sensitivity
interphase PBMC
interpolar region
interposition
    colonic i.
    i. Dacron graft
    i. flap of omentum
    ileal i.
    jejunal pouch i. (JPI)
    omental i.
    i. operation
interrogans
    Leptospira i.
interrupted
    i. manual mucomucosal absorbable
      suture
    i. seromuscular suture

intersex
    i. condition
    i. gonad
intersexual
    adult i.
intersexuality
intersphincteric
    i. anal fistula
    i. anorectal space
    i. groove
    i. perirectal abscess
    i. plane
    i. rectal dissection
    i. resection
    i. sulcus
InterStim device
interstitial
    i. brachytherapy
    i. cells of Cajal (ICC)
    i. cell tumor of testis
    i. collagenase
    i. cystitis
    I. Cystitis Data Base
      (ICDB)
    i. diffusion
    i. diode
    i. fibroblast
    i. fibrosis
    i. gastritis
    i. hernia
    i. hypercellularity
    i. immunocompetent cell
    i. inflammation
    i. irradiation
    i. laser coagulation
      (ILC)
    i. laser thermoablation
    i. mononuclear cell
    i. pancreatitis
    i. photodynamic therapy
    i. photon radiation energy
    i. rejection
    i. scarlatinal nephritis
    i. syphilitic nephritis
    i. volume
interstitium
    medullary i.
    renal i.
intersymphyseal stitch
intersymphysial bar
intertriginous region
intertrigo
    candidal i.
intertropical hypovolemia
intereureteral
intereureteric ridge
interval
    i. appendectomy
    confidence i.

I

intervention
    angiographic i.
    endoscopic i.
    urologic i.
interventional
    i. technique
    i. uroradiology
interventricular defect
interview (IV)
intestinal
    i. absorption
    i. absorptive cell
    i. adaptation
    i. amebiasis
    i. anastomosis
    i. angina
    i. anthrax
    i. antireflux valve
    i. atony
    i. atresia
    i. atrophy
    i. bacterium
    i. bag
    i. biopsy
    i. brush border (IBB)
    i. bypass
    i. calculus
    i. capillariasis
    i. channelopathy
    i. clamp
    i. colic
    i. colonization
    i. concretion
    i. contents
    i. decompression
    i. distention
    i. distomiasis
    i. diverticulum
    i. emphysema
    i. endocrine cell
    i. endoscopy
    i. enterocyte
    i. epithelial cell (IEC)
    i. fatty acid-binding protein
    (I-FABP)
    i. fistula
    i. fixation
    i. flora
    i. hemorrhage
    i. histoplasmosis
    i. immunology
    i. indigestion
    i. infarction
    i. infection
    i. intoxication
    i. intussusception
    i. ischemia
    i. juice
    i. lactase deficiency

    i. lamina propria
    i. lipodystrophy
    i. loop
    i. lumen
    i. lymphangiectasis
    i. malrotation
    i. metaplasia type I—III
    i. motility disorder
    i. mucosa
    i. mucosal mast cell
    (IMMC)
    i. myiasis
    i. myoneurosis
    i. myxoneurosis
    i. necrosis
    i. obstruction
    i. parasite
    i. peptide
    i. peptide TFF3
    i. perforation
    i. perfusion
    i. permeability
    i. permeability measurement
    i. phlebectasia
    i. pneumatosis
    i. polyposis
    i. polyposis-cutaneous pigmentation
    syndrome
    i. prolapse
    i. protozoa
    i. pseudoobstruction
    i. radiation injury
    i. schistosomiasis
    i. sedative
    i. sling
    i. sling placement
    i. spirochete
    i. stasis
    i. stasis syndrome
    i. steatorrhea
    i. stenosis
    i. stricture
    i. surgery
    i. tract
    i. transit study
    i. tuberculosis
    i. ureteral replacement
    i. viability
    i. villous architecture
    i. villus
    i. volvulus
    i. web
intestinale
    Encephalitozoon i.
intestinales (*pl. of* intestinalis)
intestinalis (*pl.* intestinales)
    arteriae intestinales
    Giardia i.
    mycosis i.

intestinalis (*continued*)
    pneumatosis cystoides i. (PCI)
    Septata i.
    trunci intestinales
intestine
    bacterial metabolism in i.
    blind i.
    Crohn small i.
    distal i.
    empty i.
    iced i.
    jejunoileal i.
    kink in i.
    malrotation of i.
    milking of i.
    papillary adenoma of large i.
    segmental i.
    small i.
    straight i.
    villous coat of small i.
intestinofugal neuron
intestinogastric reflex
intestinointestinal
intimal
    i. fibroplasia
    i. hyperplasia
intimin
intolerance
    dietary protein i.
    disaccharide i.
    fatty food i.
    fructose i.
    glucose i.
    hereditary fructose i. (HFI)
    lactose i.
intoxication
    acute methanol i.
    alcohol i.
    drug i.
    intestinal i.
    metal i.
    methanol i.
    quinidine i.
    systemic mercury i.
intraabdominal
    i. abscess
    i. actinomycosis
    i. adhesion
    i. bile leakage
    i. desmoid tumor
    i. hemorrhage
    i. ileal reservoir
    i. infection
    i. mass
    i. pressure
    i. pressure gauge
    i. sepsis (IAS)
    i. transverse testicular ectopia
    i. viscus

intraanal
    i. electromyography
    i. pressure
    i. wart
intraaortic endovascular sonography
intraappendicular
intraarterial
    i. chemotherapy
    i. chemotherapy catheter
    i. digital subtraction angiography
    i. vasopressin infusion
intraassay precision
intraballoon pressure
intrabulbar fossa
intracapillary thrombosis
intracapsular dissection
intracaval
    i. surgery
    i. tumor
intracavernosal
    i. injection therapy (ICIT)
    i. injection treatment
    i. pressure
intracavernous
    i. injection and stimulation test
    i. injection therapy
intracavitary
    i. application brachytherapy
    i. implantation
    i. radiation boost therapy
    i. topical therapy
    i. transducer
intracellular
    i. acidity
    i. acification
    i. buffering
    i. fluid (ICF)
    i. flush effect
    i. pH
    i. pool
    i. potassium
    i. signaling system
intracellulare
    Mycobacterium i.
intracholedochal
    i. manometric catheter
    i. pressure
    i. stent
intracisternal
IntraCoil nitinol stent
intracolonic Kaposi sarcoma
intracorporeal
    i. anastomosis
    i. electrohydraulic lithotripsy
    (IEHL)
    i. injection therapy
    i. laser lithotripsy (ILL)
    i. lithotripsy
    i. lithotriptor

    i. needle breakage
    i. shock wave lithotripsy (ISWL)
    i. therapy of erectile dysfunction
intracranial pressure monitoring
intracrine negative feedback modulator
intractable
    i. constipation
    i. diarrhea
    i. tumor
    i. ulcer
    i. ulcerative colitis
    i. vomiting
intracuticular suture
intracystic epithelial proliferation
intracytoplasmic
    i. calcium
    i. CMV inclusion body
    i. mucin
    i. sperm injection (ICSI)
    i. tuboreticular inclusion (TRI)
intradermal, intradermic
    i. suture
    i. tattooing technique
intradermic (*var. of* intradermal)
intradialytic
    i. hypotension (IDH)
    i. parenteral nutrition (IDPN)
    i. period
    i. symptom
intradiverticular papilla
IntraDose gel
Intraducer peritoneal cannula
intraductal
    i. cholangioscopy
    i. endoscope
    i. imaging catheter
    i. lithiasis
    i. mucin-hypersecreting neoplasm
    i. mucin-producing tumor
    i. oncocytic papillary neoplasia
    (IOPN)
    i. papillary and mucinous tumors
    i. papillary and mucinous tumors of
    pancreas
    i. papillary-mucinous neoplasm
    (IPMN)
    i. papillary-mucinous tumor
    (IPMT)
    i. papillary tumor (IPT)
    i. pressure
    i. secretin test (IDST)
    i. ultrasonography (IDUS)
    i. ultrasound (IDUS)
    i. ultrasound probe
intraduodenal lipid infusion
intraepiploic hernia
intraepithelial
    i. body
    i. cancer

    i. leukocyte (IEL)
    i. lymphocyte (IEL)
    i. lymphocytosis
intraesophageal
    i. acid test
    i. balloon distention (IEBD)
    i. peristaltic pressure
    i. pH
    i. pH monitoring (EpMH)
    i. pH test
    i. stent
    i. variceal pressure
intrafamilial clustering of *Helicobacter pylori*
intragastric (IG)
    i. acidity
    i. balloon
    i. bubble
    i. continuous pH-meter
    i. drip
    i. EGF
    i. gallstone
    i. hydrolysis
    i. pH
    i. pH mapping
    i. pH monitor record
    i. pressure
    i. volume
intraglandular fluid
intraglomerular
    i. hemodynamics
    i. hypertension
    i. mesangial cell
    i. pressure
intragraft
intrahaustral contraction ring
intrahepatic
    i. abscess
    i. antigen-dependent
    lymphocyte-hepatocyte
    i. artery-systemic shunt
    i. ascariasis
    i. atresia (IHA)
    i. AV fistula
    i. bile duct
    i. biliary cystic dilation
    i. biliary duct hypoplasia
    i. biliary stricture
    i. cholangioenterostomy
    i. cholangiojejunostomy
    i. cholelithiasis
    i. cholestasia (IHC, IHPC)
    i. cholestasis of pregnancy (ICP)
    i. ductal dilation
    i. hematoma
    i. hepatitis
    i. invasion
    i. lymphocyte
    i. portal hypertension

intrahepatic (*continued*)
  i. portal obstruction
  i. radicle
  i. sclerosing cholangitis
  i. spontaneous arterioportal fistula
  i. stone
intrailiac hernia
intrajejunal
intralesional
  i. steroid injection
  i. treatment
intralipid fat emulsion
intralobar
intralobular
  i. fibrosis
  i. inflammation
intraluminal
  i. clot
  i. cyst
  i. distention
  i. duodenal diverticulum (IDD)
  i. electrical impedance
  i. electrical impedancometry
  i. esophageal pressure
  i. filling defect
  i. gas bubble
  i. lipolysis
  i. manometry
  i. pH-pressure relationship
  i. pouch
  i. pressure recording
  i. probe
  i. proliferation
  i. radiotherapy
  i. reference electrode
  i. silastic esophageal stent
  i. stapler (ILS)
  i. stone
  i. ultrasound (ILUS)
  i. urethral pressure
intramembranous particle strand
intramesenteric
  i. abscess
  i. desmoid tumor
intramucosal
  i. cancer
  i. carcinoma
  i. metastasis
intramural
  i. air dissection
  i. aneurysm
  i. atheromatous disease
  i. colonic air
  i. diverticulum
  i. duodenal hematoma (IDH)
  i. fistulous tract
  i. ganglion
  i. incision technique
  i. intestinal hemorrhage

  i. lesion
  i. microvessel density
  i. secretory reflex
  i. ureter
intramuscular (IM)
  i. perineural stimulation graciloplasty
intranuclear CMV inclusion body
intraoperative
  i. angiography
  i. autologous transfusion
  i. biliary endoscopy
  i. cavernous nerve stimulation
  i. cholangiogram (IOC)
  i. cholangiography (IOC)
  i. complication
  i. electron beam radiotherapy
  i. enteroscopy (IOE)
  i. findings
  i. kidney hypothermia
  i. mortality
  i. penile erection
  i. phlebography
  i. radiation therapy (IORT)
  i. radiotherapy (IORT)
  i. ultrasonography (IOUS)
intrapancreatic
  i. bile duct
  i. nerve
intrapapillary terminus
intraparavariceal procedure
intraparenchymal tumor
intrapelvic
  i. filling defect
  i. somatic fiber
intraperitoneal (IP)
  i. abscess
  i. adhesion
  i. air
  i. bladder rupture
  i. cavity
  i. hemorrhage
  i. hyperthermic chemotherapy (IPHC)
  i. hyperthermic perfusion (IPHP)
  i. injection
  i. onlay mesh (IPOM)
  i. onlay mesh hernia repair (IPOM)
  i. partial cystectomy
  i. perforation
  i. tissue expander
  i. viscus
  i. volume
intraportal endovascular ultrasonography (IPEUS)
intraportally
intraprostatic
  i. characteristic variation
  i. spiral
  i. stent

i. temperature
i. temperature-guided treatment
i. temperature measurement
i. vascularization
i. vasculature
intrapulmonary shunting
intrarectal
i. intussusception
i. retroflexion
i. ultrasonography
intrarenal
i. calculus
i. chemolysis
i. collecting system
i. distribution
i. hemodynamics
i. matrix-degrading enzyme cascade
i. reflux
i. renal artery aneurysm
i. resistive index
i. vascular thrombosis
IntraSonix TULIP laser device
intrasphincteric botulinum toxin injection
intrasplenic pseudocyst
IntraStent DoubleStrut biliary endoprosthesis
intratesticular cyst
intrathecal
i. catheter
i. chemotherapy
intrathoracic
i. esophagogastroscopy
i. esophagogastrostomy
i. Nissen fundoplication
i. stomach
intratubular
i. germ cell neoplasia (ITGCN)
i. obstruction
intratumoral heterogeneity
intraurethral
i. coil
i. PGE$_1$
i. pressure
i. prostaglandin suppository (IPS)
i. swab specimen
i. therapy of erectile dysfunction
intrauterine insemination (IUI)
intravaginal
i. ejaculation latency time (IELT)
i. electrical stimulation
i. torsion
intravariceal
i. ethanolamine oleate
i. infusion
i. injection
i. injection sclerotherapy
i. pressure
intravasation

intravascular
i. instillation of hypericin
i. lipolysis
i. thrombosis
i. ultrasound (IVUS)
i. ultrasound catheter
i. volume
i. volume expansion
intravenous (IV)
i. access (IVAC)
i. albumin
botulism immune globulin i.
i. cholangiogram (IVC)
i. cholangiography (IVC)
i. cholecystography
i. drip
i. drug abuse
i. feeding
i. heme-albumin
i. H2 receptor antagonist
i. hydration
i. hyperalimentation (IVH)
i. immunoglobulin (IVIg)
i. lipid emulsion
i. nitroglycerin
i. nutrition (IVN)
i. pyelogram (IVP)
i. pyelography (IVP)
i. renal angiography
i. secretin test
i. urea infusion
i. urogram (IVU)
i. urography (IVU)
i. vasopressin infusion
intravesical
i. alum
i. alum irrigation
i. anastomosis
i. bacillus Calmette-Guérin
i. BCG
i. capsaicin
i. chemotherapy
i. electromotive drug administration
i. formalin
i. heparin
i. hyaluronic acid
i. immunotherapy
i. instillation
i. migration
i. mitomycin C (IMMC)
i. oxybutynin
i. pressure
i. silver nitrate
i. ureterocele
i. ureterolysis
intrinsic
i. enzymatic activity
i. excitatory innervation
i. factor (IF)

intrinsic (*continued*)
    i. factor secretion
    i. proteinuria
    i. reflex
    i. sensory neuron
    i. sphincter deficiency (ISD)
    i. sphincter dysfunction (ISD)
    i. striated muscle of urethra
    i. striated sphincter
    i. ureteral stricture
    i. ureteropelvic junction obstruction
    i. urethral sphincter

introducer
    Atkinson i.
    Dumon-Gilliard prosthesis i.
    Furlow i.
    i. gun
    KeyMed Nottingham i.
    LapSac i.
    i. method
    Nottingham KeyMed i.
    Nottingham semirigid i.
    pull-apart i.
    semirigid Nottingham i.
    i. set
    split-sheath i.
    Wilson-Cook prosthesis i.

introitus
Introl bladder neck support prosthesis
intromission
Intromit
Intron
    I. A multidose pen
    Rebetol with I.

Intropin
intubate
intubated ureterotomy
intubation
    balloon-assisted i.
    catheter-guidedendoscopic i. (CAGEIN)
    endotracheal i.
    enterocutaneous i.
    esophageal i.
    esophagogastric i.
    i. failure
    gastrointestinal i.
    nasal i.
    nasogastric i.
    nasotracheal i.
    oral i.
    orotracheal i.
    pyloric i.
    terminal ileum i.

intumescence
intumescent
intussuscepted
    i. ileal triple nipple
    i. nipple valve

intussusception
    agonic i.
    appendiceal i.
    bowel i.
    cecocolic i.
    colocolic i.
    double i.
    ileocecal i.
    ileocolic i.
    ileoileal i.
    intestinal i.
    intrarectal i.
    jejunogastric i.
    postmortem i.
    rectal i.
    retrograde i.
    sigmoidoanal i.
    spontaneously reducing i.
    triple i.

intussusceptum
intussuscipiens
inulin
    i. clearance
    plasma i.
    i. solution

Inutest test
invaginated membrane
invaginating ampulla of Vater
invagination
    i. of ampulla
    stomal i.
    stump i.
    i. technique

InVance male sling procedure
Invanz
invariant
    kinetically i.

invasion
    capillary-lymphatic i.
    dermatolymphatic i.
    intrahepatic i.
    neural i.
    i. of adjacent organ
    periportal i.
    stromal i.
    vascular i.
    venous i.
    Wilms tumor
      capsule i.

invasive
    i. adenocarcinoma
    i. carcinoma
    i. colorectal polyp
    i. diagnostic test
    i. enteric pathogen
    i. procedure
    i. surgery
    i. transvaginal approach

invasiveness
> minimal i.
> i. of surgery

inventory
> Ostomy Assessment I. (OAI)
> Urogenital Distress I. (UDI)

invermination

inversely proportional

Inversine

inversion
> i. appendectomy
> chromosome i.
> i. of bladder

inversion-ligation appendectomy

inversus
> abdominal situs i.
> situs i.

inverted
> i. diverticulum of colon
> i. papilloma
> i. sigmoid diverticulum
> i. testis

inverted-U
> i.-U abdominal incision
> i.-U pouch
> i.-U pouch ileal reservoir

inverted-V sign

inverter
> Mayo-Kelly appendix i.

inverting suture

investigation
> clinical i.
> Lapides cystometric i.
> radiologic i.
> urodynamic i.

investing fascia

Invicorp

InView male external catheter

involuntary
> i. guarding
> i. reflex rigidity

involution
> prostate gland i.

involvement
> mediastinal i.
> multifocal i.
> renal i.
> tubercular i.

I&O
> intake and output

IOA
> Internal Ostomy Association

IOC
> intraoperative cholangiogram
> intraoperative cholangiography

iocetamic
> i. acid
> i. acid contrast medium

Iodamoeba buetschlii

iodide
> isopropamide i.
> Lugol i.
> i. nephropathy
> propidium i.

iodinated
> i. contrast agent
> i. contrast material

iodine
> i. dye
> i. hippurate scanning
> inorganic i.
> Lugol i.
> i. scan
> i. staining

iodine-123 iodoamphetamine

iodine-125 (I-125, ^{125}I)
> i.-125 brachytherapy seed

iodine-131 (I-131, ^{131}I)
> radioactive i.-131

iodine-131-labeled metaiodobenzylguanidine

iodipamide
> i. meglumine
> i. meglumine contrast medium
> sodium i.

iodism

iodoamphetamine
> iodine-123 i.

iodoantipyrine clearance

iodochlorhydroxyquin

iodocholesterol scan

Iodoflex pad

iodoform gauze

iodohippurate

iodophor

iodopyracet

iodoquinol

Iodosorb gel

IOE
> intraoperative enteroscopy

iohexol

ion
> i. beam-assisted deposition
> calcium i.'s (Ca2+, Ca^{2+})
> i. channel
> i. chromatography
> hydrogen i.
> i. laser
> phosphate i. (PI)
> potassium i. (K+)

Ionamin

ionizing radiation

ionomycin

ionophore
> calcium i.

ion-sensitive field-effect transistor

ion-specific electrode

iontophoresis

ion-urea
    phosphate i.-u. (PI-urea)
iopamidol
    i. contrast imaging agent
    i. injection
iopanoic
    i. acid
    i. acid contrast medium
IOPN
    intraductal oncocytic papillary
    neoplasia
iopromide
IORT
    intraoperative radiation therapy
    intraoperative radiotherapy
iothalamate
    i. clearance
    i. level
    sodium i.
iothalamate-125
iothalamic acid
iotroxate
    meglumine i.
IOUS
    intraoperative ultrasonography
ioversol
ioxaglate
IP
    ileoproctostomy
    inactivated pepsin
    infusion pump
    inlet pouch
    intraperitoneal
    IP chemotherapy
IP3, IP$_3$
    inositol triphosphate
    inositol 1,4,5-triphosphate
IPAA
    ileal pouch-anal anastomosis
IPCD
    infantile polycystic disease
IPD
    incomplete pancreas divisum
ipecac
    i. abuse
    i. syrup
ipecac-induced
    i.-i. cardiotoxicity
    i.-i. myopathy
    i.-i. vomiting
IPEC-J2 cell
IPEUS
    intraportal endovascular ultrasonography
IPFC
    inflammatory polyp-fold complex
IPG
    impedance plethysmography
    implantable pulse generator

IPH
    idiopathic portal hypertension
IPHC
    intraperitoneal hyperthermic
    chemotherapy
IPHP
    intraperitoneal hyperthermic perfusion
I-Plant brachytherapy seed
IPM
    inflammatory prostatic mass
IPMN
    intraductal papillary-mucinous neoplasm
IPMT
    intraductal papillary-mucinous tumor
IPN
    infected pancreatic necrosis
ipodate contrast medium
IPOM
    intraperitoneal onlay mesh
    intraperitoneal onlay mesh hernia
    repair
      IPOM hernia repair
IPP
    inflatable penile prosthesis
ipratropium
iproniazid
iproniazid-induced jaundice
iproplatin
IPS
    intraurethral prostaglandin suppository
IPSID
    immunoproliferative small intestinal
    disease
ipsilateral adrenalectomy
IPSP
    inhibitory postsynaptic potential
IPSS
    International Prostate Symptom Score
IPT
    intraductal papillary tumor
Ir-192, ^{192}Ir
    iridium 192
    Ir-192 wire
IRA
    ileorectal anastomosis
IRF
    idiopathic retroperitoneal fibrosis
iridectomy scar
iridium
    i. 192 (Ir-192, ^{192}Ir)
    i. 192-loaded stent
    i. prosthesis
    i. ribbon
    i. seed
    i. 192 wire implant
irinotecan hydrochloride
IRIS
    intensified radiographic imaging system

IRMA
immunoradiometric assay
iron (Fe)
i. deficiency
i. deficiency anemia
i. dextran
i. gluconate
i. nephropathy
oral i.
i. overload disease
i. overload disorder
i. poisoning
serum i.
i. shuttle hypothesis
i. storage disease
i. store
i. sucrose
i. sucrose injection
iron-binding capacity (IBC)
iron-dependent oxidant
Irospan
Vitelle I.
IRP
idiopathic recurrent pancreatitis
IRPGN
idiopathic rapidly progressive
glomerulonephritis
irradiate
irradiated tumor vaccine
irradiation
i. effect
external-beam i.
i. failure
half-body i.
hemibody i.
interstitial i.
Nd:YAG laser i.
total body i. (TBI)
total lymphoid i. (TLI)
ultraviolet i.
irreducible hernia
irregular
i. amputated mucosal pattern
i. duct
i. pupil
i. rhythm
irregularity
cervical i.
irretrievable object
irrigant
Neosporin GU i.
irrigating
i. fluid
i. patient
irrigation
acetohydroxamic acid i.
bladder i.
bowel i.

catheter i.
continuous bladder i. (CBI)
copious i.
hemiacidrin i.
H-600 normothermic i.
intravesical alum i.
i. of colostomy
pulsed i.
rectal pulsed i.
rectum i.
Renacidin i.
whole-gut i.
irrigation-fluid absorption syndrome
irrigation-suction
postoperative i.-s.
irrigator
BioShield i.
Sur-Fit Natura Visi-Flow i.
irrigator/aspirator
Nezhat-Dorsey i./a.
irritable
i. bladder
i. bowel syndrome (IBS)
i. bowel syndrome
diarrhea-predominant (IBS-D)
i. colon
i. colon syndrome
i. gut syndrome
i. male syndrome
i. pouch syndrome
i. stricture
i. testis
irritant dermatitis
irritative
i. diarrhea
i. symptom
IRT
immunoreactive trypsinogen
Isaacs-Ludwig arteriole
ISC
intermittent self-catheterization
ischemia
acute gastric i.
acute occlusive mesenteric i.
atherosclerosis-induced cavernosal i.
AVF-induced renal i.
colonic i.
glomerular i.
intestinal i.
kidney i.
mesenteric i.
midgut i.
mucosal i.
myocardial i.
i. necrosis
nonocclusive mesenteric i.
i. or sloughing of flap
outer medullary i.

ischemia (*continued*)
    renal i.
    tubular i.
    visceral i.
    warm i.
ischemia-reperfusion injury
ischemic
    i. bowel
    i. bowel disease
    i. colitis
    i. fecal incontinence
    i. hepatitis
    i. insult
    i. penile gangrene
    i. tubular cell death
    i. tubular damage
ischial tuberosity
ischioanal
ischiocavernosus muscle
ischiorectal
    i. abscess
    i. anorectal space
    i. aponeurosis
    i. excavation
    i. fascia
    i. fat
    i. fistula
    i. fossa
    i. fossa plane
    i. region
ischochymia
ISD
    intrinsic sphincter deficiency
    intrinsic sphincter dysfunction
ISEL
    in situ end labeling
isethionate
    pentamidine i.
ISH
    isolated systolic hypertension
ISIS 2302
island
    buried vaginal i.
    cytotoxin-associated gene
      pathogenicity i. (cagPAI)
    i. flap procedure
    i. groin flap
    lipid i.
    mucosal i.
    i. pedicle flap
islet
    i. amyloid polypeptide
    i. cell
    i. cell adenoma
    i. cell antibody (ICA)
    i. cell carcinoma
    i. cell hyperplasia
    i. cell implant
    i. cell of Langerhans
    i. cell tumor
    Langerhans i.
Isletest-ICA
Ismelin
Is-5-Mn
    isosorbide-5-mononitrate
isoamyl alcohol
isoamylase
    salivary-type i.
Isobar barostat distention device
isobaric gastric distention
isobutyl 2-cyanoacrylate
isobutyl-methyl-xanthine (IMx)
Isocal
    I. HCN
    I. HCN liquid feeding
isocarboxazid
isodose contour
isoechogenic
isoechoic
isoenzyme, isozyme
    alkaline phosphatase i.
    CYP i.
    galactosyltransferase i. II
    LDH i. 5
    Regan i.
    serum pepsinogen i. I, II
isoflavone
isoflurane
isoform
    growth factor i.
isoiodide
isolate
isolated
    i. adenomatous lesion
    i. cortical tubule (ICT)
    i. cyst
    i. gastric varix type 1, 2 (IGV)
    i. generator
    i. granulomatous gastritis
    i. hepatocyte perfusion
    i. hypoaldosteronism
    i. renal mucormycosis
    i. retained antrum syndrome
    i. systolic hypertension (ISH)
    i. urinary tract infection
isolation defect
isoleucine
    peptide histidine i. (PHI)
isomannide
IsoMed constant-flow infusion system
isomerase
    glucose-6-phosphate i.
isometric
    i. force
    i. tubular vacuolization
Isomil
    I. SF
    I. SF formula

isomotic lavage
isoniazid
isoniazid-induced hepatitis
isoosmolar liquid
isopentane
isoperistaltic
    i. anastomosis
    i. direction
    i. ileal reservoir
    i. stricturoplasty
isoprenaline
isoprenologue
isopropamide iodide
isopropanol
isoproterenol
Isoptin
Isordil
isosorbide dinitrate
isosorbide-5-mononitrate (Is-5-Mn)
Isospora belli
isosporan parasite
isosporiasis
Isotein HN feeding
isotherm
    Langmuir adsorption i.
isothiocyanate
    fluorescein i. (FITC)
Iso-Tome papillotome
isotonic
    i. contraction
    i. feeding
    i. saline
isotope
    ^{131}I-lipiodol i.
    i. meal
    ^{99m}Tc MAG-3 i.
    i. nephrography
    i. renal scan
    i. renogram
    i. renography
    i. study
    technetium-99m
        mercaptoacetyltriglycine i.
    i. voiding cystourethrography
    (IVCU)
isotropic, isotropous
    i. probe
    i. scan
isotropous (*var. of* isotropic)
isovaleric
    i. acid
    i. acidemia
isovolemic variance
Isovue
Isovue-300
isoxazole derivative
isoxsuprine
I-Soyalac formula
isozyme (*var. of* isoenzyme)

ispaghula husk
isradipine
Israel
    I. operation
    I. retractor
ISRE
    interferon-stimulated regulatory
    element
isthmectomy
isthmi (*pl. of* isthmus)
isthmian (*var. of* isthmic)
isthmic, isthmian
isthmus, *pl.* isthmi, isthmuses
    i. prostatae
    i. urethra
isthmuses (*pl. of* isthmus)
I-Stop midurethral sling
Isuprel
ISWL
    intracorporeal shock wave lithotripsy
itch
    jock i.
    swimmer's i.
iterative bifid branching system
ITGCN
    intratubular germ cell neoplasia
ITGP
    immunotactoid glomerulopathy
Ito
    I. cell
    I. cell sarcoma
itopride
ITP
    Ifex, Taxol, Platinol
itraconazole
Itrel pulse generator
ITS balloon dilation
Iturelix
IUI
    intrauterine insemination
IU/L
    international units per liter
IV
    intravenous
        Feridex IV
        IV fluid
        IV fluid therapy
        Merrem IV
        piggybacking of IV
        IV sedation
IVAC
    intravenous access
        IVAC needleless IV system
Ivalon
    I. sponge
    I. sponge hysterosacropexy
    I. sponge rectopexy
    I. sponge-wrap operation
    I. suture

Ivanissevitch ligation
IVC
    inferior vena cava
    intravenous cholangiogram
    intravenous cholangiography
IVCU
    isotope voiding cystourethrography
Ivemark syndrome
ivermectin
IVH
    intravenous hyperalimentation
IVIg
    intravenous immunoglobulin
IVN
    intravenous nutrition

Ivor
    I. Lewis esophagogastrectomy
    I. Lewis 2-stage subtotal
    esophagectomy
IVP
    intravenous pyelogram
    intravenous pyelography
IVU
    intravenous urogram
    intravenous urography
    high-dose IVU
    1-shot IVU
IVUS
    intravascular ultrasound
    IVUS catheter

J

J chain
J line
J needle
J pelvic ileal pouch
J reservoir
J tube
J turn of scope
J wire

Jaboulay

J. button
J. gastroduodenostomy
J. procedure
J. pyloroplasty

Jaboulay-Doyen-Winkleman

J.-D.-W. hemipelvectomy
J.-D.-W. hydrocele bottleneck
technique

jackknife position
Jackson

J. esophageal bougie
J. esophagoscope
J. membrane
J. staging system
J. veil

Jackson-Pratt

J.-P. catheter
J.-P. drain

jackstone calculus
Jacobson needle holder
Jacobs-Palmer laparoscope
Jacoby test
Jaffe

J. picrate reaction
J. test

Jagged 1 gene
Jagwire guidewire
Jaksch test
jalap
Jamaican

J. morning sickness
J. vomiting sickness
J. vomiting syndrome

Jamshidi liver biopsy needle
Janeway

J. gastroscope
J. gastrostomy
J. lesion

Jansen retractor
Jansen-type metaphysial
chondrodysplasia
Janus System III
Japanese

J. cancer classification
J. classification of cancer

J. dysentery
J. schistosomiasis

japonica

cutaneous schistosomiasis j.
schistosomiasis j.

japonicum

Schistosoma j.

japonicus

Petasites j.

Jarit rotator
Jarvis

J. hemorrhoid clamp
J. hemorrhoid forceps
J. pile clamp

Jass staging for rectal carcinoma
jatrox

J. *Helicobacter pylori* test
J. Hp-test

jaundice

acholuric j.
benign postoperative j.
black j.
Budd j.
catarrhal j.
cholestatic j.
chronic idiopathic j.
cloxacillin-induced cholestatic j.
Crigler-Najjar j.
deep j.
Epping j.
familial chronic idiopathic j.
familial nonhemolytic j.
Hayem j.
hemolytic j.
hepatocanalicular j.
hepatocellular j.
hepatogenic j.
homologous serum j.
human serum j.
infectious j.
infective j.
iproniazid-induced j.
latent j.
leptospiral j.
malignant obstructive j.
mechanical j.
neonatal j.
newborn j.
nonhemolytic j.
nonobstructive j.
obstructive j.
painless j.
parenchymatous j.
physiologic j.
regurgitation j.

jaundice (*continued*)
retention j.
shrapnel-induced obstructive j.
ticrynafen-induced j.
jaundiced skin
Jaworski
J. body
J. corpuscle
J. test
jaw wiring
J/cm
joules per centimeter
J-curve effect
Jeffrey introducer set
jejunal
j. bypass
j. colonization
j. crest
j. cutaneous urinary diversion
j. diverticulosis
j. drainage and biopsy
j. feeding tube
j. gas infusion test
j. gluten challenge
j. IgA
j. interposition of Henle loop
j. limb
j. pouch
j. pouch interposition (JPI)
j. syndrome
j. tube insertion
j. tube through percutaneous
endoscopic gastrostomy (JETPEG)
j. ulcer
j. urinary conduit
j. varix
j. villus
jejunales
arteriae j.
jejunectomy
jejuni
Campylobacter j.
jejunitis
nongranulomatous j.
ulcerative j.
jejunocecostomy
ulcerative jejunitis j.
jejunocolic fistula
jejunocolostomy
jejunogastric intussusception
jejunoileal
j. atresia
j. bypass (JIB)
j. bypass surgery
j. fold pattern reversal
j. intestine
j. shunt
jejunoileitis
nongranulomatous ulcerative j.

jejunoileostomy
Roux-en-Y distal j.
jejunoileum
jejunojejunostomy
jejunoplasty
jejunorrhaphy
jejunostomy
direct percutaneous j. (DPJ)
direct percutaneous endoscopic j.
(DPEJ)
j. elemental diet feeding
endoscopic j.
laparoscopic-guided feeding j.
long Roux-en-Y pouch j.
loop j.
needle-catheter j.
percutaneous endoscopic j.
(PEJ)
Roux-en-Y j.
j. tract choledochoscopy
j. tube (J-tube)
j. tube feeding
Witzel j.
jejunotomy
jejunum
proximal j.
Roux-en-Y loop of j.
Jelco catheter
jelly
Anestacon 2% lidocaine
hydrochloride j.
carboxymethylcellulose j.
electrode j.
lidocaine hydrochloride j.
Lubraseptic j.
Snap-It lubricating j.
spermatocidal j.
Xylocaine j.
JEM-100B, -100S electron microscope
Jenamicin
Jendrassik-Grof method
Jenning-Streifeneder gastroscope
JEOL
JEOL 100 CX electron microscope
JEOL JSM 35 CF scanning
electron microscope
Jesberg esophagoscope
jet
j. nebulizer
j. stream phenomenon
ureteral j.
Jetco-Spray cannula
jetlike bleeding
JETPEG
jejunal tube through percutaneous
endoscopic gastrostomy
Jeune
J. asphyxiating thoracic dystrophy
J. syndrome

Jevity
> J. isotonic liquid nutrition
> J. tube-feeding formula

jeweler's forceps

jewel weed

Jewett
> J. bladder carcinoma classification
> J. classification of bladder carcinoma
> J. sound
> J. staging system

Jewett-Strong system

Jewett-Whitmore cancer staging system

JF-200
> JF-200 duodenoscope
> JF-200 side-viewing videoendoscope

JFB III endoscope

JF-IT20 duodenoscope

JF-20 side-viewing fiberoptic endoscope

J-hook-tip laparoscopic electrode

JIB
> jejunoileal bypass

Jin Bu Huan

J-loop ileostomy

J-Maxx stent

JNC
> Joint National Committee
> JNC VI classification of hypertension

Jobert de Lamballe suture

Job syndrome

jock itch

Joe hoe

Joel-Cohen incision

Johanson-Blizzard syndrome

Johne disease

Johns
> J. Hopkins gallbladder forceps
> J. Hopkins gallbladder retractor
> J. Hopkins prostate cancer grading system

Johnson
> J. and DeMeester score
> J. esophagogastroscopy
> J. esophagogastrostomy

Johnson-DeMeester symptom score

Johnston buttonhole arteriovenous hemodialysis fistula procedure

joint
> j. erythema
> J. National Committee (JNC)

Jolles test

Jonas
> J. implant
> J. penile prosthesis

Jones-Politano technique

Jones silver stain

Jonnesco
> J. fold

> J. fossa
> J. operation

Joseph
> J. hook
> J. syndrome

joules per centimeter (J/cm)

Joyce-Loebl Magiscan image analysis system

JP
> juvenile polyposis

J-pexy
> omental J-p.

JPI
> jejunal pouch interposition

JPS
> juvenile polyposis syndrome

JR-St cell

J-scope esophagoscope

J-shaped
> J-s. endoscope
> J-s. ileal pouch
> J-s. ileal pouch-anal anastomosis
> J-s. ileal reservoir

JT1001 prostate cancer vaccine

J-tube
> jejunostomy tube
> J-t. insertion

J-type maneuver

Jubileum 2.0 single-use gastroesophageal pH probe

Judd
> J. cystoscope
> J. pyloroplasty
> J. ventral hernia repair

Judd-Allis intestinal forceps

Judd-DeMartel gallbladder forceps

jugular

juice
> acid-peptic j.
> duodenal j.
> gastric j.
> intestinal j.
> pancreatic j.
> pure pancreatic j. (PPJ)

Julian
> J. cystoresectoscope
> J. splenorenal forceps

jumbo
> j. biopsy
> j. biopsy forceps

jumentosa

junction
> anomalous pancreatobiliary duct j. (APBDJ)
> anorectal j.
> cardioesophageal j. (CEJ)
> cardioesophageal mucosal j.
> choledochoduodenal j.
> choledochopancreatic ductal j.

junction (*continued*)
    corticomedullary j.
    costochondral j.
    cystic-choledochal j.
    cysticohepatic j.
    desmosomal j.
    detrusor muscle protrusion j.
    duodenojejunal j. (DJJ)
    esophagogastric j.
    fundic-antral j.
    gap j.
    gastroesophageal j. (GEJ)
    GE j.
    hepaticocystic j.
    hyperactive rectosigmoid j.
    ileocecal j.
    intermediate j.
    mucosal j.
    NS3/NS4 j.
    NS4/NS5 j.
    pancreaticobiliary ductal j.
    pancreaticocholedochoductal
      j.
    patulous gastroesophageal j.
    penopubic j.
    penoscrotal j.
    pharyngoesophageal j.
    prostatovesical j.
    pyloroduodenal j.
    rectosigmoid j.
    saphenofemoral j.
    squamocolumnar mucosal j.
    tracheoesophageal j.
    ureteropelvic j. (UPJ)
    ureterovesical j. (UVJ)
    urethrovesical j.

junctional
    j. cyst
    j. intestinal metaplasia
juniper
juvenile
    j. cirrhosis
    j. nephronophthisis
    j. nephronophthisis-medullary cystic
      disease
    j. polyposis (JP)
    j. polyposis coli
    j. polyposis syndrome (JPS)
    j. retention polyp
    j. xanthogranuloma
juxtacapillary process
juxtaglomerular
    j. apparatus
    j. apparatus tumor
    j. body
juxtahepatic venous injury
juxtamedullary
    j. arteriole
    j. renal corpuscle
juxtapapillary
    j. duodenal diverticulum
    j. gangliocytic paraganglioma
juxtaposed mesenteric lymph nodes
juxtapyloric ulcer
juxtaregional node
juxtavesical ureter
J-Vac
    J-V. closed wound drainage
    J-V. drain
    J-V. suction reservoir
J-wave phenomenon
J-wire guide

K+
  potassium ion
    Ca^{2+}-activated K+
K
  K antigen
  K diet
  K tube
K2
  vitamin K2
K-141
  Dianeal K-141
kabure
Kader
  K. gastrostomy
  K. operation
kala azar
Kaleorid
KAL1 **gene**
Kalginate dressing
kaliopenic nephropathy
Kaliscinski
  K. plication
  K. ureteral folding technique
kaliuretic
  k. diuretic
  k. effect
kallidin
kallikrein
  human glandular k. 3 (hk3)
  k. inheritance
  plasma k.
  tissue k.
  urinary k.
kallikreinlike gene
Kallmann syndrome
Kaltostat dressing
Kammerer-Battle incision
Kanagawa phenomenon
kanamycin nephropathy
Kane umbilical clamp
Kangaroo
  K. delivery system
  K. 200, 330 enteral feeding
    pump
  K. gastrostomy tube
kansasii
  Mycobacterium k.
Kantor-Berci videolaryngoscope
Kantor string sign
Kantrex
kanyemba
Kaodene
kaolin
Kaopectate
Kapectolin

Kaplan-Meier
  K.-M. analysis
  K.-M. curve
  K.-M. estimation
  K.-M. method
Kaposi
  K. sarcoma (KS)
  K. sarcoma-associated herpesvirus
    (KSHV)
kappa
  k. light chain
  nuclear factor k. B
    (NF-KB)
  k. receptor opioid agonist
Kapp-Beck colon clamp
Kapsinow test
karaya
  K. gum
  K. 5 paste
  k. powder
  K. ring ileostomy appliance
  K. 5 seal
Karl
  K. Storz Calcutript
  K. Storz endoscope
  K. Storz flexible ureteropyeloscope
  K. Storz instrumentation
  K. Storz-Lutzeyer lithotriptor
Karmen unit
Karnofsky
  K. index
  K. performance status scale
  K. score
Karroo syndrome
Kartagener syndrome
karyometry
karyotype
  chromosome k.
Kasabach-Merritt syndrome
Kasai
  K. classification for extrahepatic bile
    duct atresia
  K. operation
  K. peritoneal venous shunt
  K. portoenterostomy
  K. portoenterostomy procedure
Kasai-type hepatoportoenterostomy
Kashin-Beck disease
Kashiwado test
Kaslow intestinal tube
Kasugai
  chronic pancreatitis of K.
  K. pancreatitis classification
Katayama
  K. disease

K

Katayama (*continued*)
  K. fever
  K. syndrome
KATO-III cell
Kato test
Kaufman syndrome
kava kava
Kawasaki syndrome
Kaye
  K. nephrostomy tamponade balloon
  K. tamponade balloon catheter
Kayexalate enema
Kayser-Fleischer ring
KB
  ketone body
KBR
  ketone body ratio
KCl
  potassium chloride
40-kDa colonic antigen
87kDa protein
K+2 diet
32/67-kD laminin receptor
K/DOQI
  Kidney Disease Outcomes Quality
  Initiative
Kearns-Sayre syndrome
Keeler
  K. Magnalite headlamp
  K. panoramic loupe
Keen Edge disposable biopsy forceps
Keflex
Keftab
Kefzol
Kegelcisor
Kegel pelvic muscle exercise
Kehr
  K. incision
  K. sign
  K. T tube
Keith needle
Kelami penile curvature classification
Keller
  K. hydrodynamic hypothesis of
  sieving
  K. hypothesis
Kelling
  K. gastroscope
  K. test
Kelling-Madlener gastric resection procedure
Kellogg's castor oil
Kelly
  K. abdominal retractor
  K. clamp
  K. cystoscope
  K. fistula scissors
  K. forceps
  K. hemostat

  K. operation
  K. plication
  K. proctoscope
  K. rectal speculum
  K. sigmoidoscope
  K. sign
  K. sphincteroscope
  K. urethrovesical plication procedure
Kelly-Kennedy modification
Kelly-Murphy forceps
Kelly-Stoeckel operation
Kelman
  K. air cystotome
  K. double-bladed cystotome
  K. knife-cannula cystotome
  K. knife cystotome
keloid
kelotomy
Kelsey pile clamp
Kemadrin
Kendall Foley catheter
Kenguard silicone-coated Foley catheter
Kennedy disease
Kent deep surgery forceps
Keofeed
  K. enteral feeding bag
  K. 500 enteral feeding pump
  K. II enteral feeding pump
  K. II feeding tube
KeraPac device
keratin
  antibody to k.
keratinization
  single-cell k.
keratinocyte
  k. growth factor (KGF)
  k. serum-free medium culture
keratitis (kera)
  seborrheic k.
keratoacanthoma (KA)
keratoderma blennorrhagica
keratosis
  k. blennorrhagica
  k. follicularis
  lacelike k.
keratotic pseudoepitheliomatous balanitis
Kerckring
  circular folds of K.
  K. fold
  valve of K.
kerion formation
Kerlix wrap
kernicterus
Kerr kink
K562 erythroid line
Keshan disease
Kessler-Kleinert suture
ketamine
ketanserin

keto
    k. acid
    k. acid-amino acid supplement
ketoacidosis
    diabetic k. (DKA)
7-ketocholesterol
ketoconazole
ketogenesis
ketoglutaramate (KGM)
    alpha k.
ketoglutarate (KG)
    k. dehydrogenase (KGDH)
ketone
    k. body (KB)
    k. body ratio (KBR)
    k. body test
    urinary k.
ketoprofen analgesic therapy
ketorolac tromethamine
17-ketosteroid
ketosteroid
ketotifen
keyhole
    k. deformity
    k. limpet hemocyanin (KLH)
KeyMed
    K. advanced dilator
    K. advanced esophageal dilator set
    K. Atkinson endoprosthesis
    K. automatic reprocessor
    K. disposable variceal injection needle
    K. heater probe thermocoagulation
    K. Nottingham introducer
    K. unit
Key-Pred 25, 50
keystone anterior discectomy and fusion technique
KG
    ketoglutarate
KGDH
    ketoglutarate dehydrogenase
KGF
    keratinocyte growth factor
KGM
    ketoglutaramate
KHB
    Krebs-Henseleit bicarbonate
    KHB buffer
Kidd cystoscope
kidney
    abdominal k.
    k. abscess
    k. adenoma
    adipose artery of k.
    adipose capsule of k.
    k. adysplasia
    k. agenesis
    allocating cadaveric k.

    k. allograft
    amyloid k.
    k. amyloidosis
    k. angiomyolipoma
    k. aplasia
    k. arteriovenous fistula
    artificial k.
    k. ascent
    Ask-Upmark k.
    k. ballottement
    cadaver k.
    cake k.
    k. calcification
    k. calyx
    k. carbuncle
    k. carcinoma
    k. carcinosarcoma
    k. clearance
    clear cell carcinoma of k.
    k. clear cell sarcoma
    coarsely granular k.
    k. collecting system
    congenital double k.
    congested k.
    k. cortex
    crush k.
    cyanotic k.
    k. cyst
    decapsulation of k.
    K. Disease Outcomes Quality Initiative (K/DOQI)
    disk k.
    k. donor
    donor k.
    Dow hollow-fiber k. (DHFK)
    dump k.
    dwarf k.
    k. dysplasia
    dysplastic k.
    dystopic k.
    ectopic k.
    k. electrolyte clearance rate
    k. electrolyte excretion rate
    embryoma of k.
    k. failure
    fatty k.
    k. fibroma
    k. fibrosarcoma
    finely granular k.
    flea-bitten k.
    Formad k.
    k. function
    fused k.
    Gambro Lundia Minor artificial k.
    k. Gerota fascia
    k. glomerulocystic disease
    k. glomerulus
    Goldblatt k.
    gouty k.

K

kidney (*continued*)
   granular k.
   k. hematoma
   k. hemorrhage
   hind k.
   HLA-matched k.
   horseshoe k.
   hypermobile k.
   hypoplastic k.
   k. inflammation
   k. innervation
   k. internal splint/stent (KISS)
   k. internal splint/stent catheter
   k. ischemia
   lardaceous k.
   k. leiomyosarcoma
   k. liposarcoma
   living donor k.
   k. lobe
   lumbar k.
   lump k.
   k. lymphoblastoma
   Madin-Darby canine k. (MDCK)
   k. magnesium filtration
   k. malacoplakia
   malacoplakia of k.
   k. malignant fibrous histiocytoma
   k. mass
   maximal tubular excretory capacity
      of k.
   k. medulla
   medullary sponge k.
   mortar k.
   multicystic k. (MCK)
   multicystic dysplastic k. (MCDK)
   multilobar k.
   multilobular k.
   mural k.
   murine k.
   myelin k.
   myeloma k.
   k. nephroma
   non-heart-beating donor k.
   obstructed k. (OBK)
   k. oncocytoma
   k. ossifying tumor
   Page k.
   palpable k.
   pancake k.
   k. pedicle clamp
   pelvic k.
   pole of k.
   presacral ectopic k.
   primordial k.
   k. pseudotumor
   k. punch
   putty k.
   pyramid of k.
   k. rhabdomyosarcoma

   Rokitansky k.
   Rose-Bradford k.
   sacciform k.
   k. scarring
   sclerotic k.
   k. shock wave effect
   sigmoid k.
   k. size
   soapy k.
   solitary k.
   k. stone
   supernumerary k.
   thoracic k.
   k. transillumination
   k. transplant
   k. transplantation
   k. transplant recipient
   unilateral fused k.
   unipapillary k.
   k.'s, ureters, bladder (KUB)
   k.'s, ureters, bladder radiography
   K. Urology Foundation of America,
      Inc.
   k. variant
   k. vascular pedicle
   k. vasculature
   k. weight
   k. worm
KidneyScreen at Home test
kidney-sparing operation
Kids
   Florastor K.
   Resource Just for K.
Kiernan space
Kikuchi lymphadenitis
killer
   lymphokine-activated k. (LAK)
   natural k. (NK)
   natural k. T (NKT)
   k. T cell
killer-activating receptor
Killian
   K. dehiscence
   K. rectal speculum
   K. suction tube
   K. triangle
Killian-Jamieson area
Killian-Lynch laryngoscope
Kilner needle holder
KilRoid single-handed ligator
Kim Care contour briefs
Kimmelstiel-Wilson
   K.-W. disease
   K.-W. syndrome
Kimura disease
3-kinase
   phosphoinositide 3-k.
   PI 3-k.
kinase

conserved helix-loop-helix ubiquitous
k. (CHUK)
cyclin-dependent k. (CDK)
extracellular signal-regulated protein
k. (ERK)
foal adhesion k.
glucocorticoid k.
herpes simplex virus-thymidine k.
(HSV-tk)
ligand-triggered protein tyrosine k.
mitogen-activated protein k.
(MAPK)
muscle-brain isoenzyme of creatine
k. (CK-MB)
myosin light-chain k.
protein k. A (PKA)
protein k. C (PKC)
protein serine k.
protein threonine k.
protein tyrosine k.
pyruvate k.
serum k.
serum pyruvate k. (SPK)
Ste-20-related, proline-alanine-rich k.
(SPAK)
tyrosine protein k.

Kinesed

kinetic

k. gallbladder study
k. parameter

kinetically invariant

kinetics

bromodeoxyuridine cell k.
capacity-limited k.
first-order k.
gastric cell k.
gompertzian tumor k.
Michaelis-Menten k.
urea k.

Kinevac

King-Armstrong unit

King contrast venography technique

King's College ALF criteria

kinin

kink

k. in bowel
k. in intestine
Kerr k.

Kinkiang fever

kinking

Kinnier Wilson disease

ki-ras

Kirsten-ras
Ki-ras gene
Ki-ras gene mutation

Kirchner diverticulum

Kirschner abdominal retractor

Kirsten-ras (Ki-ras, K-ras)

K.-r. gene

K.-r. oncogene
K.-r. oncogene mutation

Kish urethral illuminate catheter

KISS

kidney internal splint/stent
KISS catheter

kissing

k. prostatic lobes
k. ulcers

Ki-67 stain

kit

Abbott HCV EIA 2nd generation k.
Abbott HCV test k.
Bard-Stiegmann-Goff variceal ligation
k.
Bayer Versant HCV RNA assay test
k.
BCA-1 protein assay k.
Boehringer k.
Carey-Coons biliary endoprosthesis
k.
Cavilon diabetes foot care k.
Chariker-Jeter wound sealing k.
Coloplast irrigation k.
Cytoscreen human interferon gamma
ELISA k.
DNA labeling k.
EIA k.
Enteryx GERD procedure k.
EZ Detect colorectal screening test
k.
FertilMARQ home diagnostic
screening test k.
Fix and Perm permeabilizing k.
Flexiflo Inverta-PEG gastrostomy k.
Flexiflo Lap J laparoscopic
jejunostomy k.
Flexiflo over-the-guidewire
gastrostomy k.
FlexSure in-office rapid serology
test k.
Gastrin RIA k. II
GastroPanel assay k.
Gene Clean II k.
GFX Genomic blood DNA
purification k.
Handi-Cath catheter k.
Hashizume endoscopic ligator k.
Helisal rapid blood diagnostic k.
Histofine SAB k.
Histofine SAB-PO k.
Hybritech Tandem-R assay k.
Mermaid DNA k.
Moss G-tube PEG k.
Nichols IRMA k.
OctreoScan k.
Ott/Mayo channel sampling k.
Percufix catheter cuff k.
Predicta TGF-β1 k.

K

kit (*continued*)
    propHiler urinary pH testing k.
    Pros-Check k.
    Pulse-Pak infusion k.
    Puregene DNA isolation k.
    PyloriTek *Helicobacter pylori* test k.
    QuickVue *H. pylori* gII test k.
    Random Primed DNA labeling k.
    rapid urease testing k.
    RIA k.
    Russell gastrostomy k.
    RUT k.
    Sacks-Vine gastrostomy k.
    Serodia commercial k.
    Steigmann-Goff endoscopic ligator k.
    StoneRisk diagnostic monitoring k.
    Tandem-R assay k.
    UltraTag RBC k.
    Uri-Kit culture k.
    UriSite urine collection k.
    Uri-Three culture k.
    Vectastain ABC k.
    Versa-PEG gastrostomy k.
    Vesica percutaneous bladder neck
      suspension k.
    Vitros Immunodiagnostic Products
      HBsAg confirmatory k.
    Wilson-Cook feeding tube k.
    Xtrax DNA commercial extraction
      k.
Kitano knot
Kiton red dye
Kittner dissector
Klatskin
    K. cholangiocarcinoma
    K. liver biopsy needle
    K. tumor
Klebanoff
    K. common duct bougie
    K. common duct sound
    K. gallstone scoop
Klebs disease
Klebsiella
    K. *oxytoca*
    K. *pneumoniae*
Kleinert
    K. pants
    K. Safe and Dry panty and pad
      system
Kleinschmidt appendectomy clamp
Klemm sign
Klemperer disease
Kleppinger forceps
KLF6
    Kruppel-like factor 6
    KLF6 gene
KLH
    keyhole limpet hemocyanin
KLH-ImmuneActivator

Klinefelter syndrome
Kling dressing
Klippel-Trenaunay-Weber syndrome
Klonopin
Klor-Con
    K.-C. 8, 10
    K.-C. M10, M20
Klotho **gene**
KMI 60 enteral feeding pump
knee-chest position
knee-elbow position
knife, *pl.* **knives**
    Bard-Parker k.
    k. blade
    cautery k.
    cold k.
    Collin k.
    Collings electrosurgery k.
    Desmarres paracentesis k.
    electrocautery k.
    k. electrode
    electrosurgical cutting k.
    endarterectomy k.
    flex k.
    hernia k.
    hook k.
    HPC-2 standard needle k.
    insulated-tip electrosurgical k.
    insulation-tipped electrosurgical k.
    Lempert paracentesis k.
    Mori k.
    needle k.
    optic laser k.
    optic urethrotome k.
    Orandi k.
    skin k.
    triangle-tipped k.
    urethrotome k.
knifelike pain
knives (*pl. of* knife)
knobby process
knock
    pericardial k.
Knodell
    K. component
    K. criteria for histology activity
    K. index
    K. score
knot
    Aberdeen k.
    crochet k.
    curved-needle surgeon's k.
    externally releasable k.
    friction k.
    granny k.
    half-hitch k.
    1-handed k.
    ileosigmoid k.
    Kitano k.

laparoscopic k.
prelooped intracorporeal k.
Roeder loop k.
self-tightening slip k.
square k.
surgeon's k.
Tim k.
knotting
stochastic k.
knowledge
Crohn and Colitis K. (CCKNOW)
facile working k.
knuckle of colon
Ko-Airan cystic artery hemostasis maneuver
Kocher
K. anastomosis
K. clamp
K. dilation ulcer
K. forceps
K. gallbladder retractor
K. hemostat
K. incision
K. maneuver
K. operation
K. pylorectomy
K. ureterosigmoidostomy procedure
kocherization
Koch postulate
Kock
K. continent ileostomy
K. neobladder
K. nipple
K. nipple valve
K. pouch cutaneous urinary diversion
K. pouch modified procedure
K. reservoir
K. reservoir ileostomy
K. technique
K. urinary pouch
Kockogram
Kodak Ektachem 700 machine
Koenig, König
K. syndrome
Koerte gallstone forceps
KOH
potassium chloride
potassium hydroxide
KOH smear
Koh-I-Noor Universal India ink
Kohlmeier-Degos disease
Kohlrausch valve
koilocytosis
kola
gotu k.
Kollmann dilator
Kolmogorov-Smirnov test
kolypeptic

Kommerell diverticulum
Kondremul
König (*var. of* Koenig)
Konigsberg
K. catheter
K. 5-channel solid-state catheter assembly
K. microtransducer
Konsyl
Konsyl-D
Koplik spot
Korean
K. hemorrhagic fever
K. hemorrhagic nephrosonephritis
Koro syndrome
Korsakoff syndrome
Kossa stain
Kovia ointment
Koyanagi technique for hypospadias repair
K-Pek
K-Phos Neutral
K-ras
Kirsten-ras
K-r. gene
K-r. oncogene
Kraske
K. operation
K. parasacral approach
K. position
K. roll
kraurosis
penile k.
Krause
K. arm rest
K. ligament
Krazy Glue sclerosant
Krebs
K. cycle
K. solution
Krebs-Henseleit bicarbonate (KHB)
Krebs-Ringer
K.-R. bicarbonate buffer
K.-R. solution
Kreha
polysaccharide K. (PSK)
Krentz gastroscope
Kretz
K. Combison 330 ultrasound scanner
K. granule
K. 311 ultrasound scanner
K. ultrasound system
Kringle domain
Kristalose for oral solution
kristensenii
Yersinia k.
Krokiewicz test

K

Kron
    K. bile duct dilator
    K. gall duct dilator
Krönlein hernia
Kropp
    K. bladder neck reconstruction
    K. cystourethroplasty
    K. onlay urethral lengthening
      operation
    K. technique
    K. urethral lengthening procedure
Kruger index
Krukenberg
    K. tumor
    K. vein
Kruppel-like
    K.-l. factor 11
    K.-l. factor 6 (KLF6)
    K.-l. factor 6 gene
krusei
    Candida k.
Kruskal-Wallis
    K.-W. analysis of variance
    K.-W. test
krypton laser
17-KS
    17-ketosteroid
KS
    Kaposi sarcoma
KSHV
    Kaposi sarcoma-associated
      herpesvirus
KTP
    potassium-titanyl phosphate
    KTP 532 laser
    KTP laser probe
    KTP laser prostatectomy

    Laserscope KTP 532
    KTP 532 laser system
KTP/Nd:YAG laser treatment
KTP/YAG surgical laser system
Kt/V urea
KUB
    kidneys, ureters, bladder
    KUB radiography
Kudrox
Kugel hernia patch
Kulchitsky cell
Kumar Pre-View cholangiography clamp
Kumpe catheter
kunecatechins
Kunkel syndrome
Kupffer
    K. cell
    K. cell sarcoma
Kussmaul
    K. breathing
    K. endoscope
Kutrase
Ku-Zyme
    K.-Z. HP
    K.-Z. HP pancreatic
      enzyme
Kveim test
kwashiorkor
Kwell
Kyasanur Forest
  disease
kymography
    balloon k.
kyphoscoliosis
kyphosis
Kyrle disease
Kytril

L cell
LA, L.A.
    long acting
    Los Angeles
        LA classification
        Dalalone L.A.
        Detrol LA
        Trelstar LA
LAAL
    lower anterior axillary line
Labbe
    L. syndrome
    L. triangle
labeled
    l. leukocyte scintigraphy
    l. red blood cell scan
labeling
    in situ end l. (ISEL)
    terminal uridine deoxynucleotide
        nick-end l. (TUNEL)
labetalol
labia (*pl. of* labium)
labialis
    herpes l.
labial ulceration
labile
    acid l.
labioplasty
labium, *pl.* **labia**
    l. inferius valvulae coli
    l. majus muscle
    l. minus muscle
    l. superius valvulae coli
    l. urethrae
laboratory
    l. abnormality
    surgical simulation virtual reality l.
    Venereal Disease Research L.
        (VDRL)
    l. zymogen
labyrinth
    cortical l.
    Ludwig l.
    renal l.
    Santorini l.
lacelike keratosis
laceration
    concurrent hepatic l.
    longitudinal l.
    lower pole l.
    Mallory-Weiss l.
    rectal l.
    splenic l.
    vascular l.
Lachnospira

lacrimal duct probe
lactaciduria
Lactaid
lactaris
    Ruminococcus l.
lactase
    l. deficiency
    l. enzyme
lactase-ceramidase complex
lactase-phlorizin hydrolase (LPH)
lactate
    l. dehydrogenase (LDH)
    Ringer l.
lactated Ringer solution (LRS)
lacteal vessel
lactic
    l. acid
    l. acid dehydrogenase (LDH)
    l. acidosis
Lactinex
lactobacilli (*pl. of* Lactobacillus)
lactobacillus, *pl.* **lactobacilli**
    L. acidophilus
    L. agilis
    L. bifidus
    L. bulgaricus
    L. casei
    L. GG (LGG)
    L. plantarum
    L. plantarum-fermented food
    L. plantarum-fermented oats
    L. plantarum 299v
    l. preparation
    L. reuteri
    L. rhamnosus
lactobezoar
lactobionate
    erythromycin l.
lactoferrin
    fecal l.
lacto-*N*-fucopentaose
    sialylated l.-N-f.
lactose
    disaccharide l.
    l. hydrogen breath testing (LHBT)
    l. intolerance
    l. malabsorption (LMA)
    l. maldigestor
    l. tolerance test (LTT)
lactose-associated diarrhea
lactose-free
    l.-f. diet (LFD)
    l.-f. feeding
lactovegetarian
lactovegetarianism

L

Lactrase
lactulose
    l. breath test (LBT)
    l. enema
    l. solution
lactulose-mannitol
    l.-m. permeability test
    l.-m. ratio
lacuna, *pl.* **lacunae**
    great l.
    l. magna
    Morgagni l.
    l. of muscle
    l. of urethra
    urethral l.
lacunae (*pl. of* lacuna)
lacunar abscess
lacunule
Ladd
    L. band
    L. correction of malrotation of
      bowel
    L. mobilization of intestine
      procedure
    L. operation
    L. syndrome
laddering
    DNA l.
lady's mantle
Laënnec cirrhosis
Lafora
    L. body
    L. disease
LAGB
    Lap-Band adjustable gastric banding
    LAGB system
lag phase
Lahey
    L. aneurysm needle
    L. gall duct forceps
    L. liver transplant bag
Lahey-Babcock forceps
Laidley double catheterizing
cystoscope
Laird-McMahon anorectoplasty
LAK
    lymphokine-activated killer
    LAK cell
lake
    bile l.
Lalonde hook forceps
LAMA
    laser-assisted microanastomosis
L-AmB
    liposomal amphotericin B
Lambda Plus PDL 1, 2 laser system
lamblia
    Giardia l.
lambliasis

lamina, *pl.* **laminae**
    basal l.
    l. densa
    l. muscularis mucosae
    proper l.
    l. propria
    l. propria lymphoid cell
    l. propria of buccal mucosa
    l. rara externa (LRE)
    l. rara interna (LRI)
    vascular l.
laminae (*pl. of* lamina)
laminar cortical necrosis
laminated calcification
laminectomy
laminin
    destruction of l.
    l. receptor
    l. receptor inhibition
lamivudine
lamotrigine
lamp
    low-pressure argon gas/liquid
      mercury l.
    slit l.
    Wood l.
    xenon l.
Lancereaux nephritis
lancet-shaped biopsy forceps
lancinating pain
Landau
    L. reflex
    L. trocar
landmark
    bony l.
Landzert fossa
Lane
    L. band
    L. disease
    L. gastroenterostomy catheter
    L. gastroenterostomy clamp
    L. ileorectal anastomosis
    L. intestinal clamp
    L. intestinal forceps
Lange
    L. skinfold calipers
    L. test
Langerhans
    L. cell
    L. cell histiocytosis
    L. islet
    islet cell of L.
    L. lineage
Langer line
Langhans
    L. cell
    L. line
Langmuir adsorption isotherm
Lanoxin

lanreotide
lansoprazole, amoxicillin, clarithromycin
lanthanum carbonate
Lantiseptic skin protectant
Lanza scale
Lanz point
LAP
  leucine aminopeptidase
  leukocyte alkaline phosphatase
    LAP test
lap
  lap Nissen
  lap pad
  lap sac
  lap sponge
  lap tape
laparectomy
laparocele
laparocholecystotomy
laparocolectomy
laparocolostomy
laparocystectomy
laparoendoscopy
laparoenterostomy
Laparofan
laparoflator
  Weck high-flow l.
laparogastroscopy
Laparolift system
LaparoLith
laparonephrectomy
laparorrhaphy
LaparoSAC single-use obturator and cannula
LaparoScan laparoscopic ultrasonic imaging
laparoscope
  diagnostic l.
  Foroblique optic l.
  forward optic l.
  Jacobs-Palmer l.
  Olympus l.
  operating l.
  operative l.
laparoscopic (lap)
  l. abdominoperineal excision
  l. abdominoperineal resection
  l. adjustable gastric banding
  l. adrenalectomy
  l. adrenal gland surgery
  l. Allis clamp
  l. anterior abdominal wall hernia repair
  l. antireflux surgery (LARS)
  l. appendectomy
  l. biopsy of liver
  l. bladder neck suspension
  l. bladder neck suture suspension procedure

l. Burch urethrocystopexy
l. cannula
l. cecostomy button
l. cholecystectomy
l. clip application
l. colectomy
l. colorectal cancer surgery
L. Colorectal Surgery Group
l. colposuspension technique
l. contact ultrasonography (LCU)
l. cryoablation
l. cystoplasty
l. cystourethropexy
l. dismembered pyeloplasty
l. donor nephrectomy (LDN)
l. extravesical bladder cuff
l. gastric bypass
l. grasper
l. Heller myotomy
l. hysterosalpingectomy
l. intracorporeal ultrasound (LICU)
l. knot
l. laser-assisted autoaugmentation
l. laser cholecystectomy (LLC)
l. living donor nephrectomy
l. lymphocelectomy
l. lysis
l. Mainz pouch II
l. management
l. marsupialization
l. needle colposuspension
l. needle driver
l. Nissen and Toupet fundoplication
l. orchiopexy
l. partial nephrectomy (LPN)
l. pelvic lymphadenectomy
l. pelvic lymph node dissection (LPLND)
l. photography
l. promontofixation
l. pyelolithotomy
l. radical nephrectomy (LRN)
l. radical nephroureterectomy
l. radical prostatectomy (LRP)
l. renal artery aneurysm repair
l. renal biopsy
l. retraction system
l. retroperitoneal lymph node dissection
l. retropubic colposuspension
l. scissors
l. seromyotomy
l. stapler
l. stapling
l. surgery in pediatric urology
l. suture rectopexy
l. tie clip
l. transcystic duct exploration

L

laparoscopic (*continued*)
    l. transcystic duct stenting of papilla
    l. transcystic papillotomy
    l. treatment of ureteropelvic junction obstruction
    l. trocar configuration
    l. trocar placement
    l. trocar sleeve
    l. ultralow anterior resection
    l. ultrasound (LUS)
    l. ureteral reanastomosis
    l. ureterolithotomy
    l. ureterolysis
    l. urinary diversion procedure
    l. uterolysis
    l. vagotomy
    l. varicocelectomy
    l. varicocele repair
    l. varix ligation

laparoscopically
    l. assisted colorectal resection
    l. assisted panenteroscopy
    l. guided transcystic exploration

laparoscopic-assisted
    l.-a. approach
    l.-a. hemicolectomy
    l.-a. ileocystoplasty and ileovesicostomy

laparoscopic-guided feeding jejunostomy
laparoscopist
laparoscopy
    5-aminolevulinic acid-induced fluorescence l.
    l. complication
    l. contraindication
    diagnostic l.
    double-puncture l.
    extraperitoneal hand-assisted l.
    flexible l.
    gasless l.
    gynecologic l.
    hand-assisted l. (HAL)
    inguinal l.
    l. in pediatric urology
    pulmonary gas embolism during l.
    robot-assisted l. (RAP)
    single-puncture l.
    standard l.
    subsequent diagnostic l.
    therapeutic l.

laparoscopy-assisted ileocystoplasty and ileovesicostomy
laparoscopy-guided subhepatic cholecystostomy
Laparoshield laparoscopic smoke filtration system
LaparoSonic coagulating shears
laparosplenectomy

laparotomy (lap)
    emergency l.
    exploratory l.
    negative l.
    l. pack
    l. pad
    l. pad cover
    second-look l.
    l. sponge
    l. tape

laparotyphlotomy
Lap-Band adjustable gastric banding (LAGB)
Lapides
    L. classification
    L. classification of voiding dysfunction
    L. cystometric investigation
    L. test
    L. vesicostomy

Lapides-Ball urethrocystopexy
Laplace
    L. forceps
    L. law
    law of L.

Lapra-Ty clip
Lapro-Clip
LapSac introducer
LapTie
LAR
    low anterior resection

LAR/CAA
    low anterior resection in combination with coloanal anastomosis

lardaceous kidney
large
    l. bowel
    l. common duct stone
    l. impacted ureteral stone
    l. needle size

large-bore
    l.-b. biliary endoprosthesis
    l.-b. cannula
    l.-b. catheter
    l.-b. double-pigtail stent
    l.-b. gastric lavage tube
    l.-b. heat probe
    l.-b. rigid esophagoscope
    l.-b. Tygon tubing

large-bowel
    l.-b. cancer
    l.-b. carcinoma
    l.-b. obstruction

large-cell change
large-channel
    l.-c. curvilinear videoechoendoscope
    l.-c. endoscope
    l.-c. therapeutic duodenoscope

large-diameter bougie

large-droplet fatty liver
large-forceps biopsy
large-particle biopsy
large-volume paracentesis (LVP)
L-arginine
lari
    Campylobacter l.
larkspur
Larodopa
LaRoque
    L. herniorrhaphy incision
    L. repair
    L. technique
Larrey hernia
Larrey-Weil disease
Larry
    L. rectal director
    L. rectal probe
LARS
    laparoscopic antireflux surgery
larva, *pl.* **larvae**
    anisakid l.
    l. migrans
larvae (*pl. of* larva)
larval nephrosis
laryngeal
    l. carcinoma
    l. edema
    l. jack-assisted retrograde esophageal
      membranotomy
    l. jack technique
    l. vestibule
larynges (*pl. of* larynx)
laryngitis
    reflux l.
laryngopharyngectomy
laryngoscope
    Bullard intubating l.
    Killian-Lynch l.
    Olympus ENF-P-series l.
    Ossoff-Karlan l.
laryngoscopy
    direct l.
laryngospasm
larynx, *pl.* **larynges**
laser
    l. ablation
    ADD'Stat l.
    l. adjustable silicone gastric banding
      (LASGB)
    alexandrite l.
    argon ion l.
    argon pumped-dye l.
    balloon l.
    Candela MDL 2000 l.
    Candela pulsed-dye l.
    carbon dioxide l.
    L. CHRP rigid fiberscope system
    l. clipping

CO_2 l.
l. coagulation
Coherent 90-K l.
coumarin dye l.
coumarin flashlamp-pumped
  pulsed-dye l.
l. desorption/ionization mass
  spectrometry
diode l.
Diomed l.
l. disk
l. Doppler flowmeter
l. Doppler velocimetry
dye l.
endoscopic pulsed-dye l.
erbium:YAG l.
flashlamp pumped-dye l.
FREDDY Nd:YAG l.
frequency-doubled double pulse
  ND:YAG l.
helium-neon l.
l. hemorrhoidectomy
l. hemorrhoid excision
holmium l.
holmium:YAG l.
Indigo Optima l.
l. interstitial thermal therapy (LITT)
ion l.
krypton l.
KTP 532 l.
l. laparoscopic vagotomy
Lateralase l.
lateral-firing l.
Lithognost flash-lamp pulsed-dye l.
l. lithotripsy
l. lithotriptor
l. lithotriptor basket
LX-20 l.
medical l.
Medilas fiberTome l.
l. microscope
Molectron Nd:YAG l.
Myriadlase side-fire l.
Nd:YAG l.
neodymium:yttrium-garnet l.
Olympus Nd:YAG l.
OmniPulse MAX holmium l.
l. partial nephrectomy
l. photoablation
l. photocoagulation
l. photodestruction
l. photothermolysis
l. plume
potassium-titanyl phosphate crystal l.
Prolase II lateral-firing Nd:YAG l.
l. prostatectomy
pulsed-dye l.
pulsed-dye neodymium:YAG l.
Pulsolith l.

L

laser (*continued*)
    pumped-dye l.
    Q-switched alexandrite l.
    Q-switched Nd:YAG l.
    rhodamine 6G dye l.
    l. scanning confocal microscopy
    l. sclerosis
    semiconductor l.
    Side-Fire l.
    SLT contact MTRL l.
    l. surgery
    l. technology
    l. temperature
    l. therapy
    l. thermocoagulation
    l. tissue weld
    l. tissue welding
    l. tissue-welding solder
    Trimedyne holmium l.
    tunable pulsed-dye l.
    Ultraline l.
    ultrasound-guided l.
    Urolase l.
    l. vaporization
    VersaPulse PowerSuite
      dual-wavelength l.
    VersaPulse PowerSuite holmium l.
    VersaPulse Select l.
    visual endoscopically controlled l.
    l. welding technique
    l. writer
    YAG l.
    yttrium-aluminum-garnet l.
laser-assisted
    l.-a. endoscopic myotomy
    l.-a. microanastomosis (LAMA)
    l.-a. tissue-welding technique
laser-Doppler Periflux PF-3 probe
laser-guided biopsy
laser-induced
    l.-i. fluorescence spectroscopy (LIFS)
    l.-i. fragmentation
    l.-i. intracorporeal shock wave
      lithotripsy (LISL)
LaserMed laser pointer
Laserscope
    L. KTP 532
    L. YAG 1064
LaserSonics
    L. Endoblade
    L. Nd:YAG Laserblade scalpel
laserthermia
lasertripsy
LaserTripter
    Candela MDA-200 L.
    L. MDL-3000
LASGB
    laser adjustable silicone gastric
    banding

Lashmet-Newburgh method
Lasix
L-asparaginase
Lassa hemorrhagic fever
lasso
    guidewire/basket l.
    l. snare
    l. technique
last-generation serologic ELISA test
lata
    fascia l.
    solvent-dehydrated cadaveric fascia
      l.
latamoxef sodium
Latarjet
    nerve of L.
late
    l. dumping
    l. dumping syndrome
    l. graft dysfunction
latency
    pudendal nerve terminal motor l.
      (PNTML)
latent
    l. jaundice
    l. nephritis
late-onset hepatic failure
late-period filariasis
lateral
    l. abdominal region
    l. bending technique
    l. branch
    l. chordee
    l. cutaneous paresthesia
    l. cystocele
    l. decubitus
    l. decubitus position
    l. fossa
    l. fossa of preputial space
    l. gutter
    l. internal pelvic reservoir
    l. lithotomy
    l. lobe
    l. margin
    l. node dissection
    l. oblique fascia
    l. pancreatojejunostomy
    l. prostatotomy
    l. pyelography
    l. rectal ligament
    l. reflection of colon
    l. sphincterotomy
    l. ventral hernia
    l. window technique
Lateralase laser
lateral-firing laser
lateralizing sensory deficit
lateral-lateral pouch
lateral-viewing endoscope

latex
- l. agglutination assay
- l. allergy
- l. balloon
- l. fixation test
- l. hood
- l. sclerosant

latex-base skin cement

latissimus
- l. dorsi detrusor myoplasty
- l. dorsi free flap
- l. dorsi muscle

latum
- condyloma l.
- *Diphyllobothrium l.*

Latzko
- L. partial colpocleisis
- L. technique

Laubry-Soulle syndrome

laudanum

Laugier hernia

Launois-Cléret syndrome

Laurence-Moon-Bardet-Biedl syndrome

Laurence-Moon-Biedl syndrome

Lauren gastric carcinoma classification

lavage
- abdominal l.
- l. and suction
- l. bowel preparation
- cisapride-assisted l.
- closed continuous l.
- colonic l.
- l. cytology
- Easi-Lav l.
- endoscopically guided segmental gut l.
- external biliary l.
- gastric l.
- gastrointestinal l.
- iced saline l.
- internal biliary l.
- isomotic l.
- Lazarus-Nelson peritoneal l.
- nasocystic catheter l.
- nasogastric l.
- norepinephrine l.
- oral l.
- oral colonic l. (OCL)
- PEG l.
- peritoneal l.
- polyethylene glycol-based l.
- rapid colonic l.
- l. solution
- stomach l.
- Waterpik l.

lavage-induced
- l.-i. cardiac asystole
- l.-i. pill malabsorption

law
- Bell l.
- Courvoisier l.
- Fitz l.
- Laws gastroplasty
- Laws gastroplasty with silastic collar-reinforced stoma
- Laplace l.
- Meyer-Weigert l.
- l. of Laplace
- Poiseuille l.
- Poiseuille-Hagen l.
- Salmon l.
- Tait l.
- Weigert-Meyer l.

lawn mower technique

Lawrence
- L. Add-A-Cath
- L. deep surgery forceps
- L. gastric reservoir

laxa
- cutis l.

laxation

laxative
- l. abuse
- anthracene-type l.
- anthraquinone l.
- bulk l.
- bulk-producing l.
- Ceo-Two l.
- contact l.
- emollient l.
- Fleet Phospho-soda buffered saline l.
- hyperosmotic l.
- lubricant l.
- osmotic l.
- saline l.
- sodium phosphate-based l.
- stimulant l.
- stool-softening l.
- surfactant l.
- Women's Gentle L.

LaxCaps
- Phillips L.

Laxinate 100

laxity
- ligamentous l.

Lax-Senna
- Black-Draught L.-S.

2-layer
- 2-l. enteroenterostomy
- 2-l. interrupted intestinal anastomosis
- 2-l. latex and Marlex closure technique
- 2-l. open technique

layer
- Bernard glandular l.
- echo-poor l.

L

layer (*continued*)
  fascial l.
  germ l.
  glycosaminoglycan l.
  hypoechoic ringed l.
  seromuscular l.
  sonographic l.
  subcutaneous l.
  submucosal vaginal smooth
    musculofascial l.
  submucous l.
  subserous l.
laying-open fistulotomy
lay-open method
Lazaro da Silva technique
Lazarus-Nelson
  L.-N. peritoneal lavage
  L.-N. peritoneal lavage
    technique
lazy
  l. bladder syndrome
  l. colon
LBM
  lean body mass
LBT
  lactulose breath test
LCA
  lithocholic acid
LCA-DCA
  lithocholic acid-deoxycholic acid
    LCA-DCA ratio
L-carnitine
  L-c. capsule
  L-c. tablet
LCAT
  lecithin-cholesterol acyltransferase
LCDD
  light-chain deposition disease
LC-EMR
  lift-and-cut endoscopic mucosal
    resection
LCFA
  long-chain fatty acid
LCG
  liquid chemical germicide
LCHAD
  long-chain 3-hydroxyacyl coenzyme A
    dehydrogenase
L-citrulline
lck protein
LCT
  long-chain triglyceride
LDH
  lactate dehydrogenase
  lactic acid dehydrogenase
    LDH enzyme
    LDH isoenzyme 5
    LDH level of ascitic fluid
    LDH test

LDL
  low-density lipoprotein
    LDL Direct test
    oxidized LDL
    LDL susceptibility
LDLC, LDL-C
  low-density lipoprotein cholesterol
LDLT
  living donor liver transplantation
LDP-02 antibody
LDS
  ligating and dividing stapler
LE
  lupus erythematosus
    LE cell
le
  L. Bag
  L. Bag ileocolonic pouch
  L. Bag neobladder
  L. Bag pouch reservoir
  L. Bag urinary diversion
  L. Bag urinary pouch
  L. Fort procedure
  L. Fort sound
Lea
  disialosyl L.
  monosialosyl L.
**Leach dual-imaging surgical planning
  technique**
lead
  l. citrate
  l. citrate stain
  l. colic
  l. nephropathy
  l. poisoning
  l. wire
Leadbetter
  L. and Clarke technique
  L. and Clarke ureteral anastomosis
  L. cystourethroplasty
  L. hip reduction maneuver
  L. ileal loop diversion
  L. tunneling technique
  L. ureteroplasty modification
    technique
  L. urethral reconstruction procedure
Leadbetter-Politano
  L.-P. reimplantation
  L.-P. ureteroneocystostomy
  L.-P. ureterovesicoplasty
leading bar
lead-pipe
  l.-p. appearance
  l.-p. colon
leaf
  chaparral l.
  l. of diaphragm
  l. of mesentery
leafless tree appearance

leaflike villus
leak
anastomotic l.
distal pouch l.
lymphatic l.
l. pressure
proximal pouch l.
renal calcium l.
leakage
anastomotic l.
biliary l.
bilious l.
l. bypass cable
cavernovenous l.
crural venous l.
cystic duct l.
intraabdominal bile l.
postmicturition continuous l.
postoperative biliary l.
precipitant l.
l. severity
tube l.
venous l.
leaking
leak-point pressure (LPP)
leaky gut syndrome
lean body mass (LBM)
learned enuresis
learning curve
leather-bottle stomach
Leber amaurosis
Lebsche shears
lechleri
Croton l.
lecimibide
lecithin
polyunsaturated l.
lecithin-cholesterol acyltransferase (LCAT)
lectin
hepatic l.
l. reactivity
l. staining
lecturescope
LeDuc
L. fashion
L. technique urinary diversion
L. ureteral anastomosis
L. ureteral tunneling technique
LeDuc-Camey
L.-C. ileocolostomy
L.-C. ileocystoplasty
leech
mechanical l.
leflunomide
left
l. colon
l. colonic flexure
l. gastroomental artery

l. gutter
l. hepatic duct
l. hepatic duct stricture
l. hepatic lobe
l. hepatic vein
l. lateral decubitus position
l. lower quadrant
Monti-Malone, l.
l. pancreaticogastric fold
l. upper quadrant
l. ureter
left-sided
l.-s. appendicitis
l.-s. clonus
l.-s. colitis
left-to-right subtotal pancreatectomy
Legionella pneumophila
Leigh disease
Leiner disease
leiomyoblastoma
leiomyoma, *pl.* **leiomyomas, leiomyomata**
bizarre l.
colonic l.
duodenal l.
epithelioid l.
esophageal l.
gastric l.
l. of seminal vesicle
parasitic l.
testicular l.
Zenker l.
leiomyomas (*pl. of* leiomyoma)
leiomyomata (*pl. of* leiomyoma)
leiomyosarcoma
bladder l.
gastric l.
hepatic l.
kidney l.
low-grade l.
paratesticular l.
prostate gland l.
rectal l.
small-intestine l.
spermatic cord l.
Leishmania
L. donovani chagasi
L. donovani donovani
L. donovani infantum
L. esophagitis
L. infantum
leishmanial enteritis
leishmaniasis, leishmaniosis
infantile l.
visceral l.
leishmaniosis (*var. of* leishmaniasis)
Lembert inverting seromuscular suture
lemostenosis
Lempert paracentesis knife

L

Lendrum stain
length
        anal canal l. (ACL)
        functional profile l.
        functional urethral l. (FUL)
        lower infundibular l.
        peripheral capillary filtration
          slit l.
        telomere l.
        total slit pore l.
l-ENK, L-enk
    leucine-enkephalin
Lennhoff sign
lens
        Foroblique l.
        Hopkins II rod l.
        narrow l.
        objective l.
        right-angle l.
lenta
        cholangitis l.
Lente insulin
lentigines, electrocardiographic conduction abnormalities, ocular hypertelorism, pulmonary stenosis, abnormal genitalia, retardation of growth, and deafness (LEOPARD)
Lentivirus
lentum
        Eubacterium l.
Leonard
        L. Arm
        L. deep surgery forceps
LEOPARD
    lentigines, electrocardiographic
    conduction abnormalities, ocular
    hypertelorism, pulmonary stenosis,
    abnormal genitalia, retardation of
    growth, and deafness
    LEOPARD syndrome
Leo test
leprae
        Mycobacterium l.
leprosy
leptin
        l. level
        recombinant methionyl human l.
          (r-metHuLeptin)
Leptospira interrogans
leptospiral
        l. jaundice
        l. nephritis
leptospirosis
leptum
        Clostridium l.
LES
    lesser esophageal sphincter
    lower esophageal sphincter
    LES incompetence

LES locator
LES relaxation
transient relaxation of LES
Lesch-Nyhan syndrome
Lescol
Lesgaft
        L. hernia
        L. space
        L. triangle
lesion
        acetowhite l.
        acute gastric mucosal l.
        ampullary l.
        anal squamous intraepithelial l.
          (ASIL)
        angiodysplastic l.
        Antopol-Goldman l.
        aortoostial l.
        aphthous-type l.
        apple-core l.
        Armanni-Ebstein l.
        Baehr-Lohlein l.
        bilobed polypoid l.
        blanching of l.
        bleeding l.
        bull's-eye l.
        Cameron l.
        cauda equina l.
        colonic vascular l.
        Councilman l.
        cutaneous l.
        Dieulafoy gastric l.
        doughnut l.
        duodenal l.
        dye sham intrarenal l.
        Ebstein l.
        echo-poor l.
        ectatic vascular l.
        exophytic l.
        extramural l.
        fingertip l.
        flat depressed l.
        flat elevated l.
        florid bile duct l.
        Forest I, II l.
        gastric l.
        gastrointestinal l.
        glomerular tip l. (GTL)
        gunpowder l.
        hamartomatous l.
        hepatic mass l.
        high fundal l.
        high neurological l.
        hypoechoic l.
        identifiable intrascrotal l.
        l. identification
        intramural l.
        isolated adenomatous l.
        Janeway l.

local glomerular l.
localized l.
Lohlein-Baehr l.
lower motor neuron l.
Lugol-voiding l.
lumbar spinal cord l.
lymphoepithelial l.
macroorchidism l.
macroscopic l.
Mallory-Weiss l.
mesenteric vascular l.
metachronous l.
metastatic l.
minute polypoid l.
mucosal l.
mulberry l.
multicentric l.
napkin ring anular l.
neoplastic l.
nodular l.
nonerosive gastric mucosal l.
nonneoplastic l.
ocular l.
pancreas l.
pancreatic l.
papillary l.
penile l.
perianal l.
photon-deficient l.
plaquelike l.
pliable l.
polypoid l.
precancerous l.
preoperative l.
primary glomerular l.
right-sided l.
ringlike l.
ruptured peliotic l.
satellite l.
scirrhous l.
semipedunculated l.
sessile l.
short-segment l.
significant liver l.
skip l.
space-occupying l.
stenotic l.
stress l.
subglottic l.
submucosal upper gastrointestinal
  tract l.
synchronous l.
target l.
thrombotic l.
traumatic l.
trophic l.
tubulovillous l.
uremic gastrointestinal l.
vascular l.

vasculitic l.
vegetative l.
wire-loop l.

LESP
  lower esophageal sphincter pressure
LESR
  lower esophageal sphincter relaxation
lesser
  l. celandine
  l. curvature of stomach
  l. curvature ulcer
  l. epiploon
  l. esophageal sphincter (LES)
  l. galangal
  l. omentum
  l. pancreas
  l. peritoneal sac
less morbid lower abdominal transverse
  incision
Lester Martin modification of Duhamel
  abdominoperineal pullthrough operation
lethargic
LE-TUMT
  low-energy transurethral microwave
    thermotherapy
Leube test meal
leucine
  l. aminopeptidase (LAP)
  l. aminopeptidase test
  l. metabolism
  radiolabeled l.
  l. zipper
  l. zipper sequence
leucine-enkephalin (l-ENK, L-enk)
Leucomax
leucovorin
  oxaliplatin, 5-fluorouracil, l.
  l. rescue
leu-enkephalin
leukemia
  acute lymphoblastic l. (ALL)
  acute lymphocytic l. (ALL)
  acute myelomonocytic l.
  chylous l.
  testicular l.
Leukeran
leukobilin
leukocytapheresis
leukocyte
  l. adherence inhibition test
  l. alkaline phosphatase (LAP)
  l. alkaline phosphatase test
  chemotaxis of polymorphonuclear l.
  l. common antigen
  l. esterase
  l. esterase test
  fecal l.
  intraepithelial l. (IEL)
  peritoneal l.

L

leukocyte (*continued*)
    PMN l.
    polymorphonuclear l. (PMNL)
    l. scintiphotography
    tether circulating l.
    l. trafficking
    WBC l.
leukocytoclastic vasculitis
leukocytosis
leukoencephalopathy
leukopenia
    acute l.
leukoplakia
    bladder l.
    hairy l.
    l. of penis
    oral l.
Leukotest
leukotriene
    l. A_4
    l. C_4
    cysteinyl l.
    l. D_4
leukourobilin
leu-peptide
leupeptin
Leuprogel
leuprolide
    l. acetate
    l. acetate for injectable
    suspension
    l. acetate implant
    L. Depot Neoadjuvant Prostate
    Cancer Study Group
Leutrol
Leuvectin
levamfetamine
levamisole
levan cotton
Levaquin
Levarterenol
Levatol
levator
    l. ani
    l. ani hernia
    l. ani muscle
    l. ani syndrome
    l. fascia
    l. myorrhaphy
    l. plate
    l. span
    l. veli palatini muscle
Levbid
levcromakalim
LeVeen
    L. ascites shunt
    L. catheter
    L. inflation syringe
    L. inflator

    L. inflator with pressure gauge
    L. peritoneal shunt
    L. peritoneovenous shunt
    L. valve
level
    air-fluid l.
    Albarran deflecting l.
    alpha-1 antitrypsin l.
    alpha fetoprotein l.
    ammonia l.
    AMP l.
    anti-M2 antimitochondrial
     antibody l.
    blood alcohol l. (BAL)
    blood lead l.
    blood urea l.
    breath ethane l.
    complement l.
    control l.
    des-gamma-carboxy prothrombin l.
    fasting C-peptide l.
    fasting serum gastrin l.
    fluid-debris l.
    gamma glutamyltransferase l.
    gastrin mRNA l.
    homocysteine l.
    HSP-70 messenger ribonucleoprotein
     acid l.
    25-hydroxyvitamin D l.
    iothalamate l.
    leptin l.
    lipoprotein X l.
    motilin plasma l.
    pathologic resistive index l.
    pentane excretion l.
    pepsinogen l. A, B, C
    pericardial air-fluid l.
    polyamine l.
    protein C, S l.
    red blood cell folate l.
    serum eotaxin l.
    serum gastrin l.
    serum leptin l.
    serum urate l.
    somatostatin mRNA l.
    stairstep air-fluid l.
    theophylline l.
    thyroid-stimulating hormone l.
    transferrin saturation l.
    uric acid l.
    urinary cGMP l.
    whole-blood trough l.
levetiracetam
Levin
    L. tube
    L. tube aspiration
Levitra
levocarnitine
levodopa/carbidopa

levodopa dopaminergic medication
levofloxacin
levorphanol
levothyroxine
levovirin
Levovist contrast agent
Levsinex Timecaps
Levsin/SL
levulose test
Lewis
    L. A blood group antigen
    L. acid
    L. blood group
    L. B, X, Y antigen
    L. classification for vascular
      anomalies of gastrointestinal tract
    L. cystometer
    sialyl L. A
    L. Y carbohydrate epitope
Lewis-Tanner esophagectomy
 procedure
Lewy syringe
lexipafant
Lexirin
Leyden disease
Leydig
    L. cell
    L. cell adenoma
    L. cell secretion
    L. cell secretory function
    L. cell tumor
    L. duct
leydigarche
LFS
    liver function series
LFT
    liver function tests
LG
    light guide
    lymphocytic gastritis
      LG bundle
LGD
    low-grade dysplasia
LGG
    Lactobacillus GG
LGIB
    lower gastrointestinal bleeding
L-glutamine
l-glyceric aciduria
LGV
    lymphogranuloma venereum
LH
    luteinizing hormone
LHBT
    lactose hydrogen breath testing
Lhermitte-Duclos disease
LH-FSH
    luteinizing hormone follicle-stimulating
      hormone

LHRH
    luteinizing hormone-releasing hormone
libera
    tenia l.
libidinal
libido
Librax
Libritabs
Lich
    L. extravesical technique
    L. ureteral implantation for
      neobladder construction
    L. ureterocystostomy procedure
lichen
    l. nitidus
    l. planus
    l. sclerosus
    l. sclerosus et atrophicus
    l. simplex chronicus
lichenoid reaction
Lich-Gregoire
    L.-G. anastomosis
    L.-G. repair
    L.-G. technique
    L.-G. ureterolysis
Lichtenstein
    L. hernia repair
    L. herniorrhaphy
    L. open tension-free mesh
      hernioplasty
licorice
LICU
    laparoscopic intracorporeal ultrasound
lidamidine
Liddle
    L. disease
    L. mutation
    L. syndrome
Lidex
lidocaine
    l. hydrochloride jelly
    l. topical anesthetic
    viscous l.
lidocaine-prilocaine cream
lidofenin
    ^{99m}Tc l.
Lidox
Lidoxide
Lieberkühn
    L. ampulla
    L. crypt
    L. follicle
    L. gland
Lieberman
    L. proctoscope
    L. sigmoidoscope
Liebermeister
    L. furrow
    L. groove

L

lien
    l. accessorius
    l. mobilis
lienal artery
lienalis
    arteria l.
lienculus, lienunculus
lienectomy
lienis
    pulpa l.
    trabeculae l.
lienitis
lienocele
lienomalacia
lienomedullary
lienomyelogenous
lienomyelomalacia
lienopancreatic
lienopathy
lienophrenic ligament
lienorenal ligament
lienteric
    l. diarrhea
    l. stool
lientery
lienunculus
Lieutaud uvula
LIFE
    light-induced fluorescence endoscopy
Lifecath peritoneal implant
life cycle of *Echinococcus*
LifeJet catheter
lifelong obesity
Lifemed catheter
LifeSite hemodialysis access system
lifestyle
    l. modification
    l. therapy
Life-Tech flowmeter
L-IFN
    human lymphoblastoid interferon
LIFS
    laser-induced fluorescence spectroscopy
lift
    gallbladder l.
lift-and-cut
    l.-a.-c. biopsy
    l.-a.-c. endoscopic mucosal resection
    (LC-EMR)
    l.-a.-c. method
    l.-a.-c. technique
lifting sign
LIG
    lymphocyte immune globulin
ligament
    Arantius l.
    Bellini l.
    Camper l.
    Carcassonne perineal l.

cardinal l.
cholecystoduodenal l.
Clado l.
Cooper l.
coronary l.
costovertebral l.
external l.
falciform l.
femoral l.
fissure of round l.
fundiform l.
gastrocolic l.
gastrohepatic l.
gastrolienal l.
gastropancreatic l.
gastrophrenic l.
gastrosplenic l.
gonadal l.
Helvetius l.
hepatic l.
hepatocolic l.
hepatocystocolic l.
hepatoduodenal l.
hepatogastric l.
hepatogastroduodenal l.
hepatophrenic l.
hepatorenal l.
hepatoumbilical l.
Hesselbach l.
Hey l.
Huschke l.
infundibulopelvic l.
inguinal l.
Krause l.
lateral rectal l.
lienophrenic l.
lienorenal l.
lumbodorsal l.
medial umbilical l.
median arcuate l.
mucosal suspensory l.
l. of Mackenrodt
l. of Treitz
periurethral l.
phrencolic l.
phrenicocolic l.
phrenicoesophageal l.
Poupart l.
pubocervical l.
puboprostatic l.
pubourethral l.
pubovesical l.
rectosacral l.
l. reflecting edge
reflecting edge of l.
round l.
sacrospinous l.
sacrotuberous l.
sacrouterine l.

shelving edge of Poupart l.
splenocolic l.
splenopancreatic l.
splenorenal l.
suspensory l.
triangular l.
umbilical l.
ureteropelvic l.
urethropelvic l.
uterosacral l.
vesical l.

ligamenta (*pl. of* ligamentum)
ligamentous laxity
ligamentum, *pl.* **ligamenta**
l. teres
l. teres cardiopexy
l. teres hepatis
l. venosum

ligand
l. for ELAM-1
reciprocal l.
l. recognition

ligand-dependent receptor homodimerization
ligand-gated channel
ligandin
ligand-triggered
l.-t. membrane guanylate cyclase
l.-t. protein tyrosine kinase

ligase
Thermus aquaticus DNA l.

ligated
doubly l.
suture l.

ligating and dividing stapler (LDS)
ligation
band l.
Barron l.
bidirectional l.
bile duct l. (BDL)
detachable miniloop l.
l. device
Doppler-guided hemorrhoidal artery l. (DGHAL)
elastic band l.
Endoloop l.
endoscopic band l. (EBL)
endoscopic detachable miniloop l.
endoscopic esophagogastric variceal l.
endoscopic hemorrhoid l. (EHL)
endoscopic mucosal resection with l. (EMRL)
endoscopic ultrasound-assisted band l.
endoscopic variceal l. (EVL)
endoscopic variceal band l.
esophageal band l.
gastric variceal l.

hepatic artery l.
high l.
Ivanissevitch l.
laparoscopic varix l.
loop l.
miniloop l.
needlescope laparoscopic varix l.
l. of hemorrhoid
open retroperitoneal high l.
penile vein l.
postureteral l.
retroflexed endoscopic multiple-band l. (REMBL)
rubber band l. (RBL)
spermatic vein l.
stump l.
transesophageal l.
transgastric l.
triple rubber band l.
tubal l.
variceal band l.
varix l.

ligator
Bandito single-band l.
Barron rubber band l.
DDV l.
Duette multiband variceal l.
endoscopic band l.
KilRoid single-handed l.
McGivney hemorrhoidal l.
multiband variceal l.
multiple-band l.'s
O'Regan hemorrhoid l.
RapidFire multiple-band l.
rubber band l. (RBL)
Rudd Clinic hemorrhoidal l.
Saeed multiband l.
Saeed multiple l.
Saeed 6-shooter l.
Speedband SuperView l.
Stiegmann-Goff Clearvue endoscopic l.
Stiegmann-Goff variceal l.
variceal l.

Ligat test
ligature
elastic l.
interlocking l.
pursestring l.
retroperitoneoscopic vein l.
l. sign
silk l.
Surgiwip suture l.
suture l.

light
l. and electron immunoperoxidase
l. and electron immunoperoxidase observation
bili l.

light (*continued*)
    l. cable
    Cholestyramine L.
    l. electrocautery
    l. emitter
    l. flow
    fluorescence correlation spectroscopy
      magnifying l. (FCS-ML)
    l. fluorescent intensity
    l. guide (LG)
    l. guide bundle
    l. micrographic study
    l. microscopy
    l. reflex
    ultraviolet l. C
light-chain deposition disease (LCDD)
Light-Cycler PCR
light-induced
    l.-i. autofluorescence spectroscopy
    l.-i. fluorescence endoscopy
      (LIFE)
light-monitoring probe
Lightwood syndrome
Lignac
    L. disease
    L. syndrome
Lignac-Fanconi
    L.-F. disease
    L.-F. syndrome
lignan
likelihood ratio
Likert scale
Lillie intestinal forceps
lily
    American white pond l.
limb
    afferent ileal l.
    afferent jejunal l.
    ascending l.
    blind l.
    l. deformity
    efferent l.
    jejunal l.
    Roux l.
    Roux-en-Y jejunal l.
    thick ascending l.
    thin descending l.
    vertebral, anal, cardiac,
      tracheoesophageal fistula, renal, l.
      (VACTERL)
Limberg flap repair
3-limb S pouch
limbus
LIM 2537 cell
limerence
limit dextrinosis
limited (LTD, Ltd.)
    l. economic lithotripsy
    l. intravenous pyelography

    l. obturator node dissection
    l. partnership (LP)
limiting
    l. dilution assay
    l. dilution cloning polymerase chain
      reaction (LDC-PCR)
    l. plate
    l. plate erosion
limosum
    Eubacterium l.
limy bile
Lincoln deep surgery scissors
lincomycin
lindane
line
    Aldrich-Mees l.
    anocutaneous l.
    anorectal l.
    anterior axillary l. (AAL)
    apoptosis in cell l.
    arcuate l.
    arterial l.
    B-cell l.
    Beacon surgical l.
    Brödel l.
    Cantlie l.
    CaSki cell l.
    cell l.
    central venous pressure l.
    colonic mucosal l.
    Conradi l.
    dentate l.
    Dul45 cell l.
    Freedom Clear long-seal male
      external catheter l.
    Freedom Clear LS male external
      catheter l.
    Freedom Clear sport-sheath male
      external catheter l.
    Freedom Clear SS male external
      catheter l.
    gas density l.
    Hampton l.
    hepaRV cell l.
    hep G2 cell l.
    Hilton white l.
    Hunter l.
    iliopectineal l.
    incision l.
    J l.
    K562 erythroid l.
    Langer l.
    Langhans l.
    lower anterior axillary l. (LAAL)
    lower midclavicular l. (LMCL)
    lymphoblastoid cell l.
    midaxillary l.
    midclavicular l. (MCL)
    milkman's l.

mucosal l.
murine mesangial cell l.
myelomonocytic cell l.
neuronal cell l.
l. of Douglas
l. of Toldt
pararectal l.
pectinate l.
Poupart l.
pubococcygeal l. (PCL)
pubosacral l.
Rex-Cantli-Serege l.
Richter-Monroe l.
Sergent white adrenal l.
skin l.
suture l.
T-cell l.
total parenteral nutrition l.
TPN l.
transverse umbilical l.
upper midclavicular l. (UMCL)
white anococcygeal l.
Z l.

linea, *pl.* **lineae**
l. alba
l. nigra

lineae (*pl. of* linea)

lineage
hemopoietic l.
Langerhans l.

linear
l. analog pain score
l. convex array scanner
l. erosion
l. fluorescein
l. gastric ulcer
l. mode
l. probe
l. proctotomy
l. regression
l. staple cutter
l. stapler
l. stapling device
l. streaks en face
l. ulceration

linear-array
l.-a. analog pain score
l.-a. convex array scanner
l.-a. echoendoscope
l.-a. erosion
l.-a. fluorescein
l.-a. gastric ulcer
l.-a. mode
l.-a. probe
l.-a. proctotomy
l.-a. regression
l.-a. staple cutter
l.-a. stapler
l.-a. stapling device

l.-a. streaks en face
l.-a. transducer
l.-a. ulceration

linear-oriented radial scanning echoendoscope

4-lines sign

Lingeman
L. 3-in-1 procedure drape
L. TUR drape

lingua, *pl.* **linguae**
pityriasis l.

linguae (*pl. of* lingua)

lingual lipase

linguatuliasis

lingula, *pl.* **lingulae**

lingulae (*pl. of* lingula)

linitis
l. plastica
l. plastica carcinoma

link
cytoskeletal l.

linkage
gene l.
inherent to l.

linked

Linnartz intestinal clamp

linoleic acid

linsidomine chlorohydrate

Linton
L. shunt
L. tourniquet clamp

Linton-Nachlas tube

Lioresal

Lipancreatin

liparocele

lipase
bile salt-stimulated l. (BSSL)
Cherry-Crandall method for testing serum l.
colipase-dependent l.
l. enzyme
hepatic l.
hepatic triglyceride l. (HTGL)
lingual l.
lipoprotein l. (LPL)
pancreatic l.
serum l.
l. test

lipemia

lipid
l. bilayer
biliary l.
l. emulsion
extracellular l.
l. hydroperoxide
l. infusion
inositol l.
l. island
l. maldigestion

445

lipid (*continued*)
  membrane-based l.
  l. metabolism
  l. nephrosis
  l. oxidation rate
  l. peroxidation
  sulfated l.
lipid-laden
  l.-l. clear cell
  l.-l. hepatocyte
lipid-lowering drug
lipidosis
  ceramide lactoside l.
  Schwann cell l.
lipidosterol extract
lipid-to-protein ratio
lipiduria
lipiodol
  l. injection
  l. transarterial embolization treatment
lipoblastic sarcoma
lipoblastoma
lipocalin
  neutrophil gelatinase-associated l.
    (NGAL)
lipocele
lipodystrophy
  Dunnigan-type familial partial l.
  intestinal l.
  mesenteric l.
lipofection reagent
lipofuscin
lipogranuloma
  mesenteric l.
lipogranulomatosis
lipohyperplasia
  ileocecal valve l.
lipoidal
lipoid nephrosis
lipolysis
  heparin-induced l.
  intraluminal l.
  intravascular l.
  LPL-mediated l.
lipolytic enzyme
lipoma
  colonic l.
  gastric l.
  gastrointestinal l.
  l. of cord
  submucosal ileal l.
lipomalike tissue
lipomatosis
  pelvic l.
lipomatous
  l. ileocecal valve
  l. nephritis
  l. paranephritis
  l. tissue

lipomeningocele
lipomyelocystocele
lipomyelomeningocele
lipophagic intestinal granulomatosis
lipophagy
lipopolysaccharide
lipoprotein
  apolipoprotein B-containing l.
  l. glomerulopathy
  high-density l. (HDL)
  intermediate density l. (IDL)
  intermediate low density l. (ILDL)
  l. lipase (LPL)
  liver-specific membrane l.
  low-density l. (LDL)
  l. metabolism
  oxidized low-density l. (Ox-LDL)
  triglyceride-rich l. (TRL)
  very low density l. (VLDL)
  l. X
  l. X level
liposarcoma
  bladder l.
  kidney l.
  spermatic cord l.
liposclerotic mesenteritis
liposomal
  l. amphotericin B (L-AmB)
  l. daunorubicin HCl
Liposorber System lithotriptor
Liposyn II fat emulsion solution
lipothymia
Lipoxide
lipoxin
lipoxygenase
  l. blockade
  l. inhibition
  l. inhibitor
  l. pathway
5-lipoxygenase inhibitor
Lipram-PN10
Lipshultz urology microsurgical set
liquefaciens
  Aeromonas l.
  Enterobacter l.
  Serratia l.
liquefaction
  semen l.
liquefactive necrosis
Liqui-Char
liquid (l, liq., liq)
  l. antacid
  AntaGel l.
  l. chemical germicide (LCG)
  l. chromatographic assay
  l. diarrhea
  l. diet
  EMF oral l.
  l. emptying

Enfamil Low Iron l.
l. food dysphagia
full l.'s
hyperosmolar l.
isoosmolar l.
Nutrament oral l.
Peptamen L.
Peptic Relief l.
Phenyl-Free oral l.
L. Pred
Resource Diabetic ready-to-use l.
Resource Fruit Beverage ready-to-use
l.
Resource Just for Kids ready-to-use
l.
Resource oral l.
l. scintillation spectrometer
l. stool

Liqui-Doss
Liqui-E
liquor
l. entericus
l. gastricus
l. pancreaticus
l. seminis
lisinopril
LISL
laser-induced intracorporeal shock wave
lithotripsy
listeria
L. monocytogenes
Listeria monocytogenes peritonitis
liter
international units per l. (IU/L)
millimoles per l. (mmol/L)
lithagogue
lithangiuria
lithectasy
lithectomy
lithiasis
Crixivan l.
intraductal l.
renal l.
urinary l.
lithium
l. clearance (CLi)
fractional excretion of l. (FELI)
lithocenosis
lithocholate
lithocholic
l. acid (LCA)
l. acid-deoxycholic acid (LCA-DCA)
l. acid-deoxycholic acid ratio
lithoclast
L. endoscopic lithotriptor
Swiss L.
lithoclysmia
lithocystotomy
lithodialysis

lithogenesis, lithogeny
urinary l.
lithogenic bile
lithogeny (*var. of* lithogenesis)
Lithognost flash-lamp pulsed-dye laser
lithokonion
litholabe
litholapaxy
Bigelow l.
litholysis
chemical l.
litholyte
litholytic
lithometer
lithomyl
lithonephritis
lithonephrotomy
lithophone
lithoscope
Lithostar
L. nonimmersion lithotriptor
L. Plus
L. Plus electromagnetic lithotriptor
bidimensional x-ray focusing
system
Siemens L.
Lithostat
lithostathine molecule
lithotome
lithotomist
lithotomy
bilateral lithotomies
dorsal l.
high l.
lateral l.
Marian l.
median l.
mediolateral l.
perineal l.
l. position
prerectal l.
rectovesical l.
suprapubic l.
vaginal l.
vesical l.
vesicovaginal l.
lithotresis
ultrasonic l.
lithotripsy, lithotrity
alexandrite laser l.
biliary l.
blind l.
contact l.
coumarin green tunable dye laser l.
cystoscopic electrohydraulic l.
Dornier extracorporeal shock
wave l.
Dornier MPL gallstone l.
electrohydraulic l. (EHL)

L

lithotripsy (*continued*)
  electrohydraulic shock wave l. (ESWL)
  endoscopic-controlled l.
  endoscopic electrohydraulic l.
  endoscopic Ho:YAG l.
  endoscopic metallic stent l.
  endoscopic pulsed-dye laser l.
  external shock wave l.
  extracorporeal piezoelectric l. (EPL)
  extracorporeal piezoelectric shock wave l.
  intracorporeal l.
  intracorporeal electrohydraulic l. (IEHL)
  intracorporeal laser l. (ILL)
  intracorporeal shock wave l. (ISWL)
  laser l.
  laser-induced intracorporeal shock wave l. (LISL)
  limited economic l.
  mechanical l.
  Medstone extracorporeal shock wave l.
  nonstented ureteroscopic l.
  pancreatoscopic laser l. (PSLL)
  peroral shock wave l. (PSWL)
  piezoelectric l.
  pneumatic l.
  pressure-regulated electrohydraulic l.
  l. retreatment
  shock wave l. (SWL)
  stented ureteroscopic l.
  l. table
  l. technology
  tunable dye laser l.
  ultrasonic l.
  ureteroscopic intracorporeal electrohydraulic l.
  visible-light l.
lithotripsy-induced hypertension
lithotripter (*var. of* lithotriptor)
lithotriptic
lithotriptor, lithotripter
  American Endoscopy mechanical l.
  Breakstone l.
  Calcutript electrohydraulic l.
  Circon-ACMI l.
  Diasonics Therasonic l.
  Direx Tripter X-1 l.
  DoLi S extracorporeal shock wave l.
  Dornier compact l.
  Dornier electrohydraulic l.
  Dornier gallstone l.
  Dornier MFL l.
  Dornier MPL l.
  DP-1 l.
  dual-pulse l.

Econolith l.
EDAP l.
effective l.
electrohydraulic l.
electromagnetic l.
electropneumatic endoscopic l.
extracorporeal piezoelectric l.
extracorporeal shock wave l.
HM4 l.
intracorporeal l.
Karl Storz-Lutzeyer l.
laser l.
Liposorber System l.
Lithoclast endoscopic l.
Lithostar nonimmersion l.
manual l.
Medispec Econolith spark plug l.
Medstone STS l.
Modulith SL l.
Northgate SD-3 dual-purpose l.
Olympus BML-3Q, -4Q l.
out-of-scope l.
percutaneous ultrasonic l.
piezoelectric shock wave l.
Piezolith EPL l.
pneumatic endoscopic l.
Pulsalith l.
Richard Wolf Piezolith l.
second-generation l.
shock wave l.
Siemens Lithostar Plus System C l.
Sonolith Praktis portable l.
Sonotrode l.
Swiss Lithoclast l.
Technomed Sonolith l.
Therasonics l.
third-generation l.
tubeless l.
Twinheads shock wave l.
ultrasonic l.
Waltz endoscopic l.
water cushion l.
Wilson-Cook mechanical l.
Wolf Piezolith l.
Wolf Sonolith l.
lithotriptoscope
lithotriptoscopy
lithotrite
  Lowsley l.
  Marmite l.
  Reliquet l.
  Rotolith l.
  Thompson l.
  Wolf l.
lithotrity (*var. of* lithotripsy)
lithous
Lithovac stone removal
lithoxiduria

lithuresis
lithureteria
litmus milk test
LITT
    laser interstitial thermal therapy
littoral
    l. cell
    l. cell angioma
Littré
    crypt of L.
    L. gland
    L. hernia
Livaditis circular myotomy
live
    l. attenuated virus
    BCG l.
    l. renal donation
live-donor
    l.-d. nephrectomy
    l.-d. segmental graft
liver
    l. abscess
    l. acinus
    acute fatty l.
    acute yellow atrophy of l.
    l. Ah receptor
    albuminoid l.
    alcoholic fatty l.
    ballottable l.
    bare area of l.
    l. bed
    biliary cirrhotic l.
    bioartificial l.
    l. biopsy
    l. breath
    l. cancer
    capsular cirrhosis of l.
    l. capsule
    cardiac impression on l.
    caudate eminence of l.
    caudate lobe of l.
    l. cell adenoma
    l. cell carcinoma
    l. cell dysplasia
    l. cell plate
    centrilobular region of l.
    l. cirrhosis
    cirrhotic l.
    colic impression on l.
    cutdown l.
    cut surface of l.
    l. cyst infection
    l. death
    l. deposit
    l. dialysis system
    l. dialysis unit
    diaphragmatic surface of l.
    l. diet
    l. distribution

dome of l.
l. dullness
duodenal impression on l.
l. eater
echogenic l.
l. edge
l. engorgement
l. enzyme
l. failure
fatty l.
fatty infiltration of l.
l. fibrosis
fibrous appendage of l.
fibrous capsule of l.
fibrous tunic of l.
finely fatty foamy l.
l. flap
l. flap sign
l. fluke
foamy l.
focal fatty infiltration of l.
focal nonfatty infiltration of l.
l. function profile
l. function series (LFS)
l. function tests (LFT)
gastric impression on l.
l. hilum
hobnail l.
l. hydatid disease
l. impression
l. iron store
l., kidneys, spleen (LKS)
laparoscopic biopsy of l.
large-droplet fatty l.
lobe of l.
lobular architecture of l.
l. lymphoma
macrovesicular fatty l.
l. meal
l. membrane antigen
l. metastasis
nodular l.
l. nodule
noncirrhotic l.
nonparasitic cyst of l.
nutmeg l.
L. Panel Plus 9
l. parenchyma
phlegmonous alcoholic fatty l.
polycystic disease of l. (PDL)
polylobar l.
potato l.
l. protein store
pyogenic l.
quadrate lobe of l.
renal impression on l.
l. resection
sagittal fissure of l.
l. scan

L

liver (*continued*)
    segmentectomy of l.
    shock l.
    shrunken l.
    l. sinusoid
    l. sinusoidal endothelial cell
    small-droplet fatty l.
    l. span
    stasis l.
    subacute atrophy of l.
    subchronic atrophy of l.
    suprarenal area of l.
    tender l.
    l. transplant
    l. transplantation
    l. transplantation preservation injury
    l. trauma
    undersurface of l.
    undifferentiated embryonal sarcoma of l. (UESL)
    venoocclusive disease of l.
    l. volume
    wandering l.
    yellow atrophy of l.
liver-adipose tissue cycle
liver-deprived epithelial clonic cell
liver-directed autoreactivity
liver-kidney
    l.-k. microsomal antibody
    l.-k. microsome (LKM)
liver-specific
    l.-s. antigen
    l.-s. membrane lipoprotein
    l.-s. protein (LSP)
liver-spleen scan
liverwort
    American l.
living
    l. adult-to-adult donor
    l. donor
    l. donor kidney
    l. donor liver transplantation (LDLT)
    l. donor transplant
    l. related donor (LRD)
    l. unrelated donor (LURD)
Livingston triangle
livor mortis
LKB Optiphase 2 scintillation fluid
LKB-Wallac scintillation counter
LKM
    liver-kidney microsome
    LKM specificity
LKS
    liver, kidneys, spleen
LLC
    laparoscopic laser cholecystectomy
    MedSlant LLC

LLC-PK1-FBPase+ cell
LLC-PK renal tubular cell
Lloyd-Davies
    L.-D. stirrup
    L.-D. Trendelenburg position
Lloyd-Davis
    L.-D. knee and leg holder
    L.-D. sigmoidoscope
Lloyd sign
LMA
    lactose malabsorption
LMCL
    lower midclavicular line
LMP **gene**
LMW
    low molecular weight
LMWH
    low molecular weight heparin
LMWP
    low molecular weight protein
LND
    lymph node dissection
L-NAME
    N^G-nitro-arginine methyl ester
L-N-monomethyl-arginine
load
    osmotic l.
    virus l.
loading
    differential l.
    methionine l.
    peripheral l.
    uniform l.
    water l.
lobar
    l. atrophy
    l. nephronia
lobatum
    hepar l.
lobe
    caudate l.
    l. graft
    Home l.
    kidney l.
    kissing prostatic l.'s
    lateral l.
    left hepatic l.
    median l.
    l. of liver
    predominant median l.
    quadrate l.
    renal l.
    Riedel l.
    right l.
lobectomy
    hepatic l.
lobi (*pl. of* lobus)
lobucavir

lobular
- l. architecture
- l. architecture of liver
- l. hepatitis
- l. inflammatory infiltrate
- l. mononuclear cell infiltrate
- l. necroinflammation

lobulated
- l. border
- l. filling defect
- l. mass

lobulation
- portal l.

lobule
- l. of pancreas
- portal l.

lobuli (*pl. of* lobulus)
lobulization
lobulose
lobulus, *pl.* **lobuli**
- lobuli testis

lobus, *pl.* **lobi**
local
- l. alcohol instillation effect
- l. anesthesia
- l. depot injection
- l. glomerular lesion
- l. recurrence
- l. scarring

localization
- bleeding site l.
- manometric l.
- pancreatic tumor l.
- target l.

localized
- l. amyloidosis
- l. lesion
- l. pain

localizing tenderness
locally
- l. acting paracrine effector
- l. made rapid urease test (LRUT)

location
- distant pH probe l.
- tumor l.

locator
- LES l.
- lower esophageal sphincter l.

LoCholest
loci (*pl. of* locus)
locker room syndrome
locking suture
lock stitch
lock-stitch suture
Lockwood-Allis intestinal forceps
LOCM
- low osmolar contrast medium

locomotor
Locteron

locus, *pl.* **loci**
- hereditary prostate cancer 1 l. (HPC-1)
- tellurite resistance loci

Loewe (*see also* **Löwe**)
Lofenalac formula
logarithmic rate
Logen
logger
- Digitrapper Gold MK III solid-state data l.

logistic regression analysis
log-rank test
Lohlein-Baehr lesion
Lohlein nephritis
loin
- l. pain
- l. pain hematuria syndrome (LPHS)

lollipop tree sign
Lomanate
lomefloxacin
- l. HCl
- l. hydrochloride
- l. TMP-SMX

Lomotil
lomustine
Lonalac
- L. feeding
- L. formula

Lone
- L. Star retractor
- L. Star self-retractor

long
- l. acting (LA, L.A.)
- l. anal sphincter
- L. 45 endocutter
- l. incubation hepatitis
- l. intestinal tube
- l. intestinal tube decompression
- l. Roux-en-Y pouch jejunostomy
- l. seal
- l. terminal repeat
- l. vascular needle driver

longa
- *Curcuma* l.

long-chain
- l.-c. acyl-CoA dehydrogenase deficiency
- l.-c. fatty acid (LCFA)
- l.-c. 3-hydroxyacyl coenzyme A dehydrogenase (LCHAD)
- l.-c. triglyceride (LCT)

longitudinal (l, long.)
- l. band of colon
- l. choledochotomy
- l. colostomy
- l. enterotomy
- l. esophageal stricture
- l. fasciculus of colon

longitudinal (*continued*)
- l. fissure
- l. image
- l. laceration
- l. myotomy
- l. nephrotomy of Boyce
- l. pancreatojejunostomy
- l. subepithelial venous plexus
- l. ulcer
- l. view

longitudinalis
- plica l.

long-jaw disposable forceps
long-limb surgical bypass
Longmire operation
long-neck diverticulum
long-nosed
- l.-n. retriever snare
- l.-n. sphincterotome

Longo hemorrhoidectomy
long-segment
- l.-s. Barrett esophagus (LSBE)
- l.-s. CLE

long-term
- l.-t. antibiotic
- l.-t. catheter use
- l.-t. effect of metabolic acidosis
- l.-t. followup data
- l.-t. graft destruction
- l.-t. indwelling catheter
- l.-t. low-dose maintenance chemoprophylaxis
- l.-t. outcome
- l.-t. outcome of urethroplasty
- l.-t. renal functional effect
- l.-t. result
- l.-t. survival of renal allograft

longum
- *Bifidobacterium l.*

Lonox
3-loop
- 3-l. ileal pouch
- 3-l. technique

loop
- afferent l.
- air-filled l.
- alpha-sigmoid l.
- autocrine reinforcing l.
- Biebl l.
- bipolar urological l.
- blind l.
- bowel l.
- Bradley l.
- brainstem-sacral l.
- C l.
- l. caliber
- cerebral-sacral l.
- l. choledochojejunostomy
- closed afferent l.

closed efferent l.
- colonic l.
- contiguous l.
- Cordonnier ureteroileal l.
- Davis l.
- diathermic l.
- l. diuretic
- double reverse alpha-sigmoid l.
- duodenal C l.
- efferent l.
- l. end ileostomy
- l. esophagojejunostomy
- l. forearm graft
- gamma transverse colon l.
- l. gastrojejunostomy
- Heiss l.
- Henle l.
- ileal l.
- intestinal l.
- jejunal interposition of Henle l.
- l. jejunostomy
- l. ligation
- Maxon l.
- N l.
- N-shaped sigmoid l.
- l. of Henle
- l. of redundant colon
- ostomy l.
- l. ostomy bridge
- polyglactin monofilament l.
- polyglyconate monofilament l.
- puborectalis l.
- resectoscope l.
- reverse alpha sigmoid l.
- Roeder l.
- Roux-en-Y l.
- sentinel l.
- sigmoid l.
- l. stoma
- Surgitite ligating l.
- l. suture
- transverse l.
- l. transverse colostomy
- Vapor Cut l.
- vesical-sacral-sphincter l.
- Wedge l.

looped cautery
looping of endoscope
2-loop J-shaped ileal pouch
loopogram
loopography
- ileal l.
- retrograde l.

loop-tipped electrode
loop-type
- l.-t. snare forceps
- l.-t. stone-crushing forceps

Looser-Milkman stria
loose stool

loosestrife
>   purple l.

loperamide
Lopez enteral valve
Lopid
Lopressor
LoPressure panendoscope
LoPresti
>   L. fiberoptic endoscope
>   L. fiberoptic esophagoscope

Lopurin
Lorabid
loracarbef
Lorad StereoGuide
lorazepam
Lord
>   L. dilation
>   L. dilation of hemorrhoid
>   L. method of hemorrhoidectomy
>   L. procedure

Lorenzo oil
Lortat-Jacob hepatic resection
Los
>   L. Angeles (LA, L.A.)
>   L. Angeles classification
>   L. Angeles classification grade A,
>   B, C, D esophagitis
>   L. Angeles classification of GERD

losartan
Losec
LoSo
>   L. Prep
>   L. Prep bowel cleansing solution

Losotron Plus
losoxantrone
loss
>   autoimmune sensorineural hearing l.
>   chronic gastrointestinal blood l.
>   chronic GI blood l.
>   cortical l.
>   electrolyte l.
>   estimated blood l. (EBL)
>   fluid l.
>   ganglion cell l.
>   graft l.
>   negligible blood l.
>   nephron l.
>   obligatory dialysate protein l.
>   l. of heterozygosity
>   l. of sigmoid curve
>   penile skin l.
>   psoas l.
>   sensory l.
>   weight l.

Lotheissen-McVay technique
Lotrel
Lotrimin
Lotrisone
Lotronex tablet

lotus
loupe
>   Keeler panoramic l.
>   surgical l.
>   wide-angled l.

lovastatin
Lovelace forceps
Lovenox
low
>   l. anterior resection (LAR)
>   l. anterior resection in combination
>   with coloanal anastomosis
>   (LAR/CAA)
>   l. available carbohydrate diet
>   l. coloanal anastomosis
>   l. intermittent suction
>   l. intersphincteric anal fistula
>   l. molecular weight (LMW)
>   l. molecular weight heparin
>   (LMWH)
>   l. molecular weight protein
>   (LMWP)
>   l. molecular weight protein
>   ribonuclease
>   l. osmolar contrast medium
>   (LOCM)
>   l. recurrence rate
>   l. salt
>   l. small-bowel obstruction
>   l. sodium
>   l. tonicity
>   l. transverse incision
>   l. urethral pressure (LUP)
>   l. vaginal confluence

low-affinity
>   l.-a. high-capacity system
>   l.-a. transporter

low-calcium dialysate
low-calorie diet
low-compliance
>   l.-c. balloon
>   l.-c. bladder
>   l.-c. perfusion pump
>   l.-c. perfusion system
>   l.-c. pneumohydraulic pump

low-density
>   l.-d. lipoprotein (LDLP, LDL)
>   l.-d. lipoprotein cholesterol (LDLC)
>   l.-d. lipoprotein susceptibility

low-dose
>   l.-d. HpD
>   l.-d. interferon

Lowe (*see also* **Löwe**)
>   L. syndrome

Löwe (*see also* **Loewe**)
>   L. disease

low-energy
>   l.-e. program
>   l.-e. protocol

L

low-energy (*continued*)
   l.-e. transurethral microwave thermotherapy (LE-TUMT)
   l.-e. TUMT
lower
   l. abdominal reoperation
   l. abdominal transverse incision
   l. anterior axillary line (LAAL)
   l. energy treatment
   l. esophageal B ring
   l. esophageal contraction ring
   l. esophageal mucosal ring
   l. esophageal sphincter (LES)
   l. esophageal sphincter circular muscle
   l. esophageal sphincter locator
   l. esophageal sphincter pressure (LESP)
   l. esophageal sphincter relaxation (LESR)
   l. esophageal sphincter tone
   L. gall duct forceps
   l. gastrointestinal bleeding (LGIB)
   l. gastrointestinal hemorrhage
   l. GI bleeding
   l. GI tract foreign body
   l. infundibular diameter
   l. infundibular length
   l. infundibulum
   l. midclavicular line (LMCL)
   l. motor neuron bladder disorder
   l. motor neuron lesion
   l. nephron nephrosis
   l. panendoscopy
   l. pole laceration
   l. pole stone
   l. ureter
   l. ureteric calculus
   l. urinary tract dysfunction (LUTD)
   l. urinary tract obstruction (LUTO)
   l. urinary tract symptom (LUTS)
   l. urinary tract symptomatology
Lowery method
lowest clearance
Lowe syndrome (LS)
low-fat diet
low-fiber diet
low-flow priapism
low-flux
   l.-f. cuprophane membrane
   l.-f. dialysis membrane
   l.-f. polysulfone membrane
low-grade
   l.-g. dysplasia (LGD)
   l.-g. fever
   l.-g. leiomyosarcoma
   l.-g. positive smear
low-lactose diet

low-loop cutaneous ureterostomy
low-lying rectal cancer
low-magnification electron micrograph
Lown criteria
low-oxalate diet
low-pitched bowel sounds
low-power photomicrograph
low-pressure
   l.-p. argon gas/liquid mercury lamp
   l.-p. bladder substitute
   l.-p. cardiopulmonary baroreceptor
   l.-p. low-flow voiding dysfunction
   l.-p. pouch
   l.-p. venous system
low-pulsatility arterial waveform
low-residue
   l.-r. diet
   l.-r. feeding
low-roughage diet
Lowsium
Lowsley
   L. lithotrite
   L. operation
   L. retractor
   L. tractor
Lowsley-Peterson cystoscope
low-sodium diet
low-tyrosine, low-phenylalanine diet
low-volume
   l.-v. PEG
   l.-v. sclerotherapy
loxiglumide
lozenge
   tetracaine l.
Lozol
LP
   limited partnership
   lymphomatous polyposis
      AstraZeneca Pharmaceuticals LP
l-PAM
   l-phenylalanine mustard
LPH
   lactase-phlorizin hydrolase
l-phenylalanine mustard (l-PAM)
LPHS
   loin pain hematuria syndrome
LPL
   lipoprotein lipase
LPL-mediated lipolysis
LPLND
   laparoscopic pelvic lymph node dissection
LPN
   laparoscopic partial nephrectomy
LPP
   leak-point pressure
LRE
   lamina rara externa
L-rhamnose

LRI
　　lamina rara interna
LRN
　　laparoscopic radical nephrectomy
LRP
　　laparoscopic radical prostatectomy
LRS
　　lactated Ringer solution
LRUT
　　locally made rapid urease test
LSBE
　　long-segment Barrett esophagus
LSC 7000 curved-array transducer
LSD
　　lysosomal storage disease
L-selectin
LSP
　　liver-specific protein
LTBR
　　lymphotoxin beta receptor
LTD, Ltd.
　　limited
　　　　Given Imaging Ltd.
LTT
　　lactose tolerance test
Lubb syndrome
lubiprostone
Lubraseptic jelly
lubricant
　　l. laxative
　　Surgilube l.
Lubri-Flex ureteral stent
lucent cyst
Lucey-Driscoll syndrome
Luder-Sheldon syndrome
Ludwig labyrinth
Luer
　　L. hemorrhoid forceps
　　L. syringe
Luer-Lok
　　L.-L. connector
　　L.-L. syringe
lues
Lugol
　　L. chromoendoscopy
　　L. dye spray chromoendoscopy
　　L. iodide
　　L. iodine
　　L. iodine solution
　　L. solution stain
Lugol-combined upper gastrointestinal videoendoscopy
Lugol-voiding lesion
Lukes-Collins classification
lumbar
　　l. appendicitis
　　l. artery
　　l. kidney
　　l. nephrectomy

　　l. nephrotomy
　　l. plexus
　　l. spinal cord lesion
　　l. spine bone mineral density
　　l. vein
lumbocolostomy
lumbocolotomy
lumbocostoabdominal triangle
lumbodorsal
　　l. fascia
　　l. incision
　　l. ligament
lumbosacral
　　l. fascia
　　l. plexus
　　l. trunk
lumbotomy
　　dorsal l.
　　l. incision
　　posterior l.
lumbricoides
　　Ascaris l.
lumen, *pl.* **lumina, lumens**
　　bile duct l.
　　bowel l.
　　cystic duct l.
　　duct l.
　　duodenal l.
　　esophageal l.
　　gastroduodenal l.
　　Lumina guidewire
　　intestinal l.
　　l. of seminiferous tubule
　　rectal l.
　　scalloped bowel l.
　　single l.
8-lumen catheter assembly
lumens (*pl. of* lumen)
lumen-seeking catheter
lumen-to-bath sodium flux
4-lumen tube
lumina (*pl. of* lumen)
luminal
　　l. acid
　　l. acid clearance
　　l. amoxicillin
　　l. antigliadin
　　l. bulge
　　l. candesartan
　　l. CCK-releasing factor
　　l. contents
　　l. contrast study
　　l. Crohn disease
　　l. diameter
　　l. EGF
　　l. glucose
　　l. HCO_3^{-}
　　l. hypoacidity
　　l. narrowing

luminal (*continued*)
    l. nutrition
    l. secretagogue
    l. sodium
    l. stenosis
Luminexx stent
luminol-enhanced chemiluminescence
luminometer
Lumi-Phos 530
lump kidney
Lunar DPX total-body scanner
lunata
    Curvularia l.
lunatus
    penis l.
Lunderquist guidewire
Lunderquist-Ring torque guide
Lundh
    L. meal
    L. test
lung
    l. cancer
    l. disease
    l. dysplasia
    farmer's l.
    l. purpura
LUP
    low urethral pressure
lupoid hepatitis
Lupron Depot
lupus
    l. anticoagulant
    l. erythematosus (LE)
    l. nephritis
LURD
    living unrelated donor
LUS
    laparoscopic ultrasound
Luschka
    accessory duct of L.
    L. crypt
    L. cystic gland
    L. duct
lusoria
    arteria l.
    dysphagia l.
lusorian artery
LUTD
    lower urinary tract dysfunction
luteinized granulosa-theca cell tumor
luteinizing
    l. hormone (LH)
    l. hormone follicle-stimulating hormone (LH-FSH)
    l. hormone follicle-stimulating hormone-releasing factor
    l. hormone-releasing hormone (LHRH)
    l. hormone-releasing hormone antagonist
Lütkens sphincter
LUTO
    lower urinary tract obstruction
LUTS
    lower urinary tract symptom
Lutz automatic reprocessor
luxation
Luy segregator
LVP
    large-volume paracentesis
lwoffii
    Acinetobacter l.
LX-20 laser
lyase
    cystathionine gamma l.
    gamma l.
Lycopodium serratum
lye ingestion
Lyell disease
Lyme disease
lymph
    l. channel
    l. node
    l. node adenopathy
    l. node dissection (LND)
    l. node metastasis
    l. scrotum
    subcarinal l.
lymphadenectomy
    endocavitary pelvic l. (ECPL)
    endoscopic transgastric l.
    extended pelvic l.
    2-field l.
    3-field l.
    inguinal l.
    laparoscopic pelvic l.
    mediastinal l.
    mesorectal l.
    minilaparotomy staging pelvic l.
    paraaortic l.
    pelvic l.
    prophylactic l.
    retroperitoneal l.
    thoracoabdominal retroperitoneal l.
lymphadenitis
    Kikuchi l.
lymphadenopathy
    cervical l.
    inguinal l.
    malignant peribiliary l.
    mediastinal l.
    perihepatic l.
    l. syndrome
lymphangiectasia (*var. of* lymphangiectasis)
lymphangiectasis, lymphangiectasia
    congenital renal l.
    intestinal l.

pancreatic l.
peritoneal l.
primary intestinal l. (PIL)
lymphangiogram
lymphangiography
lymphangioma
scrotal l.
lymphangitic streak
lymphangitis
penile sclerosing l.
sclerosing l.
lymphapheresis
lymphatic
l. channel
l. leak
l. metastasis
l. microcyst
l. obstruction
l. package
l. transport
l. vessel
lymphatica
folliculus l.
lymphedema
filarial l.
lymphoblast homing
lymphoblastoid
l. cell line
l. interferon alfa
lymphoblastoma
kidney l.
renal l.
lymphocele
l. aspiration
l. internal drainage
l. percutaneous drainage
l. spontaneous regression
lymphocelectomy
laparoscopic l.
pelvic l.
lymphocyst
lymphocyte
B l.
CD8 l.
CD8+ T l.
CD45RO l.
l. costimulatory molecule
l. count
crypt intraepithelial l. (cIEL)
cytolytic T l. (CTL)
l. cytotoxicity
cytotoxic T l. (CTL)
l. immune globulin (LIG)
intraepithelial l. (IEL)
intrahepatic l.
l. migration
naive B and T l.'s
peripheral blood l. (PBL)
sinusoidal l.

T l.
l. target cell
thymus-derived l.
total l.'s
tumor-infiltrating l. (TIL)
virgin l.
WBC l.
lymphocyte-hepatocyte
intrahepatic antigen-dependent l.-h.
lymphocytic
l. colitis
l. gastritis (LG)
l. vasculitis
lymphocytosis
intraepithelial l.
lymphocytotoxic antibody
lymphocyturia
lymphoepithelial lesion
lymphogenic metastasis
lymphogranuloma venereum (LGV)
lymphography
lymphohemangioma
bladder l.
lymphohistiocytic infiltration
lymphoid
l. aggregate
l. cholangitis
l. component
l. follicle
l. interstitial pneumonia
l. nodule
l. polyp
l. tumor
lymphokine-activated
l.-a. killer (LAK)
l.-a. killer cell
lymphokine production
lymphoma
benign l.
bladder l.
Burkitt l.
colorectal l.
cutaneous T-cell l.
duodenal l.
enteropathy-associated T-cell l.
(EATCL)
gastric l.
hepatosplenic T-cell l.
histiocytic l.
infiltrative l.
liver l.
MALT l.
marginal zone l.
Mediterranean l.
mucosa-associated lymphoid tissue l.
(MALToma)
nodular l.
non-Hodgkin l. (NHL)
penis l.

L

lymphoma (*continued*)
  polypoid l.
  primary B-cell l.
  primary gastric l. (PGL)
  primary hepatosplenic l. (PHSL)
  prostate gland l.
  retroperitoneal l.
  seminal vesicle l.
  small-intestinal malignant l.
  small noncleaved-cell l.
  T-cell l.
  testicular l.
  ulcerative l.
lymphomatosis
lymphomatous
  l. nodule
  l. polyposis (LP)
lymphomononuclear cell
lymphonodular hyperplasia
lymphonodulus
lymphoplasmacytosis
lymphoproliferative
  l. disorder
  l. syndrome
lymphosarcoma
lymphoscintigraphy
lymphotoxin beta receptor (LTBR)
lymphovascular permeation
Lynch syndrome II
Lynx midurethral sling
Lyofoam dressing

Lyon
  L. ring
  L. ring constrictive band
lyophilized dura mater for pubovaginal sling
Lyphocin
lysate
  depleted l.
lyse
lysine
lysinuria
lysis
  colon tumor cell l.
  CTL-mediated l.
  laparoscopic l.
  mesangial l.
  l. of adhesions
  tumor cell l.
lysolecithin
lysosomal
  l. accumulation
  l. enzyme
  l. membrane
  l. storage disease (LSD)
  l. swelling
lysosome
  hepatocyte l.
lysozyme
lysyl-bradykinin
lytic cocktail
Lytren electrolyte solution

M

   M antibody
   M cell
   M phase

M1

   antibody to Leu M1
   glutathione S-transferase M1

M2A

   M2A capsule/Given imaging
     capsule
   M2A swallowable imaging capsule

MAA

   macroaggregated albumin
   MAA adduct
   ^{99m}Tc MAA

Maalox

   M. antacid/calcium supplement
   M. Anti-Gas Extra-Strength oral
     suspension
   M. HRF
   M. Plus
   M. Quick Dissolve chewable tablet
   M. spray
   M. Therapeutic Concentrate

MAb

   monoclonal antibody
   anticlass II MAb
   MAb IOT2-recognizing monomorphic
     DR determinant

MABP

   mean arterial blood pressure

Macalister

   valve of M.

Macaluso stent remover
MacConkey agar
Macdonald test
MACE

   Malone antegrade continence enema

Macewen

   M. hernia operation
   M. herniorrhaphy

MACH1

   metronidazole, amoxicillin,
     clarithromycin, *H. pylori*, 1-week
     therapy
   MACH1 study

Machado-Guerreiro test
Machida

   M. choledochoscope
   M. FCS-ML II magnifying
     colonoscope

machine

   ABGII hemodialysis m.
   Acuson-128 color flow Doppler m.
   Belzer m.

   endoscopic sewing m.
   Endotek m.
   Fresenius hemodialysis m.
   Gambro m.
   gastric hypothermia m.
   Kodak Ektachem 700 m.
   MOX portable renal preservation m.
   Narco esophageal motility m.
   Nova II m.
   perfusion m.
   Phillips ultrasound m.
   portable renal preservation m.
   Primus prostate m.

Mackenrodt

   ligament of M.

Mackenzie

   M. disease
   M. point

MacLean test
Maclet magnetic ring
macroaggregated albumin (MAA)
macroalbuminuria
macroamylase
macroamylasemia
macroangiodynamic
macroangiopathic hemolytic anemia
Macrobid
macrocephalia (*var. of* macrocephaly)
macrocephaly, macrocephalia
macrocrystal
macrocyclic triene
macrocyst

   adrenocortical m.

macrocystic pancreatic cystadenoma
Macrodantin
macrogenitosomia
macroglobulinemia

   Waldenström m.

macrolide

   m. antibiotic
   m. antimicrobial

macromolecular

   m. secretion
   m. uronate (MMUA)

macromolecule

   radiolabeled m.

macronidia
macronodular cirrhosis
macroorchidism lesion
macropenis
macrophage

   bile-laden m.
   ceroid-laden m.
   m. colony-stimulating factor
     (M-CSF)

M

macrophage (*continued*)
    hemosiderin-laden m.
    parasitizing m.
    peritoneal m.
macrophage-rich inflammatory response
macrophage-TGF-beta axis
macrophallus
Macroplastique
    M. implant
    M. implantation device
    M. injectable
    M. soft tissue synthetic bulking agent
macroprolactinoma
macroproteinuria
macroregenerative nodule
macroscopic
    m. hematuria
    m. lesion
    m. liver cyst
macrosomia
    fetal m.
macrosteatosis
macrothrombocyte
macrovascular disease
macrovesicular
    m. fat
    m. fatty liver
    m. steatosis
macula, *pl.* **maculae**
    m. densa
    m. densa cell
maculae (*pl. of* macula)
macule
maculopapular
Madayag biopsy needle
Madden
    M. hernia repair
    M. incisional herniorrhaphy
    M. intestinal clamp
    M. modified radical mastectomy technique
    M. repair of incisional hernia
Maddrey discriminant function
Madelung disease
Mad Hatter syndrome
Madigan prostatectomy
Madin-Darby canine kidney (MDCK)
Madsen-Iversen
    M.-I. scale
    M.-I. scoring system
Madsen symptom score
mafenide acetate
Maffucci syndrome
MAG
    multifocal atrophic gastritis

MAG-3
    mercaptoacetyltriglycine
    MAG-3 renal scan
    TechneScan MAG-3
magaldrate
Magic Lite chemiluminometric immunoassay
magna
    arteria pancreatica m.
    Fascioloides m.
    lacuna m.
Magnacal liquid feeding
Magnascanner
    Picker Vista M.
magnesia
    citrate of m.
    milk of m. (MOM)
    Phillips Milk of M.
magnesium
    m. ammonium phosphate
    m. ammonium phosphate urolithiasis
    m. carbonate
    m. citrate (mag cit)
    m. deficiency
    esomeprazole m.
    m. hydroxide
    m. metabolism
    m. oxide
    m. salt
    m. trisilicate
magnesium-induced diarrhea
magnet
    endoscopic gastroenteric anastomosis with m.'s
magnetic
    m. bore
    m. compression anastomosis
    m. endoscopic imaging
    m. internal ureteral stent
    m. resonance (MR)
    m. resonance angiography (MRA)
    m. resonance cholangiography (MRC)
    m. resonance cholangiopancreatography (MRCP)
    m. resonance colonography (MRC)
    m. resonance imaging (MRI)
    m. resonance imaging thermometry
    m. resonance pancreatography (MRP)
    m. resonance spectroscopy (MRS)
    m. resonance urography (MRU)
    m. stimulation
    m. susceptibility test
magnetization prepared-rapid gradient echo (MP-RAGE)
magnetoencephalography (MEG)
magnetometry

magnification
>   m. chromoendoscopy
>   m. endoscopy
>   m. endoscopy with acetic acid
>   spraying

magnifying
>   m. colonoscope
>   m. colonoscopy
>   m. endoscope
>   m. endoscopy with narrow-band
>   image system
>   m. enteroscope
>   m. pharmacoendoscopy

Mag-OX 400

MAGP
>   microfil-associated glycoprotein
>   MAGP microfibrillar protein

MAGPI
>   meatal advancement and glansplasty
>   meatal advancement, glanuloplasty,
>   penoscrotal junction meatotomy
>   MAGPI operation

Magsal tablet

mahogany-colored stool

Mahurkar catheter

MAI
>   *Mycobacterium avium-intracellulare*

main
>   m. pancreatic duct (MPD)
>   m. pancreatic duct stent

Maine
>   M. Medical Assessment Program
>   (MMAP)
>   M. Medical Assessment Program
>   index

Mainstay urologic soft tissue anchor

maintenance treatment

Mainz
>   M. enterocystoplasty
>   M. pouch augmentation
>   M. pouch cutaneous urinary
>   diversion
>   M. pouch I continent urinary
>   diversion
>   M. pouch II
>   M. pouch III
>   M. pouch urinary reservoir
>   M. urinary pouch

Mainz-type ureterocolostomy

maitre
>   tour de m.

Maixner cirrhosis

major
>   curvatura gastrica m.
>   curvatura ventriculi m.
>   m. deceleration injury
>   m. GI surgery
>   globus m.

>   m. histocompatibility complex
>   (MHC)
>   m. papilla
>   papilla duodeni m.

majus
>   *Chelidonium m.*
>   omentum m.

Makkas operation

Makler
>   M. cannula
>   M. counting chamber
>   M. insemination device
>   M. sperm-counting device

malabsorption
>   bile acid m. (BAM)
>   m. disease
>   D-xylose m.
>   folate m.
>   folic acid m.
>   glucose-galactose m.
>   iatrogenic m.
>   idiopathic bile acid m.
>   lactose m. (LMA)
>   lavage-induced pill m.
>   m. syndrome
>   vitamin B$_{12}$ m.

malabsorptive diarrhea

malacia
>   tracheobronchial m.

malacoplakia, malakoplakia
>   bladder m.
>   kidney m.
>   m. of kidney
>   m. vesicae

malacotomy

maladaptive response

Malakit *Helicobacter pylori* Biolab

malakoplakia (*var. of* malacoplakia)

malaria
>   algid m.
>   bilious remittent m.
>   dysenteric algid m.
>   falciparum m.
>   gastric m.
>   malignant tertian m.
>   pernicious m.
>   *Plasmodium falciparum* m.
>   quartan m.

malariae
>   *Plasmodium m.*

malarial
>   m. dysentery
>   m. hepatitis
>   m. nephropathy

malate

malayi
>   *Brugia m.*

maldescended testicle

maldescent

M

maldigestion
    lipid m.
maldigestion-absorption syndrome
maldigestive diarrhea
maldigestor
    lactose m.
male
    m. catheter
    m. epispadias
    m. escutcheon
    m. genitalia melanoma
    m. pelvis
    m. perineum
    m. predominance of urinary tract
      calculi
    m. sterility
    m. Turner syndrome
maleate
    methysergide m.
    perhexiline m.
    tegaserod m.
Malecare
Malecot
    M. gastrostomy tube
    M. nephrostomy tube
    M. reentry catheter
    M. suprapubic catheter
malemission
malformation
    anorectal m.
    anus m.
    arteriovenous m. (AVM)
    bronchopulmonary foregut m.
    Chiari m.
    cloacal m.
    Dieulafoy vascular m.
    dysraphic m.
    gastric arteriovenous m.
    mermaid m.
    polypoid vascular m.
    pulmonary arteriovenous m.
    scrotal arteriovenous m.
    sink-trap m.
    submucosal arterial m.
    submucosal vascular m.
    vascular m.
malignancy
    bulky m.
    de novo m.
    detection of m.
    esophageal m.
    esophagocardial m.
    extracolonic m. (ECM)
    hepatic m.
    hepatobiliary m.
    humoral hypercalcemia of m.
      (HHM)
    hypercalcemia of m.
    nonskin m.

    pancreaticobiliary m.
    paratesticular m.
    periampullary m.
    peritoneal m.
malignancy-associated cellular marker
malignant
    m. acanthosis nigricans
    m. ascites
    m. atrophic papulosis
    m. B-cell syndrome
    m. biliary obstruction
    m. biliary obstructive disease
    m. cachexia
    m. carcinoid syndrome
    m. dysentery
    m. dysphagia
    m. dysplasia
    m. esophagopericardial fistula
    m. histiocytosis
    m. hyperthermia
    m. malnutrition
    m. melanoma
    m. mesenchymal tumor
    m. mesenchymoma
    m. nephrosclerosis
    m. nuclear structure
    m. obstructive jaundice
    m. pancreatic neoplasm
    m. peribiliary lymphadenopathy
    m. pheochromocytoma
    m. polyp
    m. potential
    m. pseudoachalasia
    m. rectal stricture
    m. renal mass
    m. seeding
    m. serous cystic neoplasm of
      pancreas
    m. stenosis
    m. teratoma
    m. tertian malaria
    m. ulcer
maljunction
    pancreaticobiliary m.
mall
    space of M.
Mallard incision
malleability
    pelvic m.
malleable
    m. blade
    m. implant
    m. prosthesis
    m. retractor
    m. scoop
Mallinckrodt catheter
Mallory
    M. hyalin
    M. hyaline body

Mallory-Azan stain
Mallory-Weiss
    M.-W. laceration
    M.-W. lesion
    M.-W. mucosal rupture
    M.-W. syndrome
    M.-W. tear
mallow
    high m.
    musk m.
malnourished
malnutrition
    index of m.
    malignant m.
    protein-calorie m. (PCM)
    protein-energy m. (PEM)
malnutrition-related diabetes mellitus (MRDM)
malodorous
    m. fluid
    m. stool
malondialdehyde (MDA)
malondialdehyde-acetaldehyde adduct
Malone
    M. antegrade colonic enema
    M. antegrade colonic enema stoma procedure
    M. antegrade continence enema (MACE)
    M. antegrade continence enema
    M. antegrade continence enema channel
    M. cecostomy
    M. conduit
    M. continent appendicostomy
    M. principle
Maloney
    M. bougie
    M. dilation
    M. mercury-filled esophageal dilator
    M. tapered-tip dilator
Maloney-Hurst dilator
malpighian
    m. body
    m. corpuscles
    m. glomerulus
malpighii
    acinus renalis m.
    acinus renis m.
    stratum m.
Malpighi pyramid
malrotation
    intestinal m.
    midgut volvulus with m.
    m. of intestine
MALT
    mucosa-associated lymphoid tissue
    MALT lymphoma

maltase glucoamylase
Maltese cross
MALToma
    mucosa-associated lymphoid tissue lymphoma
maltophilia
    Stenotrophomonas m.
    Xanthomonas m.
maltose tetrapalmitate
Maltsupex
Maly test
mammalgia
mammalian
    m. cell membrane
    m. transgenesis
mammillated
mammillation
mammilliform
mammose
management
    antibiotic m.
    conservative m.
    endoscopic m.
    endourologic m.
    foreign body m.
    laparoscopic m.
    mechanical endoscopic m.
    m. of adult urinary tract trauma
    open m.
    seton m.
    stone m.
Manchester-Fothergill uterine suspension
Manchester virus
Manchurian hemorrhagic fever
Mancke flex-rigid gastroscope
Mandelamine
mandelate
    methenamine m.
mandelic acid
mandible
mandril set
maneuver
    alpha-loop m.
    avoidance m.
    bunching m.
    Credé placental removal m.
    experimental m.
    Fowler-Stephens spermatic vessel ligation m.
    Heimlich m.
    Hoguet hernial sac conversion m.
    Hueter m.
    J-type m.
    Ko-Airan cystic artery hemostasis m.
    Kocher m.
    Leadbetter hip reduction m.
    Mattox m.
    Mendelsohn m.

M

maneuver (*continued*)
Müller esophageal varices m.
peroral m.
Prentiss cryptorchidism repair m.
Pringle liver hemorrhage m.
straightening m.
suppressive m.
U-turn m.
Valsalva m.
mangafodipir trisodium
manifestation
extrahepatic m.
frequent joint m.
hepatobiliary m.
otolaryngologic m.
tissue m.
Manifold II slot-blot apparatus
manipulation)
antegrade ureteroscopic m.
direct m.
endoscopic stone m.
pancreatic duct m.
postureteroscopic m.
transurethral endoscopic m.
manipulator
endoscopic m.
mannan
yeast strain m.
Mann-Bollman fistula
Manning criteria
mannitol
mannose-specific adhesion
mannosidase
alpha-delta m.
Mann-Whitney rank sum test
Mann-Williamson
M.-W. operation
M.-W. ulcer
manofluorography (MFG)
manometer
manometric
m. criteria
m. evaluation
m. feature
m. finding
m. localization
m. pattern
m. sensor
m. study
manometry
ambulatory m.
anal vector m.
aneroid m.
anorectal m.
antral m.
antroduodenal m.
antroduodenojejunal m.
balloon reflex m.

biliary m.
m. catheter
colonic m.
computer-aided ambulatory gastrojejunal m.
dry swallow on esophageal m.
endoscopic sphincter of Oddi m.
ERCP m.
esophageal m.
InSIGHT m.
intraluminal m.
papillary m.
perendoscopic m.
PIP on esophageal m.
point of respiratory reversal on esophageal m.
pullthrough m.
rectosigmoid m.
sphincter of Oddi m.
transileostomy m.
Manson
M. disease
M. schistosomiasis
mansonelliasis
mansoni
Schistosoma m.
schistosomiasis m.
Mansson
M. operation
M. urinary pouch
Mantel-Haenszel test
mantle
lady's m.
manual lithotriptor
MAO
maximal acid output
MAOI
monoamine oxidase inhibitor
MAP
mean arterial pressure
MAP kinase signaling cascade
MAPK
mitogen-activated protein kinase
maple syrup urine disease (MSUD)
mapping
anal m.
bladder m.
cavernous nerve m.
intragastric pH m.
maprotiline
Maquet endoscopy table
Maranon syndrome
marasmus
Marblen
Marburg virus
Marcaine block
marcescens
Serratia m.

Marchand adrenals
Marchiafava-Micheli
    M.-M. disease
    M.-M. syndrome
Marcillin
Mardis soft stent
Mardi test
Marechal-Rosen test
Marezine
Marfan
    M. epigastric puncture
    M. syndrome
marfanoid habitus
margin
    anal m.
    cell-positive m.
    circumferential m.
    convex m.
    costal m.
    crenate m.
    cristate m.
    dentate m.
    disk m.
    dissection m.
    echogenic duct m.
    lateral m.
    medial m.
    obtuse m.
    positive m.
    subcostal m.
    superior m.
marginal
    m. artery of Drummond
    m. kidney donor
    m. ulcer
    m. zone lymphoma
margines (pl. of margo)
margo, pl. margines
Marian
    M. lithotomy
    M. operation
marianum
    Silybum m.
Marie-Strümpell disease
marigold
    burr m.
marihuana (var. of marijuana)
marijuana, marihuana
marina
    Anisakis m.
Marinesco-Sjögren syndrome
Marinol
marinus
    vomitus m.
Marion disease
marjoram
    sweet m.
mark
    crosshatch m.

    diathermy m.
    M. IV Moss decompression feeding
      catheter
marked
    m. deterioration
    m. tube
marker
    anthropometric m.
    antigen m.
    biochemical m.
    biologic m.
    bone turnover m.
    B5 tumor m.
    CA 1-18 tumor m.
    CA 72-4 tumor m.
    cell cycle m.
    C100-3 hepatitis C m.
    chromosomal m.
    m. chromosome
    chromosome m.
    claudin-7 intestinal m.
    D4S231 m.
    D4S414 m.
    D16S84 m.
    D16S283 m.
    D16S291 m.
    Dupan-2 tumor m.
    fecal m.
    fluid phase m.
    m. for cancer
    genetic m.
    hepatitis serologic m.
    HLA-DQ2 m.
    HLA-DQ8 m.
    HMB-45 monoclonal
      antibody m.
    inflammation m.
    interleukin-1b urinary m.
    malignancy-associated cellular m.
    molecular m.
    novel molecular m.
    OA-519 prognostic prostate
      carcinoma m.
    p-ANC genetic m.
    pancreatic cancer m.
    plasma membrane m.
    polycationic m.
    radiopaque m.
    serologic m.
    serum m.
    Spot endoscopic m.
    m. stitch
    surrogate m.
    tape m.
    m. transit study
    tumor m.
    vascular endothelial cell m.
    viral hepatitis m.
    XL784 renal damage m.

M

marking
>> haustral m.
>> red wale m.

Markov model

Marlen
>> M. double-faced adhesive disk
>> M. Gas Relief drainage pouch
>> M. Neoprene All-Flexible
>> faceplate
>> M. Odor-Ban ileostomy pouch
>> M. Solo ileostomy pouch
>> M. Ultramax 1-piece disposable
>> ostomy system
>> M. Zip Klosed pouch

Marlex
>> M. band
>> M. graft
>> M. hernia repair
>> M. mesh
>> M. mesh abdominal rectopexy
>> M. plug technique

Marmite lithotrite
marneffei
>> *Penicillium m.*

Marogen
maroon blood
maroon-colored stool
marrow transplant recipient
MARS
>> molecular adsorbent recirculating
>> system

Marseille pancreatitis classification
Marshall
>> M. and Tanner pubertal staging
>> M. test
>> M. U-stitch suture

Marshall-Bonney test
Marshall-Marchetti-Birch operation
Marshall-Marchetti-Krantz (MMK)
>> M.-M.-K. cystourethropexy
>> M.-M.-K. operation
>> M.-M.-K. retropubic
>> cystourethrography suspension
>> procedure
>> M.-M.-K. urethrocystopexy

Marshall-Marchetti test
Marsh classification
marshmallow
>> barium-coated m.
>> barium-impregnated m.
>> m. bolus

marsupialization
>> epididymis m.
>> laparoscopic m.
>> renal cyst m.

marsupium
Martel clamp
Martin
>> M. anoplasty

>> M. gastrostomy
>> M. operation

Martin-Davis rectal speculum
Martius
>> M. fascial sling
>> M. fat pad
>> M. graft
>> M. labial fat pad flap
>> M. operation
>> M. scarlet blue stain

Martius-Harris operation
Martorell hypertensive ulcer
MAS
>> multiple anal sphincterotomies

masculinae
>> crista urethralis m.
>> ostium urethrae externum m.

masculinizing genitoplasty
masculinum
>> ovarium m.

masculinus
>> uterus m.
>> utriculus m.

MASE
>> microsurgical extraction of sperm from
>> epididymis

mask
>> Bili m.
>> m. phenomenon
>> Prohibit antifog face m.

Mason
>> M. abdominal transsphincteric
>> resection
>> M. needle holder
>> M. operation
>> M. vertical banded gastroplasty

mass (m, M)
>> abdominal wall m.
>> adjusted body m. (ABM)
>> adnexal m.
>> adrenal gland m.
>> appendiceal m.
>> asymptomatic m.
>> body cell m. (BCM)
>> colonic m.
>> colorectal m.
>> congenital renal m.
>> cul-de-sac m.
>> cystic m.
>> discrete m.
>> duodenal m.
>> dysplasia-associated lesion or m.
>> (DALM)
>> esophageal m.
>> exophytic m.
>> expansile abdominal m.
>> extramucosal m.
>> extrarenal m.
>> extrinsic m.

flank m.
fluctuant m.
gastric m.
hilar m.
inflammatory prostatic m. (IPM)
inflammatory renal m.
inhomogeneous hyperechoic m.
intraabdominal m.
kidney m.
lean body m. (LBM)
lobulated m.
malignant renal m.
mediastinal m. (MM)
mushroom-shaped m.
neoplastic renal m.
palpable m.
parapancreatic m.
parovarian m.
periampullary m.
perirectal m.
m. peristalsis
phlegmonous m.
pleural m.
polypoid m.
pulsatile m.
rectal m.
renal m.
salivary m.
scrotal m.
soft tissue m.
submucosal m.
testicular m.
m. transfer area coefficient (MTAC)
transformary m.
traumatic renal m.
tubular excretory m.
vaginal m.
vascular renal m.

massage
prostatic m.

masse
colostomy shift en m.
reduction en m.

masseter strength
Masset test
massive
m. bowel resection syndrome
m. colonic diverticular bleeding
m. epithelial cell necrosis
m. hepatic necrosis
m. malignant infiltration

Masson
M. trichrome
M. trichrome stain
M. trichrome staining technique

Masson-Fontana stain
mast
m. cell
m. cell degranulation

master
m. duodenoscope
m. IG bundle
m. image guide

MasterFlex pump
Masters intestinal clamp
Masters-Schwartz liver clamp
masticatory-salivary reflex
Mastisol liquid surgical adhesive
mastocytosis
systemic m.

mastoiditis
masturbation
traumatic m.

Masugi nephritis
matairesinol
matching
donor/recipient race m.
HLA-DR m.
optimizing HLA m.
optimizing human leukocyte antigen m.

material
anastomotic m.
biocompatible m.
coarse m.
coffee-grounds m. (CGM)
congophilic m.
Conray 60, 70, 280 contrast m.
extravasated iodinated contrast m.
fecal m.
implantation of prosthetic m.
iodinated contrast m.
methods and m.'s
microcrystalline m.
polyglactin suture m.
proteinaceous cast m.
purulent m.
suture m.
Triangle gelatin-sealed sling m.

maternal
m. age as risk factor
m. morbidity

Mathews rectal speculum
Mathieu
M. hypospadias repair technique
M. island onlay flap

Mathieu-Horton-Devine flip-flap
Mathieu-Righini hypospadias procedure
matico
matrices (*pl. of* matrix)
Matrigel
Matritech NMP22 test for bladder cancer
matrix, *pl.* **matrices**
m. calculus
m. deposition
extracellular m. (ECM)
glomerular extracellular m.

M

matrix (*continued*)
 m. metalloproteinase (MMP)
 m. metalloproteinase-7 (MMP-7)
 m. metalloproteinase-9
  (MMP-9)
 nuclear m.
 Oasis wound m.
 pericellular m. (PCM)
 prostate gland tissue m.
 m. protein
 TissueMend soft tissue
  repair m.
 m. urolithiasis
Matson operation
matted node
Mattox maneuver
mattress
 Bedge antireflux m.
 Home Care Simplimatt Plus zoned
  foam m.
 ProCair One dynamic
  pressure-relieving m.
 ProCair Two dynamic
  pressure-relieving m.
 m. suture
Matts grade 1–4
maturation
 collagen m.
 mucosal barrier m.
 normal m.
 osteoclast m.
 stone m.
mature teratoma
maturing the stoma
maturity-onset diabetes of youth
 (MODY)
matutinus
 vomitus m.
Mauch double-sheathed plastic wash
 pipe
Maunoir hydrocele
Maunsell-Weir coloanal anastomosis
Maxamine
Maxaquin
Max-EPA capsule
Maxeran
MaxForce
 M. TTS biliary balloon dilation
  catheter
 M. TTS high-performance balloon
  dilation catheter
Maxgel hydrogel
maximal
 m. acid output (MAO)
 m. androgen blockade (MAB)
 m. toleration
 tubular m.
 m. tubular excretory capacity of
  kidney

maximum
 m. anal resting pressure
  (MRP)
 m. bladder capacity
 m. coagulative necrosis
 m. cystometric capacity
 m. detrusor pressure
 m. diameter
 m. free-flow rate
 m. squeeze pressure (MSP)
 m. tolerable volume (MTV)
 m. urethral closure pressure
  (MUCP)
 m. urinary flow rate
 m. vasal pressure (MVP)
maximus
 gluteus m.
Maxipime
Maxisal with vitamin C
Maxisorb test plate
Maxolon
Maxon
 M. loop
 M. suture
Maxorb dressing
Maxum reusable forceps
Maxzide
Maydl
 M. colostomy procedure
 M. hernia
 M. operation
 M. ureterocolostomy
Mayer
 M. acid alum hematoxylin
  stain
 M. hematoxylin solution
May-Grünwald-Giemsa stain
Mayo
 M. abdominal clamp
 M. abdominal retractor
 M. bladder
 M. Clinic system for primary
  biliary cirrhosis
 M. common duct probe
 M. common duct scoop
 M. common duct spoon
 M. gallstone scoop
 M. grading system
 M. operation
 M. scissors
 M. stand
 M. trocar-point needle
Mayo-Adams appendectomy retractor
Mayo-Blake gallstone forceps
Mayo-Hegar needle holder
Mayo-Kelly appendix inverter
Mayo-Noble dissecting scissors
Mayo-Ochsner suction trocar
 cannula

Mayo-Péan forceps
Mayo-Robson
>   M.-R. gallstone scoop
>   M.-R. intestinal clamp
>   M.-R. intestinal forceps
>   M.-R. position

Mays operation
Mazicon
mazindol
Mazzariello-Caprini forceps
MBS
>   modified barium swallow

MCAD
>   medium-chain acyl-CoA
>   dehydrogenase

McArdle syndrome
McBurney
>   M. incision
>   M. point
>   M. retractor
>   M. sign

MCC
>   mutated colorectal carcinoma
>   *MCC* gene

McCall culdoplasty
McCarthy
>   M. electrode
>   M. evacuator
>   M. Foroblique panendoscope
>   cystoscope

McCarthy-Campbell miniature
cystoscope
McCleery-Miller intestinal clamp
McCormack gastric mucosal sign
McCort sign
McCrea
>   M. cystoscope
>   M. sound

McCune-Albright syndrome
MCD
>   metastatic Crohn disease

MCDK
>   multicystic dysplastic kidney

McDonald
>   M. cerclage
>   M. stone dissector

McDougal prostatectomy clamp
MCFA
>   medium-chain fatty acid

MCF-7 tumor
McGaw
>   M. plastic bottle
>   M. volumetric pump

McGill
>   M. forceps
>   M. pain questionnaire

McGivney
>   M. hemorrhoidal ligator
>   M. hemorrhoid forceps

M-CH
>   mitomycin adsorbed onto activated
>   charcoal

MCH
>   mean corpuscular hemoglobin
>   methacholine
>   microfibrillar collagen hemostat
>   Endo-Avitene MCH
>   *MCH* gene

MCHC
>   mean corpuscular hemoglobin
>   concentration

***m*-chlorophenyl-piperazine**
McIndoe vaginal construction procedure
McIntyre reverse cystotome
MCK
>   multicystic kidney

MCKD
>   multicystic kidney disease

MCL
>   midclavicular line
>   MCL port

McLean pile clamp
McNealey-Glassman-Mixter forceps
McNeer gastric carcinoma classification
McNemar ascites test
MCP
>   monocyte chemoattractant protein
>   monocyte chemotactic protein

MCP-1
>   monocyte chemoattractant protein-1

M-CSF
>   macrophage colony-stimulating factor

MCT
>   mean colonic transit
>   medium-chain triglyceride
>   medullary carcinoma of thyroid
>   MCT oil

MCU
>   micturating cystourethrogram
>   micturating cystourethrography

MCUG
>   micturating cystourethrogram

MCV
>   methotrexate, cisplatin, vinblastine

McVay
>   M. herniorrhaphy
>   M. inguinal hernial repair
>   M. operation

M.D. Anderson grade
MDCK
>   Madin-Darby canine kidney
>   MDCK epithelial cell

MD-60 contrast medium
MDL-3000
>   LaserTripter MDL-3000

MDLO
>   metoclopramide, dexamethasone,
>   lorazepam, ondansetron

M

MDM2 gene
MDP
> methylene diphosphonate
> ^{99m}Tc MDP

MDR
> minimum daily requirement

MDR1
> multidrug-resistance gene
>   *MDR1* gene

MDRD
> modification of diet in renal disease

MDS
> membrane-spanning domain

MDT
> mean dissolution time
> median detection threshold
>   MDT renogram

meadowsweet
Meadox Surgimed Doppler probe
MeAIB
> methylaminoisobutyric acid

MEA-I, -II
> multiple endocrine adenomatosis type I, II

meal
> barium m.
> Boas test m.
> Boyden test m.
> butter m.
> Dock test m.
> double-contrast barium m.
> Ehrmann alcohol test m.
> Ewald test m.
> fatty m.
> Fischer test m.
> isotope m.
> Leube test m.
> liver m.
> Lundh m.
> motor test m.
> ^{99m}Tc sulfur colloid egg m.
> normal saline m.
> opaque m.
> pH standardized m.
> retention m.
> Riegel test m.
> Salzer test m.
> small-bowel m.
> solid egg-white m.
> standard fatty m.
> test m.

meal-related secretion pattern
meal-stimulated
> m.-s. acid output (MSAO)
> m.-s. pancreatic secretion

mean
> m. allograft survival
> m. arterial blood pressure (MABP)
> m. arterial pressure (MAP)
> m. colonic transit (MCT)
> m. corpuscular hemoglobin (MCH)
> m. corpuscular hemoglobin concentration (MCHC)
> m. corpuscular volume
> m. dissolution time (MDT)
> m. distal contraction amplitude (MDCA)
> m. electrosurgical resistance
> m. energy
> m. input time (MIT)
> m. prostatic volume
> m. renal volume
> m. resistance time (MRT)
> m. shunt index
> m. TIMP-1/GAPDH rate
> m. TIMP-3/GAPDH ratio
> m. transit time (MTT)
> m. treatment duration
> m. venous outflow (MVO)

Meares-Stamey chronic prostatitis technique
measure
> antiendotoxin m.
> cGy radiation m.
> temporizing m.

measurement
> anorectal m.
> anthropometric m.
> bulbocavernous reflex latency m.
> Doppler ultrasound intestinal blood flow m.
> intestinal permeability m.
> intraprostatic temperature m.
> microfluorometric m.
> physiologic m.
> planimetric m.
> plasma bile acid m.
> pressure m.
> quantitative m.
> rectal compliance m.
> RigiScan m.
> serum bile acid m.
> standard m.
> m. test
> urethral pressure m.
> Vector volume m.
> velocity m.
> voiding urethral pressure m. (VUPM)

measuring-mounting (MM)
> m.-m. catheter

meatal
> m. advancement
> m. advancement and glansplasty (MAGPI)

m. advancement, glanuloplasty,
  penoscrotal junction meatotomy
  (MAGPI)
m. atresia
m. spreader
m. stenosis
m. stenosis after circumcision
meatal-based flap procedure
meat impaction
meatoplasty
  Stacke m.
  V-flap m.
meatorrhaphy
meatoscope
meatoscopy
  ureteral m.
meatotome
meatotomy
  meatal advancement, glanuloplasty,
    penoscrotal junction m. (MAGPI)
  m. scissors
  ureteral m.
  ventral m.
  Y-V m.
meatus (M)
  retrusive m.
  urethral m.
  m. urinarius
mebendazole
mebeverine
mebrofenin
mecamylamine
mecasermin
mechanical
  m. anastomosis
  m. assist system
  m. biliary obstruction
  m. cystitis
  m. diarrhea
  m. duct obstruction
  m. endoscopic management
  m. extrahepatic obstruction
  m. ileus
  m. intestinal obstruction
  m. jaundice
  m. leech
  m. lithotripsy
  m. product
  m. radial scanning instrument
  m. rotating probe
  m. small-bowel obstruction
  m. stress wave
  m. ureteral dilation
  m. variceal compression
  m. ventilation
mechanism
  Albarran m.
  antireflux flap-valve m.
  cell-mediated m.

countercurrent m.
cyclooxygenase-dependent m.
deglutition m.
deranged hemostatic m.
flap-valve m.
Mitrofanoff m.
neuroparacrine m.
nonimmune m.
peptidergic m.
pinchcock m.
renal autoregulatory m.
sphincteric m.
swallowing m.
T-cell-dependent m.
tubuloglomerular feedback m.
urethral closure m.
mechanoreceptor dysfunction
Mecholyl
mecillinam
Meckel
  M. diverticulitis
  M. diverticulum
  M. ileitis
  M. rod
  M. scan
  M. syndrome
Meckel-Gruber syndrome
meclizine, meclozine
meclofenamate
  sodium m.
meclozine (*var. of* meclizine)
meconium
  m. hydrocele
  m. ileus
  m. ileus equivalent (MIE)
  m. peritonitis
  m. plug
  m. plug syndrome
Mectra tissue sample retainer
Medena tube
media (*pl. of* medium)
medial
  m. fibroplasia
  m. margin
  m. preoptic area
  m. umbilical ligament
median
  m. arcuate ligament
  m. bar formation
  m. bar of Mercier
  m. detection threshold (MDT)
  m. followup
  m. furrow of prostate
  m. incision
  m. lithotomy
  m. lobe
  m. lobe hyperplasia
  m. operative time
  m. raphe cyst

M

mediastinal
- m. crunch
- m. histoplasmosis
- m. involvement
- m. lymphadenectomy
- m. lymphadenopathy
- m. lymph node sampling
- m. mass
- m. pleura
- m. shift
- m. thickening
- m. tube
- m. tumor
- m. widening

mediastinitis

mediastinum
- m. germ cell tumor
- m. testis

mediated
- integrin m.
- plasmid m.

mediation
- autoimmune immunoglobulin m.

mediator
- mesenchymal inductive m.
- secreted m.

medical
- m. castration
- Conway Stuart M. (CSM)
- m. dilation
- m. evaluation
- m. food
- m. laser
- m. prevention
- m. prophylaxis
- m. resource
- m. therapy
- M. Therapy of Prostatic Symptoms (MTOPS)
- M. Therapy of Prostatic Symptoms trial
- m. vagotomy

medically induced achlorhydria

medicamentosus
- pseudopolyposis m.

Medicated Urethral System for Erection (MUSE)

medication
- m. allergy
- anticholinergic m.
- m. bezoar
- bromocriptine dopaminergic m.
- carbidopa dopaminergic m.
- dopaminergic m.
- levodopa dopaminergic m.
- pergolide dopaminergic m.
- psychopharmacologic m.
- psychotropic m.
- m. teratogenesis

medication-associated
- m.-a. erection
- m.-a. suppression of gastric secretion

medication-induced injury

medicine
- American College of Physicians-American Society of Internal M. (ACP-ASIM)
- complementary and alternative m. (CAM)
- nuclear m.
- renal m.
- teratogenic m.

MediClenze hygiene and water therapy system

Medicone

Medicon-Jackson rectal forceps

medicus
- furor m.

Medicut
- M. cannula
- M. catheter

Mediflex-Gazayerli retractor

Mediflex MD-7 endoscopic video system

Medi-Ject

Medi-Jector Choice

Medilas fiberTome laser

Medina
- M. ileostomy catheter
- M. tube

mediolateral lithotomy

Mediplex Ultra tabule

medisect

Medisense Pen 2 glucose meter

Medispec Econolith spark plug lithotriptor

Medi-Tech
- M.-T. bipolar catheter
- M.-T. bipolar probe
- M.-T. steerable catheter

Mediterranean
- M. fever
- M. lymphoma

Meditron EL-100 Endolav

medium, *pl.* **media**
- *Aeromonas media*
- arteria colica media
- arteria rectalis media
- Balch 1 broth m.
- Baricon contrast m.
- Baroflave contrast m.
- Barosperse contrast m.
- Biligrafin contrast m.
- Biliscopin contrast m.
- Bilivist contrast m.
- Bilopaque contrast m.
- Biloptin contrast m.
- Campy-BAP culture m.

Cary-Blair m.
Cheetah radiopaque contrast m.
chocolate agar m.
Cholebrine contrast m.
Cholografin contrast m.
contrast m.
culture m.
dissociated m.
Dulbecco modified Eagle m.
 (DMEM)
Eagle minimal essential m. (EMEM)
Earle m.
extravasation of contrast m.
Gastrografin contrast m.
Gastrovist contrast m.
Ham F12 m.
Hypaque contrast m.
inoculated m.
iocetamic acid contrast m.
iodipamide meglumine contrast m.
iopanoic acid contrast m.
ipodate contrast m.
low osmolar contrast m. (LOCM)
MD-60 contrast m.
meglumine diatrizoate contrast m.
meglumine iotroxate contrast m.
Niopam contrast m.
OCT m.
Oragrafin contrast m.
Reno-M contrast m.
RPMI-1640 contrast m.
Selenite-F enrichment m.
serum-free conditional m.
Skirrow m.
sodium iodipamide contrast m.
Solu-Biloptin contrast m.
sorbitol-MacConkey m.
Telepaque contrast m.
Thorotrast contrast m.
tyropanoate contrast m.
Urografin 290 contrast m.
Varibar oral contrast m.
water-soluble contrast m.
medium-chain
 m.-c. acyl-CoA dehydrogenase
  (MCAD)
 m.-c. acyl-CoA dehydrogenase
  deficiency
 m.-c. fatty acid (MCFA)
 m.-c. triglyceride (MCT)
medium-power photomicrograph
medium-term result
Medivator automatic reprocessor
Medoc-Celestin
 M.-C. endoprosthesis
 M.-C. pulsion tube
medorrhea
**Medrad MRInnervu endorectal colon
 probe**

Medralone
Medrol
medronate
 ^{99m}Tc m.
medroxyprogesterone acetate
MEDS
 microsurgical extraction of ductal
 sperm
MedSlant
 M. LLC
 M. therapeutic pillow
Medstone
 M. extracorporeal shock wave
  lithotripsy
 M. IRIS system
 M. STS lithotripsy system
 M. STS lithotriptor
 M. STS shock wave generator
Medtrax urology database
**Medtronic thin flexible antimony
 electrode**
medulla, *pl.* **medullae**
 adrenal m.
 m. glandulae suprarenalis
 inner m.
 kidney m.
 microcystic disease of renal m.
 m. of suprarenal gland
 outer m.
 renal m.
 suprarenal m.
medullae (*pl. of* medulla)
medullaris
 conus m.
medullary
 m. carcinoma of thyroid (MCT)
 m. collecting duct
 m. cystic disease
 m. interstitial osmolality
 m. interstitium
 m. oxygenation
 m. pyramid
 m. sponge kidney
 m. thyroid carcinoma
medullation
medullectomy
medulloadrenal
medulloblastoma
medulloid
medullosuprarenoma
medusa, *pl.* **medusae**
 caput medusae
 M. head
medusae (*pl. of* medusa)
Meeker gallbladder clamp
mefenamic acid
mefloquine
Mefoxin
Mefoxin-saline solution

M

MEG
  magnetoencephalography
megabladder
megacalycosis
megacaryocyte (*var. of* megakaryocyte)
Megace
megacolon
  acquired functional m.
  acute m.
  aganglionic m.
  congenital m.
  m. congenitum
  idiopathic m.
  toxic m.
megacystic
  m. mucinous neoplasm
  m. syndrome
megacystis
  bladder congenital m.
megacystis-megaureter
  m.-m. association
  m.-m. syndrome
megacystis-microcolon-intestinal hypoperistalsis syndrome
megaduodenum
megaesophagus
  chagasic m.
megakaryocyte, megacaryocyte
megalin
Megalink biliary stent
megaloblastic anemia
megalocystis
megaloesophagus
megalogastria
megalopenis
megalophallus
megaloureter (*var. of* megaureter)
megalourethra
megameatus hypospadias repair
megameatus-intact prepuce (MIP)
megamitochondria
megarectum
  idiopathic m.
megasigmoid syndrome
megaureter, megaloureter
  m. classification
  obstructive m.
  primary obstructive m.
  primary refluxing m.
  secondary refluxing m.
  unilateral m.
megaurethra
megavitamin
megestrol acetate
meglumine
  m. diatrizoate
  m. diatrizoate contrast medium
  m. diatrizoate enema

  iodipamide m.
  m. iotroxate
  m. iotroxate contrast medium
  Urovist M.
MEIA
  microparticle enzyme immunoassay
Meissner plexus
mekongi
  Schistosoma m.
  schistosomiasis m.
melan A staining
melaninogenicus
  Bacteroides m.
melanogaster
  Drosophila m.
melanoma
  adrenal gland m.
  bladder malignant m.
  familial atypical multiple-mole m. (FAMMM)
  m. intratumor pressure
  male genitalia m.
  malignant m.
  metastatic m.
melanorrhagia
melanorrhea
melanosis
  m. coli
  penile m.
melanotic neuroectodermal tumor of infancy (MNTI)
melas
  icterus m.
MELAS
  mitochondrial encephalomyopathy, lactic acidosis and strokelike episodes
  MELAS syndrome
melasma
  m. addisonii
  m. suprarenale
melatonin
Melchior ileal neobladder
MELD
  Model for End-Stage Liver Disease
  MELD model
  MELD score
melena
  m. neonatorum
  m. spuria
  m. vera
melenemesis
melenic stool
Melgisorb dressing
melitensis
  Brucella m.
melituria
Melkersson-Rosenthal syndrome
mellitus
  diabetes m.

insulin-dependent diabetes m. (IDDM)

malnutrition-related diabetes m. (MRDM)

noninsulin-dependent diabetes m. (NIDDM)

posttransplant diabetes m. (PTDM)

prevalence of diabetes m.

risk factors of posttransplant diabetes m.

streptozotocin-induced diabetes m.

type 2 diabetes m.

meloxicam

melphalan

MELS

molecular extracorporeal liver support MELS system

Meltzer

M. sign

M. triad

Meltzer-Lyon test

membranate

membrane

abdominal m.

antiglomerular basement m. (anti-GBM)

antitubular basement m.

antral m.

apical m.

basement m.

basolateral m. (BLM)

biocompatible m.

bioincompatible m.

brush-border m. (BBM)

m. catheter technique

cell m.

cellulose-based m.

cellulose diacetate m.

Chwalla m.

cloacal m.

m. cofactor protein

congenital pyloric m.

croupous m.

cuprophane m.

m. current

Debove m.

dialyzer m.

dry mucous m.'s

m. effect

elastic silicone m.

false m.

filtration slit m.

glomerular basement m. (GBM)

Hemophan m.

Hibond N+ nylon m.

high-flux dialysis m.

high-flux polysulfone m.

m. hyperpolarization

invaginated m.

Jackson m.

low-flux cuprophane m.

low-flux dialysis m.

low-flux polysulfone m.

lysosomal m.

mammalian cell m.

microvillous m.

moist mucous m.'s

MSI nylon m.

mucous m.

Na/K-ATPase m.

nuclear m.

m. oxygenator

m. permeability

m. peroxidation

phrenoesophageal m.

polymethylmethacrylate m.

polysulfone m.

porous filter m.

posttransplant antiglomerular basement m.

Preclude peritoneal m.

prostate-specific m. (PSM)

Seprafilm bioresorbable m.

serous m.

small-intestinal m.

thin basement m.

Toldt m.

m. trafficking

m. transport protein

tubular basement m. (TBM)

urea-impermeable m.

urothelial basement m. (UBM)

membrane-attack complex

membrane-based lipid

membrane-bound multicomponent enzyme complex

membrane-coated SEMS

membrane-covered stent

membranectomy

endoscopic m.

membrane-spanning

m.-s. domain (MDS)

m.-s. integrin

membranolysis

membranoproliferative glomerulonephritis type I, II (MPGN)

membranotomy

laryngeal jack-assisted retrograde esophageal m.

membranous

m. glomerulonephritis (MGN)

m. nephropathy

m. neuropathy

m. urethra

m. urethral stricture

membrum virile

Memokath catheter

M

memory
    m. impairment
    m. T cell
    m. wire
Memotherm
    M. colorectal stent
    M. endoscopic biliary stent
    M. Flexx biliary stent
    M. nitinol stent
MEN
    multiple endocrine neoplasia
    MEN I syndrome
menaquinone
mendelian pattern
Mendelsohn maneuver
Mendez ultrasonic cystotome
Ménétrier disease
Menghini
    M. liver biopsy needle
    M. technique
    M. technique for percutaneous liver
      biopsy
Menghini-type coring bevel
Meni-D
Ménière disease
meningismus
meningitis
    pyogenic m.
meningomyelocele
meningosepticum
    Flavobacterium m.
meniscus sign
Menkes
    M. disease
    M. disease gene
menouria
mentagrophytes
    Trichophyton m.
Mentor
    M. Alpha 1 inflatable penile
      prosthesis
    M. Bioflex cylinder
    M. GFS penile prosthesis
    M. gun
    M. IPP penile prosthesis
    M. malleable penile prosthesis
    M. Mark II penile prosthesis
    M. nonhydrophilic PVC catheter
    M. straight catheter
**Menuet Compact urodynamic testing
  device**
MEOS
    microsomal ethanol oxidizing
    system
mepenzolate bromide
meperidine
    m. conscious sedation
    m. hydrochloride

mephentermine
Mepilex
    M. Border Lite dressing
    M. Transfer dressing
mepiperphenidol
meprobamate
mercaptan
mercaptoacetyltriglycine (MAG-3)
mercaptoethane sulfonate
2-mercaptoethanesulfonic acid (mesna)
6-mercaptopurine (6-MP)
Mercedes Benz sign
Mercier
    M. bar
    median bar of M.
    M. operation
mercurialism
mercurial nephrosis
mercuric
    m. chloride-induced ARF
    m. chloride-induced nephritis
    m. chloride nephrotoxicity
    m. oxide
    m. oxide battery ingestion
mercury
    m. bougienage treatment
    m. chloride (HgCl2)
    M. herb
    millimeters of m. (mmHg)
    m. poisoning
mercury-containing balloon
mercury-filled dilator
mercury-weighted
    m.-w. dilator
    m.-w. rubber bougie
    m.-w. tube
Meridia
merimepodib
Merindino operation
Meritene liquid feeding
mermaid
    M. DNA kit
    m. malformation
meropenem for injection
Merrem IV
Mersilene
    M. for pubovaginal sling
    M. mesh
    M. strut
    M. suture
    M. tape
**merthiolate fresh stool
  examination**
merycism
MESA
    microepididymal sperm aspiration
    microsurgical epididymal sperm
    aspiration

mesalamine (FIV-ASA)
    m. enema
    m. rectal suppository
    m. sodium
mesalazine
mesangial
    m. angle
    m. cell
    m. deposit
    m. hypercellularity
    m. lysis
    m. matrix expansion
    m. nephropathy
    m. pattern
    m. proliferation
    m. volume fraction
mesangiocapillary glomerulonephritis
mesangiolysis
mesangiolytic change
mesangioproliferative glomerulonephritis (MPGN)
mesangium
    extraglomerular m. (EGM)
    glomerular m.
mesaraic (*var. of* mesenteric)
mesaraica
    tabes m.
mesareic (*var. of* mesenteric)
Mesavance
mesenchymal
    m. change
    m. hamartoma
    m. inductive mediator
    m. protein
    m. stem cell
mesenchyme
    metanephrogenic m.
mesenchymoma
    benign m.
    malignant m.
mesenterectomy
mesenteric, mesaraic, mesareic
    m. adenitis
    m. angiogram
    m. apoplexy
    m. arterial embolism
    m. arterial thrombosis
    m. arteriography
    m. arteriovenous fistula
    m. artery
    m. artery constriction
    m. attachment
    m. attachment of colon
    m. circulation
    m. cyst
    m. defect
    m. fat stranding

    m. fibromatosis
    m. hematoma
    m. hernia
    m. infarction
    m. inflammatory venoocclusive disease (MIVOD)
    m. ischemia
    m. lipodystrophy
    m. lipogranuloma
    m. lymph node (MLN)
    m. panniculitis
    m. rupture
    m. sensory receptor
    m. steal syndrome
    m. tear
    m. triangle
    m. tumefaction
    m. varix
    m. vascular disease
    m. vascular lesion
    m. vascular occlusion
    m. vasculitis
    m. vein
    m. vein thrombosis (MVT)
    m. window
mesenterica
    tabes m.
mesentericoparietal hernia
mesenteriolum
mesenteriopexy
mesenteriorrhaphy
mesenteriplication
mesenteritis
    liposclerotic m.
    retractile m.
    sclerosing m.
mesenterium
mesenteroaxial gastric volvulus
mesenterorenal bypass
mesentery
    leaf of m.
    small-intestine m. (SIM)
mesentorrhaphy
mesh
    Bard Visilex m.
    m. bolster
    Dacron m.
    Dexon polyglycolic acid m.
    IntePro polypropylene m.
    intraperitoneal onlay m. (IPOM)
    Marlex m.
    Mersilene m.
    PelviSoft m.
    polypropylene m.
    polytetrafluoroethylene m.
    m. sling procedure
    Sperma-Tex preshaped m.
    m. stent

M

mesh (*continued*)
    m. stent prosthesis
    Surgipro m.
    synthetic m.
    Trelex m.
    TyRx bioresorbable polymer m.
    Vicryl m.
    Visilex m.
meshed graft
mesher
    Collin m.
mesh-plug hernioplasty
mesna
    2-mercaptoethanesulfonic acid
Mesnex
mesnili
    Chilomastix m.
mesoappendicitis
mesoappendix
mesoblastic nephroma
mesocaval
    m. anastomosis
    m. H-graft shunt
    m. interposition shunt
mesocecum
mesocolic
    m. band
    m. hernia
    m. shelf
mesocolica
    tenia m.
mesocolon
mesocolonic vessel
mesocolopexy
mesocoloplication
mesodermal ingrowth
mesogastric
mesogastrium
    dorsal m.
    ventral m.
mesoileum
mesometrium
mesonephric
    m. adenoma
    m. duct
    m. hyperplasia
    m. nephron
    m. remnant
    m. tubule
mesonephricus
    ductus m.
mesonephroi (*pl. of* mesonephros)
mesonephros, *pl.* **mesonephroi**
    caudal m.
    cranial m.
    genital m.
mesopexy
mesophilic bacterium
mesorectal

m. excision
m. lymphadenectomy
m. tissue
mesorectum
mesoridazine
mesorrhaphy
mesosigmoid colon
mesosigmoidopexy
mesothelial
    m. hyperplasia
    m. metaplasia
mesothelioma
    benign cystic m.
    diffuse malignant m.
    giant fibrous m.
    peritoneal m.
    well-differentiated papillary m.
mesotrypsin
message-2
    testosterone-repressed prostate m.-2
    (TRPM-2)
messenger
    m. ribonucleic acid (mRNA)
    m. RNA (mRNA)
    m. RNA molecule
    T-cell second m.
    ureteral peristalsis second m.
Messerklinger endoscope
Mestinon
mesylate
    doxazosin m.
    gabexate m.
    hycanthone m.
    imatinib m.
    nafamostat m.
metaanalysis
metaanalytic review
metabolic
    m. abnormality
    m. acidosis
    m. alkalosis
    m. balance
    m. bone survey
    m. calculus
    m. complication
    m. consequence
    m. derangement
    m. disorder
    m. effect
    m. evaluation
    m. liver disease
    m. predictor
    m. range
    m. rate
    m. stone
    m. stone disease
    m. therapy
metabolism
    albumin m.

basal m.
bile salt m. (BSM)
calcium m.
citrate m.
cortisol m.
cystine m.
drug m.
first-pass m. (FPM)
gas m.
gastric first-pass m. (GFPM)
glomerular m.
glutathione m.
hepatic m.
inborn error of m.
leucine m.
lipid m.
lipoprotein m.
magnesium m.
oxalate m.
phosphorus m.
protein m.
sulfur amino acid m.
tryptophan m.

metabolite
arachidonic acid m.
cyclooxygenase m.
cytochrome P450 m.
reactive oxygen m.
toxic m.

metachromatic dye
metachronous
m. adenoma
m. colon cancer
m. contralateral hernias
m. lesion
m. neoplasia
m. small-bowel adenocarcinoma
m. tumor

metadysentery
MetaFluor system
Metagonimus yokogawai
Metahydrin
metaicteric
metaiodobenzylguanidine (MIBG)
iodine-131-labeled m.

metal
m. ball-tip catheter
m. bar retractor
m. clip
m. intoxication
m. olive
m. olive dilator
m. sound
m. wing clamp
m. Z stent

metallic
m. biliary stent
m. biliary stent migration
m. embolus

self-expanding m. (SEM)
m. staple
m. stent placement

metallic-tip catheter
metalloenzyme
metalloproteinase
m. inhibitor
matrix m. (MMP)
tissue inhibitor of m. (TIMP)

metalloproteinase-1
tissue inhibitor of m.-1 (TIMP-1)

metalloproteinase-2
tissue inhibitor of m.-2 (TIMP-2)

metalloproteinase-7
matrix m.-7 (MMP-7)

metalloproteinase-9
matrix m. (MMP-9)

metallothionein
metal-tipped stent pusher
metal-weighted silastic feeding tube
metamorphosis
fatty m.

Metamucil
metanephric
m. tubule
m. vesicle

metanephrine
metanephrogenic mesenchyme
metanephros
metaplasia
agnogenic myeloid m.
Barrett m.
bladder squamous m.
cardia intestinal m. (CIM)
colonic m.
columnar m.
gastric intestinal m.
glandular m.
goblet cell m.
intestinal m. type I-III
junctional intestinal m.
mesothelial m.
myeloid m.
osseous m.
pancreatic acinar m. (PAM)
pyloric m. (PYME)
specialized intestinal m. (SIM)

metaplasia-dysplasia-carcinoma sequence
metaplastic
m. atrophic gastritis
m. epithelium
m. gastric fundic gland
m. ossification
m. polyp

metaproterenol
metaraminol
metastases (*pl. of* metastasis)

M

metastasis, *pl.* **metastases**
    bleeding jejunal m.
    bone m.
    brain m.
    colonic m.
    cutaneous m.
    diffuse m.
    disseminated m.
    distant m.
    duodenal m.
    extrahepatic m. (EHM)
    extralymphatic m.
    m. gene
    hematogenic m.
    implantation m.
    intramucosal m.
    liver m.
    lymphatic m.
    lymph node m.
    lymphogenic m.
    neoplasm m.
    paraesophagogastric lymph node m.
    percutaneous image-guided thermal
      ablation of hepatic m.
    port site m.
    m. suppression
    tumor, nodes, metastases (TNM)
metastatic
    m. adenocarcinoma
    m. cancer
    m. carcinoid syndrome
    m. cascade
    m. cholangiocarcinoma
    m. complication
    m. Crohn disease (MCD)
    m. dissemination
    m. fat necrosis
    m. implantation
    m. lesion
    m. melanoma
    m. neuroblastoma
    m. orchitis
    m. prostatic carcinoma
    m. renal cell carcinoma (MRCC)
Metastron
metasulfobenzoate
    prednisolone m.
metasynchronous bacterial urinary tract infection
Metatensin
metaxalone
met-enkephalin
    methionine-enkephalin
meteorism
meter
    Aleo m.
    Fisher Accumet pH m.
    integrating spherical power m.
    Medisense Pen 2 glucose m.

    One Touch blood glucose m.
    Synectics 6000 digital pH m.
metformin
methacholine (MCH)
methadone
methamphetamine
methane excretor
methanethiol
Methanobrevibacter smithii
methanogen
methanogenesis
methanogenic archaea
methanol intoxication
methantheline bromide
methapyrilene
methdilazine
Methedrine
methemalbumin
methemoglobinemia
methenamine
    m. hippurate
    m. mandelate
methicillin
methicillin-resistant *Staphylococcus aureus* **(MRSA)**
methimazole
Methiodal
methionine-enkephalin (met-enkephalin)
    immunoreactive m.-e. (IRME)
    m.-e. peptide
    plasma m.-e.
methionine loading
methionine-rich food
methixene
method
    ablate-and-chip m.
    acid guanidine
      thiocyanate-phenol-chloroform m.
    acid hematin m.
    Addis m.
    Albert-Lembert m.
    m.'s and materials
    anthrone m.
    avidin-biotin-peroxidase complex m.
    barostat m.
    Beck m.
    Bence Jones protein m.
    Benedict and Franke m.
    Benedict-Talbot body surface area m.
    Bertrand m.
    Biogenex antigen retrieval m.
    Brown and Wickham pressure
      profile m.
    cap m.
    cholesterol-cholesteroloxidase-phenol
      4-aminophenazone m.
    cinefluoroscopic m.
    Cockroft m.
    2-devices-in-1-channel m.

double-endoscope m.
dye scattering m.
efficacious noninvasive
 anesthesia-independent first-line m.
ellipsoid m.
endoscopic mucosal resection, cap
 m. (EMRC)
endoscopic mucosal resection, tube
 m. (EMRT)
Esbach m.
Essed plication m.
Fishberg m.
Folin-Benedict-Myers m.
Folin-Denis m.
Folin gravimetric m.
Genta m.
Giemsa m.
Halsted m.
Hanley m.
Hasson m.
Hybritech m.
imaging m.
immunohistochemical m.
introducer m.
Jendrassik-Grof m.
Kaplan-Meier m.
Lashmet-Newburgh m.
lay-open m.
lift-and-cut m.
Lowery m.
Metzer-Boyce m.
microwave-assisted streptavidin-biotin
 peroxidase m.
Morison m.
noninvasive m.
m. of Gates
Okamoto m.
Papanicolaou m.
Parker-Kerr suture-closed m.
partial hood-assisted lift-and-cut m.
Patterson-Parker m.
pause-squeeze m.
Payr m.
percutaneous sampling m.
Permutit m.
phosphotungstic acid-magnesium
 chloride precipitation m.
pull m.
Quimby m.
radiochromium-labeled erythrocyte m.
Reddick-Saye m.
Rehfuss m.
Schwartz m.
Shohl-Pedley m.
Sjöqvist m.
Stachrom AT III routine
 chromogenic m.
standard radioenzymatic m.
suck-and-cut m.

Sumner m.
technically elaborate m.
thermally active m.
thiourea-resorcinol m.
trapezoid m.
triangulation stapling m.
turn-and-suction m.
Volhard-Fahr m.
Warthin-Starry m.
Waterston aorto-to-right-pulmonary
 artery closure m.
Wheeless m.
Woolf m.
methotrexate (MTX)
 m., cisplatin (MC)
 m., cisplatin, vinblastine (MCV)
 m., Oncovin, fluorouracil (MOF)
 m., vinblastine, Adriamycin, cisplatin
  (MVAC, M-VAC)
 m., vinblastine, epirubicin, cisplatin
  (M-VEC)
methotrimeprazine
methoxamine
methoxsalen
methoxyflurane anesthesia
methoxyphenamine
methscopolamine bromide
methyclothiazide
methyl
 m. red test
 m. salicylate
methylaminoisobutyric acid (MeAIB)
methylate
 phentolamine m.
methylatropine nitrate
methylbromide
 anisotropine m.
 homatropine m. (HMB-45, HMB,
  HMB45)
methyl-CCNU
 fluorouracil, Adriamycin, m.-C.
methylcellulose
 hydroxypropyl m.
methylcitric
2-methylcitric acid
5-methyl cytosine
methyldopa
 parenteral m.
methyldopate
methylene
 m. blue
 m. blue chromoendoscopy
 m. blue dye
 m. blue enema
 m. blue stain
 m. diphosphonate (MPD)
5,10-methylene-tetrahydrofolate reductase
 (MTHFR)
methylhistamine

M

3-methylhistidine
    urinary 3-m.
methylmalonic acid
methylnaltrexone (MNTX)
methylnitrate
    atropine m.
methylparatyrosine
    alpha m.
methylphenidate
1-methyl-4-phenyl-1,2,3,6-
  tetrahydropyridine
  (MTPT)
6-methylprednisolone
methylprednisolone acetate
methylsulfate
    diphemanil m.
    neostigmine m.
methyl-*tert*-butyl
    m.-*t*.-b. ether (MTBE)
    m.-*t*.-b. ether therapy
methyltestosterone
methyltestosterone-induced cholestasia
methysergide maleate
Meticorten
meticulous dissection
Metizol
metoclopramide
    m., dexamethasone, lorazepam,
      ondansetron (MDLO)
    m. premedication
metocurine
metolazone
metoprolol tartrate
metreleptin
Metricide disinfectant
metrifonate
metrizamide
metrizoate
MetroGel
metronidazole
    m., amoxicillin, clarithromycin, *H.*
      pylori, 1-week therapy (MACH1)
    omeprazole, amoxicillin, m.
      (OAM)
metronidazole-resistant strain
Metryl 500
metschnikovii
    Vibrio m.
metyrapone stimulation test
metyrosine
Metzenbaum scissors
Metzer-Boyce method
Meulengracht diet
Mevacor
Mewissen infusion catheter
Mexican
    M. hat sign
    M. Scammony root
mexiletine

Meyenburg complex
Meyer-Weigert law
mezlocillin
MFG
    manofluorography
MGN
    membranous glomerulonephritis
MGUS
    monoclonal gammopathy of
      undetermined significance
MHC
    major histocompatibility complex
    MHC class I, II antigen
    MHC molecule
MHC-bound
MHV
    middle hepatic vein
Mi-Acid
Miami pouch
MIB-1
    monoclonal antibody MIB-1
    MIB-1 staining
MIBG
    metaiodobenzylguanidine
MIC
    minimal inhibitory concentration
    MIC gastroenteric tube
    MIC gastrostomy tube
micaceous growth of penis
mica operation
micellar solubilization
micelle formation
Michaelis constant (Km)
Michaelis-Gutmann body
Michaelis-Menten kinetics
Michal
    M. II technique
    M. procedure I, II
Michel clip
Michigan
    M. intestinal forceps
    M. Kidney Registry
Mick
    M. applicator
    M. prostate template
MIC-Key
    M.-K. G gastrostomy tube
    M.-K. J gastrostomy tube
miconazole
Micral urine dipstick test
microabscess
microacinus
microadenoma
microaerophilic organism
microalbuminuria
microanastomosis
    laser-assisted m. (LAMA)
microaneurysm
microangiopathic renal injury

microangiopathy
    diabetic m.
    tacrolimus-associated m.
    thrombotic m.
microarray
    protein m.
microarray-based study
microballoon probe
microbial
    m. approach
    m. biofilm
    m. ecology
microbiliary inflammation
microbiology
microbiota
    fecal m.
microcalcification
microcalculi (*pl. of* microcalculus)
microcalculus, *pl.* **microcalculi**
microcalix
microcatheter
    FasTracker 325 coaxial m.
Microcell chamber
microcephalia (*var. of* microcephaly)
microcephaly, microcephalia
microchimerism
    donor hematopoietic cell m.
    donor-type m.
microchromoendoscopy
microclimate
    acid m.
Micrococcus
microcoil
    Intercept esophagus m.
    Intercept prostate m.
    Intercept urethra m.
Microcoleus
microcolitis
microcolon
microcrystal
microcrystalline material
microcyst
    lymphatic m.
microcystic disease of renal medulla
microdensitometer
    Vickers M85a m.
microdissection testicular sperm extraction
microdroplet fat deposition
Microelectrode
    M. MI-506 small-caliber pH electrode
    M. MI-506 small-caliber probe
microemulsion
    cyclosporine for m.
microenvironment
    gastric m.
microepididymal sperm aspiration (MESA)

microerosion
microexplosive generator
microfibril
microfibrillar
    m. collagen hemostat (MCH)
    m. protein
microfilament bundle
microfilariasis
microfil-associated glycoprotein (MAGP)
microfilter
    Minnpure m.
microflora
    colonic m.
microfluorometric measurement
microfold cell
microgastria
microgenitalism
Microglass pH electrode
microglobulin
    beta-2 m.
microgram (mcg)
micrograph
    low-magnification electron m.
Microgyn II urinary incontinence device
microhamartoma
    biliary m.
microhematuria
microimplant
    silicone m.
microlens cystourethroscope
microlith
microlithiasis
    common bile duct m. (CBDM)
    pulmonary alveolar m.
    testicular m.
microlithiasis-induced pancreatitis
MicroLyzer
    M. gas analyzer
    QuinTron M.
micromanipulation
    gamete m.
    oocyte m.
micrometastases (*pl. of* micrometastasis)
micrometastasis, *pl.* **micrometastases**
    hematogenic m.
Micronase
microneedle holder
micronidia
micronized flavonidic fraction
micronodular cirrhosis
microparticle enzyme immunoassay (MEIA)
micropenis
microperforation
microperfusion study
microphallus
micropipet (*var. of* micropipette)
micropipette, micropipet
microprocessor-controlled electrosurgery

M

micropuncture
>epididymis m.
>m. technique

microrchidia

micros
>*Peptostreptococcus m.*

microsatellite
>m. instability (MSI)
>m. stable (MSS)

microscope
>dual-axis confocal m.
>Elmiskop 101 electron m.
>JEM-100B, -100S electron m.
>JEOL 100 CX electron m.
>JEOL JSM 35 CF scanning
>electron m.
>laser m.
>Olympus BH2 epifluorescence m.
>Olympus BH2-RFCA reflecting m.
>Olympus BHT-2 m.
>Olympus CBK fluorescence m.
>Phillips CM 12 electron m.
>real-time confocal scanning
>laser m.
>scanning electron m.
>Zeiss Axiophot m.
>Zeiss IDO3 phase-contrast m.
>Zeiss S9 electron m.

microscopic, microscopical
>m. colitis
>m. colitis syndrome
>m. epididymal sperm aspiration
>m. hematuria
>m. polyangiitis (MPA)
>m. urine examination

microscopical (*var. of* microscopic)

microscopy
>atomic force m.
>confocal laser scanning m.
>electron m.
>epifluorescence m.
>immune electron m.
>immunofluorescence m.
>in vivo m.
>laser scanning confocal m.
>light m.
>paraffin-section light m.
>polarization m.
>rotary shadowing electron m.
>scanning electron m.
>scanning force m. (SFM)
>single-fiber confocal m.
>transmission electron m. (TEM)
>urinalysis sediment m.

microseminoprotein
>beta m.

MicroSkin ostomy pouch

microsomal
>m. damage

>m. ethanol oxidizing system
>(MEOS)

microsome
>m. antibody (MCHA)
>antiliver kidney m. (anti-LKM)
>liver-kidney m. (LKM)

microsphere
>biodegradable m.
>^{99m}Tc albumin m.
>Super-Bright m.

Microspike approximator clamp

Microsporidia

microsporidian

microsporidiasis (*var. of* microsporidiosis)

microsporidiosis, microsporidiasis

microsurgery
>rectal expander-assisted transanal
>endoscopic m. (RE-TEM)
>transanal endoscopic m.
>(TEM)

microsurgical
>m. denervation of spermatic cord
>m. epididymal sperm aspiration
>(MESA)
>m. epididymal sperm aspiration
>procedure
>m. epididymovasostomy (MSEV)
>m. extraction of ductal sperm
>(MEDS)
>m. extraction of sperm from
>epididymis (MASE)
>m. inguinal varicocelectomy

microsuture
>Sharpoint m.

microtelangiectasia

microtendon

microtip
>m. sensor catheter
>m. transducer catheter

microtitration plate reader

**microtrabecular hepatocellular
carcinoma**

microtransducer
>imbedded m.
>Konigsberg m.
>m. technique

microtubule (MT)

Micro-6 ureteroscope

microvascular
>m. anastomosis
>m. clamp
>m. flap
>m. needle holder

Microvasive
>M. Altertome
>M. angled hydrophilic guidewire
>M. ASAP 18
>M. balloon catheter
>M. biliary stent system

M. CRE esophageal dilator
M. disposable alligator-shaped forceps
M. Geenen Endotorque guidewire
M. Glidewire guidewire
M. Gold probe bipolar electrocautery device
M. instrumentation
M. minisnare
M. papillotome
M. radial-jaw large-capacity biopsy forceps
M. retrieval balloon
M. Rigiflex balloon dilator
M. Rigiflex through-the-scope balloon
M. sclerotherapy needle
M. Ultraflex esophageal stent system
M. Ultratome

microvesicular
    m. fat
    m. steatosis
microvilli (*pl. of* microvillus)
microvillous membrane
microvillus, *pl.* **microvilli**
    m. inclusion disease
microvolt (mcV)
microwave
    m. ablation
    m. applicator
    endoscopic m.
    m. hyperthermia
    m. nonsurgical treatment
    m. therapy
    m. thermotherapy
    m. tissue coagulation
    m. tissue coagulator
microwave-assisted streptavidin-biotin peroxidase method
microwell plate
miction
MIC-TJ transgastric jejunal tube
micturating
    m. cystogram
    m. cystourethrogram (MCU, MCUG)
    m. cystourethrography (MCU)
micturition
    m. cystourethrogram
    m. phase
    m. problem
    m. reflex
    m. reflex inhibition
    m. reflex manual initiation
midabdominal
    m. abscess
    m. transverse incision
    m. wall

Midamor
midaxillary line
midazolam
    m. conscious sedation
    m. hydrochloride
midclavicular line (MCL)
midcolon
middle
    m. adrenal artery
    m. colic artery (MCA)
    m. extrahepatic bile duct
    m. gland
    m. hemorrhoidal artery
    m. hepatic vein (MHV)
    m. hypospadias
    m. rectal fold
    m. rectal vein
    m. rectal venous plexus
    m. stomach
    m. ureter
midepigastric area
midepigastrium
midesophageal diverticulum
midesophagus
midgastric electrode
midgut
    m. ischemia
    m. volvulus
    m. volvulus with malrotation
midline
    m. abdominal crease
    m. lower abdominal incision
    m. upper abdominal incision
midodrine
midrectal area
midregion PTH
midsigmoid colon
midstomach
midstream
    m. specimen of urine (MSU)
    m. urinalysis
midtransverse segment
midureteral calculus
midurethral
    m. sling
    m. support
MIE
    meconium ileus equivalent
Miescher cheilitis granulomatosa
mifepristone
miglitol
migraine
    abdominal m.
migrans
    larva m.
    visceral larva m.
migrating
    m. motor complex (MMC)
    m. myoelectric complex

M

migration
    aboral m.
    calculus m.
    electrode m.
    gallstone m.
    gastrostomy tube m.
    m. inhibition factor
      (MIF)
    intravesical m.
    lymphocyte m.
    metallic biliary stent m.
    retrograde m.
    stent m.
    tube m.
Mikulicz
    M. bag
    M. clamp
    M. colostomy
    M. drain
    M. drain technique
    M. gastroscope
    M. gastrostomy tube
    M. operation
    M. packing
    M. pad
    M. peritoneal forceps
    M. procedure
    M. pyloroplasty
    M. retractor
mild
    m. distress
    m. hyperoxaluria
    m. idiopathic adulthood biliary
      ductopenia
    m. tubulitis
Miles
    M. abdominoperineal resection
    M. operation
    M. V.I.P. 300 vacuum infiltration
      processor
milia (*pl. of* milium)
miliaria rubra
miliary tuberculosis
milium, *pl.* **milia**
milk
    acidophilus m.
    m. diet
    m. of calcium
    m. of calcium sign
    m. of magnesia (MOM)
    m. protein antibody
    m. sickness
    m. thistle
milk-alkali syndrome
milking of intestine
Milkinol
milkman's line
milk-of-calcium bile
milk-sensitive colitis

milkweed
    giant m.
milky
    m. ascites
    m. fluid
    m. urine
Millard mouth gag
Millar urodynamic catheter
Millen technique retropubic
   prostatectomy
Miller
    M. cystoscope
    M. Fisher syndrome
    M. rectal forceps
    M. rectal scissors
Miller-Abbott intestinal tube
milleri
    Streptococcus m.
Miller-Senn retractor
Millex-GS pore-size filter
Millex-GV filter
Millie female urinal
Milligan-Morgan
    M.-M. hemorrhoidectomy
    M.-M. operation
    M.-M. technique for hemorrhoid
      treatment
milligram (mg)
millijoule (mJ)
milliliter (mL)
millimeters of mercury (mmHg)
millimolar concentration
millimoles per liter (mmol/L)
Millin
    M. bladder retractor
    M. forceps
    M. T clamp
milliosmole/kilogram (mosm/kg)
Millipore filter
milliwatt (mW)
Mill-Rose
    M.-R. flexible endoscopic overtube
    M.-R. RiteBite biopsy forceps
milrinone
Milroy disease
miltiorrhiza
    Salvia m.
MILTS
    Multicentre International Liver Tumor
    Study
mimic
    endocrine m.
mind-bladder syndrome
mineral
    divalent m.
    m. oil (M-O)
mineralocorticoid
mineralocorticoid-independent factor
Ming gastric carcinoma classification

miniature
  m. probe
  m. ultrasound suction device
miniaturized
  m. sheath
  m. ultrasound catheter probe
MiniBard catheter
minicap
  Coloplast flange m.
minigenome
Miniguard adhesive patch
minihelical basket
minilaparoscope
  m. cholecystectomy
  Storz m.
minilaparotomy (minilap)
  m. approach
  m. incision
  m. pelvic lymph node dissection
  m. restorative proctocolectomy
  m. staging pelvic lymphadenectomy
miniloop
  m. ligation
  Olympus HX-21L detachable m.
minimal
  m. distending pressure
  m. inhibitory concentration (MIC)
  m. invasiveness
  m. transurethral resection of prostate (M-TURP)
minimal-access
  m.-a. surgery
  m.-a. surgical skill
minimal-change
  m.-c. disease
  m.-c. nephrotic syndrome
minimal-lesion nephrotic syndrome
minimally
  m. invasive approach
  m. invasive surgery
  m. invasive therapy
  m. invasive treatment
minimicrosphere
minimize patient morbidity
minimum daily requirement (MDR)
minipapillotome
miniperc technique
minipercutaneous nephrolithotomy
mini-Pfannenstiel incision
minipouch
  Assura closed m.
  Coloplast m.
  Sur-Fit m.
Minipress
miniprobe
  high-frequency m.
minipump
  Alzer osmotic m.

miniscope
  Candela M.
  Circon-ACMI m.
  Wolfe m.
minisnare
  Microvasive m.
mink cell bioassay
Minnesota
  M. antilymphocyte globulin
  M. tube
Minnpure microfilter
Minocin
minocycline
minor
  m. calyx
  m. cognitive motor disorder (MCMD)
  curvatura gastrica m.
  curvatura ventriculi m.
  globus m.
  m. papilla
  papilla duodeni m.
  m. papilla sphincterotomy
minoxidil
mint
  wild m.
Mintezol
minus
  omentum m.
minute
  m. bleeding
  counts per m. (cpm, CPM)
  m. polypoid lesion
1-minute endoscopy room test
30-minute
  30-m. transurethral microwave thermotherapy
  30-m. TUMT
minutissimum
  Corynebacterium m.
MIP
  megameatus-intact prepuce
mirabilis
  Proteus m.
MiraLax
Mirizzi syndrome
mirror-image artifact
misakiensis
  Streptomyces m.
miscellaneous urolithiasis
mismatch
  HLA m.
misonidazole
misoprostol protection
misperfusion
  gastroduodenal m.
misplaced gland
missed diagnosis
missense mutation

M

Mission
>M. vacuum constriction device
>M. vacuum erection device
>M. VCD
>M. VED

Missouri catheter

Misstique female external urinary collector

Mistifier spray catheter

mistletoe
>European m.

MIT
>mean input time

Mitchell
>M. technique
>M. technique for epispadias repair

Mitek bone anchor

Mithracin

mithramycin

mitis
>nephritis m.

mitochondrial
>m. antibody
>m. complex
>m. encephalomyopathy, lactic acidosis and strokelike episodes (MELAS)
>m. ethanol oxidase system
>m. fatty acid beta oxidation
>m. glutamate dehydrogenase pathway
>m. immunologic study
>m. injury
>m. neurogastrointestinal encephalomyopathy (MNGIE)
>m. neurogastrointestinal encephalomyopathy syndrome
>m. phosphate-dependent glutaminase

mitogen

mitogen-activated protein kinase (MAPK)

mitogenic
>m. effect
>m. stimulation
>m. stimulus

mitomycin
>m. adsorbed onto activated charcoal (M-CH)
>m. C
>5-fluorouracil, Adriamycin, m. C (FAM)
>intravesical m. C (IMMC)
>m. transarterial embolization treatment

mitosis count

mitosis-karyorrhexis index (MKI)

mitotane

mitotic
>m. activity
>m. index

mitoxantrone (DHAD)

Mitrofanoff
>M. appendicovesicostomy
>M. appendicovesicostomy procedure
>M. catheterizable channel
>M. catheterizable stoma
>M. conduit
>M. continent urinary diversion technique
>M. continent urinary stoma
>M. mechanism
>M. neourethra
>M. principle
>M. solution
>M. tube
>M. valve

Mitrolan

Mitscherlich test

mittelschmerz

mivacurium chloride

MIVOD
>mesenteric inflammatory venoocclusive disease

mixed
>m. cholesterol gallstone
>m. cirrhosis
>m. connective tissue disorder
>m. essential cryoglobulinemia
>m. germ cell-sex cord stromal tumor
>m. germ cell tumor
>m. gonadal dysgenesis
>m. growth on culture
>m. hemorrhoids
>m. hyperlipidemia
>m. hyperplastic-adenomatous gastric polyp
>m. incontinence
>m. intralobular fibrosis
>m. leukocyte culture (MLC)
>m. rhabdomyosarcoma
>m. structure
>m. urinary incontinence (MUI)

Mixter
>M. clamp
>M. dilating probe
>M. dissector
>M. gallstone forceps
>M. hemostat

mixture
>amino acid-glucose m.
>citric acid bladder m.
>eutectic m.
>sodium citrate and potassium citrate m.

Miyazaki-Bonney test for stress incontinence
mizoribine
mJ
    millijoule
MKII automated scanner
mL
    milliliter
MLC
    mixed leukocyte culture
        allogenic MLC
MLH1 gene
MLN
    mesenteric lymph node
MLP
    multiple lymphomatous polyposis
MM
    measuring-mounting
        MM catheter
MMAP
    Maine Medical Assessment Program
        MMAP index
MMC
    migrating motor complex
    murine mesangial cell
MMF
    mycophenolate mofetil
mmHg
    millimeters of mercury
MMK
    Marshall-Marchetti-Krantz
mmol/L
    millimoles per liter
MMP
    matrix metalloproteinase
MMP-7
    matrix metalloproteinase-7
MMP-9
    matrix metalloproteinase-9
MMUA
    macromolecular uronate
MN
    mononuclear
        MN cell
        MN infiltrate
MNB
    monomicrobial nonneutrocytic
    bacterascites
MNE
    monosymptomatic nocturnal enuresis
MNGIE
    mitochondrial neurogastrointestinal
    encephalomyopathy
MNTI
    melanotic neuroectodermal tumor of
    infancy
MNTX
    methylnaltrexone

M-O
    mineral oil
        Haley's M-O
Moban
Mobigesic
mobile gallbladder
mobilis
    lien m.
mobility
    electrophoretic m.
mobilization
    anorectal m.
    total urogenital m.
    urogenital m.
    urogenital sinus m.
Mobin-Uddin umbrella
Moctanin
modality
    current treatment m.
    dialysis m.
    ever-expanding armamentarium of
      therapeutic m.'s
    indispensable diagnostic m.
    therapeutic m.
Modane
    M. Soft
    M. Versabran
mode
    autosomal-recessive m.
    linear m.
    linear-array m.
    radial m.
model
    ablation m.
    Cox regression m.
    dominant inheritance m.
    M. for End-Stage Liver Disease
      (MELD)
    in vitro m.
    Markov m.
    MELD m.
modeling
    penile m.
    urea kinetic m. (UKM)
moderate
    m. distress
    m. proteinuria
moderately differentiated adenoma
modification
    Al-Ghorab m.
    evidence-based dietary/fluid m.
    Goligher m.
    high-energy m.
    Kelly-Kennedy m.
    lifestyle m.
    Muzsnai m.
    m. of diet in renal disease
      (MDRD)

M

modification (*continued*)
    M. of Diet in Renal Disease trial
    posttranslational m.
    pylorus-preserving Whipple m.
    Pugh m.
    Raz m.
    recent technical m.
    Walsh surgical m.

modified
    m. aspirating catheter
    m. barium swallow (MBS)
    m. Barthel degree of disability index
    m. Bismuth-Corlette classification
    m. Cantwell technique
    m. caulking gun
    m. Essed-Schroeder corporoplasty
    m. Gibson incision
    m. Hassan open technique
    m. Hetzel-Dent scale
    m. ileocecal valve
    m. Ingelman-Sundberg procedure
    m. Lich-Gregoir ureteroneocystostomy
    m. liver diet
    m. Lloyd-Davies position
    m. method of Pugh
    m. Minnesota tube
    m. Nesbit procedure
    m. Norfolk procedure
    m. penectomy
    m. Pereyra bladder neck suspension
    m. polyethylene dilator
    m. Sacks-Vine push-pull technique
    m. sham feeding
    m. thermal nitinol electrode
    m. Thiersch-Duplay technique
    m. transduodenal rendezvous procedure
    m. Vest technique
    m. Whitehead hemorrhoidectomy
    m. Young urethroplasty
    m. Z stent

modifier
    biologic response m. (BRM)

modulation
    antigenic m.
    obstruction-induced m.
    pressure amplitude m.

modulator
    intracrine negative feedback m.

Modulith
    M. device for ESWL
    M. SL lithotriptor
    Storz M. SL20

Moduretic

MODY
    maturity-onset diabetes of youth

Moersch esophagoscope

MOF
    methotrexate, Oncovin, fluorouracil
    multiple-organ failure

mofetil
    mycophenolate m. (MMF)

Mogen clamp

Mohr test

Mohs microsurgery technique

moiety
    steroid m.

moist
    m. laparotomy pack
    m. mucous membranes
    m. necrosis
    m. papule

Moi-Stir

molar pregnancy

mole
    hydatid m.
    hydatidiform m.

Molectron Nd:YAG laser

molecular
    m. adsorbent recirculating system (MARS)
    m. basis of proteinuria
    m. cloning
    m. cloning and sequencing
    m. extracorporeal liver support (MELS)
    m. extracorporeal liver support system
    m. genetic alteration
    m. marker
    m. study
    m. typing
    m. weight (mol wt)

molecule
    adhesion m.
    CD4 m.
    CD8 m.
    cell-adhesion m.
    class I, II MHC m.
    extracellular matrix m.
    HLA-DQ2 m.
    immunoglobulin superfamily adhesion m.
    lithostathine m.
    lymphocyte costimulatory m.
    messenger RNA m.
    monocyte adhesion m.
    neural cell-adhesive m. (NCAM)
    retinoid-related m.

molecule-1
    endothelial leukocyte adhesion m.-1 (ELAM-1)
    intercellular adhesion m.-1 (ICAM-1)
    vascular cell adhesion m.-1 (VCAM-1)

molgramostim
molimina
molindone
mollusc
  bivalve m.
molluscum
  m. contagiosum
  m. contagiosum virus (MCV)
Molnar disk
mol wt
  molecular weight
MOM
  milk of magnesia
Monarc urethral sling
Mondor phlebitis
Monfort
  M. abdominal wall reconstruction
  M. abdominoplasty
mongolian spot
Monilia esophagitis
monilial
  m. esophagitis
  m. infection
moniliasis
Monistat
monitor
  Bravo pH m.
  Contimed II pelvic floor
    muscle m.
  Deltatrac metabolic m.
  Dinamap Plus m.
  Dobbhoff biofeedback m.
  gastric pH m.
  Gould pressure m.
  24-hour ambulatory gastric pH m.
  Ingold M3, M4 glass electrode pH
    m.
  inline blood gas m.
  Interceptor M3 triple-channel
    solid-state m.
  m. peptide
  return electrode m.
  RigiScan penile tumescence and
    rigidity m.
  television m.
  video m.
monitoring
  ambulatory intraesophageal
    bilirubin m.
  ambulatory intraesophageal pH
    m.
  ambulatory urodynamic m.
  Bravo pH m.
  clinical m.
  cystometrographic m.
  endoscopic m.
  esophageal pH m.
  fluoroscopic m.
  heart rate m.

  24-hour ambulatory esophageal pH
    m.
  24-hour spectrophotometric bilirubin
    m.
  intracranial pressure m.
  intraesophageal pH m.
  multichannel intraluminal impedance
    m.
  nocturnal penile tumescence m.
  NPT m.
  pH m.
  prescription-event m. (PEM)
  tumescence m.
  wireless pH m.
monitor/recorder
  Gastroreflex ambulatory
    pH m./r.
monoamine oxidase inhibitor
  (MAOI)
Monocal tablet
monocapsule
  bismuth triple m.
Monocid
monoclonal
  m. antibody (MAb)
  m. antibody BR96
  m. antibody ED1
  m. antibody MIB-1
  m. antibody scintigraphic scan
  m. antibody therapy
  m. anti-DNA antibody
  m. antigen
  m. anti-HBc
  m. gammopathy
  m. gammopathy of undetermined
    significance (MGUS)
  m. IgM
  m. light chain
  m. proliferation
monoclonality by genetic analysis
Monocryl suture
monocrystant antimony pH catheter
monocyte
  m. adhesion molecule
  m. chemoattractant protein
    (MCP)
  m. chemoattractant protein-1
    (MCP-1)
  m. chemotactic protein (MCP)
  WBC m.
monocytes/macrophages
monocytogenes
  Listeria m.
  m. peritonitis
Monodox
Monodral
monoethanolamine oleate
monoethylglycinexylidide (MEGX)
  m. liver function tests

M

491

monofilament
 m. absorbable suture
 m. nylon suture
 m. snare wire
monofocal papillary carcinoma
Mono-Gesic
monohydrate
 cefadroxil m.
 doxycycline m.
 sodium phosphate monobasic m.
monohydroxy bile salt
monokine
monolayer
 cobblestonelike m.
monomer
 tissue m.
monomicrobial nonneutrocytic bacterascites (MNB)
mononephrous
mononuclear (MN)
 m. cell recruitment
 m. dyspepsia
 m. histiocytic portal infiltrate
mononucleotide
 flavin m.
monooctanoin infusion
monooxygenase pathway
monophosphate
 adenosine m. (AMP)
 5′-cyclic adenosine m. (cAMP)
 cyclic adenosine m. (AMP-c, cAMP)
 5′-cyclic guanosine m.
 cyclic guanosine m. (cGMP)
 guanosine m. (GMP)
5′-monophosphate
 guanosine 5′.-m.
monopodial
monopolar
 m. coagulation
 m. electrocautery
 m. electrocoagulation
 m. probe
 m. triple-hook active needle
monopole
monopolypoid adenoma
monosaccharide
Monoscopy locking trocar with Woodford spike
monosialoganglioside
monosialosyl Lea
monosodium urate
Monospot
monosymptomatic nocturnal enuresis (MNE)
monoterpene
monotherapy
 androgen ablative m.
 bicalutamide m.

 nonsteroidal antiandrogen m.
 sirolimus m.
mons
 m. plasty
 m. veneris
Montague
 M. proctoscope
 M. sigmoidoscope
Montezuma revenge
Montgomery
 M. abdominal strap
 M. salivary bypass tube
 M. strap dressing
 M. tape
Monti-Malone, left
Monti procedure
Monti-Yang ileovesicostomy
Monurol
moon
 m. facies
 M. rectal retractor
Moore
 M. classification for vascular anomalies of gastrointestinal tract
 M. gallstone scoop
MOP-Videoplan morphometric system
Moraxella
 M. bovis
 M. nonliquefaciens
morbidity
 febrile m.
 maternal m.
 minimize patient m.
 m. of percutaneous nephrolithotomy
 operative m.
 perioperative m.
 postoperative m.
 reflux m.
 m. risk
 treatment m.
 uncorrected maternal m.
 uncorrected reflux m.
morbid obesity
morbus
 cholera m.
morcellated nephrectomy
morcellation
 m. operation
 m. technique
 vaginal m.
morcellator
 Cook tissue m.
 electric tissue m.
 high-speed electrical tissue m.
 tissue m.
Moreno gastroenterostomy clamp
Morgagni
 M. appendix
 M. caruncle

column of M.
M. crypt
foramen of M.
fossa of M.
M. fovea
frenum of M.
M. hernia
M. hydatid
M. lacuna
M. retinaculum
M. valve

morganii
Proteus m.

Morganstern
M. aspiration/injection system
M. continuous-flow operating
cystoscope

moribund
moricizine
Mori knife
Morison
hepatorenal space of M.
M. method
M. pouch

morning
m. diarrhea
m. glory

Moro-Heisler diet
morphea
morphine
m. cholescintigraphy
m. narcotic analgesic therapy

morphine-neostigmine test
morphogenesis
morphogenetic process
morphologic, morphological
m. change
m. stage
m. study of renal biopsy

morphological (*var. of* morphologic)
morphology
chromosome m.
closed m.
crystal m.
Dogiel type I, II m.
filamentous m.
glomerular m.
gram-stain m.
open m.

morphomate
Zeiss m. M30

morphometric criteria
morphometry
nuclear m.

morrhuate
m. sclerosant
sodium m.

mortality
cardiovascular m.

intraoperative m.
overall m.
prostate cancer-specific m.
(PCSM)
risk-adjusted m.

mortar kidney
mortis
livor m.
rigor m.

mosaic duodenal mucosal pattern
Moschcowitz
M. culdoplasty procedure
M. operation
M. vaginal prolapse repair

Moscontin
MOSD
multiple-organ system dysfunction

MOSF
multiorgan system failure
multiple-organ system failure

Mosher
M. bag
M. dilator
M. esophagoscope

mosm/kg
milliosmole/kilogram

mosquito
m. forceps
m. hemostat
m. hemostatic clamp

moss
club m.
M. gastrostomy tube
M. G-tube
M. G-tube PEG kit
Iceland m.
M. Mark IV tube
M. T-anchor introducer gun

Mosse syndrome
Mostofi-grade prostate cancer
mother
m. cyst
m. endoscopic retrograde
cholangiopancreatoscopy system

mother-baby
m.-b. endoscope system
m.-b. scope system

mother-daughter endoscope
mother-infant dyad
**mother-to-infant transmission of hepatitis
C virus**
motif
coiled-coil m.
Patterson-Parker m.

motilide
motilin
m. agonist
basal release of m.
m. plasma level

M

motility
    m. agent
    altered sperm m.
    antropyloroduodenal m.
    colonic m.
    colorectal m.
    m. disorder
    disordered m.
    esophageal m.
    gastrointestinal m.
    ineffective esophageal m. (IEM)
    interdigestive antroduodenal m.
    neurohumoral control of m.
    prefreeze m.
    reduced m.
    sequential m.
    spermatozoon m.
    m. test
Motilium
motion
    brownian m.
    paradoxical m.
    m. sickness
motogenesis
motogenic
motoneuron (*var. of* motor
  neuron)
motor
    m. activity
    m. endplate
    m. examination
    m. neuron
    m. oil peritoneal fluid
    m. syringe
    m. test meal
    m. unit action potential
    m. urgency
Moto-Tool
    Dremel M.-T.
Motrin
mottled testis
moulage sign
mound
    infraumbilical m.
mountain flax
Moure esophagoscope
mouse
    peritoneal m.
**Mousseau-Barbin prosthetic
  tube**
mouth
    m. breathing
    Ceylon sore m.
    m. gag
mouthgag (*var. of* mouth gag)
mouthguard
    oxygenating m.
    Oxyguard oxygenating m.

movable testis
Moveen bedside night bag
movement
    bowel m. (BM)
    dyscoordinate hyoid m.
    pelvic floor m.
    segmentation m.
    symmetric face m.
    tongue m.
    urethral catheter m.
    vermicular m.
MoviPrep
moxalactam
moxisylyte injection
**MOX portable renal preservation
  machine**
Moynihan
    M. artery forceps
    M. bile duct probe
    M. clamp
    M. gall duct forceps
    M. gallstone probe
    M. gallstone scoop
    M. technique
    M. test
6-MP
    6-mercaptopurine
MPA
    microscopic polyangiitis
MPD
    main pancreatic duct
    methylene diphosphonate
    MPD stent
MPEC
    multipolar electrocoagulation
MPGN
    mesangioproliferative glomerulonephritis
MP-RAGE
    magnetization prepared-rapid gradient
    echo
MPTP
    1-methyl-4-phenyl-1,2,3,6-
    tetrahydropyridine
MR
    magnetic resonance
      MR hydrography
MRA
    magnetic resonance angiography
MRC
    magnetic resonance cholangiography
    magnetic resonance colonography
MRCC
    metastatic renal cell carcinoma
MRCP
    magnetic resonance
    cholangiopancreatography
      MRCP using HASTE with
      phased-array coil

MRDM
    malnutrition-related diabetes mellitus
MRI
    magnetic resonance imaging
        endorectal surface coil MRI
        fast spin-echo acquisition MRI
        rectal coil MRI
        MRI scan
        ultrafast MRI
mRNA
    messenger ribonucleic acid
    messenger RNA
        AR mRNA
        clusterin mRNA
        cotransporter mRNA
        COX mRNA
        cyclooxygenase mRNA
        gastrin mRNA
        glomerular fibronectin mRNA
        hepcidin mRNA
        HSP-70 mRNA
        IGF-binding protein-1 mRNA
        IGF-1R mRNA
        preproEt-1 mRNA
        taurine cotransporter mRNA
        TCT mRNA
MRP
    magnetic resonance pancreatography
    maximum anal resting pressure
MRP2
    multidrug resistance-associated protein-2
MRS
    magnetic resonance spectroscopy
MRSA
    methicillin-resistant *Staphylococcus
    aureus*
MRT
    mean resistance time
MRU
    magnetic resonance urography
MS
    multiple sclerosis
MS-8
    Pancrecarb MS-8
MSAO
    meal-stimulated acid output
MS Classique balloon dilation catheter
M-scope multibending scope
MSEV
    microsurgical epididymovasostomy
MS-1, -2 hepatitis
MSH2 **gene**
MSI
    microsatellite instability
        MSI nylon membrane
MSOF
    multiple-system organ failure
    multisystem organ failure

MSP
    maximum squeeze pressure
MSU
    midstream specimen of urine
MSUD
    maple syrup urine disease
MTAC
    mass transfer area coefficient
MTBE
    methyl-*tert*-butyl ether
        MTBE gallstone dissolution
        MTBE therapy
99mTc, ^{99m}Tc
    technetium-99m
^{99m}Tc
        ^{99m}Tc albumin colloid
        ^{99m}Tc albumin microsphere
        ^{99m}Tc DISIDA
        ^{99m}Tc DISIDA contrast
        injection
        ^{99m}Tc DMSA
        ^{99m}Tc DTPA aerosol
        ^{99m}Tc DTPA renal scan
        ^{99m}Tc GHP
        ^{99m}Tc GSA
        ^{99m}Tc GSA scintigraphy
        ^{99m}Tc HIDA
        ^{99m}Tc HMPAO-labeled leukocyte
        scan
        ^{99m}Tc IDA scan
        ^{99m}Tc lidofenin
        ^{99m}Tc MAA
        ^{99m}Tc MAG-3 isotope
        ^{99m}Tc MDP
        ^{99m}Tc MDP nuclear isotope bone
        scan
        ^{99m}Tc medronate
        ^{99m}Tc pertechnetate scan
        ^{99m}Tc pertechnetate scintigraphy
        ^{99m}Tc PIPIDA
        ^{99m}Tc polyphosphate
        ^{99m}Tc PYP
        ^{99m}Tc RBC bleeding scan
        ^{99m}Tc sodium pertechnetate
        ^{99m}Tc SPP
        ^{99m}Tc sulfur colloid
        (^{99m}Tc SC)
        ^{99m}Tc sulfur colloid egg meal
        ^{99m}Tc sulfur colloid scan
^{99m}Tc-DTPA
    technetium-99m diethylenetriamine
    pentaacetic acid
        ^{99m}Tc-DTPA renal scan
^{99m}Tc-labeled
        ^{99m}Tc-l. Amberlite pellet
        ^{99m}Tc-l. anti-alpha fetoprotein
        ^{99m}Tc-l. stannous methylene
        diphosphonate

M

^{99m}Tc-phytate liquid state esophageal transit study

^{99m}Tc-SC
technetium-99m sulfur colloid

m-tetrahydroxyphenyl chlorin photodynamic therapy

MTHFR
5,10-methylene-tetrahydrofolate reductase

m-THP-Chlorin

MTOPS
Medical Therapy of Prostatic Symptoms
MTOPS trial

MTPT
1-methyl-4-phenyl-1,2,3,6-tetrahydropyridine

MTS1 gene

MTS2 gene

Mt. Sinai classification

MTT
mean transit time

M-TURP
minimal transurethral resection of prostate

MTV
maximum tolerable volume

MUC
mucosal ulcerative colitis

MUC-1 gene

mucilaginous

mucin
m. granule
intracytoplasmic m.
m. polymer

mucin-hypersecreting
m.-h. carcinoma
m.-h. tumor

mucinous
m. adenocarcinoma
m. adenoma
m. carcinoma
m. cystadenoma
m. cystic neoplasm
m. cystic tumor
m. ductal ectasia (MDE)
m. pancreatic tumor
m. tumor nodule

mucin-producing
m.-p. adenocarcinoma
m.-p. cancer
m.-p. tumor

mucin-type glycolipid

Muckle-Wells syndrome

mucocele
appendiceal m.
m. of gallbladder

mucociliary clearance

mucocolitis

mucocutaneous
m. hemorrhoid
m. pigmentation of Peutz-Jeghers syndrome

mucoenteritis

mucoepidermoid carcinoma

mucoid
m. secretion
m. stool

mucolipidosis

mucolytic agent

mucolytic-antifoam solution

mucomembranous enteritis

Mucomyst

mucopolysaccharide

mucoprotein
Tamm-Horsfall m. (THM)

mucopurulent
m. cervicitis
m. exudate

Mucorales

Mucor corymbifera

Mucoreae

mucormycosis
m. esophagitis
gastric m.
isolated renal m.
pulmonary m.

mucorrhea

mucosa, *pl.* mucosae
antral m.
antral-type m.
antrofundal m.
biopsy of gastric m.
blanching of m.
buccal m.
burned-out m.
cardiac stomach m.
cardiac-type m.
cobblestone m.
cobblestoning of m.
colitic m.
colorectal m.
columnar m.
congested m.
denuded m.
duodenal m.
dysplastic m.
ectopic gastric m.
edematous hyperemic m.
esophageal m.
foveolar gastric m.
friable m.
frog-spawnlike m.
fundic m.
gastric muscularis m.
gastroduodenal m.
gastrosuccorrhea m.
giant hypertrophy of gastric m.

heterotopic gastric m.
honeycomb m.
hyperemic m.
inflamed m.
inlet patch m.
intestinal m.
lamina muscularis mucosae
lamina propria of buccal m.
multifocal ectopic gastric m.
muscularis mucosae
neoanal m.
normal-appearing m.
oxyntic m.
pyloric m.
rectal m.
rose thorn ulcer of m.
sloughing of m.
tethering of m.
thumbprinting of m.
tunica m.
urothelial m.
vaginal m.

mucosa-associated
    m.-a. lymphoid tissue (MALT)
    m.-a. lymphoid tissue lymphoma
      (MALToma)

mucosae (*pl. of* mucosa)

mucosal
    m. abnormality
    m. abrasion
    m. adenocarcinoma
    m. aneuploidy
    m. angiography
    m. atrophy
    m. background
    m. banding
    m. barrier maturation
    m. biopsy
    m. bleeding
    m. blood flow
    m. blood hemoglobin
    m. border
    m. break
    m. bridge
    m. bridging
    m. cell proliferation
    m. cobblestoning
    m. detachment
    m. diverticulum
    m. dysplasia
    m. electrosensitivity (MES)
    m. elevation
    m. erosion
    m. esophageal ring
    m. fatty acid
    m. fold
    m. gastric ulcer
    m. graft
    m. guideline pattern

m. hexosamine content
m. homogenate
m. ileal diaphragm
m. ileostomy
m. imaging
m. injury
m. integrity
m. ischemia
m. island
m. junction
m. lesion
m. lesion of acid peptic disease
m. line
m. lymphoid follicle
m. nodularity
m. pallor
m. pit
m. plexus
m. PMN grade
m. polyp
m. proctectomy
m. prolapse
m. prolapse syndrome
m. prostaglandin synthesis
m. protective drug
m. sleeve resection
m. stripping
m. suspensory ligament
m. tear
m. tongue
m. ulcerative colitis (MUC)
m. urease
m. vaccine
m. vascular dilation
m. vascular permeability
m. washout
m. web

mucosanguineous, mucosanguinolent
mucosanguinolent (*var. of*
  mucosanguineous)
mucosa-to-mucosa anastomosis
mucosectomy
    aspiration m.
    m. cap-assisted ampullectomy
    endoanal m.
    endoscopic oblique aspiration m.
    negative pressure-method ambulatory
      endoscopic esophageal m.
    rectal m.
    suck-and-cut m.
mucosector
    oblique aspiration m.
mucoserous
mucositis
mucous
    m. colic
    m. colitis
    m. crypt
    m. crypt of duodenum

M

mucous (*continued*)
    m. diarrhea
    m. enteritis
    m. fistula
    m. gel thickness
    m. gland
    m. lake of stomach
    m. membrane
    m. membrane pemphigoid
    m. neck cell
    m. papule
    m. patch
    m. stool
    m. tunic
mucoviscidosis
MUCP
    maximum urethral closure pressure
mucronata
    Bertiella m.
mucus
    m. depletion
    excess m.
    extruding m.
    gastric m.
    m. secretagogue
mucus-secreting
    m.-s. cell
    m.-s. gland
mud
    biliary m.
Mueller-Hinton-supplemented agar plate
muelleri
    ductus m.
mugwort
MUI
    mixed urinary incontinence
Muira puama
Muir hemorrhoid forceps
Muir-Torre syndrome
Mui Scientific pressurized capillary infusion system
mulberry
    black m.
    m. calculus
    m. gallstone
    m. lesion
    m. stone
Mulholland sphincterotomy
muliebris
    urethra m.
mullein
Müller esophageal varices maneuver
müllerian
    m. capsule
    M. duct
    m. duct cyst
    m. duct derivation syndrome

    m. duct, unilateral renal agenesis, and anomalies of cervicothoracic somites (MURCS)
    m. inhibiting factor
    m. remnant
multiacinar regenerative nodule
multiband
    m. ligating device
    m. variceal ligator
Multibite biopsy forceps
multicenter
    m. outcome
    m. prospective trial
    m. study
Multicentre International Liver Tumor Study (MILTS)
multicentricity
multicentric lesion
multichannel
    m. cystometry
    m. intraluminal impedance monitoring
    m. recorder
multiclip device
multicystic
    m. dysplastic kidney (MCDK)
    m. kidney (MCK)
    m. kidney disease (MCKD)
    m. renal dysplasia
multidetector spiral computed tomography enteroclysis
multidrug
    m. regimen
    m. resistance-associated protein
    m. resistance-associated protein-2 (MRP2)
multidrug-resistance gene (MDR1)
multifiber catheter
Multifire
    M. clip applicator
    M. Endo GIA stapling device
Multi-Flex stent
multiflorum
    Polygonum m.
multifocal
    m. atrophic gastritis (MAG)
    m. bladder tumor
    m. ectopic gastric mucosa
    m. involvement
multiforme
    erythema m.
    glioblastoma m.
Multifunctional Opus surgical table
multigenic origin
Multikine
multiligand receptor
multiloaded clip applier
multiload occlusive clip applicator
multilobar kidney

multilobular
>m. cirrhosis
>m. kidney

multilocular
>m. crypt
>m. cyst
>m. cystic nephroma

multilocularis
>*Echinococcus m.*

multiloculated cyst

multilumen
>m. manometric catheter
>m. probe

multimodal protocol

multinucleated giant cell

multiorgan
>m. hernia
>m. system failure (MOSF)

multiple
>m. acute rejection episodes
>m. anal sphincterotomies (MAS)
>m. band ligators
>m. biopsies
>m. calices
>m. concentric rings sign
>m. data testing
>m. endocrine adenomatosis type I,
>II (MEA-I, −II)
>m. endocrine neoplasia (MEN)
>m. endocrine neoplasia 1, 2A, 2B
>m. endocrine neoplasia syndrome
>(MENS)
>m. endoscopic biopsy specimens
>m. hamartoma syndrome
>m. hepatitis virus infections
>m. intraluminal impedancometries
>m. lymphomatous polyposis (MLP)
>m. myeloma
>m. nodules
>m. recurrent renal colic
>m. sclerosis (MS)
>m. stones
>m. surgical procedures
>m. testing of data
>m. vasovasostomies
>m. vitamins for infusion

multiple-band ligator

multiple-organ
>m.-o. failure (MOF)
>m.-o. failure syndrome
>m.-o. system dysfunction
>(MOSD)
>m.-o. system failure (MOSF)

multiple-sidehole manometric assembly

multiple-system
>m.-s. atrophy
>m.-s. organ failure (MSOF)

multiplication
>countercurrent m.

multiplier
>countercurrent m.

multipolar
>m. coagulation
>m. electrocautery
>m. electrocoagulation (MPEC)
>m. neuron

Multipulse laser system

multiseptate gallbladder

multiseries
>*Pseudo-nitzschia m.*

multispecific organic anion transporter

multisynaptic pathway

multisystem organ failure (MSOF)

multitargeted antifolate

multivariable logistic regression analysis

multivariate
>m. analysis
>m. analysis of hematocrit

multocida
>*Pasteurella m.*

MU-3 monoclonal antibody

mumps
>m. epididymitis
>m. pancreatitis

Munchausen syndrome

Munich inclusion criteria

Munk disease

Munro point

mural
>m. kidney
>m. thrombus

MURCS
>müllerian duct, unilateral renal
>agenesis, and anomalies of
>cervicothoracic somites
>MURCS association

murine
>m. B16 cell
>m. hepatitis
>m. kidney
>m. lymphoid cell
>m. mesangial cell (MMC)
>m. mesangial cell line
>m. Peyer patch
>m. proximal tubule cell

muris
>*Cryptosporidium m.*
>*Trichuris m.*

murmur
>continuous m.
>Cruveilhier-Baumgarten m.
>systolic m.

muromonab-CD3

Murphy
>M. button
>M. common duct dilator
>M. drip
>M. gallbladder retractor

M

Murphy (*continued*)
    M. kidney punch
    M. sign
    M. treatment
muscarine
muscarinic
    m. activity
    m. blockade
    m. cholinergic agonist
    m. receptor
muscimol
muscle
    adductor brevis m.
    adductor longus m.
    aryepiglottic m.
    m. atrophy
    Bell m.
    bladder neck detrusor m.
    bladder smooth m.
    Braune m.
    bulbospongiosus m.
    circular m.
    coccygeus m.
    colonic circular m.
    cremaster m.
    cremasteric m.
    cricopharyngeus m.
    dartos m.
    diaphragmatic m.
    digastric anterior m.
    digastric posterior m.
    electromyography of penile corpus
      cavernosum m.
    external anal sphincter m.
    external oblique m.
    external sphincter ani
      profundus m.
    m. filling
    gastrointestinal smooth m.
    Gavard m.
    geniohyoid m.
    gracilis m.
    m. guarding
    Houston m.
    m. hypertrophy
    iliacus m.
    iliococcygeus m.
    interfoveolar m.
    internal oblique m.
    ischiocavernosus m.
    labium majus m.
    labium minus m.
    lacuna of m.
    latissimus dorsi m.
    m. layer disease
    levator ani m.
    levator veli palatini m.
    lower esophageal sphincter circular
      m.

mylohyoid m.
oblique arytenoid m.
obturator internus m.
Ochsner m.
organic m.
palatoglossus m.
palatopharyngeus m.
paraspinous m.
pectoralis m.
pelvis m.
perineal m.
periurethral striated m.
piriformis m.
pleuroesophageal m.
psoas m.
puboanalis m.
pubococcygeus m.
puborectal m.
puborectalis m.
pubovisceral m.
pyramidal m.
rectococcygeus m.
rectourethral m.
rectourethralis m.
rectus abdominis m.
rhabdosphincter m.
sacrospinalis m.
m. sensory receptor
serratus posterior m.
smooth m.
m. spasm
styloglossus m.
stylohyoid m.
stylopharyngeus m.
submucosal vaginal m.
superficial trigonal m.
suspensory m.
tendinous arch of levator ani m.
tensor veli palatini m.
thyroarytenoid m.
thyrohyoid m.
transversus abdominis m.
transversus perinei m.
urogenital sphincter m.
vascular smooth m.
visceral m.
m. wasting
Wilson m.
muscle-alginate complex
muscle-brain isoenzyme of creatine
  kinase (CK-MB)
muscle-cutting incision
muscle-filling procedure
muscle-splitting
    m.-s. incision
    m.-s. technique
muscular
    m. coat
    m. dystrophy

m. esophageal ring
m. tunic
muscularis
m. externa
fibrae obliquae tunicae m.
m. mucosae
m. propria
tunica m.
m. tunnel closure
muscularization of vein
musculature
electrophysiology of gastric m.
paraspinal m.
musculocutaneous flap
musculomucoid intimal hyperplasia
musculotropic relaxant
MUSE
Medicated Urethral System for Erection
MUSE urethral suppository
mushroom
Amanita m.
m. catheter
Coprinus m.
m. poisoning
mushroom-and-stem appearance
mushroom-shaped mass
mushy stool
musical bowel sounds
musk mallow
Musshoff modification of Ann Arbor classification
mustard
l-phenylalanine m. (I-PAM)
m. seed
Mustarde
M. hypospadias repair
M. procedure
mutagenic effect
Mutamycin
mutated colorectal carcinoma (MCC)
mutation
C282Y m.
deletion m.
endogenous m.
germline m.
H63D m.
insertion m.
Ki-ras gene m.
Kirsten-ras oncogene m.
Liddle m.
m. mismatch repair
missense m.
nontruncating m.
p53 m.
splice-cite m.
transition m.
transversion m.

MutL **gene**
MutS **gene**
Muzsnai modification
muzzled sperm
MVAC, M-VAC
methotrexate, vinblastine, Adriamycin, cisplatin
M-VEC
methotrexate, vinblastine, epirubicin, cisplatin
MVP
maximum vasal pressure
MVT
mesenteric vein thrombosis
acute MVT
mW
milliwatt
myasthenia
m. gastrica
m. gravis
mycelial
m. antibody
m. phase
mycetism, mycetismus
m. gastrointestinalis
mycetismus (*var. of* mycetism)
Mycin
mycobacteria (*pl. of* mycobacterium)
mycobacterial
m. antibody
m. disease
m. spheroplast
mycobacteriology
mycobacterium, *pl.* **mycobacteria**
M. avium
M. avium complex
M. avium-intracellulare (MAI)
M. bovis
M. bovis BCG
M. fortuitum
M. genavense
M. gordonae
M. infection
M. intracellulare
M. kansasii
M. leprae
M. paratuberculosis
M. phlei cellular extract
Runyon group III mycobacteria
M. smegmatis
M. tuberculosis
M. xenopi
mycogastritis
Mycolog-II
mycology
mycophenolate
m. area
m. mofetil (MMF)
m. mofetil capsule

M

mycophenolate (*continued*)
    m. mofetil intravenous for injection
    m. mofetil oral suspension
    m. mofetil tablet
mycoplasma
    M. hominis
    m. urethritis
mycoplasmal
mycoses (*pl. of* mycosis)
mycosis, *pl.* **mycoses**
    endemic deep m.
    m. fungoides
    gastric m.
    m. intestinalis
Mycostatin
mycotic
    m. aneurysm
    m. gastritis
    m. prostatitis
Mycotrim triphasic culture system
Mycromesh biomaterial
myectomy
    anorectal m.
    detrusor m.
myelin kidney
myelocele
myelocystocele
myelodysplasia
myelofibrosis
    primary m.
myelography
myeloid
    m. dendritic cell
    m. metaplasia
myelolipoma
    adrenal gland m.
myeloma
    IgA kappa-chain m.
    m. kidney
    multiple m.
    plasmablastic m.
    m. protein
myelomeningocele
myelomonocytic cell line
myelopathy
    HTLV-I-associated m.
myeloperoxidase
myeloperoxidase-H2O2-halide system
myelophthisic splenomegaly
myeloproliferative
    m. disease
    m. disorder
myelosuppression
myenteric
    m. ganglion cell
    m. plexus
    m. potential oscillation
    m. reflex

myentericus
    plexus m.
Myers bunching technique
Myers-Fine test
Mygel II
myiasis
    intestinal m.
Mylanta-II
Myles hemorrhoidal clamp
Mylicon
Mylius test
mylohyoid muscle
myoblastic myoma
myoblastoma
    bladder granular cell m.
    granular cell m.
myocardial
    m. infarction
    m. ischemia
myocelialgia
myoclonic encephalopathy
myoclonus
myoclonus-opsoclonus syndrome
myocutaneous flap
myoelectric activity
myoelectrical
myofibroblast
myofibroma
myogenic tumor
myoglobinuria
myointimal
    m. cell
    m. hyperplasia
Myojector
myolysis
myoma
    ball m.
    myoblastic m.
    red degeneration of uterine m.
myoneurosis
    colic m.
    intestinal m.
myopathy
    childhood visceral m. (CVM)
    familial visceral m. (FVM)
    hereditary internal anal sphincter m.
    ipecac-induced m.
    nemaline m.
    nonfamilial visceral m.
    schistosomal pelvic floor m.
    sporadic hollow visceral m.
myoplasty
    latissimus dorsi detrusor m.
myorrhaphy
    levator m.
myosin
    m. crossbridge
    detrusor muscle m.
    m. light-chain kinase

myotomy
 circular m.
 cricoid m.
 cricopharyngeal m.
 esophageal m.
 Heller m.
 laparoscopic Heller m.
 laser-assisted endoscopic m.
 Livaditis circular m.
 longitudinal m.
Myotonachol
myotonic muscular dystrophy
MyoTrac EMG
Myotrophin
Myphentol

Myriadlase side-fire laser
myringotomy tube
myrtle
Mytelase
myxedema ascites
myxocystitis
myxofibroma
myxoglobulosis
 appendicitis
myxomembranous
 m. colitis
 m. enteritis
myxoneurosis
 intestinal m.
myxorrhea gastrica

M

N

Alferon N
N loop

NAB

nocturnal acid breakthrough

Nabi-HB

NABS

normoactive bowel sounds

nabumetone

***N*-acetylated alpha-linked dipeptidase**

***N*-acetyl-beta-D-glucosaminidase**

***N*-acetyl-beta-glucosaminidase (NAG)**

***N*-acetylcysteine**

***N*-acetyl-p-benzoquinoneimine (NAPQI)**

***N*-acetyltransferase 2**

Nachlas gastrointestinal tube

Nachlas-Linton esophagogastric balloon tamponade device

NaCl cotransporter (NCC)

Naclerio

N. sign
V sign of N.

NADH

nicotinamide adenine dinucleotide

nadolol group

NADPH

nicotinamide adenine dinucleotide phosphate
NADPH diaphorase stain
NADPH oxidase

NAE

net acid excretion

naeslundii

Actinomyces n.

naevus (*var. of* nevus)

nafamostat mesylate

nafcillin

NAFLD

nonalcoholic fatty liver disease

nafoxidine

NAG

N-acetyl-beta-glucosaminidase
NAG lysosomal marker enzyme

nagging pain

NA+-glucose cotransporter

Na+/H+

Na+/H+ antiporter
Na+/H+ antiporter activity

naive B and T lymphocytes

Nakao snare I, II

Na/K-ATPase

Na/K-A. activity
Na/K-A. membrane

Nakayama test

Na-KCl cotransporter (NKCC)

naked fat sign

nalbuphine

Naldecon

nalidixic acid

NA+-linked cotransport system

Nallpen

nalmefene

naloxone hydrochloride

nana

Hymenolepis n.

NANB

non-A non-B
NANB hepatitis

NANC

nonadrenergic noncholinergic
NANC inhibitory transmitter

nandrolone decanoate

nanocrystalline silver-containing dressing

naphazoline

naphthylamine

naphthylurea

polysulfonated n.

napkin ring anular lesion

nappe

NAPQI

N-acetyl-p-benzoquinoneimine

NapraPAC

Naprosyn

naproxen sodium

Naqua

Narcan

Narco

N. Bio-Systems MMS 200 physiograph tracing
N. Bio-Systems rectilinear recorder
N. esophageal motility machine

narcotic

n. analgesic
n. bowel syndrome

Nardil

Nardi test

nares (*pl. of* naris)

naris, *pl.* **nares**

narrow

n. albumin gradient ascites
n. band imaging (NBI)
n. lens
n. substrate

narrow-band

n.-b. imaging
n.-b. imaging endoscopy system

N

narrow-caliber duct
narrowing
    bird-beak n.
    discrete n.
    hourglass n.
    luminal n.
nasal
    Concentraid N.
    n. deformity
    n. discharge
    n. feeding
    n. intubation
    n. polyp
    n. trumpet
Nasalcrom
Nasalide
nascent macula densa
Nascobal nasal spray
NASH
    nonalcoholic steatohepatitis
nasobiliary
    n. drain (NBD)
    n. drainage
    n. drainage catheter
    n. drain cholangiography
    n. tube
nasocystic
    n. catheter
    n. catheter lavage
    n. drain
    n. drainage tube
nasoduodenal feeding tube
nasoenteric
    n. feeding
    n. feeding tube
nasogastric (NG)
    n. aspirate
    n. decompression
    n. drainage
    n. feeding tube
    n. intubation
    n. lavage
    n. suction
    n. tube (NGT)
nasoileal tube
nasojejunal (NJ)
    n. feeding
    n. feeding tube
nasopancreatic
    n. catheter
    n. drainage
nasopharyngeal
    n. angiofibroma
    n. reflux
nasotracheal intubation
nasovesicular
    n. catheter
    n. catheter
     technique

NASPGN
    North American Society for Pediatric
    Gastroenterology and Nutrition
natalizumab
nateglinide
Nathanson liver retractor
national
    N. Association of Anorexia Nervosa
    and Associated Disorders
    N. Cooperative Dialysis Study
    N. general purpose cystoscope
    N. Health and Nutrition
    Examination Survey (NHANES)
    N. Hospital Discharge Survey
    database
    N. Institute of Diabetes, Digestive
    and Kidney Disease (NIDDK)
    N. Institutes of Health (NIH)
    N. Institutes of Health Chronic
    Prostatitis Symptom Index
    (NIH-CPSI)
    N. Kidney Foundation (NKF)
    N. Kidney Foundation-Data
    Outcomes Quality Initiative
    (NKF-DOQI)
    N. Pancreas Foundation
    N. Prostate Cancer Coalition
    N. Prostatic Cancer Project
    N. Prostatic Cancer Treatment
    Group (NPCTG)
    N. Wilms Tumor Study Group
    (NWTSG)
native
    n. kidney function
    n. pancreatic secretin receptor
    n. renal biopsy
    n. urethra
NA+ transport system
natriuresis
    pressure n.
natriuretic peptide receptor (NPR)
natural
    n. immunity
    n. killer (NK)
    n. killer cell
    n. killer T (NKT)
    N. stool formula
Natura ostomy system
nature
    Gentle N.
Naturetin
Naturlose
nausea
    n. and vomiting (N&V)
    chemotherapy-induced n.
    epidemic n.
    postprandial n.
    nausea, vomiting, diarrhea (NVD)
nauseant

nauseate
nauseated
nauseous
Navane
navel
blue n.
navicular abdomen
navicularis
valvula fossae n.
Navigator flexible endoscope
Navy single-layer everting anastomosis
NBC
nephroblastomatosis complex
nonbacterial cystitis
NBD
nasobiliary drain
nucleotide-binding domain
N-benzoyl-L-tyrosyl-P-aminobenzoic
N-b.-L-t.-P-a. acid
N-b.-L-t.-P-a. acid excretion test
NBNC CLD
non-B non-C chronic liver disease
NBP
nonbacterial prostatitis
NBT
nitroblue tetrazolium
NBT-PABA
nitroblue tetrazolium-paraaminobenzoic
acid
NBT-PABA test
N-butyl cyanoacrylate
N-butyl-2-cyanoacrylate injection
N-cadherin
NCAM
neural cell-adhesive molecule
NCC
NaCl cotransporter
NCCP
noncardiac chest pain
NCGN
necrotizing crescentic glomerulonephritis
NCompass multiwire nitinol stone
extractor
NCPF
noncirrhotic portal fibrosis
N-demethylation
NDI
Nepean Dyspepsia Index
nephrogenic diabetes insipidus
X-linked recessive NDI
Nd:YAG
neodymium:yttrium-aluminum-garnet
Nd:YAG laser
Nd:YAG laser irradiation
Nd:YAG laser photoablation
Nd:YAG laser therapy
near-infrared
n.-i. electronic endoscope
n.-i. Raman spectroscopy

nebulizer
jet n.
nebulous urine
NEC
necrotizing enterocolitis
Necator americanus
necatoriasis
neck
bladder n.
infundibular n.
n. of pancreas
tonic n.
transurethral incision of bladder n.
(TUIBN)
vesical n.
necroinflammation
lobular n.
necroinflammatory activity
necrolysis
toxic epidermal n. (TEN)
necrolytic
n. migratory erythema
n. migratory erythema syndrome
necropsy, necroscopy
necropurulent appendicitis
necroscopy (*var. of* necropsy)
necrosectomy
necroses (*pl. of* necrosis)
necrosis, *pl.* **necroses**
acute sclerosing hyaline n. (ASHN)
acute tubular n. (ATN)
arterial wall n.
avascular n.
Balser fatty n.
biliary piecemeal n.
bowel n.
bridging hepatic n.
calpain in acute tubular n.
caseating n.
cecal n.
cell n.
central n.
centrilobular acidophilic n.
centrizonal n.
cheesy n.
coagulation n.
coagulative n.
colliquative n.
colonic n.
confluent hepatic n.
distal renal tubular n.
drug-induced acute tubular n.
electrocoagulation n.
enzymatic fat n.
ethanol-induced tumor n. (ETN)
fatty n.
fibrinoid n.
fibrosing piecemeal n.
focal hepatocellular n.

N

necrosis (*continued*)
gangrenous n.
glomerular n.
gummatous n.
heme pigment-induced acute tubular n.
hepatocellular n.
hepatocyte n.
icteric n.
infected pancreatic n. (IPN)
infectious pancreatic n.
intestinal n.
ischemia n.
laminar cortical n.
liquefactive n.
massive epithelial cell n.
massive hepatic n.
maximum coagulative n.
metastatic fat n.
moist n.
nephrotoxic tubular n.
n. of renal papilla
pancreatic glandular n.
papillary n.
patchy n.
penile n.
pericentral n.
peripancreatic n.
peripheral n.
perivenular confluent n.
piecemeal n.
postischemic tubular n.
pressure n.
progressive emphysematous n.
puromycin aminonucleoside n.
renal coagulation n.
renal papillary n. (RPN)
renal tubular n. (RTN)
renocortical n.
scrotal fat n.
septic n.
spinal cord n.
spontaneous penile ischemic n.
sterile pancreatic n.
strangulation n.
subacute hepatic n. (SHN)
submassive hepatic n.
tissue n.
tubular n.
tumor n.
necrospermia
necrotic
n. cirrhosis
n. hemorrhagic colitis
n. hemorrhoid
n. tissue
n. ulceration
necroticans
enteritis n.

necrotizing
n. bowel vasculitis
n. crescentic glomerulonephritis (NCGN)
n. enterocolitis (NEC)
n. fasciitis
n. fasciitis of scrotum
n. infection
n. pancreatitis
n. vasculitis of bowel
necrozoospermia
needle
n. ablation
Articulator injection n.
ASAP channel-cut automated biopsy n.
ASAP prostate biopsy n.
aspirating n.
n. aspiration biopsy (NABX)
n. aspiration cytology
Baldwin perineum n.
Bassini n.
B-D Safety-Gard n.
bicurve n.
n. biopsy diagnosis
Biopty cut n.
BIP high-speed multibiopsy n.
n. bladder neck suspension
blunt n.
butterfly n.
Carr-Locke injection n.
CE-24 n.
Chiba n.
Childs-Phillips intestinal plication n.
circle n.
Colapinto n.
concentric n.
n. core biopsy (NCB)
Corson n.
n. count
curved transjugular n.
cutting LR n.
DiaCan fistula n.
diathermic precut n.
n. driver
Durrani dorsal vein complex ligation n.
EchoTip Ultra endoscopic n.
n. electrode
n. electrode electromyography
electrosurgical n.
Emmett n.
EUSN-1 EchoTip n.
Ferguson n.
fine n.
flexible aspiration n.
Franseen n.
French-eye n.
GAN-19 n.

gastrointestinal n.
GIP/MEDI-Globe n.
Gittes n.
Greenwald n.
Grice suture n.
Hemoject n.
n. holder
Howell n.
n. hydrophone
J n.
Jamshidi liver biopsy n.
Keith n.
KeyMed disposable variceal
  injection n.
Klatskin liver biopsy n.
n. knife
Lahey aneurysm n.
Madayag biopsy n.
Mayo trocar-point n.
Menghini liver biopsy n.
Microvasive sclerotherapy n.
monopolar triple-hook active n.
noncutting n.
Nottingham colposuspension n.
Olympus NM-K-series sclerotherapy
  n.
Olympus NM-L-series n.
Olympus reusable oval-cup forceps
  with n.
optic n.
n. papillotome
Pentax prototype n.
Pereyra n.
pneumoperitoneum n.
Promex biopsy n.
PS-2 n.
Quick-Core biopsy n.
reusable forceps with n.
n. root
Safety AV fistula n.
sclerotherapy n.
Securcut aspiration biopsy n.
Seldinger gastrostomy n.
Silverman n.
Silverman-Boeker n.
single-use maximum-capacity radial
  jaw with n.
skinny Chiba n.
smaller gauge n.
Spinelli biopsy n.
Stamey n.
Stifcore transbronchial
  aspiration n.
Sure-Cut biopsy n.
n. suspension procedure
suture-release n.
swaged n.
swaged-on n.
tapered n.

through-the-scope injection n.
n. tracheoesophageal puncture
n. tract
Tru-Cut biopsy n.
Tru Taper Ethalloy n.
TT-3 n.
Turner-Warwick n.
Variject n.
Veress n.
Vim-Silverman biopsy n.
Williams n.
winged steel n.
Yang n.
needle-catheter jejunostomy
needle-knife
  n.-k. electrocautery (NKE)
  n.-k. endoscopic pancreatic
    sphincterotomy
  n.-k. fistulotome
  n.-k. fistulotomy (NKF)
  n.-k. papillotome
  n.-k. papillotomy (NKP)
  n.-k. precut papillotomy (NKPP)
  n.-k. sphincterotome
  n.-k. technique
  n.-k. wire
needleless system
needlescope
  n. device
  n. laparoscopic varix ligation
needlescopic
  n. laparoscopic adrenalectomy
  n. transperitoneal radical
    nephroureterectomy
needle-tip
  n.-t. catheter
  n.-t. laparoscopic electrode
needle-tipped sphincterotome
needle-track seeding
nefazodone hydrochloride
negative
  n. anatomical factor
  n. chemotaxis
  n. core biopsy specimen
  false n.
  n. immunofluorescence
  n. laparotomy
  n. nitrogen balance
  n. predictive value (NPV)
  n. pressure-method ambulatory
    endoscopic esophageal
    mucosectomy
negative-pressure
  n.-p. overtube
  n.-p. tube
  n.-p. wound therapy
negative-pressure-controlled tube
NegGram
negligible blood loss

N

negro
    vomito n.
Negus rigid esophagoscope
Neil-Moore electrode
Neisseria gonorrhoeae
Neisser syringe
Neivert polyp hook
Nélaton
    N. catheter
    N. fold
    N. rubber tube drain
    N. sphincter
nelfinavir
Nellcor Durasensor adult oxygen transducer
Nelson
    N. forceps
    N. scissors
nemaline myopathy
nematode infection
nematodiasis
Nembutal
NEMD
    nonspecific esophageal motility disorder
neoadjuvant
    n. androgen derivation therapy
    n. antiandrogenic treatment
    n. chemoradiation
    n. chemotherapy
    n. hormonal ablation therapy
    n. hormonal deprivation
    n. total androgen ablation
neoanal
    n. function
    n. mucosa
    n. sphincter
neobladder
    Camey n.
    decompensated n.
    gastric n.
    Hautmann ileal n.
    hemi-Kock n.
    ileal n.
    ileocolic n.
    Kock n.
    Le Bag n.
    Melchior ileal n.
    orthotopic ileal n.
    sigmoid n.
    Studer n.
    T-pouch ileal n.
    W-stapled ileal n.
neobladder-urethra anastomosis
neocholangiole
Neocholex
neocystostomy
    ureteral n.
    ureteroileal n.

neodymium:YAG laser therapy
neodymium:yttrium-aluminum-garnet (Nd:YAG)
neodymium:yttrium-garnet laser
neoformans
    Candida n.
    Cryptococcus n.
neointimal hyperplasia
Neo-Lax
Neoloid
neomeatus
Neomed electrocautery
neomembrane
neomycin
neonatal
    n. adrenal gland hemorrhage
    n. arginine vasopressin
    n. cholestasia
    n. circumcision
    n. conjugated hyperbilirubinemia
    n. exstrophic bladder repair
    n. hepatitis
    n. jaundice
    n. oliguria
neonate
    amino acid excretion in n.
    aminoaciduria in n.
neonatorum
    icterus n.
    melena n.
    volvulus n.
neopenis
neophallus
neoplasia
    anal intraepithelial n. (AIN)
    cervical intraepithelial n. (CIN)
    colonic n.
    distal n.
    high-grade prostatic intraepithelial n.
    intraductal oncocytic papillary n. (IOPN)
    intratubular germ cell n. (ITGCN)
    metachronous n.
    multiple endocrine n. (MEN)
    multiple endocrine n. 1, 2A, 2B
    penile intraepithelial n.
    predictor of proximal n.
    preinvasive urothelial n.
    prostatic intraepithelial n. (PIN)
    n. risk
    vascular n.
neoplasm
    anal n.
    bladder n.
    colorectal n.
    extragonadal germ cell n.
    genitourinary n.
    germ cell n.
    intraductal mucin-hypersecreting n.

intraductal papillary-mucinous n. (IPMN)
malignant pancreatic n.
megacystic mucinous n.
n. metastasis
mucinous cystic n.
nonseminomatous germ cell n.
paratesticular n.
periampullary n.
prostatic n.
retroperitoneal n.
n. staging
stomach n.
urothelial n.

neoplastic
n. cell proliferation
n. cyst
n. disease
n. lesion
n. origin
n. polyp
n. potential
n. renal mass
n. tissue
n. transformation

Neopterin
Neoral
neorectal emptying
neorectum
neoscrotum
NeoSoft nephrostomy drainage catheter
neosphincter
Acticon n.
gracilis n.
stimulated gracilis n.
Neosporin GU irrigant
neostigmine methylsulfate
neostomy
neoterminal ileum
neotransformation
papillomatous n.
neoumbilicus
neourethra
Mitrofanoff n.
NeoVadrin
neovagina
n. construction
gracilis myocutaneous n.
skin graft n.
neovascular bundle
neovascularization
Nepean Dyspepsia Index (NDI)
nephelometry
nephradenoma
nephralgia
idiopathic n.
nephralgic
NephrAmine

nephrectomize
nephrectomized
nephrectomy
abdominal n.
adjunctive n.
adjuvant n.
n. allograft
anterior n.
apical polar n.
Balkan n.
bilateral nephrectomies
cytoreductive n.
difficult n.
donor n.
extracorporeal partial n.
extraperitoneal laparoscopic n.
extraperitoneal supracostal live-donor n.
flank n.
hand-assisted laparoscopic donor n.
hand-assisted laparoscopic partial n.
laparoscopic living donor n.
laparoscopic partial n. (LPN)
laparoscopic radical n. (LRN)
laser partial n.
live-donor n.
lumbar n.
morcellated n.
palliative n.
paraperitoneal n.
partial polar n.
perifascial n.
polar segmental n.
posterior n.
radical n.
retroperitoneoscopic n.
segmental polar n.
simple n.
subcapsular n.
transperitoneal laparoscopic n. (TLN)
transperitoneal simple n.
transplant n.
unilateral n.
nephredema
nephrelcosis
nephremia
nephremphraxis
nephric
nephridium
nephritic
n. calculus
n. edema
n. sediment
n. syndrome
nephritides (*pl. of* nephritis)
nephritis, *pl.* **nephritides**
acute focal bacterial n. (AFBN)
acute interstitial n. (AIN)

N

511

nephritis (*continued*)

    acute serum sickness n.
    acute suppurative n.
    albuminous n.
    allergic interstitial n.
    anaphylactoid purpura n.
    antiglomerular basement membrane
      antibody n.
    antiglomerular basement
      membrane-negative crescentic
      glomerular n.
    anti-Thy-1 n.
    autoimmune interstitial n.
    bacterial n.
    Balkan n.
    capsular n.
    n. caseosa
    caseous n.
    catarrhal n.
    cheesy n.
    chloroazotemic n.
    clostridial n.
    crescentic n.
    croupous n.
    degenerative n.
    diffuse suppurative n.
    n. dolorosa
    dropsical n.
    embolic n.
    epidemic n.
    exudative n.
    familial n.
    fibrolipomatous n.
    fibrous n.
    focal bacterial n.
    glomerulocapsular n.
    n. gravidarum
    hemorrhagic n.
    hereditary n.
    Heymann n.
    hydremic n.
    hydropigenous n.
    hypogenetic n.
    ICR strain-derived glomerular n.
    idiopathic hypocomplementemic
      interstitial n.
    immune-mediated interstitial n.
    indurative n.
    infection-related interstitial n.
    interstitial scarlatinal n.
    interstitial syphilitic n.
    Lancereaux n.
    latent n.
    leptospiral n.
    lipomatous n.
    Lohlein n.
    lupus n.
    Masugi n.
    mercuric chloride-induced n.

    n. mitis
    nephrotoxic antiglomerular basement
      membrane antibody n.
    nephrotoxic serum n.
    n. of pregnancy
    parenchymatous n.
    passive Heymann n. (PHN)
    pauciimmune glomerular n.
    phenacetin n.
    pneumococcus n.
    potassium-losing n.
    productive n.
    salt-losing n.
    saturnine n.
    scarlatinal n.
    serum n.
    shunt n.
    silent lupus n.
    Steblay n.
    subacute n.
    suppurative cortical n.
    syphilitic n.
    tartrate n.
    transfusion n.
    trench n.
    tuberculous n.
    tubulointerstitial n. (TIN)
    vascular n.
    Volhard n.
    war n.
    water-losing n.

nephritogenic

    n. antigen
    n. epitope

nephroabdominal
nephroangiosclerosis
nephroblastoma
nephroblastomatosis complex (NBC)
nephrocalcin
nephrocalcinosis

    calcium phosphate n.

nephrocapsectomy
nephrocardiac
nephrocele
nephrocolic
nephrocolopexy
nephrocoloptosis
nephrocystanastomosis
nephroerysipelas
nephrogastric
nephrogenetic (*var. of* nephrogenic)
nephrogenic, nephrogenetic

    n. adenoma
    n. ascites
    n. cord
    n. diabetes insipidus (NDI)
    n. rest
    n. ridge
    n. zone

nephrogenous
n. albuminuria
n. dialysis ascites
n. proteinuria
nephrogram
delayed n.
diffuse patchy n.
rim n.
soap-bubble n.
nephrography
isotope n.
nephrohemia
nephrohydrosis
nephrohypertrophy
nephroid
nephrolith
nephrolithiasis
autosomally inherited form of n.
calcium oxalate n.
N. Clinical Guidelines Panel
glucocorticoid-induced hypercalcemic n.
hypercalcemic n.
iatrogenic hypercalcemic n.
indinavir-induced n.
percutaneous n.
X-linked recessive n. (XRN)
nephrolitholapaxy
percutaneous n.
nephrolithotomies (*pl. of* nephrolithotomy)
nephrolithotomy, *pl.* **nephrolithotomies**
anatrophic n.
minipercutaneous n.
morbidity of percutaneous n.
percutaneous n.
simultaneous bilateral percutaneous n.'s (SBPN)
nephrolithotripsy
percutaneous n.
nephrologist
nephrology
American Society of N.
nephrolysin
nephrolysis
nephrolytic
nephroma
congenital mesoblastic n.
cystic n.
embryonal n.
kidney n.
mesoblastic n.
multilocular cystic n.
nephromalacia
nephromegaly
nephron
aldosterone-sensitive distal n.
n. loss
mesonephric n.
n. plasma flow

proximal n.
n. segment
n. transport
n. underdosing
nephroncus
nephronia
lobar n.
nephronophthisis (*var. of* nephrophthisis)
familial juvenile n.
juvenile n.
nephron-sparing surgery
nephroparalysis
nephropathia (*var. of* nephropathy)
n. epidemica
nephropathic
nephropathy, nephropathia
acute hypokalemic n.
acute urate n.
acute uric acid n.
Adriamycin n.
amphotericin B n.
amyloid n.
analgesic n.
Balkan n.
Berger n.
bismuth n.
cadmium n.
carbon tetrachloride n.
cast n.
chronic allograft n.
chronic hypokalemic n.
chronic urate n.
cisplatin n. (CPN)
copper n.
C1q n.
Danubian endemic familial n.
diabetic n.
dropsical n.
epidemic n.
gold n.
human immunodeficiency virus-associated n. (HIVAN)
hypazoturic n.
hypercalcemic n.
hypochloruric n.
hypokalemic n.
IgA n.
IgM n.
immunoglobulin A n.
incipient n.
iodide n.
iron n.
kaliopenic n.
kanamycin n.
lead n.
malarial n.
membranous n.
mesangial n.
nonnephrotic immunoglobulin A n.

N

nephropathy (*continued*)
    obstructive n.
    n. of potassium depletion
    overt n.
    oxalate n.
    phenacetin n.
    polymyxin n.
    proteinuric n.
    puromycin aminonucleoside n.
     (PAN)
    Ramipril Efficacy in N. (REIN)
    reflux n.
    salt-losing n.
    sickle cell n.
    silver n.
    sodium-wasting n.
    streptomycin n.
    sulfonamide n.
    tetracycline n.
    toxic n.
    tropical n.
    tubular n.
    tubulointerstitial n.
    urate n.
    uric acid n.
    vascular n.
nephropexy
nephrophagiasis
nephrophthisis, nephronophthisis
nephropoietic
nephropoietin
nephroptosia (*var. of* nephroptosis)
nephroptosis, nephroptosia
nephropyelitis
nephropyelography
nephropyelolithotomy
nephropyeloplasty
nephropyosis (*var. of* pyonephrosis)
nephrorrhagia
nephrorrhaphy
nephrosclerosis
    arteriolar n.
    benign n.
    hyaline arteriolar n.
    hyperplastic arteriolar n.
    hypertensive n. (HN)
    intercapillary n.
    malignant n.
    senile n.
nephroscope
    flexible n.
    rigid n.
    n. sheath
    steerable n.
    Storz n.
    Wolf percutaneous universal n.
nephroscopy
    anatrophic n.
    antegrade n.

    flexible n.
    second-look flexible n.
nephrosis
    acute n.
    Adriamycin-induced n.
    amyloid n.
    cholemic n.
    congenital n.
    Epstein n.
    familial n.
    glycogen n.
    Heymann n.
    hydropic n.
    hypokalemic n.
    infectious avian n.
    larval n.
    lipid n.
    lipoid n.
    lower nephron n.
    mercurial n.
    osmotic n.
    pure n.
    puromycin aminonucleoside n. (PAN)
    steroid-dependent idiopathic n.
    steroid-resistant idiopathic n.
    steroid-sensitive idiopathic n.
    vacuolar n.
    n. with hypovolemia
    n. without hypovolemia
nephrosonephritis
    hemorrhagic n.
    Korean hemorrhagic n.
nephrosplenopexy
nephrostogram
nephrostolithotomy
    percutaneous n. (PCNL)
nephrostomy
    n. catheter
    percutaneous n.
    retrograde n.
    n. tract
    n. tube
nephrotic
    n. edema
    n. syndrome
nephrotomic cavity
nephrotomogram
nephrotomography
    infusion n.
nephrotomy
    abdominal n.
    anatrophic n.
    lumbar n.
    n. tube
nephrotoxic
    n. acute renal failure
    n. antiglomerular basement
     membrane antibody nephritis
    n. antiserum

n. serum nephritis
n. tubular necrosis
nephrotoxicity
cadmium-induced n.
cyclosporine n.
mercuric chloride n.
nephrotoxin
nephrotropic
nephrotuberculosis
nephrotyphoid
nephroureteral stent
nephroureterectasis
nephroureterectomy
Beer n.
bilateral nephroureterectomies
hand-assisted laparoscopic n.
(HALNU)
laparoscopic radical n.
needlescopic transperitoneal radical
n.
radical n.
retroperitoneal laparoscopic n.
transperitoneal laparoscopic n.
transperitoneal radical n.
n. with en bloc removal of cuff of
bladder
nephroureterocystectomy
nephroureteroscopy
virtual n.
nephrourography
nephrovesical stent
Nephrox suspension
Nepro diet supplement
Neptune girdle
NERD
nonerosive reflux disease
Nernst equation
nerve
afferent renal n.
anterior scrotal n.
n. block
cavernosal n.
cavernous n.
n. conduction study
n. cooling
criminal n.
n. entrapment syndrome
extrapudendal pelvic n.
femoral n.
genitofemoral n.
gluteal n.
n. growth factor (NGF)
n. growth factor receptor (NGFR)
n. hook
hypogastric n.
iliohypogastric n.
ilioinguinal n.
inferior anal n.
inferior rectal n.

intrapancreatic n.
noncholinergic n.
obturator n.
n. of Grassi
n. of Latarjet
pelvic autonomic n.
perineal n.
posterior scrotal n.
postganglionic cholinergic n.
postganglionic sympathetic n.
pudendal pelvic n.
rectal n.
renal afferent n.
renal sympathetic n.
saphenous n.
sciatic n.
somatic peripheral n.
splanchnic n.
subcostal n.
transcutaneous n.
n. transection
vagus n.
nerve-sparing
n.-s. lymph node dissection
n.-s. radical retropubic prostatectomy
nervi (*pl. of* nervus)
nervosa
anorexia n.
bulimia n.
dysphagia n.
nervous
n. bladder
n. dyspepsia
n. eructation
n. gut
n. indigestion
n. urine
n. vomiting
nervus, *pl.* **nervi**
nervi erigentes
Nesbit
N. congenital curvature of penis
operation
N. corporeal plication
N. cystoscope
N. technique
N. technique ureterocolonic
anastomosis
N. tuck penis straightening
procedure
nesidiectomy
nesidioblastoma
nest
Brunn epithelial n.
net
n. acid excretion (NAE)
rotatable Roth retrieval n.
Roth polyp retrieval n.
ureteral retrieval n.

N

NET
    neuroendocrine tumor
netilmicin
Netromycin
nettle
    Indian n.
    stinging n.
network
    capillary n.
    Florida Prostate Cancer N.
    Pentax EndoNet digital endoscopy n.
    trans-Golgi n.
    vascular collateral n.
Neubauer and Fischer test
Neukomm test
Neu-Laxova syndrome
Neu oncoprotein
neural
    n. cell-adhesive molecule (NCAM)
    n. control
    n. growth factor receptor (NGFR)
    n. invasion
    n. nodule
    n. pathway
    n. plexus
neuraminidase
neuraminidase-treated sheep erythrocyte
neurapraxia
neurasthenia
    gastric n.
neurectomy, neuroectomy
    gastric n.
neurinoma
neuroaminidase
neuroanatomy
neuroblastoma
    cervical n.
    metastatic n.
    olfactory bulb n.
    paravertebral n.
    pediatric n.
    presacral n.
    n. staging
    n. subcutaneous nodule
neuroblockage
neurodegenerative disorder
neuroectodermal dysplasia
neuroectomy (*var. of* neurectomy)
neuroendocrine
    n. cell
    n. tumor (NET)
neuroendocrinology
    gastrointestinal n.
neurofibroma
    bladder n.
    duodenal n.

    gastrointestinal n.
    plexiform n. (PN)
    von Recklinghausen gastric n.
neurofibromatosis (NF)
    familial intestinal n.
    von Recklinghausen n.
neurofilament protein triplet
neurogastroenterology
neurogenetic (*var. of* neurogenic)
neurogenic, neurogenetic, neurogenous
    n. bladder
    n. bladder disease
    n. diabetes insipidus
    n. disorder
    n. dysphagia
    n. erectile dysfunction
    n. hyperreflexia
    n. intestinal obstruction
    n. refractory urge incontinence
    n. secretory diarrhea
    n. sphincteric incompetence
    n. tumor
neurogenous (*var. of* neurogenic)
neurogram
    pudendal n.
neurohumoral
    n. control of motility
    n. disease
    n. excitation state
    n. factor
neurohumoral-immune axis
neurohypophysis
neuroimmune dysfunction
neurokinin A, B
neurologic, neurological
    n. complication
    n. deficit
    n. disorder
neurological (*var. of* neurologic)
neurolysis
    celiac plexus n. (CPN)
    CT-guided celiac plexus n.
    endoscopic ultrasound-guided celiac plexus n. (EUS-CPN)
    endosonography-guided celiac plexus n.
    EUS-guided celiac plexus n.
neurolytic
    n. celiac plexus block
    n. drug
neuroma, *pl.* **neuromata, neuromas**
neuromas (*pl. of* neuroma)
neuromata (*pl. of* neuroma)
neuromedin U
neuromodulation
    chronic sacral n.
    efficacy of n.
    percutaneous sacral nerve root n.
    sacral nerve n.

sacral root n.
subchronic sacral n.
n. work
neuron, neurone
adrenergic n.
afferent n.
alpha motor n.
argyrophilic and argyrophobic n.'s
bipolar n.
cholinergic n.
enteric excitatory motor n.
enteric inhibitory motor n.
enteric vasodilator n.
final motor n.
gamma aminobutyric acidergic n.
intestinofugal n.
intrinsic sensory n.
motor n.
multipolar n.
nonadrenergic n.
noncholinergic n.
parasympathetic postganglionic n.
parasympathetic preganglionic n.
peptidergic n.
S n.
sensory n.
serotoninergic n.
unipolar n.
upper motor n.
vagal input n.
vagal preganglionic n.
neuronal cell line
neurone (*var. of* neuron)
neuron-specific enolase (NSE)
neuroparacrine mechanism
neuropathic
n. bladder
n. cystinosis
n. voiding dysfunction
neuropathy
autonomic n.
cyclosporine-induced optic n.
diabetic autonomic n.
familial visceral n. (FVN)
idiopathic nonfamilial visceral n.
IgA n.
immunoglobulin n.
membranous n.
optic n.
pigment n.
polyradicular n.
pudendal n.
reflux n.
topical n.
vasculitic n.
visceral n.
neuropeptide Y (NPY)
neuropharmacology
neurophysiologic recording

neurophysiology
pelvic floor n.
neuroplasticity
neuropsychotropic drug
neurosis
bladder n.
neurosteroid
neurostimulation
root n.
sacral n.
transcutaneous sacral n.
neurotensin
neurotensinoma
neurotransmitter
noncholinergic n.
neurotrophin
neurotropic
neuroureterectomy
neurourlogical (*var. of* neurourologic)
neurourologic, neurourlogical
neurturin
neutral
n. endopeptidase
n. gadolinium chelate
K-Phos N.
n., protamine Hagedorn (NPH)
neutralophile
Neutra-Phos
Neutra-Phos-K
Neutrexin
neutrocytic ascites
neutron
neutropenia
neutropenic
n. colitis
n. typhlitis
neutrophil, neutrophile
n. chemotactic peptide
n. dysfunction
n. elastase
n. gelatinase-associated lipocalin (NGAL)
polymorphonuclear n. (PMNN)
segmented n.
WBC n.
neutrophil-activating protein of
Helicobacter pylori **(HP-NAP)**
neutrophile (*var. of* neutrophil)
neutrophilia
neutrophilic
n. cryptitis
n. dermatosis
n. gastroduodenitis
n. infiltration
n. satellitosis
neutropic virus
nevi (*pl. of* nevus)
Neville tracheal reconstruction prosthesis
nevirapine

N

nevus, naevus, *pl.* **nevi**
    n. flammeus
    inguinal crease compound n.
    pigmented n.
    spider n.
new
    n. chemotherapy combinations for
      advanced bladder cancer
    n. differentiation factor (NDF)
newborn
    n. hepatitis
    n. jaundice
newcastle
    Shigella n.
Newman proctoscope
newport
    Salmonella n.
NexACT
Nexavar
Nexium triple therapy
nexus, *pl.* **nexus**
Nezhat-Dorsey irrigator/aspirator
NF
    neurofibromatosis
NFAT
    nuclear factor of activated T cells
NF-KB
    nuclear factor kappa B
***N*-formyl-methionyl-leucyl-phenylalanine**
  (fMLP)
NG
    nasogastric
      NG suction
NGAL
    neutrophil gelatinase-associated
      lipocalin
NGF
    nerve growth factor
NGFR
    nerve growth factor receptor
    neural growth factor receptor
^{15}N-glutamine
NGT
    nasogastric tube
NGU
    nongonococcal urethritis
NHANES
    National Health and Nutrition
    Examination Survey
      NHANES III
NHD
    nocturnal hemodialysis
NHL
    non-Hodgkin lymphoma
NH2-terminal SH2 domain
***N*-2-hydroxyethyl-piperazine-*N*-2-ethane-**
  sulfonic acid (HEPES)
niacin deficiency
Niagara temporary dialysis catheter

nialamide
Niaouli oil
Nibblit
nicardipine
niche sign
Nichols-Condon bowel preparation
Nichols IRMA kit
nick end-labeling
niclosamide
Nicolet SM-300 stimulator
Nicorette
nicotinamide
    n. adenine dinucleotide (NADH)
    n. adenine dinucleotide phosphate
      (NADPH)
nicotine therapy
nicotinic
    n. agonist
    n. receptor
    n. receptor blocker
NIDDK
    National Institute of Diabetes,
      Digestive and Kidney Disease
NIDDM
    noninsulin-dependent diabetes
      mellitus
nidogen
Niemann-Pick disease
Niemeier gallbladder perforation
nifedipine
    n. extended release
    n. ointment
    topical n.
Niferex-150
Niflex PEG-based lavage fluid
nifurtimox
niger
    Aspergillus n.
    vomitus n.
nigericin
night-blooming cereus
nightly intermittent peritoneal dialysis
  (NIPD)
nightshade
    black n.
nighttime
    n. polyuria
    n. reflux
nigra
    linea n.
nigricans
    acanthosis n.
    malignant acanthosis n.
NIH
    National Institutes of Health
      NIH Classification Category I acute
        bacterial prostatitis
      NIH Classification Category II
        chronic bacterial prostatitis

NIH Classification Category III
inflammatory and noninflammatory
chronic pelvic pain
NIH Classification Category I–IV
NIH Classification Category IV
asymptomatic inflammatory
prostatitis
NIH Classification System for
Prostatitis
NIH-CPSI
National Institutes of Health Chronic
Prostatitis Symptom Index
NIH-CPSI prostatitis classification
NIH-CPSI type I–IV
NIHF
nonimmune hydrops fetalis
nihonkaiense
Diphyllobothrium n.
Nilandron
nil disease
Nilstat
nilutamide
nimesulide
nimodipine
Ninhydrin
Niopam contrast medium
NIPD
nightly intermittent peritoneal
dialysis
niperotidine
nipple
antireflux n.
antirefluxing n.
continence n.
n. discharge
ileum n.
intussuscepted ileal triple n.
Kock n.
pigmented n.
split-cuff n.
ureteral split-cuff n.
n. valve
nippled stoma
Nippostrongylus brasiliensis
nipradilol
Nipride
niridazole
Nisbet
N. chancre
N. disease
nisoldipine
N-isopropyl-p-iodoamphetamine
biodistribution of N-i.-p-i.
Nissen
N. antireflux operation
N. fundoplication
N. fundoplication wrap
N. fundus repair
N. gall duct forceps

lap N.
N. laparoscopic fundoplication
Nissenkorn stent
nitazoxanide (NTZ)
nitidus
lichen n.
nitinol
n. basket
n. mesh-covered frame
n. mesh stent
n. wire
nitisinone
Niti-S stent
nitrate
gallium n.
intravesical silver n.
methylatropine n.
organic n.
silver n.
nitrate-induced venodilation
nitrazepam
nitrendipine
nitric
n. oxide
n. oxide-blocked sphincter
relaxation
n. oxide donor
n. oxide-releasing nonsteroidal
antiinflammatory drugs
(NO-NSAIDs)
n. oxide-releasing NSAIDS
n. oxide synthase
n. oxide synthase inhibitor
nitrite
amyl n.
dietary n.
n. test
4-nitrobiphenyl
nitroblue
n. tetrazolium (NBT)
n. tetrazolium-paraaminobenzoic acid
(NBT-PABA)
9-nitrocamptothecin
nitrocellulose filter
nitrofigilis
Arcobacter n.
nitroflurbiprofen
nitrofuran
nitrofurantoin hepatotoxicity
nitrofurazone Foley
nitrogen
n. balance (NB)
blood urea n. (BUN)
glutamine n.
high n. (HN)
high calorie and n. (HCN)
n. overload
n. partition test
n. retention test

N

nitrogen (*continued*)
    serum urea n. (SUN)
    total body n. (TBN)
    total urinary n.
     (TUN)
    urea n. (UN)
    urine urea n. (UUN)
nitrogenous waste
nitroglycerin
    intravenous n.
    n. ointment
    vasopressin with n.
nitroimidazole
2-nitropropane hepatotoxicity
nitroprusside
    sodium n.
4-nitroquinolin-1-oxide-induced tumor
  (4NOQ)
nitrosamine
    carcinogenic n.
nitroso compound
nitrosourea
Nitrostat
nitrous
    n. oxide
    n. oxide insufflator
nizatidine
Nizoral
NJ
   nasojejunal
    NJ feeding tube
NK
   natural killer
NKCC
   Na-KCl cotransporter
NKE
   needle-knife electrocautery
NKF
   National Kidney Foundation
   needle-knife fistulotomy
NKF-DOQI
   National Kidney Foundation-Data
   Outcomes Quality Initiative
NK1, NK2 tachykinin receptor
NKP
   needle-knife papillotomy
NKPP
   needle-knife precut papillotomy
NKT
   natural killer T
    N. cell
    N. cell
NLH
   nodular lymphoid
   hyperplasia
N-linked glycoprotein
NLV
   Norwalk-like virus
NM23 **gene**

NMP22, NMP-22
   nuclear matrix protein-22
    NMP22 BladderChek test
NMR
   nuclear magnetic resonance
N-myc oncogene
N-nitrosamine
NNRTI
   nonnucleoside reverse transcription
   inhibitor
Noble
   N. bowel plication
   N. surgical plication of bowel
Nocardia otitidiscaviarum
nociceptin/orphanin FQ (N/OFQ)
nociceptive
   n. sensory input
   n. stimulation
   n. structure
nociceptor
nocte
   ranitidine n.
nocturia, nycturia
   age-related n.
nocturnal
   n. acid breakthrough (NAB)
   n. acid reflux
   n. diarrhea
   n. emission
   n. enuresis
   n. erection
   n. gastric reflux
   n. heartburn
   n. hemodialysis (NHD)
   n. incontinence
   n. pain
   n. penile tumescence (NPT)
   n. penile tumescence monitoring
   n. polyuria
   n. regurgitation
   n. tumescence self-monitoring
node
   celiac lymph n.
   n. dissection
   n. distribution
   Ewald n.
   hypogastric n.
   inguinal lymph n.
   intermediate mesenteric lymph n.
   juxtaposed mesenteric lymph n.'s
   juxtaregional n.
   lymph n.
   matted n.
   mesenteric lymph n. (MLN)
   obturator lymph n.
   n. of Cloquet
   Osler n.
   pelvic lymph n.
   perigastric n.

retrorectal lymph n.
sentinel n.
shotty lymph n.'s
Sister Mary Joseph lymph n.
subcarinal n.
succulent mesenteric lymph n.
Troisier n.
Virchow sentinel n.
Virchow-Troisier n.
NOD2 gene
nodosa
    periarteritis n.
    polyarteritis n.
    vasitis n.
nodose ganglion (NG)
nodosum
    erythema n.
nodular
    n. hyperplasia of prostate
    n. lesion
    n. liver
    n. lymphoid hyperplasia (NLH)
    n. lymphoma
    n. pancreatitis
    n. regenerative hyperplasia (NRH)
    n. transformation
    n. transitional cell carcinoma
nodularity
    antral n.
    coarse n.
    mucosal n.
    surface n.
nodulated
nodulation
nodule
    cecal mucosal n.
    colonic lymphoid n.
    daughter n.
    discrete n.
    Gamna n.
    Gandy-Gamna n.
    gelatinous n.
    hyperplastic n.
    liver n.
    lymphoid n.
    lymphomatous n.
    macroregenerative n.
    mucinous tumor n.
    multiacinar regenerative n.
    multiple n.'s
    neural n.
    neuroblastoma subcutaneous n.
    pentastomum denticulatum n.
    peritoneal n.
    prostatic n.
    regenerative cirrhotic n.
    siderotic n.
    Sister Mary Joseph n.
    spindle cell n.

    surface n.
    thyroid n.
    yellow n.
nodule-in-nodule pattern
N/OFQ
    nociceptin/orphanin FQ
nolatrexed dihydrochloride
Nolvadex
nomenclature
    anorectal n.
nomogram
    A Bayesian n.
    Abrams-Griffith n.
    Schäfer n.
    Siroky n.
non-A
    n.-A non-B (NANB)
    n.-A non-B hepatitis
    n.-A non-B non-C hepatitis
    n.-A non-B posttransfusion hepatitis
nonabsorbable
    n. disaccharide
    n. suture
nonadherent clot
nonadhesive dressing
nonadrenergic
    n. neuron
    n. noncholinergic (NANC)
    n. noncholinergic inhibitory
      transmitter
non-A–E hepatitis
non-A–G
    n.-A. chronic liver disease
    n.-A. fulminant hepatitis
nonagglutinable
nonalcoholic
    n. fatty liver disease (NAFLD)
    n. steatohepatitis (NASH)
nonalpha nonbeta pancreatic islet cell
nonamyloid glomerulopathy
nonaneuploid tumor
nonanion gap metabolic acidosis
nonantibiotic colitis
nonantigen-expressing target cell
nonantral endocrine cell hyperplasia
nonapoptotic pathway
NO-naproxen
nonatrophic pangastritis
**nonautoimmune fundic atrophic
  gastritis**
nonazotemic
    n. cirrhosis
    n. patient
non-B
    chronic active viral hepatitis non-A
    n.-B (CAVH-NAB)
    enterically transmitted non-A n.-B
    (ENANB)
    n.-B islet cell tumor

N

non-B (*continued*)
    non-A n.-B (NANB)
    n.-B non-C chronic liver disease
      (NBNC CLD)
    n.-B non-C CLD
    persistent viral hepatitis non-A n.-B
      (PVH-NANB)
nonbacterial
    n. cystitis (NBC)
    n. gastroenteritis
    n. prostatitis (NBP)
nonbench surgery
nonbilious vomitus
nonbiodegradable
nonbleeding visible vessel
nonbloody stool
nonbreath-hold MR cholangiography
nonbuckling erection
noncalcareous renal calculus
noncalcified stone
noncalculous disease
noncardiac chest pain (NCCP)
noncaseating tubcrclelike granuloma
noncerebral vasculopathy
non-CH4 excretor
noncholecystokinin substance
noncholinergic
    n. nerve
    n. neuron
    n. neurotransmitter
    nonadrenergic n. (NANC)
nonchylous ascites
noncirrhotic
    n. liver
    n. portal fibrosis (NCPF)
    n. portal hypertension
noncleaved B cell
noncollagen protein
noncommunicating
    n. biliary cyst
    n. diverticulum
    n. hydrocele
    n. polycystic disease
noncompliance
nonconductive guidewire
nonconfluent
noncontrast
    n. computerized tomography
    n. helical computed tomography
noncontributory
noncrushing bowel clamp
noncutting needle
nondiabetic
    n. gastroparesis
    n. neurogenic erectile dysfunction
    n. proteinuric renal disease
nondilating reflux
nondismembered anastomosis
nondisseminated intestinal threadworm

nondistended abdomen
nondistensible
nonenzymatic, nonenzymic
nonenzymic (*var. of* nonenzymatic)
    n. glycosylation
    n. reaction
nonepithelial cyst
nonerosive
    n. esophagitis
    n. gastric mucosal lesion
    n. gastroesophageal reflux
    disease
    n. nonspecific gastritis
    n. reflux disease (NERD)
nonestrogen supplemented
nonfamilial
    n. gastrointestinal polyposis
    n. intestinal pseudoobstruction
    n. visceral myopathy
nonferromagnetic MR endoscope
nonfixed cancer
nonfluctuant
nonfunction
    primary graft n.
nonfunctional pituitary tumor
nonfunctioning gallbladder
nonfusion
nonganglionated plexus
nongangrenous sigmoid volvulus
nongas-forming liver abscess
nongene carrier
nongenomic
nongerm cell carcinoma
nonglomerular hematuria
nonglycated albumin
nongonococcal urethritis (NGU)
nongranulomatous
    n. jejunitis
    n. ulcerative jejunoileitis
nonhealing ulcer
non-heart-beating
    n.-h.-b. donor kidney
    n.-h.-b. donor protocol
nonhemolytic
    n. jaundice
    n. *Streptococcus*
nonhemolyzed blood
non-HFE hemochromatosis
non-Hodgkin lymphoma (NHL)
nonhyperfunctioning adrenocortical
adenoma
nonicteric
    n. sclerae
    n. skin
nonimmune
    n. factor
    n. hydrops
    n. hydrops fetalis (NIHF)
    n. mechanism

nonimmunocompromised
nonimmunologic immunity
nonimmunosuppressed
noninflamed peripheral tissue
noninsulin-dependent diabetes mellitus
  (NIDDM)
nonintussuscepted valve
noninvasive
  n. assessment of urinary flow
  n. diagnosis
  n. diagnostic test
  n. intraanal electromyography
  n. method
  n. tumor
  n. urodynamic test
nonionizing radiation
nonirrigating
  n. descending colostomy
  n. patient
nonischemic tubule
nonkeratinizing squamous epithelium
nonliquefaciens
  Moraxella n.
nonmalleable pelvis
nonmalodorous fluid
nonmetallic
nonmyeloablative
  n. allogeneic peripheral blood stem
    cell transplantation
  n. stem cell therapy
nonnecrotizing granuloma
nonnegligible number
Nonnenbruch syndrome
nonneoplastic
  n. lesion
  n. polyp
nonnephrotic immunoglobulin A
  nephropathy
nonnephrotoxic drug
nonneurogenic
  n. neurogenic bladder
  n. voiding dysfunction
nonnuclear fraction
nonnucleoside reverse transcription
  inhibitor (NNRTI)
NONOate
  spermine N.
nonobstructive
  n. hepatic parenchymal
    disease
  n. jaundice
nonocclusive
  n. intestinal infarction
  n. mesenteric ischemia
  n. mesenteric thrombosis
nonoliguric acute renal failure
nonorgan-confined disease
nonorganic dyspepsia
nonoxynol-9

nonpalpable
  n. cryptorchidism
  n. testicle
nonparametric Wilcoxon statistic
nonparasitic
  n. cyst of liver
  n. splenic cyst
nonparticulate radiation
nonpathogenic *Escherichia coli*
nonpeptidyl agonist
nonperforated
  n. appendicitis
  n. appendix
nonpitting
nonpliable
nonplicated appendicocystostomy
nonpolar region
nonpolypoid adenoma
nonpolyposis colorectal cancer
nonpruritic
nonradioactive ^{13}C test
nonreactive pupil
nonreflux esophagitis
nonrefluxing colon conduit
nonrehydrated
  n. guaiac examination
  n. guaiac examination of rectum
nonrosetted cell
NO-NSAIDs
  nitric oxide-releasing nonsteroidal
  antiinflammatory drugs
nonsecreting pituitary tumor
nonsecretory sigmoid cystoplasty
nonseminomatous
  n. germ cell neoplasm
  n. germ cell tumor (NSGCT)
  n. testicular carcinoma
nonskin malignancy
nonsmall cell lung carcinoma
nonspecific
  n. colitis
  n. erosive gastritis
  n. esophageal motility disorder
    (NEMD)
  n. esophagitis
  n. gas pattern
  n. reactive hepatitis
  n. ulcerative proctitis
  n. urethritis (NSU)
nonstented ureteroscopic lithotripsy
nonsteroidal
  n. antiandrogen monotherapy
  n. antiinflammatory agent (NSAIA)
  n. antiinflammatory drug (NSAID)
  n. antiinflammatory drug gastropathy
  n. antiinflammatory drug-induced
    intestinal stricture
nonstrenuous activity
nonstructural protein 4

N

nonstruvite
>n. calculus
>n. stone

nonsulfated bile acid
nonsuppurative destructive cholangitis
nonswallow-associated relaxation
nontarget tissue
non-T-cell fraction
nontoxic goiter
nontransected pancreatic duct
nontranslated region
nontropical sprue
nontruncating mutation
nontuberculous mycobacteria-associated
  enterocolitis
nontumorous epithelium
nontyphoidal
>n. *Salmonella*
>n. salmonellosis

nonulcer
>n. dyspepsia (NUD)
>n. dysplasia

nonulcerative interstitial cystitis
nonvariceal upper GI hemorrhage
nonvenereal bubo
nonviable tissue
nonvisualization of gallbladder
nonvoiding patient
noose
>Dormia n.

4NOQ
>4-nitroquinolin-1-oxide-induced
>tumor

noradrenaline
>serum n.

no rejection
norepinephrine lavage
norethandrolone
Norflex
norfloxacin
Norfolk phalloplasty technique
normal
>n. anatomy
>n. appendix
>n. asymptomatic volunteer
>bowel sounds n. (BSN)
>n. carrier hepatitis
>n. detrusor contractility
>eversion n.
>n. flora
>n. maturation
>palpably n.
>n. penile size
>n. saline meal
>n. saline solution

normal-appearing mucosa
normal-caliber duct
normalized
>n. protein catabolic rate (NPCR)

>n. protein nitrogen appearance
>(nPNA)

normeperidine
Normiflo
Nor-Mil
normoacidity
normoactive bowel sounds (NABS)
normoamylasemia
normocephalic
normochlorhydria
normochromic
normocytic
Normodyne
normoglycemia
normokalemia, normokaliemia
normokaliemia (*var. of* normokalemia)
normoproliferative
Normosol-M IV infusion
normospermatogenic sterility
normotensive
Normotest test
normothermia
normothermic effect
Noroxin
Norplant
Norpramin
Nor-tet Oral
North American Society for Pediatric
  Gastroenterology and Nutrition
  (NASPGN)
Northern blot analysis
Northgate
>N. SD-3 dual-purpose lithotriptor
>N. SD-100 EHL generator

nortriptyline
Norvasc
Norwalk
>N. agent
>N. gastroenteritis
>N. virus

Norwalk-like virus (NLV)
Norwegian cholestasia
Norwich
Norwood rectal snare
no-scalpel
>n.-s. vasectomy
>n.-s. vasectomy fixator ring clamp
>forceps
>n.-s. vasectomy instrument set

nosocomial
>n. fungal infection
>n. urinary tract infection

nostras
>cholera n.

nostril blood
notch
>gastric n.
>n. of gallbladder
>splenic n.

note
    percussion n.
notification of tumor
Nottingham
    N. colposuspension needle
    N. KeyMed introducer
    N. KeyMed introducing device
    N. One-Step tapered dilator
    N. semirigid introducer
    N. ureteral dilator
Nova II machine
Novamine amino acid
Novantrone
Novarel
novel
    N. erythropoiesis-stimulating protein
    n. molecular marker
    n. tissue ablation technology
novo
    de n.
Novocain
NovolinPen device
NPCR
    normalized protein catabolic rate
NPCTG
    National Prostatic Cancer Treatment
    Group
NPH
    neutral, protamine Hagedorn
    NPH insulin
nPNA
    normalized protein nitrogen
    appearance
NPR
    natriuretic peptide receptor
NPT
    nocturnal penile tumescence
    NPT monitoring
NPY
    neuropeptide Y
NRH
    nodular regenerative hyperplasia
NSAIA
    nonsteroidal antiinflammatory agent
NSAID
    nonsteroidal antiinflammatory drug
    NSAID gastropathy
NSAID-induced
    N.-i. gastric injury
    N.-i. intestinal injury
NS5B protein coding sequence
NSGCT
    nonseminomatous germ cell tumor
N-shaped sigmoid loop
NS3/NS4 junction
NS4/NS5 junction
NS2, NS3, NS4, NS5 protein
NSU
    nonspecific urethritis

N-terminal
    N-t. fragment
    N-t. propeptide of type III
    procollagen
Ntrap device
***N*-trimethylsilylimidazole**
NTS
    nucleus tractus solitarii
    nucleus tractus solitarius
NTZ
    nitazoxanide
    NTZ Long-Acting nasal solution
Nuck
    canal of N.
    diverticulum of N.
    N. hydrocele
nuclear
    n. bleeding scan
    n. enema
    n. factor kappa B (NF-KB)
    n. factor kappa B transcription
    factor protein
    n. factor of activated T cells (NFAT)
    n. fraction
    n. fragment
    n. hepatobiliary imaging
    n. hyperchromasia and pleomorphism
    n. isotope scan
    n. magnetic resonance (NMR)
    n. matrix
    n. matrix alteration
    n. matrix protein-22 (NMP-22,
    NMP22)
    n. medicine
    n. medicine scan
    n. membrane
    n. morphometry
    n. protein cyclin proliferating cell
    nuclear antigen
    n. roundness factor
    n. sclerosis
    n. transcriptional activation
nuclear-tagged
    n.-t. cell
    n.-t. red blood cell bleeding study
nuclear-to-cytoplasmic size ratio
nucleation
    epitaxial n.
    homogeneous n.
    n. time
nuclei (*pl. of* nucleus)
nucleic
    n. acid
    n. acid hybridization
    n. acid testing (NAT)
nucleocapsid
    n. antigen-specific
    n. antigen-stimulated interferon
    gamma

N

nucleocapsid-derived peptide
nucleoside
nucleosome
nucleotidase
    5′ n.
5′ nucleotidase
nucleotide
    adenosine n.
    guanine n.
nucleotide-binding domain (NBD)
nucleus, *pl.* **nuclei**
    n. ambiguus
    cigar-shaped hyperchromatic n.
    elongated pseudostratified n.
    hyperchromatic n.
    n. of solitary tract
    Onuf n.
    paraventricular n.
    pyknotic n.
    n. raphe obscurus
    n. solitarius
    n. tractus solitarii (NTS)
    n. tractus solitarius (NTS)
NUD
    nonulcer dyspepsia
Nu-Hope
    N.-H. adhesive waterproof skin
      barrier
    N.-H. cleaning solvent
    N.-H. convex insert
    N.-H. hole cutter
    N.-H. ileostomy pouch
    N.-H. Karaya powder
    N.-H. neonatal and preemie pouch
    N.-H. Nu-Self drainable pouch
    N.-H. pouch cover
    N.-H. protective skin barrier
    N.-H. tubing
    N.-H. urinary pouch
    N.-H. urine collection bottle
    N.-H. urostomy pouch
NuLev orally disintegrating tablet
null cell tumor
Nullo deodorant tablet
NuLYTELY enema
number
    nonnegligible n.
    shock n.
numbness
numerous plant extracts
Nupercainal ointment
Nuport PEG tube
nurse
    n. cell formation
    enterostomal therapy n.
nurse-administered propofol sedation
Nurses' Health Study (NHS)
Nursoy formula
Nussbaum

    N. experiment
    N. intestinal clamp
    N. intestinal forceps
nut
    betel n.
nutcracker
    n. esophagus
    n. syndrome
Nu-Tetra
Nu-Tip laparoscopic scissors
nutmeg liver
nutraceutical, nutriceutical
Nutrament oral liquid
Nutramigen formula
NutraPrep
    N. bowel cleansing solution
    N. colonoscopy preparation
    N. food
    N. preprocedure meal plan
nutriceutical (*var.* of nutraceutical)
Nutricia
NutriCran GI fruit powder
nutrient enema
nutrition
    enteral n.
    European Society of Pediatric
      Gastroenterology, Hepatology, and
      N. (ESPGHAN)
    home parenteral n. (HPN)
    intradialytic parenteral n. (IDPN)
    intravenous n. (IVN)
    Jevity isotonic liquid n.
    luminal n.
    North American Society for
      Pediatric Gastroenterology and N.
      (NASPGN)
    Nutri-Vent liquid n.
    parenteral n.
    Peptamen liquid n.
    perioperative n.
    Replete liquid n.
    support parenteral n. (SPN)
    total enteral n. (TEN)
    total parenteral n. (TPN)
    total peripheral parenteral n. (TPPN)
nutritional
    n. assessment
    n. cirrhosis
    n. deficiency
    n. dropsy
    n. index
    n. pancreatitis
    n. status
    n. support
    n. therapy
nutritive
nutriture
Nutri-Vent liquid nutrition
Nutromat Pad S feeding pump

Nutropin
Nuttall liver retractor
Nuvion
Nuviva
nux vomica
N&V
    nausea and vomiting
NVD
    nausea, vomiting, diarrhea
NWTSG
    National Wilms Tumor Study Group

nycturia (*var. of* nocturia)
Nyhus-Nelson gastric decompression and
  jejunal feeding tube
Nyhus procedure
nylidrin
nylon tissue biopsy bag
Nymox urinary test
nystagmus
nystatin suspension
Nystex
Nytilax

N

O

O antigen
O ring

O₂, O2

oxygen
fMLP-stimulated O_2
PMA-stimulated O_2

OAB

overactive bladder

OAC

omeprazole, amoxicillin,
clarithromycin

OAE

open-access endoscopy

OAI

Ostomy Assessment Inventory

OAM

omeprazole, amoxicillin, metronidazole

OA-519 prognostic prostate carcinoma marker

Oasis

O. stent
O. tube system
O. wound matrix

OASIS

One Action Stent Introduction System

oasthouse urine disease

oat

o. cell
o. cell carcinoma
Lactobacillus plantarum-fermented
o.'s

oatmeal

colloidal o.

OBA

oral bile acid

OB-10 Comfort bite block

O'Beirne sphincter

obesity

adult-onset o.
alimentary o.
endogenous o.
exogenous o.
hyperplastic o.
hypertrophic o.
o. hypoventilation syndrome (OHS)
o. index
lifelong o.
morbid o.

obeum

Ruminococcus o.

OB **gene**

object

foreign o.
ingested foreign o.

irretrievable o.
radiolucent o.

objective

o. lens
o. vertigo

objectivity

degree of o.

OBK

obstructed kidney

obligate anaerobe

obligatory dialysate protein loss

oblique

aponeurosis of external o.
aponeurosis of internal o.
o. arytenoid muscle
o. aspiration mucosector
external o.
o. fibers of stomach
o. fluoroscopy
o. forward-viewing instrument
o. gastric fiber
o. incision
internal o.
o. mucosectomy device tip
o. obturator
o. viewing echoendoscope
o. viewing endoscope

obliterans

appendicitis o.
arteriosclerosis o.
balanitis xerotica o. (BXO)
endophlebitis hepatica o.

obliterated varix

obliteration

balloon-occluded retrograde
transvenous o. (B-RTO)
cicatricial o.
o. of psoas shadow
percutaneous transhepatic o.

obscured ureteral orifice

obscure gastrointestinal bleeding

obscurus

nucleus raphe o.

observation

electron immunoperoxidase o.
light and electron immunoperoxidase
o.

observational followup study

obsolescent glomerulus

obstetric injury

obstipation

obstipum

abdomen o.

obstructed

o. collecting system

O

obstructed (*continued*)
    o. kidney (OBK)
    o. pelvis
    o. testis
obstructing
    o. cancer
    o. rectosigmoidal carcinoma
obstruction (obst)
    acquired ureteropelvic junction o.
    acute extrarenal o.
    adynamic intestinal o.
    airflow o.
    airway o.
    benign prostatic o. (BPO)
    bilateral ureteral o. (BUO)
    biliary tract o.
    bladder neck o.
    bladder outflow o.
    bladder outlet o. (BOO)
    bowel o.
    bronchial o.
    Brugia lymphatic o.
    calyx o.
    cerumen o.
    closed-loop intestinal o.
    clot-induced urinary tract o.
    colonic o.
    common bile duct o.
    complete bowel o.
    congenital ureteropelvic junction o.
    ductal o.
    duodenal o.
    o. duodenum
    ejaculatory duct o.
    epididymis o.
    esophageal o.
    extrahepatic bile duct o.
    extrahepatic biliary o.
    extrahepatic portal vein o.
      (EHPVO)
    extrinsic ureteral o.
    extrinsic ureteropelvic junction o.
    false colonic o.
    fecal o.
    food bolus o.
    functional cystic duct o.
    gastric outlet o. (GOO)
    gastroduodenal outflow o. (GOO)
    hepatic venous outflow o. (HVOO)
    high-grade o.
    high small-bowel o.
    idiopathic o.
    o. index
    infravesical prostatic o.
    intermittent o.
    intestinal o.
    intrahepatic portal o.
    intratubular o.
    intrinsic ureteropelvic junction o.

    laparoscopic treatment of
      ureteropelvic junction o.
    large-bowel o.
    lower urinary tract o. (LUTO)
    low small-bowel o.
    lymphatic o.
    malignant biliary o.
    mechanical biliary o.
    mechanical duct o.
    mechanical extrahepatic o.
    mechanical intestinal o.
    mechanical small-bowel o.
    neurogenic intestinal o.
    o. of bile flow
    oliguric o.
    outflow o.
    outlet o.
    palliation of malignant
      large-bowel o.
    paralytic colonic o.
    paralytic intestinal o.
    partial bile outflow o.
    partial bowel o.
    partial ureteral o.
    portal vein o. (PVO)
    postoperative ureteral o.
    posturethral suspension o.
    primary ureteropelvic junction o.
    prolonged partial ureteral o.
    prostatic outlet o. (POO)
    pyloric outlet o.
    pyloroduodenal o.
    renal o.
    renovascular o.
    secondary ureteropelvic junction o.
    seminal vesicle o.
    shrapnel-induced biliary o.
    simple mechanical o.
    small-bowel o. (SBO)
    splenic vein o. (SVO)
    strangulated bowel o.
    tubular o.
    unilateral ureteral o. (UUO)
    ureteral o.
    ureteropelvic junction o.
    ureterovesical o.
    urethral o.
    urinary o.
    urodynamic o.
    vas deferens o.
obstruction-induced modulation
obstructive
    o. anuria
    o. appendicitis
    o. biliary cirrhosis
    o. change
    o. cholangitis
    o. defecation
    o. dysfunctional ileitis

o. gastroduodenal Crohn disease
o. jaundice
o. megaureter
o. nephropathy
o. pancreatitis
o. uropathy

OBT

FlexSure OBT

obtunded
obturation
obturator

Alcock-Timberlake o.
o. artery
blunt-tipped o.
Endopath Optiview laparoscopic o.
o. hernia
o. internus muscle
o. lymphatic chain
o. lymph node
o. nerve
oblique o.
Optiview o.
o. shelf cystourethropexy
o. sign
o. test
Timberlake o.
o. vein

obtuse margin
occipital
occiput
occluded shunt
occludens

zonula o.

occlusion

o. balloon
balloon ureteral o.
o. cholangiogram
enteromesenteric o.
hepatic vein o.
mesenteric vascular o.
o. of TIPS
portal triad o.
retinal artery o.
retinal vein o.
tourniquet o.
urethral o.

occlusive

o. azoospermia
o. clamp
o. collodion dressing
o. ileus
o. infarction

occult

o. blood
o. filariasis
o. gastrointestinal bleeding
o. hepatitis
o. levator ani hernia
o. pancreatobiliary reflux

occupational

o. toxin
o. toxin exposure

OCG

oral cholecystogram

Ochoa syndrome
Ochsner

O. clamp
O. flexible spiral gallstone probe
O. forceps
O. gallbladder probe
O. gallbladder trocar
O. hemostat
O. muscle
O. retractor
O. ring
O. treatment

Ockerblad-Boari ureteral flap
OCL

oral colonic lavage
OCL bowel preparation

10 o'clock selector catheter
O'Connor drape
OCP

ova, cysts, and parasites

OCT

optic coherence tomography
OCT medium

octahedral-shaped dihydrate
Octamide
octanoic acid breath test
octapeptide

cholecystokinin o. (CCK-8, CCK-OP)

OctreoScan

O. kit
O. scintigraphy

octreotide

o. acetate
o. acetate for injectable suspension
o. effect
somatostatin analogue o.

octreotide-induced hepatic toxicity
OCTT

orocecal transit time

2-octyl cyanoacrylate injection
Ocuflox
ocular

o. abnormality
o. lesion

oculocerebrorenal

o. dystrophy
o. syndrome

oculopharyngeal muscular dystrophy
OD

once daily
overdose
Xatral OD

O

ODC
>   ornithine decarboxylase

Oddi
>   denervated sphincter of O.
>   sphincter of O.

O'Donoghue cystourethroscope

odor
>   breath o.
>   foul-smelling o.
>   fruity o.

odorant

O'Duffy criteria

odynophagia

OEC-Diasonics 9400 fluoroscopy C-arm system

OEIS
>   omphalocele, exstrophy of bladder, imperforate anus, and spinal abnormality
>   OEIS complex

Oerskovia

OES
>   Olympus endoscopy system
>   OES 4000 resectoscope

Oettingen abdominal retractor

office-based esophageal screening

offset-lens ureteroscope

ofloxacin

Ogen

Ogilvie syndrome

O'Hanlon intestinal clamp

Ohara disease

O'Hara forceps

OHS
>   obesity hypoventilation syndrome

oil
>   arachis o.
>   castor o.
>   cottonseed o.
>   fish o.
>   Fleet enema mineral o.
>   Fleet flavored castor o.
>   Kellogg's castor o.
>   Lorenzo o.
>   MCT o.
>   mineral o. (M-O)
>   Niaouli o.
>   olive o.
>   pennyroyal o.
>   peppermint o.
>   radiopaque iodized o.
>   o. red O stain
>   o. retention enema
>   seabuckthorn seed o.
>   silicone-based o.

oily stool

ointment
>   Calmoseptine o.
>   Collagenase Santyl o.
>   Ethezyme debriding o.
>   Fougera Vitamin A+D o.
>   Kovia o.
>   nifedipine o.
>   nitroglycerin o.
>   Nupercainal o.
>   Panafil o.
>   Pazo Hemorrhoidal o.
>   Puer-castor oil-trypsin o.
>   Sween Peri-Care moisture barrier o.
>   Tucks o.
>   Xenaderm o.
>   Ziox o.

Okadaella gastrococcus **infection**

okadaic acid

Okamoto method

OK432 picibanil streptococcal suspension

OKT3
>   Ortho-Kung T3
>   Orthoclone OKT3

OKT4
>   Ortho-Kung T4
>   OKT4 cell

OKT8
>   Ortho-Kung T8
>   OKT8 cell

Okuda
>   O. staging system
>   O. transhepatic obliteration of varix

Olbert balloon dilator

Oldfield syndrome

Olean

oleandomycin

oleate
>   intravariceal ethanolamine o.
>   monoethanolamine o.

oleic acid

Olestra fat substitute

oleyl estrone

olfactory bulb neuroblastoma

OLGC
>   osteoclast-like giant cell

OLGC cell

oligo
>   oligonucleotide

oligoasthenospermia

oligoasthenoteratospermia

oligoasthenoteratozoospermia

oligoazoospermia

oligocholia

oligochylia

oligochymia

oligocilia

oligohydramnios complex

oligohydruria

oligomeganephronia

oligomerization

oligomerize

oligometric complex

oligonecrospermia
oligonephronic hypoplasia
oligonucleotide (oligo)
    antisense o.
    o. probe
    specific o.
oligopepsia
oligopeptide
oligophosphaturia
oligosaccharidase
oligosaccharide
oligosaccharide-binding membrane protein
oligospermatic
oligospermatism (*var. of* oligospermia,
  oligozoospermia)
oligospermia, oligospermatism
oligosymptomatic ADPKD
oligosynaptic pathway
oligoteratoasthenozoospermia (OTA)
    o. syndrome
oligozoospermatism (*var. of*
  oligozoospermia)
oligozoospermia, oligospermia,
  oligospermatism, oligozoospermatism
oliguresia (*var. of* oliguria)
oliguresis (*var. of* oliguria)
oliguria, oliguresis, oliguresia
    neonatal o.
oliguric
    o. obstruction
    o. renal failure
olive
    Eder-Puestow o.
    expandable o.
    metal o.
    o. oil
    o. over guidewire
    palpable pyloric o.
    Savary-Gilliard metal o.
    o. shaped
olive-tipped
    o.-t. catheter
    o.-t. plastic dilator
OLS
    ouabainlike substance
olsalazine sodium
Olsen cholangiogram clamp
OLT
    orthotopic liver transplantation
oltipraz
Olympus
    O. adapter
    O. alligator-jaw endoscopic forceps
    O. Aloka EU-MI ultrasound
    gastrointestinal fiberscope
    O. Aloka GF-EU-series endoscope
    O. automatic reprocessor
    O. basket-type endoscopic forceps
    O. BH2 epifluorescence microscope

O. BH2-RFCA reflecting microscope
O. BHT-2 microscope
O. BML-3Q, -4Q lithotriptor
O. camera with enlarging adapter
O. catheter echoprobe
O. CBK fluorescence microscope
O. CD-20Z heater probe
O. CD-Z-series heat probe
  thermocoagulator
O. CF 2301 endoscope
O. CF-20 fibercolonoscope
O. CF-HM-series magnifying
  colonoscope
O. CF-L-series flexible
  sigmoidoscope
O. CF-MB/LB colonoscope
O. CF-MB-M colonoscope
O. CF-MB-series colonoscope
O. CF-OSF-series flexible
  sigmoidoscope
O. CF24OZI colonoscope
O. CF-PL-series colonoscope
O. CF-P20S fiberoptic colonoscope
O. CF100S sigmoidoscope
O. CF-1T100L colonoscope
O. CF-TL-series forward-viewing
  videocolonoscope
O. CF100TL videocolonoscope
O. CF-1T100L videocolonoscope
O. CF-T-series colonoscope
O. CF-TVL-series colonoscope
O. CF-UHM-series colonoscope
O. CF-UM3 colonoscope
O. CF-UM3 flexible
  echocolonoscope
O. CF-UM-series echoendoscope
O. CF-UM20 ultrasonic endoscope
O. CF-UM20 ultrasound endoscope
O. CF-VL-series colonoscope
O. CF-200Z colonoscope
O. CF-200Z endoscope
O. CG-P-series colonofiberscope
O. cholangioscope
O. choledochoscope
O. clip-fixing device
O. CLV10 fiberscope light source
O. CLV-series fiberoptic system
O. CLV-U 20 endoscopic halogen
  light source
O. continuous-flow resectoscope
O. CV-series colonoscope
O. CV-series endoscope
O. cystofiberscope
O. cytology brush
O. DES-series endoscope
O. EF-series esophagoscope
O. endoscopy system (OES)
O. endotherapy disposable biopsy
  forceps

O

Olympus (*continued*)

O. ENF-P2 scope
O. ENF-P-series laryngoscope
O. EUM-20 echoendoscope
O. EUM-20 endoscope
O. EU-M30S endoscopic ultrasonography receiver
O. EU-M-series endosonography image processor
O. Europe ETD automated endoscope washer
O. EUS-series endoscope
O. EVIS 140
O. EVIS color computer chip system
O. EVIS Q-series endoscope
O. EVIS Q-200V
O. EVIS 140Q videoendoscope
O. EVIS videocolonoscope
O. EW-series fiberoptic duodenoscope
O. FB-20C endoscopic forceps
O. FB-25K endoscopic forceps
O. FB-24U biopsy forceps
O. FG-12U wide-mouth forceps
O. fiberoptic cystoscope
O. FK-13-1 biopsy forceps
O. FS-K-series endoscopic suture-cutting forceps
O. gastrostomy
O. GF-EU1 gastrointestinal fiberscope
O. GF-series videoendoscope
O. GFT gastroscope
O. GF-UC30P echoendoscope
O. GF-UCT30P linear-array echoendoscope
O. GF-UM30P echoendoscope
O. GF-UM30P endoscope
O. GF-UM30P linear scanning probe
O. GF-UM29 radial scanner echoendoscope
O. GF-UM20 radial scanning endoscope
O. GF-UM3 ultrasonic endoscope
O. GF-UM20 ultrasound endoscope
O. GF-UM3, -UM20 system
O. GIF-D2 endoscope
O. GIF-D-series panendoscope
O. GIF20 echoendoscope
O. GIF-EUM2 echoendoscope
O. GIF-HM-series endoscope
O. GIF-J-series endoscope
O. GIF-K-series gastroscope
O. GIF-P endoscope
O. GIF-Q200 endoscope
O. GIF-Q30 fiberscope

O. GIF-series double-channel therapeutic videoendoscope
O. GIF-series echoendoscope
O. GIF-SQ-series videoendoscope
O. GIF-1T10 echoendoscope
O. GIF-2T10 endoscope
O. GIF-2T200 endoscope
O. GIF-T-series endoscope
O. GIF-T-series videoendoscope
O. GIFxP10 gastroscope
O. GIF-XP-series endoscope
O. GIF-XQ240 endoscope
O. GIF-XQ30 flexible gastroscope
O. GIF-XQ-series panendoscope
O. GIF-XQ230 videogastroscope
O. GIF-XQ240 videogastroscope
O. GIF-XQ200 videogastroscope
O. GIF-XV-series endoscope
O. GIF-200Z videoendoscope
O. grasping rat-tooth forceps
O. GTF-A gastrocamera
O. heater probe unit
O. heat probe
O. high-definition endoscope
O. hot biopsy forceps
O. HX-21L detachable miniloop
O. injector
O. intracavity transducer
O. JF-series videoduodenoscope
O. JF-series videoendoscope
O. JF1T endoscope
O. JF1T10 fiberoptic duodenoscope
O. JF-T-series endoscope
O. JF-TV-series endoscope
O. JF-UM20 echoendoscope
O. JF-V-series endoscope
O. JF-V-series videoduodenoscope
O. JT-series videoduodenoscope
O. laparoscope
O. large-channel endoscope GIF1T130
O. linear-array echoendoscope
O. LUS-1 rigid device
O. LUS-2 ultrasonic energy rigid device
O. magnetic extractor forceps
O. MAJ363 FNA needle system
O. minisnare forceps
O. monopolar cannula
O. Nd:YAG laser
O. needle-knife papillotome
O. NM-K-series sclerotherapy needle
O. NM-L-series needle
O. OES fiberscope
O. OM-1 reflex camera
O. OM-series endoscopic camera
O. One-Step button gastrostomy tube
O. OSF flexible sigmoidoscope
O. OSF scope

O. OSP fluorescence measuring system
O. OTV S-series miniature camera
O. P20
O. PCF-130L videocolonoscope
O. PCF-100 pediatric colonoscope
O. PCF-130 pediatric colonoscope
O. PCF-series pediatric colonoscope
O. pelican-type endoscopic forceps
O. PJF endoscope
O. PJF-series pediatric duodenoscope
O. PJF-series pediatric endoscope
O. PSD-10 electrosurgical blend current
O. P-series endoscope
O. PW-1L wash catheter
O. PW-5V spray catheter
O. Q200 videoendoscope
O. rat-tooth endoscopic forceps
O. reusable oval-cup forceps
O. reusable oval-cup forceps with needle
O. rubber-tip endoscopic forceps
O. SCA series endoscopic camera
O. SD-5L semicircular snare
O. shark-tooth endoscopic forceps
O. SIF-10 enteroscope
O. SIF-M magnifying colonoscope
O. SIF-M-series videoenteroscope
O. SIF-Q240 enteroscope
O. SIF-SW fiberoptic endoscope
O. SIF-SW-series videoenteroscope
O. SIF-100 video push endoscope
O. SIF-100 video push enteroscope
O. SIG-100L videoenteroscope
O. sphincterotome
O. spray catheter PW-5V
O. SP-series image analyzer
O. S-20-20R probe
O. SSIF-series videoendoscope
O. SSIF-series videoenteroscope
O. 1-Step Button
O. 1-Step Button gastrostomy tube
O. stone retrieval basket
O. 2T100 endoscope
O. TJF-10, -100, -200 duodenoscope
O. TJF-100 endoscope
O. translaparoscopic choledochofiberscope
O. tripod-type endoscopic forceps
O. 2T-2000 twin-channel therapeutic gastroscope
O. UES-series snare cautery device
O. ultrasonic esophagoprobe
O. ultrathin balloon-fitted ultrasound probe
O. UM-F30-20R probe
O. UM-20 radial echoendoscope
O. UM-2R, -3R probe

O. UM-R-series miniature ultrasonic probe
O. UM-series endoscope
O. UM-S30-25R probe
O. UM-1W endoscopic probe
O. UM-W-series endoscopic probe
O. URF type P2 flexible ureteroscope
O. videoendoscopy system
O. videourology procedure system
O. V-series endoscope
O. VU-M2 echoendoscope
O. W-shaped endoscopic forceps
O. XCF-XK-series endoscope
O. XGF-UCT30 endoscope
O. XIF-UM3 echoendoscope
O. XK-series oblique-viewing flexible fiberscope
O. XP-series endoscope
O. XQ230 gastroscope
O. XQ-200, XQ-230 videoendoscope
O. XSIF-series videoenteroscope
O. Zoom endoscope

omapatrilat
Ombrédanne
O. forceps
O. operation

OMC
omeprazole, metronidazole, clarithromycin

OmegaPort access port
omega-shaped
o.-s. epiglottis
o.-s. incision

omenta (*pl. of* omentum)
omental
o. adhesion
o. band
o. bursitis
o. cyst
o. enterocleisis
o. foramen
o. hammock
o. infarction
o. interposition
o. J-pexy
o. patch
o. pedicle
o. pedicle flap
o. pedicle flap graft
o. plug
o. studding
o. tuberosity
o. vein
o. wrapping

omentale
foramen o.

omentalis
tenia o.

omentectomy
omentitis
omentofixation
omentopexy
omentoplasty
    pedicled o.
    pelvic o.
omentorrhaphy
omentovolvulus
omentum, *pl.* **omenta**
    bowel adherent to o.
    colic o.
    gastric o.
    gastrocolic o.
    gastrohepatic o.
    gastrosplenic o.
    greater o.
    incarcerated o.
    interposition flap of o.
    lesser o.
    o. majus
    o. majus flap procedure
    o. minus
    pancreaticosplenic o.
    pedicled o.
    splenogastric o.
omeprazole
    o., amoxicillin, clarithromycin (OAC)
    o., amoxicillin, metronidazole (OAM)
    o., metronidazole, clarithromycin (OMC)
    o. test
    o. therapy
omeprazole/amoxicillin
omeprazole-clarithromycin-amoxicillin therapy
Omnicef
Omnicide disinfectant
Omni-LapoTract support system
Omnilink biliary stent
Omnipaque
Omnipen
Omnipen-N
OmniPhase penile prosthesis
OMNI Prep
OmniPulse MAX holmium laser
Omnitract retractor
omphalectomy
omphalocele
    o., exstrophy of bladder, imperforate anus, and spinal abnormality (OEIS)
    o. repair
once daily (OD)
Onchocerca volvulus
onchocerciasis
oncoantigen 519

oncocytoma
    kidney o.
    renal o.
oncocytomatosis
oncofetal protein
oncogene
    c-jun o.
    c-met o.
    c-*myc* o.
    HER-2/neu o.
    o. inactivation
    Kirsten-ras o.
    K-ras o.
    N-myc o.
    polyoma middle T o.
    ras p21 o.
    sarcoma virus o.
oncogene-induced carcinogenesis
oncologic, oncological
    o. outcome
    o. principle
    o. radicality
oncological (*var. of* oncologic)
On-Command catheter
oncoprotein
    c-ErbB-2/Neu o.
    Neu o.
    viral o.
OncoScint
    O. CR/OV
    O. CR/OV carcinoma localization scintigraphy
OncoSeed
OncoSpect
ondansetron
    metoclopramide, dexamethasone, lorazepam, o. (MDLO)
one
    O. Action Stent Introduction System (OASIS)
    O. Touch blood glucose meter
one-piece
    o.-p. disposable plug
    o.-p. ostomy pouch
one-session crossover study
one-shot
one-stage
    o.-s. hypospadias repair
    o.-s. procedure
    o.-s. reaction
    o.-s. urethroplasty
one-step
    o.-s. button (OSB)
    O.-S. gastric button
    Surgitek O.-S. (SOS)
onion-skinning
onlay
    o. bulbar urethroplasty
    o. island flap

o. island flap urethroplasty
o. technique
onlay-tube-onlay urethroplasty technique
online hemodiafiltration
onset
o. of dysphagia
o. of pain
ontogeny
Onuf nucleus
Oochoristica
oocyst
Cryptosporidium o.
oocyte micromanipulation
oolemma
oophorectomy
ooplasm
ooze
oozing blood
O&P
ova and parasites
O&P test
opacification
opacified
organs o.
opacify
opaque
o. meal
Sur-Fit Natura closed-end pouch, o.
open
o. adrenalectomy
o. biopsy
bowels not o. (BNO)
o. cystotomy
o. drainage
o. electrocautery snare
o. hemorrhoidectomy
o. injury
o. management
o. mesh-plug hernioplasty
o. morphology
o. pyelolithotomy
o. pyelotomy
o. radical prostatectomy
o. renal descent
o. retroperitoneal high ligation
o. sphincterotome
o. stone surgery
o. testis biopsy
o. transurethral resection
o. ulcer
o. wound
open-access endoscopy (OAE)
open-ended
o.-e. ostomy pouch
o.-e. ureteral catheter
o.-e. vasectomy
open-end flow-through radiopaque tip
opener
potassium channel o.

opening
appendiceal o.
epispadiac o.
open-label Gelusil
operating
o. frequency
o. laparoscope
operation
Abbe small-bowel o.
Aldridge o.
Alexander-Adams o.
Allingham o.
Amussat o.
Andrews o.
antireflux o.
Aylett o.
Bacon-Babcock rectovaginal fistula o.
Baldy-Webster o.
Ball o.
bariatric o.
Bassini o.
Bates o.
Battle o.
Belfield o.
Belsey Mark IV antireflux o.
Belsey Mark V o.
Bennett o.
Bergenhem o.
Best o.
Bevan o.
Bigelow o.
Billroth I, II o.
Bloodgood o.
Boari o.
Bottini o.
bottle o.
Bozeman o.
Bricker o.
Browne o.
Brunschwig o.
Calot o.
Camey I, II detubalarized neobladder o.
Cecil o.
Child o.
Civiale o.
Clark o.
Cock o.
Collis antireflux o.
Crespo o.
Deming o.
Denis Browne o.
Dittel o.
Doppler o.
Doyen o.
Duhamel o.
Duplay o.
Edebohls o.

O

operation (*continued*)
- Everett-TeLinde o.
- eversion o.
- Finney o.
- Foley o.
- Franco o.
- Frank o.
- Fredet-Ramstedt o.
- Freyer o.
- Fuller o.
- Furlow-Fisher modification of Virag 1 erectile failure microsurgical o.
- Gauderer-Ponsky PEG o.
- Gil-Vernet o.
- Hagner o.
- Halsted o.
- Hartmann o.
- Heineke-Mikulicz o.
- Heller o.
- Hess o.
- Hill antireflux o.
- Hochenegg o.
- Hofmeister o.
- Horton-Devine o.
- Huggins o.
- interposition o.
- Israel o.
- Ivalon sponge-wrap o.
- Jonnesco o.
- Kader o.
- Kasai o.
- Kelly o.
- Kelly-Stoeckel o.
- kidney-sparing o.
- Kocher o.
- Kraske o.
- Kropp onlay urethral lengthening o.
- Ladd o.
- Lester Martin modification of Duhamel abdominoperineal pullthrough o.
- Longmire o.
- Lowsley o.
- Macewen hernia o.
- MAGPI o.
- Makkas o.
- Mann-Williamson o.
- Mansson o.
- Marian o.
- Marshall-Marchetti-Birch o.
- Marshall-Marchetti-Krantz o.
- Martin o.
- Martius o.
- Martius-Harris o.
- Mason o.
- Matson o.
- Maydl o.
- Mayo o.
- Mays o.
- McVay o.
- Mercier o.
- Merindino o.
- mica o.
- Mikulicz o.
- Miles o.
- Milligan-Morgan o.
- morcellation o.
- Moschcowitz o.
- Nesbit congenital curvature of penis o.
- Nissen antireflux o.
- Ombrédanne o.
- orthotopic hemi-Kock o.
- Payne o.
- Petersen o.
- Pickrell o.
- Pólya o.
- pubovaginal o.
- Ramstedt o.
- Raz sling o.
- repeat o.
- restorative proctocolectomy o.
- Rigaud o.
- Ripstein rectal prolapse o.
- Roux-en-Y o.
- Rovsing o.
- Scott o.
- scrotal pouch o.
- second-look o.
- sling o.
- Smith-Boyce o.
- Soave o.
- sphincter-preserving o. (SPO)
- Spivack o.
- Ssabanejew-Frank o.
- staging o.
- Steinach o.
- Stoppa o.
- string o.
- Swenson o.
- Tanner stomach devascularization o.
- Thal fundic patch o.
- Thiersch anal incontinence o.
- Torek o.
- transection and devascularization o.
- Tuffier o.
- Turnbull ostomy o.
- Turner-Warwick o.
- van Hook o.
- Vidal o.
- Virag o.
- Vogel o.
- Volkmann o.
- Voronoff o.
- Wangensteen o.
- Waugh-Clagett o.
- Wheelhouse o.
- Whipple o.

White o.
Whitehead o.
Wood o.
Young o.
Young-Dees-Leadbetter o.
operative
    o. cholangiogram
    o. cholangiography
    o. choledochoscopy
    o. decompression
    o. laparoscope
    o. morbidity
    o. mortality rate
    o. staging
    o. time
ophthalmoplegia
opiate
    o. antagonist
    o. receptor
opioid
    o. antagonist
    o. antidiarrheal
    antisecretory o.
    endogenous o.
    o. peptide
    o. receptor agonist (ORA)
opioid-mediated pruritus
opisthorchiasis
Opisthorchis
    O. felineus
    O. sinensis
    O. viverrini
Opitz-Frias syndrome
opium
    o. antidote
    deodorized tincture of o. (DTO)
Opmilas 144 Plus laser system
opportunistic
    o. complication
    o. infection
opposure
Op-Site dressing
opsonic activity
opsonization
opsonized zymosan
Optase wound care gel
optic, optical
    o. coherence tomography (OCT)
    o. crystallography
    o. esophagoscope
    o. fiber
    o. laser knife
    o. multichannel analyzer system
    o. needle
    o. neuropathy (ON)
    o. switch
    o. ureterotome
    o. urethrotome knife
optical (*var. of* optic)

optics
    Wappler cystoscope with microlens o.
Optifoam dressing
Optilume prostate balloon dilator
optimal
    O. Regimen Cures *Helicobacter*-Induced Dyspepsia (ORCHID)
    o. shock wave rate
Optimental
optimization
optimizing
    o. HLA matching
    o. human leukocyte antigen matching
optimum cooling range
option
    therapeutic o.
Optiray
Optiview obturator
Opti-Vue plastic barrel
Opus
    O. 1
    Ausonics O. 1
ORA
    opioid receptor agonist
Oracit
orad
    o. propagation
    o. side
Oragrafin contrast medium
oral
    o. alkalinization
    Ansaid O.
    o. barium suspension
    o. bile acid (OBA)
    Cartrol O.
    Ceftin O.
    o. cholecystogram (OCG)
    o. cholecystography (OCG)
    o. colonic lavage (OCL)
    o. disease
    o. dissolution therapy
    o. intubation
    o. iron
    o. iron preparation
    o. lavage
    o. leukoplakia
    Nor-tet O.
    Permitil O.
    Protostat O.
    o. purge
    o. rehydration
    o. rehydration solution (ORS)
    o. rehydration therapy (ORT)
    o. suction catheter
    Sumycin O.
    o. therapy of erectile dysfunction

O

oral (*continued*)
    o. thermometer
    o. thrush
    o. tolerance
    o. transmission
    o. ulcer
    Wilpowr O.
Oralgen
Oramide
Orandi
    O. knife
    O. vascularized flap technique
orange
    o. bezoar
    bitter o.
    sweet o.
orange-colored tonsil
Orasone
OraSure salivary collection device
Orathecin
OraVax vaccine
orbiculare
    Pityrosporon o.
orbital
Orcein stain
orchalgia (*var. of* orchialgia)
orchectomy (*var. of* orchiectomy)
orchialgia, orchalgia, orchioneuralgia,
  orchidalgia, testalgia
orchichorea
ORCHID
    Optimal Regimen Cures
    Helicobacter-Induced Dyspepsia
    ORCHID study
orchidalgia (*var. of* orchialgia)
orchidectomy (*var. of* orchiectomy)
orchidic
orchiditis (*var. of* orchitis)
orchidoepididymectomy
orchidometer, orchiometer
    Prader o.
    punched-out o.
    test-size o.
orchidopexy (*var. of* orchiopexy)
    laparoscopic o.
orchidoptosis
orchidorrhaphy (*var. of* orchiorrhaphy,
  orchiopexy)
orchidotherapy
orchidotomy (*var. of* orchiotomy)
orchiectomy, orchidectomy, orchectomy,
  testectomy
    inguinal o.
    partial o.
    prophylactic o.
    radical inguinal o.
    subcapsular o.
    subepididymal o.
orchiencephaloma

orchiepididymitis
orchilytic
orchiocatabasis
orchiocele
orchiococcus
orchiometer (*var. of* orchidometer)
orchiomyeloma
orchioncus
orchioneuralgia (*var. of* orchialgia)
orchiopathy
orchiopexy, orchidopexy, orchidorrhaphy
    Bevan o.
    Cabot-Nesbit o.
    eversion o.
    Fowler-Stephens laparoscopic o.
    inguinal o.
    laparoscopic o.
    Prentiss o.
    prophylactic o.
    scrotal pouch o.
    staged o.
    standard o.
    2-step o.
    Torek o.
    transperitoneal o.
    transseptal o.
    vasal pedicle o.
orchioplasty
orchiorrhaphy, orchidorrhaphy
orchiotherapy
orchiotomy, orchotomy, orchidotomy
orchis, *pl.* **orchises**
orchises (*pl. of* orchis)
orchitic
orchitis, orchiditis, testitis
    filarial o.
    metastatic o.
    o. parotidea
    Salmonella enteritidis o.
    spermatogenic granulomatous o.
    traumatic o.
    o. variolosa
orchitolytic (*var. of* orchilytic)
orchotomy (*var. of* orchiotomy)
orciprenaline
O'Regan
    O. hemorrhoid ligator
    O. procedure
Oresus Potentest test
Oretic
Oreticyl
Orfadin capsule
organ
    accessory digestive o.
    o. allocation policy
    artificial o.
    o. donation
    o. function
    invasion of adjacent o.

o. of Giraldes
o. of Zuckerkandl
o.'s opacified
O. Procurement Program
radiosensitive o.
o. transplantation
well-matched o.
organelle
organic
    o. conditioning film
    o. impotence
    o. muscle
    o. neurologic disease
    o. nitrate
organism
    Campylobacter-like o. (CLO)
    enteropathic o.
    gram-positive o.
    Helicobacter pylori-like o.
     (HPLO)
    microaerophilic o.
    pyogenic o.
    resistant o.
    terrestrial o.
    urea splitting o.
organization
    World Health O. (WHO)
organized germinal center
organoaxial gastric volvulus
organogenesis
organomegaly
organoscopy
orgastic impotence
Oriental
    O. cholangiohepatitis
    O. schistosomiasis
orienting reflex (OR)
orifice
    appendiceal o.
    bell-shaped o.
    biliary o.
    duodenal o.
    epispadiac o.
    fistulous o.
    obscured ureteral o.
    pancreatic o.
    papillary o.
    sharp-edged o.
    ureteral o.
orificia (*pl. of* orificium)
orificial
orificium, *pl.* **orificia**
origin
    GI bleeding of obscure o.
    multigenic o.
    neoplastic o.
    O. trocar
Orion ion analyzer
orlistat

Ormond
    O. disease
    O. syndrome
ornidazole
ornithine
    o. aspartate
    o. carbamoyl transferase deficiency
    o. decarboxylase (ODC)
orocecal transit time (OCTT)
oroesophageal overtube
orogastric Ewald tube
oropharyngeal
    o. carcinoma
    o. damage
    o. dysphagia
    o. tube
ororespiratory tract
orosomucoid
orotracheal intubation
orphenadrine
Orr
    O. automatic reprocessor
    O. gall duct forceps
    O. rectal prolapse repair
Orr-Loygue transabdominal proctopexy
ORS
    oral rehydration solution
ORT
    oral rehydration therapy
Ortho
    O. Diagnostic System
    O. HCV 2.0 ELISA test system for
     hepatitis C
    O. HCV ELISA test system second
     generation
orthochromatic dye
Orthoclone OKT3
Orthohepadnavirus
Ortho-Kung
    O.-K. T3 (OKT3)
    O.-K. T4 (OKT4)
    O.-K. T8 (OKT8)
Orthopara-DDD
orthophosphate
orthoplasty
    penile o.
orthostatic
    o. change
    o. proteinuria
orthostatism
orthotopic
    o. appendicocystostomy
    o. bladder
    o. bladder augmentation
    o. bladder substitution
    o. colonic reservoir
    o. continent reservoir
    o. hemi-Kock operation
    o. ileal neobladder

O

orthotopic (*continued*)
    o. liver transplantation (OLT)
    o. reconstruction
    o. remodeled ileocolonic reservoir
    o. ureterocele
    o. urinary diversion
    o. voiding
    o. voiding pouch
Orthotripter
    OssaTron O.
orthovoltage teletherapy
Orthoxine
Orudis
Orzel
OSB
    one-step button
    OSB gastrostomy device
Osbon
    O. ErecAid VCD
    O. pressure-point tension
       ring
Os-Cal
oscheal
oscheitis
oschelephantiasis
oscheocele
oscheohydrocele
oscheolith
oscheoma
oscheoncus
oscheoplasty
oscillation
    myenteric potential o.
oscillatory potential
oscilloscope
    Tektronix digital o.
Osler
    O. II syndrome
    O. node
Osler-Weber-Rendu
    O.-W.-R. disease
    O.-W.-R. syndrome
    O.-W.-R. telangiectasia
Osmette osmometer
osmium tetroxide (OsO4)
osmoceptor (*var. of* osmoreceptor)
Osmoglyn
osmolality
    body fluid o.
    diurnal urine o.
    medullary interstitial o.
    plasma o.
    urine o.
osmolar clearance
osmolarity
    o. gap
    o. of ink
    serum o.
    urine o. (Uosm)

Osmolite HN enteral feeding
osmolyte
osmometer
    Osmette o.
    vapor pressure o.
OsmoPrep
osmoreceptor, osmoceptor
Osmo reverse osmosis unit
osmotherapy
osmotic
    o. cathartic
    o. demyelination syndrome
    o. diarrhea
    o. diuresis
    o. diuretic
    o. laxative
    o. load
    o. nephrosis
    o. stimulus
    o. threshold for thirst
OsO4
    osmium tetroxide
OssaTron
    O. Orthotripter
    O. shock wave therapy
osseous metaplasia
ossification
    metaplastic o.
Ossoff-Karlan laryngoscope
osteitis pubis
osteoarthropathy
osteoblast-derived
osteoblast-like proliferation
osteocalcin
osteoclast
    acid phosphate o.
    o. maturation
osteoclast-activating factor
osteoclast-like giant cell (OLGC)
osteodystrophia (*var. of* osteodystrophy)
osteodystrophy, osteodystrophia
    Albright hereditary o.
    azotemic o.
    hepatic o.
    renal o. (ROD)
osteogenetic (*var. of* osteogenic)
osteogenic, osteogenetic
    o. differentiation
    o. sarcoma
osteomalacia
    dialysis o.
osteomyelitis
osteoonychodysplasia
    hereditary o.
osteophyte
    esophageal o.
osteopontin
osteosarcoma
    bladder o.

osteotomy
    anterior innominate o.
    Dickson o.
    pelvic o.
ostia (*pl. of* ostium)
ostial
    o. artery atherosclerosis
    o. atherosclerotic plaque
ostiomeatal
ostium, *pl.* **ostia**
    o. appendicis vermiformis
    o. ileocecale
    o. pyloricum
    o. urethrae externum feminae
    o. urethrae externum masculinae
    o. urethrae internum
ostomate
ostomy
    o. appliance
    O. Assessment Inventory (OAI)
    o. bag
    ConvaTec Durahesive Wafer o.
    o. loop
    o. skin
    o. takedown
ostreotoxism
**O'Sullivan-O'Connor abdominal
retractor**
O'Sullivan scoring system
OTA
    oligoteratoasthenozoospermia
**12-O-tetradecanoylphorbol-13-acetate
(TPA, tPA)**
    phorbol ester 12-O-t.-13-a.
Otis
    O. anoscope
    O. sound
    O. urethrotome
    O. urethrotomy
otitidiscaviarum
    Nocardia o.
otolaryngologic manifestation
Otrivin
Ott/Mayo channel sampling kit
OTW
    over-the-wire
ouabain
ouabainlike substance (OLS)
out
    coring o.
outcome
    o. and process assessment
    o. equivalent to open surgery
    favorable o.
    health o.
    impact of microwave antenna on
      treatment o.
    long-term o.
    multicenter o.

    o. of cadaveric renal allograft
    oncologic o.
    poor long-term o.
    o. predictor
    primary o.
    short-term survival o.
outer
    o. cortical blood flow
    o. crossbar
    o. diameter
    o. inflammatory protein
    o. medulla
    o. medullary collecting duct
    o. medullary ischemia
outflow
    hepatic venous o.
    mean venous o.
    o. obstruction
    pulmonary o.
    o. tract
    vagal efferent o.
outlet
    bladder o.
    o. delay
    o. dysfunction
    gastric o.
    o. obstruction
    o. obstruction constipation
    pyloric o.
outlier syndrome
outline
    gastric o.
out-of-scope lithotriptor
outpatient endoscopy
output
    basal acid o. (BAO)
    bile phospholipid o. (BPO)
    bile salt o. (BSO)
    biliary cholesterol o. (BCO)
    cardiac o.
    intake and o. (I&O)
    maximal acid o. (MAO)
    meal-stimulated acid o. (MSAO)
    peak acid o. (PAO)
    pulse-induced contour cardiac o.
    urinary o.
outstanding anatomical detail
ova (*pl. of* ovum)
oval
    o. fat body
    o. open esophagoscope
    o. snare
ovalbumin
oval-form colonic groove
ovalis
    fossa o.
ovaria (*pl. of* ovarium)
ovarian
    o. artery

O

ovarian (*continued*)
    o. cancer
    o. carcinoma
    o. dermoid cyst
    o. disease
    o. endometrioma
    o. enlargement
    o. fibroma
    o. hyperstimulation syndrome
    o. overstimulation syndrome
    o. remnant syndrome
    o. teratoma
    o. vein syndrome
ovarii
    stroma o.
    struma o.
    tunica albuginea o.
ovarium, *pl.* ovaria
    o. masculinum
ovary
    streak o.
ovatus
    Bacteroides o.
overactive bladder (OB)
overactivity
    detrusor muscle o.
overall
    o. mortality
    o. survival
over-and-over suture
overdistension (*var. of* overdistention)
overdistention, overdistension
    bladder o.
overdose (OD)
    acetaminophen o.
overdosing
overexpression
    p53 o.
overflow
    o. aminoaciduria
    o. fecal incontinence
    o. proteinuria
    o. theory
overgrowth
    bacterial o.
    candidal o.
    gastric bacterial o. (GBO)
    small-intestine bacterial o. (SIBO)
    tube o.
    tumor o.
    yeast o.
overlapping sphincteroplasty
overlap syndrome
overload
    African iron o.
    hepatic copper o.
    nitrogen o.
    transfusional iron o.
    volume o.

overlying clot
overproduction
    oxalate o.
overreactive puborectalis
oversedation
over-the-endoscope Witzel dilator
over-the-scope bougie
over-the-wire (OTW)
    o.-t.-w. balloon catheter
    o.-t.-w. set
    o.-t.-w. technique
overt nephropathy
overtube
    Christopher-Williams o.
    flexible endoscopic o.
    Guardian o.
    Guardus o.
    Mill-Rose flexible endoscopic o.
    negative-pressure o.
    oroesophageal o.
    rotational colonoscope o.
    o. sheath
    split o.
    Steigmann-Goff endoscopic ligature o.
    Williams varix injection o.
oviductal fluid
oviduct epithelium
ovoid fungus
ovotestes (*pl. of* ovotestis)
ovotestis, *pl.* ovotestes
ovum, *pl.* ova
    ova and parasites (O&P)
    ova, cysts, and parasites (OCP)
oxacillin
oxacillin-associated anicteric hepatitis
oxalate
    calcium o.
    o. calculus
    o. crystal
    dietary o.
    o. intestinal absorption
    o. metabolism
    o. nephropathy
    o. overproduction
    urinary o.
oxalic acid
oxaliplatin, 5-fluorouracil, leucovorin
oxaloacetate
Oxalobacter formigenes
oxalosis
    primary o.
oxaluria
    calcium o.
    enteric o.
oxamniquine

oxandrolone treatment
oxaprozin
oxatomide
oxazepam
oxcarbazepine
ox-eye daisy
oxidant
    o. injury
    iron-dependent o.
oxidant-trapping potential
oxidase
    o. cytosolic factor
    diamine o.
    fatty acyl CoA o.
    NADPH o.
    xanthine o.
oxidation
    arachidonic acid o.
    mitochondrial fatty acid beta o.
    substrate o.
    xanthine o.
oxidative
    o. burst
    o. cell injury
    o. phosphorylation
    slow-twitch o.
    o. stress
oxidative-glycolytic fiber
oxide
    deuterium o.
    donor of nitric o.
    endothelium-derived nitric o.
    (EDNO)
    ethylene o. (ETO)
    magnesium o.
    mercuric o.
    nitric o.
    nitrous o.
    propylene o.
    ultrasmall superparamagnetic iron o.
    (USPIO)
oxidized
    o. LDL
    o. low-density lipoprotein (Ox-LDL)
oxidoreductase activity
oxime
    sugar o.

oximetry
    pulse o.
oxine
Ox-LDL
    oxidized low-density lipoprotein
oxpentifylline
oxybutynin
    o. ATD gel
    o. chloride
    intravesical o.
    o. transdermal patch
    o. transdermal system
Oxycel cotton
oxychlorosene sodium
oxycodone
oxygen ($O2$, O_2)
    blood gas on o.
    o. desaturation
    fractional percentage of inspired o.
    (FIO_2)
    hyperbaric o. (HBO)
    o. radical
    o. saturation
    o. saturation index (ISO_2)
oxygen-15
oxygenating mouthguard
oxygenation
    medullary o.
oxygenator
    membrane o.
oxygen-derived free radical
oxygen-free radical
Oxyguard oxygenating mouthguard
oxymorphone
oxyntic
    o. cell
    o. gland
    o. mucosa
    o. mucosal gastritis
oxyphenbutazone
oxyphencyclimine hydrochloride
oxyphenonium
oxytoca
    Klebsiella o.
oxytocin
Oxytrol transdermal system
Oxyuris

O

P

P blood group system
P cell

P-32, ^{32}P

phosphorus-32

P450

cytochrome P450
P450 function

p53

p53 allelotyping
p53 antibody
p53 assay
p53 expression
p53 gene
p53 immunohistochemical
stain
p53 immunohistochemistry
p53 mutation
p53 nuclear protein
p53 nuclear staining
p53 overexpression
p53 protein
p53 protooncogene
p53 reactivity
p53 tumor-suppressor gene
analysis

PAA

periampullary adenoma

10Pa Amicon chamber

PAb

protein antibody

PABA

paraaminobenzoic acid
PABA test

PACAP

pituitary adenylate cyclase-activating
polypeptide

paced rhythm

pacemaker

p. cell
Enterra gastrointestinal p.

pachycholia

pachychymia

pacificum

Diphyllobothrium p.

pacinian corpuscle

**Pacis BCG bladder cancer
immunotherapy**

pack

gauze p.
laparotomy p.
moist laparotomy p.
petrolatum gauze p.
Rheumatrex dose p.

package

GastroSoft data reduction and
prognostic software p.
lymphatic p.

Packard Auto-Gamma analyzer

packed red blood cells (PRBC)

packet

single-dose p.

packing

Adaptic p.
p. forceps
p. fraction
gelatin sponge p.
Mikulicz p.

paclitaxel

polyglutamate p.

Pacquin ureterolysis

pad

abdominal fat p.
abdominal laparotomy p.
Active Living incontinence p.
antimesenteric fat p.
bed p.
bulbocavernosus fat p.
p. cover
dinner p.
esophagogastric fat p.
fat p.
ileocecal fat p.
Iodoflex p.
lap p.
laparotomy p.
Martius fat p.
Mikulicz p.
perineal p.
Sani-Pads medicated cleansing p.
p. test for urinary incontinence
p. testing
p. urinary incontinence test

padding

absorbent p.
Spenco p.

Padua

P. bladder urinary pouch
P. ileal bladder

Paecilomyces

PAF

platelet-activating factor

Pagano

P. technique ureterocolonic
anastomosis
P. ureteral anastomosis

PAGE

polyacrylamide gel electrophoresis

Page kidney

Pagenstecher circle

P

Paget
  P. disease of perianal area
  P. extramammary disease
  P. perianal disease
pagetoid
Pagitane
PAH
  paraaminohippurate
  paraaminohippuric
    PAH acid
    PAH clearance
PAI-1, -2
  plasminogen activator inhibitor-1, -2
pain
  abdominal p.
  acute flank p.
  biliary tract p. (BTP)
  bladder p.
  boring p.
  burning p.
  chest p.
  colicky abdominal p.
  constricting p.
  p. control
  crampy abdominal p.
  deep p.
  diffuse p.
  drug-induced p.
  dull p.
  epicritic p.
  epigastric p.
  exacerbation of p.
  exertion-induced p.
  exquisite p.
  p. fiber
  flank p.
  functional p.
  gnawing p.
  hunger p.
  inevitable postoperative p.
  intermittent p.
  knifelike p.
  lancinating p.
  localized p.
  loin p.
  nagging p.
  NIH Classification Category III
    inflammatory and noninflammatory
    chronic pelvic p.
  nocturnal p.
  noncardiac chest p. (NCCP)
  onset of p.
  palliation of p.
  parietal p.
  perianal p.
  perirectal p.
  poorly localized p.
  postligation p.
  postprandial p.

  posture-dependent p.
  protopathic p.
  radiating p.
  rebound p.
  recurrent abdominal p.
    (RAP)
  referred p.
  remission of p.
  retrosternal chest p.
  sciatica-like p.
  scrotal p.
  severe p.
  somatic p.
  steady p.
  sudden onset of p.
  tearing p.
  testicular p.
  triangle of p.
  unrelenting p.
  unrelieved p.
  unremitting p.
  visceral p.
pain-associated disability syndrome
painful
  p. defecation
  p. hematuria
painless
  p. hematuria
  p. jaundice
  p. rectal bleeding
**pain-predominant irritable bowel
  syndrome**
paint
  Castellani p.
painter's colic
Pak
  Trovan/Zithromax Compliance P.
palate
  cleft p.
  smoker's p.
palatine pillar
palatinus
  torus p.
palatoglossus muscle
palatopharyngeal fold
palatopharyngeus muscle
Palco enuretic alarm system
pale
  p. cell
  spermatogonium p. type A
  p. stool
Paleolithic diet
palindrome
palindromic rheumatism
palisade-type vein
palisade vessel
palladium-103
  p.-103 seed implant
  transperineal p.-103

palliation
  p. of malignant large-bowel
    obstruction
  p. of pain
palliative
  p. cystectomy
  p. decompression
  p. exeresis
  p. nephrectomy
  p. surgery
  p. therapy
  p. urinary diversion
pallidum
  Treponema p.
pallidus
  raphe p.
pallor
  cachectic p.
  mucosal p.
palmar
  p. erythema
  p. grasp
palmaris
  tylosis p.
palmatus
  penis p.
Palmaz
  P. balloon-expandable
    stent
  P. Blue stent
  P. Corinthian biliary stent and
    delivery system
  P. Corinthian stent
Palmaz-Schatz biliary stent
Palmer acid test for peptic ulcer
palmetto
  saw p.
palmin, palmitin
  p. test
palmitin (*var. of* palmin)
Palomo
  P. approach
  P. varicocelectomy
  P. varicocelectomy
    procedure
  P. varicocele ligation
    technique
palonosetron
palpable
  p. adenopathy
  p. cord
  p. gallbladder
  p. kidney
  p. mass
  p. pyloric olive
  p. rib diastasis
  p. stool
palpably normal
palpating probe

palpation
  bladder p.
  p. in epigastrium
  p. tenderness
palpatory proteinuria
palpebrae
  paraphimosis p.
palsy
  cerebral p.
PAM
  pancreatic acinar metaplasia
Pamelor
Pamine Forte
Pamisyl
pamoate
  pyrantel p.
pampiniformis
  plexus p.
pampiniform plexus
pampinocele
PAN
  puromycin aminonucleoside nephropathy
  puromycin aminonucleoside nephrosis
panacinar
  p. disease
  p. emphysema
Panafil
  P. ointment
  P. SE spray emulsion
pan-bud anomaly
p-ANC
  perinuclear antineutrophil cytoplasmic
  p-ANC genetic marker
p-ANCA, PANCA, P-ANCA
  perinuclear antineutrophil cytoplasmic
    antibody
pancake kidney
pancolectomy
pancolitis
  steroid-responsive p.
pancolonoscopy
pancreas
  aberrant p.
  p. accessorium
  accessory p.
  acinarization of p.
  anlage of p.
  anular p.
  Aselli p.
  capsule of p.
  Christmas tree appearance of p.
  divided p.
  p. divisum (PD)
  ectopic p.
  endoscopic retrograde
    parenchymography of p. (ERPP)
  exocrine p.
  fibrocystic disease of p.
  fibrofatty infiltration of p.

P

pancreas (*continued*)
    head of p.
    heterotopic p.
    heterotopic-aberrant p.
    intraductal papillary and mucinous
      tumors of p.
    p. lesion
    lesser p.
    lobule of p.
    malignant serous cystic neoplasm of p.
    neck of p.
    solid and cystic tumors of p.
      (SCTP)
    tail of p.
    p. transplantation
    unciform p.
    uncinate process of p.
    Willis p.
    Winslow p.
Pancrease MT 4, 10, 16, 20
pancreas-kidney transplant
pancreatalgia
pancreatectomy, pancreectomy
    distal p.
    en bloc distal p.
    endoscopic transgastric distal p.
      (ETDP)
    left-to-right subtotal p.
    partial p.
    subtotal p.
    total p.
pancreatic
    p. acinar cell
    p. acinar cell carcinoma
    p. acinar metaplasia (PAM)
    p. acinus
    p. agenesis
    p. alpha-amylase
    p. ascariasis
    p. ascites
    p. bladder
    p. blood flow
    p. calcification
    p. calculus
    p. cancer
    p. cancer marker
    p. carcinoma (PCA)
    p. cholera
    p. cholera syndrome
    p. colic
    p. cutaneous fistula
    p. cyst
    p. diabetes
    p. diastase
    p. disease
    p. diverticulum
    p. duct
    p. ductal hypertension
    p. ductal morphological change

p. duct-choledochus channel
p. duct disruption
p. duct encasement
p. duct manipulation
p. ductogram
p. duct pressure (PDP)
p. duct sphincter (PDS)
p. duct sphincterotomy
p. duct stent
p. duct stone
p. duct stricture
p. duct to pseudocyst
p. endopeptidase
p. endoprosthesis
p. enema
p. enzyme replacement therapy
  (PERT)
p. exocrine dysfunction
p. exocrine insufficiency
p. exopeptidase
p. fibrosis
p. flare
p. fluid collection (PFC)
p. glandular necrosis
p. hamartoma
p. head
p. injury
p. intraluminal radiation therapy
p. islet cell
p. islet cell carcinoma
p. islet cell transplantation (PICT)
p. islet cell tumor
p. isoamylase enzyme
p. juice
p. lesion
p. lipase
p. lipase deficiency
p. lymphangiectasis
p. mucinous cystadenocarcinoma
p. oncofetal antigen (POA)
p. orifice
p. papillary stenosis
p. parenchyma
p. phlegmon
p. polypeptide
p. polypeptide-secreting tumor
  (PPoma)
p. polypeptide stain
p. pseudocyst
p. pseudocyst abscess
p. pseudocystogastrostomy
p. rendezvous
p. rest
p. sarcoidosis
p. secretory flow rate (PSFR)
p. secretory test
p. secretory trypsin inhibitor (PSTI)
p. sepsis
p. sepsis in acute pancreatitis

p. sphincteroplasty
p. steatorrhea
p. stone protein (PSP)
p. tail resection
p. transpapillary stenting
p. trauma
p. tree
p. tumor diagnosis
p. tumor localization
pancreatica
achylia p.
diarrhea p.
p. magna artery
sialorrhea p.
pancreaticobiliary, pancreatobiliary
p. canal
p. common channel
p. disease
p. ductal junction
p. ductal system
p. endoscopy
p. malignancy
p. maljunction
p. reflux
p. region
p. septum
p. sphincter
p. stricture
p. tract
p. tree
pancreaticocholedochoductal junction
pancreaticocystostomy
pancreaticoduodenal, pancreatoduodenal
anterosuperior p. (ASPD)
p. arteriography
p. cancer
p. transplantation
p. vein
p. venous drainage
pancreaticoduodenectomy (*var. of* pancreatoduodenectomy)
pylorus-sparing p.
pancreaticoduodenostomy (*var. of* pancreatoduodenostomy)
pancreaticogastric anastomosis
pancreaticogastrostomy (*var. of* pancreatogastrostomy)
pancreaticohepatic syndrome
pancreaticojejunostomy (*var. of* pancreatojejunostomy)
pancreaticopleural fistula
pancreaticosplenic omentum
pancreatic-portal vein fistula
pancreaticus
ansa p.
ductus p.
hemosuccus p.
liquor p.
succus p.

pancreatin
pancreatis
arteria caudae p.
caput p.
corpus p.
pancreatitis
acquired p.
acute edematous p. (AEP)
acute gallstone p. (AGP)
acute hemorrhagic p. (AHP)
acute recurrent p. (ARP)
acute relapsing p.
alcoholic p.
alcohol-induced p.
biliary p.
calcareous p.
calcific p.
calcifying p.
capsula p.
centrilobular p.
chronic p. (CP)
chronic alcoholic p. (CAP)
chronic alcohol-induced p.
chronic calcifying p. (CCP)
chronic fibrosing p.
chronic relapsing p. (CRP)
coagulopathy p.
diffuse p.
drug-induced acute p.
edematous p.
endoscopic sphincterotomy-induced p.
familial p.
focal p.
fulminating p.
gallstone p.
Glasgow criteria for severity of p.
groove p.
hemoductal p.
hemorrhagic necrotizing p.
hereditary p.
idiopathic fibrosing p.
idiopathic recurrent p. (IRP)
inflammatory p.
interstitial p.
microlithiasis-induced p.
mumps p.
necrotizing p.
nodular p.
nutritional p.
obstructive p.
pancreatic sepsis in acute p.
pentamidine-induced p.
perilobar p.
phlegmonous p.
postendoscopic retrograde cholangiopancreatography p.
post-ERCP-induced p.
postprocedure p.
purulent p.

P

551

pancreatitis (*continued*)
    Ranson criteria for severity of p.
    recurrent p.
    relapsing acute p.
    segmentary p.
    tropical calcific p.
    ventral chronic calcific p.
pancreatitis-related
    p.-r. bleeding
    p.-r. hemorrhage
pancreatobiliary (*var. of* pancreaticobiliary)
pancreatocholangiography
    retrograde p.
pancreatocholecystostomy
pancreatoduodenal (*var. of*
  pancreaticoduodenal)
pancreatoduodenectomy,
  pancreaticoduodenectomy
    pylorus-preserving p. (PPPD)
    Whipple p.
pancreatoduodenostomy,
  pancreaticoduodenostomy
    Child p.
    Dennis-Varco p.
    Waugh-Clagett p.
    Whipple p.
pancreatogastrostomy,
  pancreaticogastrostomy
pancreatogenic, pancreatogenous
pancreatogenous (*var. of* pancreatogenic)
    p. diarrhea
pancreatogram
    rat-tail appearance on p.
    retrograde p.
pancreatography
    3-dimensional CT p. (3DCTP)
    dye-injection endoscopic retrograde
      p.
    endoscopic digital p. (EDP)
    endoscopic retrograde p.
      (ERP)
    magnetic resonance p. (MRP)
    retrograde p.
pancreatoicoduodenal cancer
pancreatojejunostomy,
  pancreaticojejunostomy
    caudal p.
    cystolateral p.
    Duval distal p.
    lateral p.
    longitudinal p.
    Puestow p.
    Puestow-Gillesby p.
    retrocolic end-to-end p.
    Roux-en-Y p.
    p. stenosis
pancreatolith, pancreolith
pancreatolithectomy (*var. of*
  pancreatolithotomy)

pancreatolithiasis
pancreatolithotomy, pancreatolithectomy
pancreatolysis, pancreolysis
pancreatolytic, pancreolytic
pancreatomegaly
pancreatomy (*var. of* pancreatotomy)
pancreatopathy, pancreopathy
pancreatoscope
    peroral electronic p. (PEPS)
    ultrathin p.
pancreatoscopic laser lithotripsy (PSLL)
pancreatoscopy, pancreoscopy
    infragastric p.
    peroral p. (POPS)
pancreatotomy, pancreatomy
Pancrecarb MS-8
pancreectomy (*var. of* pancreatectomy)
pancrelipase
pancreolith (*var. of* pancreatolith)
pancreolysis (*var. of* pancreatolysis)
pancreolytic (*var. of* pancreatolytic)
pancreopathy (*var. of* pancreatopathy)
pancreoprivic
pancreoscopy (*var. of* pancreatoscopy)
pancreozymin
Pancrex
pancuronium
Panda gastrostomy feeding tube
pandysautonomia
panel
    Nephrolithiasis Clinical Guidelines P.
panel-reactive antibody
panendoscope
    cap-fitted p.
    flexible forward-viewing p.
    LoPressure p.
    Olympus GIF-D-series p.
    Olympus GIF-XQ-series p.
    Storz p.
    Wolf rigid p.
panendoscopy
    fiberoptic p.
    lower p.
    primary p.
    upper gastrointestinal p.
panenteroscopy
    laparoscopically assisted p.
Paneth cell
pangastritis
    atrophic p.
    nonatrophic p.
panitumumab
panlobular emphysema
panmalabsorption
panmucosal inflammatory cell
  infiltration
panmural cystitis
Panmycin
panni (*pl. of* pannus)

panniculalgia
panniculectomy
panniculi (*pl. of* panniculus)
panniculitis
    mesenteric p.
    scrotal p.
panniculus, *pl.* **panniculi**
    hanging p.
pannus, *pl.* **panni**
panostotic fibrous dysplasia
Panoview rod-lens ureteroscope
panproctocolectomy
pantaloon hernia
Pantoloc+
Pantoloc tablet
Pantopaque
pantoprazole
    p. sodium
    p. sodium delayed-release tablet
pantothenic
    p. acid
    p. acid deficiency-induced colitis
pants
    Ashton p.
    Dignity incontinence p.
    Endo p.
    Holyoke p.
    Kleinert p.
    Suretys p.
    Ultrafem p.
pants-over-vest
    p.-o.-v. hernia repair
    p.-o.-v. herniorrhaphy
panurethral stricture
Panvac-VF
Panzer gallbladder scissors
PAO
    peak acid output
PAOGRP
    peak acid output after gastrin-releasing
    peptide
PAOPg
    peak acid output after pentagastrin
    stimulation
PAP
    prostatic acid phosphatase
    pulmonary artery pressure
Pap
    Papanicolaou
    Pap smear
papain, papainase
    p., urea, chlorophyllin copper
      complex sodium spray emulsion
papainase (*var. of* papain)
Papanicolaou (Pap)
    P. method
    P. smear (Pap smear)
    P. stain
    P. test

papaverine
    p. hydrochloride
    p. injection
PAP-HT25 cell
papilla, *pl.* **papillae**
    balloon dilation of p.
    ballooning of p.
    bile p.
    bulging p.
    duodenal p.
    p. duodeni major
    p. duodeni minor
    foliate papillae
    frenulum of duodenal p.
    fungiform p.
    glans penis p.
    ileal p.
    p. ilealis
    ileocecal p.
    intradiverticular p.
    laparoscopic transcystic duct stenting
      of p.
    major p.
    minor p.
    necrosis of renal p.
    p. of Santorini
    p. of Vater
    patulous p.
    renal p.
    sloughed p.
    Suda classification type I, II, III of
      p.
    vallate p.
papillae (*pl. of* papilla)
papillary, papillate
    p. adenocarcinoma
    p. adenoma
    p. adenoma of large intestine
    p. cystitis
    p. gastric carcinoma
    p. hyperplasia
    p. lesion
    p. manometry
    p. necrosis
    p. orifice
    p. renal cancer
    p. renal cell carcinoma
    p. stenosis
    p. tip
    p. transitional cell carcinoma
papillate (*var. of* papillary)
papillation
papillectomy
    balloon catheter-assisted endoscopic
      snare p.
papilledema
papilliferous
papilliform
papillitis

P

papilloma
> bladder inverted p.
> esophageal squamous p.
> gingival p.
> hirsutoid p.
> inverted p.
> p. of renal pelvis
> sporadic gingival p.
> squamous cell p.
> p. venereum
> villous p.

papilloma-carcinoma sequence
papillomatosis
> biliary p.
> p. of intrahepatic bile duct

papillomatous neotransformation
papillomavirus
> genital human p.
> human p. (HPV)

papillotome
> 30-30 p.
> Accuratome precurved p.
> Bard Companion p.
> Classen-Demling p.
> Cremer-Ikeda p.
> double-lumen tapered-tip p.
> dual-lumen p.
> Erlangen p.
> Frimberger-Karpiel 12 o'clock p.
> Howell Rotatable BII p.
> Huibregtse-Katon p.
> Iso-Tome p.
> Microvasive p.
> needle p.
> needle-knife p.
> Olympus needle-knife p.
> Piggyback needle-knife p.
> precut p.
> shark-fin p.
> Swenson p.
> traction-type p.
> Wilson-Cook p.
> Wiltek p.

papillotome/sphincterotome
> Zimmon p./s.

papillotomy
> access p.
> endoscopic p.
> Erlangen pull-type precut p.
> laparoscopic transcystic p.
> needle-knife p. (NKP)
> needle-knife precut p. (NKPP)
> precut p.

Pap-Kaps
papular acrodermatitis of childhood
papule
> Bowen p.
> moist p.

mucous p.
> pearly penile p.

papulosis
> bowenoid p.
> malignant atrophic p.

papulosquamous disorder
papulous gastropathy
Paque
> E-Z P.

Paquin
> P. repair
> P. ureteral reimplantation
> P. ureterocystoneostomy technique

paraaminobenzoic acid (PABA)
paraaminohippurate (PAH)
> p. clearance

paraaminohippuric (PAH)
> p. acid

paraaminosalicylate hypersensitivity
para-ANC antibody
paraaortic
> p. lymphadenectomy
> p. region

parabola
paracancerous tissue
paracecal appendix
paracellular
> p. flux
> p. pathway
> p. route

paracentesis
> abdominal p.
> diagnostic p.
> large-volume p. (LVP)

paracervical tenderness
paracetamol
> p. absorption
> p. absorption test
> p. acute liver failure

parachute reflex
Paracoccidioides brasiliensis
paracoccidioidomycosis
paracolic
> p. abscess
> p. groove
> p. gutter

paracollicular biopsy
paracolostomy
> p. hernia
> p. herniation

paraconal fascia
paracrine
> p. cell
> p. factor
> p. peptide

paradigm
> Sternberg p.

paradoxic, paradoxical
    p. diarrhea
    p. motion
    p. puborectalis contraction
    p. renal response
    p. sphincter reaction
paradoxical (*var. of* paradoxic)
    p. incontinence
paraduodenal
    p. fold
    p. hernia
    p. pseudocyst
paradysenteriae
    Shigella p.
paraesophageal
    p. collateral vein
    p. diaphragmatic hernia
    p. hernia type I, II
    p. hiatal hernia
    p. varix
paraesophagogastric
    p. devascularization
    p. lymph node metastasis
paraesthesia (*var. of* paresthesia)
paraexstrophy skin flap
paraffin-embedded
    p.-e. specimen
    p.-e. tissue
paraffinoma
paraffin-section light microscopy
paraformaldehyde
parafrenal abscess
paraganglioma
    juxtapapillary gangliocytic p.
paragastric pseudocyst
paragenitalis
paraglobulinuria
parahaemolyticus
    Vibrio p.
parahiatal hernia
paraileostomal hernia
paraisopropyliminodiacetic acid (PIPIDA)
parakeratosis
parallel plate dialyzer
paralyses (*pl. of* paralysis)
paralysis, *pl.* **paralyses**
    esophageal p.
paralytic
    p. colonic obstruction
    p. ileus
    p. incontinence
    p. intestinal obstruction
    p. secretion
    p. shellfish poisoning
paralytica
    dysphagia p.
paralyticus
    ileus p.
paramagnetic contrast agent

parameatal-based flap
paramedian incision
parameter
    anthropomorphic p.
    chronobiological p.
    clinical p.
    clotting p.
    DIC p.
    individual p.
    kinetic p.
    prostate-specific antigen-based p.
    PSA-based p.
    quality-of-life p.
    specific clinical p.
    urodynamic p.
    valuable additional p.
    vascular p.
    voiding p.
paraneoplastic
    p. dermatomyositis
    p. syndrome
paranephric abscess
paranephritis
    lipomatous p.
paranephroma
paranitroaniline release
paranitrophenol phosphate
parapancreatic mass
paraparesis
    spastic p.
    tropical spastic p.
parapelvic cyst
paraperitoneal nephrectomy
paraphimosis palpebrae
paraplegia
paraproctitis
paraprostatitis
paraproteinemia
parapubic hernia
paraquat
paraquat-induced upper gastrointestinal injury
pararectal
    p. abscess
    p. fistula
    p. line
    p. pouch
pararectus incision
pararotovirus
parasagittal plane
parasite
    p. examination
    hemoflagellate p.
    intestinal p.
    isosporan p.
    ova and p.'s (O&P)
    ova, cysts, and p.'s (OCP)
    protozoan p.
    stool for ova and p.'s

P

parasitemia
parasitic
    p. chylocele
    p. cyst
    p. infection
    p. infestation
    p. leiomyoma
    p. liver disease
    p. peritonitis
    p. prostatitis
parasitizing macrophage
parasitology
paraspinal musculature
paraspinous
    p. aspect
    p. muscle
parastomal hernia
parasympathetic
    p. postganglionic neuron
    p. preganglionic neuron
    p. projection
parasympatholytic drug
parasympathomimetic
    p. agent
    p. anticholinesterase
    p. drug
paratesticular
    p. fat
    p. leiomyosarcoma
    p. malignancy
    p. neoplasm
    p. rhabdomyosarcoma
    p. tumor
parathyroid
    p. disease
    p. hormone (PTH)
    p. hormone-related polypeptide
    p. hyperplasia
    p. imaging
paratuberculosis
    Mycobacterium p.
paratyphi
    Salmonella p. A, B, C
paraumbilical
    p. vein
    p. vein tumor (PUVT)
paraureteric
paraurethra
paraurethral
    p. cyst
    p. gland
paraurethrales
paraurethritis
paravaginal
    p. fascial repair
    p. pedicle
paravariceal
    p. fibrosis
    p. injection

    p. sclerotherapy
paraventricular nucleus
paravertebral neuroblastoma
paravesical
    p. fossa
    p. pouch
paregoric
parenchyma
    allograft p.
    hepatic p.
    inhomogeneity of p.
    liver p.
    pancreatic p.
    renal p.
parenchymal (*var. of* parenchymatous)
parenchyma-sparing surgery
parenchymatous, parenchymal
    p. acute renal failure
    p. atrophy
    p. collapse
    p. damage
    p. hematoma
    p. inflammation
    p. jaundice
    p. liver disease
    p. nephritis
    p. tissue
    p. tumor
parenchymography
    endoscopic retrograde p.
parenteral
    p. alimentation
    p. diarrhea
    p. feeding
    p. guanethidine
    p. hyperalimentation
    p. immunization
    p. methyldopa
    p. nutrition
paresthesia, paraesthesia
    lateral cutaneous p.
paretic impotence
pargyline
paricalcitol
paries, *pl.* parietes
parietal
    p. cell
    p. cell index
    p. cell vagotomy (PCV)
    p. epithelium
    p. fistula
    p. hernia
    p. pain
    p. peritoneum
parietes (*pl. of* paries)
Parietex composite mesh for hernia surgery
parietitis
parietocolic fold

parietography
gastric p.
parietosplanchnic
Pariet therapy
Paris renal adenocarcinoma
Parker-Kerr
P.-K. closed method of end-to-end enteroenterostomy
P.-K. intestinal clamp
P.-K. suture
P.-K. suture-closed method
Parker retractor
Parkinson disease
parkinsonian gait
Parks
P. ileal reservoir
P. ileoanal anastomosis
P. ileoanal reservoir
P. ileostomy pouch
P. method of anal fistulotomy
P. partial sphincterotomy
P. retractor
P. staged fistulotomy
Parnate
paromomycin
paromphalocele
paronychia
parorchidium
parotidea
orchitis p.
parotid gland enlargement
parovarian
p. cyst
p. mass
paroxetine
paroxysmal
p. anal hyperkinesis
p. motor disease
p. nocturnal hemoglobinemia
p. nocturnal hemoglobinuria (PNH)
Parsidol
parsley
fool's p.
partial
p. adrenalectomy
p. bile outflow obstruction
p. bladder denervation
p. bowel obstruction
p. cystectomy
p. enterocele
p. external biliary diversion
p. fasting
p. fundoplication
p. gastrectomy
p. hepatectomy
p. hood-assisted lift-and-cut method
p. ileal bypass (PIB)

p. nephrectomy
p. nephrogenic diabetes insipidus phenotype
p. orchiectomy
p. pancreatectomy
p. penectomy
p. polar nephrectomy
p. thromboplastin time (PTT)
p. ureteral obstruction
p. villous atrophy (PVA)
p. water bath and water cushion
p. zonal dissection (PZD)
partial-occlusion clamp
particle
core p.
Dane p.
food p.
viruslike p.
particulate
p. radiation
p. silicone
p. stool
Partington-Rochelle procedure
Partin table
partition
gastric p.
partitioning
abdominal p.
partnership
limited p. (LP)
paruresis
parvum
Corynebacterium p.
Cryptosporidium p.
Diphyllobothrium p.
PAS
periodic acid-Schiff
PAS stain
PAS test
PAS-AB
periodic acid-Schiff-Alcian blue
pasque flower
pass
guided fine-needle p.
passage
biliary p.
P. biliary dilation catheter
guidewire p.
incomplete p.
p. of flatus per vagina
p. of stool
p. pressure
spontaneous fragment p.
spontaneous stone p.
passer
Carter-Thomason suture p.
Protect-a-Pass suture p.
passion flower

P

passive
- p. chest drainage
- p. congestion
- p. Heymann nephritis (PHN)
- p. incontinence

Passport balloon-on-a-wire dilation catheter

paste
- Anatrast barium sulfate p.
- barium p.
- Coloplast skin barrier p.
- Hollister Premium p.
- iLEX skin protectant p.
- Karaya 5 p.
- sandy skin-prepping p.
- Stomahesive p.

Pasteurella multocida

patch
- Androderm testosterone transdermal p.
- aortic p.
- bladder p.
- Bowen p.
- Carrel aortic p.
- cecal red p.
- p. clamp technique
- colic p.
- colonic p.
- estradiol transdermal p.
- Gore-Tex Acuseal cardiovascular p.
- Gore-Tex soft tissue p.
- p. graft
- p. graft urethroplasty
- herald p.
- inlet p.
- Kugel hernia p.
- Miniguard adhesive p.
- mucous p.
- murine Peyer p.
- omental p.
- oxybutynin transdermal p.
- periappendiceal red p.
- Peyer p.
- Rutkow sutureless plug and p.
- schistosomiasis sandy p.
- shagreen p.
- Testoderm p.
- testosterone p.
- vein p.
- white p.

patchiness
- endoscopic p.
- histologic p.

patchy
- p. colitis
- p. colonic ulceration
- p. necrosis

patency
- biliary stent p.
- p. rate
- stent p.

patent
- p. airway
- p. processus vaginalis
- p. urachus
- p. urethra

Paterson-Kelly syndrome

pathergy phenomenon

Pathfinder
- P. exchange guidewire
- P. wire

Pathilon

pathogen
- bloodborne p.
- enteric p.
- invasive enteric p.
- prokaryotic p.
- protozoan p.
- zoonotic foodborne p.

pathogenesis
- bacterial p.
- p. of hyperreflexia

pathogenetic factor

pathogenic bacterium

pathogenicity

pathognomonic feature

pathologic, pathological
- p. diagnosis
- p. hypersecretory condition
- p. reflux
- p. resistive index level
- p. substaging

pathological (*var. of* pathologic)

pathology
- extravesical p.
- renal p.
- thoracic aortic p.

pathomechanism

pathophysiology of condition

pathway
- activation of programmed cell death p.
- antigen-dependent p.
- antigen-independent p.
- beta-oxidation p.
- care p.
- cholehepatic shunt p.
- cyclooxygenase p.
- gluconeogenic p.
- glutamine aminotransferase p.
- guanosine monophosphate p.
- lipoxygenase p.
- mitochondrial glutamate dehydrogenase p.
- monooxygenase p.
- multisynaptic p.
- neural p.
- nonapoptotic p.

oligosynaptic p.
paracellular p.
polyol p.
receptor-mediated endocytosis p.
renal transduction p.
replication p.
signal transduction p.
transcellular p.
transduction p.
Wnt/wingless signaling p.

PATI
Penetrating Abdominal Trauma Index
patient
American Association of Kidney P.'s
p. analgesia
asymptomatic hemodialysis p.
Child class A–C p.
cholestasia p.
cystinuric p.
diabetic p.
endoscopically normal p.
European primary sclerosing
cholangitis p.
p. factor
factors influencing colonic
involvement in p.'s
false-negative rate in high-risk p.
gastrectomized p.
hemodialysis p.
highly selective group of p.'s
hypoalbuminemic p.
hypochondriacal p.
immunophenotypical profiling of p.
immunosuppressed p.
institutionalized p.
irrigating p.
nonazotemic p.
nonirrigating p.
nonvoiding p.
p. positioning
posttransplant p.
renal transplant p.
seminal oxidative stress in p.
shock p.
stone-forming p.
tube-fed p.
unobstructed p.
patient-controlled
p.-c. analgesia (PCA)
p.-c. sedation (PCS)
pattern
abdominal wall venous p.
anhaustral colonic gas p.
circadian testosterone p.
cobblestone p.
colonic mucosal p.
complex calyceal p.
crow's-foot p.
cytometric p.

DNA ploidy p.
echo p.
fasted-to-fed p.
fasting motor p.
fed motor p.
fine gastric mucosal p.
fine reticular p.
fold p.
gallstone p.
gas p.
haustral p.
hindgut p.
histochemical p.
honeycomb p.
irregular amputated mucosal p.
manometric p.
meal-related secretion p.
mendelian p.
mesangial p.
mosaic duodenal mucosal p.
mucosal guideline p.
nodule-in-nodule p.
nonspecific gas p.
propulsive motor p.
punctate fluorescence p.
Quimby p.
reticulonodular p.
rugal p.
sausage-string p.
segment-specific expression p.
snakeskin mucosal p.
sonographic gallstone p.
spongy p.
trabecular sinusoidal p.
vascular p.
venous p.
Wilms tumor tubuloglomerular p.
Patterson-Parker
P.-P. method
P.-P. motif
patulous
p. anus
p. cardia
p. gastroesophageal junction
p. hiatus
p. papilla
p. pylorus
patupilone
Pauchet gastrectomy procedure
pauciimmune
p. antineutrophil cytoplasmic
antibody-associated
glomerulonephritis
p. crescentic glomerulonephritis
p. glomerular nephritis
paucity
bile duct p.
p. of clinical data
Paul-Mikulicz staged bowel resection

P

PDE
 peritoneal dialysis effluent
 phosphodiesterase
PDE5
 phosphodiesterase 5
  PDE5 inhibitor
PDE-I
 phosphodiesterase inhibitor
PDGF
 platelet-derived growth factor
PDH
 pyruvate dehydrogenase
PDL
 polycystic disease of liver
PDP
 pancreatic duct pressure
PDS
 pancreatic duct sphincter
 polydioxanone suture
  PDS Vicryl suture
PDT
 photodynamic therapy
  Photofrin PDT
PDUR
 postdialysis urea rebound
PE
 pharyngoesophageal
 platinum, etoposide
peak
 p. acid output (PAO)
 p. acid output after gastrin-releasing
  peptide (PAOGRP)
 p. acid output after pentagastrin
  stimulation (PAOPg)
 p. flow
 p. flow rate (PFR)
 p. pressure
 pressure p.
 p. response
 p. secretory flow rate (PSFR)
 p. secretory flow rate test
 p. urinary flow study
 p. uroflow
Péan
 P. clamp
 P. forceps
peanut
 p. agglutinin (PNA)
 p. dissector
 p. sponge
pearly
 p. papule of penis
 p. penile papule
Pearson
 P. product correlation
 P. syndrome
pea soup stool
PEB
 platinum, etoposide, bleomycin

pecqueti
 receptaculum p.
pecten
 anal p.
 p. analis
 p. band
 p. of anal canal
pectenitis
pectenotomy
pectin
pectinate line
pectin-based skin barrier
pectiniforme
 septum p.
pectoralis muscle
pedal
 p. control venography
 p. edema
 suction foot p.
Pedialyte RS electrolyte solution
Pediapred
PediaSure with Fiber
pediatric
 p. carcinoma
 p. colonoscope
 p. colonoscopy
 P. Crohn Disease Activity Index
  (PCDAI)
 P. Crohn's and Colitis Association,
  Inc.
 p. cryptococcal epididymoorchitis
 p. cryptorchidism
 p. endoscope
 p. endoscopy
 p. endstage liver disease (PELD)
 p. esophagogastroduodenoscopy
 p. feeding tube
 p. fiberscope
 p. gastroscope
 p. nasogastric tube
 p. neuroblastoma
 P. Peritoneal Dialysis Study
  consortium
 p. renal allotransplantation
 p. stirrup
 p. stone disease
 p. urinary tract infection
 p. urolithiasis
 p. urology
 p. voiding dysfunction
Pediazole
pedicle
 p. clamp
 p. flap urethroplasty
 p. graft
 p. island flap
 kidney vascular p.
 p. muscle flap
 omental p.

P

pedicle (*continued*)
    paravaginal p.
    renal p.
    vascular p.
pedicled
    p. omental graft
    p. omentoplasty
    p. omentum
    p. penile skin urethroplasty
pediculicide
pediculosis pubis
Pedi PEG tube
pedunculated
    p. angiodysplasia
    p. polyp
pedunculation
peel-away introducer sheath
peeping testis
Pee Wee low-profile gastrostomy tube
pefloxacin
PEG
    percutaneous endoscopic gastrostomy
    polyethylene glycol
      Bard PEG
      PEG bumper
      complete replacement PEG
      CT-guided PEG
      PEG insertion
      PEG lavage
      low-volume PEG
      Ponsky-Gauderer-type PEG
      PEG pull
      PEG push
      replacement PEG
      Sacks-Vine-type PEG
      Sandoz Caluso super PEG
      PEG tube
peg
    rete p.
PEG-assisted decompression
Pegasys
PEG-ELS
    polyethylene glycol electrolyte lavage
    solution
PEG-interferon
    PEG-i. alfa-2a
    PEG-i. alfa-2b powder for
      injection
PEG-intron
    PEG-I. powder for injection
    PEG-I. Redipen
PEG-J
    percutaneous endoscopic
    gastrojejunostomy
PEG-JET
    percutaneous endoscopic gastrostomy
    and jejunal extension tube
      PEG-JET placement
PEG-3500 solution

PEGstim
PEG-400 tube
pegylated interferon
pegylation
PEI
    percutaneous ethanol injection
    polyethylenimine
      PEI therapy
PEJ
    percutaneous endoscopic jejunostomy
      PEJ tube
PELD
    pediatric endstage liver disease
      PELD score
pelican biopsy forceps
Pelikan brand India ink
peliosis
    hepatic p.
    p. hepaticus
    p. hepatis
pellagra
    infantile p.
pellagroid
pellagrous
pellet
    p. artifact
    ^{99m}Tc-labeled Amberlite p.
    radiopaque p.
pelleted stool
pellicular enteritis
pellucida
    zona p.
pelves (*pl. of* pelvis)
pelvic
    p. abscess
    p. adhesion
    p. anatomy
    p. appendicitis
    p. autonomic nerve
    p. brim
    p. colon
    p. colonic surgery
    p. colon of Waldeyer
    p. diaphragm
    p. discontinuity
    p. evisceration
    p. exenteration
    p. fascia
    p. floor
    p. floor descent
    p. floor disorder
    p. floor dysfunction
    p. floor dyssynergia
    p. floor electrical stimulation
    p. floor electromyography
    p. floor exercise (PFE)
    p. floor movement
    p. floor muscle exercise (PFME)
    p. floor neurophysiology

p. floor rehabilitation
p. floor relaxation
p. floor syndrome
p. girdle relaxation (PGR)
p. ileal reservoir construction
p. ileal reservoir volume
p. inflammatory disease
  (PID)
p. kidney
p. lipomatosis
p. lymphadenectomy
p. lymph node
p. lymph node dissection
  (PLND)
p. lymphocelectomy
p. malleability
p. muscle strength
p. muscle training
p. nerve plexus
p. omentoplasty
p. organ prolapse
p. organ prolapse quantification
  (POP-Q)
P. Organ Prolapse Urinary
  Incontinence Sexual Questionnaire
p. osteotomy
p. peritoneum
p. phased-array coil
p. pole
p. pouch
p. pouchoscopy
p. pouch procedure
p. prolapse
p. sepsis
p. sidewall
p. stone
p. ultrasonography
p. ureter
p. ureterostomy
pelvicaliceal (*var. of* pelvicalyceal)
pelvicalyceal, pelvicaliceal
p. stasis
p. system
pelvicus
plexus p.
pelviectasis
pelvilithotomy (*var. of* pyelolithotomy)
pelvioileoneocystostomy
pelviolithotomy (*var. of* pyelolithotomy)
pelvioneocystostomy
pelvioneostomy
pelvioperitonitis, pelviperitonitis
pelvioplasty (*var. of* pyeloplasty)
pelvioradiography, pelviradiography
pelviostomy
pelviotomy, pelvitomy
pelviperitonitis (*var. of* pelvioperitonitis)
pelviradiography (*var. of*
  pelvioradiography)

pelvirectal
p. abscess
p. achalasia
p. fistula
pelvis, *pl.* **pelves**
arcus tendineus fasciae p.
bifid renal p.
bony p.
cavum p.
coccygeal p.
extrarenal renal p.
fascia p.
female p.
p. fracture
p. innervation
male p.
p. muscle
nonmalleable p.
obstructed p.
papilloma of renal p.
pseudospider p.
renal p.
spider p.
split p.
subepithelial hematoma of renal p.
pelviscope
pelviscopic clip ligation technique
PelviSoft mesh
pelvitomy (*var. of* pelviotomy)
pelviureteroradiography (*var. of*
  pyelography)
pelvocaliectasis
PEM
protein-energy malnutrition
Pemberton sigmoid clamp
pemoline
pemphigoid
benign mucous membrane p.
  (BMMP)
bullous p.
mucous membrane p.
pemphigus
benign familial p.
p. foliaceus
p. vulgaris
PE-MV balloon dilation catheter
pen
Intron A multidose p.
penbutolol
pencil
cautery p.
electrocautery p.
pencillike stool
pencil-tipped electrode
pendetide
satumomab p.
pendulous
p. abdomen
p. urethra

P

penectomy
    modified p.
    partial p.
    subcutaneous p.
penes (*pl. of* penis)
Penetrak
penetrating
    p. abdominal trauma
    P. Abdominal Trauma Index (PATI)
    p. pancreatic trauma
    p. penile trauma
    p. ulcer
    p. wound
penetration
    capsular p.
    splenic p.
Penetrex
Pen-F half-frame camera
penial (*var. of* penile)
penicillamine (PCA)
penicilli (*pl. of* penicillus)
penicilliary
penicillin
    benzathine p.
    beta-lactamase-resistant p.
    procaine p.
penicillin-streptomycin
Penicillium
    P. citrinum
    P. marneffei
penicillus, *pl.* **penicilli**
penile, penial
    p. amputation
    p. anomaly
    p. arterial reconstruction
    p. arteriography
    p. artery
    p. biothesiometry
    p. blood pressure
    p. body
    p. carcinoma
    p. clamp
    p. crus
    p. curvature
    p. cyst
    p. deformity
    p. disassembly
    p. Doppler
    p. duplex ultrasonography
    p. edema
    p. enlargement
    p. epispadias
    p. erection
    p. extensibility
    p. fibromatosis
    p. fibrosis
    p. hypospadias
    p. implant
    p. incarceration

    p. injection testing
    p. injection therapy
    p. intraepithelial neoplasia
    p. island flap
    p. kraurosis
    p. lesion
    p. melanosis
    p. modeling
    p. necrosis
    p. orthoplasty
    p. plethysmography
    p. prosthesis
    p. prosthesis implantation
    p. prosthesis mechanical problem
    p. prothesis reliability
    p. pulse volume recording
    p. raphe
    p. reconstruction
    p. reconstructive surgery
    p. reflex
    p. replantation
    p. revascularization
    p. root
    p. rupture
    p. schwannoma
    p. sclerosing lymphangitis
    p. sensitivity
    p. shaft degloving
    p. skin loss
    p. synechia
    p. torsion
    p. trauma
    p. tuberculosis
    p. tumescence
    p. urethra
    p. vascular function assessment
    p. vein ligation
    p. vein occlusion therapy
    p. venous ligation surgery
    p. vibratory stimulation
penile-brachial
    p.-b. index (PBI)
    p.-b. pressure index (PBPI)
penis, *pl.* **penes**
    adolescent p.
    albuginea p.
    angiofibroma of p.
    bifid p.
    bulbus p.
    buried p.
    p. captivus
    carcinoma in situ of glans p.
    chorda p.
    clubbed p.
    collum glandis p.
    concealed p.
    corona glandis p.
    corpus spongiosum p.
    crus p.

cutaneous horn of p.
dorsal nerve of p.
dorsum of p.
double p.
dystrophic p.
emissary vein of p.
flaccid p.
p. fracture
frenulum preputii p.
glans p.
hirsute papilloma of p.
inconspicuous p.
leukoplakia of p.
p. lunatus
p. lymphoma
micaceous growth of p.
p. palmatus
pearly papule of p.
p. plastica
preputium p.
prosthetic p.
pseudoepitheliomatous micaceous
  growth of p.
psoriasis of p.
radix p.
raphe p.
p. reconstruction
p. reflex
retractile concealed p.
p. sarcoma
scapus p.
septum of glans p.
trabeculae of corpora cavernosa of
  p.
trabeculae of corpus spongiosum of
  p.
trapped p.
venae cavernosae p.
ventrum of p.
webbed p.
penischisis
penitis
Penn
   P. pouch
   P. umbilical scissors
Pennington
   P. clamp
   P. forceps
   P. rectal speculum
pennyroyal oil
penoplasty
penopubic
   p. epispadias
   p. junction
penoscrotal
   p. hypospadias
   p. junction
   p. transposition
   p. transposition complex

p. trapping
p. webbing
penotomy
Penrose
   P. seton
   P. sump drain
pentagastrin (PG)
   p. gastric secretory test
   p. infusion
   p. infusion test
   p. provocative test
   p. stimulated analysis test
pentamidine-induced pancreatitis
pentamidine isethionate
pentane excretion level
pentapiperium
Pentasa
pentastomiasis
pentastomum
   p. denticulatum
   p. denticulatum nodule
pentavalent
   rotavirus vaccine, live oral p.
Pentax
   P. duodenoscope
   P. EC-series videoendoscope
   P. EG-2901, -2940, -3800
     endoscope
   P. EG-2900 videogastroscope
   P. EndoNet
   P. EndoNet digital endoscopy
     network
   P. endoscopic camera
   P. ESI-2000 fiberoptic endoscope
   P. EUP-EC124 ultrasound
     gastroscope
   P. FC-series colonoscope
   P. FD-series videoendoscope
   P. FG-32UA
   P. FG-36-UX linear-array
     echoendoscope
   P. FG-38X endoscope
   P. fiberscope
   P. FS-series flexible fiberoptic
     videosigmoidoscope
   P. linear-array echoendoscope
   P. prototype needle
   P. VSB-2000 fiberoptic endoscope
   P. VSB-P2900 pediatric colonoscope
   P. VSB-P-series enteroscope
Pentax/Hitachi FG-32UA
pentazocine
pentetreotide
   In-111 p.
   indium p.
   indium-111 p.
penthienate
pentolinium
pentopril

P

pentosan
    p. polysulfate
    p. polysulfate sodium
    p. sulfate
pentose phosphate shunt
pentosuria
pentoxifylline
Pento-X syndrome
peony
    European p.
peotomy
Pepcid
    P. AC
    P. Complete
    P. RPD
PEPCK
    phosphoenolpyruvate carboxykinase
peplomycin
pepo
    Cucurbita p.
peppermint oil
peppertree
    California p.
PEPS
    peroral electronic pancreatoscope
pepsic (*var. of* peptic)
pepsin
    inactivated p. (IP)
    p. secretion
pepsinogen
    p. A-C ratio
    p. level A, B, C
pepstatin
Peptamen
    P. Liquid
    P. liquid nutrition
Peptavlon stimulation test
peptic, pepsic
    p. cell
    p. cell receptor
    p. disease
    p. esophageal stricture
    p. esophagitis
    p. reflux
    p. reflux disease
    P. Relief
    P. Relief chewable tablet
    P. Relief liquid
    p. ulcer
    p. ulcer bleeding
    p. ulcer disease (PUD)
peptidase
    signal peptide p. (SPP)
peptide
    adrenomedullin 52-amino acid p.
    28-amino acid p.
    antibody to core p. 9 (anti-CP9)
    antibody to core p. 10 (anti-CP10)
    antral p.

    atrial natriuretic p. (ANP)
    brain-gut p.
    brain natriuretic p. (BNP)
    calcitonin gene-related p. (CGRP)
    Cathelin-related antimicrobial p.
      (CRAMP)
    cellular p.
    chemotactic p.
    C-type atrial natriuretic p.
      (C-ANP)
    C-type natriuretic p. (CNP)
    gastric inhibitory p. (GIP)
    gastrin-releasing p. (GRP)
    gastrointestinal regularity p.
    glucose-dependent insulinotropic p.
      (GIP)
    p. HI
    p. histidine isoleucine (PHI)
    p. hormone
    intestinal p.
    p. mass fingerprinting
    methionine-enkephalin p.
    monitor p.
    neutrophil chemotactic p.
    nucleocapsid-derived p.
    opioid p.
    paracrine p.
    peak acid output after
      gastrin-releasing p. (PAOGRP)
    plasma atrial natriuretic p.
    posttranslational processing of p.
    regulatory p.
    somatostatin p.
    trefoil p.
    trypsinogen activation p.
    p. tyrosine
    urinary trypsinogen activation p.
    vasoactive intestinal p. (VIP)
    vasoconstrictor p.
    p. YY (PYY)
peptide/bombesin
    gastrin-releasing p./b.
peptidergic
    p. mechanism
    p. neuron
Pepto-Bismol
peptone
Peptostreptococcus micros
per
    p. anum
    p. anum bleeding
    p. anum intersphincteric rectal
      dissection
    p. rectal portal scintigraphy
    p. rectum
Perceived Stress Scale (PSS)
percent
    p. reduction in urea (PRU)
    p. transferrin saturation

percentage
    p. frequency of bacteremia
    p. of hypochromic red cells (%HYPO)
Percival gastric balloon
Percodan
Percoll
    P. bead
    P. filter
Percufix catheter cuff kit
Percuflex
    P. Amsterdam stent
    P. biliary stent
    P. catheter
    P. endopyelotomy stent
    P. Plus ureteral stent
percussion
    dullness to p.
    p. note
    p. tenderness
percutaneous
    p. abscess drainage
    p. antegrade biliary drainage
    p. antegrade pyelography
    p. antegrade urography
    p. bacille Calmette-Gúerin administration
    p. balloon aspiration
    p. balloon dilation
    p. biliary bypass
    p. biliary drainage (PBD)
    p. bladder neck stabilization (PBNS)
    p. bladder neck suspension (PBNS)
    p. catheter cecostomy
    p. cholecystolithotomy (PCCL)
    p. choledochoscopy
    p. CT-guided aspiration
    p. debulking
    p. drainage of epididymal abscess
    p. embolization therapy
    p. endopyeloplasty
    p. endopyeloureterotomy
    p. endoscopic cecostomy
    p. endoscopic gastrojejunostomy (PEG-J)
    p. endoscopic gastrostomy (PEG)
    p. endoscopic gastrostomy and jejunal extension tube (PEG-JET)
    p. endoscopic gastrostomy and jejunal extension tube placement
    p. endoscopic jejunostomy (PEJ)
    p. endoscopic placement of jejunal tube
    p. endoscopic removal
    p. epididymal sperm aspiration (PESA)
    p. ethanol injection (PEI)
    p. ethanol injection therapy
    p. femoral vein catheter
    p. fetal cystoscopy

    p. fine-needle pancreatic biopsy
    p. gastroenterostomy (PGE)
    p. gastrostomy
    p. hepatobiliary cholangiography
    p. image-guided thermal ablation of hepatic metastasis
    p. liver biopsy (PLB)
    p. native renal biopsy
    p. needle aspiration
    p. nephrolithiasis
    p. nephrolitholapaxy
    p. nephrolithotomy (PCN, PCNL, PNL)
    p. nephrolithotripsy (PCNL)
    p. nephrostolithotomy (PCNL)
    p. nephrostomy
    p. nephrostomy Malecot catheter
    p. nephrostomy tube placement
    p. nerve evaluation (PNE)
    p. pancreas biopsy
    p. pressure ureteral perfusion test
    p. procedure
    p. radical cryosurgical ablation of prostate
    p. radiofrequency ablation
    p. removal of bezoar
    p. renal access
    p. resection
    p. sacral nerve root neuromodulation
    p. sampling method
    p. stent
    p. Stoller afferent nerve stimulation
    p. stone removal
    p. testis biopsy
    p. testosterone gel
    p. transcatheter perfusion
    p. transhepatic approach
    p. transhepatic biliary drainage (PTBD)
    p. transhepatic biliary drainage catheter
    p. transhepatic cholangiodrainage (PTCD)
    p. transhepatic cholangiogram (PTC, PTHC)
    p. transhepatic cholangiography (PTC, PTHC)
    p. transhepatic cholangioscopy (PTCS)
    p. transhepatic cholecystolithotomy (PCTCL)
    p. transhepatic cholecystoscopy (PTCC)
    p. transhepatic cholecystostomy
    p. transhepatic decompression
    p. transhepatic drainage (PTD)
    p. transhepatic liver biopsy with tract embolization
    p. transhepatic obliteration

P

percutaneous (*continued*)
    p. transhepatic obliteration of esophageal varix
    p. transhepatic pigtail catheter
    p. transhepatic portography (PTP)
    p. transluminal angioplasty (PTA)
    p. transluminal balloon angioplasty
    p. transluminal renal angioplasty (PTRA)
    p. transperineal seed implantation
    p. ultrasonic lithotriptor
    p. vasectomy
    p. vasography
Percy intestinal forceps
Percy-Wolfson gallbladder retractor
Perdiem Plain
perendoscopic manometry
Pereyra
    P. bladder neck suspension
    P. ligature carrier
    P. needle
    P. procedure
Pereyra-Raz cystourethropexy
PerFix Marlex mesh plug
perflubron
perforate
perforated
    p. acid peptic ulcer
    p. appendicitis
    p. appendix
    p. carcinoma
    p. cholecystitis
    p. diverticulum
    p. nasal septum
    p. ulcer disease
    p. viscus
perforating
    p. aneurysm
    p. diverticulitis
    p. forceps
    p. ulcer
perforation
    appendiceal p.
    barogenic p.
    bladder p.
    bowel p.
    cecal p.
    colonic p.
    ductal system p.
    duodenal ulcer p. (DUP)
    endoscopic sphincterotomy-induced duodenal p.
    eosinophilic ileal p.
    esophageal p.
    gastric p.
    iatrogenic tumor p.
    intestinal p.
    intraperitoneal p.
    Niemeier gallbladder p.

    p. of colon
    p. of gallbladder
    peritoneal p.
    polyethylene p.
    prepyloric p.
    pyloroduodenal p.
    resistant to electrosurgical p.
    retroduodenal p.
    retroperitoneal p.
    stercoraceous p.
perforin
performance
    cellulose acetate high p. (CAHP)
    p. characteristic
Performa ultrasound system
perfringens
    Clostridium p.
perfusate
    p. bag
    esophageal p.
    hyperosmolar p.
    p. solution
perfusion
    allogenic liver p.
    p. cannula
    CCD p.
    con A/anti-con A p.
    continuous hypothermic pulsatile p.
    p. cooling
    extracorporeal liver p. (ECLP)
    extracorporeal whole-organ p.
    ex vivo p.
    heterologous liver p.
    p. hypothermia technique
    hypothermic pulsatile p.
    intestinal p.
    intraperitoneal hyperthermic p. (IPHP)
    isolated hepatocyte p.
    p. machine
    percutaneous transcatheter p.
    plasma p.
    skin p.
    p. study
    transcatheter p.
    transvenous p.
    trickle p.
    ventilation p. (V/Q)
pergolide dopaminergic medication
perhexiline maleate
Periactin
periadventitial tissue
periampullary
    p. adenoma (PAA)
    p. carcinoma
    p. duodenal diverticulum
    p. duodenal tumor
    p. malignancy
    p. mass

p. neoplasm
p. pseudotumor
perianal
p. and enterourethral fistulae
p. anorectal space
p. area
p. condyloma
p. Crohn disease
P. Crohn Disease Activity Index (PCDAI)
p. edema
p. fistula
p. fistula abscess
p. hematoma
p. hygiene
p. infection
p. lesion
p. pain
p. region
p. sepsis
p. skin tag
p. soak
p. wart
periappendiceal red patch
periappendicitis decidualis
periarteritis
p. gummosa
p. nodosa
pericapillary diffusion
pericardial
p. air-fluid level
p. decompression
p. knock
pericarditis
constrictive p.
pericecal abscess
pericellular matrix (PCM)
pericentral
p. cholestasia
p. fibrosis
p. hypoxia
p. necrosis
p. pyridine nucleotide fluorescence
pericholangiolar
pericholangitis
pericholecystic
p. abscess
p. edema
p. stranding
pericholecystitis
gaseous p.
perichromatin granule
Peri-Colace
pericolic, pericolonic
p. abscess
p. fat
p. membrane syndrome
p. phlegmon
pericolitis

pericolonic (*var. of* pericolic)
pericolostomy area
pericostal suture
pericrypt eosinophilic enterocolitis
pericystectomy
RF-assisted cystectomy and p.
pericystitis
perididymis
perididymitis
peridiverticular
peridiverticulitis
phlegmonous p.
periductal
p. adenopathy
p. fibrosis
p. gland
periesophageal collateral vein
periesophagitis
chronic p.
perifascial nephrectomy
perigastric node
periglandular nonspecific inflammatory reaction
periglomerular space
perihepatic
p. adhesion
p. lymphadenopathy
perihepatitis syndrome
perihilar cholangiocarcinoma
periileal
perikaryon
perilobar pancreatitis
perilobular
p. duct
p. fibrosis
perimedial fibroplasia
perimesangial GBM
perimolysis, perimylolysis
perimylolysis (*var. of* perimolysis)
perinatal
p. hemochromatosis
p. torsion
p. urology
perindopril
perinea (*pl. of* perineum)
perineal
p. abscess
p. approach
p. body
p. Crohn disease
p. dermatitis
p. descent
p. drain
p. fascia
p. flexure
p. hypospadias
p. impact trauma
p. incision
p. infection

P

perineal (*continued*)
  p. lithotomy
  p. muscle
  p. nerve
  p. nerve terminal motor latency test
  p. pad
  p. polyp
  p. pouch
  p. prostatectomy
  p. raphe
  p. rectosigmoidectomy
  p. region
  p. section
  p. sensation
  p. sinus
  p. sinus tract
  p. skin tag
  p. tendon
  p. ulcer
  p. urethrostomy
  p. urethrotomy
  p. urinary fistula
perinei
  raphe p.
perineobulbar
  p. detrusor facilitative reflex
  p. detrusor inhibitory reflex
perineodetrusor inhibitory reflex
perineometer
  Peritron Precision p.
perineometry
perineorrhaphy
perineostomy
perineotomy
perinephria (*pl. of* perinephrium)
perinephric
  p. abscess
  p. fat
  p. fluid collection
  p. hematoma
  p. stranding
  p. tissue
perinephritic fibrosis
perinephrium, *pl.* **perinephria**
perineum, *pl.* **perinea**
  anterior p.
  bulging of p.
  female p.
  male p.
  posterior p.
  raphe of p.
  watering-can p.
  water pot p.
perinuclear
  p. antineutrophil cytoplasmic
    (p-ANC)
  p. antineutrophil cytoplasmic
    antibody (p-ANCA)
  p. intracellular staining

period
  dwell p.
  intradialytic p.
  pH-monitoring p.
periodic
  p. abdominalgia
  p. acid-Schiff (PAS)
  p. acid-Schiff-Alcian blue
    (PAS-AB)
  p. acid-Schiff-Alcian blue
    combination stain
  p. acid-Schiff stain
  p. acid-Schiff test
  p. peritonitis
  p. polyserositis
  p. vomiting
periodicity
  circadian p.
perioperative
  p. antibiotic
  p. data
  p. morbidity
  p. nutrition
  p. risk
  p. vomiting
peripancreatic
  p. area
  p. fibrosis
  p. fluid
  p. fluid collection
  p. necrosis
peripapillary diverticulum
peripartum
  p. endoscopy
  p. symphysis separation
peripelvic
  p. cyst
  p. extravasation
  p. fat
peripenial
peripheral
  p. acinar vein
  p. adrenergic agent
  p. arterial vasodilation theory
  p. arthritis
  p. bile duct
  p. bladder denervation
  p. blood lymphocyte (PBL)
  p. blood mononuclear cell (PBMC)
  p. capillary filtration slit length
  p. cholangiocarcinoma (PCC)
  p. extremity edema
  p. hyperalimentation
  p. intrahepatic cholangiocarcinoma
  p. intravenous alimentation
  p. leukocyte count
  p. loading
  p. necrosis
  p. nerve evaluation (PNE)

p. nerve evaluation test
p. T cell
p. vascular resistance
p. vasodilation
p. venipuncture
p. venous thrombosis
p. zone

periphery
hypoechoic p.

Periplast sealant
peripolesis
periportal
p. area
p. cirrhosis
p. fibrosis
p. hepatocyte
p. inflammation
p. invasion
p. pyridine nucleotide fluorescence
p. sinusoidal dilation

periportal-perisinusoidal fibrosis
periprandial
periprostatic
p. block
p. tissue

perirectal
p. abscess
p. fat
p. fat infiltration
p. fistula
p. mass
p. pain

perirenal
p. abscess
p. fascia
p. fat
p. hematoma

perisigmoid colon
perisinusoidal
p. cell
p. fibrin deposition
p. fibrosis
p. space

perispermatitis serosa
perisplenitis
fibropurulent p.

peristalsis
absent p.
antegrade p.
antral p.
decreased p.
disrupted p.
esophageal p.
high-amplitude p. (HAP)
mass p.
retrograde p.
reversed p.
secondary p.
visible p.

peristaltic
p. anastomosis
p. contraction
p. pump
p. reflex
p. rush
p. unrest
p. wave

peristomal, peristomatous
p. area
p. infection
p. skin
p. varix

peristomatous (*var. of* peristomal)
Peri-Strips
peritomy
peritonea (*pl. of* peritoneum)
peritoneal
p. access
p. adenocarcinoma
p. adhesion
p. anatomy
p. aspiration
p. attachment
p. autoplasty
p. band
p. biopsy
p. blastomycosis
p. button
p. carcinoma
p. carcinomatosis
p. cavity
p. cavity abscess
p. deposit
p. dialysate
p. dialysis (PD)
p. dialysis catheter (PDC)
p. dialysis creatinine clearance
target
p. dialysis effluent (PDE)
p. dialysis urea removal
p. dropsy
p. encapsulation
p. equilibration test (PET)
p. fluid
p. friction rub
p. fungal infection
p. lavage
p. leukocyte
p. loose body
p. lymphangiectasis
p. macrophage
p. malignancy
p. membrane permeability
p. membrane solute transport
capacity
p. membrane transport
p. mesothelial cell
p. mesothelioma

P

peritoneal (*continued*)
 p. mouse
 p. nodule
 p. perforation
 p. reflection
 p. sac
 p. seeding
 p. sign
 p. soilage
 p. solute transport
 p. space
 p. studding
 p. tap
 p. toilet
 p. transfusion
 p. tuberculosis
 p. vein
 p. window
peritoneal-anal distance
peritoneal-atrial shunt
peritonealgia
peritonealis
 cavitas p.
peritonealize, peritonize
peritonectomize
peritonei
 carcinomatosis p.
 pseudomyxoma p.
peritoneocaval shunt
peritoneocentesis
peritoneoclysis
peritoneogram
peritoneography
peritoneojugular shunt (PJS)
peritoneopathy
peritoneopexy
peritoneoplasty
peritoneoscope
peritoneoscopy
peritoneotomy
peritoneovenous
 p. shunt (PVS)
 p. shunt patency scan
peritoneum, *pl.* **peritonea**
 abdominal p.
 parietal p.
 pelvic p.
 visceral p.
peritonism
peritonitis
 adhesive p.
 bacterial p.
 barium p.
 benign paroxysmal p.
 bile p.
 Candida p.
 chemical p.
 chylous p.

 coccidioidal p.
 Coccidioides immitis p.
 p. deformans
 exudative p.
 fecal p.
 fungal p.
 generalized p.
 granulomatous p.
 Listeria monocytogenes p.
 meconium p.
 parasitic p.
 periodic p.
 postsclerotherapy bacterial p.
 primary p.
 sclerosing encapsulating p.
 secondary bacterial p.
 Sgambati test for p.
 spontaneous bacterial p. (SBP)
 starch granulomatous p.
 sterile p.
 subacute nonspecific p.
 tuberculous p.
peritonize (*var. of* peritonealize)
Peritron Precision perineometer
peritubular
 p. capillary
 p. fluid
 p. HCO_3^-
 p. myoid cell
 p. sodium
perityphlitis actinomycotica
periumbilical
 p. port
 p. region
periureteral, periureteric
 p. abscess
 p. fibrosis
 p. stone
 p. stranding
periureteric (*var. of* periureteral)
periureteritis plastica
periurethral
 p. abscess
 p. bulking agent
 p. collagen injection
 p. gland
 p. injection therapy
 p. ligament
 p. spongiofibrosis
 p. striated muscle
 p. vein
periurethral-transurethral microwave thermotherapy (P-TUMT)
periurethritis
perivascular
 p. fibroblast
 p. plexus
 p. sheath
perivascularis

perivenular
    p. confluent necrosis
    p. fibrosis
perivesical fat
perivesicular
perivesiculitis
periwinkle
Perkin-Elmer
    P.-E. 5000 atomic absorption
      spectrophotometer
    P.-E. thermal cycler
Perls
    P. reaction
    P. stain
Perma-Hand silk suture
Permalume covering
permanent
    p. end colostomy
    p. loop ileostomy
    p. section
    p. stoma
permanganate
    potassium p.
PermCath
    P. dual-lumen catheter
    Quinton P.
permeability
    capillary p.
    colonic p.
    increased bladder p.
    intestinal p.
    membrane p.
    mucosal vascular p.
    peritoneal membrane p.
    tight junction p.
    urea p.
    water p.
permeable
permeation
    lymphovascular p.
permethrin
Permitil Oral
Permixon group
permselectivity
Permutit method
pernasal cholangiogram
pernicious
    p. anemia
    p. malaria
    p. vomiting
    p. vomiting of pregnancy
peroral
    p. approach
    p. bougienage
    p. cholangiopancreatoscopy (PCPS)
    p. cholangioscopy (PCS)
    p. electronic pancreatoscope (PEPS)
    p. endoprosthesis
    p. endoscopy

    p. esophageal dilation
    p. gastroscope
    p. jejunal biopsy
    p. maneuver
    p. pancreatoscopy (POPS)
    p. pneumocolon examination
    p. retrograde pancreaticobiliary
      ductography
    p. shock wave lithotripsy (PSWL)
peroxidase
    cholesterol oxidase phenol
      4—aminoantipyrine p.
      (CHOD-PAP)
    endogenous p.
    glutathione p.
    p. stain
peroxidase-conjugated streptavidin
peroxidation
    lipid p.
    membrane p.
peroxide
    hydrogen p.
peroxisome proliferator-activated receptor (PPAR)
peroxynitrite-induced colitis
perphenazine
PerQ SANS
PerQ SANS system
Perry bag
PerryMeter anal electromyographic sensor EPS-21
Persantine
persimmon bezoar
persistent
    p. chronic hepatitis
    p. cloaca
    p. müllerian duct syndrome
    p. postmolar gestational trophoblastic
      tumor
    p. proteinuria
    p. pylorospasm
    p. symptom
    p. viral hepatitis (PVH)
    p. viral hepatitis non-A non-B
      (PVH-NANB)
    p. viral hepatitis type B (PVH-B)
    p. vomiting
personal
    P. EMG trainer
    p. experience
    p. preference
    P. Scanner TM 18 bedside real-time
      ultrasonography system
personality
    histrionic p.
    ulcer-prone p.
personalized program
PERT
    pancreatic enzyme replacement therapy

P

pertechnetate
  ^{99m}Tc sodium p.
  technetium-99m p.
Pertik diverticulum
Pertofrane
pertussin
  p. toxin
  p. toxin-sensitive G protein
pertussis
PERV
  porcine endogenous retrovirus
perversion
  taste p.
perversus
  situs p.
perverted appetite
PESA
  percutaneous epididymal sperm
  aspiration
pessary
  bladder neck support p.
  Gellhorn p.
  Smith-Hodge p.
pestis
  Yersinia p.
PET
  positron emission tomography
  PET scan
Petasites japonicus
petechia, *pl.* **petechiae**
  gastric p.
petechiae (*pl. of* petechia)
petechial
  p. angioma
  p. rash
Petersen
  P. bag
  P. operation
pethidine premedication
Petit triangle
petrificans
  urethritis p.
petrolatum
  p. gauze pack
  white soft p.
Pettenkofer test
Petz clamp
Peumus boldus
Peutz-Jeghers
  P.-J. gastrointestinal polyposis
  P.-J. hamartoma
  P.-J. polyp
  P.-J. syndrome (PJS)
Peyer
  aggregated lymphatic follicles of P.
  P. patch
Peyronie
  P. disease
  P. plaque

Pezzer
  P. catheter
  P. drain
Pfannenstiel incision
PFC
  pancreatic fluid collection
PFE
  pelvic floor exercise
PFIC
  progressive familial intrahepatic
  cholestasia
PFME
  pelvic floor muscle exercise
PFR
  peak flow rate
PFS
  pressure-flow study
  Adriamycin PFS
Pfuhl sign
PG
  pentagastrin
  prostaglandin
  Amogel PG
  serum PG
PG1, PG₁
  prostaglandin 1
PGE
  percutaneous gastroenterostomy
  prostaglandin E
PGE1, PGE₁
  prostaglandin E1
  intraurethral PGE1
PGE2, PGE₂
  prostaglandin E2
  exogenous PGE2
  ratio of PGF2-alpha PGE2
p15 **gene**
p16 **gene**
p18 **gene**
PGF
  prostaglandin F
PGF2-alpha
  prostaglandin F2-alpha
PGG
  prostaglandin G
PGG2
  prostaglandin G2
  PGG2 endoperoxide
PGH
  prostaglandin H
PGH2
  prostaglandin H2
  PGH2 endoperoxide
PGI2
  prostaglandin I2
PGL
  primary gastric lymphoma
PGN
  proliferative glomerulonephritis

PGR
  pelvic girdle relaxation
    symptom-giving PGR
PGV
  proximal gastric vagotomy
pH
  hydrogen ion concentration
    blood pH
    pH electrode placement
    gastric luminal pH
    pH holding time
    intracellular pH
    intraesophageal pH
    intragastric pH
    pH monitoring
    pH probe
    pH recording
    pH standardized meal
    pH test
    pH threshold
    urinalysis pH
    urinary pH
Phadebas angiotensin-I test
phage type
phagocyte
  bactericidal function of p.
  p. respiratory burst
phagocytic
  p. respiratory burst oxidase complex
  p. stellate cell
phagocytosis
phagosome
phallalgia
phallanastrophe
phallaneurysm
phallectomy
phalli (*pl. of* phallus)
phallic construction
phallitis
phalloarteriography
phallocampsis
phallocrypsis
phallodynia
phalloncus
phalloplasty
  reconstructive p.
  Shaeer augmentation p.
phalloplethysmography (PPG)
phallorrhagia
phallorrhea
phallotomy
phallus, *pl.* **phalli**
phantom
    P. 5 Plus ST balloon dilation
      catheter
    p. ulcer
pharmacoangiography
pharmacoarteriography
pharmacocavernosogram

pharmacocavernosography
pharmacocavernosometry
pharmacoduplex ultrasonography
pharmacodynamic
pharmacoendoscopy
  magnifying p.
pharmacokinetic
  everolimus p.'s
  famotidine p.'s
pharmacologic, pharmacological
  p. agent
  p. treatment
pharmacological (*var. of* pharmacologic)
pharmacologically induced erection
pharmacomechanical coupling
PharmaSeed
  P. I-125 brachytherapy
  P. iodine-125 seed
  P. palladium-103 seed
pharyngeal
  p. anesthesia
  p. diverticulum
  p. exudate
  p. pouch
  p. pouch syndrome
  p. tear
  p. tunic
  p. wall
pharyngeal-UES incoordination
pharynges (*pl. of* pharynx)
pharyngitis
  herpes p.
pharyngobasilar tunic
pharyngoesophageal (PE)
  p. diverticulectomy
  p. diverticulum
  p. function
  p. junction
  p. sphincter
  p. tear
pharyngoesophagogastroduodenoscopy
pharyngolaryngoesophagectomy
pharynx, *pl.* **pharynges**
phase (ph)
  complement-independent autologous
    p.
  hepatic arterial-dominant p.
    (HAP)
  p. II contraction
  p. II, III marrow transplant
    recipient
  lag p.
  M p.
  micturition p.
  mycelial p.
  predialysis p.
  pre-S p.
  prolonged expiratory p.
  4 phases of swallowing

P

phase (*continued*)
  reservoir p.
  skin graft imbibition p.
  skin graft inoculation p.
phasic
  p. contractile activity
  p. contraction
  p. fluctuation on squeeze
  p. wave duration
  p. wave sequence
phasic-free tone variation
Phazyme
Phazyme-95, -125
Phazyme-PB
phenacetin
  p. nephritis
  p. nephropathy
phenazopyridine
  p. hydrochloric acid
  p. hydrochloride
  sulfamethoxazole and p.
  sulfisoxazole and p.
phencyclidine abuse
phendimetrazine
phenelzine
Phenergan
phen-fen diet
phenindamine
phenindione hypersensitivity
phenmetrazine
phenobarbital
phenol
  aqueous p.
  p. II
  p. red chromoendoscopy
Phenolax
phenolphthalein
phenolsulfonphthalein (PSP)
**phenoltetrachlorophthalein
  test**
phenomena (*pl. of
  phenomenon*)
phenomenon, *pl.* **phenomena**
  bicalutamide withdrawal p.
  capillary leak p.
  cloud p.
  common cavity p.
  disappearing p.
  dystonic p.
  first-set p.
  Goldblatt p.
  Hayflick p.
  jet stream p.
  J-wave p.
  Kanagawa p.
  mask p.
  pathergy p.
  Schramm p.
  second-set p.

vanishing cancer p.
  walking stick p.
  yo-yo weight fluctuation p.
phenothiazine
phenotype
  antigenic p.
  B cellular p.
  CD4 p.
  CD8 p.
  codominant p.
  colonic p.
  HLA class II p.
  p.'s of mast cells
  partial nephrogenic diabetes
    insipidus p.
  Potter p.
  replication error p.
  slow bilirubin glucuronidation p.
  ZZ p.
phenotypic
  p. expression
  p. sex
  p. study
Phenoxine
phenoxodiol
phenoxybenzamine hydrochloride
phenoxymethylpenicillin
phenprocoumon
phentermine
phentolamine
  p. methylate
  p. test
phenylacetate
phenylalanine
phenylbutazone hepatotoxicity
phenylephrine
phenylethyl alcohol agar
Phenyl-Free oral liquid
phenylhydrazine
phenyl-methane-sulfonyl fluoride
phenylpropanolamine
phenylpropylmethylamine
phenytoin
pheochromocytoma
  bilateral p.'s
  bladder p.
  ectopic p.
  familial p.
  malignant p.
  retroperitoneal laparoscopic
    adrenalectomy for p.
PHG
  portal hypertensive gastropathy
PH-I, II
  primary hyperoxaluria
  type I, II
Philadelphia chromosome
philippinensis
  Capillaria p.

Phillips
- P. catheter
- P. CM 12 electron microscope
- P. LaxCaps
- P. Milk of Magnesia
- P. rectal clamp
- P. ultrasound machine

phimoses (*pl. of* phimosis)
phimosiectomy
phimosis, *pl.* **phimoses**
- adult p.

phimotic
pH-Informer Deltron probe
pHisoHex scrub
PHIV
- portal hypertensive intestinal vasculopathy

PHLA
- postheparin lipolytic activity

phlebectasia
- intestinal p.

phlebitis
- enterocolic lymphocytic p. (ELP)
- Mondor p.

phlebography
- intraoperative p.

phlebolith
phleborheography
- Cranley p.

phlebosclerosis
- chronic ischemic colonic lesion caused by p. (CICLP)

phlegmon
- diverticular p.
- pancreatic p.
- pericolic p.

phlegmonous
- p. abscess
- p. adenitis
- p. alcoholic fatty liver
- p. change
- p. enteritis
- p. gastritis
- p. mass
- p. pancreatitis
- p. peridiverticulitis

phlorizin
pH-manometry probe
pH-meter
- intragastric continuous pH-m.

pH-metric testing
pH-metry
- esophagogastric pH-m.
- 24-hour ambulatory pH-m.
- 24-hour home pH-m.

pH-monitoring period
PHN
- passive Heymann nephritis

pholedrine

phonoenterography
- computerized p.

phonorenogram
phorbol
- p. ester
- 12-O-tetradecanoylphorbol-13-acetate
- p. ester TPA
- p. myristate acetate (PMA)

PhosLo
Phosphaljel
phosphatase
- alkaline p. (ALP, AP)
- alkaline phosphatase-antialkaline p. (APAAP)
- p. and tensin homologue deleted on chromosome 10
- Bessey-Lowry unit for alkaline p.
- bone alkaline p. (BAP)
- bone-specific alkaline p. (BALP)
- leukocyte alkaline p. (LAP)
- phosphorylase p.
- placental alkaline p.
- prostate-specific acid p.
- prostatic acid p. (PAP)
- protein tyrosine p.
- total serum prostatic acid p. (TSPAP)

phosphate
- aluminum p.
- p. binder therapy
- calcium hydrogen p.
- cellulose p.
- chloroquine p.
- p. crystal
- dexamethasone sodium p.
- dietary p.
- disopyramide p. (DP, D.P.)
- elemental p.
- p. enema
- estramustine p.
- fludarabine p.
- Hexadrol P.
- p. ion (PI)
- p. ion-urea (PI-urea)
- magnesium ammonium p.
- nicotinamide adenine dinucleotide p. (NADPH)
- paranitrophenol p.
- phosphatidylinositol p. (PI4P)
- potassium p.
- potassium-titanyl p. (KTP)
- pyridoxal p.
- renal p.
- serum p.
- sodium p. (NaP)
- sodium cellulose p.

phosphate-buffered
- p.-b. saline (PBS)
- p.-b. saline solution

phosphate-dependent glutaminase (PDG)

P

577

phosphate-independent glutaminase (PIG)
phosphatidylethanolamine
phosphatidylinositol (PI)
    p. 4,5-bisphosphate (PI4,5P2)
    p. phosphate (PI4P)
phosphatidylserine
phosphaturia
phosphodiester
phosphodiesterase (PDE)
    p. 5 (PDE5)
    p. inhibitor (PDE-I)
phosphoenolpyruvate carboxykinase (PEPCK)
phosphofructokinase
phosphoglucomutase
phosphoinositide 3-kinase
phosphokinase
    creatine p. (CPK)
phospholipase
    p. A2 (PLA2)
    p. A2 catalytic activity
    p. C (PLC)
    p. D (PLD)
phospholipid
    p. bilayer
    gG p. (GPL)
    p. ratio
    serum p.
phospholipid-bound choline concentration
phospholipidosis
phosphonoformate
phosphopeptidomannan (PPM)
phosphoprotein
    glycosylated p.
phosphoramidite chemistry
phosphoribosyltransferase
    adenine p. (APRT)
    hypoxanthine-guanine p. (HGPRT)
phosphorous-31 magnetic resonance spectroscopy
phosphorus
    dietary p.
    p. metabolism
    p. poisoning
    serum p.
    tubular reabsorption of p.
phosphorus-32 (P-32, ^{32}P)
phosphorylase
    brain-type glycogen p. (BGP)
    glycogen p.
    p. phosphatase (PP)
    uridine p.
phosphorylated growth factor receptor
phosphorylation
    host tyrosine p.
    oxidative p.

    protein p.
    p. protein
    src p.
    tyrosine p.
phosphorylcholine
Phospho-soda
    P.-s. enema
    Fleet P.-s.
phosphotungstic acid-magnesium chloride precipitation method
phosphotyrosine antibody
phosphotyrosine-SH2 binding
phosphotyrosyl protein profile
photoablation
    laser p.
    Nd:YAG laser p.
photoaffinity
photochemical ablation
photochemotherapy
photocoagulation
    infrared p.
    laser p.
    transendoscopic laser p.
    p. treatment
photodestruction
    laser p.
photodiode
photodocumentation
photodynamic
    p. diagnosis
    p. imaging
    p. therapy (PDT)
Photofrin
    P. derivative
    P. PDT
photogastroscope
photography
    endoscopic p.
    instant p.
    laparoscopic p.
    television p.
photoirradiation
photometer
    Anthos ht II automatic p.
    TUR-Cue p.
photometry
    flame p.
photomicrograph
    high-power p.
    low-power p.
    medium-power p.
    p. of colonoscopic biopsy specimen
    p. of specimen staining
photomicrography
photomultiplier tube
photon-deficient lesion
photophobia
photoradiation therapy
Photoscan-3 hematoporphyrin derivative

photoselective vaporization of prostate (PVP)
photosensitivity
photosensitizer
  porphyrin p.
photosensitizing hemoporphyrin derivative
photothermal laser ablation
photothermolysis
  laser p.
PHP
  pseudohypoparathyroidism
PH30 protein
phrenalgia
phrencolic ligament
phrenectomy (*var. of* phrenicectomy)
phrenemphraxis
phrenic artery
phrenicectomize
phrenicectomy, phrenectomy, phrenicoexeresis, phreniconeurectomy
phreniclasia, phreniclasis, phrenicotripsy
phreniclasis (*var. of* phreniclasia)
phrenicocolic, phrenocolic
  p. ligament
phrenicoesophageal ligament
phrenicoexeresis (*var. of* phrenicectomy)
phreniconeurectomy
phrenicosplenic, phrenosplenic
phrenicotomy
phrenicotripsy (*var. of* phreniclasia)
phrenocolic (*var. of* phrenicocolic)
phrenocolopexy
phrenodynia
phrenoesophageal membrane
phrenogastric
phrenoglottic
phrenohepatic
phrenoplegia
phrenoptosia, phrenoptosis
phrenoptosis
phrenospasm
phrenosplenic (*var. of* phrenicosplenic)
phrygian
  p. cap
  p. cap deformity
pH-sensitive radiotelemetry capsule
PHS I, II
PHSL
  primary hepatosplenic lymphoma
  B-cell PHSL
PHTN
  portal hypertension
Phycomycetes
phycomycosis
phyllodes
  cystosarcoma p.
phylloquinone, phylloquinone K
phylogenetic tree

physalopteriasis
physical
  p. examination
  p. examination finding
  p. inactivity
physician
  treating p.
Physicians' Health Study I, II
Physick pouch
physicochemical basis of gallstone formation
physiograph
physiologic, physiological
  p. condition
  p. gastrectomy
  p. jaundice
  p. measurement
  p. pH solution
  p. reflux test (PRT)
  p. role in acid secretion
  p. salt solution
  p. scaling
  p. testosterone replacement therapy
  p. trophic effect
physiological (*var. of* physiologic)
physiology
  anorectal p.
  renal p.
  p. testing
physiotherapy
  chest p.
physostigmine
phytobezoar
phytochemical
phytoestrogen
phytoestrogen-induced menstrual cycle disturbance
phytohemagglutinin
phytonadione
phytopharmaceutical
phytosterolemia
phytotherapy
phytyl group
PI
  phosphate ion
  phosphatidylinositol
    PI 3-kinase
    PI surgical stapler
PIB
  partial ileal bypass
PIC
  polysaccharide-iron complex
pica
Picchini syndrome
pick
  P. cell
  P. testicular adenoma
  P. tubular adenoma
  tubular adenoma of P.

P

Picker Vista Magnascanner
picket fence appearance
Pickrell operation
pickwickian syndrome
picobirnavirus
Picolax
Picoprep-3
Picornaviridae
picornavirus
picosulfate
    sodium p.
picrorrhiza
PICT
    pancreatic islet cell transplantation
PID
    pelvic inflammatory disease
PI-90 double-headed stapler
piecemeal
    p. necrosis
    p. polypectomy
    p. resection
2-piece ostomy pouch
Pierre Robin syndrome
Piersol point
piezoelectric
    p. crystal
    p. generator
    p. lithotripsy
    p. shock wave
    p. shock wave lithotriptor
    p. transducer
piezoelectrically generated ultrasound
Piezolith
    P. EPL
    P. EPL lithotriptor
    P. lithotriptor
piggyback
    p. liver transplantation
    P. needle-knife papillotome
piggybacking of IV
pigment
    Dubin-Johnson p.
    gastric p.
    p. neuropathy
    p. stone
pigmentary cirrhosis
pigmentation
pigmented (pigm)
    p. gallstone
    p. histiocyte
    p. nevus
    p. nipple
    p. protuberance
pigment-laden Kupffer cell
pigmentosa
    urticaria p.
pigmenturia
PIGN
    postinfectious glomerulonephritis

pIgR
    polyimmunoglobulin receptor
pigtail
    p. biliary stent
    p. catheter
    p. endoprosthesis
    p. nephrostomy tube
3/4-pigtail plastic endoprosthesis
PIL
    primary intestinal lymphangiectasis
pile
    bleeding p.
    prostatic p.
    sentinel p.
    thrombosed p.
pilimiction
pili torti et canaliculus
pill
    p. esophagitis
    video p.
pillar
    palatine p.
PillCam
    P. ESO capsule endoscope
    P. ESO capsule endoscopy
    P. ESO videocamera
pill-induced
    p.-i. esophageal injury
    p.-i. esophagitis
pillow
    Bedge p.
    MedSlant therapeutic p.
    Sand-Eze EGD p.
    p. sign
pilonidal
    p. cyst
    p. cystectomy
    p. perirectal abscess
    p. sinus
    p. sinus disease
pilosicoli
    Serpulina p.
pilot study
pimagedine
pimelorrhea
PIN
    prostatic intraepithelial neoplasia
pinacidil
pinch
    p. biopsy
    diaphragmatic p.
    p. forceps
    p. injury
pinchcock
    diaphragmatic p.
    p. effect
    p. mechanism
pindolol
pineapple test

pine cone appearance of
  bladder
pineoblastoma
pinguecula, pinguicula
pinguicula (*var. of* pinguecula)
P15/INK4B gene
pinocytosis
    fluid-phase p.
    p. vacuole
pinpoint pupil
Pin-Rid
pinus bark
pinwheel appearance
pinworm
Pin-X
PI4P
    phosphatidylinositol phosphate
PIP
    pressure inversion point
    PIP on esophageal manometry
PI4,5P2
    phosphatidylinositol 4,5-bisphosphate
pipe
    endoscopic washing p.
    Mauch double-sheathed plastic
      wash p.
pipecuronium
pipenzolate
piperacillin sodium
piperazine citrate
piperidolate
piperoxan
pipestem
    p. cirrhosis
    p. stool
PIPIDA
    paraisopropyliminodiacetic
      acid
    PIPIDA hepatobiliary scan
    ^{99m}Tc PIPIDA
Pippi
    P. Salle technique
    P. Salle urethral lengthening
      procedure
Pipracil
Pipsissewa
PIR
    pressure increment rate
pirenzepine
piretanide
piriform, pyriform
    p. fossa
    p. pooling
    p. sinus
piriformis, pyriformis
    p. artery
    p. muscle
piritramide
piritrexim

piroxicam
PI-30 stapler
piston-type syringe
pit
    anal p.
    p. cell
    clathrin-coated p.
    colonic p.
    Frey gastric p.
    gastric p.
    mucosal p.
    postanal p.
pitcher plant
pitfall
    potential p.
Pitres sign
Pitressin
pitting
    anal p.
    colonic p.
    p. edema
    gastric p.
pituitary
    p. adenoma
    p. adenylate cyclase-activating
      polypeptide (PACAP)
pituitary-gonadal axis
pityriasis
    p. lingua
    p. rotunda
Pityrosporon orbiculare
PI-urea
    phosphate ion-urea
pivalate derivative
PIVKA
    protein in vitamin K absence
PIVKA-II
    prothrombin induced by vitamin K
      absence or antagonist-II
    PIVKA-I. antagonist
    PIVKA-I. EIA kit for hepatocellular
      carcinoma
PIVOT
    Prostate Cancer Intervention Versus
      Observation Trial
pivoxil
    cefditoren p.
PiZZ alpha-1-antitrypsin deficiency
PJS
    peritoneojugular shunt
    Peutz-Jeghers syndrome
PKA
    protein kinase A
PKC
    protein kinase C
PKD1, PKD2 gene
P27Kip1 gene
PLA2
    phospholipase A2

P

placebo
  p. effect
  p. therapy
placebo-controlled trial
placement
  band p.
  dilator p.
  electrode p.
  endoscopic biliary stent p.
  endotracheal tube p.
  feeding tube p.
  graft p.
  intestinal sling p.
  laparoscopic trocar p.
  metallic stent p.
  PEG-JET p.
  percutaneous endoscopic gastrostomy
    and jejunal extension tube p.
  percutaneous nephrostomy
    tube p.
  pH electrode p.
  4-port diamond p.
  5-port fan p.
  posttreatment p.
  radiologic biliary stent p.
  tube p.
  ultrasound-assisted PEG p.
  ureteral stent p.
  wire-guided p.
placental alkaline phosphatase
Placer guidewire
plain
  p. abdominal radiography
  p. catgut suture
  p. film
  p. film of abdomen
  p. gut
  p. gut suture
  Perdiem P.
  p. radiograph
plan
  NutraPrep preprocedure meal p.
planar
  p. imaging
  p. xanthoma
plane
  Addison clinical p.'s
  Camper p.
  cleavage p.
  intersphincteric p.
  ischiorectal fossa p.
  p. of dissection
  p. of Treves
  parasagittal p.
planimeter
planimetric measurement
planimetry
  impedance p.
  rectal impedance p.

planktonic bacterium
plant
  castor oil p.
  pitcher p.
Plantago ovata **seed**
plantain
  English p.
plantar grasp
plantaris
  hyperkeratosis palmaris et p.
  tylosis palmaris et p.
plantarum
  Lactobacillus p.
  Lactobacillus plantarum 299v
planuria
planus
  lichen p.
plaque
  atherosclerotic p.
  augmentation p.
  p. excision
  Hollenhorst p.
  p. incision
  ostial atherosclerotic p.
  Peyronie p.
  Randall p.
  stone p.
plaquelike
  p. lesion
  p. linear defect
  p. thickening
plasm (*var. of* plasma)
plasma, plasm
  p. albumin
  p. ammonia
  p. androgen
  p. apo B-48
  p. atrial natriuretic peptide
  p. bile acid measurement
  p. bubble
  p. caffeine concentration
  p. catecholamine
  p. cell
  p. cell balanitis
  p. cell granuloma
  p. cell hepatitis (PCH)
  p. cell portal infiltration
  p. clearance
  p. cloud
  p. cortisol
  p. creatinine
  cryoprecipitated p.
  dialysis to p.
  p. enzyme
  p. exchange
  p. fibronectin
  p. flow
  fresh frozen p. (FFP)
  gastric p.

p. gastrin concentration
p. homocysteine
p. inulin
p. ionized calcium
p. kallikrein
p. membrane marker
p. methionine-enkephalin
p. norepinephrine concentration
p. oncotic pressure
p. osmolality
p. parathyroid hormone
p. perfusion
p. protein
p. protein fraction
p. renin
p. renin activity
p. renin activity captopril test
p. renin concentration
p. tonicity
p. ultrafiltrate
p. urea
p. urea concentration
p. viscosity
p. volume
p. volume depletion
p. volume expansion

plasma-activated
p.-a. complement 3 (C3a)
p.-a. complement 4 (C4a)
p.-a. complement 5 (C5a)

plasmablastic myeloma
plasmacellularis
balanitis circumscripta p.

plasmacytoma, plasmocytoma
bladder p.
extramedullary p.
gastric p.
radioresistant gastric p.

plasmacytosis
plasma-free choline concentration
PlasmaKinetic
P. radiofrequency energy
delivery
P. surgery

plasmalogen
Plasma-Lyte
Plasmanate
plasmapheresis
therapeutic p.

plasmid
p. mediated
p. profile
p. profile role

plasminogen
p. activator
p. activator inhibitor
p. activator inhibitor type 1, 2
(PAI-1, -2)
functional p.

plasmocytoma (*var. of* plasmacytoma)
plasmodium
encapsulated p.
P. falciparum
P. falciparum malaria
P. malariae

Plastibell circumcision
plastica
linitis p.
penis p.
periureteritis p.
rectal linitis p. (RLP)

plastic endoprosthesis
plasty
bladder neck Y-V p.
Foley Y-V p.
mons p.
posterior bladder flap p.
V-Y p.
Y-V p.

plate
anal p.
bladder p.
blood agar p.
bowel p.
brain-heart infusion p.
cloacal p.
exstrophic bladder p.
hilar p.
levator p.
limiting p.
liver cell p.
Maxisorb test p.
microwell p.
Mueller-Hinton-supplemented
agar p.
Skirrow agar p.
trigonal p.
tubularized incised p.
urethral p.

plateau
dieting p.
p. response

platelet
p. abnormality
p. activation
p. count
p. dysfunction
p. factor 4
p. glycoprotein 2b3a receptor
antagonist
p. transfusion

platelet-activating factor (PAF)
platelet-derived growth factor (PDGF)
Platinol
etoposide, Adriamycin, P. (EAP)
5-fluorouracil, Adriamycin, P. (FAP)
fluorouracil, leucovorin rescue,
Adriamycin, P. (FLAP)

P

Platinol (*continued*)
      Ifex, Taxol, P. (ITP)
      VePesid, ifosfamide with mesna
      rescue, P. (VIP)
platinum
      cyclophosphamide, Velban,
      actinomycin D, bleomycin, p.
      p., etoposide (PE)
      p., etoposide, bleomycin (PEB)
      Velban, actinomycin D,
      bleomycin, p.
      p., Velban, bleomycin (PVB)
platinum-based consolidation
  chemotherapy
platysma
PLB
      percutaneous liver biopsy
PLC
      phospholipase C
PLC-50 linear stapler
PLC/PRF5 cell
PLD
      phospholipase D
      polycystic liver disease
pleating of small bowel
Pleatman sac
Plegine
pleiotropic
Plenaxis powder for IM injection
pleomorphic
      p. destructive cholangitis
      p. rhabdomyosarcoma
pleomorphism
      nuclear hyperchromasia and p.
Plesiomonas shigelloides
plethora
plethoric
plethysmography
      impedance p. (IPG)
      penile p.
pleura, *pl.* **pleurae**
      mediastinal p.
pleurae (*pl. of* pleura)
pleural
      p. mass
      p. rub
      p. tube
pleuritis
      bile p.
pleurobiliary fistula
pleurocholecystitis
pleuroesophageal muscle
pleuroperitoneal
      p. canal
      p. foramen
      p. sinus
pleurovisceral
plexiform neurofibroma (PN)
plexus (plx), *pl.* **plexus, plexuses**

Auerbach and Meissner p.
Auerbach mesenteric p.
biliary p.
celiac p.
colonic myenteric p.
cystic p.
deep muscular p.
distal venous p.
esophageal p.
extrapancreatic nerve p.
fundic p.
ganglionated p.
gastric p.
gastroesophageal variceal p.
gastrointestinal myenteric p.
hemorrhoidal p.
hypogastric p.
ileocolic p.
inferior anal p.
inferior hypogastric p.
p. interiliacus
longitudinal subepithelial venous p.
lumbar p.
lumbosacral p.
Meissner p.
middle rectal venous p.
mucosal p.
myenteric p.
p. myentericus
neural p.
nonganglionated p.
pampiniform p.
p. pampiniformis
pelvic nerve p.
p. pelvicus
perivascular p.
preprostatic p.
prostaticovesical p.
p. prostaticus
proximal venous p.
rectal p.
p. renalis
sacral p.
Santorini venous p.
spermatic p.
p. spermaticus
submucosal venous p.
submucous p.
submuscular p.
suburothelial nerve p.
superior hypogastric nerve p.
superior rectal venous p.
suprarenal p.
testicular p.
p. testicularis
thyreoideus impar p.
ureteral p.
p. uretericus
vascular p.

p. venosus
vesical p.
p. vesicalis
vesicoprostatic p.
plexuses (*pl. of* plexus)
pliable lesion
plica, *pl.* **plicae**
plicae circulares
p. duodenalis inferior
p. duodenalis superior
p. epigastrica
p. ileocecalis
p. longitudinalis
p. pubovesicalis
Rathke p.
p. umbilicalis
p. vesicalis transversa
plicae (*pl. of* plica)
plicamycin
plicated appendicocystostomy
plication
Bard endoscope transesophageal
endoscopic p.
Childs-Phillips bowel p.
dorsal curve p.
fundal p.
Graham p.
Kaliscinski p.
Kelly p.
Nesbit corporeal p.
Noble bowel p.
Rehne-Delorme p.
Starr p.
p. suture
suture p.
transesophageal endoscopic p.
(TEP)
transgastric p.
transmesenteric p.
tunica albuginea p.
plicator
His-Wiz device endoscopic p.
ploidy
p. analysis
chromosome p.
plot
Eadie-Hofstee p.
pluck technique
plug
bile p.
canalicular bile p.
Coloplast Conseal p.
p. gastrostomy
meconium p.
omental p.
one-piece disposable p.
PerFix Marlex mesh p.
protein p.
urethral p.

plugged liver biopsy
plumbism
plume
laser p.
Plummer
P. bag
P. dilator
P. treatment
Plummer-Vinson syndrome
pluripotent, pluripotential
pluripotential (*var. of* pluripotent)
plus
Bayer P.
Charcoal P.
Ensure P.
HCV QuantaSure P.
Lithostar P.
Liver Panel P. 9
Losotron P.
Maalox P.
Pyridium P.
Resource P.
Riopan P.
RX Herculink P.
Therevac P.
Titralac P.
PMA
phorbol myristate acetate
PMA-stimulated O$_2$
PMC
pontine micturition center
pseudomembranous colitis
PMMA
polymethylmethacrylate
PMMA bead
PMME
primary malignant melanoma of
esophagus
PMN
polymorphonuclear
PMN cell
PMN chemotaxis assay
PMN infiltrate
PMN leukocyte
PMN oxidative burst capacity
uremic PMN
PMN-elastase
fecal PMN-e.
**PMN-mediated endothelial cell
injury**
PMNN
polymorphonuclear neutrophil
P-Mod-S factor
PMP
postmenopausal
PMR
polymorphic reticulosis
PN
pyelonephritis

P

PNE
  percutaneous nerve evaluation
  peripheral nerve evaluation
  PNE test
pneumatic
  p. bag
  p. bag dilation of esophagus
  p. bag esophageal dilation
  p. balloon catheter dilation
  p. balloon dilator
  p. compression device (PCD)
  p. endoscopic lithotriptor
  p. leg pump
  p. lithotripsy
pneumatinuria (*var. of* pneumaturia)
pneumatocele
  scrotal p.
pneumatosis
  p. cystoides coli (PCC)
  p. cystoides intestinalis (PCI)
  intestinal p.
pneumaturia, pneumatinuria
pneumocholecystitis
pneumococcal infection
pneumococcus nephritis
pneumocolon
  spiral computed tomography p.
Pneumocystis
  P. carinii (PC)
  P. carinii pneumonia (PCP)
pneumocystosis
  gastric p.
pneumodissection
pneumoenteritis
pneumogastrography
pneumography
  retroperitoneal p.
pneumohydraulic capillary infusion system
pneumohydroperitoneum
pneumokidney
pneumomediastinum
pneumonectomy
pneumonia
  aspiration p.
  lymphoid interstitial p.
  Pneumocystis carinii p. (PCP)
  Proteus p.
  Pseudomonas aeruginosa p.
  Pseudomonas pseudomallei p.
pneumoniae
  Klebsiella p.
pneumonitis
  radiation p.
pneumopenis
pneumopericardium
pneumoperitoneum
  benign p.
  p. needle

  stent-induced p.
  tension p.
pneumoperitonitis
pneumophila
  Legionella p.
pneumopyelography
pneumoradiography
  retroperitoneal p.
pneumoretroperitoneum
pneumoscrotum
Pneumo Sleeve
pneumostatic dilation
pneumothoraces (*pl. of* pneumothorax)
pneumothorax, *pl.* **pneumothoraces**
  iatrogenic p.
  tension p.
PNH
  paroxysmal nocturnal hemoglobinuria
PNI
  prognostic nutritional index
POA
  pancreatic oncofetal antigen
  POA test
Pockel cell
pocketed calculus
pod
  bean p.
podocalyxin
podocin
podocyte
  glomerular p.
  p. glycocalyx
podocyte-specific protein
podofilox solution
podophyllin
podophyllotoxin
POEMS
  polyneuropathy, organomegaly, endocrinopathy, monoclonal protein, and skin changes
  POEMS syndrome
poikilocyte
  teardrop p.
point
  Addison p.
  APACHE-II p.
  bleeding p.
  Boas p.
  Brewer p.
  Cannon p.
  Chauffard p.
  Desjardins p.
  dorsal p.
  F2 focal p.
  Griffith p.
  Halle p.
  Hartmann p.
  Lanz p.
  Mackenzie p.

McBurney p.
Munro p.
p. of respiratory reversal on
esophageal manometry
Piersol p.
pressure inversion p. (PIP)
Ramond p.
respiratory inversion p.
(RIP)
Robson p.
Sudeck critical p.
p. tenderness
Voillemier p.
point-counting image
pointed condyloma
pointer
LaserMed laser p.
Poiseuille-Hagen law
Poiseuille law
poison
poisoning
ackee fruit p.
acute lead p.
acute mercury p.
Amanita phalloides mushroom p.
bacterial food p.
chronic lead p.
chronic mercury p.
ciguatera fish p.
excitotoxic food p.
ferrous salt p.
food p.
histamine fish p.
iron p.
lead p.
mercury p.
mushroom p.
paralytic shellfish p.
phosphorus p.
scombroid fish p.
Staphylococcus food p.
thallium p.
Poisson regression
Polachrome slide system
polar
p. artery
p. body
P. enteral feeding bag
p. region
p. segmental nephrectomy
p. sheathed flagellum
Polaris grasper
polarization microscopy
polarized
p. glucose transporter
p. standing reflex
polarographic study
Polaroid
P. camera

P. endocamera
P. with ACMI adapter
pole
caudal p.
cranial p.
inferior p.
p. of kidney
pelvic p.
Polhemus-Schafer-Ivemark syndrome
policy
organ allocation p.
polidocanol
p. injection
p. injection therapy
p. sclerosant
poliomyelitis
POLIP
polyneuropathy, ophthalmoplegia,
leukoencephalopathy, and intestinal
pseudoobstruction
POLIP syndrome
Politano-Leadbetter
P.-L. anastomosis
P.-L. technique
P.-L. tunnel creation
P.-L. ureterolysis
P.-L. ureteroneocystostomy
polka fever
Pollack ureteral catheter
pollakiuria
pollen extract
Pólya
P. anastomosis
P. gastrectomy
P. gastroduodenal anastomosis
technique
P. gastroenterostomy
P. operation
polyacrylamide
p. gel
p. gel electrophoresis (PAGE)
polyamine
p. level
p. spermine
polyangiitis
microscopic p. (MPA)
polyanion
GBM p.
polyantibiotic chemotherapy
polyarteritis nodosa
polyarthritis
seronegative p.
polycationic
p. histochemical probe
p. marker
polychemotherapy
polychloruria
Polycillin-N
Polycitra

P

polyclonal
    p. epidermal growth factor antibody
    p. IgG
Polycose glucose supplement
polycystic
    p. chronic esophagitis
    p. disease of liver (PDL)
    p. kidney disease (PCKD)
    p. liver disease (PCLD, PLD)
polycystin-1, -2
polycythemia vera (PCV)
Polydek suture
polydimethylsiloxane
polydioxan
polydioxanone suture (PDS)
polydipsia
    psychogenic p.
polyester-reinforced Dacron tape
polyestradiol phosphate therapy
polyethylene
    p. balloon dilator
    p. cannula
    p. catheter
    p. endoprosthesis
    p. glycol (PEG)
    p. glycol 600
    p. glycol-based lavage
    p. glycol electrolyte lavage solution (PEG-ELS)
    p. perforation
    p. stent
    p. tube
polyethylenimine (PEI)
Polyflex esophageal stent
Poly GIA stapler
polyglactin
    p. monofilament loop
    p. suture
    p. suture material
polyglecaprone 25 suture
polyglutamate
    p. folate
    p. paclitaxel
polyglycolic
    p. acid
    p. acid collar
    p. acid suture
polyglyconate
    p. monofilament loop
    p. staple
    p. suture
polygonal hepatocyte
Polygonum multiflorum
polyhydramnios
polyimmunoglobulin receptor (pIgR)
polylactide coglycolide
poly-l-lysine-coated glass slide

polylobar liver
polymer
    Enteryx injectable p.
    mucin p.
    silicone p.
polymerase
    p. chain reaction (PCR, PRC)
    p. chain reaction-based single-stranded conformation polymorphism (PCR-SSCP)
    p. chain reaction technology
    DNA p.
    HBV-associated DNA p.
    Taq p.
polymerization
    IgA p.
polymethylmethacrylate (PMMA)
    p. membrane
polymicrobial
    p. bacterascites
    p. biofilm
    p. infection
polymorphic
    p. gene
    p. reticulosis (PMR)
polymorphism
    ACE gene p.
    aldosterone synthase p.
    angiotensin-converting enzyme gene p.
    angiotensin I-converting enzyme insertion/deletion p.
    CARD15 p.
    deletion p.
    DNA p.
    polymerase chain reaction-based single-stranded conformation p. (PCR-SSCP)
    restriction fragment length p. (RLP)
    single nucleotide p.
polymorphonuclear (PMN)
    p. cell
    p. inflammatory infiltrate
    p. leukocyte (PMNL)
    p. neutrophil (PMNN)
Polymox
polymyositis
polymyositis-dermatomyositis
polymyxin
    p. B
    p. nephropathy
polyneuropathy
    arsenical p.
    familial amyloid p. (FAP)
    polyneuropathy, ophthalmoplegia, leukoencephalopathy, and intestinal pseudoobstruction (POLIP)

polyneuropathy, organomegaly,
  endocrinopathy, monoclonal protein,
  and skin changes (POEMS)
polynuclear leukocyte
polyol pathway
polyoma middle T oncogene
Polyomavirus **infection**
polyorchidism (*var. of* polyorchism)
polyorchism, polyorchidism
polyostotic fibrous dysphasia
polyp
  adenomatous p. (AP)
  adenomatous colorectal p.
  adenomatous gastric p.
  antral p.
  benign adenomatous p.
  bleeding p.
  broad-based p.
  cervical p.
  cholesterol p.
  cloacogenic p.
  colonic p.
  colorectal p.
  diminutive adenomatous p.
  diminutive colonic p.
  diminutive hyperplastic p.
  duodenal p.
  elusive p.
  eroded p.
  esophageal p.
  fibroblastic p.
  fibroid p.
  fibrovascular p.
  filiform p.
  fundic gland p.
  gastric antral sessile p.
  gastric hyperplastic p.
  gastric inflammatory fibroid p.
  gastrointestinal hamartomatous p.
  giant gastric p.
  p. grasper
  hamartomatous gastric p.
  hyperplasiogenic p.
  hyperplastic p. (HP)
  hyperplastic adenomatous p.
  hyperplastic epithelial gastric p.
  hyperplastic gastric p.
  inflammatory fibroid p. (IFP)
  invasive colorectal p.
  juvenile retention p.
  lymphoid p.
  malignant p.
  metaplastic p.
  mixed hyperplastic-adenomatous
    gastric p.
  mucosal p.
  nasal p.
  neoplastic p.

nonneoplastic p.
pedunculated p.
perineal p.
Peutz-Jeghers p.
polypoid p.
postinflammatory p.
prepyloric p.
prostatic urethral p.
rectal p.
p. relocation
retention p.
sentinel hyperplastic p.
sessile p.
small inflammatory p.
p. stalk
synchronous p.
tuberculosis p.
tubular p.
tubulovillous p.
villoglandular p.
villous p.
polypectomized
polypectomy
  colonoscopic p.
  duodenal endoscopic p.
  electrosurgical snare p.
  endoscopic sessile p.
  gastric p.
  incomplete p.
  piecemeal p.
  saline-assisted p. (SAP)
  snare p.
  p. snare
  p. stump
polypeptide
  gastric inhibitory p. (GIP)
  p. growth factor
  islet amyloid p.
  pancreatic p.
  parathyroid hormone-related p.
  pituitary adenylate cyclase-activating
    p. (PACAP)
  vasoactive intestinal p. (VIP)
polyphagia
polyphosphate
  ^{99m}Tc p.
polyphosphoinositide
polypiform (*var. of* polypoid)
polypoid, polypiform
  p. cancer
  p. carcinoma
  p. colorectal cavernous hemangioma
  p. dysplasia
  p. excrescence
  p. exophytic nonulcerating
    carcinosarcoma
  p. filling defect
  p. gastric rugal hyperplasia

P

polypoid (*continued*)
    p. lesion
    p. lymphoid hyperplasia
    p. lymphoma
    p. lymphomatous hyperplasia
    p. mass
    p. polyp
    p. tumor
    p. urethritis
    p. vascular malformation
polyposa
    colitis p.
    enteritis p.
    gastritis cystica p.
polyposis
    adenomatous p.
    cap p.
    p. coli
    colonic p.
    dense p.
    diffuse hyperplastic p.
    diffuse mucosal p.
    duodenal p.
    familial adenomatous p. (FAP)
    familial colorectal p.
    familial gastrointestinal p.
    familial hamartomatous p.
    familial intestinal p.
    familial juvenile p. (FJP)
    filiform p.
    florid p.
    gastric p.
    gastrointestinal p. (GIP)
    hamartomatous p.
    hyperplastic p.
    intermediate p.
    intestinal p.
    juvenile p. (JP)
    lymphomatous p. (LP)
    multiple lymphomatous p.
    nonfamilial gastrointestinal p.
    Peutz-Jeghers gastrointestinal p.
    pseudolipomatosis p.
    sparse p.
    p. syndrome
    p. ventriculi
polypous gastritis
polyprenoic acid
Polyprep centrifugation
polypropylene
    p. mesh
    suprapubic approach to suburethral p. (SPARC)
    p. suture
polypus
    p. cysticus
    p. hydatidosus
polypyrimidine

    p. tract binding (PTB)
    p. tract-binding protein
polyradicular neuropathy
polyribosome
polysaccharide
    p. antigen
    p. capsule
    p. hyaluronan
    p. Kreha (PSK)
polysaccharide-iron complex (PIC)
polyserositis
    familial paroxysmal p. (FPP)
    familial recurrent p.
    periodic p.
polysome
    endoplasmic reticulum-bound p.
polyspermia (*var. of* polyspermy)
polyspermism (*var. of* polyspermy)
polyspermy, polyspermia, polyspermism
polysplenia syndrome
polystyrene sodium sulfonate
polysulfate
    pentosan p.
    sodium pentosan p.
polysulfonated naphthylurea
polysulfone
    p. dialyzer
    F60S p.
    high-flux p.
    p. membrane
polysynaptic reflex
Polytef injection
polytetrafluoroethylene (PTFE)
    p. mesh
    p. paste injection
    p. periurethral injection
    p. sock
Polytrac Gomez retractor
polytropous enteronitis
polyunsaturated lecithin
polyurethane
    p. nasoenteric catheter
    p. stent
polyurethane-covered metallic stent
polyuria
    nighttime p.
    nocturnal p.
polyvinyl
    p. alcohol
    p. alcohol sponge
    p. alcohol sponge hysterosacropexy
    p. bougie
    p. chloride (PVC)
    p. chloride catheter
    p. dilator
    p. manometric catheter
    p. tubing
pomegranate
Pompe disease

Pondimin
Ponka
  P. herniorrhaphy
  P. technique for herniorrhaphy anesthesia
  P. technique for local anesthesia
pons hepatis
Ponsky
  P. pull
  P. technique
Ponsky-Gauderer-type PEG
ponticulus hepatis
pontine micturition center (PMC)
pontine-sacral reflex
POO
  prostatic outlet obstruction
pool
  abdominal p.
  bile acid p.
  gastric p.
  intracellular p.
pooled
  p. glomeruli
  p. saliva
Poole suction tube
pooling
  piriform p.
  vallecular p.
  venous p.
poor
  p. long-term efficacy
  p. long-term outcome
  p. long-term result
  p. risk
  p. surgical risk case
poorly
  p. compliant bladder
  p. differentiated adenoma
  p. localized pain
popliteal
  p. swelling
  p. tenderness
pop-off suture
Poppel sign
poppy seed
POP-Q
  pelvic organ prolapse quantification
POPS
  peroral pancreatoscopy
population
  challenging patient p.
  gluten-dependent p.
  hemodialysis p.
  susceptible p.
population-based control group
popule
  Puritan LiquiShield p.
porcelain gallbladder
porcine

  p. carboxypeptidase B
  p. dermis for pubovaginal sling
  p. endogenous retrovirus (PERV)
  p. hepatocyte
pore, porus
  filtration slit p.
  shuntlike p.
porfimer
  p. sodium
  p. sodium photodynamic therapy
Porges catheter
porin channel protein
pork tapeworm
porotomy
porous filter membrane
porphobilinogen (PBG)
  p. deaminase (PBG-D)
porphyria
  acute intermittent p. (AIP)
  p. cutanea tarda (PCT)
  hepatic p.
  variegate p.
porphyrin photosensitizer
porphyrinuria, porphyruria
porphyruria (*var. of* porphyrinuria)
port
  BardPort implanted p.
  Fastrac gastric access p.
  inlet p.
  MCL p.
  OmegaPort access p.
  periumbilical p.
  p. site metastasis
  subcostal p.
  suprapubic p.
  umbilical p.
porta
  p. hepatis
  p. renis
portable
  p. digital data recorder
  p. perfused manometric system
  p. renal preservation machine
Port-A-Cath catheter
portacaval, portocaval
  p. anastomosis (PCA)
  p. H graft
  p. H-graft shunt
  p. shunt (PCS)
  p. transposition (PCT)
Portagen
  P. diet
  P. feeding
  P. formula
Port-A-Germ anaerobic transport vial
portal
  p. block
  p. canal

P

portal (*continued*)
    p. cannula
    p. catheter
    p. circulation
    p. cirrhosis
    p. decompression
    p. embolization
    p. eosinophilic inflammation
    p. fissure
    p. hypertension (PHT, PHTN)
    p. hypertensive gastropathy
      (PHG)
    p. hypertensive intestinal
      vasculopathy (PHIV)
    p. hypotensive drug
    p. lobulation
    p. lobule
    p. perfusion defect
    p. plasma cell infiltration
    p. portography
    p. pyemia
    p. repermeation
    p. shunt index (PSI)
    p. tract
    p. tract fibrosis
    p. tract inflammation
    p. triad
    p. triaditis
    p. triad occlusion
    p. trunk
    p. vascular bed
    p. vein
    p. vein blood flow velocity
    p. vein congestive index (PVCI)
    p. vein obstruction (PVO)
    p. vein thrombosis (PVT)
    p. vein thrombus
    p. venous pressure (PVP)
    p. venous system
    p. venous velocity (PVV)
    p. venule
    p. zone
    p. zone granuloma
portal-collateral circulation
portal-systemic (*var. of* portosystemic)
portal-to-portal
    p.-t.-p. bridging
    p.-t.-p. fibrosis
4-port diamond placement
Porter duodenal forceps
5-port fan placement
portocaval (*var. of* portacaval)
portoenterostomy
    Kasai p.
portography
    arterial p.
    computed tomography arterial p.
    computed tomography during arterial
      p. (CTAP)

    CT during arterial p. (CTAP)
    percutaneous transhepatic p.
      (PTP)
    portal p.
    splenic p.
    transhepatic p.
    umbilical p.
    wedged retrograde p.
portopulmonary
    p. hypertension
    p. shunt
portosystemic, portal-systemic
    p. encephalopathy (PSE)
    p. shunt
    p. shunting (PSS)
    p. shunt surgery
PortSaver PercLoop device
Portsmouth predictor equation
porus (*var. of* pore), *pl.* **pori**
    p. galeni
position
    anterior oblique p.
    body p.
    Buie p.
    cervical p.
    curved flank p.
    decubitus p.
    dorsal lithotomy p.
    dorsosacral p.
    Edebohls p.
    Elliot p.
    final p.
    flank p.
    forward-viewing p.
    Fowler p.
    frogleg p.
    Gil-Vernet p.
    greater curve p.
    jackknife p.
    knee-chest p.
    knee-elbow p.
    Kraske p.
    lateral decubitus p.
    left lateral decubitus p.
    lithotomy p.
    Lloyd-Davies Trendelenburg p.
    Mayo-Robson p.
    modified Lloyd-Davies p.
    prone split-leg p.
    reverse Trendelenburg p.
    right anterior oblique p.
    Robson p.
    Scultetus p.
    semioblique p.
    Sims p.
    ski p.
    subclavian p.
    supine p.
    Trendelenburg p.

positional obstructive uropathy
positioner
> gallbladder bag p.

positioning
> automated endoscopic system for optimal p. (AESOP)
> flank roll p.
> patient p.

positive
> antigen p.
> p. bowel sounds
> p. chemotaxis
> p. culture result
> extradomain A p. (EDA+)
> false p.
> p. family history
> FOBT p.
> HBeAg p.
> p. margin
> p. nitrogen balance
> p. predictive value (PPV)
> p. secretin stimulation study

positive-pressure urethrography (PPUG)
Positrap
> P. miniretrieval basket
> P. 3-prong nonretracting grasping forceps
> P. retriever

positron
> p. camera
> p. emission tomography (PET)
> p. emission tomography scan
> P. Plus cushion

Posner attention test
post
> p. hoc test
> p. jejunoileal bypass hepatic disease
> p. rubber band sepsis

postage stamp penile tumescence test
postanal
> p. dimpling
> p. pit
> p. repair

postatrophic hyperplasia
postauricular Wolfe graft
postautoclave contamination
postbiopsy
> p. fistula
> p. vascular complication

postbulbar duodenal ulcer
postcaval ureter
postcecal abscess
postchemotherapy surgery
postcholangitic stricture
postcholecystectomy
> p. flatulent dyspepsia
> p. syndrome (PCS)

postcholecystitis adhesion

postcibal symptom
postcoagulation syndrome
postcoital test
postcolonoscopy distention syndrome
postcricoid
> p. area
> p. web

postdialysis urea rebound (PDUR)
postdilation meglumine diatrizoate
postdystrophic scarring
postendoscopic
> p. cholangitis
> p. retrograde cholangiopancreatography pancreatitis

postendoscopy
postenteritis syndrome
post-ERCP-induced pancreatitis
posterior
> p. abdominal wall
> anterior and p. (A&P)
> arteria caecalis p.
> arteria gastrica p.
> arteria pancreaticoduodenalis superior p.
> p. bladder flap plasty
> p. duodenal ulcer
> p. extremity
> p. fissure
> p. flap vaginoplasty
> p. hypospadias
> p. lumbar approach
> p. lumbotomy
> p. mediastinal adenopathy
> p. nephrectomy
> p. pararenal compartment
> p. pelvic exenteration
> p. perineum
> p. rectopexy
> p. rectus sheath
> p. renal fascia
> p. sagittal and 3-flap anoplasty
> p. sagittal anorectoplasty (PSARP)
> p. scrotal nerve
> p. transthoracic incision
> p. urethra
> p. urethral valve surgery
> p. urethral valve type I—IV
> p. urethral valve [type I-IV] (PUV)

posteroinferior
> ventral p. (VPI)

posterolateral
posterorsuperior pancreaticoduodenal artery
postevacuation
> p. film
> p. view

post-fatty meal cholecystography
postfundoplication syndrome

P

postganglionic
    p. cholinergic nerve
    p. sympathetic nerve
postgastrectomy
    p. bleed
    p. cancer
    p. dysfunction
    p. gastritis
    p. hemorrhage
    p. stasis
    p. syndrome
postglomerular arteriole
postheparin lipolytic activity (PHLA)
posthepatic
posthepatitic cirrhosis
posthepatitis aplastic anemia
posthetomy
posthioplasty
posthitis
postholith
posthysterectomy vaginal prolapse
postictal
postinfectious glomerulonephritis (PIGN)
postinfective glomerulonephritis
postinflammatory
    p. contracture
    p. polyp
    p. traction
postischemic
    p. acute renal failure
    p. tubular necrosis
postligation
    p. discomfort
    p. pain
    p. ulcer
postmenopausal (PMP)
postmicturition
    p. continuous leakage
    p. dribble
postmortem intussusception
postmyotomy reflux
postnasal drip
postnecrotic
    p. cirrhosis
    p. scarring
postnephrectomized
postobstructive diuresis
postoperative
    p. abscess
    p. adhesion
    p. advance
    p. alloantigen-dependent
    p. analgesia requirement
    p. anticoagulation therapy
    p. autologous transfusion
    p. biliary leakage
    p. cholangiography
    p. choledochoscopy

    p. cholesterol embolism
    p. complication
    p. evaluation
    p. gastritis
    p. hydrocele
    p. ileus
    p. irrigation-suction
    p. irrigation-suction drainage
    p. morbidity
    p. pleurobiliary fistula
    p. recurrent bleeding rate
    p. reflux
    p. regimen for oral early feeding (PROEF)
    p. retroperitoneal fibrosis
    p. stricture
    p. ureteral obstruction
    p. urinary retention
    p. vomiting
postoperatively
    fluid intake p.
postparacentesis circulatory dysfunction (PCD)
postpartum constipation
postperfusion
postpolypectomy
    p. bleed
    p. coagulation syndrome
    p. hemorrhage
postprandial
    p. distention
    p. fullness
    p. hypoglycemia
    p. nausea
    p. pain
    p. portal hyperemia
    p. vomiting
postprocedure pancreatitis
postprostatectomy
    p. hemostatic catheter
    p. incontinence
postpyloric feeding tube
postreceptor signaling of parietal cell
postrema
    area p.
postrenal
    p. albuminuria
    p. anuria
    p. proteinuria
postsclerotherapy bacterial peritonitis
postsecretory processing
postshunt encephalopathy
postsphincterotomy
    p. ductography
    p. ERCP cannulation
postsplenectomy infection
poststreptococcal
    p. acute glomerulonephritis
    p. glomerulonephritis (PSGN)

postsurgical
    p. change
    p. endoscopy
    p. gastric stasis
    p. recurrent ulcer
posttest score
postthaw sperm motility index
postthrombotic syndrome
posttransfusion hepatitis
posttranslational
    p. modification
    p. processing of peptide
posttransplant
    p. antiglomerular basement
      membrane
    p. diabetes mellitus (PTDM)
    p. immunosuppression
    p. immunosuppression therapy
    p. lymphoproliferative disorder
      (PTLD)
    p. patient
    p. renal dysfunction
posttransplantation
    p. cholangitis
    p. survival rate
**posttransurethral microwave
thermotherapy prostatitis-like
syndrome**
posttraumatic
    p. autotransplantation
    p. incontinence
    p. pancreatic-cutaneous fistula
    p. posterior urethral stricture
posttreatment
    p. discomfort
    p. placement
post-TUMT prostatitis-like syndrome
posttussive vomiting
postulate
    Koch p.
postural
    p. quantitative analysis of acid
      exposure
    p. regurgitation
    p. stimulation test (PST)
posture-dependent pain
postureteral ligation
postureteroscopic manipulation
posture test
posturethral suspension obstruction
posturing
    decerebrate p.
    decorticate p.
posturography
    computerized dynamic p. (CDP)
post-UUO time
Pos-T-Vac
    P.-T-V. vacuum erection device
    P.-T-V. VCD

postvagotomy
    p. diarrhea (PVD)
    p. dysphagia
    p. gastroparesis
    p. syndrome
postvoid
    p. dribble
    p. dribbling of urine
    p. incontinence
    p. radiography
    p. residual (PVR)
    p. residual urine
postvoiding cystogram (PVC)
Potaba
potassium
    aminobenzoate p.
    p. balance
    p. bicarbonate
    p. channel
    p. channel opener
    p. chloride (KCl)
    p. citrate
    p. conductance
    p. cyanide
    p. deficiency
    p. depletion
    dietary p.
    p. electrolyte
    extracellular p.
    fractional excretion of p. (FEFEK)
    p. hydroxide (KOH)
    p. hydroxide smear
    intracellular p.
    p. ion (K+)
    p. permanganate
    p. phosphate
    p. sensitivity test (PST)
potassium-binding resin
potassium-canrenoate antagonist
potassium-losing nephritis
potassium-sparing diuretic
potassium-titanyl
    p.-t. phosphate (KTP)
    p.-t. phosphate crystal laser
potato
    African p.
    p. liver
potency
    erectile p.
    failed recovery of p.
    recovery of sexual p.
    sexual p.
potential
    p. complication
    p. difference (PD)
    evoked p.
    excitatory junction p. (EJP)
    excitatory postsynaptic p. (EPSP)
    p. fusion protein

P

potential (*continued*)
 inhibitory postsynaptic p. (IPSP)
 malignant p.
 motor unit action p.
 neoplastic p.
 oscillatory p.
 oxidant-trapping p.
 p. pitfall
 pudendal evoked p.
 redox p.
 resting membrane p.
 p. role for simethicone in bowel
  preparation
 short-lasting afterhyperpolarizing p.
 spike p.
 stromal tumor of unknown
  malignant p. (STUMP)
 threshold p.
 p. toxicity
 visual evoked p.
potentiation
 alcohol p.
 p. of drug hepatotoxicity
Potentilla
Potter
 P. disease
 P. facies
 P. phenotype
 P. syndrome
Potts
 P. forceps
 P. scissors
Potts-Smith
 P.-S. forceps
 P.-S. scissors
pouch
 abdominovesical p.
 anal p.
 Assura convex drainable p.
 Assura convex urostomy p.
 Assura pediatric p.
 Assura standard drainable p.
 banded gastroplasty with divided
  p.
 Bard closed-end adhesive p.
 Bard drainage adhesive p.
 Bard Extra Ileo B p.
 Bard security p.
 Barnett p.
 Benchekroun p.
 p. biopsy
 bladder replacement urinary p.
 blind upper esophageal p.
 Bricker p.
 bulky colonic p.
 Camey urinary p.
 catheterization p.
 closed-end ostomy p.
 colon p.

colonic J p.
Coloplast closed p.
Coloplast drainable p.
Coloplast flange p.
coloplasty p.
p. configuration
continent ileal reservoir
 catheterization p.
ConvaTec colostomy p.
ConvaTec Sur-Fit Little Ones p.
ConvaTec Sur-Fit 2-piece p.
Cymed Micro Skin 1-piece drainage
 p.
Dansac Karaya Seal 1-piece
 drainage p.
Dansac Standard Ileo p.
Denis Browne p.
double-loop p.
Douglas p.
drainable ostomy p.
Duke p.
endorectal ileal p.
p. excision
p. failure
First-Choice drainable p.
p. fistula
Florida urinary p.
Fobi p.
p. former
fundal p.
gastric p.
Graham closure with omental p.
Greer EZ Access drainage p.
Hartmann p.
haustral p.
Heidenhain p.
hemi-Kock p.
hernia p.
Hollister First Choice p.
Hollister Holligard p.
Hollister Karaya 5 ostomy p.
Hollister Karaya Seal p.
Hollister Premium p.
Hunt-Lawrence p.
ileal J p.
ileal low-pressure bladder substitute
 p.
ileal neobladder urinary p.
ileal S p.
ileal W p.
p. ileitis
ileoanal p.
ileocecal p.
ileocolic p.
Incise p.
Indiana urinary p.
inlet p. (IP)
intraluminal p.
inverted-U p.

jejunal p.
J pelvic ileal p.
J-shaped ileal p.
Kock urinary p.
laparoscopic Mainz p. II
lateral-lateral p.
Le Bag ileocolonic p.
Le Bag urinary p.
3-limb S p.
3-loop ileal p.
2-loop J-shaped ileal p.
low-pressure p.
Mainz p. II
Mainz p. III
Mainz urinary p.
Mansson urinary p.
Marlen Gas Relief drainage p.
Marlen Odor-Ban ileostomy p.
Marlen Solo ileostomy p.
Marlen Zip Klosed p.
Miami p.
MicroSkin ostomy p.
Morison p.
Nu-Hope ileostomy p.
Nu-Hope neonatal and
    preemie p.
Nu-Hope Nu-Self drainable p.
Nu-Hope urinary p.
Nu-Hope urostomy p.
one-piece ostomy p.
open-ended ostomy p.
orthotopic voiding p.
Padua bladder urinary p.
pararectal p.
paravesical p.
Parks ileostomy p.
pelvic p.
Penn p.
perineal p.
pharyngeal p.
Physick p.
2-piece ostomy p.
protease p.
RapiSeal p.
rectal p.
rectouterine p.
rectovaginal p.
rectovesical p.
renal p.
right colon p.
Rowland p.
S p.
sigma rectum p.
sigmoid p.
sigmoid-rectum p.
S pelvic ileal p.
S-shaped p.
Studer p.
superficial inguinal p.

Sur-Fit Natura flexible wafer and
    drainable p.
Sur-Fit Natura urostomy p.
Tena p.
terminal ileal p.
triple-loop p.
U p.
UCLA catheterization p.
p. ulceration
United Bongort Lifestyle p.
United Max-E drainable p.
United Surgical Bongort Lifestyle p.
United Surgical Featherlite ileostomy
    p.
United Surgical Shear Plus drainable
    p.
United Surgical Soft Secure p.
vesica ileale p.
vesicouterine p.
VPI nonadhesive open-end p.
W p.
Willis p.
W pelvic ileal p.
W-shaped p.
Zenker p.
pouch-anal anastomosis
pouched ileostomy
pouchitis
chronic active p.
collagenous p.
P. Disease Activity Index (PDAI)
episode of p.
refractory p.
wastebasket p.
pouchocele
pouchogram
pouchography
evacuation p.
pouchoscopy
pelvic p.
pouch-specific complication
Poupart
P. ligament
P. ligament shelving edge
P. line
**Pourchez XpressO hemodialysis
    catheter**
povidone-iodine
p.-i. enema
p.-i. wash
powder
BCAD 2 p.
BC Cold P.
karaya p.
Nu-Hope Karaya p.
NutriCran GI fruit p.
p. pyelogram
Resource Arginaid p.
Secretin-Ferring p.

P

powder (*continued*)
    Seidlitz p.
    Sween Micro Guard p.
power
    p. Doppler ultrasound
    p. grip
pp65
    pp65 antigenemia
    pp65 antigenemia assay
PPAF
    progressive perivenular alcoholic
    fibrosis
PPAR
    peroxisome proliferator-activated
    receptor
PPC
    prostatic pressure coefficient
p47, p67 cytosolic protein
PPD
    purified protein derivative
    PPD immunologic study
    PPD test
p$_2$ penile-brachial index
PPG
    phalloplethysmography
PPI
    proton pump inhibitor
    PPI triple therapy
PP-immunoreactive cell
PPM
    phosphopeptidomannan
PPoma
    pancreatic polypeptide-secreting tumor
    pure PPoma
PPPD
    pylorus-preserving
    pancreaticoduodenectomy
PPSH
    pseudovaginal perineoscrotal
    hypospadias
PPTT
    prepubertal testicular tumor
PPUG
    positive-pressure urethrography
PPV
    positive predictive value
PPW
    pylorus-preserving Whipple
    PPW modification
Prader orchidometer
Prader-Willi syndrome
praeacutus
    Bacteroides p.
praecox
    ejaculatio p.
    icterus p.
praeputii
    smegma p.

Praktis
    Sonolith P.
pralidoxime
pramlintide
Prandase
Prandin
Pratt
    P. anoscope
    P. bivalve retractor
    P. crypt hook
    P. rectal hook
    P. rectal probe
    P. rectal scissors
    P. rectal speculum
pravastatin
praziquantel
prazosin hydrochloride
PRBC
    packed red blood cells
preampullary portion of bile duct
preauricular
prebiotic
precaliceal canalicular ectasia
precancerous lesion
prechylomicron transport vesicle
precipitancy
precipitant
    p. leakage
    p. urination
precipitation
    glucagon p.
precirrhosis
precirrhotic hemochromatosis
precision
    p. grip
    intraassay p.
    P. Isotein HN powdered feeding
    P. Isotonic powdered feeding
    P. LR powdered feeding
    P. office TUNA system
    P. QID glucose monitoring system
    P. SpeedTac transvaginal anchor
    system
    P. Tack transvaginal anchor system
    P. Twist transvaginal anchor system
Precision-HN, -LR
Precisor
    P. Direct Bite biopsy forceps
    P. disposable biopsy forceps
Preclude peritoneal membrane
precordium
    hyperdynamic p.
precore mutant strain
Precose
precursor
    androgen p.
    benign neoplastic p.
    T-helper p.

precut
- p. incision
- p. papillotome
- p. papillotomy
- p. sphincterotome
- p. sphincterotomy

Pred
- Liquid P.

predialysis
- p. phase
- p. plasma phosphate concentration

Predicta TGF-β1 kit
predictive value
predictor
- independent p.
- metabolic p.
- p. of proximal neoplasia
- outcome p.

predigested protein formula
predigestion
- diastase p.

predisposition
- familial p.
- genetic p.

prednisolone
- p. enema
- p. metasulfobenzoate

prednisone
prednisone-colchicine combination
predominant
- p. hyperparathyroid bone disease (PHBD)
- p. median lobe

preeclamptic liver disease
preendoscopy
preesophageal dysphagia
preexisting
- p. discomfort
- p. disease

preference
- personal p.

preferential heating
prefreeze
- p. motility
- p. semen analysis

PreGenPlus stool DNA test
Pregestimil formula
preglomerular
- p. arteriole
- p. vasculature

pregnancy
- abdominal ectopic p.
- acute fatty liver of p. (AFLP)
- cholestasis of p.
- ectopic sigmoid p.
- fatty liver of p.
- heartburn of p.
- intrahepatic cholestasis of p. (ICP)
- molar p.
- nephritis of p.
- pernicious vomiting of p.
- pyelonephritis of p.
- recurrent molar p.
- subacute fatty liver of p.
- toxemia of p.
- tubal ectopic p.
- ureteral calculus in p.
- voluntary interruption of p. (VIP)
- p. wastage

pregnant uterus
pregnenolone
Prehn sign
preinvasive urothelial neoplasia
prekallikrein
Prelief
preliminary
- p. baseline descriptive statistic
- p. finding

Prelone
prelooped intracorporeal knot
Preludin
Premarin
Premasol
premature
- p. ejaculation
- p. stop codon

prematurity
premedication
- metoclopramide p.
- pethidine p.
- viscous lidocaine p.

premenarchal
premicturition pressure
Premier
- P. Platinum HpSA
- P. Platinum HpSA test

Premium
- P. Barrier
- P. CEEA circular stapler
- P. Plus CEEA disposable stapler

Premix-Slip
Prempree modification staging system
prenatal
- p. diagnosis
- p. fetal hydronephrosis
- p. ultrasonography

Prentice-Wilcoxon test
Prentiss
- P. cryptorchidism repair maneuver
- P. orchiopexy

preop
- preoperative

P

preoperative (preop)
    p. advance
    p. antibiotic
    p. function
    p. lesion
    p. tumor treatment
prep
   preparation
    LoSo Prep
    OMNI Prep
    Sween Prep
    United Skin Prep
prepancreatic anlage
prepapillary bile duct
preparation (prep)
    bowel p.
    Brown dietary method for
     colon p.
    colonic purge p.
    Colonlite bowel p.
    Colyte bowel p.
    cytocentrifuge p.
    Dulcolax bowel p.
    electrolyte p.
    Emulsoil bowel p.
    Evac-Q-Kwik bowel p.
    Fleet bowel p.
    galenic p.
    GoLYTELY bowel p.
    P. H
    inadequate bowel p.
    lactobacillus p.
    lavage bowel p.
    Nichols-Condon bowel p.
    NutraPrep colonoscopy p.
    OCL bowel p.
    oral iron p.
    potential role for simethicone in
     bowel p.
    renal proximal tubule p.
    Touch p.
    Tridrate bowel p.
    X-Prep bowel p.
prepatent-period filariasis
prepenile dislocation of scrotum
preperfusion
preperitoneal
    p. abscess
    p. anesthesia
    p. approach
    p. distention balloon
     (PDB)
    p. fat
    p. space
    transabdominal p. (TAPP)
preproenkephalin
preproEt-1 mRNA
preprostatic
    p. plexus

    p. sphincter
    p. urethra
prepubertal testicular tumor (PPTT)
prepuce
    hooded p.
    megameatus-intact p. (MIP)
    ventral apron p.
preputia (*pl. of* preputium)
preputial
    p. adhesion
    p. calculus
    p. collar
    p. continent vesicostomy
    p. gland
    p. stenosis
    p. transverse island flap and glans
     channel
preputiotomy
preputium, *pl.* **preputia**
    p. clitoridis
    p. penis
prepyloric
    p. antral diaphragm
    p. antrum
    p. atresia
    p. gastric ulcer
    p. perforation
    p. polyp
    p. sphincter
prerectal lithotomy
prerenal
    p. anuria
    p. azotemia
presacral
    p. cyst
    p. ectopic kidney
    p. neuroblastoma
    p. rectopexy
    p. space
    p. teratoma
    p. tumor
presbyesophagus
prescribed clearance
prescription-event monitoring
presentation
    rectocele p.
    specific stone p.
    trismus p.
preservation
    bladder p.
    cadaver renal p.
    extracorporeal renal p.
    p. of uterus
    renal p.
    simple cold storage p.
    p. time
    p. time effect
presinusoidal intrahepatic portal
hypertension

pre-S phase
pressure
    abdominal leak-point p. (ALPP)
    ambulatory blood p. (ABP)
    p. amplitude modulation
    anal sphincter squeeze p.
    basal anal canal p.
    basal anal sphincter p.
    bile duct p.
    biliary tract p.
    bladder intravesical p.
    blood p. (BP)
    cavernosal systolic p.
    cavernous artery occlusion p.
    central venous p. (CVP)
    cerebral perfusion p. (CPP)
    choledochal basal p.
    closing p.
    colloid osmotic p.
    cybernetic regulation of blood p.
    detrusor muscle leak-point p.
    p. diverticulum
    p. dressing
    dynamic closure p.
    end-expiratory intragastric p.
    end-filling p.
    esophageal peristaltic p.
    p. flow analysis
    free hepatic venous p. (FHVP)
    glomerular capillary p.
    hepatic vein wedge p.
    hepatic venous p.
    high intraluminal p.
    high resting anal p.
    hydrostatic p.
    p. increment rate (PIR)
    intraabdominal p.
    intraanal p.
    intraballoon p.
    intracavernosal p.
    intracholedochal p.
    intraductal p.
    intraesophageal peristaltic p.
    intraesophageal variceal p.
    intragastric p.
    intraglomerular p.
    intraluminal esophageal p.
    intraluminal urethral p.
    intraurethral p.
    intravariceal p.
    intravesical p.
    p. inversion point (PIP)
    leak p.
    leak-point p. (LPP)
    lower esophageal sphincter p.
      (LESP)
    low urethral p. (LUP)
    maximum anal resting p. (MRP)
    maximum detrusor p.

    maximum squeeze p. (MSP)
    maximum urethral closure p.
      (MUCP)
    maximum vasal p. (MVP)
    mean arterial p. (MAP)
    mean arterial blood p. (MABP)
    p. measurement
    melanoma intratumor p.
    minimal distending p.
    p. natriuresis
    p. necrosis
    pancreatic duct p. (PDP)
    passage p.
    peak p.
    p. peak
    penile blood p.
    plasma oncotic p.
    portal venous p. (PVP)
    premicturition p.
    proximal p.
    pulmonary artery p. (PAP)
    pulmonary capillary wedge p.
      (PCW)
    renal perfusion p.
    resting anal sphincter p.
    sinusoidal capillary p.
    p. sore (PS, P/sore)
    sphincter of Oddi p.
    splanchnic capillary p.
    squeeze p.
    static closure p.
    p. study
    systemic arterial p.
    p. transducer
    transglomerular hydrostatic filtration
      p.
    transmembrane hydraulic p.
    p. transmission ratio
    ureteral p.
    urethral closure p. (UCP)
    Valsalva leak-point p. (VLPP)
    variceal p.
    vesical leak point p. (VLPP)
    voiding p.
    wedge p.
    wedged hepatic venous p.
      (WHVP)
    Whitaker perfusion p.
pressure-flow
    p.-f. electromyography study
    p.-f. micturition study
    p.-f. study (PFS)
pressure-injected bovine collagen
pressure-point tension ring
pressure-regulated electrohydraulic
  lithotripsy
pressure-specific bladder capacity
prestomal ileitis
presumed circle area ratio

P

presumptive sphincter
presurgical medical evaluation
presynaptic inhibition
preternatural anus
pretest global rating score
pretransplant evaluation
pretreatment serum creatinine
preureteral iliac artery
preurethritis
Prevacare Total Solution skin care
  spray
Prevacid Packet powder for oral
  suspension
Prevail protective underwear
prevalence
    cholelithiasis p.
    p. of diabetes mellitus
    p. of low glomerular filtration rate
Prevalite
preventing urinary tract infection
prevention
    acute pancreatitis p.
    Centers for Disease Control and P.
     (CDC)
    medical p.
    p. of first bleeding
    somatostatin p.
preventive intravesical therapy
prevertebral fascia
previous in vitro result
Prevpac triple therapy
PrHPT
    primary hyperparathyroidism
priapism
    arterial p.
    drug-induced p.
    high-flow p.
    low-flow p.
    secondary p.
    stuttering p.
    Winter shunt for p.
priapitis
priapus
prilocaine
Prilosec
primaquine
primary
    p. adrenal insufficiency
    p. advantage of self-management
    p. anastomosis
    p. antiphospholipid syndrome
    p. arteriovenous fistula
    p. B-cell lymphoma
    p. biliary cirrhosis (PBC)
    p. case
    p. ciliary dyskinesia
    p. closure
    p. colorectal cancer (PCRC)
    p. contraction

p. diagnostic endoscopy
p. fistulotomy
p. gastric lymphoma (PGL)
p. gastric lymphoma staging
p. glomerular disease
p. glomerular lesion
p. graft nonfunction
p. hepatosplenic lymphoma
  (PHSL)
p. hyperaldosteronism
p. hyperoxaluria type I, II
  (PH-I, -II)
p. hyperoxaluria type I, II
  (PH-I, -II)
p. hyperparathyroidism (PrHPT)
p. indication
p. infection of ascetic fluid
p. intestinal lymphangiectasis (PIL)
p. malignant melanoma of
  esophagus (PMME)
p. myelofibrosis
p. obstructive megaureter
p. outcome
p. oxalosis
p. panendoscopy
p. perineal hypospadias surgery
p. peristaltic wave
p. peritonitis
p. procedure
p. prophylaxis
p. pseudoobstruction syndrome
p. refluxing megaureter
p. renal calculus
p. sclerosing cholangitis (PSC)
p. sclerosing cholangitis
  inflammatory bowel disease
  (PSC-IBD)
p. spermatocyte
p. staging of testicular tumor
p. sterility
p. suture
p. syphilis
p. transitional cell carcinoma
p. tuberculosis
p. ureteropelvic junction obstruction
p. urinary diversion
p. vesicoureteral reflex
primed cell
primidone
priming
    androgen p.
primitive neuroectodermal tumor
  (PNET)
primordial kidney
Primus
    P. prostate machine
    P. transrectal thermography
principal cell
Principen

principle

    Boari-Ockerblad p.
    continent catheterizable
      appendicovesicostomy using
      Mitrofanoff p.
    countercurrent multiplier p.
    detubularization p.
    Fick p.
    flap-valve p.
    Goodwin cup-patch p.
    Heineke-Mikulicz p.
    Malone p.
    Mitrofanoff p.
    oncologic p.
    Sarfeh p.
    Seldinger p.
    Yang-Monti p.

Pringle liver hemorrhage maneuver
prior negative inguinal exploration
Priscoline
privilege

    bathroom p.

pro

   prothrombin
   pro time

proapoptotic effect
probability

    progression-free p.

probable long-term kidney damage
Probactrix
proband
Pro-Banthine
probe

    AcuNav steerable phased
      vector-array ultrasound catheter p.
    Aloka MP-PN ultrasound p.
    ambulatory p.
    p. and groove director
    antisense RNA p.
    Bakes p.
    Barr fistula p.
    Beckman pH p.
    beta-actin cDNA p.
    BICAP bipolar hemostasis p.
    BICAP electrocoagulation p.
    BICAP electrode p.
    BICAP endoscopic p.
    BICAP monopolar p.
    biliary balloon p.
    Bilitec intraluminal fiberoptic p.
    biotinylated DNA p.
    biplane sector p.
    bipolar cautery p.
    bipolar circumactive p. (BICAP)
    Bipolar EndoStasis p. (BESP)
    bipolar hemostasis p.
    blunt p.
    Bravo pH p.
    Buie fistula p.

    bullet p.
    caliber p.
    Cameron-Miller monopolar p.
    catheter p.
    catheter-based ultrasound p.
    cDNA p.
    8-channel cross-sectional anal
      sphincter p.
    coagulation p.
    CO_2 laser p.
    contact p.
    continuously perfused p.
    Corson needle electrosurgical p.
    C-Trak p.
    cystic fibrosis gene p.
    Desjardins gallbladder p.
    Desjardins gall duct p.
    Desjardins gallstone p.
    p. dilator
    Dobbhoff bipolar coagulation p.
    Doppler p.
    dot-plotted p.
    Earle rectal p.
    EHL p.
    electrode p.
    electrohydraulic lithotripsy p.
    electrosurgical monopolar spatula p.
    endfire transrectal p.
    endoanal p.
    endorectal p.
    endoscopic BICAP p.
    endoscopic Doppler p.
    endoscopic heat p.
    endoscopic ultrasound p.
    EndoSound ultrasound p.
    Fenger gallbladder p.
    fistula p.
    Fluhrer rectal p.
    Fogarty biliary p.
    front-loading ultrasound p. (FLUP)
    gallstone p.
    galvanic p.
    genomic DNA p.
    Gold P.
    p. gorget
    heat p.
    heater p. (HP)
    high-density endocavity p.
    24-hour esophageal pH p.
    human apo A-I DNA p.
    human fibronectin cDNA p.
    human gastrin p.
    p. image
    injection gold p.
    intraductal ultrasound p.
    intraluminal p.
    isotropic p.
    Jubileum 2.0 single-use
      gastroesophageal pH p.

P

probe (*continued*)
KTP laser p.
lacrimal duct p.
large-bore heat p.
Larry rectal p.
laser-Doppler Periflux PF-3 p.
light-monitoring p.
linear p.
linear-array p.
Mayo common duct p.
Meadox Surgimed Doppler p.
mechanical rotating p.
Medi-Tech bipolar p.
Medrad MRInnervu endorectal
colon p.
microballoon p.
Microelectrode MI-506 small-caliber
p.
miniature p.
miniaturized ultrasound catheter p.
Mixter dilating p.
monopolar p.
Moynihan bile duct p.
Moynihan gallstone p.
multilumen p.
Ochsner flexible spiral gallstone p.
Ochsner gallbladder p.
oligonucleotide p.
Olympus CD-20Z heater p.
Olympus GF-UM30P linear scanning
p.
Olympus heat p.
Olympus S-20-20R p.
Olympus ultrathin balloon-fitted
ultrasound p.
Olympus UM-F30-20R p.
Olympus UM-2R, -3R p.
Olympus UM-R-series miniature
ultrasonic p.
Olympus UM-S30-25R p.
Olympus UM-1W endoscopic p.
Olympus UM-W-series endoscopic p.
palpating p.
pH p.
pH-Informer Deltron p.
pH-manometry p.
polycationic histochemical p.
Pratt rectal p.
Radiometer pH p.
rectal p.
reflectance spectrophotometric p.
RNA p.
rotating Bruel and Kjaer p.
Sandhill pH antimony p.
silver p.
Sonocath ultrasound p.
stimulation p.
tactile p.
through-the-scope catheter p.

Transonics Systems flow p.
transrectal p.
triple-balloon p.
tumor p.
ultrasonic lithotriptor p.
ultrasound catheter p. (UCP)
virtual colonoscopy Side Fire APC
p.
water p.
probenecid
probenecid-containing solution
**probenecid-inhibited organic anion
transport system**
probiotic
p. therapy
VSL#3 p.
Probiotica
problem
bone marrow transplantation-related
p.
clinical p.
micturition p.
penile prosthesis mechanical p.
probucol
procainamide
**procainamide-induced systemic lupus
erythematosus**
procaine
p. hydrochloride
p. penicillin
ProCair
P. One dynamic pressure-relieving
mattress
P. Two dynamic pressure-relieving
mattress
Pro-Cal-Sof
Procaltrol
procarbazine
Procardia XL
procedure (*see also* **operation, repair**)
abdominal p.
abdomino-Peña pullthrough p.
ACE p.
Acucise retrograde p.
Acucise RP outpatient p.
Al-Ghorab p.
Altemeier perineal rectal pullthrough
p.
alternative endourological p.
antegrade continence enema p.
antiincontinence p.
antireflux p.
Asopa p.
auxiliary p.
Ball p.
Barcat p.
basket p.
Belsey Mark IV p.
Bengt-Johansson p.

bladder chimney p.
Bloodgood p.
Boari bladder flap p.
bowel refashioning p.
Boyce-Vest bladder exstrophy p.
Burch p.
butterfly endoluminal gastroplasty p.
bypass p.
Camey total gastrectomy p.
Campbell p.
Cantwell-Ransley hypospadias
  repair p.
CaverMap p.
cecal imbrication p.
Cecil hypospadias repair p.
Chester-Winter urinary stress
  incontinence repair p.
Cleveland Clinic weighted scale of
  endoscopic p.'s
Cohen antireflux p.
colon p.
complex renal p.
coring-out p.
corporal plication p.
corporal rotation p.
dartos pouch p.
DAWG p.
Delorme rectal prolapse repair p.
Devine-Devine p.
Duckett tubularized neourethra p.
Duhamel pullthrough p.
Duval pancreaticojejunostomy p.
Ebbehoj penile
  straightening-reinforcing p.
endorectal pullthrough p.
endoscopy p.
endourological p.
Enteryx p.
esophageal sling p.
Essed surgical p.
flap-valve antireflux p.
flip-flap p.
Fowler-Stephens spermatic vessel
  division p.
Frykman-Goldberg p.
full Monti p.
Fungi-Fluor p.
gastric neobladder p.
Gilchrist urinary diversion p.
Gil-Vernet ileocecocystoplasty p.
Gittes-Loughlin needle bladder
  suspension p.
Gittes urethral suspension p.
glans approximation p. (GAP)
Goulding p.
Gregoir-Lich ureteroneocystostomy p.
Halban culdoplasty p.
Hanley rectal bladder p.
Hartmann resection of intestine p.

Heitz-Boyer p.
Heller-Dor p.
hemi-Kock p.
hemi-T augmentation p.
Hinman stress incontinence p.
Hodgson technique of modified Lich
  p.
Hodgson XX p.
Hofmeister gastrectomy p.
Horton-Devine hypospadias flip-flap
  p.
hydrocelectomy bottle p.
hydrocelectomy dartos pouch p.
ileoanal pullthrough p.
imaging-guided minimally invasive
  p.
infrarenal template p.
intraparavariceal p.
InVance male sling p.
invasive p.
island flap p.
Jaboulay p.
Johnston buttonhole arteriovenous
  hemodialysis fistula p.
Kasai portoenterostomy p.
Kelling-Madlener gastric resection p.
Kelly urethrovesical plication p.
Kocher ureterosigmoidostomy p.
Kock pouch modified p.
Kropp urethral lengthening p.
Ladd mobilization of intestine p.
laparoscopic bladder neck suture
  suspension p.
laparoscopic urinary diversion p.
Leadbetter urethral reconstruction p.
Le Fort p.
Lewis-Tanner esophagectomy p.
Lich ureterocystostomy p.
Lord p.
Malone antegrade colonic enema
  stoma p.
Marshall-Marchetti-Krantz retropubic
  cystourethrography suspension p.
Mathieu-Righini hypospadias p.
Maydl colostomy p.
McIndoe vaginal construction p.
meatal-based flap p.
mesh sling p.
Michal p. I, II
microsurgical epididymal sperm
  aspiration p.
Mikulicz p.
Mitrofanoff appendicovesicostomy p.
modified Ingelman-Sundberg p.
modified Nesbit p.
modified Norfolk p.
modified transduodenal rendezvous
  p.
Monti p.

P

procedure (*continued*)

Moschcowitz culdoplasty p.
multiple surgical p.'s
muscle-filling p.
Mustarde p.
needle suspension p.
Nesbit tuck penis straightening p.
Nyhus p.
omentum majus flap p.
one-stage p.
O'Regan p.
Palomo varicocelectomy p.
Partington-Rochelle p.
Pauchet gastrectomy p.
pelvic pouch p.
percutaneous p.
Pereyra p.
Pippi Salle urethral lengthening p.
primary p.
promontofixation p.
ProstRcision p.
pubovaginal allograft sling p.
Puestow p.
pullthrough p.
Raz bladder neck suspension p.
Reichel-Pólya stomach p.
repeat p.
retropubic needle suspension p.
Richardson p.
Righini p.
Ripstein prolapsed rectum repair p.
Rives-Stoppa p.
routine outpatient p.
Roux-en-Y gastrointestinal system p.
Schoemaker transscrotal orchiopexy
p.
Schwartz-Pregenzer urethropexy p.
Secca p.
selective tubal occlusion p.
(STOP)
simultaneous Malone antegrade
continent enema and Mitrofanoff
p.'s
sling p.
Snow p.
Soave abdominal pullthrough p.
Spence urethral diverticulum p.
sphincter-saving p.
Stamey p.
Stamey-Martius antiincontinence p.
Sting p.
Stretta radiofrequency for GERD p.
Studer pouch ileal neobladder p.
suburethral rectus fascial sling p.
Sugiura esophageal varix p.
surgical p.
takedown of pelvic sling p.
tension-free vaginal tape p.
Thiersch anus p.

Thiersch-Duplay proximal tube
urethroplasty p.
Thompson cleft lip repair p.
TIPS p.
Toupet antireflux p.
transhepatic antegrade biliary
drainage p.
transjugular intrahepatic portacaval
shunt p.
transvaginal Burch p.
TVT p.
untethering p.
upper gastrointestinal p.
ureteral patch p.
vaginal flap reconstruction and
pubovaginal sling p.
vaginal needle suspension p.
vaginal wall sling p.
Van de Kamer fecal fat p.
Vesica sling p.
Walsh p.
Whipple radical
pancreatoduodenectomy p.
Winkleman p.
Winter priapism repair p.
Womack portal systemic
shunting p.
xenograft sling p.
York-Mason repair of postoperative
rectoprostatic-urethral fistula p.
Young-Dees bladder neck repair
p.

process

epithelial regenerative p.
fingerlike epithelial p.
foot p.
glycosylation p.
juxtacapillary p.
knobby p.
morphogenetic p.
signal transduction p.
sodium-linked p.
spinous p.
transverse p.
uncinate p.

processing

image p.
postsecretory p.
swim-up p.

processor

Miles V.I.P. 300 vacuum infiltration
p.
Olympus EU-M-series
endosonography image p.
ThinPrep p.
Video Image P.

processus vaginalis
prochlorperazine suppository
ProCide disinfectant

procidentia
    anal p.
    internal p.
    rectal p.
    p. recti
procoagulant
procollagen
    C-terminal propeptide of type I p.
    N-terminal propeptide of
      type III p.
Procon incontinence device
Procrit
proctalgia fugax
proctectasia
proctectomy
    mucosal p.
proctitis
    acute p.
    allergic p.
    bleeding p.
    chronic radiation p.
    chronic ulcerative p.
    Dean stage I, II radiation p.
    diversion p.
    epidemic gangrenous p.
    factitial p.
    glutaraldehyde-induced p.
    gonococcal p.
    gonorrheal p.
    idiopathic p.
    nonspecific ulcerative p.
    radiation p.
    traumatic p.
    ulcerative p.
proctoclysis
proctocolectomy
    minilaparotomy restorative p.
    restorative p. (RP, RPC)
    single-stage total p.
    totally stapled restorative p.
      (TSRPC)
proctocolitis
    aphthoid p.
    idiopathic p.
    radiation p.
    venereal p.
proctocolonoscopy
Proctocort
    P. cream
    P. suppository
ProctoCream-HC
proctocystocele
proctocystoplasty
proctocystotomy
ProctoFoam
ProctoFoam-HC
proctogram
    balloon p.
    defecating p.

proctography
    dynamic p.
    evacuation p.
    quantitative scintigraphic evacuation
      p.
proctopathy
    chronic radiation-induced p.
proctoperineoplasty
proctopexy
    Orr-Loygue transabdominal p.
proctoplasty
proctoptosis
Proctor-Livingston
    P.-L. endoprosthesis
    P.-L. tube
proctorrhaphy
proctoscope
    Boehm p.
    Gabriel p.
    Kelly p.
    Lieberman p.
    Montague p.
    Newman p.
    Salvati p.
    Vernon-David p.
proctoscopy
    rigid p.
proctosigmoidectomy
proctosigmoiditis
    refractory p.
proctosigmoidoscope
    ACMI fiberoptic p.
proctosigmoidoscopy
    rigid p.
proctospasm
proctostenosis
proctotomy
    external p.
    internal p.
    linear p.
    linear-array p.
proctovalvotomy
procyclidine
Prodium
prodromal symptom
prodrome, prodromus
prodromus (*var. of* prodrome)
prodrug
    GSH p.
product
    Amadori p.
    Biomedical Instruments and P.'s
      (BIP)
    ConvaTec Little Ones pediatric
      ostomy p.
    fibrin/fibrinogen degradation p.
      (FDP)
    fibrinogen degradation p. (FDP)
    fibrin split p. (FSP)

P

product (*continued*)
    mechanical p.
    secretory p.
    thermodynamic solubility p.
production
    ammonia p.
    autoantibody p.
    chylomicron p.
    creatinine p.
    hydrogen ion p.
    lymphokine p.
    spermatozoon p.
    superoxide p.
    unilateral renin p.
productive nephritis
productus
    Ruminococcus p.
prodynorphin gene
PROEF
    postoperative regimen for oral early
    feeding
proenkephalin gene
profile
    Astra p.
    cytokine p.
    emerging p.
    gut-hormone p.
    ideal patient p.
    liver function p.
    P. pediatric polypectomy snare
    phosphotyrosyl protein p.
    plasmid p.
    resting urethral pressure p.
    sickness impact p.
    side-effect p.
    spicule in p.
    StoneRisk diagnostic p.
    stress urethral pressure p.
    urethral closure pressure p. (UCPP)
    urethral pressure p. (UPP)
profiled dialysis
ProfileR
    PCA3 P.
profilometry
    urethral pressure p. (UPP)
profound acid reduction
profunda
    colitis cystica p. (CCP)
    fascia penis p.
    gastritis cystic p.
profuse vomiting
progenitalis
    herpes p.
progestational agent
progesteronal agent
progesterone
progesterone-associated colitis
prognostic
    p. factor

    p. indicator
    p. nutritional index (PNI)
    p. significance
    p. tool
prograde technique
Prograf
program
    instituted GI bleeding management
    p.
    low-energy p.
    Maine Medical Assessment P.
    (MMAP)
    Organ Procurement P.
    personalized p.
    Stat-View computer p.
    stone-prevention p.
    surveillance p.
    Synectics computer p.
    VariSeed 7.0 software computer p.
programming
    in utero p.
progression
    p. factor
    renal p.
progression-free
    p.-f. probability (PFP)
    p.-f. survival
progressive
    p. diet
    p. dysphagia
    p. emphysematous necrosis
    p. familial cirrhosis
    p. familial intrahepatic cholestasia
    (PFIC)
    p. perivenular alcoholic fibrosis
    (PPAF)
    p. renal dysfunction
    p. renal insufficiency
    p. suppurative cholangitis
    p. systemic sclerosis (PSS)
    p. toxicity
ProGuide chronic dialysis catheter
Prohibit antifog face mask
proinflammatory cytokine
project
    Captopril Prevention P. (CAPPP)
    National Prostatic Cancer P.
projectile vomiting
projection
    afferent p.
    parasympathetic p.
    single-shot voxel p.
    sympathetic p.
prokaryotic pathogen
prokinetic
    p. agent
    p. drug
    p. effect
    p. therapy

prolactin
Prolamine
prolapse
    anal p.
    bladder p.
    concomitant p.
    Cytocare P. II
    Delorme operation for rectal p.
    external anorectal mucosal p.
    Frykman-Goldberg operation for
      rectal p.
    gastric mucosal p.
    p. gastropathy
    genitourinary p.
    hemorrhoidal p.
    incarcerated p.
    incomplete rectal p.
    intestinal p.
    mucosal p.
    pelvic organ p.
    posthysterectomy vaginal p.
    rectal p.
    stomal p.
    sudden valve p.
    ureterocele p.
    urethral p.
    urogenital p.
    vaginal p.
    valve p.
    Well operation for rectal p.
prolapsed
    p. bowel
    p. internal hemorrhoid
    p. rectum
    p. stoma
prolapsing fourth-degree
  hemorrhoid
Prolase II lateral-firing Nd:YAG
laser
Pro-Lax
Prolene suture
Proleukin
Prolieve microwave therapy system
proliferans
    angiocholitis p.
    cholecystitis glandularis p.
proliferating
    p. state
    p. tubular cell
proliferation
    bile duct p.
    cell p.
    cellular p.
    colonic epithelial p.
    cystic epithelial p.
    diffuse mesangial p.
    DNA p.
    extraglandular endocrine cell p.
    glomerular cell p.

    index of cell p.
    intracystic epithelial p.
    intraluminal p.
    mesangial p.
    monoclonal p.
    mucosal cell p.
    neoplastic cell p.
    p. of gastric epithelium
    p. of prostatic tissue
    osteoblast-like p.
    rectal cell p.
proliferative, proliferous
    p. glomerulonephritis (PGN)
    p. hypertrophic gastritis
    p. inflammatory atrophy
proliferous (var. of proliferative)
prolinuria
    glycyl p.
Prolixin
prolonged
    p. expiratory phase
    p. partial ureteral obstruction
Proloprim
prolyl endopeptidase
promazine
promethazine
Prometheus
    P. device
    P. First Step inflammatory bowel
      disease screening assay
Promex biopsy needle
promontofixation
    laparoscopic p.
    p. procedure
promontorium (var. of promontory), pl.
  promontoria
promontory, promontorium
    sacral p.
promoter
    basic core p. (BCP)
    growth hormone p. (GHP)
promotor hypermethylation
prompt GI consult
promulgated
Pronase
pronation
pronephroi (pl. of pronephros)
pronephros, pl. pronephroi
prone split-leg position
Pronestyl
3-pronged
    3-p. grasper
    3-p. grasping forceps
    3-p. polyp retriever
4-pronged polyp grasper
pronucleus
proopiomelanocortin gene
propafenone
propagated antroduodenal contraction

P

propagation
> p. of contractions
> orad p.

propantheline bromide

propendens
> venter p.

proper
> p. hepatic artery
> p. lamina
> p. tunic

properitoneal
> p. fat
> p. flank stripe
> p. hernia

property
> similar psychometric p.'ss
> structural p.

prophecy
> self-fulfilling p.

propHiler urinary pH testing kit

prophylactic
> p. antibiotic
> p. antibiotic treatment
> p. cephalosporin
> p. cholecystectomy
> p. device
> p. gamma globulin
> p. lymphadenectomy
> p. orchiectomy
> p. orchiopexy
> p. sclerotherapy
> p. urethritis

prophylaxes (*pl. of* prophylaxis)

prophylaxis, *pl.* **prophylaxes**
> antibiotic p.
> antimicrobial p.
> continuous p.
> medical p.
> primary p.
> secondary p.
> stress ulcer p.
> stricture p.

propidium iodide

propionate
> testosterone p.

Propionibacterium acnes

propiverine

propofol

proportion
> increased in p.

proportional
> inversely p.

proportionate reduction

propoxyphene hydrochloride

propranolol

propria, *pl.* **propriae**
> arteria hepatica p.
> intestinal lamina p.
> lamina p.

muscularis p.
ratio of mucosa to submucosa to
> muscularis p.
tunica p.
underlying muscularis p.

propriae (*pl. of* propria)

Propulsid

propulsion
> colonic p.
> ineffective colonic p.

propulsive
> p. motor pattern
> p. wave

propylene oxide

propylhexedrine

prorenin
> serine protease-activated p.

Proscan
> P. ultrasound imaging system
> P. ultrasound unit

Proscar

Pros-Check
> P.-C. kit
> P.-C. PSA assay

Prosed/DS

Proshield Plus skin protectant

ProSobee liquid formula

prospective
> p. blind study of diagnostic
> esophagoscopy
> p. clinical trial
> p. comparison
> p. evaluation
> p. multicenter randomized trial
> p. multicenter study
> p. randomized controlled trial

prospermia

Prostacoil stent

prostacyclin

prostaglandin (PG)
> p. 1 (PG1, PG_1)
> p. analogue
> colonic p.
> cytoprotective p.
> p. E (PGE)
> p. E1 (PGE1, PGE_1)
> p. E2 (PGE2, PGE_2)
> p. F (PGF)
> p. F2-alpha (PGF2-alpha)
> p. G (PGG)
> p. G2 endoperoxide (PGG2
> endoperoxide)
> p. H (PGH)
> p. H2 endoperoxide (PGH2
> endoperoxide)
> p. I2 (PGI2)
> renal vasodilator p.
> p. supplementation
> p. synthesis

Prostakath urethral stent
Prostalase laser system
ProstaLund
    P. CoreTherm system
    P. feedback treatment
ProstaMark early prostate cancer antigen (ProstaMark EPCA)
prostanoid
    p. formation
    p. synthesis
ProstaScint scan
ProstaSeed I-125 seed
prostatae
    isthmus p.
prostatalgia
prostate
    atypical small acinar proliferation of p. (ASAP)
    p. balloon dilator
    boggy p.
    p. cancer
    P. Cancer Intervention Versus Observation Trial (PCIVOT, PIVOT)
    p. cancer-specific mortality (PCSM)
    carcinoma of p. (CAP)
    coagulation and hemostatic resection of p. (CHRP)
    contact laser vaporization of p. (CLVP)
    Costello laser ablation of p.
    cryosurgical ablation of p. (CSAP)
    ductal adenocarcinoma of p.
    enlarged p.
    ethanol injection therapy of p. (EIP)
    funnel-neck p.
    p. gland benign hyperplasia
    p. gland biopsy
    p. gland C3 complement
    p. gland color flow Doppler examination
    p. gland cross-section
    p. gland cytoskeleton
    p. gland electrovaporization
    p. gland hypoplasia
    p. gland innervation
    p. gland involution
    p. gland leiomyosarcoma
    p. gland lymphoma
    p. gland needle ablation
    p. gland peripheral zone
    p. gland periurethral zone
    p. gland prostate-specific membrane antigen
    p. gland sarcoma
    p. gland secretion
    p. gland small cell carcinoma
    p. gland stroma

    p. gland stromal cell
    p. gland tissue matrix
    p. gland transition zone
    p. gland transurethral balloon dilation
    p. gland transurethral resection
    holmium laser ablation of p. (HoLAP)
    holmium laser resection of p. (HoLRP)
    median furrow of p.
    minimal transurethral resection of p. (M-TURP)
    nodular hyperplasia of p.
    percutaneous radical cryosurgical ablation of p.
    photoselective vaporization of p. (PVP)
    prostatisme sans p.
    P. Px clinical test
    p. rhabdomyosarcoma
    salvage cryoablation of p.
    thick-loop transurethral resection of p.
    total transurethral resection of p. (T-TURP)
    transurethral electrovaporization of p. (TUEP, TUEVP)
    transurethral ethanol ablation of p. (TEAP)
    transurethral evaporation of p. (TUEP)
    transurethral grooving of p.
    transurethral incision of p. (TUIP)
    transurethral laser incision of p.
    transurethral needle ablation of p.
    transurethral resection of p. (TURP)
    transurethral vaporization of p. (TUVP)
    transurethral vaporization-resection of p. (TUVRP)
    visual laser ablation of p. (VLAP)
    p. volume
prostatectomy
    anatomic radical retropubic p.
    cavernosal nerve-sparing radical p.
    KTP laser p.
    laparoscopic radical p.
    laser p. (LRP)
    Madigan p.
    Millen technique retropubic p.
    nerve-sparing radical retropubic p.
    open radical p.
    perineal p.
    pubic p.
    radical perineal p. (RPP)
    radical retropubic p. (RRP)
    radical transcoccygeal p.
    retropubic ascending radical p.

P

prostatectomy (*continued*)
  salvage p.
  Stanford radical retropubic p.
  suprapubic p.
  total perineal p.
  transurethral ablative p.
  transurethral balloon laserthermia p.
  transurethral ultrasound-guided
    laser-induced p. (TULIP)
  Vattikuti Institute p.
  visual laser-assisted p. (VLAP)
  Walsh radical retropubic p.
prostate-specific
  p.-s. acid phosphatase
  p.-s. antigen (PSA)
  p.-s. antigen-based parameter
  p.-s. antigen bound to alpha-1
    antichymotrypsin
  p.-s. antigen density (PSAD)
  p.-s. antigen density of transition
    zone (PSA-TZ, PSATZ)
  p.-s. antigen velocity (PSAV)
  p.-s. membrane (PSM)
  p.-s. membrane antigen (PSMA)
Prostathermer
  Biodan P.
  P. device
  P. prostatic hyperthermia system
prostatic
  p. abscess
  p. acid phosphatase (PAP)
  p. adenocarcinoma
  p. adenoma
  p. antibacterial factor
  p. artery
  p. block
  p. calculus
  p. capsule
  p. catheter
  p. chip
  p. cryptococcosis
  p. fascia
  p. fossa
  p. hyperplasia
  p. hypertrophy
  p. intraepithelial neoplasia (PIN)
  p. massage
  p. mesonephric remnant
  p. neoplasm
  p. nodule
  p. outlet obstruction (POO)
  p. pile
  p. pressure coefficient (PPC)
  p. sinus
  p. stent
  p. thermal treatment
  p. tuberculosis
  p. urethra
  p. urethral polyp

  p. urethral transitional cell
    carcinoma
  p. utricle
  p. volume
prostatica
  ductus p.
  vesica p.
prostatici
  ductuli p.
  ductus p.
prostaticovesical plexus
prostaticovesiculectomy
prostaticus
  plexus p.
  utriculus p.
prostatism
  silent p.
  vesical p.
prostatisme sans prostate
prostatitic
prostatitis
  bacterial p.
  chemical p.
  chronic abacterial p.
  chronic bacterial p. (CBP)
  chronic nonbacterial p. (CNP)
  diagnosis of bacterial p.
  granulomatous p.
  mycotic p.
  NIH Classification Category I acute
    bacterial p.
  NIH Classification Category II
    chronic bacterial p.
  NIH Classification Category IV
    asymptomatic inflammatory p.
  NIH Classification System for P.
  nonbacterial p. (NBP)
  parasitic p.
  tuberculous p.
prostatocystitis
prostatocystotomy
prostatodynia
prostatography
prostatolith
prostatolithotomy
prostatomegaly
prostatometer
prostatomy (*var. of* prostatotomy)
prostatomyomectomy
prostatorrhea
prostatoseminal vesiculectomy
prostatotomy, prostatomy
  lateral p.
prostatotoxin
prostatourethral fistula
prostatourethral-rectal fistula
prostatovesical junction
prostatovesiculectomy
prostatovesiculitis

Prostatron
P. microwave system
P. transurethral thermotherapy device
prostatropin
prostheses (*pl. of* prosthesis)
prosthesis, *pl.* **prostheses**
Alpha I inflatable penile p.
Ambicor penile p.
AMS controlled-expansion penile p.
AMS Hydroflex penile p.
AMS inflatable penile p.
AMS malleable penile p.
AMS 3-piece inflatable penile p.
AMS Sphincter 800 urinary p.
Amsterdam-type p.
AMS Ultrex penile p.
Angelchik antireflux p.
Angelchik ring p.
antireflux p.
Atkinson p.
balloon tamponade p.
biliary p.
bilioduodenal p.
bladder neck support p.
Celestin p.
composite p.
covered self-expanding p.
CXM p.
CX Plus p.
Dacron p.
Dilamezinsert penile p.
double-pigtail p.
Dura-II positionable penile p.
Duraphase inflatable penile p.
Dynaflex penile p.
ERCP conventional p.
EsophaCoil p.
esophageal p.
Finney Flexirod penile p.
Flexi-Flate I, II penile p.
Flexirod penile p.
GFS Mark II inflatable penile p.
Gianturco expandable self-expanding metallic biliary p.
glass penile p.
hydraulic hinge penile p.
Hydroflex penile p.
inflatable penile p. (IPP)
Introl bladder neck support p.
iridium p.
Jonas penile p.
malleable p.
Mentor Alpha 1 inflatable penile p.
Mentor GFS penile p.
Mentor IPP penile p.
Mentor malleable penile p.
Mentor Mark II penile p.
mesh stent p.
Neville tracheal reconstruction p.
OmniPhase penile p.
penile p.
Scott AMS inflatable penile p.
silicone donut p.
silicone self-expanding p.
Small-Carrion penile p.
Subrini penile p.
testicular p.
Ultraflex esophageal p.
Ultrex Plus penile p.
Uni-Flate 1000 penile p.
Unitary inflatable penile p.
urethral stent p.
UroLume Endourethral Wallstent p.
UroLume urethral p.
valved voice p.
Wallstent esophageal p.
Wilson-Cook plastic p.
prosthesis-related seroma formation
prosthetic
p. arterial graft
p. bladder
p. penis
p. testis
p. utricle cyst
prosthetist
Prosthex sponge
Prostigmin
Prostiva RF therapy system
ProstRcision
P. procedure
P. treatment
ProTack
P. stapler
P. tacking device
Protalba-R
protamine
p. sulfate
p. zinc insulin
Protandim antioxidant therapy
protease
p. inhibitor
p. pouch
serine p.
V8 p.
protease-activated receptor
proteasome
Protect
Baza Cleanse and P.
protectant
Lantiseptic skin p.
Proshield Plus skin p.
Protect-a-Pass suture passer
protection
antibody-mediated p.
gastroduodenal mucosal p.
misoprostol p.
P. Plus male guard
protective probiotic flora

P

protector plus wire
protein

A-4 p.
acute phase p.
acylation stimulating p.
adenovirus-12 viral p.
agouti-related p.
aldosterone-induced p. (AIP)
androgen-binding p. (ABP)
p. antibody (PAb)
antibody to c100 p.
anti-Tamm-Horsfall p.
ascitic fluid total p. (AFTP)
bactericidal/permeability-increasing p.
band 3 p.
basement membrane p.
Bence Jones p.
bladder cancer-specific nuclear
  matrix p.
p. C
cagA p.
calcium-binding p.
calcium-regulated p.
calcium-specific binding p.
p. catabolic rate (PCR)
CD2-associated p.
CDC42 p.
CD3, CD4, CD8 p.
cholesterol ester transfer p. (CETP)
claudin p.
c-met p.
complement regulatory p.
copper-binding p. (CBP)
C-reactive p. (CRP)
p. C, S deficiency
CSF p.
p. C, S level
cytoplasmic adaptor p.
cytotoxin-associated gene A p.
p. depletion
dietary p.
dipstick p.
downstream signaling p.
E1 p.
E1b p.
E2 p.
E2F p.
E6 p.
enzymatic p.
eosinophil cationic p.
eosinophilic major basic p.
EP2-EP3 p.
estramustine-binding p.
EZH2 p.
fatty acid-binding p. (FABP)
fibronectin-binding p.
fyn p.
G p.
Gal 4 p.

green fluorescent p.
GTPase-activating p. (GAP)
GTP-dependent signaling p.
GTP-regulatory p.
guanine nucleotide-regulatory p.
HCV p.
heat shock p. (HSP)
helix-loop-helix p.
helix-turn-helix p.
hepatocellular p.
heptahelical receptor p.
heterodimeric p.
heterotrimeric G p.
H-related p.
IkBa p.
intestinal fatty acid-binding p.
  (I-FABP)
p. in vitamin K absence (PIVKA)
87kDa p.
p. kinase A (PKA)
p. kinase C (PKC)
lck p.
liver-specific p. (LSP)
low molecular weight p. (LMWP)
MAGP microfibrillar p.
matrix p.
membrane cofactor p.
membrane transport p.
mesenchymal p.
p. metabolism
p. microarray
microfibrillar p.
monocyte chemoattractant p.
  (MCP)
monocyte chemotactic p. (MCP)
multidrug resistance-associated p.
myeloma p.
noncollagen p.
nonstructural p. 4
Novel erythropoiesis-stimulating p.
NS2, NS3, NS4, NS5 p.
nuclear factor kappa B transcription
  factor p.
oligosaccharide-binding membrane p.
oncofetal p.
outer inflammatory p.
p53 p.
pancreatic stone p. (PSP)
pertussin toxin-sensitive G p.
PH30 p.
p. phosphorylation
phosphorylation p.
plasma p.
p. plug
p53 nuclear p.
podocyte-specific p.
polypyrimidine tract-binding p.
porin channel p.
potential fusion p.

p47, p67 cytosolic p.
PTB p.
p21/Waf1 p.
pyrimidine tract binding p.
rac p.
ras-related p.
Rb p.
receptor-associated p. (RAP)
replacement enzyme p.
p. restriction
retinoid binding p.
retinol-binding p. (RBP)
rho p.
p. S
S-100 p.
salt-transporting p.
scrapie p.
p. serine kinase
p. serine/threonine kinase activity
serum core p.
p. solder
StAR p.
stress p.
p. supplement
surface p.
p. synthesis (PS)
Tamm-Horsfall p. (THP)
TATA-binding p.
T-cell-specific p.
testicular androgen-binding p.
p. threonine kinase
tight junction membrane p.
toll-interleukin 1 receptor
  domain-containing adapter p.
total p.
transmembrane p.
triglyceride-rich p.
p. tubular reabsorption
p. tyrosine kinase
p. tyrosine phosphatase
urinary marker p.
uronic acid-rich p.
vitamin D-binding p.
protein-1
insulinlike growth factor-binding p.-1
  (IGFBP-1)
monocyte chemoattractant p.-1
  (MCP-1)
protein-2
multidrug resistance-associated p.-2
  (MRP2)
protein-3
insulinlike growth factor-binding p.-3
  (IGFBP-3)
protein-22
nuclear matrix p.-2. (NMP-22,
  NMP22)
protein-70
heat shock p.-7. (HSP-70)

proteinaceous
p. cast
p. cast material
proteinase
p. enzyme
p. inhibitor
protein-bound homocysteine
**protein-calorie malnutrition
  (PCM)**
protein-crystal interaction
**protein-energy malnutrition
  (PEM)**
protein-glutathione-S-transferase
receptor-associated p.-g.-S-t.
protein-losing
p.-l. enteropathy
p.-l. gastroenteropathy
p.-l. gastropathy
protein-mediated tubular toxicity
protein-overload proteinuria
protein-protein assay
proteinuria
asymptomatic p.
Bence Jones p.
BSA-induced overload p.
cardiac p.
colliquative p.
cyclic p.
emulsion p.
febrile p.
globular p.
glomerular p.
gouty p.
hematogenic p.
incipient p.
intermittent p.
intrinsic p.
moderate p.
molecular basis of p.
nephrogenous p.
orthostatic p.
overflow p.
palpatory p.
persistent p.
postrenal p.
protein-overload p.
residual p.
p. test
transient p.
tubular p.
proteinuric
p. glomerulopathy
p. nephropathy
p. state
proteoglycan
p. biglycan
p. decorin
heparan sulfate p. (HSPG)
proteolysis

P

proteolytic
- p. degradation
- p. digestion
- p. enzyme

proteomics

Proteus
- *P. mirabilis*
- *P. morganii*
- *P.* pneumonia
- *P. rettgeri*
- *Vibrio cholerae* biotype *P.*
- *P. vulgaris* (Pv)

prothrombin (pro)
- des-gamma-carboxy p. (DCP)
- p. induced by vitamin K absence or antagonist-II (PIVKA-II)
- p. time (pro time, PT)
- p. time/partial thromboplastin time (PT/PTT)

Protilase

protocol
- p. biopsy
- CISCA p.
- clinical p.
- Costello p.
- ELF chemotherapy p.
- Eulexin plus LHRH-A chemotherapy/radiation therapy p.
- high-energy p.
- low-energy p.
- multimodal p.
- non-heart-beating donor p.
- salvage p.
- Stanford p.
- surveillance p.
- treatment p.
- VAB6 chemotherapy p.

PROTOCO$_2$L insufflator

Protocult test

proton
- p. flux
- p. magnetic resonance spectroscopy
- p. pump
- p. pump blocker
- p. pump inhibition therapy
- p. pump inhibitor (PPI)

protonated

proton-induced release of secretin

Protonix
- P. delayed-release tablet
- P. IV powder for infusion

protooncogene
- *c-fos* p.
- *c-jun* p.
- *c-kit* p. (CD117)
- *c-myc* p.
- p53 p.
- RET p.

protopathic pain

protoporphyria
- erythropoietic p. (EPP)

protoporphyrin-9

Protostat Oral

prototype cholangioscope

protozoa (*pl. of* protozoon)

protozoal (*var. of* protozoan)

protozoan, protozoal
- p. abscess
- p. disease
- p. dysentery
- p. enteritis
- p. parasite
- p. pathogen

protozoon, *pl.* **protozoa**
- intestinal protozoa

Protractor

protriptyline

protruding fat

protrusion
- anal p.

protuberance
- pigmented p.

protuberant
- p. abdomen
- p. carcinoma

Provera

Providencia
- *P. alcalifaciens*
- *P. rettgeri*
- *P. stuartii*

Provir

provocation
- edrophonium p.

provocative
- P. sensitivity balloon
- p. test
- p. testing

provoked cystometry

ProXeed dietary supplement

proxetil
- cefpodoxime p.

proximal
- p. bile duct
- p. convoluted tubule (PCT)
- p. gastrectomy
- p. gastric vagotomy (PGV)
- p. human colonic flora
- p. jejunum
- p. muscle weakness
- p. nephron
- p. pouch leak
- p. pressure
- p. renal tubular acidosis
- p. splenorenal shunt
- p. straight tubule (PST)
- p. superior mesenteric artery

p. tubular cell
p. tubular secretion of angiotensin
p. tubule function
p. ureteral calculus
p. venous plexus
Proximate
P. flexible linear stapler
P. ILS circular stapler
P. intraluminal stapler
P. linear cutter
Prozac
PRT
physiologic reflux test
PRU
percent reduction in urea
prucalopride
Prudoxin cream
Pruitt anoscope
Prulet
prune-belly syndrome category I-III
prune juice peritoneal fluid
prunetin
pruning
p. abnormality
p. sign
pruritic
pruritus
p. ani
opioid-mediated p.
p. scroti
uremic p.
PSA
prostate-specific antigen
PSA doubling time
free PSA (fPSA)
PSA free/total index
free-to-total PSA
F:T PSA
PSA RT-PCR
total PSA (tPSA)
PSA-based parameter
PSAD
prostate-specific antigen density
PSA4 prostate cancer test
PSARP
posterior sagittal anorectoplasty
PSA-TZ, PSATZ
prostate-specific antigen density of
transition zone
PSAV
prostate-specific antigen velocity
PSC
primary sclerosing cholangitis
PSC-IBD
primary sclerosing cholangitis
inflammatory bowel disease
PSE
portosystemic encephalopathy

Pseudallescheria boydii
pseudoachalasia
malignant p.
pseudoalcoholic liver disease
pseudoallergy
pseudoaneurysm
p. formation
ruptured p.
pseudoaneurysmal roof
pseudobile canaliculus
pseudo-Billroth I appearance
pseudocapsule
pseudocholangiocarcinoma sign
pseudochylous ascites
pseudocirrhosis
cholangiodysplastic p.
pseudocolitis
pseudocolor fluorescence of Fura ed
pseudocryptorchism
pseudo-Cushing syndrome
pseudocyst
p. communication
drainage-resistant p.
endosonography-guided drainage of
pancreatic p.
extramural p.
extrapancreatic p.
giant nonpancreatic p.
heterogeneous p.
infected p.
intrasplenic p.
pancreatic duct to p.
paraduodenal p.
paragastric p.
p. puncture
retrogastric p.
small p.
uriniferous p.
pseudocystobiliary fistula
pseudocystogastrostomy
pancreatic p.
pseudodefecation
pseudodeficiency rickets
pseudodelicatissima
Pseudo-nitzschia p.
pseudodiverticulosis
esophageal intramural p.
pseudodiverticulum
urethral p.
pseudoductular transformation of
hepatocyte
pseudodysentery
pseudodyssynergia
pseudoephedrine hydrochloride
pseudoepitheliomatous micaceous growth
of penis
pseudoesophageal colic
pseudoexstrophy

P

pseudogout
pseudohermaphroditism
pseudohydronephrosis
pseudohyperkalemia
    familial p.
pseudohypha
pseudohypoaldosteronism
    type I, II p.
pseudohyponatremia
pseudohypoparathyroidism
 (PHP)
pseudoileus
pseudoleukemia gastrointestinalis
pseudolipomatosis polyposis
pseudolithiasis
    ceftriaxone p.
pseudolymphoma
    gastric p.
pseudomelanosis
pseudomembrane
pseudomembranous
    p. colic
    p. colitis (PMC)
    p. enteritis
    p. enterocolitis
    p. gastritis
pseudomicrolithiasis
pseudomigration
Pseudomonas
    P. aeruginosa
    P. aeruginosa pneumonia
    P. exotoxin A
    P. pseudomallei pneumonia
pseudomononucleosis
pseudomyxoma peritonei
pseudoneurogenic bladder
Pseudo-nitzschia
    P.-n. australis
    P.-n. multiseries
    P.-n. pseudodelicatissima
    P.-n. pungens
pseudoobstruction
    acute colonic p. (ACPO)
    bowel p.
    chronic idiopathic intestinal p.
     (CIIP)
    chronic intestinal p.
     (CIP, CIPO)
    colonic p.
    dolichocolon with p.
    familial intestinal p.
    idiopathic intestinal p.
    intestinal p.
    nonfamilial intestinal p.
    polyneuropathy, ophthalmoplegia,
     leukoencephalopathy, and intestinal
     p. (POLIP)
    p. syndrome
pseudopancreatic cholera syndrome

pseudoparallel channel sign
pseudopelade
pseudoperoxidase
pseudophimosis
pseudophytobezoar
pseudopodia
    tumorous p.
pseudopolyp
    chili-bean p.
pseudopolyposis medicamentosus
pseudoprune-belly syndrome
pseudo-pseudohypoparathyroidism
pseudoresistance
pseudosac
pseudosacculation
pseudosarcoid
pseudosarcoma
    bladder p.
    p. of esophagus
pseudospider pelvis
pseudospiralis
    Trichinella p.
pseudostone
pseudostricture
pseudotubercle
pseudotuberculosis
    Yersinia p.
pseudotumor
    p. appearance
    helminthic p.
    helmintic p.
    inflammatory p.
    kidney p.
    periampullary p.
    urethral p.
pseudovaginal perineoscrotal hypospadias
 (PPSH)
pseudowatermelon esophagus
pseudo-Whipple disease
pseudoxanthoma elasticum
PSFR
    pancreatic secretory flow rate
    peak secretory flow rate
     PSFR test
PSGN
    poststreptococcal glomerulonephritis
PSI
    portal shunt index
psittaci
    Chlamydia p.
PSK
    polysaccharide Kreha
PSLL
    pancreatoscopic laser lithotripsy
PSM
    prostate-specific membrane
PSMA
    prostate-specific membrane antigen
PS-2 needle

psoas
  p. abscess
  p. fascia
  p. hitch
  p. loss
  p. muscle
  p. shadow
  p. sign
psorenteritis
psoriasis of penis
psoriatic arthropathy
Psorospermium haeckelii
PSP
  pancreatic stone protein
PSS
  portosystemic shunting
  progressive systemic sclerosis
PST
  postural stimulation test
  potassium sensitivity test
  proximal straight tubule
PSTI
  pancreatic secretory trypsin
  inhibitor
psuedocystolonic fistula
PSWL
  peroral shock wave lithotripsy
psychic, psychical
  p. dysuria
  p. impotence
psychical (*var. of* psychic)
psychogenetic (*var. of* psychogenic)
psychogenic, psychogenetic
  p. constipation
  p. erectile dysfunction
  p. erection
  p. impotence
  p. polydipsia
  p. vomiting
  p. water drinking
psychologic (*var. of* psychological)
psychological, psychologic
  p. disorder
  p. dysfunction
  p. enuresis
  p. factor
  p. nonneuropathic bladder
  p. support
psychometric test
psychometry
psychopharmacologic medication
psychophysiologic
  p. disorder
  p. testing
psychosexual
  p. history
  p. support
  p. therapy
psychoses (*pl. of* psychosis)

psychosis, *pl.* **psychoses**
psychosomatic disorder
psychotropic
  p. drug
  p. medication
psychrophore
psyllium
  p. husk fiber
  p. seed
PT
  prothrombin time
PTA
  percutaneous transluminal angioplasty
PTB
  polypyrimidine tract binding
  PTB protein
PTBD
  percutaneous transhepatic biliary
  drainage
  PTBD catheter
PTC
  percutaneous transhepatic cholangiogram
  percutaneous transhepatic
  cholangiography
PTCC
  percutaneous transhepatic
  cholecystoscopy
PTCD
  percutaneous transhepatic
  cholangiodrainage
PTC-guided biopsy
PTCS
  percutaneous transhepatic
  cholangioscopy
PTD
  percutaneous transhepatic drainage
PTDM
  posttransplant diabetes mellitus
PTEN suppressor gene function
pteroylglutamic acid
pterygium
pterygoid depression
PTFE
  polytetrafluoroethylene
PTH
  parathyroid hormone
  carboxyterminal PTH
  intact PTH
  midregion PTH
PTHC
  percutaneous transhepatic cholangiogram
  percutaneous transhepatic
  cholangiography
  PTHC catheter
pthiriasis
Pthirus pubis
PTLD
  posttransplant lymphoproliferative
  disorder

P

ptosis
    renal p.
PTP
    percutaneous transhepatic
      portography
PT/PTT
    prothrombin time/partial thromboplastin
      time
PTQ implant
PTRA
    percutaneous transluminal renal
      angioplasty
PTT
    partial thromboplastin time
P-TUMT
    periurethral-transurethral microwave
      thermotherapy
PT141 with Viagra
ptyocrinous cell
P-type amylase
puama
    Muira p.
puberty
pubes, *pl.* **pubes**
pubic
    p. arch
    p. diastasis
    p. fixation
    p. hairline
    p. prostatectomy
    p. ramus
    p. symphysis
    p. tubercle
pubis
    body of p.
    osteitis p.
    pediculosis p.
    Pthirus p.
    symphysis p.
    symphysis ossium p.
published comparative trial
puboanalis muscle
pubocervical
    p. fascia
    p. ligament
pubococcygeal
    p. line (PCL)
    p. muscle training
pubococcygeus muscle
puboprostatic
    p. ligament
    p. sling
puborectalis
    p. dysfunction
    dyskinetic p.
    p. loop
    p. muscle
    p. muscle function

    overreactive p.
    p. sling
    p. syndrome
puborectal muscle
pubosacral line
pubourethral
    p. ligament
    p. sling
pubovaginal
    p. allograft sling procedure
    p. autologous fascial sling
    p. operation
pubovesicalis
    plica p.
pubovesical ligament
pubovesicocervical fascia
pubovisceral muscle
Pucci-Seed
    P.-S. hook
    P.-S. spatula
PUD
    peptic ulcer disease
pudding
    Ensure p.
    Sustacal p.
puddle sign
puddling on barium enema
pudenda (*pl. of* pudendum)
pudendal
    p. artery
    p. canal
    p. evoked potential
    p. nerve function
    p. nerve terminal motor latency
      (PNTML)
    p. neurogram
    p. neuropathy
    p. pelvic nerve
    p. vein
    p. vessel
pudendal-anal reflex
pudendi
    rima p.
pudendum, *pl.* **pudenda**
Puer-castor oil-trypsin ointment
puerperal septic pelvic vein
    thrombophlebitis
puerperia (*pl. of* puerperium)
puerperium, *pl.* **puerperia**
Puestow
    P. pancreatojejunostomy
    P. procedure
Puestow-Gillesby pancreatojejunostomy
Pugh
    P. liver disease classification
    P. modification
    P. modification of Child criteria
    modified method of P.

Pugh-Child scoring system
pull
    complete PEG p.
    p. enteroscopy
    p. method
    PEG p.
    Ponsky p.
pull-apart introducer
pullthrough
    endorectal ileal p.
    ileal p.
    ileoanal endorectal p.
    p. manometry
    p. procedure
    rapid p. (RPT)
    sacroabdominoperineal p.
    Soave endorectal p.
    station p. (SPT)
    Swenson abdominal p.
    p. technique
pull-type sphincterotomy
pulmonary
    p. alveolar microlithiasis
    p. arteriovenous malformation
    p. artery pressure (PAP)
    p. aspiration
    p. bile embolism
    p. capillaritis
    p. capillary wedge pressure
    p. cavitation
    p. complication
    p. disorder
    p. edema
    p. embolus
    p. gas embolism during laparoscopy
    p. granuloma
    p. methane excretion
    p. mucormycosis
    p. outflow
pulp, pulpa
    p. lienis
    splenic p.
    p. splenica
pulpa (*var. of* pulp)
pulpar cell
pulpy testis
Pulsalith lithotriptor
pulsatile
    p. hematoma
    p. mass
pulsatility index
pulse
    abdominal p.
    abrupt p.
    Altmann p.
    atrial liver p.
    Corrigan p.
    p. fluoroscopy

    frequency-doubled double p.
      (FREDDY)
    intermittent p.
    p. oximetry
    Quincke p.
    p. repetition frequency (PRF)
    p. spray catheter
    thready p.
    p. volume recording
pulsed
    p. Doppler
    p. Doppler ultrasound
    p. irrigation
    p. Solu-Medrol
pulsed-dye
    p.-d. laser
    p.-d. laser therapy
    p.-d. neodymium:YAG laser
pulsed-field gel electrophoresis (PFGE)
pulse-induced contour cardiac output
Pulse-Pak infusion kit
pulse-width analysis
pulsion
    enterocele p.
Pulsolith laser
pulsus abdominalis
pulverizer
    Thermovac tissue p.
Pulvules
    Cinobac P.
    Compound-65 P.
    Darvon Compound-65 P.
pump
    Abbott LifeCare p.
    acid p.
    AS-800 p.
    Asid Bonz PP infusion p.
    bile salt export p. (BSEP)
    Biosearch 7000 enteral feeding p.
    Bluemle p.
    calcium ATPase p.
    centrifugal p.
    Companion feeding p.
    Compat enteral feeding p.
    Cub R-200 enteral feeding p.
    Endolav lavage p.
    EnteraLite Infinity feeding p.
    Enteroport feeding p.
    Felig insulin p.
    Flexiflo Companion enteral feeding
      p.
    Flexiflo II enteral feeding p.
    Flocare 500 feeding p.
    Flo-Gard p.
    Frenta Mat feeding p.
    Frenta System II feeding p.
    Harvard p.
    hepatic artery infusion p.

P

pump (*continued*)
  HK-ATPase proton p.
  Holter pediatric p.
  IMED 430 enteral feeding p.
  Infusaid chemotherapy implantable p.
  Infusaid hepatic p.
  infusion p. (IP)
  Kangaroo 200, 330 enteral feeding
   p.
  Keofeed 500 enteral feeding p.
  Keofeed II enteral feeding p.
  KMI 60 enteral feeding p.
  low-compliance perfusion p.
  low-compliance pneumohydraulic p.
  MasterFlex p.
  McGaw volumetric p.
  Nutromat Pad S feeding p.
  peristaltic p.
  pneumatic leg p.
  proton p.
  retroperistaltic p.
  reverse osmosis p.
  roller p.
  Sarns Siok II blood p.
  sodium p.
  Space Saver volumetric p.
  stomach p.
  subcutaneous morphine p. (SQMP)
  suction p.
  Tonkaflo p.
  VTR-300 enteral feeding p.
  xenobiotic p.
pumped-dye laser
punch
  aortic p.
  p. biopsy
  biopsy p.
  kidney p.
  Murphy kidney p.
  Turkel p.
punched-out
  p.-o. orchidometer
  p.-o. ulcer
  p.-o. ulceration
punctata
  Aeromonas p.
punctate
  p. area
  p. fluorescence pattern
  p. ulcer
puncture
  calyceal p.
  calyx p.
  cecal ligation and p. (CLP)
  cystic p.
  diathermic p.
  direct cautery p.
  endoscopic fine-needle p.
  epididymis percutaneous p.
  epigastric p.
  Marfan epigastric p.
  needle tracheoesophageal p.
  pseudocyst p.
  suprapubic p.
  tracheoesophageal p. (TEP)
pungens
  Pseudo-nitzschia p.
pure
  p. cholestasia
  p. cutting current
  p. nephrosis
  p. pancreatic juice (PPJ)
  p. PPoma
  p. red cell aplasia (PRCA)
Puregene DNA isolation kit
purgation
purgative
purge
  oral p.
purging
  bingeing and p.
  self-induced p.
purified
  p. HBeAg
  p. protein derivative (PPD)
  p. T cell
Purilon
  Comfeel P.
purine
  dietary p.
  p. synthesis inhibitor
purinergic
Puritan
  P. DM Stick wound measuring
   device
  P. LiquiShield popule
puromycin
  p. aminonucleoside
  p. aminonucleoside necrosis
  p. aminonucleoside nephropathy
   (PAN)
  p. aminonucleoside nephrosis
   (PAN)
purple
  p. gromwell
  p. loosestrife
purpose-built silicone rubber multilumen manometric assembly
purpura
  p. abdominalis
  anaphylactoid p.
  Henoch-Schönlein p. (HSP)
  idiopathic thrombocytopenic p. (ITP)
  lung p.
  Schönlein-Henoch p.
  thrombocytopenic p.
  thrombotic thrombocytopenic p.
   (TTP)

purpurea
> *Echinacea p.*

purpureum
> tinea p.

pursestring
> p. ligature
> p. suture

pursestringed

Pursuer
> P. CBD helical stone basket
> P. minihelical stone basket

purulent
> p. appendicitis
> p. debris
> p. discharge
> p. gastritis
> p. material
> p. pancreatitis

puruloid

pus
> p. collection
> frank p.

push
> complete PEG p.
> p. enteroscope
> p. enteroscopy
> PEG p.
> p. technique

push-and-pull enteroscopy

pusher
> p. catheter
> Clarke-Reich knot p.
> Endo-Assist reusable knot p.
> Gazayerli knot p.
> metal-tipped stent p.
> p. tube

push-pull T technique

push-type enteroscopy

pustule

putative
> p. anion transporter
> p. hepatotrophic factors insulin/glucagon
> p. host restriction
> p. transmitter

putredinis
> *Bacteroides p.*

putrefactive diarrhea

putrescine

putty kidney

PUV
> posterior urethral valve type I–IV
> PUV type I–IV

PUVT
> paraumbilical vein tumor

P&V
> pyloroplasty and vagotomy

PVA
> partial villous atrophy

PVB
> platinum, Velban, bleomycin

PVC
> polyvinyl chloride
> postvoiding cystogram
> PVC catheter

PVCI
> portal vein congestive index

PVD
> postvagotomy diarrhea

PVH
> persistent viral hepatitis

PVH-B
> persistent viral hepatitis type B

PVH-NANB
> persistent viral hepatitis non-A non-B

PVO
> portal vein obstruction

PVP
> photoselective vaporization of prostate
> portal venous pressure

PVR
> postvoid residual

PVS
> peritoneovenous shunt

PVT
> portal vein thrombosis

PVV
> portal venous velocity

p21/waf1
> *P21/WAF1* gene
> p21/waf1 protein

PW-5V
> Olympus spray catheter PW-5V

pyelectasia (*var. of* pyelectasis)

pyelectasis, pyelectasia

pyelic

pyelitic

pyelitis
> calculous p.
> p. cystica
> defloration p.
> p. glandularis
> hematogenic p.
> incrusted p.
> urogenous p.

pyelocaliceal (*var. of* pyelocalyceal)

pyelocalicotomy

pyelocaliectasis (*var. of* caliectasis)

pyelocalyceal, pyelocaliceal
> p. cyst

pyelocutaneostomy
> pyelotransverse p.

pyelocystitis

pyelocystostomosis

pyelofluoroscopy

pyelogenic renal cyst

P

pyelogram, pyeloureterogram
    antegrade p.
    dragon p.
    hydrated p.
    intravenous p. (IVP)
    powder p.
    retrograde p.
pyelography, pelviureteroradiography,
  pyeloureterography, ureteropyelography
    air p.
    antegrade p.
    ascending p.
    p. by elimination
    excretion p.
    infusion p.
    intravenous p. (IVP)
    lateral p.
    limited intravenous p.
    percutaneous antegrade p.
    respiration p.
    respiratory p.
    retrograde p.
    washout p.
pyeloileal anastomosis
pyeloileocutaneous anastomosis
pyelointerstitial
pyelolithotomy, pelvilithotomy,
  pelviolithotomy
    coagulum p.
    extended p.
    Gil-Vernet extended p.
    laparoscopic p.
    open p.
    standard p.
pyelolymphatic backflow
pyelolysis
pyelometer
pyelometry
pyelonephritis (PN)
    acute nonobstructive p.
    ascending p.
    asymptomatic p.
    chronic p. (CP, CPN)
    chronic bacterial p.
    cryptococcal p.
    emphysematous p.
    fungal p.
    hematogenic p.
    p. of pregnancy
    xanthogranulomatous p. (XGP)
pyelonephrosis
pyelopathy
pyeloplasty, pelvioplasty
    Anderson-Hynes dismembered p.
    capsular flap p.
    Culp-DeWeerd spiral flap p.
    Culp spiral flap p.
    disjoined p.
    dismembered p.

    Fenger nondismembered p.
    Foley V-V p.
    Foley Y-plasty p.
    Foley Y-V p.
    laparoscopic dismembered p.
    robotically assisted laparoscopic
      dismembered p.
    Scardino-Prince vertical flap p.
    Scardino vertical flap p.
    Thompson capsule flap p.
pyeloplication
pyelorenal
    p. backflow
    p. reflux
pyeloscopy
pyelosinus
    p. backflow
    p. extravasation
pyelostomy
    cutaneous p.
pyelotomy
    p. closure
    extended p.
    p. incision
    open p.
    slash p.
pyelotubular
    p. backflow
    p. reflux
pyeloureteral catheter
pyeloureterectasis
pyeloureteritis cystica
pyeloureterogram (*var. of* pyelogram)
pyeloureterography (*var. of* pyelography)
pyeloureterolysis
pyeloureteroplasty
pyeloureterostomy
pyelovenous backflow
pyelovesical stent
pyelovesicostomy
pyemesis
pyemia
    portal p.
pygeum
    P. africanum
    p. extract
pyknotic nucleus
pylephlebitic abscess
pylephlebitis
pyloralgia
pylorectomy
    Kocher p.
pylori (*pl. of* pylorus)
pyloric
    p. atresia
    p. autotransplantation
    p. canal
    p. cap
    p. channel

p. channel ulcer
p. dilation
p. fullness
p. gland
p. insufficiency
p. intubation
p. metaplasia (PYME)
p. mucosa
p. outlet
p. outlet obstruction
p. pressure wave
p. ring
p. sphincter
p. spreader
p. stenosis
p. stricture
p. string sign
p. tone
pyloricum
antrum p.
ostium p.
Pylorid
PyloriScreen test
Pyloriset EIA-G test
pyloristenosis, pylorostenosis
pyloritek
P. *Helicobacter pylori*
test kit
P. rapid urease test
P. reagent strip
pylorodiosis
pyloroduodenal
p. junction
p. obstruction
p. perforation
p. segment
pylorogastrectomy
pyloromyotomy
endoscopic p.
Fredet-Ramstedt p.
Ramstedt p.
Ramstedt-Fredet p.
pyloroplasty
p. and vagotomy (P&V)
double p.
Finney p.
Heineke-Mikulicz p.
Horsley p.
Jaboulay p.
Judd p.
Mikulicz p.
Ramstedt p.
reconstructive p.
truncal vagotomy and p.
vagotomy and p. (V&P)
Weinberg modification of p.
pyloroptosia (*var. of* pyloroptosis)
pyloroptosis, pyloroptosia
pyloroscopy

pylorospasm
congenital p.
persistent p.
reflex p.
pylorostenosis (*var. of* pyloristenosis)
pylorostomy
pylorotomy
pylorus, *pl.* **pylori**
cagA-negative *Helicobacter pylori*
cagA-positive *Helicobacter pylori*
Campylobacter pylori
closed p.
coccoid form of *Helicobacter
pylori*
double p.
Helicobacter pylori (HP)
hypertrophic p.
intrafamilial clustering of
Helicobacter pylori
neutrophil-activating protein of
Helicobacter pylori (HP-NAP)
patulous p.
Pylori Stat assay test
pylorus-preserving
p.-p. pancreaticoduodenectomy
(PPPD)
p.-p. Whipple (PPW)
pylorus-sparing pancreaticoduodenectomy
PYME
pyloric metaplasia
PyNPase activity
pyocalix (*var. of* pyocalyx)
pyocalyx, pyocalix
pyocele
pyochezia
pyocystis
pyoderma gangrenosum
pyogenes
Streptococcus p.
pyogenetic (*var. of* pyogenic)
pyogenic, pyogenetic, pyogenous
p. bacterium
p. cholangitis
p. granuloma
p. liver
p. liver abscess
p. meningitis
p. organism
pyogenicum
granuloma p.
pyogenous (*var. of* pyogenic)
pyohydronephrosis
pyonephritis
pyonephrolithiasis
pyonephrosis, nephropyosis
pyonephrotic
pyopneumocholecystitis
pyopneumohepatitis
pyopneumoperitoneum

P

pyopneumoperitonitis
pyopyelectasis
pyosemia, pyospermia
pyospermia (*var. of* pyosemia)
pyostomatitis vegetans
pyoureter
pyovesiculosis
PYP
> pyrophosphate
> ^{99m}Tc PYP

pyramid
> base of renal p.
> Malpighi p.
> medullary p.
> p. of kidney
> renal p.

pyramidal
> p. muscle
> p. trocar

pyramides (*pl. of* pyramis)
Pyraminyl
pyramis, *pl.* **pyramides**
pyrantel pamoate
pyrazinamide
pyrazinoisoquinoline
pyrexia
pyrexial
Pyribenzamine
pyridinoline
> serum p.

Pyridium
> P. Plus
> P. test of vaginal drainage

Pyridorin XR
pyridostigmine
pyridoxal
> p. phosphate
> p. 5′-phosphate deficiency

pyridoxamine
pyridoxine
pyriform (*var. of* piriform)
pyriformis (*var. of* piriformis)
pyrilamine
Pyrilinks-D urinary assay
pyrimethamine
pyrimidine
> p. synthesis
> p. tract binding protein

pyrogen
> endogenous p.

pyrophosphate (PYP)
> stannous p. (SPP)

pyrosis
pyrrolidinedithiocarbamate
pyruvate
> p. dehydrogenase (PDH)
> p. kinase

PYtest urea breath test
pyuria
> abacterial p.

pyxigraphic device
PYY
> peptide YY

PYY-like immunoreactivity
PZD
> partial zonal dissection

Q

Q cell
Q fever

QAD1

Doppler QAD1
QAD1 sonography unit

QDR 1000 densitometer/absorptiometer
Q200 gastroscope
QHS

quantitative hepatobiliary scintigraphy

QID

Quantum inflation device

Q-Maxx side-firing laser device
QOLRD

Quality of Life in Reflux and
Dyspepsia
QOLRD score

Q-switched

Q-s. alexandrite laser
Q-s. Nd:YAG laser

Q-tip test
Q-TWIST

quality-adjusted time without symptoms
or toxicity

Quad-Lumen drain
Quadra-Coil ureteral stent
QuadraFoam dressing
quadrant

both lower q.'s
both upper q.'s
left lower q.
left upper q.
right lower q.
right upper q.

4-quadrant

4-q. incision
4-q. jumbo biopsy
4-q. tattooing

quadrant-sampling technique
quadrate

q. lobe
q. lobe of liver

quadriplegia
quadruple therapy
quadruplicate well
qualitative

q. fecal fat test
q. microculture assay

quality

assessment of bowel preparation q.
q. of kidney graft
Q. of Life in Reflux and
Dyspepsia (QOLRD)
Q. of Life in Reflux and
Dyspepsia score

**quality-adjusted time without symptoms
or toxicity (Q-TWIST)**
quality-of-life

q.-o.-l. instrument
q.-o.-l. parameter

quantification

pelvic organ prolapse q. (POP-Q)

quantified protein excretion
**Quantikine quantitative
immunoenzymatometric sandwich
technique**
quantitation

fat q.

quantitative

q. angiography
q. fecal fat test
q. hepatobiliary scintigraphy
(QHS)
q. liquid hybridization
q. measurement
q. scintigraphic evacuation
proctography
q. stool collection
q. ultrasound (QUS)

Quantum

Q. inflation device (QID)
Q. TTC balloon dilator
Q. TTC biliary balloon

quartan malaria
3-quarter circle electrode
**Quartey pedicled penile flap
urethroplasty technique**
quartz waveguide
Quarzan
quasispecies
quassia
quaternary ammonium ion
quazepam
queasiness
queasy
quercetin
Quervain abdominal retractor
query
questionnaire

Biliary Symptoms Q. (BSQ)
Bowel Disease Q.
Chronic Liver Disease Q. (CLDQ)
q. data
Diabetes Bowel Symptom Q.
(DBSQ)
Inflammatory Bowel Disease Q.
(IBDQ)
McGill pain q.
Pelvic Organ Prolapse Urinary
Incontinence Sexual Q.

questionnaire (*continued*)
    Sexual Function Inventory Q.
    (SFIQ)
    Short Inflammatory Bowel Disease
    Q. (SIBDQ)
Questran
Quetelet BMI index
Queyrat erythroplasia
QuickClip
Quick-Core biopsy needle
quick-dissolving crystal
Quick-Tap paracentesis system
Quick test
QuickVue
    Q. *H. pylori* gII test kit
    Q. One-Step *H. pylori* test
Quidel QuickVue *H. pylori* test
quiescent
    q. hepatitis
    q. human fibroblast
Quiess
quiet bowel sounds
quill sheath
quilted suture
Quimby
    Q. method
    Q. pattern
quinacrine
Quinaglute

quinapril
quince
Quincke
    Q. pulse
    Q. triad
quinidine
    q. gluconate
    q. intoxication
    q. sulfate
quinine urea hydrochloride
Quinlan test
quinolone
Quinton
    Q. catheter
    Q. PermCath
    Q. single-port scissors valve
    Q. suction biopsy instrument
    Q. tube
Quinton-Mahurkar dual-lumen peritoneal catheter
Quinton-Scribner shunt
QuinTron
    Q. AlveoSampler
    Q. MicroLyzer
    Q. MicroLyzer 12 chromatograph
Quire mechanical finger forceps
Quixil spray
QUS
    quantitative ultrasound

RAAA
> ruptured abdominal aortic aneurysm

RAAS
> renin-angiotensin-aldosterone system

rabbit
> r. polyclonal antibody
> r. stool

rabeprazole sodium
Rabuteau test
RAC
> ranitidine bismuth citrate, amoxicillin, clarithromycin

racephedrine
RackBeta scintillation counter
rac **protein**
radial
> r. examination
> r. groove
> r. immunodiffusion
> r. incision
> R. Jaw hot biopsy forceps
> R. Jaw III Max Capacity 1589 biopsy forceps
> R. Jaw III Max Capacity needle biopsy forceps
> R. Jaw III single-use biopsy forceps
> r. mode
> r. suture track

radial-flow bioreactor
radial-sector scanning echoendoscope
radiata
> corona r.

radiating pain
radiation
> r. colitis
> r. cystitis
> r. dosage
> effective dose-equivalent r.
> endocavitary r.
> r. enteritis
> r. enterocolitis
> r. enteropathy
> r. esophagitis
> r. exposure
> 5-fluorouracil, mitomycin C r. (FUMIR)
> r. gastritis
> r. hepatopathy
> r. injury
> ionizing r.
> nonionizing r.
> nonparticulate r.
> particulate r.
> r. pneumonitis
> r. proctitis
> r. proctocolitis
> radiotracer half-life r.
> rectosigmoid r.
> r. sensitizer
> r. stenosis
> r. telangiectasia
> r. therapy

radiation-induced
> r.-i. angiosarcoma
> r.-i. angiosclerosis
> r.-i. colitis
> r.-i. disease
> r.-i. obliterative arteritis
> r.-i. sterility
> r.-i. ulceration
> r.-i. ureteral stricture
> r.-i. vesicovaginal fistula

radical
> r. cystectomy
> r. en bloc removal
> free r.
> r. hemorrhoidectomy
> hydroxyl r.
> r. inguinal orchiectomy
> r. nephrectomy
> r. nephroureterectomy
> oxygen r.
> oxygen-derived free r.
> oxygen-free r.
> r. perineal prostatectomy (RPP)
> r. resection group
> r. retropubic prostatectomy (RRP)
> superoxide r.
> r. surgery
> r. transcoccygeal prostatectomy

radicality
> oncologic r.

radices (*pl. of* radix)
radiciform
radicle
> biliary r.
> intrahepatic r.
> right hepatic r.
> tertiary r.

radiculitis
radii (*pl. of* radius)
radioactive
> r. carbon-14 test
> r. cholesterol
> r. detection
> r. iodine-131
> r. seed
> r. seed implantation

radioallergosorbent test (RAST)

radioautography
    thaw-mount r.
radiobiology
radiocephalic fistula
radiochemotherapy
radiochromium-labeled erythrocyte method
radiocolloid
radiocontrast-induced
    r.-i. acute renal failure
    r.-i. renal vasoconstriction
radiocystitis
radiodensity
radioenzymatic assay
radiofrequency
    r. ablation
    r. interstitial tissue ablation
radiograph
    plain r.
radiographic
    r. situation
    r. triad
radiography
    abdominal r.
    barium contrast r.
    calculus r.
    double-contrast r.
    kidneys, ureters, bladder r.
    KUB r.
    plain abdominal r.
    postvoid r.
    single-contrast r.
    skeletal r.
radioimmunoassay (RIA)
    Cyclotrac-SP r.
    hepatitis A virus r. (HAVAB)
    homogeneous r.
    solid-phase r.
    Yang PSA r.
radioimmunodetection
radioimmunofocus inhibition test (RIFIT)
radioimmunoguided surgery (RIGS)
radioimmunoinhibition assay
radioimmunoprecipitation modified assay
radioiodination
radioisotope
    r. capsule
    r. renal excretion test
    r. renogram test
    r. renography
    r. scan
    r. scanning
    r. scintigraphy
radiolabeled
    r. imaging
    r. leucine
    r. macromolecule
radiologic, radiological
    r. biliary stent placement

    r. castration
    r. investigation
    r. portacaval shunt
    r. study
radiological (*var. of* radiologic)
radiolucent
    r. gallstone
    r. object
Radiometer
    R. 85 instrument
    R. pH probe
radionecrosis
radionuclide
    r. cholescintigraphy
    r. cystography
    r. esophageal emptying time
    [^{123}I] iodoamphetamine r.
    r. renal imaging
    r. scan
    r. scintigraphy
    r. ^{99}Tc scintiscanning
    r. therapy
    r. transit study
    r. voiding cystourethrography
radiopaque
    r. density
    r. dye
    r. ERCP catheter
    r. iodized oil
    r. marker
    r. pellet
radioresistant gastric plasmacytoma
radioscintigraphy
radioscopically
radiosensitive organ
radiotelemetering capsule
radiotherapy, radiation therapy
    infradiaphragmatic r.
    intraluminal r.
    intraoperative r. (IORT)
    intraoperative electron beam r.
radiotracer half-life radiation
radius, *pl.* **radii**
    R. enteral feeding tube
    r. of varix
    thrombocytopenia-absent r. (TAR)
radix, *pl.* **radices**
    r. penis
RAEB
    refractory anemia with excess blasts
ragged red fiber
railroading
railroad track scars
RAIR
    rectoanal inhibitory reflex
rake
    r. retractor
    r. ulcer
Ralks adapter

Raman
    R. scattering
    R. spectroscopic system
    R. spectroscopy
rami (*pl. of* ramus)
ramification
ramipril
    R. Efficacy in Nephropathy (REIN)
    R. Efficacy in Nephropathy study
Ramirez
    R. shunt
    R. silastic cannula
Ramond point
ramosum
    Absidia r.
    Clostridium r.
ramotomy
    superior pubic r.
Rampley sponge-holding forceps
Ramstedt
    R. operation
    R. pyloric stenosis dilator
    R. pyloromyotomy
    R. pyloroplasty
Ramstedt-Fredet pyloromyotomy
ramus, *pl.* **rami**
    pubic r.
ranarum
    Basidiobolus r.
Randall
    R. plaque
    R. stone forceps
Randolph abdominoplasty
random
    r. bladder biopsy
    r. flap
    R. Primed DNA labeling kit
    r. stool sample
randomized clinical trial data
Rand Short Form-36 survey
Ranfac
    R. cholangiographic catheter
    R. cholangiography catheter
range
    arrhythmic frequency r.
    chromatofocusing pH r.
    dilation r.
    hapatotoxic r.
    metabolic r.
    optimum cooling r.
ranitidine
    r. bismuth citrate (RBC)
    r. bismuth citrate, amoxicillin, clarithromycin (RAC)
    r. bismuth citrate, metronidazole, tetracycline (RMT)
    r. hydrochloride
    r. nocte
    r. therapy

rank
    Spearman r.
Rankin clamp
Ransley-Cantwell epispadias repair
Ranson
    R. acute pancreatitis classification
    R. criteria
    R. criteria for severity of pancreatitis
    R. grading system
RAP
    receptor-associated protein
    recurrent abdominal pain
Rapamune
    R. oral solution
    R. tablet
rapamycin
    r. inhibitor
    treatment with r.
raphe
    anococcygeal r.
    r. of perineum
    r. of scrotum
    r. pallidus
    penile r.
    r. penis
    perineal r.
    r. perinei
    scrotal r.
    r. scroti
Rapicide
rapid (RPD)
    r. acquisition fast spin-echo sequence
    r. alternating recorder exchange in capsule endoscopy
    r. colonic lavage
    r. emptying of dye
    r. enzyme immunoassay
    r. exchange (RX)
    r. exchange technique for therapeutic endoscopy
    r. gastric emptying
    r. pullthrough (RPT)
    r. pullthrough esophageal manometry technique
    r. serum amylase test
    R. Strand implant
    r. urease test (RUT)
    r. urease testing kit
    r. viral response
RapidFire multiple-band ligator
Rapid-hyb buffer
rapidly progressive glomerulonephritis (RPGN)
RapiSeal pouch
Rapoport test
Rappaport classification
Rapunzel syndrome

RARS
    refractory anemia with ringed
      sideroblasts
ras
    r. p21 oncogene
RAS
    renin-angiotensin system
    RAS blocker
    RAS effector RASSF2
      tumor-suppressor gene
rasburicase
rash
    butterfly r.
    discoid r.
    genital r.
    petechial r.
    scarlatiniform r.
raspatory
    Doyen r.
***ras*-related protein**
RAST
    radioallergosorbent test
rate
    albumin excretion r. (AER)
    alcohol elimination r. (AER)
    allograft survival r.
    amphotericin B-induced reduction
      glomerular filtration r.
    average flow r.
    basal carbohydrate oxidation r.
    basal metabolic r. (BMR)
    basal secretory flow r. (BSFR)
    blood flow r. (BFR)
    crude incidence r.
    demonstrated hypertensive r.
    detection r.
    erythrocyte sedimentation r. (ESR)
    exponential r.
    flow r.
    gallbladder ejection r. (GBER)
    glomerular filtration r. (GFR)
    high failure r.
    high false-positive r.
    kidney electrolyte clearance r.
    kidney electrolyte excretion r.
    lipid oxidation r.
    logarithmic r.
    low recurrence r.
    maximum free-flow r.
    maximum urinary flow r.
    mean TIMP-1/GAPDH r.
    metabolic r.
    normalized protein catabolic r.
      (NPCR)
    operative mortality r.
    optimal shock wave r.
    pancreatic secretory flow r. (PSFR)
    patency r.
    peak flow r. (PFR)

    peak secretory flow r. (PSFR)
    postoperative recurrent bleeding r.
    posttransplantation survival r.
    pressure increment r. (PIR)
    prevalence of low glomerular
      filtration r.
    protein catabolic r. (PCR)
    r. ratio
    rebleeding r.
    recurrence r.
    reduced graft survival r.
    reintervention r.
    reoperation r.
    respiratory r. (RR)
    retreatment r.
    seroconversion r.
    seroprevalence r.
    single-nephron glomerular filtration r.
     (SNGFR)
    stone-free r.
    stone recurrence r.
    survival r.
    transcapillary escape r.
    urine flow r.
    voiding flow r. (VFR)
Rathke
    R. duct
    R. plica
**Rating Form of Inflammatory Bowel
Disease Patient Concerns (RFIPC)**
ratio
    adenoma hyperplastic polyp r.
    adenoma to nonadenoma r.
    aldosterone-to-renin r.
    albumin-globulin ratio (A/G)
    amylase/creatinine clearance r. (A:C)
    androstenedione-to-testosterone r.
    apolipoprotein CII/CIII r.
    AST/ALT r.
    BCAA/AAA plasma r.
    bile salt-phospholipid r.
    BUN-to-creatinine r.
    calcium-creatinine r.
    CD4+ — CD8+ T-cell r.
    chloride-to-phosphate r.
    CO_2-CO_2 abundance r.
    decreased postprandial-to-fasting
     power r.
    dialysate-to-plasma r.
    distribution r. (DR)
    distribution r. 2 (DR2)
    distribution r. 3 (DR3)
    distribution r. 4 (DR4)
    distribution r. 5 (DR5)
    distribution r. 7 (DR7)
    D-P urea r.
    foveola-gland r.
    free-to-total PSA r.
    G:D-cell r.

R

ketone body r. (KBR)
lactulose-mannitol r.
LCA-DCA r.
likelihood r.
lipid-to-protein r.
lithocholic acid-deoxycholic acid r.
mean TIMP-3/GAPDH r.
nuclear-to-cytoplasmic size r.
r. of mucosa to submucosa to
   muscularis propria
r. of PGF2-alpha PGE2
pepsinogen A-C r.
phospholipid r.
pressure transmission r.
presumed circle area r.
rate r.
renal vein renin r.
serum pepsinogen I/II r.
signal-to-cutoff r.
somatostatin mRNA-D-cell density r.
standardized incidence r.
surface-to-volume r.
UA/C r.
urea reduction r. (URR)
urinary protein-urinary creatinine r.
urine-plasma r.
Valsalva r.
Xc/R r.
rational allocation strategy
rationing
Ratliff-Blake gallstone forceps
Ratliff-Mayo forceps
rat-tail
r.-t. appearance on pancreatogram
r.-t. configuration
r.-t. sign
rat-tooth Olympus FG 8L grasping forceps
Rauber
hepatic funiculus of R.
Raudixin
Rautina
Rauval
Rauwolfia
Rauzide
raw
r. milk-associated diarrhea
r. surface of liver bed
Rayer disease
Raz
R. anterior vaginal wall sling
R. bladder neck suspension
R. bladder neck suspension
   procedure
R. 4-corner vaginal wall sling
R. double-prong ligature carrier
R. modification
R. needle bladder suspension
R. 4-quadrant suspension

R. sling operation
R. urethral suspension
razor
r. blade
r. blade ingestion
Rb
rubidium
Rb gene
Rb influx
Rb protein
RBC
ranitidine bismuth citrate
red blood cell
technetium-99m pyrophosphate-tagged
   RBC
RBF
renal blood flow
RBL
rubber band ligation
rubber band ligator
RBP
retinol-binding protein
RCC
renal cell carcinoma
RCF
Ross carbohydrate-free
   RCF formula
RCRC
recurrent colorectal cancer
RCT
rectal carcinoid tumor
RCU
recurrent calcium urolithiasis
RDA
recommended daily allowance
RDG
retrograde duodenogastroscopy
Reabilan HN tube-feeding formula
reabsorption
fractional proximal r.
HCO^{3-} r.
implant r.
protein tubular r.
sodium r.
spontaneous cyst r.
tubular sodium r.
reactance (Xc)
r. and resistance (Xc/R)
reaction
acrosome r.
allergic r.
amplification refractory mutation
   system-polymerase chain r.
   (ARMS-PCR)
anaphylactic r.
Bittorf r.
cholestatic r.
desmoplastic r.
drug r.

reaction (*continued*)
>Ehrlich diazo r.
>Feulgen r.
>fixed drug r.
>foreign body r.
>Haber-Weiss r.
>hypersensitivity r.
>immune-mediated r.
>inflammatory r.
>insulin r.
>Jaffe picrate r.
>lichenoid r.
>limiting dilution cloning polymerase chain r. (LDC-PCR)
>nonenzymic r.
>one-stage r.
>paradoxic sphincter r.
>periglandular nonspecific inflammatory r.
>Perls r.
>polymerase chain r. (PCR)
>reversed passive hemagglutination r.
>reverse transcriptase r.
>reverse transcriptase-polymerase chain r. (RT-PCR)
>scar tissue r.
>Schmorl r.
>specific polymerase chain r. (SP-PCR)
>sphincter r.
>T-lymphocyte-mediated cytotoxic r.
>urticarial r.
>van den Bergh r.
>Weiss r.

reactive
>r. arthritis
>r. hyperemia
>r. inflammatory vascular dermatosis
>r. oxygen metabolite
>r. oxygen species

reactivity
>Goodpasture r.
>lectin r.
>p53 r.

reader
>microtitration plate r.

reagent
>ABC r.
>Chemstrip bG r.
>CHOD-PAP cholesterol r.
>Ehrlich r.
>Folin phenol r.
>lipofection r.
>SAB r.

real focus shock wave
real-time
>r.-t. confocal scanning laser microscope
>r.-t. 3D biplanar transperineal prostate implantation
>r.-t. endoscopic ultrasound-guided fine-needle aspiration
>r.-t. fine-needle aspiration (RTFNA)
>r.-t. gallbladder ultrasound
>r.-t. sonographic unit
>r.-t. spectral analysis
>r.-t. transmission (RTX)
>r.-t. ultrasonography (RUS)
>r.-t. videoprocessor

reanastomosis
>end-to-end branch r.
>laparoscopic ureteral r.
>Roux-en-Y r.

reapproximate
reassignment
>gender r.

Rebetol
>R. capsule
>R. with Intron

Rebetron combination therapy
rebleeding rate
rebound
>gastric acid r.
>r. pain
>postdialysis urea r. (PDUR)
>r. sign
>r. tenderness

recanalization
>endoscopic laser r.
>r. of clogged biliary stent
>spontaneous r.
>umbilical vein r.

receiver
>Olympus EU-M30S endoscopic ultrasonography r.
>r. operating characteristic (ROC)

receiving
>external r.

recent
>r. clinical trial
>r. technical modification

receptacula (*pl. of* receptaculum)
receptaculum, *pl.* **receptacula**
>r. chyli
>r. pecqueti

receptive
>r. anal intercourse
>r. relaxation

receptor
>ability of glucocorticoid r.
>adhesive protein r.
>adrenergic r.
>alpha-1 adrenergic r.
>alpha-2 adrenergic r.
>alpha-adrenergic r.
>androgen r.
>r. and signal transduction
>angiotensin II r.
>ANP r.

antiasialoglycoprotein r.
antidiuretic arginine vasopressin
    V2 r. (AVPR2)
asialoglycoprotein r.
beta-adrenergic r.
bladder muscarinic r.
bombesin r.
cardiac beta r.
C3 r.
C3b r.
C4b r.
C5 r.
CC-chemokine r. 2
cell surface r.
chemokine r.
cholinergic r.
c-met r.
corpus cavernosum muscarinic r.
r. crosstalk
endothelin A r.
epidermal growth factor r. (EGFR)
estrogen r.
EtA r.
EtB r.
expression of hemin r.
farnesoid X r.
fMLP chemoattractant r.
formyl peptide r.
gastric mucosal laminin r.
gastric oxyntic cell r.
gastrin r.
growth hormone secretagogue r.
    (GHSR)
H2 r.
high-affinity r.
histaminergic type 2 r.
hormone r.
5-HT3 r.
human motilin r.
human PDGF r.
IL-2, -3, -4, -6, -8 r.
insulin receptor-related r.
32/67-kD laminin r.
killer-activating r.
laminin r.
liver Ah r.
lymphotoxin beta r. (LTBR)
mesenteric sensory r.
multiligand r.
muscarinic r.
muscle sensory r.
native pancreatic secretin r.
natriuretic peptide r. (NPR)
nerve growth factor r. (NGFR)
neural growth factor r. (NGFR)
nicotinic r.
NK1, NK2 tachykinin r.
opiate r.
peptic cell r.

peroxisome proliferator-activated r.
    (PPAR)
phosphorylated growth factor r.
polyimmunoglobulin r. (pIgR)
protease-activated r.
recombinant pancreatic secretin r.
retinoid X r.
sensory r.
serotonergic type 3 r.
smooth muscle motilin r.
soluble recombinant
    complement r. 1
soluble transferrin r. (sTf-R)
somatostatin r.
steroid r.
stretch r.
T-cell r. (TCR, TcR)
toll-interleukin 1 r.
toll-like r.
transferrin r.
transferrin r. 2
tyrosine kinase growth-factor r.
umami taste r.
uroepithelial glycoid r.
vasopressin type 2 r.
vitamin D r.
receptor-associated
    r.-a. protein (RAP)
    r.-a. protein-glutathione-S-transferase
receptor-blocker
    H2 r.-b.
receptor-mediated endocytosis pathway
recess, recessus
    duodenojejunal r.
    splenorenal r.
recession
    clitoral r.
recessive polycystic kidney disease
recessus (*var. of* recess), *pl.* **recessus**
recipient
    r. hepatectomy
    kidney transplant r.
    marrow transplant r.
    phase II, III marrow transplant r.
    relationship of r.
    renal allograft r.
    renal transplant r.
    unsensitized transplant r.
recipient-derived anti-HLA antibody
reciprocal ligand
recirculation
    enterohepatic r.
Reclomide
recognition
    ligand r.
    stone-tissue r. (STR)
recombinant
    r. capsid protein of Norwalk virus
    (rNV)

recombinant (*continued*)
  r. growth hormone
  r. HBcAg (rHBcAg)
  r. hepatitis C antigen
  r. HGF
  r. human alfa interferon
  r. human erythropoietin (rh-EPO)
  r. human gelsolin
  r. human relaxin
  r. IL-10
  r. immunoblot assay (RIBA)
  r. immunoblot assay-2
  r. immunoblot assay-2 test
  r. interferon alfa (rIFN-alfa)
  r. interferon alfa-2a
  r. interleukin-2
  r. methionyl human leptin
    (r-metHuLeptin)
  r. pancreatic secretin receptor
  r. tissue transglutaminase radioligand
    assay
  r. tTG radioligand assay
recombination fraction
Recombivax HB
recommendation
  criteria for grading of clinical
    studies and r.'s
recommended daily allowance (RDA)
reconstruction
  anal sphincter r.
  biliary r.
  Billroth I, II gastrointestinal r.
  bladder neck r.
  bladder outlet r.
  corporeal r.
  dural patch r.
  functional r.
  genital r.
  Kropp bladder neck r.
  Monfort abdominal wall r.
  orthotopic r.
  penile r.
  penile arterial r.
  penis r.
  Roux-en-Y r.
  sphincter r.
  synchronous bladder r.
  Tanagho bladder neck r.
  r. technique
  total anorectal r.
  tubularized bladder neck r.
  urethral surgical r.
  urinary r.
  Young-Dees bladder neck r.
  Young-Dees-Leadbetter bladder neck
    r.
reconstructive
  r. endourology
  r. phalloplasty

  r. pyloroplasty
  r. surgery
record
  initial in-plan r.
  intragastric pH monitor r.
recorder
  Digitrapper MK III portable digital
    r.
  multichannel r.
  Narco Bio-Systems rectilinear r.
  portable digital data r.
  Rectigraph-8K r.
  rectilinear r.
  Sandhill-800 TDS chart r.
  Sekomic SS-100F r.
  Toshiba ERVF 1A video floppy r.
  video r.
RecorderBelt
recording
  bipolar esophageal r.
  cutaneous r.
  external r.
  intraluminal pressure r.
  neurophysiologic r.
  penile pulse volume r.
  pH r.
  pulse volume r.
recovery
  complete anatomical r.
  detrusor r.
  r. of sexual potency
recreational drug
recrudescence
recruitment
  mononuclear cell r.
recta (*pl. of* rectum)
rectal
  r. abscess
  r. air suctioning
  r. akinesia
  r. alimentation
  r. ampulla
  r. amyloidosis
  r. artery
  r. augmentation
  r. balloon
  r. balloon expulsion
  r. barostat
  r. barostat study
  r. biopsy
  r. bladder urinary diversion
  r. bleeding
  r. cancer
  r. capacity
  r. carcinoid tumor (RCT)
  r. cell proliferation
  r. cisapride
  r. coil MRI
  r. column

r. compliance
r. compliance measurement
r. cream
r. descensus
r. digital stimulation
r. dilation
r. dilator
r. disease
r. dissection
r. distention
r. emptying
r. endoscopic ultrasonography (REU, REUS)
r. endosonography
r. epithelial cell
r. evacuation
r. evacuatory disorder (RED)
r. examination
r. expander
r. expander-assisted transanal endoscopic microsurgery (RE-TEM)
r. fascia
r. feedback trigger
r. filling
r. fistula
r. fold
r. foreign body
r. fossa
r. gluten challenge
r. gonorrhea
r. hyposensitivity
r. hypotonia
r. impaction
r. impedance
r. impedance planimetry
r. incontinence
r. inhibitory reflex
r. injury
r. innervation
r. intussusception
r. laceration
r. leiomyosarcoma
r. linitis plastica (RLP)
r. linitis plastica colorectal carcinoma
r. lumen
r. mass
r. motor complex
r. mucosa
r. mucosectomy
r. muscle cuff
r. myogenic tumor
r. nerve
r. plexus
r. polyp
r. pouch
r. probe
r. probe electroejaculation
r. procidentia

r. prolapse
r. pulsed irrigation
r. reservoir
r. sensation
r. shelf
r. sinus
r. snare
r. sparing
r. spasm
r. speculum
r. sphincter
r. stenosis
r. stricture
r. stump
r. suppository
r. telangiectasia density
r. tenderness
r. tenesmus
r. thermometer
r. trauma
r. tube
r. ulcer
r. valve
r. valvotomy
r. varix
r. vault
r. vein
r. villous adenoma
r. visceral sensitivity

rectale
   Eubacterium r.
rectales
   columnae r.
recti (*pl. of* rectus)
Rectigraph-8K recorder
rectilinear recorder
rectoabdominal
rectoanal
   r. dyssynergia
   r. function
   r. inhibitor
   r. inhibitory reflex (RAIR)
rectocele
   r., cystocele, enterocele
   r. presentation
rectoclysis
rectococcygeus muscle
rectocystotomy
rectogenital septum
rectoischiadic excavation
rectolabial fistula
rectoneovaginal fistula
rectopexy
   abdominal r.
   anterior r.
   Ivalon sponge r.
   laparoscopic suture r.
   Marlex mesh abdominal r.
   posterior r.

rectopexy (*continued*)
    presacral r.
    Ripstein anterior sling r.
    suture r.
    Teflon sling r.
    Wells posterior r.
rectoplasty
    vertical reduction r.
Rector-Gordon-Healey-Mendoza-Spitzer type IV renal tubular acidosis
rectorrhagia
rectosacral
    r. fascia
    r. ligament
rectosigmoid
    r. anastomosis
    r. cancer
    r. colon
    r. function
    r. junction
    r. manometry
    r. radiation
    r. region
    r. varix
rectosigmoidectomy
    Altemeier perineal r.
    perineal r.
rectosigmoidoscopy
rectosphincteric
    r. abnormality
    r. dyssynergia
    r. reflex (RSR)
rectosphincter manometric study
rectotomy
rectourethral
    r. fistula
    r. muscle
rectourethralis muscle
rectourinary fistula
rectouterina
    excavatio r.
rectouterine
    r. pouch
    r. pouch of Douglas
rectovaginal
    r. fistula
    r. pouch
    r. septum
    r. surgery
    r. surgical treatment
rectovesical
    r. center
    r. fascia
    r. fistula
    r. lithotomy
    r. pouch
    r. septum
rectovesicalis
    excavatio r.

rectovestibular fistula
rectovulvar fistula
rectum, *pl.* **rectums, recta**
    ampulla of r.
    augmented valved r.
    benign lymphoma of r.
    bleeding per r.
    blood per r. (BPR)
    bright red blood per r. (BRBPR)
    gastric mucosal ectopia in r. (GMER)
    Hartmann closure of r.
    horizontal folds of r.
    r. irrigation
    nonrehydrated guaiac examination of r.
    per r.
    prolapsed r.
    transverse folds of r.
    valved r.
    vasa recta
    watermelon r.
rectums (*pl. of* rectum)
rectus, *pl.* **recti**
    r. abdominis
    r. abdominis hematoma
    r. abdominis muscle
    r. abdominis musculocutaneous flap
    ampulla recti
    r. diastasis
    r. fascia
    r. fascial wrap
    r. fascia sling
    r. femoris flap
    flexura perinealis recti
    flexura sacralis recti
    folliculi lymphatici recti
    procidentia recti
    r. sheath
    r. sheath hematoma (RSH)
recurrence
    anastomotic r.
    local r.
    r. rate
    short-term prostate-specific antigen r.
    source of r.
    Wilms tumor r.
recurrent (rec, recur)
    r. abdominal pain (RAP)
    r. appendicitis
    r. bleeding
    r. bouts of vomiting
    r. calcium-containing stones
    r. calcium stone formation
    r. calcium urolithiasis (RCU)
    r. cholestasia
    r. colonic histoplasmosis
    r. colorectal cancer (RCRC)
    r. cystitis

r. episodes of *Clostridium difficile*
disease
r. focal sclerosing glomerulonephritis
r. molar pregnancy
r. pancreatitis
r. pyogenic cholangiohepatitis (RPC)
r. stress incontinence
r. stricture
r. ulcer
r. urinary calculus
r. urinary tract infection

red
r. blood cell (RBC)
r. blood cell cast
r. blood cell count
r. blood cell extravasation
r. blood cell folate
r. blood cell folate level
r. bryony
r. cell distribution width
r. color sign
r. degeneration of uterine myoma
r. flag sign
r. ring sign
r. rubber Robinson catheter
ruthenium r.
r. wale marking

RED
rectal evacuatory disorder

Reddick cystic duct cholangiogram catheter

Reddick-Saye
R.-S. method
R.-S. screw

Redfield infrared coagulator

Redipen
Peg-Intron R.

Redivac suction drain

Rediwash skin cleanser

Redman approach

redness
diffuse r.

Redo intestinal clamp

Redon drain

red-out

redox potential

reduced
r. graft survival rate
r. liver transplant (RLT)
r. motility
r. rejection episode

reduced-size
r.-s. graft
r.-s. liver transplant (RSLT)

reducible hernia

reducing
r. diet
r. substance
r. substances test

reductase
aldose r.
HMG-CoA r.
5,10-methylene-tetrahydrofolate r.
(MTHFR)

reduction
air pressure enema r.
barium enema r.
dissimilatory sulfate r.
r. en masse
gastric acidity r.
hemorrhoid r.
hepatic venous pressure gradient r.
profound acid r.
proportionate r.
sigmoid loop r.
volvulus r.

redundant sac tissue

Redux

Redy hemodialysis system

REE
resting energy expenditure

reefing
stomach r.

reentry

reexamined
retrospectively r.

reexploration

refeeding
casein r.
r. syndrome

reference value

referred pain

refill
capillary r.
delayed capillary r.

refined carbohydrate complex

refining surgical technique

reflectance
r. analysis
endoscopic r.
r. spectrophotometer
r. spectrophotometric probe
r. spectrophotometry
r. spectroscopy
r. spectrum analyzer

reflecting edge of ligament

reflection
colon medial r.
hepatoduodenal r.
hepatoduodenal-peritoneal r.
peritoneal r.
total internal r.

reflex
absent gag r.
anal r.
anocutaneous r.
axon r.
Babinski r.

reflex (*continued*)
 Barrington third r.
 bladder cooling r.
 blinking r.
 bulbocavernosus r. (BCR)
 cardioesophageal r.
 celiac plexus r.
 consensual r.
 corneal r.
 cremasteric r.
 cutaneous r.
 deglutition r.
 descending inhibitory r.
 detrusodetrusor facilitative r.
 r. detrusor contraction
 detrusosphincteric inhibitory r.
 detrusourethral inhibitory r.
 diminished gag r.
 r. dyspepsia
 emetic r.
 enteric neuronal r.
 enterogastric r.
 epigastric r.
 r. erection
 esophagosalivary r.
 fencing r.
 gag r.
 Galant r.
 gastrocolic r.
 gastroileac r.
 gastropancreatic r.
 glabella r.
 guarding r.
 gustatory-salivary r.
 r. HPV test
 ileogastric r.
 r. incontinence
 infant r.
 inhibitory intestinointestinal r.
 intestinogastric r.
 intramural secretory r.
 intrinsic r.
 Landau r.
 light r.
 masticatory-salivary r.
 micturition r.
 myenteric r.
 r. neurogenic bladder
 r. neuropathic bladder
 orienting r.
 parachute r.
 penile r.
 penis r.
 perineobulbar detrusor facilitative r.
 perineobulbar detrusor inhibitory r.
 perineodetrusor inhibitory r.
 peristaltic r.
 polarized standing r.
 polysynaptic r.

 pontine-sacral r.
 primary vesicoureteral r.
 pudendal-anal r.
 r. pylorospasm
 rectal inhibitory r.
 rectoanal inhibitory r. (RAIR)
 rectosphincteric r. (RSR)
 renal r.
 renointestinal r.
 renorenal r.
 Roger r.
 rooting r.
 scrotal r.
 secondary vesicoureteral r.
 secretory r.
 sexual r.
 skin-CNS-bladder r.
 somatic nociceptive flexion r.
 somatointestinal r.
 spinobulbospinal micturition r.
 r. splanchnic vasoconstriction
 stepping r.
 swallowing r.
 sympathetic enteroenteric
  inhibitory r.
 sympathetic sphincter constrictor r.
 thermal sphincteric r.
 urethrodetrusor facilitative r.
 urethrosphincteric guarding r.
 urethrosphincteric inhibitory r.
 urethrosphincteric recruitment r.
 urinary continence r.
 vasovagal r.
 vesicoanal r.
 vesicointestinal r.
 virile r.
 visceral traction r.
 viscerosensory r.
 r. voiding
 r. voiding dysfunction
 von Mering r.
 wake r.
 wink r.
reflexogenic erection
reflux
 acid r.
 antiperistaltic r.
 bile r.
 r. bile gastritis
 cecoileal r.
 cholangiovenous r.
 contralateral r.
 delayed vesicoureteral r.
 r. disease
 duodenal gastroesophageal r.
  (DGER)
 duodenobiliary r.
 duodenogastric r. (DGR)
 duodenogastroesophageal r. (DGER)

duodenopancreatic r.
r. dyspepsia
ejaculatory duct r.
esophageal r.
r. esophagitis
r. esophagitis classification I—IV
exertion-associated gastroesophageal
  r. (EAGER)
free r.
gastroesophageal r. (GER)
gastrointestinal r.
GE r.
hepatojugular r. (HJR)
Hinman r.
ileal r.
intrarenal r.
r. laryngitis
r. morbidity
nasopharyngeal r.
r. nephropathy
r. neuropathy
nighttime r.
nocturnal acid r.
nocturnal gastric r.
nondilating r.
occult pancreatobiliary r.
pancreaticobiliary r.
pathologic r.
peptic r.
postmyotomy r.
postoperative r.
pyelorenal r.
pyelotubular r.
Roux gastric r.
scintigraphic r.
r. small-bowel examination
r. symptom
ureterorenal r.
vesicoileal r.
vesicoureteral r. (VUR)
vesicoureteric r.
vesicourethral r.

refluxant
refluxate
refluxing ileourethral anastomosis
refluxlike dyspepsia
reflux-related stricture
refraction
refractory
r. anemia with excess blasts
  (RAEB)
r. anemia with ringed sideroblasts
  (RARS)
r. ascites
r. duodenal ulcer
r. esophagitis
r. hypertension
r. motor urge incontinence
r. pouch inflammation

r. pouchitis
r. proctosigmoiditis
r. sideroblastic anemia
r. sprue
r. variceal hemorrhage

refrigerant diuretic
Refsum disease
Regan isoenzyme
regeneration
bladder r.
carbon tetrachloride-induced liver r.
tubular r.
regenerative cirrhotic nodule
regimen
antireflux r.
bismuth triple r.
bowel-emptying r.
calcineurin inhibitor-free
  immunosuppressive r.
dietetic r.
3-drug r.
immunosuppressive r.
multidrug r.
sequential quadruple-drug r.
Shorr r.
region
abdominal r.
antropyloroduodenal r.
capsid-encoding r.
choledochal r.
floor of inguinal r.
gastric pacemaker r.
genitourinary r.
hepatic hilar r.
hydrophobic binding r.
hypervariable r. 1
hypochondriac r.
hypogastric r.
ileocecal r.
inframammary r.
interferon sensitivity determining r.
  (ISDR)
interpolar r.
intertriginous r.
ischiorectal r.
lateral abdominal r.
nonpolar r.
nontranslated r. (NTR)
pancreaticobiliary r.
paraaortic r.
perianal r.
perineal r.
periumbilical r.
polar r.
rectosigmoid r.
retroperitoneal r.
substernal r.
suprainguinal r.
suprapubic r.

region (*continued*)
    umbilical r.
    untranslated r.
    ureteropelvic r.
    urogenital r.
regional
    r. colitis
    r. enteritis
    r. enterocolitis
    r. heparinization
    r. ileitis
    R. Organ Procurement Agency
    (ROPA)
registration
    transcutaneous r.
registry
    Michigan Kidney R.
Regitine
Reglan
Regressin
regression
    r. analysis
    linear r.
    linear-array r.
    lymphocele spontaneous r.
    Poisson r.
    spontaneous r.
Regroton
regucalcin
regular diet
regulation
    autocrine r.
    follicle-stimulating hormone
    inhibin r.
    growth r.
regulator
    cystic fibrosis transductance r.
    cystic fibrosis transmembrane
    conductance r. (CFTR)
regulatory
    r. peptide
    steroidogenic acute r. (StAR)
Regulax SS
regurgitant
regurgitation
    acid r.
    chronic r.
    r. jaundice
    nocturnal r.
    postural r.
    vesicoureteral r.
Regutol
rehabilitation
    pelvic floor r.
    renal r.
    sexual r.
Rehfuss
    R. duodenal tube
    R. method

    R. stomach tube
    R. test
Rehne abdominal retractor
Rehne-Delorme plication
Rehydralyte
rehydrating solution (RS)
rehydration
    oral r.
    r. therapy
Reichel-Pólya
    R.-P. stomach procedure
    R.-P. stomach resection
Reichert
    R. FLPS-series flexible fiberoptic
    sigmoidoscope
    R. MS-series flexible fiberoptic
    sigmoidoscope
    R. SC-series flexible fiberoptic
    sigmoidoscope
Reichmann
    R. disease
    R. rod
    R. syndrome
Reich-Nechtow forceps
Reifenstein syndrome
reimplantation
    aortorenal r.
    Cohen cross-trigonal r.
    end-to-side r.
    extravesical r.
    Leadbetter-Politano r.
    Paquin ureteral r.
    ureteral r.
REIN
    Ramipril Efficacy in Nephropathy
    REIN study
reinforcement
    Gore-Tex sling r.
    responsibility r.
reinforcing suture
Reinke crystal
reinsertion
reintervention rate
reintroduction
reintubation
Reitan Trail-Making test
Reiter
    R. disease
    R. syndrome
Reitman-Frankel test
rejection
    accelerated transplant r.
    acute cellular r.
    acute humoral renal allograft r.
    acute vascular r.
    allograft r.
    r. cholangitis
    chronic allograft r.
    chronic transplant r.

clinical r.
delayed hyperacute transplant r.
ductopenic r.
higher incidence of r.
hyperacute r.
incidence of acute r.
interstitial r.
no r.
renal allograft r.
renal transplantation r.
steroid-resistant r.
subclinical r.
transmural r.
transplant r.
tubulointerstitial r.
vascular r.
xenograft r.

relapsing
r. acute pancreatitis
r. appendicitis

related
human leukocyte antigen-D r.
(HLA-DR)
incontinence r.
r. living donor (RLD)

relationship
dyadic r.
endoscope-body position r.
intraluminal pH-pressure r.
r. of recipient

relative
first-degree R.
r. sterility
r. supersaturation (RSs)

relatively minimal complication

relaxant
cGMP-mediated r.
musculotropic r.
smooth muscle r.

relaxation
adaptive r.
bladder stress r.
cardioesophageal r.
endothelial-dependent r.
esophageal sphincter r.
incomplete r.
LES r.
lower esophageal sphincter r.
(LESR)
nitric oxide-blocked
sphincter r.
nonswallow-associated r.
pelvic floor r.
pelvic girdle r. (PGR)
receptive r.
stress r.
r. suture
r. technique
transient LES r.

transient lower esophageal sphincter
r. (TLESR)
upper esophageal sphincter r.
(UESR)
vagovagally mediated receptive r.

relaxatory response

relaxin
recombinant human r.

relaxing incision

Relay suture delivery system

release
extended r. (ER, XL, XR)
G-cell gastrin r.
nifedipine extended r.
paranitroaniline r.
renin r.
static pressure r. (SPR)
stimulated r.
tethered-cord r.
twin-pulse shock wave r.

Release-NF catheter

relevant gastroduodenal finding

reliability
interobserver r.
penile prothesis r.

reliable percutaneous renal access

Relia-Flow device

Reliance urinary control insert

ReliaSeal skin barrier

Relia-Vac drain

relief
Peptic R.

Reliquet lithotrite

relocation
polyp r.

REMBL
retroflexed endoscopic multiple-band
ligation

Remedy advanced skin care

Remegel soft chewable antacid

remethylation

Remicade IV infusion

remission of pain

remnant
cloacal r.
gastric r.
mesonephric r.
müllerian r.
prostatic mesonephric r.

removal
colonoscopic r.
cut-and-push method of PEG tube
r.
endoscopic stone r.
forceps r.
foreign body r.
gastric coin r.
Lithovac stone r.
percutaneous endoscopic r.

removal (*continued*)
    percutaneous stone r.
    peritoneal dialysis urea r.
    radical en bloc r.
    small polyp r.
    through-the-scope balloon r.
    tube r.
    ureteral stoma r.
remover
    Detachol adhesive r.
    Macaluso stent r.
Renacidin irrigation
Renaflo hollow-fiber dialyzer
Renagel tablet
renal
    r. absorption of calcium
    r. acid excretion
    r. adenocarcinoma
    r. afferent arteriolar resistance
    r. afferent nerve
    r. agenesis
    r. allograft
    r. allograft infection
    r. allograft recipient
    r. allograft rejection
    r. allograft rupture
    r. allograft survival
    r. allotransplantation
    r. aminoaciduria
    r. ammonium excretion
    r. amyloidosis
    r. angiography
    r. angiomyolipoma
    r. anuria
    r. arterial occlusive disease
    r. arteriography
    r. arteriole
    r. arteriovenous fistula
    r. artery
    r. artery aneurysm
    r. artery cholesterol embolization
    r. artery diameter
    r. artery embolectomy
    r. artery embolism
    r. artery graft
    r. artery stenosis
    r. artery stent
    r. artery thrombosis
    r. autoregulation
    r. autoregulatory ability
    r. autoregulatory mechanism
    r. autotransplantation
    r. baroreceptor
    r. biopsy
    r. blastema
    r. blood flow (RBF)
    r. bone disease
    r. calcium leak
    r. capsular flap

    r. capsule
    r. capsulotomy
    r. carbuncle
    r. carcinosarcoma
    r. cell carcinoma (RCC)
    r. cholesterol embolus
    r. clearance
    r. coagulation necrosis
    r. colic
    r. collecting duct cell
    r. complication
    r. concentrating defect
    r. congestion
    r. corpuscle
    r. cortex
    r. corticoadrenal
    r. cryoablation
    r. cryptococcosis
    r. cyst decortication
    r. cystectomy
    r. cyst hemorrhage
    r. cystic disease
    r. cyst infection
    r. cyst marsupialization
    r. descensus
    r. deterioration
    r. dialysis
    r. duplication
    r. echinococcosis
    r. ectopia
    r. endarterectomy
    r. endothelin
    r. epistaxis
    r. excretion of acid
    r. excretion of calcium
    r. exploration
    r. failure
    r. failure index
    r. Fanconi-like syndrome
    r. fascia
    r. fibroma
    r. fibromuscular disease
    r. function
    r. function study (RFS)
    r. gallium-67 scintigraphy
    r. glomerulus
    r. glucosuria
    r. hamartoma
    r. helical CT (RHCT)
    r. helical CT imaging
    r. hemangioma
    r. hematoma
    r. hematuria
    r. hemodynamics
    r. hemophilia
    r. hilar dissection
    r. hilum
    r. histologic section
    r. histopathology

R

r. homotransplantation
r. hydatid disease
r. hydatidosis
r. hypercalciuria
r. hyperchloremia acidosis
r. hyperfiltration
r. hypertension
r. hypertrophy
r. hypoperfusion
r. hyposthenuria
r. hypothermia
r. impression
r. impression on liver
r. injury repair
r. insufficiency
r. interstitium
r. involvement
r. ischemia
r. kallikrein-kinin system
r. labyrinth
r. lithiasis
r. lobe
r. lymphoblastoma
r. mass
r. medicine
r. medulla
r. messenger ribonucleic acid
r. messenger ribonucleoprotein acid
r. morphometric analysis
r. obstruction
r. oncocytoma
r. osteodystrophy (ROD)
r. papilla
r. papillary necrosis (RPN)
r. parenchyma
r. parenchymal damage
r. pathology
r. pedicle
r. pelvis
r. pelvis calculus
r. percutaneous transluminal angioplasty
r. perfusion pressure
r. perfusion pressure-flow study
r. perfusion scintigraphy
r. phosphate
r. phosphate excretion
r. physiology
r. plasma flow (RPF)
r. pouch
r. preservation
r. preservation-perfusion system
r. progression
r. proximal tubular cell
r. proximal tubule preparation
r. ptosis
r. pyramid
r. reflex
r. rehabilitation

r. replacement therapy
r. resistive index (RRI)
r. revascularization
r. rhabdomyosarcoma
r. rickets
r. sarcoidosis
r. scan
r. scanning
r. scarring
r. segmental renal dysplasia
r. sinus
r. sinus cyst
r. sodium
r. sodium excretion
r. sodium retention
r. sodium wasting
r. sonography
r. stab wound
r. stone
r. stone formation
r. structural damage
r. sympathetic activity
r. sympathetic nerve
r. sympathetic nerve activity recording electrode
R. System filter
r. thromboendarterectomy
r. tissue kallikrein expression
r. toxicity
r. transduction pathway
r. transplant
r. transplantation
r. transplantation rejection
r. transplant patient
r. transplant recipient
r. trauma
r. tuberculosis
r. tubular acidosis (RTA)
r. tubular acidosis type I–IV
r. tubular epithelium
r. tubular fluid
r. tubular metabolic acidosis
r. tubular necrosis (RTN)
r. tubular sodium handling
r. tubule
r. tubule epithelial cell
r. tumorlike pyonephrosis with foreign body
r. ultrasonogram
r. urate excretion
r. vasculitis
r. vasoconstriction
r. vasodilation
r. vasodilator
r. vasodilator prostaglandin
r. vein
r. vein renin
r. vein renin activity (RVRA)
r. vein renin assay (RVRA)

renal (*continued*)
    r. vein renin concentration (RVRC)
    r. vein renin ratio
    r. vein thrombosis (RVT)
    r. venogram
    r. venography
    r. venous outflow compression
    vertebral, anal, tracheoesophageal fistula, r. (VATER)
    r. volume
    r. xanthine oxidase-xanthine dehydrogenase activity

renale
    hilum r.

renales
    columnae r.

renal-hepatic steal syndrome
Renalin dialyzer
renalis
    fascia r.
    hilum r.
    plexus r.

renal-ocular syndrome
renal-retinal syndrome
renal-sparing surgery
Renalyzer
Renatron dialyzer
Renax film-coated caplet
rendezvous
    pancreatic r.
    r. technique
    r. technique for treatment of choledocholithiasis

Rendu-Osler-Weber
    R.-O.-W. disease
    R.-O.-W. syndrome

Renese
Renessa
renewal
    epithelial restitution and r.
    tissue r.

renicapsule
renicardiac
reniculi (*pl. of* reniculus)
reniculus, *pl.* **reniculi**
renin
    active r.
    r. inhibition
    plasma r.
    r. release
    renal vein r.
    r. secretion
    r. stimulation test
    r. synthesis

renin-aldosterone system
renin-angiotensin
    r.-a. system (RAS)
    r.-a. system blocker

renin-angiotensin-aldosterone
    r.-a.-a. axis
    r.-a.-a. system (RAAS)

renin-mediated renovascular hypertension
reninoma
renin-secreting juxtaglomerular cell tumor
renipelvic transitional cell carcinoma
reniportal anastomosis
renipuncture
renis
    capsula adiposa r.
    capsula fibrosa r.
    porta r.
    venulae rectae r.

Rennes variant galactosemia
renocortical
    r. abscess
    r. adenoma
    r. malondialdehyde content
    r. necrosis
    r. scintigraphy
    r. tubule cell

renogastric fistula
Renografin
renogram
    captopril r.
    furosemide washout r.
    isotope r.
    MDT r.

renography
    captopril r.
    captopril-enhanced r.
    diethylenetriamine pentaacetic acid r.
    diuretic nuclear r.
    DTPA r.
    isotope r.
    radioisotope r.

renointestinal reflex
Reno-M contrast medium
renomedullary
    r. carcinoma
    r. interstitial cell (RMIC)

renomegaly
renopathy
renoprival
renoprotective agent
renopulmonary
Renoquid
renorenal reflex
renorrhaphy
renotrophic, renotropic
renotrophin, renotropin
renotropic (*var. of* renotrophic)
renotropin (*var. of* renotrophin)
renovascular
    r. disease
    r. hypertension (RVH)
    r. hypertrophy

R

r. injury
r. obstruction
r. resistance (RVR)
r. resistance index (RVRI)
r. surgery
r. tone
Renovist injection
Renovue 65
Renu enteral feeding
renzapride
reoperation
lower abdominal r.
r. rate
reoperative ureteroneocystostomy
reovirus
reoxygenation
repaglinide
repair (*see also* operation,
  procedure)
Alliston GE reflux r.
Altemeier r.
anal sphincter r.
anastomotic r.
Asopa hypospadias r.
Barcat-Redman hypospadias r.
Bassini inguinal hernia r.
Belsey Mark IV r.
Belt-Fuqua hypospadias r.
Boari ureteral flap r.
Boerema hernia r.
bulboprostatic r.
bulbourethral stricture r.
Cantwell-Ransley epispadias r.
Cecil r.
cloacal exstrophy 1-stage r.
cloacal exstrophy 2-stage r.
Collis r.
cross-trigonal r.
Delorme rectal prolapse r.
Devine-Horton flip-flap for
  hypospadias r.
Devine hypospadias r.
double-faced island flap for
  hypospadias r.
DualMesh hernia r.
end-to-end anastomotic r.
epispadias r.
extracorporeal r.
Halsted-Bassini hernia r.
hernia r.
Hill esophageal antireflux r.
Hill hiatus hernia r.
Hill median arcuate r.
Horton-Devine flip-flap
  hypospadias r.
hydrocele r.
intraperitoneal onlay mesh hernia r.
  (IPOM)
IPOM hernia r.

Judd ventral hernia r.
Koyanagi technique for
  hypospadias r.
laparoscopic anterior abdominal wall
  hernia r.
laparoscopic renal artery aneurysm
  r.
laparoscopic varicocele r.
LaRoque r.
Lich-Gregoire r.
Lichtenstein hernia r.
Limberg flap r.
Madden hernia r.
Marlex hernia r.
McVay inguinal hernial r.
megameatus hypospadias r.
Mitchell technique for epispadias r.
Moschcowitz vaginal prolapse r.
Mustarde hypospadias r.
mutation mismatch r.
neonatal exstrophic bladder r.
Nissen fundus r.
omphalocele r.
one-stage hypospadias r.
Orr rectal prolapse r.
pants-over-vest hernia r.
Paquin r.
paravaginal fascial r.
postanal r.
Ransley-Cantwell epispadias r.
renal injury r.
reverse sigma penoscrotal
  transposition r.
Rives-Stoppa sublay incisional
  hernia r.
Rodney Smith biliary stricture r.
slipped Nissen r.
sphincter r.
2-stage r.
Stoppa r.
1st-stage r.
TAPP hernia r.
tension-free cystocele r.
TEP hernia r.
Thal esophageal stricture r.
Thiersch-Duplay r.
tight Nissen r.
timing of r.
totally extraperitoneal hernia r.
transabdominal preperitoneal
  hernia r.
transvaginal enterocele r.
transvaginal mesh cystocele r.
ureteropelvic junction obstruction r.
vaginal r.
varicocele r.
vascular laceration r.
vest-over-pants hernia r.
VVF r.

repair (*continued*)
    Young-Dees bladder neck r.
    Young epispadias r.
repeat
    direct r.
    r. exploration
    long terminal r.
    r. operation
    r. procedure
    r. sequence
    terminal r.
repens
    Serenoa r.
reperfusion injury
reperitonealization
repermeation
    portal r.
Repetabs
    Trinalin R.
replaced hepatic vessel
replacement
    antegrade stent r.
    bladder r.
    buccal mucosal urethral r.
    r. enzyme protein
    gastric bladder r.
    intestinal ureteral r.
    r. PEG
    tube r.
    tunica r.
    volume r.
replantation
    penile r.
Replete liquid nutrition
replication
    r. error phenotype
    gastric epithelial cell r.
    r. pathway
    viral r.
replicator
    Steers r.
Repliform dermal allograft
Replogle tube
repopulation
    clonogenic r.
report
    human case r.
reposable device
Rep-Pred
repreparation
representative electrophoretic mobility shift assay
reprocessor
    American Endoscopy automatic r.
    automatic endoscopic r. (AER)
    Bard automatic r.
    Custom Ultrasonic automatic r.
    ECI automatic r.
    KeyMed automatic r.

    Lutz automatic r.
    Medivator automatic r.
    Olympus automatic r.
    Orr automatic r.
    Steris automatic r.
reproduction
    assisted r.
reproductive
    r. axis
    r. system
reptilase acid
required transfusion
requirement
    analgesic r.
    minimum daily r. (MDR)
    postoperative analgesia r.
re-reflux
rescinnamine
rescue
    fluorouracil, Adriamycin, methotrexate with leucovorin r. (FAMTX)
    leucovorin r.
    r. therapy
    uridine r.
research
    r. application
    Hirshberg Foundation for Pancreatic Cancer R.
    Vioxx Gastrointestinal Outcomes R. (VIGOR)
resectable
resection
    abdominoperineal r. (APR)
    abdominosacral r.
    anterior r.
    antral r.
    bladder neck transurethral r.
    Bloch-Paul-Mikulicz extraperitoneal colon r.
    bowel r.
    cap-assisted endoscopic mucosal r.
    cold cup r.
    colon cancer r.
    colorectal r.
    colosigmoid r.
    continence-preserving r.
    curative tumor r.
    cutting endoscopic mucosal r. (C-EMR)
    cylindrical mucosal r.
    diathermic r.
    duodenum-preserving pancreatic head r.
    ejaculatory duct transurethral r.
    elective r.
    electrocautery r.
    en bloc endoscopic r.
    en bloc vein r.

endoscopic full-thickness r. (EFTR)
endoscopic mucosal r. (EMR)
endoscopic snare r.
esophageal r.
fluidjet technology-assisted mucosal r.
free r.
gastric r.
hepatic r.
ileal r.
ileocecal r.
ileocolic r.
intersphincteric r.
laparoscopic abdominoperineal r.
laparoscopically assisted colorectal r.
laparoscopic ultralow anterior r.
lift-and-cut endoscopic mucosal r. (LC-EMR)
liver r.
Lortat-Jacob hepatic r.
low anterior r. (LAR)
Mason abdominal transsphincteric r.
Miles abdominoperineal r.
mucosal sleeve r.
open transurethral r.
pancreatic tail r.
Paul-Mikulicz staged bowel r.
percutaneous r.
piecemeal r.
prostate gland transurethral r.
Reichel-Pólya stomach r.
second r.
segmental colonic r.
snare r.
spermatocele r.
strip r.
suture rectopexy with sigmoid r.
terminal ileal r.
r. time
transanal endoscopic microsurgical r.
transhiatal r.
transurethral r. (TUR)
transverse r.
wedge r.
Whipple pancreatic r.
resectional therapy
resective colostomy
resectoscope
continuous-flow r.
Foroblique r.
Iglesias fiberoptic r.
r. loop
OES 4000 r.
Olympus continuous-flow r.
r. sheath
Storz r.
transurethral r.
Wolf r.
resectoscopy

resedation
reserpine
hydrochlorothiazide and r.
reserpine-induced ulcer
reservoir
Camey r.
catheterizable r.
catheterization r.
colonic J-pouch r.
continent catheterization r.
continent cutaneous r.
continent ileal r.
detubularized right colon r.
double-barrel r.
double J-shaped r.
double-stapled ileal r.
fecal r.
Florida pouch urinary r.
Hadera continent r.
Hoffmann-Steinberg gastric r.
Hunt-Limo-Basto gastric r.
ileal low-pressure r.
ileoanal r.
ileocecal continent urinary r.
Indiana continent r.
intraabdominal ileal r.
inverted U-pouch ileal r.
isoperistaltic ileal r.
J r.
J-shaped ileal r.
J-Vac suction r.
Kock r.
lateral internal pelvic r.
Lawrence gastric r.
Le Bag pouch r.
Mainz pouch urinary r.
r. mucosal absorption
r. of underdiagnosed and misdiagnosed interstitial cystitis
orthotopic colonic r.
orthotopic continent r.
orthotopic remodeled ileocolonic r.
Parks ileal r.
Parks ileoanal r.
r. phase
rectal r.
S r.
sigmoid colon r.
spherical r.
S-shaped r.
Studer crossfolded ileal r.
W-stapled urinary r.
reset osmostat syndrome
Resident Assessment Protocol for incontinence
residua (*pl. of* residuum)
residual
r. albuminuria
r. barium

residual (*continued*)
 r. chordee
 r. fragment
 postvoid r. (PVR)
 r. proteinuria
 r. rectoperineal fistula
 r. stone
 r. stool
 r. urine
 r. urine volume (RUV)
residue
 dibasic amino acid r.
 fecal r.
 food r.
 histidine r.
 sialic acid r.
 sialyl r.
residuum, *pl.* **residua**
 gastric r.
resin
 anion exchange r.
 bile salt-binding r.
 cation exchange r.
 Epon 812 r.
 potassium-binding r.
resinifera
 Euphorbia r.
resiniferatoxin therapy
resipump
resiquimod
resistance
 activated protein C r. (APCR)
 amphotericin B r.
 antimicrobial r.
 basal renovascular r.
 cancer drug r.
 drug r.
 hepatic arterial vascular r.
 insulin r.
 mean electrosurgical r.
 r. monomicrobial biofilm
 peripheral vascular r.
 reactance and r. (X/R)
 renal afferent arteriolar r.
 renovascular r. (RVR)
 retrospective analysis of
  antimicrobial r.
 systemic vascular r. (SVR)
 tissue r.
 transhepatic vascular r.
 urethral r.
 vesical neck r.
 vitamin D r.
resistant
 r. ascites
 r. organism
 r. to electrosurgical perforation
resistin
resistive index

Resol electrolyte solution
resolution
 R. Clip device
 spatial r.
 spontaneous r.
**RESOLVE: The National Infertility
 Association**
resonance
 endoscopic magnetic r. (EMR)
 gadolinium-enhancement magnetic r.
 hydatid r.
 magnetic r. (MR)
 nuclear magnetic r. (NMR)
 tympanitic r.
 vesiculotympanitic r.
 wooden r.
resonant abdomen
resorbable thread clip applicator
resorption
 tubular r.
resorptive hypercalciuria
resource
 R. Arginaid powder
 R. Diabetic
 R. Diabetic ready-to-use
  liquid
 R. enteral feeding
 R. Fruit Beverage
 R. Fruit Beverage ready-to-use
  liquid
 R. Just for Kids
 R. Just for Kids ready-to-use liquid
 medical r.
 R. oral liquid
 R. Plus
respiration pyelography
respiratory
 r. acidosis
 r. alkalosis
 r. burst
 r. burst activity
 r. depression
 r. distress
 r. embarrassment
 r. excursion
 r. failure
 r. inversion point (RIP)
 r. pyelography
 r. rate
 r. symptoms (RS)
respiratory-esophageal fistula
response
 alloantigen r.
 ameliorated vasodilating r.
 antibody-directed cytotoxic r.
 apoptotic r.
 arterial buffer r.
 bellow r.
 cell-mediated immunohistological r.

cellular immune r.
cytotoxic T-cell r.
desmoplastic r.
desmopressin r.
dose r.
dysregulated immune r.
early virologic r. (EVR)
effector r.
fed r.
gag r.
humoral antibody r.
hypercontractile external sphincter r.
immune r.
inflammatory r.
macrophage-rich inflammatory r.
maladaptive r.
paradoxical renal r.
peak r.
plateau r.
rapid viral r.
r. rate to chemotherapy
relaxatory r.
sacral evoked r.
skin sympathetic r.
sustained virologic r. (SVR)
sympathetic skin r.
Th1 r.
therapeutic r.
unfolded protein r.

responsibility reinforcement
responsiveness
vasculature r.
rest
adrenal r.
bowel r.
ectopic adrenal r.
gut r.
Krause arm r.
nephrogenic r.
pancreatic r.
testicular adrenal r.
total bowel r.
restaging of cancer
restenosis
resting
r. anal sphincter pressure
r. energy expenditure (REE)
r. membrane potential
r. tremor
r. urethral pressure profile
restoration
foreskin r.
restorative
r. proctocolectomy (RP, RPC)
r. proctocolectomy and ileal pouch anal anastomosis (RP/IPAA)
r. proctocolectomy operation
Restore briefs
Restoril

restricted
HLA class II r.
restriction
dietary protein r.
r. endonuclease
r. enzyme
fluid r.
r. fragment length polymorphism (RLP)
protein r.
putative host r.
sodium r.
result
contradictory r.
long-term r.
medium-term r.
poor long-term r.
positive culture r.
previous in vitro r.
short-term r.
Surveillance, Epidemiology, and End R.'s (SEER)
tactile feedback r.
tissue destruction r.
transurethral microwave thermotherapy functional r.
transurethral resection of prostate functional r.
TUMT functional r.
TURP functional r.
resuscitation
fluid r.
retained
r. antrum
r. antrum syndrome
r. barium
r. bladder syndrome
r. feces
r. foreign body (RFB)
r. gallstone
r. testicle
r. testis
retainer
Mectra tissue sample r.
retardata
ejaculatio r.
retardation
triad of adenoma sebaceum, epilepsy, and mental r.
Wilms tumor, aniridia, genitourinary abnormalities, and mental r. (WAGR)
retch
retching, vomiturition
rete, *pl.* **retia**
r. peg
r. ridge
r. testis
r. testis adenocarcinoma

R

RE-TEM
rectal expander-assisted transanal endoscopic microsurgery

retention
acute urinary r. (AUR)
r. band
barium r.
BSP r.
chronic urinary r. (CUR)
crystal r.
r. cyst
r. enema
r. esophagitis
gastric r.
r. jaundice
r. meal
r. polyp
postoperative urinary r.
renal sodium r.
sodium r.
stool r.
r. suture
r. uremia
urinary r.
r. vomiting

retethering

retia (*pl. of* rete)

retial

reticula (*pl. of* reticulum)

reticularis
formatio r.
zona r.

reticulated poikilodermatous hyperpigmentation

reticulin antigen

reticulocyte hemoglobin content

reticuloendothelial system

reticulonodular pattern

reticulosis
polymorphic r. (PMR)

reticulum, *pl.* **reticula**
endoplasmic r.
rough endoplasmic r.
sarcoplasmic r.

retinacula (*pl. of* retinaculum)

retinaculum, *pl.* **retinacula**
Morgagni r.

retinal
r. artery occlusion
r. vein occlusion

retinitis
albuminuric r.

retinoblastoma

retinoic acid

retinoid
acyclic r.
r. binding protein
r. chaperone

r. transport
r. X receptor

retinoid-related molecule

retinol-binding protein (RBP)

retinol concentration

retinyl ester clearance

RET protooncogene

retracted stoma

retractile
r. concealed penis
r. mesenteritis
r. testis

retraction
bladder r.
downward r.
foreskin manual r.

retractor
Airlift balloon r.
Army-Navy r.
Aronson esophageal r.
baby Balfour r.
Balfour abdominal r.
Balfour self-retaining r.
Barr rectal r.
Beardsley esophageal r.
B.E. Glass abdominal r.
Berens esophageal r.
Berkeley-Bonney r.
Bookwalter-Goulet r.
Bookwalter-Hill-Ferguson rectal r.
Bookwalter ring r.
Bookwalter-St. Mark deep pelvic r.
Breisky-Navratil straight r.
Buie-Smith r.
Christie gallbladder r.
Cole duodenal r.
Collin abdominal r.
Collin intestinal r.
Crile angle r.
Crile malleable r.
Cushing vein r.
Deaver r.
DeBakey-Cooley r.
Denis Browne abdominal r.
Doyen abdominal r.
fan elevator r.
fan-type laparoscopic r.
Farabeuf r.
Ferguson anal r.
Ferguson-Moon rectal r.
Finochietto r.
fixed ring r.
Foerster abdominal ring r.
Forder r.
Foss bifid gallbladder r.
Foss biliary duct r.
Franz abdominal r.

Friedman perineal r.
Fritsch r.
gallows-type r.
Gazayerli endoscopic r.
Gelpi self-retaining r.
Gibson-Balfour abdominal r.
Gil-Vernet r.
Goelet r.
Goligher r.
Gosset appendectomy r.
Grant gallbladder r.
Greene r.
Greishaber self-retaining r.
handheld r.
Harrington Deaver r.
Harrington splanchnic r.
Heaney r.
hilar r.
Hill-Ferguson rectal r.
Hill rectal r.
illuminated St. Mark r.
Israel r.
Jansen r.
Johns Hopkins gallbladder r.
Kelly abdominal r.
Kirschner abdominal r.
Kocher gallbladder r.
Lone Star r.
Lowsley r.
malleable r.
Mayo abdominal r.
Mayo-Adams appendectomy r.
McBurney r.
Mediflex-Gazayerli r.
metal bar r.
Mikulicz r.
Miller-Senn r.
Millin bladder r.
Moon rectal r.
Murphy gallbladder r.
Nathanson liver r.
Nuttall liver r.
Ochsner r.
Oettingen abdominal r.
Omnitract r.
O'Sullivan-O'Connor abdominal r.
Parker r.
Parks r.
Percy-Wolfson gallbladder r.
Polytrac Gomez r.
Pratt bivalve r.
Quervain abdominal r.
rake r.
Rehne abdominal r.
ribbon r.
Richards abdominal r.
Richardson appendectomy r.
Rigby appendectomy r.
ring abdominal r.

Robin-Masse abdominal r.
Roux r.
Sawyer rectal r.
Scott r.
self-retaining ring r.
Senn r.
Senn-Kanavel r.
Smith-Buie rectal r.
Smith rectal r.
Space-OR flexible internal r.
spoon r.
spring-wire r.
Stamey dorsal vein apical r.
T-bar r.
Theis self-retaining r.
Tuffier abdominal r.
Upper Hands r.
U.S. Army double-ended r.
vein r.
Volkmann rake r.
Walker gallbladder r.
Webb-Balfour abdominal r.
Weinberg vagotomy r.
Weitlaner r.
Wesson perineal r.
Wexler r.
Wickham r.
Wilkinson abdominal r.
Wishbone Omni-Track r.
Wolfson gallbladder r.
Wylie splanchnic r.
Young prostatic r.
Yu-Holtgrewe prostatic r.

retransplantation
retreatment
lithotripsy r.
r. rate
retrieval
r. balloon
r. basket
specimen r.
spermatozoon r.
retriever
Positrap r.
3-pronged polyp r.
snail-headed catheter r.
Soehendra stent r.
stone r.
retrocaval ureter
retrocecal
r. abscess
r. appendicitis
r. appendix
retrocecalis tumor thrombus
retrocolic
r. anastomosis
r. end-to-end pancreatojejunostomy
r. end-to-side choledochojejunostomy
r. fossa

R

retroduodenal
    r. artery
    r. artery severance
    r. perforation
retroesophageal abscess
retroflected (*var. of* retroflexed)
retroflection (*var. of* retroflexion)
retroflexed, retroflected
    r. cystoscopy sheath
    r. endoscopic multiple-band ligation
    (REMBL)
    r. scope
    r. uterus
    r. view
retroflexion, retroflection
    endoscopic r.
    intrarectal r.
    success in r.
retrogastric pseudocyst
retrograde
    r. approach
    r. balloon rupture
    r. cannulation
    r. cholangiogram
    r. cholangiography
    r. contrast study
    r. cystogram
    r. cystography
    r. cystourethrogram
    r. duodenogastroscopy (RDG)
    r. ejaculation
    r. endopyelotomy
    r. fashion
    r. flow on barium enema
    r. genitography
    r. hernia
    r. instrumentation
    r. intrarenal surgery
    r. intussusception
    r. loopography
    r. migration
    r. nephrostomy
    r. occlusion balloon catheter
    r. pancreatocholangiography
    r. pancreatogram
    r. pancreatography
    r. peristalsis
    r. pyelogram (RPG)
    r. pyelography
    r. small-bowel examination
    r. sphincterotomy
    r. technique
    r. ureteropyelogram
    r. urethrogram (RUG)
    r. urethrography (RUG)
    r. urogram
    r. urography
    r. vascularization of superior
    mesenteric artery

retrohepatic vena cava
retroileal
    r. appendicitis
    r. appendix
retroiliac ureter
Retromax endopyelotomy stent
retropancreatic tunnel
retroperistaltic pump
retroperitoneal
    r. abscess
    r. approach
    r. area
    r. calcification
    r. carbon dioxide insufflation study
    r. cavity
    r. cutaneous ureterostomy
    r. fat
    r. fibrosis (RPF)
    r. fistula
    r. hematoma
    r. hemorrhage (RPH)
    r. hernia
    r. iliopsoas abscess
    r. infection
    r. laparoscopic adrenalectomy for
    pheochromocytoma
    r. laparoscopic nephroureterectomy
    r. lymphadenectomy
    r. lymph node dissection (RLND)
    r. lymphoma
    r. neoplasm
    r. perforation
    r. pneumography
    r. pneumoradiography
    r. region
    r. seminoma
    r. space
    r. surgery
    r. tumor
    r. varicocelectomy
retroperitoneoscopic
    r. adrenalectomy
    r. nephrectomy
    r. vein ligature
retroperitoneoscopy
retroperitoneum sarcoma
retroperitonitis
    idiopathic fibrous r.
retropexy
    abdominal r.
retropneumoperitoneum
retropubic
    r. ascending radical prostatectomy
    r. colposuspension
    r. implant
    r. Lapides-Ball bladder neck
    suspension
    r. needle suspension procedure
    r. space

r. urethrolysis
r. urethroscopy
retrorectal
r. cyst
r. lymph node
r. space
retrospective
r. analysis
r. analysis of antimicrobial
resistance
retrospectively reexamined
retrosternal
r. chest pain
r. hernia
retrourethral catheterization
retroversion
retroverted uterus
retrovesical vesiculectomy
retroviral genome
retrovirus
r. infection
porcine endogenous r. (PERV)
retrusive meatus
rettgeri
Proteus r.
Providencia r.
return
r. electrode monitor
total predicted r.
retzii
cavum r.
Retzius
R. space
space of R.
R. vein
REU, REUS
rectal endoscopic
ultrasonography
reusable
r. forceps with needle
r. laparoscopic electrode
reuse syndrome
reuteri
Lactobacillus r.
**Reuter suprapubic trocar and cannula
system**
revascularization
penile r.
renal r.
revenge
Montezuma r.
reverberation artifact
Reverdin abdominal spatula
reversal
jejunoileal fold pattern r.
r. of jejunoileal bypass surgery
vasectomy r.
reverse
r. alpha sigmoid loop

r. cystotome
r. dot hybridization
r. osmosis pump
r. sigma penoscrotal transposition
repair
r. sphincterotome
r. transcriptase (RT)
r. transcriptase-polymerase chain
reaction (RT-PCR)
r. transcriptase reaction
r. transcription
r. Trendelenburg position
reversed
r. anorexia syndrome
r. Mercedes Benz sign
r. passive hemagglutination
reaction
r. peristalsis
r. reimplanted appendicocystostomy
reversible
r. blockade
r. vasectomy
review
comprehensive r.
r. factor
metaanalytic r.
technological r.
Rex-Cantli-Serege line
Reye syndrome (RS)
Rezipas
Rezulin
**RF-assisted cystectomy and
pericystectomy**
RFB
retained foreign body
RFIPC
Rating Form of Inflammatory Bowel
Disease Patient Concerns
RFS
renal function study
RFS 2000
rhabdoid Wilms tumor
rhabdomyoblastic differentiation
rhabdomyolysis
exertional r.
hypoxia-induced r.
rhabdomyoma
rhabdomyomatous
**rhabdomyosarcoma (RMS),
rhabdosarcoma**
alveolar r.
bladder r.
childhood r.
interlabial r.
kidney r.
mixed r.
r. of vagina
paratesticular r.
pleomorphic r.

rhabdomyosarcoma (*continued*)
    prostate r.
    renal r.
    treatment of r.
rhabdosarcoma (*var. of*
  rhabdomyosarcoma)
rhabdosphincter
    r. electromyography
    r. muscle
rhagades
rhamnosus
    Lactobacillus r.
rHBcAg
    recombinant HBcAg
RHCT
    renal helical CT
    RHCT imaging
Rheaban
Rhein anthrone
rhenium 186
Rheomacrodex
rh-EPO
    recombinant human erythropoietin
rhesus rotavirus-tetravalent vaccine
  (RRV-TV)
rheumatica
    scarlatina r.
rheumatic disease
rheumatism
    palindromic r.
rheumatoid
    r. arthritis
    r. vasculitis
Rheumatrex dose pack
rhinosporidiosis
Rhinosporidium seeberi
Rhizopus
rhizotomy
    dorsal r.
    sacral posterior root r.
    selective sacral r.
rhodamine
    alexandrite and r.
    r. 6G dye
    r. 6G dye laser
    r. stain
Rhodesian trypanosomiasis
rhodesiense
    Trypanosoma r.
Rhodes Inventory of Nausea and
  Vomiting
rho protein
rhubarb test
rhythm
    biphasic diurnal r.
    circadian r.
    gallop r.
    irregular r.
    paced r.

    r. strip
    ultradian r.
rhythmicity
    circadian r.
rhythmometry
    cosinor r.
RIA
    radioimmunoassay
    RIA kit
RIBA
    recombinant immunoblot assay
    RIBA test
RIBA-2 test
ribavirin capsule
ribavirin-induced anemia
ribbon
    iridium r.
    r. retractor
    r. stool
rib cutter
riboflavin deficiency
ribonuclease (RNASe, RNase)
    low molecular weight protein r.
ribonucleic
    r. acid (RNA)
    r. acid interference (RNAi)
ribonucleoprotein (RNP)
riboprobe
    complementary single-stranded
    antisense r.
    ^{35}S antisense fibronectin r.
ribose-1-phosphate
ribose-5-phosphate
ribosome
    free r.
rice-flour breath test
rice-fruit diet
Rice-Lyte
rice-water stool
Richard
    R. Wolf Piezolith lithotriptor
    R. Wolf ultrasonic energy rigid
    device
    R. Wolf videoresectoscope
Richards abdominal retractor
Richardson
    R. appendectomy retractor
    R. procedure
Richet fascia umbilicus
Richner-Hanhart syndrome
Richter hernia
Richter-Monroe line
ricin
rickets
    celiac r.
    hypophosphatemic r.
    pseudodeficiency r.
    renal r.
Rickettsia conorii

Rider-Moeller
　　R.-M. dilator
　　R.-M. glossitis
ridge
　　interureteric r.
　　nephrogenic r.
　　rete r.
　　ureteral r.
ridged convoluted villus
Riedel lobe
Riegel test meal
Rieger syndrome
Riepe-Bard gastric balloon
Rieux hernia
rifabutin
Rifadin
rifampicin (*var. of* rifampin)
rifampin, rifampicin
rifamycin, rifomycin
rifaximin
RIFIT
　　radioimmunofocus inhibition test
rIFN-A, rIFN-alfa
　　recombinant interferon alfa
rifomycin (*var. of* rifamycin)
Rigaud operation
Rigby appendectomy retractor
Righini procedure
right
　　r. anterior oblique position
　　r. anterior pararenal space
　　r. colon
　　r. colonic flexure
　　r. colon pouch
　　r. gastroomental artery
　　r. gutter
　　r. hepatic duct
　　r. hepatic radicle
　　r. hepatic vein (RHV)
　　r. inguinal hernia (RIH)
　　r. lobe
　　r. lower quadrant
　　r. ovarian vein syndrome
　　r. upper quadrant
　　r. ureter
right-angle
　　r.-a. clamp
　　r.-a. electrode
　　r.-a. end-to-side anastomosis
　　r.-a. lens
right-sided
　　r.-s. clonus
　　r.-s. lesion
rigid
　　r. abdomen
　　r. endoscope
　　r. esophagoscopy
　　r. nephroscope
　　r. proctoscopy

　　r. proctosigmoidoscopy
　　r. scoop
　　r. scope
　　r. sigmoidoscope
　　r. ureteroscope
　　r. ureteroscopy
rigidity
　　abdominal r.
　　boardlike r.
　　flexural r.
　　involuntary reflex r.
Rigiflator handheld inflation/deflation device
Rigiflex
　　R. ABD balloon dilation catheter
　　R. achalasia balloon
　　R. achalasia dilator
　　R. biliary balloon dilation catheter
　　R. esophageal TTS balloon catheter
　　R. OTW balloon dilation catheter
　　R. pneumatic dilation
　　R. TTS balloon
　　R. TTS balloon dilation catheter
　　R. TTS balloon dilator
RigiScan
　　R. device
　　R. measurement
　　R. penile tumescence and rigidity monitor
　　R. testing
Rigler
　　classic triad of R.
　　R. sign
　　triad of R.
rigor mortis
RIGS
　　radioimmunoguided surgery
RIGScan CR49 test for colorectal cancer detection
Riley-Day
　　R.-D. syndrome
　　R.-D. syndrome of familial dysautonomia
riluzole
rim
　　r. calcification
　　r. nephrogram
　　r. of fascia
　　r. sign
rima, *pl.* **rimae**
　　r. pudendi
　　r. vulva
Rimactane
rimae (*pl. of* rima)
rind
ring
　　A r.
　　abdominal inguinal r.
　　r. abdominal retractor

ring (*continued*)
    anorectal r.
    apex of external r.
    B r.
    R. biliary drainage catheter
    biofragmentable anastomotic r.
      (BAR)
    Cannon r.
    Coloplast skin barrier r.
    confidence r.
    constriction r.
    continence r.
    deep abdominal r.
    distal esophageal r.
    elastic O r.
    esophageal A, B r.
    esophageal contractile r.
    esophageal mucosal r.
    esophageal muscular r.
    estradiol-releasing silicone
      vaginal r.
    Estring estradiol vaginal r.
    external abdominal r.
    external inguinal r.
    finger r.
    r. forceps
    ilioinguinal r.
    iliopsoas r.
    inguinal r.
    inositol r.
    internal abdominal r.
    internal inguinal r.
    intrahaustral contraction r.
    Kayser-Fleischer r.
    lower esophageal B r.
    lower esophageal contraction r.
    lower esophageal mucosal r.
    Lyon r.
    Maclet magnetic r.
    mucosal esophageal r.
    muscular esophageal r.
    O r.
    Ochsner r.
    Osbon pressure-point tension r.
    pressure-point tension r.
    pyloric r.
    rust r.
    Schatzki r.
    r. shadow
    silastic r.
    silicone elastomer r.
    Smith r.
    sphincter contraction r.
    superficial abdominal r.
    sutureless biofragmentable r.
ringed esophagus
Ringer lactate
ringlike
    r. contraction

    r. lesion
    r. stricture
ring-type rigidity measuring device
Rink modification of Casale continent
  catheterizable vesicostomy
rinse
    SaliCept oral r.
Riopan Plus
RIPA
    radioimmunoprecipitation assay
Ripstein
    R. anterior sling rectopexy
    R. prolapsed rectum repair
      procedure
    R. rectal prolapse operation
risedronate
risk
    r. adjustment
    r. evaluation
    r. factors of posttransplant diabetes
      mellitus
    Goldman classification of operative
      r.
    morbidity r.
    neoplasia r.
    r. of bacteremia
    perioperative r.
    poor r.
risk-adjusted mortality
Ritalin
RiteBite biopsy forceps
ritonavir
RIVA HCV 2.0 Strip immunoassay
Rives-Stoppa
    R.-S. incisional hernia repair
      technique
    R.-S. procedure
    R.-S. sublay incisional hernia repair
RJL bioelectrical impedance analyzer
RLND
    retroperitoneal lymph node dissection
RLP
    rectal linitis plastica
    restriction fragment length
      polymorphism
      RLP colorectal carcinoma
RLT
    reduced liver transplant
RMS
    rhabdomyosarcoma
    Ruvalcaba-Myhre-Smith
      RMS syndrome
      RMS voltage
RMT
    ranitidine bismuth citrate,
      metronidazole, tetracycline
RNA
    ribonucleic acid
      albumin messenger RNA

GBV-C/HGV RNA
GB virus C/hepatitis G virus RNA
guide RNA (gRNA)
hepatitis C virus RNA (HCV RNA)
IGF-1R RNA
messenger RNA (mRNA)
RNA probe
RNA-based findings
RNAse, RNase
ribonuclease
RNase digestion
RNase inhibitor
RNP
ribonucleoprotein
rNV
recombinant capsid protein of Norwalk virus
Roadmapper
FluoroPlus R.
Roadrunner wire
Robaxisal
Robbers forceps
Robert
herb R.
Roberts
R. folding esophagoscope
R. oval esophagoscope
R. syndrome
Robertson
R. sign
R. TM urethroscope
Robin-Masse abdominal retractor
Robinow syndrome
robin's egg-blue gallbladder
Robinson catheter
Robinson-Kepler-Power water test
Robinul Forte
Roboprep G instrument
robot-assisted laparoscopy
robotically assisted laparoscopic dismembered pyeloplasty
robotic automated assist device
Robson
R. intestinal forceps
R. point
R. position
ROC
receiver operating characteristic
ROC XS suture fastener
Rocaltrol
Rocephin IM
Roche
R. Elecsys free prostate-specific antigen assay
R. sign
Rochester-Carmalt forceps
Rochester gallstone forceps
Rochester-Mixter forceps
Rochester-Ochsner forceps

Rochester-Péan
R.-P. forceps
R.-P. hemostat
Rockall score
Rockey-Davis incision
rod
colostomy r.
gram-negative r.
ileostomy r.
Meckel r.
Reichmann r.
Sur-Fit Natura loop ostomy r.
ROD
renal osteodystrophy
rod-lens system
rodless end-loop stoma
Rodney Smith biliary stricture repair
Roeder
R. loop
R. loop knot
Roenigk
R. grade
R. score
roentgen finding
roentgenography
double-contrast r.
rofecoxib
Roferon-A
Roger
R. cirrhosis
R. reflex
R. syndrome
Rokitansky
R. disease
R. diverticulum
R. hernia
R. kidney
Rokitansky-Aschoff
R.-A. sinus
R.-A. sinus hyperplasia
Rokitansky-Cushing ulcer
Rolaids
role
additional unproven r.
r. of diet in therapy
r. of resistive index
r. of ureteroscopy
plasmid profile r.
roll
iliac r.
Kraske r.
rollerball electrode
roller pump
rolling hiatal hernia
Romazicon
Rome
R. criteria I, II
R. I, II criteria for irritable bowel syndrome

Rommelaere sign
roof
    pseudoaneurysmal r.
    r. strip
rooperi
    Hypoxis r.
Roosevelt clamp
root
    r. abscess
    angelica r.
    Bennet r.
    black r.
    ginger r.
    r. mean square voltage
    Mexican Scammony r.
    needle r.
    r. neurostimulation
    penile r.
    sacral nerve r.
rooting reflex
rootlet
    ventral sacral r.
ROPA
    Regional Organ Procurement Agency
Rosch-Uchida transjugular liver access set
rose
    r. bengal sodium ^{131}I biliary scan
    r. bengal sodium ^{131}I radioactive agent
    r. bengal test
    dog r.
    r. thorn ulcer
    r. thorn ulcer of mucosa
Rose-Bradford kidney
rosebud stoma
Roseburia
rosemary
Rosenbach-Gmelin test
Rosenbach sign
Rosen cyst
Rosenthal test
rosette
    r. appearance of anus
    Homer Wright r.
rosetted
    E r.
Rosewater syndrome
rosiglitazone
Rossbach disease
Ross carbohydrate-free (RCF)
Rosser crypt hook
Rossetti modification of Nissen fundoplication
Roswell Park Memorial Institute-1640 (RPMI-1640)
rotary shadowing electron microscopy
rotatable Roth retrieval net
RotaTeq

rotating
    r. Bruel and Kjaer probe
    r. endoprobe
    r. endoscissors
    r. sphincterotome
rotation
    external r.
    internal r.
rotational colonoscope overtube
rotator
    Jarit r.
    R. polypectomy snare
rotavirus
    r. diarrhea
    r. gastroenteritis
    group C r.
    r. infection
    r. tetravalent vaccine
    r. vaccine, live oral pentavalent
rotavirus-associated diarrhea
Rotazyme test
Roth
    R. Grip-Tip suture guide
    R. polyp retrieval net
    R. spot
Rothmund-Thomson syndrome
Roticulator stapling device
Rotolith lithotrite
Rotor syndrome
rotunda
    pityriasis r.
rotund abdomen
roughage
rough endoplasmic reticulum
round
    r. ligament
    r. ulcer
round-leafed wintergreen
roundworm
Rous sarcoma virus
route
    fecal-oral r.
    paracellular r.
    sodium entry r.
routine
    r. neonatal circumcision
    r. outpatient procedure
    r. ureteral stenting
Roux
    R. gastric reflux
    R. limb
    R. limb emptying
    R. limb stasis
    R. retractor
    R. stasis syndrome
Roux-en-Y
    R.-e.-Y anastomosis
    R.-e.-Y biliary bypass with antrectomy

R

R.-e.-Y chimney surgical technique
R.-e.-Y choledochojejunostomy
R.-e.-Y cystojejunostomy
R.-e.-Y distal jejunoileostomy
R.-e.-Y esophagojejunostomy
R.-e.-Y gastric bypass
R.-e.-Y gastroenterostomy
R.-e.-Y gastrointestinal system
  procedure
R.-e.-Y hepaticojejunostomy
R.-e.-Y jejunal limb
R.-e.-Y jejunostomy
R.-e.-Y limb enteroscopy
R.-e.-Y loop
R.-e.-Y loop of jejunum
R.-e.-Y operation
R.-e.-Y pancreatojejunostomy
R.-e.-Y procedure with vagotomy
R.-e.-Y reanastomosis
R.-e.-Y reconstruction
Roux-type gastroduodenal anastomosis
Roux-Y chimney
Rovighi sign
Rovsing
  R. operation
  R. sign
  R. syndrome
Rowasa enema
Rowland pouch
roxatidine acetate
Roxicodone
roxithromycin
RP
  restorative proctocolectomy
RPC
  recurrent pyogenic cholangiohepatitis
  restorative proctocolectomy
RPD
  rapid
    Pepcid RPD
RPF
  renal plasma flow
RPG
  retrograde pyelogram
RPGN
  rapidly progressive glomerulonephritis
RPH
  retroperitoneal hemorrhage
RP/IPAA
  restorative proctocolectomy and ileal
    pouch anal anastomosis
RPMI-1640
  Roswell Park Memorial Institute-1640
    RPMI-1640 contrast medium
RPN
  renal papillary necrosis
RPP
  radical perineal prostatectomy

RP3 stain
RPT
  rapid pullthrough
    RPT technique
RRI
  renal resistive index
RRP
  radical retropubic prostatectomy
RS
  rehydrating solution
  respiratory symptoms
  Reye syndrome
    RS associated with GERD
RSH
  rectus sheath hematoma
RSLT
  reduced-size liver transplant
RSR
  rectosphincteric reflex
RSs
  relative supersaturation
RT
  reverse transcriptase
RTA
  renal tubular acidosis
RTFNA
  real-time fine-needle aspiration
RTN
  renal tubular necrosis
RT-PCR
  reverse transcriptase-polymerase chain
    reaction
    PSA RT-PCR
RTX
  real-time transmission
    automated counter Technicon H.3
      RTX
rub
  peritoneal friction r.
  pleural r.
rubber
  r. band ligation (RBL)
  r. band ligation of hemorrhoid
  r. band ligator (RBL)
  r. dam
rubber-sheathed clamp
rubber-shod clamp
rubella
rubeola
rubidium (Rb)
Rubin-Quinton small-bowel biopsy tube
Rubin tube
rubitecan
rubor
  dependent r.
rubra
  Arenaria r.
  miliaria r.
Rubratope-57 radioactive agent

rubrum
    tinea r.
    Trichophyton r.
ructus
Rudd
    R. Clinic hemorrhoidal forceps
    R. Clinic hemorrhoidal ligator
rudiment
    hepatic r.
rudimentary testis syndrome
Rud syndrome
Rue hepatic encephalopathy
RUG
    retrograde urethrogram
    retrograde urethrography
ruga, *pl.* **rugae**
    r. gastrica
    rugae of stomach
    rugae of urinary bladder
    rugae zone
rugae (*pl. of* ruga)
rugal
    r. fold
    r. hypertrophy
    r. pattern
rugate
rugitus
rugose, rugous
rugous (*var. of* rugose)
rule
    Goodsall r.
    Weigert-Meyer r.
ruler catheter
Rulox No. 1, 2
rumble
rumbling bowel sounds
Rumel tourniquet
rumen
rumination
Ruminococcus
    R. lactaris
    R. obeum
    R. productus
runner's diarrhea
running suture
runny stool
runting syndrome
Runyon group III mycobacteria
rupture
    acute hepatic r.
    bladder r.
    catheterization pouch r.
    ERCP-induced splenic r.
    esophageal r.
    extraperitoneal bladder r.
    gastric r.
    hepatic r.
    hydatid cyst intrahepatic r.

    intraperitoneal bladder r.
    Mallory-Weiss mucosal r.
    mesenteric r.
    penile r.
    renal allograft r.
    retrograde balloon r.
    splenic r.
    spontaneous r.
    traumatic r.
    umbilical hernia r.
    uterine r.
ruptured
    r. abdominal aortic aneurysm
    (RAAA)
    r. appendiceal cystadenoma
    r. appendix
    r. hepatic tumor
    r. peliotic lesion
    r. pseudoaneurysm
    r. sigmoid diverticulum
RUS
    real-time ultrasonography
Rusch stent
Rusconi anus
rush
    peristaltic r.
rushing
Russell
    R. gastrostomy kit
    R. peel-away sheath dilator
    R. percutaneous endoscopic
    gastrostomy
    R. sign
    R. technique
    R. viper venom time
Russell-Silver syndrome
Russian tissue forceps
rust ring
RUT
    rapid urease test
    RUT kit
ruthenium red
Rutkow sutureless plug and patch
Rutzen ileostomy bag
RUV
    residual urine volume
Ruvalcaba-Myhre-Smith (RMS)
    R.-M.-S. syndrome
Ru-Vert-M
Ruysch
    R. disease
    R. glomerulus
    R. vein
RVH
    renovascular hypertension
RVR
    renovascular resistance

RVRA
    renal vein renin activity
    renal vein renin assay
RVRC
    renal vein renin concentration
RVRI
    renovascular resistance index
RVT
    renal vein thrombosis
R-wave
    R-w. coordination
    R-w. triggering

RX
    rapid exchange
        RX Herculink 14
        RX Herculink 14 biliary stent
        system
        RX Herculink Plus
        RX Herculink Plus biliary stent
        system
        RX stent delivery system
ryanodine binding
rye whole-grain
Ryle tube

R

S
- S cell
- S cord
- S neuron
- S pelvic ileal pouch
- S pouch
- S reservoir

S-100
- S-100 immunohistochemical stain
- S-100 protein
- S-100 staining

SAA
- serum amyloid A
- splenic artery aneurysm

SAAG
- serum-ascites albumin gradient

Saathoff test

SAB
- serum albumin
- SAB reagent

saber stroke

Sabouraud glucose agar

sabre
- coup de s.
- en coup de s.

saburra

saburral colic

sac
- enterocele s.
- entrapment s.
- fluid-filled s.
- greater peritoneal s.
- hernia s.
- high ligation of hernia s.
- indirect hernia s.
- lap s.
- lesser peritoneal s.
- peritoneal s.
- Pleatman s.
- wide-mouth s.
- yolk s.

saccharate

saccharin

saccharomyces
- *S. boulardii*
- *S. cerevisiae*
- yeast s.

sacciform kidney

Saccomanno
- S. fixative
- S. solution

saccular
- s. aneurysm
- s. colon

sacculated bladder

sacculation
- cecal s.
- colic s.
- s. of colon
- tubular narrowing and s.

saccule

sacculi (*pl. of* sacculus)

sacculiform

sacculus, *pl.* **sacculi**
- sacculi of Beale

Sachse
- S. urethrotome
- S. urethrotomy

Sachs solution

Sacks
- S. QuickStick catheter
- S. Single-Step catheter

Sacks-Vine
- S.-V. feeding gastrostomy tube
- S.-V. gastrostomy kit
- S.-V. PEG system
- S.-V. PEG tube
- S.-V. technique

Sacks-Vine-type PEG

sacral
- s. afferent fiber
- s. agenesis
- s. artery
- s. edema
- s. evoked response
- s. nerve neuromodulation
- s. nerve root
- s. nerve stimulation (SNS)
- s. nerve stimulation therapy
- s. neurostimulation
- s. plexus
- s. posterior root rhizotomy
- s. promontory
- s. reflex arc
- s. root neuromodulation
- s. vein

sacroabdominoperineal pullthrough

sacrococcygeal
- s. pilonidal cyst
- s. pilonidal sinus tract
- s. region germ cell tumor
- s. teratoma

sacrocolpopexy
- abdominal s.

sacrofixation

sacroiliitis

sacrospinalis
- s. ligament vaginal fixation
- s. muscle

S

sacrospinous
> s. ligament
> s. ligament vaginal fixation

sacrotuberous ligament

sacrouterine ligament

sacrum

S-adenosylmethionine (SAMe)
> S-a. deficiency

Saeed
> S. esophageal banding technique
> S. multiband ligator
> S. multiple ligator
> S. 6-shooter
> S. 10-shooter
> S. 6-shooter ligator

safe
> S. and Dry panty and pad system
> s. gastrocutaneous fistula tract

Safe-T-Flex enteral feeding container

safe-tract technique

safety
> S. AV fistula needle
> s. pin ingestion
> s. wire

safflower

saffron stain

SAGB
> Swedish adjustable gastric band

SAGES
> Society of American Gastrointestinal and Endoscopic Surgeons

saginata
> *Taenia s.*

sagittal
> s. fissure of liver
> s. image

sago-grain stool

sagrada
> cascara s.

Sahli glutoid test

Sahli-Nencki test

saint (St.)

Salem
> S. duodenal sump tube
> S. sump double-lumen polyvinyl tube

SALF
> subacute liver failure

Salflex

SaliCept
> S. freeze-dried dressing
> S. oral rinse

salicylate
> s. abuse
> methyl s.

salicylazosulfapyridine

saline
> buffered s.
> s. cleansing enema

> s. continence test
> s. cystometry
> s. flush
> half-normal s.
> heparinized s.
> hypertonic s.
> iced s.
> indigo carmine-stained normal s.
> s. infusion
> s. injection therapy
> isotonic s.
> s. laxative
> s. load test
> phosphate-buffered s. (PBS)
> s. slush
> s. suppression test

saline-assisted polypectomy (SAP)

saline-epinephrine
> hypertonic s.-e. (HSE)

saline-filled cholangiocatheter

saline-moistened sponge

saliva
> s. bicarbonate
> pooled s.
> s. substitute

salivarius
> *Streptococcus s.*

Salivart solution

salivary
> s. amylase
> s. calculus
> s. epidermal growth factor (sEGF)
> s. epidermal growth factor-1
> s. gland enlargement
> s. gland scan
> s. hypersecretion
> s. mass
> s. tenderness
> s. testing

salivary-type isoamylase

salivation

Salkowski-Schipper test

Salmon
> S. backcut incision
> S. law

salmonella
> *S. agona*
> *S. choleraesuis*
> *S. colitis*
> *S. enteritidis*
> *S. enteritidis* orchitis
> *S. hartford*
> *S. heidelberg*
> *S. hirschfeldii*
> *S. infantis*
> *S. newport*
> nontyphoidal *S.*
> *S. paratyphi* (A, B, C)
> *S. stanley*

S. typhi
S. typhimurium
S. typhimurium enterocolitis
S. typhimurium R5
salmonellosis
nontyphoidal s.
salmonicida
Aeromonas s.
Salomon test
salpinges (*pl. of* salpinx)
salpingitis
salpinx, *pl.* **salpinges**
salt
amphipathic bile s.
artificial Carlsbad s.
artificial Kissingen s.
artificial Vichy s.
bile s. (BS)
bismuth s.
Cheatle s.
s. consumption
dihydroxy s.
fura-2 pentapotassium s.
gold s.
low s.
magnesium s.
monohydroxy bile s.
structural effect of dietary s.
trihydroxy s.
salt-and-pepper duodenal erosion
salt-losing
s.-l. nephritis
s.-l. nephropathy
salt-sensitive hypertension
salt-transporting protein
saluresis
Saluron
salutary
Salutensin
salvage
s. brachytherapy
s. cryoablation
s. cryoablation of prostate
s. cystectomy
s. cystoprostatectomy
s. cytology
s. cytology technique
s. prostatectomy
s. protocol
s. surgery
s. therapy
Salvanios pH 10 disinfectant solution
Salvati proctoscope
Salvia miltiorrhiza
Salzer test meal
samarium
SAMe
S-adenosylmethionine
SAMe nutritional supplement

sample
arterial blood s.
aspirated s.
Bethesda System for cervicovaginal s.
blood s.
random stool s.
serum s.
stool s.
urine s.
venous blood s.
sampling
adrenal vein aldosterone s.
arterial stimulation venous s.
(ASVS)
s. gate
InSure brush s.
mediastinal lymph node s.
tissue s.
transhepatic portal venous s.
Sam Roberts esophagoscope
sand
hydatid s.
urinary s.
sandarac
sandbag
Sanders incision
Sand-Eze EGD pillow
Sandhill pH antimony probe
Sandhill-800 TDS chart recorder
Sandifer syndrome
Sandimmune
Sandostatin LAR Depot
Sandoz
S. balloon replacement tube
S. Caluso PEG tube
S. Caluso super PEG
S. feeding/suction tube
sandwich
s. staghorn calculus therapy
s. technique
sandy skin-prepping paste
sanguineous
s. drainage
s. fluid
sanguis
Streptococcus s.
Sani-Pads medicated cleansing pad
Sani-Supp
Sanorex
SANS
Stoller afferent nerve stimulation
PerQ SANS
Sansert
santa
yerba s.
Santiani-Stone pancreas head gunshot
classification
^{35}S antisense fibronectin riboprobe
santonin test

Santorini
  accessory duct of S.
  S. canal
  duct of S.
  S. labyrinth
  papilla of S.
  S. sphincter
  S. venous plexus
santorinicele
SAP
  saline-assisted polypectomy
  serum amyloid P
saphenofemoral junction
saphenous
  s. nerve
  s. vein
saponifiable fecal bile acid
saponification
Sappey
  accessory portal system
    of S.
Sapporo virus
saprophyticus
  Staphylococcus s.
saprophytism
saquinavir
saralasin
sarcocele
sarcocystosis
sarcoidosis
  epididymal s.
  hepatic s.
  hepatobiliary s.
  pancreatic s.
  renal s.
  urethral s.
sarcoma
  appendiceal Kaposi s.
  bladder s.
  Boeck s.
  botryoid s.
  s. botryoid
  clear cell s.
  Ewing s.
  gastric Kaposi s.
  gastrointestinal Kaposi s.
  granulocytic s.
  hemangioendothelial s.
  intracolonic Kaposi s.
  Ito cell s.
  Kaposi s. (KS)
  kidney clear cell s.
  Kupffer cell s.
  lipoblastic s.
  osteogenic s.
  penis s.
  prostate gland s.
  retroperitoneum s.
  seminal vesicle s.

  testis s.
  vasoablative endothelial s.
    (VABES)
  s. virus oncogene
sarcomatoid squamous cell carcinoma
sarcomatous
sarcomphalocele
sarcoplasmic reticulum
Sarcoptes scabiei
Sarfeh principle
Sarisol No. 2
Sarns Siok II blood pump
Sarot needle holder
sarsaparilla
  German s.
SART
  standard acid reflux test
Sassone score
satellite lesion
satellitosis
  neutrophilic s.
Satietrol
satiety
  early s.
  s. test
Satinsky clamp
satisfactory continence
Satoyoshi syndrome
satraplatin
satumomab pendetide
saturated fatty acid (SFA)
saturation
  arterial s.
  s. index (SI)
  oxygen s.
  percent transferrin s.
  s. riboprobe concentration
  transferrin s.
saturnine
  s. colic
  s. nephritis
saturnism
satyri
  Bertiella s.
saucerization
saucerized biopsy
Saundby test
Saunders disease
sausage digit
sausagelike appearance
sausage-string pattern
Savage perineal body
Savary
  S. bougie
  S. bronchoscope
  complete S.
  S. tapered thermoplastic dilator
Savary-Gilliard
  S.-G. dilating system

S.-G. esophagitis grade I, II
S.-G. metal olive
S.-G. over-the-wire dilator
S.-G. silastic flexible bougie
S.-G. wire-guided bougie

Savary-Miller
S.-M. criteria
S.-M. grade I-III erosive esophagitis
S.-M. grade I-III reflux esophagitis
S.-M. II grade

saver
Cell S.

saw palmetto

sawtooth
s. appearance sign
s. irregularity of bowel contour

sawtoothed appearance

Sawyer
S. rectal retractor
S. rectal speculum

saxitoxin

S-B
Sengstaken-Blakemore
S-B tube

SBE
small-bowel enteroscopy

SBFT
small-bowel followthrough

SBO
small-bowel obstruction

SBP
spontaneous bacterial peritonitis

SBPN
simultaneous bilateral percutaneous
nephrolithotomies

SC
sieving coefficient
sulfur colloid

scabiei
Sarcoptes s.

scabies
genital s.

scale
Charrière catheter size s.
children's coma s.
ECOG performance status s.
Flint colon injury s. (FCIS)
French s.
Gastrointestinal Symptom Rating S.
(GSRS)
Goldberg Anorectic Attitude s.
gray s.
Hetzel-Dent s.
Karnofsky performance status s.
Lanza s.
Likert s.
Madsen-Iversen s.
modified Hetzel-Dent s.
Perceived Stress S. (PSS)

scaling
physiologic s.

scalloped
s. antimesenteric border
s. bowel lumen

scalpel
s. blade
harmonic s.
LaserSonics Nd:YAG Laserblade s.
ultrasonic s.

scan
acetyl triglycine renal s.
bone s.
cholecystokinin dimethyl
iminodiacetic acid s. (CCK-HIDA)
colloid shift on liver-spleen s.
CT s.
diethylenetriamine pentaacetic acid
renal s.
dimercaptosuccinic acid renal s.
dimethyl iminodiacetic acid s.
DISIDA s.
DMSA s.
DTPA renal s.
dual-energy CT s.
endoanal ultrasound s.
esophageal transit s.
fluorescence-activated cell sorter s.
(FACScan)
gallbladder s.
gallium s.
gastric emptying s.
gastroesophageal reflux s.
GI bleeding s.
hepatic blood pool s.
hepatobiliary s.
HIDA s.
Hybritech PSA s.
indium-labeled leukocyte s.
indium 64-labeled white blood
cell s.
indium leukocyte s.
intercostal s.
iodine s.
iodocholesterol s.
isotope renal s.
isotropic s.
labeled red blood cell s.
liver s.
liver-spleen s.
MAG-3 renal s.
Meckel s.
monoclonal antibody scintigraphic s.
MRI s.
^{99m}Tc DTPA renal s.
^{99m}Tc HMPAO-labeled leukocyte s.
^{99m}Tc IDA s.
^{99m}Tc MDP nuclear isotope bone s.
^{99m}Tc pertechnetate s.

S

scan (*continued*)
^{99m}Tc RBC bleeding s.
^{99m}Tc sulfur colloid s.
nuclear bleeding s.
nuclear isotope s.
nuclear medicine s.
peritoneovenous shunt patency s.
PET s.
PIPIDA hepatobiliary s.
positron emission tomography s.
ProstaScint s.
radioisotope s.
radionuclide s.
renal s.
rose bengal sodium ^{131}I biliary s.
salivary gland s.
SPECT s.
splenic perfusion measurement by
  dynamic CT s.
sulfur colloid liver s.
tagged red blood cell bleeding s.
technetium-labeled autologous red
  blood cell s.
technetium-99m diethylenetriamine
  pentaacetic acid s.
technetium-99m HIDA s.
technetium radionuclide s.
s. test
transabdominal s.
transrectal s.
transvesical s.
UJ13A nuclear isotope bone s.
ultrasound s.
scan-directed biopsy
scanner
BladderScan ultrasound s.
Bruel-Kjaer s.
conventional static s.
CT Twin s.
General Electric Signa s.
high-resolution real-time s.
Kretz Combison 330
  ultrasound s.
Kretz 311 ultrasound s.
linear-array convex array s.
linear convex array s.
Lunar DPX total-body s.
MKII automated s.
sector s.
Tesla GE Signa whole-body s.
scanning
captopril-DTPA s.
s. electron microscope
s. electron microscopy
endoscopic magnetic resonance s.
fluorescent gene s.
s. force microscopy (SFM)
iodine hippurate s.
radioisotope s.

renal s.
transrectal ultrasound s. (TRUS)
scaphoid abdomen
scapus penis
scar
Billroth II anastomotic s.
chest tube s.
episiotomy s.
iridectomy s.
railroad track s.'s
sternotomy s.
thoracotomy s.
s. tissue formation
s. tissue reaction
scarce bowel sounds
Scardino
S. ureteropyeloplasty
S. vertical flap pyeloplasty
S. vertical pyeloplasty flap
Scardino-Prince
S.-P. ureteropyeloplasty
S.-P. vertical flap pyeloplasty
scarf-ring sign
scarified duodenum
scarlatinal nephritis
scarlatina rheumatica
scarlatiniform rash
Scarpa
S. fascia
S. triangle
scarring
duodenum deformed by s.
gastrostomy s.
kidney s.
local s.
postdystrophic s.
postnecrotic s.
renal s.
scatoma
scattered fluorescein
scatter factor
scattering
Raman s.
scavenger
free radical s.
hydroxyl radical s.
SCBE
single-contrast barium enema
SCC
squamous cell carcinoma
S-CCK-Pz
secretin-cholecystokinin-pancreatozymin
S-CCK-Pz stimulation
S-CCK-Pz test
SCFA
short-chain fatty acid
Schachowa spiral tube
Schäfer nomogram
Schatzki ring

Schaumann body
Scheffe-F test
schematic diagram
schenckii
> *Sporothrix s.*

Scheuer staging
Schiff
> S. biliary cycle
> S. stain
> S. test

Schilder disease
Schiller-Duval body
Schilling test
Schindler
> S. disease
> S. esophagoscope
> S. peritoneal forceps
> S. semiflexible gastroscope

schisandra
> false s.

Schistosoma
> *S. haematobium*
> *S. intercalatum*
> *S. japonicum*
> *S. mansoni*
> *S. mekongi*

schistosomal
> s. cervicitis
> s. dysentery
> s. liver disease
> s. pelvic floor myopathy

schistosomiasis
> active s.
> acute s.
> Asiatic s.
> bladder s.
> colon s.
> colonic s.
> ectopic s.
> hepatic s.
> inactive s.
> intestinal s.
> Japanese s.
> s. japonica
> Manson s.
> s. mansoni
> s. mekongi
> Oriental s.
> s. sandy patch
> ureteral s.
> urinary s.
> vesical s.

Schmidt
> S. diet
> S. syndrome

Schmitz bacillus
schmitzii
> *Shigella s.*

Schmorl reaction

Schneider stent
Schnidt
> S. gall duct forceps
> S. thoracic forceps

Schoemaker
> S. anastomosis
> S. gastroenterostomy
> S. transscrotal orchiopexy procedure

Schoemaker-Billroth II technique
Schoenberg intestinal forceps
SchonCath chronic dialysis catheter
Schönlein-Henoch
> S.-H. disease
> S.-H. purpura

Schramm phenomenon
Schuchardt relaxing incision
Schultz
> S. angina
> S. disease
> S. syndrome

Schwann
> S. cell
> S. cell lipidosis

schwannian spindle cell
schwannoma
> penile s.

Schwartz
> S. clamp
> S. method
> S. test

Schwartz-Jampel syndrome
Schwartz-Pregenzer
> S.-P. urethropexy procedure
> S.-P. urethroplasty

Schweizer-Foley Y-plasty
sciatic
> s. hernia
> s. nerve

sciatica-like pain
ScI-70 autoantibody
SCID
> severe combined immunodeficiency

scintigram
> technetium-99m dimercaptosuccinic
> acid s.

scintigraph
scintigraphic
> s. balloon
> s. balloon topography
> s. diagnosis
> s. emptying study
> s. reflux

scintigraphy
> aberration by s.
> adrenal s.
> antral s.
> dimercaptosuccinic acid s.
> direct vesicoureteral s. (DVS)
> diuretic renal s.

S

scintigraphy (*continued*)
    DMSA s.
    gastric emptying s.
    gastroesophageal s.
    hepatobiliary s.
    labeled leukocyte s.
    ^{99m}Tc GSA s.
    ^{99m}Tc pertechnetate s.
    OctreoScan s.
    OncoScint CR/OV carcinoma
     localization s.
    per rectal portal s.
    quantitative hepatobiliary s. (QHS)
    radioisotope s.
    radionuclide s.
    renal gallium-67 s.
    renal perfusion s.
    renocortical s.
    somatostatin receptor s. (SRS)
    tagged erythrocyte s.
    technetium-labeled red blood cell s.
    technetium-99m red cell s.
    whole-gut transit s. (WGTS)
scintillation vial
scintiphotography, scintography
    leukocyte s.
scintiphotosplenoportography
scintirenography
scintiscan
    biliary s.
    false-positive s.
    gastroesophageal s.
scintiscanning
    radionuclide ^{99}Tc s.
scintography (*var. of* scintiphotography)
scirrhous
    s. adenocarcinoma
    s. carcinoma
    s. lesion
scissors
    Buie rectal s.
    Busch umbilical s.
    Church deep surgery s.
    cold s.
    Crafoord thoracic s.
    curved Mayo s.
    Deaver operating s.
    diathermy s.
    dissection s.
    s. dissection
    Doyen abdominal s.
    Duffield deep surgery s.
    electrosurgical curved s.
    endoscopic s.
    Ferguson abdominal s.
    Graham deep surgery s.
    Harrington-Mayo s.
    Heiss flexible endoscopic s.
    hook s.

    Hooper deep surgery s.
    insulated curved s.
    insulated straight s.
    Kelly fistula s.
    laparoscopic s.
    Lincoln deep surgery s.
    Mayo s.
    Mayo-Noble dissecting s.
    meatotomy s.
    Metzenbaum s.
    Miller rectal s.
    Nelson s.
    Nu-Tip laparoscopic s.
    Panzer gallbladder s.
    Penn umbilical s.
    Potts s.
    Potts-Smith s.
    Pratt rectal s.
    Snowden-Pencer s.
    strabismus s.
    Strulle s.
    Super-Cut s.
    surgical s.
    suture s.
    Sweet esophageal s.
    Thorek-Feldman gallbladder s.
    Thorek gallbladder s.
    umbilical s.
    s. valve
    Vezien abdominal s.
    Westcott tenotomy s.
    Willauer thoracic s.
Scivoletto test
SCIWORA
    spinal cord injury without radiographic
    abnormality
sclera (sc), *pl.* **sclerae**
    anicteric sclerae
    icteric sclerae
    nonicteric sclerae
sclerae (*pl. of* sclera)
scleral icterus
sclerodactylia (*var. of* sclerodactyly)
sclerodactyly, sclerodactylia
scleroderma
    s. bowel disease
    esophageal s.
    s. of esophagus
    s. renal crisis
    s. sine scleroderma
Scleromate sclerosant
sclerosant
    absolute alcohol s.
    bucrylate s.
    s. dosage
    esophageal variceal s.
    ethanolamine oleate s.
    s. injection
    Krazy Glue s.

latex s.
morrhuate s.
polidocanol s.
Scleromate s.
sodium tetradecyl sulfate s.
s. solution
Sotradecol s.
variceal s.
sclerosant-contrast solution
sclerose
scleroses (*pl. of* sclerosis)
sclerosing
s. adenosis
s. agent
s. cholangitis
s. encapsulating peritonitis
s. hepatic carcinoma (SHC)
s. lymphangitis
s. mesenteritis
s. solution
s. therapy
sclerosis, *pl.* **scleroses**
alcohol s.
biliary s.
central hyaline s.
diffuse mesangial s. (DMS)
endoscopic injection s.
esophageal variceal s.
focal s.
gastric s.
global s.
glomerular s.
hepatic s.
hepatoportal s.
injection s.
laser s.
multiple s. (MS)
nuclear s.
progressive systemic s. (PSS)
systemic duodenal s.
tetracycline s.
tuberous s.
variceal s.
sclerosus
lichen s.
sclerotherapist
sclerotherapy
antegrade scrotal s.
bismuth s.
colonoscopic s.
s. complication
endoscopic injection s. (EIS)
endoscopic retrograde s.
esophageal variceal s. (EVS)
ethanol s.
fiberoptic injection s. (FIS)
hemorrhoidal s.
injection s.
intravariceal injection s.

low-volume s.
s. needle
paravariceal s.
prophylactic s.
ultralow-volume s.
variceal s.
sclerotic
s. atrophy
s. kidney
s. stomach
s. tuft
SCO
Sertoli cell-only
SCO syndrome
scoleces (*pl. of* scolex)
scolex, *pl.* **scoleces, scolices**
scolices (*pl. of* scolex)
scoliosis
scombroid fish poisoning
scoop
Beck abdominal s.
Desjardins gallbladder s.
Desjardins gallstone s.
Ferguson gallstone s.
Ferris common duct s.
gallbladder s.
Klebanoff gallstone s.
malleable s.
Mayo common duct s.
Mayo gallstone s.
Mayo-Robson gallstone s.
Moore gallstone s.
Moynihan gallstone s.
rigid s.
scope
baby s.
flexible s.
J turn of s.
M-scope multibending s.
Olympus ENF-P2 s.
Olympus OSF s.
retroflexed s.
rigid s.
torquing of s.
Scopinaro pancreaticobiliary bypass
scopolamine
scopolia
scorbutic dysentery
score
activity s.
APACHE-II s.
Baylor bleeding s.
Beppu s.
Boyarsky BPH symptom s.
Brunt s.
CCKNOW s.
Child-Pugh s.
Cleveland Clinic incontinence s.
DeMeester acid s.

S

score (*continued*)
 Emory s.
 fibrin s.
 fibrosis s.
 Glasgow alcoholic hepatitis s.
 Glasgow Dyspepsia Severity S.
  (GDSS)
 Gleason s.
 hostility s.
 incontinence s.
 International Autoimmune Hepatitis
  Group s.
 International Prognostic Index s.
 International Prostate Symptom S.
  (IPSS)
 Johnson and DeMeester s.
 Johnson-DeMeester symptom s.
 Karnofsky s.
 Knodell s.
 linear analog pain s.
 linear-array analog pain s.
 Madsen symptom s.
 MELD s.
 PELD s.
 posttest s.
 pretest global rating s.
 QOLRD s.
 Quality of Life in Reflux and
  Dyspepsia s.
 Rockall s.
 Roenigk s.
 Sassone s.
 sexual function s.
 SOFA s.
 symptom s.
 total corrected incremental s.
  (TCIS)
 visceroperception s.
Scotch broom
Scott
 S. AMS inflatable penile
  prosthesis
 S. jejunoileal bypass
 S. operation
 S. retractor
scrapie protein
scraping brush
screen
 Biosafe PSA4 s.
 ChemTrak AccuMeter s.
 ENA s.
 genomewide s.
screening
 cancer s.
 catatonic trypsinogen DNA s.
 colon cancer s.
 colonoscopy s.
 colorectal cancer s.
 s. cystometry

 early preimplantation cell s.
  (EPICS)
 endocrine s.
 s. endoscopy
 office-based esophageal s.
screw
 Reddick-Saye s.
Scribner shunt
scrota (*pl. of* scrotum)
scrotal
 s. agenesis
 s. angiokeratoma
 s. arteriovenous malformation
 s. calcification
 s. encroachment
 s. fat necrosis
 s. fixation
 s. hemangioma
 s. hematoma
 s. hernia
 s. hyperplasia
 s. hypospadias
 s. inclusion cyst
 s. lymphangioma
 s. mass
 s. orchiopexy
 s. pain
 s. panniculitis
 s. pneumatocele
 s. pouch operation
 s. pouch orchiopexy
 s. raphe
 s. reflex
 s. septum
 s. swelling
 s. tenderness
 s. trauma
 s. varicocelectomy
 s. violation
scrotal-perineal artery
scrotectomy
 total s.
scroti
 elephantiasis s.
 pruritus s.
 raphe s.
scrotitis
scrotocele
scrotoplasty
scrotoscopy
scrotum, *pl.* scrota, scrotums
 acute s.
 angiokeratoma of s.
 s. avulsion injury
 bifid s.
 s. calcification
 s. cyst
 ectopic s.
 lymph s.

necrotizing fasciitis of s.
prepenile dislocation of s.
raphe of s.
sebaceous cyst of s.
septum of s.
watering-can s.

scrotums (*pl. of* scrotum)

scrub
Betadine s.
pHisoHex s.

SCTAT
sex cord tumors with annular tubules

SCTP
solid and cystic tumors of pancreas

Scudder
S. intestinal clamp
S. intestinal forceps

SCUF
slow continuous ultrafiltration

Scultetus position

scybala (*pl. of* scybalum)

scybalous stool

scybalum, *pl.* **scybala**

SDH
sorbitol dehydrogenase
SDH enzyme

SDS
sodium dodecyl sulfate

SDS-PAGE
sodium dodecyl sulfate-polyacrylamide gel electrophoresis

sea anemone ulcer

sea-blue histiocyte syndrome

seabuckthorn seed oil

seal
fibrin s.
Karaya 5 s.
long s. (LS)

sealant
Beriplast fibrin s.
Crosseal fibrin s.
fibrin s.
Hemaseel APR kit fibrin s.
Periplast s.
Tisseel fibrin s.

searcher
stone s.

Sears Wee Alert

sebaceous, sebaceus
s. cyst
s. cyst of scrotum

sebaceum
adenoma s.

sebaceus (*var. of* sebaceous)

seborrheic
s. dermatitis
s. keratitis

seborrheica

secalin

Secca
S. procedure
S. radiofrequency system

secobarbital

secoisolariciresinol

secondary
s. achalasia
s. amyloidosis
s. bacterial peritonitis
s. bile acid
s. biliary cirrhosis
s. biliary fibrosis
s. case
s. closure
s. contraction
s. cyst
s. enterocele
s. hyperaldosteronism
s. hyperparathyroidism (sHPT)
s. hypertension
s. impotence
s. incontinence
s. jejunal ulcer
s. metastatic carcinoma
s. peristalsis
s. peristaltic wave
s. priapism
s. prophylaxis
s. pseudoobstruction syndrome
s. refluxing megaureter
s. renal calculus
s. sclerosing cholangitis
s. spermatocyte
s. sterility
s. surgery
s. suture
s. syphilis
s. tumor
s. ureteropelvic junction obstruction
s. vesicoureteral reflux
s. volvulus

second-cuff implantation

second-generation
s.-g. cephalosporin
s.-g. enzyme immunoassay (EIA-2)
s.-g. lithotriptor
s.-g. recombinant immunoblot assay

second-line drug

second-look
s.-l. flexible nephroscopy
s.-l. laparotomy
s.-l. operation

second resection

second-set phenomenon

secosteroid hormone

SecreFlo

secretagogue
> luminal s.
> mucus s.
> somatostatin s.

secreted
> s. autotransporter toxin
> s. mediator

secretin
> proton-induced release of s.
> s. provocation test
> s. stimulation
> s. stimulation test
> synthetic porcine s.
> s. ultrasonography

secretin-CCK stimulation test
secretin-cholecystokinin-pancreatozymin (S-CCK-Pz)
Secretin-Ferring powder
secretin-glucagon-vasoactive intestinal peptide family
secretin-pancreozymin stimulation test
secretion
> acid s.
> basal acid s.
> biliary cholesterol s.
> chloride s.
> chylomicron s.
> epididymis s.
> estrogen testicular s.
> follicle-stimulating hormone s.
> gastric acid s.
> gonadotropin-releasing hormone pulsatile s.
> hydrochloric acid s.
> idiopathic gastric acid s.
> intrinsic factor s.
> Leydig cell s.
> macromolecular s.
> meal-stimulated pancreatic s.
> medication-associated suppression of gastric s.
> mucoid s.
> paralytic s.
> pepsin s.
> physiologic role in acid s.
> prostate gland s.
> renin s.
> toxin-mediated intestinal s.
> vas deferens s.

secretory
> s. canaliculus
> s. cell
> s. coil
> s. component
> s. diarrhea
> s. IgA (sIgA)
> s. immunoglobulin A
> s. leukocyte proteinase inhibition (SLPI)

> s. product
> s. reflex

section
> abdominal s.
> adrenal gland microscopic s.
> cryostat tissue s.
> distal shave s.
> frozen s.
> Giemsa-stained s.
> perineal s.
> permanent s.
> renal histologic s.
> ultrathin araldite s.

sectioning
> celiac plexus s.
> thin-shave s.

sector scanner
Sectral
Securcut aspiration biopsy needle
SED
> semielemental diet

sedation
> benzodiazepine conscious s.
> conscious s.
> IV s.
> meperidine conscious s.
> midazolam conscious s.
> nurse-administered propofol s.
> patient-controlled s. (PCS)
> terminal s.

sedation-induced hypoventilation
sedative
> anxiolytic s.
> gastric s.
> intestinal s.

sediment
> nephritic s.
> spun urine s.
> urinary s.

sedimentation
> Ficoll-Hypaque gradient s.

sedoanalgesia
seeberi
> *Rhinosporidium s.*

seed
> BrachySeed brachytherapy s.
> croton s.
> EchoSeed radioactive iodine-125 brachytherapy s.
> iodine-125 brachytherapy s.
> I-Plant brachytherapy s.
> iridium s.
> mustard s.
> PharmaSeed iodine-125 s.
> PharmaSeed palladium-103 s.
> *Plantago ovata* s.
> poppy s.
> ProstaSeed I-125 s.
> psyllium s.

radioactive s.
SeedNet ice s.
Symmetra I-125 brachytherapy s.
seeding
    instrument-track s.
    malignant s.
    needle-track s.
    peritoneal s.
    tumor s.
SeedNet
    S. cryotherapy system
    S. Gold ultrathin cryoneedle
    S. ice seed
seepage
    fecal s.
SEER
    Surveillance, Epidemiology, and End
    Results
    SEER database
sEGF
    salivary epidermal growth factor
segment
    afferent tubular isoperistaltic s.
    Ask-Upmark renal s.
    Barrett s.
    demucosalized augmentation with
      gastric s. (DAWG)
    digital stream s.
    distal nephron s.
    ileal s.
    ileocecal s.
    midtransverse s.
    nephron s.
    pyloroduodenal s.
    S3 s.
    tumor-bearing s.
segmenta (*pl. of* segmentum)
segmental
    s. appendicitis
    s. bile duct fibrosis
    s. change
    s. colectomy
    s. colitis associated with diverticular
      disease
    s. colonic adenomatous polyposis
      syndrome
    s. colonic resection
    s. colonic tuberculosis
    s. enteritis
    s. glomerulosclerosis
    s. ileal infarction
    s. intestine
    s. ischemic colitis
    s. liver graft
    s. polar nephrectomy
    s. testicular infarction
    s. ureterectomy
segmentary pancreatitis
segmentation movement

segmentectomy
    hepatic s.
    s. of liver
segmented neutrophil
segment-specific expression pattern
segmentum, *pl.* **segmenta**
segregator
    Cathelin s.
    Harris s.
    Luy s.
Segura basket
Segura-Dretler laser basket
SeHCAT
    selenium-labeled homocholic acid
    conjugated with taurine
    SeHCAT test
Seidlitz powder
Seitzinger tripolar cutting forceps
seizure
    autonomic s.
    s. disorder
Sekomic SS-100F recorder
^{75}Se-labeled bile acid test
SelCID
Seldinger
    S. cystic duct catheterization
    S. gastrostomy needle
    S. principle
    S. technique
selectin
selective
    s. bladder activation
    s. catheterization
    s. ductal cannulation
    s. endothelin A
    s. gut decontamination
    s. intestinal decontamination
      (SID)
    s. jejunal hyperalgesia
    s. left gastric arteriography
    s. mesenteric angiography
    s. paracellular conductance
    s. proximal vagotomy (SPV)
    s. sacral rhizotomy
    s. targeting
    s. tubal occlusion procedure
      (STOP)
selectivity
selenite
    insulin-transferrin-sodium s.
Selenite-F enrichment medium
selenium-75
selenium-labeled homocholic acid
  conjugated with taurine (SeHCAT)
selenomethionine radioactive agent
self-antigen
self-bougienage treatment
self-catheterization
    intermittent s.-c. (ISC)

S

Self-Cath hydrogel intermittent urinary catheter
self-channelization
    urethral s.-c.
self-drainage catheter
self-expandable
    s.-e. metallic stent
    s.-e. stainless steel braided endoprosthesis
self-expanding
    s.-e. biliary metal stent
    s.-e. coil stent
    s.-e. metallic (SEM)
    s.-e. metallic stent (SEMS)
    s.-e. plastic stent (SEPS)
self-fulfilling prophecy
self-heal
self-induced
    s.-i. purging
    s.-i. vomiting
self-injection therapy
self-management
    primary advantage of s.-m.
self-MHC
self-monitoring
    nocturnal tumescence s.-m.
self-obturation
    intermittent s.-o.
self-poisoning
self-retaining
    s.-r. catheter
    s.-r. coil stent
    s.-r. ring retractor
self-retraction clamp
self-retractor
    Lone Star s.-r.
self-test
    ColoScreen s.-t.
self-tightening slip knot
Seltzer
    Bromo S.
SEM
    self-expanding metallic
    SEM stent
semantic conditioning
Semb ligature carrier
semen
    s. analysis
    s. analysis test
    s. coagulation
    s. collection
    s. liquefaction
    s. round cell
    s. sperm concentration
    s. viscosity
    s. volume
semenuria, seminuria, spermaturia
semicircular line of Douglas

semiconductor laser
semielemental
    s. diet (SED)
    s. enteral feeding
semiflexible endoscope
semiformed stool
Semilente insulin
semilunar-shaped fold
seminal
    s. colliculus
    s. fluid
    s. oxidative stress in patient
    s. plasma C3
    s. plasma cholesterol
    s. plasma choline
    s. plasma citrate
    s. plasma citric acid
    s. plasma fructose
    s. plasma Zn-alpha 2-glycoprotein
    s. tract washout
    s. vesicle
    s. vesicle abscess
    s. vesicle adenocarcinoma
    s. vesicle agenesis
    s. vesicle amyloid deposit
    s. vesicle aplasia
    s. vesicle aspiration
    s. vesicle atrophy
    s. vesicle calculus
    s. vesicle carcinoid
    s. vesicle hydatid cyst
    s. vesicle infection
    s. vesicle innervation
    s. vesicle lymphoma
    s. vesicle obstruction
    s. vesicle sarcoma
    s. vesicle weight
    s. vesiculography (SVG)
    s. vesiculotomy
seminalis
    colliculus s.
    ductus excretorius vesiculae s.
    vesicula s.
semination
seminiferous
    s. tubule
    s. tubule blood-testis barrier
    s. tubule epithelium
    s. tubule gonocyte
    s. tubule peritubular structure
    s. tubule Sertoli cell
seminis
    liquor s.
seminogelin
seminologist
seminology
seminoma
    anaplastic s.

retroperitoneal s.
testicular s.
seminomatous
seminoprotein
gamma s.
seminuria (*var. of* semenuria)
semioblique position
semiopen hemorrhoidectomy
semipedunculated
s. lesion
s. tumor
semiquantitative culture
semirigid
s. endoscope
s. fiberoptic ureteroscope
s. Nottingham introducer
s. sigmoidoscope
semisolid stool
Semken tissue forceps
SEMS
self-expanding metallic stent
membrane-coated SEMS
SEN
SEN virus (SENV)
SEN virus variant D (SENV-D)
SEN virus variant H (SENV-H)
senburi
Senecio
senescence
accelerated s.
senescent cell
Sengstaken-Blakemore (S-B)
S.-B. esophageal balloon
S.-B. tamponade
S.-B. tube
S.-B. tube insertion
senile nephrosclerosis
Senior-Loken syndrome
senktide
SennaPrompt
Senn-Kanavel retractor
Senn retractor
Senokot-S
Senokot X-Prep
Sensa
Hemoccult S.
sensation
bladder s.
burning s.
esophageal globus s.
foreign body s.
globus s.
perineal s.
rectal s.
S. Short Throw snare
threshold of rectal s.
SensiCare synthetic powder-free surgical glove

Sensipar
sensitive and specific ELISA
sensitivity
anaphylactoid food s.
culture and s. (C&S)
esophageal acid s.
gluten s.
interpersonal s.
penile s.
rectal visceral s.
soy protein s.
sensitizer
radiation s.
sensor
anal EMG PerryMeter s.
anterior esophageal s. (AES)
bladder pressure s.
Dentsleeve sleeve s.
fiberoptic s.
manometric s.
S. Medics pressure transducer sleeve s.
ultrasonic tactile s.
sensorium change
sensory
s. array
s. biofeedback
s. finding
s. loss
s. nervous terminal
s. neuron
s. receptor
s. urgency
s. voiding dysfunction
sentinel
s. clot
s. fold
s. hyperplastic polyp
s. loop
s. node
s. pile
s. tag
sentry system
SENV
SEN virus
SENV-D
SEN virus variant D
SENV-H
SEN virus variant H
separation
peripartum symphysis s.
separator
Benson pylorus s.
Sepet artificial liver support device
Sephacryl S-300 HR gel
Sepharose 4B-coupled protein-A column
Seprafilm bioresorbable membrane
Sepramesh

S

SEPS
  self-expanding plastic stent
  subfascial endoscopic perforator surgery
sepsis
  anal s.
  anorectal s.
  biliary s.
  enterococcal s.
  gram-negative s.
  gram-positive s.
  intraabdominal s. (IAS)
  pancreatic s.
  pelvic s.
  perianal s.
  post rubber band s.
  staphylococcal s.
  s. syndrome
Sepsis-Related Organ Failure Assessment (SOFA)
septa (*pl. of* septum)
septal hematoma
Septata intestinalis
septate vagina
septation
  cloaca s.
  internal s.
septectomy
septic
  s. cholangitis
  s. necrosis
  s. shock
  s. wound
septicemia
Septisol
Septopal
  S. bead
  S. implant
septotomy
  endoscopic transpancreatic
    ampullary s.
Septra DS
septula (*pl. of* septulum)
septulum, *pl.* **septula**
  s. testis
septum, *pl.* **septa**
  s. bulbi urethrae
  cloacal s.
  fibrous s.
  s. glandis
  interhaustral s.
  s. of glans penis
  s. of scrotum
  s. of testis
  pancreaticobiliary s.
  s. pectiniforme
  perforated nasal s.
  rectogenital s.
  rectovaginal s.
  rectovesical s.

  scrotal s.
  tracheoesophageal s.
  transverse vaginal s.
  urethrovaginal s.
  urorectal s.
sequela, *pl.* **sequelae**
  clinical s.
sequelae (*pl. of* sequela)
sequence
  adenoma-carcinoma s.
  adenomatous polyp-cancer s.
  contrast-enhanced fast s.
    (CE-FAST)
  cryptdin-related s. (CRS)
  dysplasia-to-carcinoma s.
  esophageal manometric s. (EMS)
  flanking s.
  genomic s.
  HASTE s.
  leucine zipper s.
  metaplasia-dysplasia-carcinoma s.
  NS5B protein coding s.
  papilloma-carcinoma s.
  phasic wave s.
  rapid acquisition fast spin-echo s.
  repeat s.
  turbo spin-echo s.
  ZIRTL s.
sequenced
  automatically s.
sequence-sequence oligonucleotide hybridization
sequencing
  s. analysis
  molecular cloning and s.
sequential
  s. counterstaining
  s. motility
  s. multiple analyzer (SMA)
  s. quadruple-drug regimen
  s. ultrafiltration hemodialysis
  s. videoconverter
sequestrant
  bile acid s.
sequestration
  fluid s.
Serenoa
  S. *repens*
  S. *repens* extract
Serentil
Sergent white adrenal line
serial
  s. cholangiograms
  s. dilution
series
  acute abdominal s. (AAS)
  barium GI s.
  gallbladder s. (GBS)
  Gastrografin GI s.

liver function s. (LFS)
upper GI s.
serine
    s. protease
    s. protease-activated prorenin
    s. threonine kinase gene 11
Seriola dumerili
seroconversion
    eAb s.
    s. rate
Serodia commercial kit
seroepidemiologic study
seroepidemiology
serologic
    s. diagnosis
    s. marker
    s. test
    s. test for syphilis (STS)
serology
    IgG s.
    specific anti-Hp s.
seromuscular
    s. colocystoplasty
    s. enterocystoplasty lined with
      urothelium (SELU)
    s. intestinal patch graft
    s. layer
    s. Lembert suture
seromyectomy
    duodenal s.
seromyotomy
    laparoscopic s.
seronegative polyarthritis
seropositive
seroprevalence rate
seroprotection
serosa
    cecal s.
    gastric s.
    perispermatitis s.
    tunica s.
serosal
    s. afferent innervation
    s. blood vessel
    s. creeping fat
    s. infiltration
    s. surface
    s. tear
serosanguineous
    s. drainage
    s. fluid
serositis
    uremic s.
serotonergic
    s. drug
    s. type 3 receptor
serotonin
    s. antagonist treatment
    s. cell

s. receptor antagonist
s. reuptake transporter
serum s.
s. stain
serotoninergic neuron
serous
    s. diarrhea
    s. membrane
Serpasil-Esidrix
serpiginosa
    elastosis perforans s.
serpiginous
    s. microcystic duct
    s. ulcer
    s. ulceration
Serpulina
    S. hyodysenteriae
    S. innocens
    S. pilosicoli
serrated adenoma
Serratia
    S. liquefaciens
    S. marcescens
serratum
    Lycopodium s.
serratus posterior muscle
serrefine clamp
Sertina
Sertoli
    S. cell
    S. cell secretory function
    S. cell tumor (SCT)
Sertoli-cell-only (SCO)
    S.-C.-O. syndrome
Sertoli-Leydig cell
sertraline serotonin reuptake inhibitor
serum
    s. albumin (SAB)
    s. alpha$_1$-protease inhibitor
    s. ammonia
    s. amylase
    s. amylase test
    s. amyloid A (SAA)
    s. amyloid P (SAP)
    s. amyloid P component
    s. bicarbonate
    s. bile acid measurement
    s. bilirubin
    s. bilirubin test
    s. blocking factor
    s. calcitonin
    s. calcium
    s. calcium concentration
    calibrator s.
    s. carotene
    s. ceruloplasmin
    s. chloride
    s. cholesterol
    s. cholinesterase activity

S

serum (*continued*)
   s. chromogranin A
   s. core protein
   s. creatinine (SCr)
   s. creatinine test
   s. cytokine analysis
   s. elastase 1
   s. eotaxin level
   s. ferritin
   s. ferritin concentration
   s. folate
   s. gamma-glutamyltransferase (SGGT)
   s. gastrin
   s. gastrin level
   s. glutamic-oxaloacetic transaminase (SGOT)
   s. glutamic-pyruvic transaminase (SGPT)
   s. haptoglobin
   s. hepatitis
   s. hyaluronic acid
   immune s.
   s. inducible factor A
   s. interleukin-2
   s. interleukin-6
   s. interleukin-8
   s. iron
   s. iron test
   s. kinase
   s. leptin level
   s. lipase
   s. marker
   s. metabolic evaluation
   s. nephritis
   s. noradrenaline
   s. osmolarity
   s. pepsinogen I/II ratio
   s. pepsinogen isoenzyme I, II
   s. PG
   s. phosphate
   s. phospholipid
   s. phosphorus
   s. protein electrophoresis (SPEP)
   s. protein test
   s. pyridinoline
   s. pyruvate kinase (SPK)
   s. RIBA-2 test
   s. sample
   s. serotonin
   s. sickness
   s. sicknesslike syndrome
   s. testosterone
   s. thrombotic accelerator
   s. transferrin
   s. triglyceride
   s. urate level
   s. urea nitrogen (SUN)
   s. uric acid
   s. virus antibody
serum-ascites albumin gradient (SAAG)
serum-free conditional medium
Serutan
servomechanism sphincter
sesame
SES-CD
   Simple Endoscopic Score for Crohn Disease
sesquioxide
   chromium s.
sessile
   s. adenoma
   s. lesion
   s. nodular carcinoma
   s. polyp
set
   Assura deluxe irrigation s.
   Assura economy irrigation s.
   Boehm rectal diagnostic and treatment s.
   Brunner ligature s.
   Coloplast ostomy irrigation s.
   Conseal ostomy irrigation s.
   cytocentrifuge s.
   Dansac ostomy irrigation s.
   dilating s.
   Eliminator nasobiliary catheter s.
   Freiburg biopsy s.
   French introducer s.
   Greene renal implant stent s.
   Heyer-Schulte Small-Carrion sizing s.
   introducer s.
   Jeffrey introducer s.
   KeyMed advanced esophageal dilator s.
   Lipshultz urology microsurgical s.
   mandril s.
   no-scalpel vasectomy instrument s.
   over-the-wire s.
   Rosch-Uchida transjugular liver access s.
   Sur-Fit Natura night drainage container s.
   Sur-Fit Natura Visi-Flow irrigation starter s.
   United Ostomy irrigation s.
   urology s.
Setguard antireflux valve
Sethotope radioactive agent
seton
   s. management
   Penrose s.
   silk s.
   s. treatment of high anal fistula
setophobia

set-point theory

sevelamer
    s. hydrochloride
    s. hydrochloride tablet

severance
    retroduodenal artery s.

severe
    s. acute respiratory syndrome coronavirus infection (SARS-CoV infection)
    s. aldosterone excess
    s. combined immunodeficiency (SCID)
    s. erosive esophagitis
    s. gastritis
    s. hematochezia
    s. macrovesicular steatosis
    s. morbid illness
    s. pain
    s. recurrent bladder neck contracture
    s. reflux esophagitis
    s. secretory diarrhea
    s. ureteral stricture
    s. variceal bleeding

severity
    Crohn Disease Endoscopic Index of S. (CDEIS)
    leakage s.
    S. of Dyspepsia Assessment (SODA)

sevoflurane

sex
    s. accessory tissue
    s. assignment by fetal ultrasonography
    s. cord-mesenchyme tumor
    s. cord tumors with annular tubules (SCTAT)
    s. hormone-binding globulin (SHBG)
    phenotypic s.
    s. reversal syndrome
    s. therapy

sextant
    s. technique
    s. transrectal ultrasound-guided biopsy

sexual
    s. abuse
    s. differentiation
    s. dysfunction androgyny
    s. evaluation
    s. function
    S. Function Index (SFI)
    S. Function Inventory Questionnaire (SFIQ)
    s. function score
    s. infantilism
    s. potency
    s. reflex
    s. rehabilitation
    s. stimulation testing

sexually
    s. related intestinal disease
    s. transmitted colitis
    s. transmitted disease (STD)
    s. transmitted disease contact tracing

Seyd-Neblett perineal template

SF
    sucrose-free
    Isomil SF

SF-9 baculovirus-insect cell system

SFI
    Sexual Function Index

SFIQ
    Sexual Function Inventory Questionnaire

SFU
    Society for Fetal Urology

Sgambati
    S. reaction test
    S. test for peritonitis

SGGT
    serum gamma-glutamyltransferase

SGOT
    serum glutamic-oxaloacetic transaminase
    SGOT test

SGP-2
    sulfated glycoprotein-2

SGPT
    serum glutamic-pyruvic transaminase
    SGPT test

shadow
    arc s.
    dumbbell-shaped s.
    obliteration of psoas s.
    psoas s.
    ring s.

shadowing
    hyperechoic s.

Shaeer augmentation phalloplasty

shaft
    Eder-Puestow dilator s.

shaggy tumor

shagreen patch

sham
    s. feeding
    s. feeding test
    s. injection
    s. surgery
    s. treatment

Shambaugh fistula hook

shape
    double-wing s.
    s. memory alloy stent

shaped
    olive s.

S

ShapeLock endoscopic guide
shape-locking
    s.-l. device
    s.-l. guide
sharing
    United Network for Organ S.
    (UNOS)
Shark disposable biopsy forceps
shark-fin papillotome
shark-tooth forceps
sharp
    s. dissection
    s. spoon
sharp-edged
    s.-e. orifice
    s.-e. tip
Sharpoint
    S. cutting instrument
    S. microsuture
shave biopsy
SHBG
    sex hormone-binding globulin
SH2-binding domain
SHC
    sclerosing hepatic carcinoma
SHE
    subclinical hepatic
    encephalopathy
shears
    Bethune s.
    harmonic scalpel coagulating s.
    LaparoSonic coagulating s.
    Lebsche s.
    UltraCision harmonic laparoscopic
    cutting s.
sheath
    Acucise access s.
    Amplatz s.
    anterior rectus s.
    fibrous s.
    Futura resectoscope s.
    miniaturized s.
    nephroscope s.
    overtube s.
    peel-away introducer s.
    perivascular s.
    posterior rectus s.
    quill s.
    rectus s.
    resectoscope s.
    retroflexed cystoscopy s.
    sport s. (SS)
    Teflon s.
    Universal s.
    ureterorenoscope procedure s.
    ureteroscope s.
    Waldeyer s.
    water-filled balloon s.
    working s.

sheathed
    s. cytology brush
    s. flexible sigmoidoscope
shedding
    virus s.
sheet
    Dacron-impregnated silastic s.
sheetlike adenoma
shelf, *pl.* **shelves**
    Blumer rectal s.
    mesocolic s.
    rectal s.
shell vial culture
shelves (*pl. of* shelf)
shelving edge of Poupart ligament
shepherd's
    s. hook catheter
    s. hook-shaped angiographic
    catheter
shield
    Active Living incontinence s.
    CapSure continence s.
    Exuderm odor s.
    Fuller rectal s.
    syringe s.
shift
    fluid s.
    mediastinal s.
shifting dullness
Shiga
    S. bacillus
    S. dysentery
    S. toxin (Stx)
    S. toxin-producing *Escherichia coli*
    (STEC)
shigae
    Shigella s.
Shiga-like toxin (SLT)
Shigella
    S. ambigua
    S. arabinotarda type A, B
    S. boydii
    S. colitis
    S. dysenteriae
    S. dysentery
    S. flexneri
    S. newcastle
    S. paradysenteriae
    S. schmitzii
    S. shigae
    S. sonnei
shigelloides
    Plesiomonas s.
shigellosis
shim
    step-up s.
Shimadzu RF-5301 PC spectrometer
Shiner tube
Shirodkar cervical cerclage

SHN
  subacute hepatic necrosis
shock
  extracorporeal s.
  hypovolemic s.
  s. liver
  s. number
  s. patient
  septic s.
  spinal s.
  s. wave (SW)
  s. wave-gas bubble interaction
  s. wave lithotripsy (SWL)
  s. wave lithotripsy cavitation
    component
  s. wave lithotripsy failure
  s. wave lithotriptor
  s. wave treatment
Shoemaker intestinal clamp
Shohl-Pedley method
Shohl solution
shooter
6-shooter
  Saeed 6-s.
  Wilson-Cook 6-s.
10-shooter
  Saeed 10-s.
  Wilson-Cook 10-s.
Shorr regimen
short
  s. band stenosis
  s. daily dialysis
  s. incubation hepatitis
  S. Inflammatory Bowel Disease
    Questionnaire (SIBDQ)
  s. urethra
short-bowel syndrome
short-chain fatty acid (SCFA)
short-dwell hypertonic exchange
shortened prep time
short-gut syndrome
short-lasting afterhyperpolarizing
  potential
short-segment
  s.-s. Barrett epithelium
  s.-s. Barrett esophagus (SSBE)
  s.-s. CLE
  s.-s. lesion
short-term
  s.-t. prostate-specific antigen
    recurrence
  s.-t. result
  s.-t. survival outcome
sho-saiko-to
1-shot
  1-s. intravenous urography
  1-s. IVU
shotty lymph nodes
shoulder girdle

Shouldice inguinal herniorrhaphy
shower
  uric acid s.
sHPT
  secondary hyperparathyroidism
shrapnel-induced
  s.-i. biliary obstruction
  s.-i. obstructive jaundice
shrunken liver
shunt
  Al-Ghorab modification s.
  Allen-Brown s.
  angiographic portacaval s.
  arterioportal venous s.
  arteriovenous s. (AVS)
  biliopancreatic s.
  Brescia-Cimino s.
  Buselmeier s.
  cavernosal-venous s.
  cavernospongiosum s.
  cavernosum-dorsal vein s.
  cavoatrial s.
  cerebral fluid s.
  chloride s.
  congenital portacaval s.
  Cordis-Hakim s.
  cystoperitoneal s.
  Denver peritoneovenous s.
  Denver pleuroperitoneal s.
  dialysis s.
  distal splenorenal s. (DSRS)
  Drapanas s.
  end-to-side portacaval s.
  esophageal s.
  extrahepatic s.
  gastric venacaval s.
  gastrorenal s.
  glans-cavernosal s.
  Gott s.
  Hashmat s.
  Hashmat-Waterhouse s.
  hepatofugal arterioportal s.
  hepatofugal portosystemic venous s.
  Hyde s.
  s. index via inferior mesenteric vein
  s. index via superior mesenteric
    vein
  intrahepatic artery-systemic s.
  jejunoileal s.
  Kasai peritoneal venous s.
  LeVeen ascites s.
  LeVeen peritoneal s.
  LeVeen peritoneovenous s.
  Linton s.
  mesocaval H-graft s.
  mesocaval interposition s.
  s. nephritis
  occluded s.
  pentose phosphate s.

S

shunt (*continued*)
    peritoneal-atrial s.
    peritoneocaval s.
    peritoneojugular s. (PJS)
    peritoneovenous s. (PVS)
    portacaval s. (PCS)
    portacaval H-graft s.
    portopulmonary s.
    portosystemic s.
    proximal splenorenal s.
    Quinton-Scribner s.
    radiologic portacaval s.
    Ramirez s.
    Scribner s.
    side-to-side s.
    small-bowel s.
    splenorenal bypass s.
    spontaneous portosystemic s. (SPSS)
    stenotic s.
    surgical portosystemic s.
    Thomas s.
    transhepatic portacaval s.
    transjugular intrahepatic
      portosystemic s. (TIPS, TIPSS)
    s. tubing
    ventriculoperitoneal s. (VPS)
    vesicoamniotic s.
    VP s.
    Warren splenorenal s.
    Winter s.
shunting
    arterioportal vein s.
    intrapulmonary s.
    portosystemic s. (PSS)
shuntlike pore
Shwachman-Diamond syndrome
Shwachman syndrome
Shy-Drager syndrome
SI
    saturation index
    serum iron
    SI of bile
SIADH
    syndrome of inappropriate secretion of
      antidiuretic hormone
sialic
    s. acid
    s. acid residue
sialidase
sialoadenectomy
sialoglycoprotein
sialomucin
    acidic s.
sialorrhea pancreatica
sialosyl-Tn antigen
sialyl
    s. Lewis A
    s. Lewis A antigen
    s. residue

sialylated
    s. derivative
    s. lacto-*N*-fucopentaose
sialylation
    cell-surface s.
sialyllactose
sialyl-Tn antigen
SIBDQ
    Short Inflammatory Bowel Disease
      Questionnaire
sibling
    HLA-identical s.
SIBO
    small-intestine bacterial
      overgrowth
sibutramine HCl
sicca
    cholera s.
    s. syndrome
sicchasia
sick
    s. cell syndrome
    s. euthyroid state
sickle
    s. cell anemia
    s. cell disease
    s. cell nephropathy
    s. hemoglobinopathy
sickling
    erythrocyte s.
sickness
    black s.
    Gambian sleeping s.
    s. impact profile
    Indian s.
    Jamaican morning s.
    Jamaican vomiting s.
    milk s.
    motion s.
    serum s.
SID
    sucrose-isomaltase
      deficiency
side
    s. branch
    high-lying s.
    host s.
    orad s.
side-effect profile
Side-Fire
    S.-F. laser
    S.-F. reflecting dish
sideroblast
    refractory anemia with ringed s.'s
      (RARS)
sideropenic dysphagia
siderotic
    s. nodule
    s. splenomegaly

side-to-side
- s.-t.-s. anastomosis
- s.-t.-s. isoperistaltic stricturotomy (SSIS)
- s.-t.-s. shunt

side-viewing
- s.-v. endoscope
- s.-v. fiberoptic duodenoscope
- s.-v. fiberscope
- s.-v. videoduodenoscope

sidewall
- pelvic s.

Siegel-Cohen dilating catheter
Siegel stent
Sielaff gastroscope
Siemens
- S. Endo-P endorectal transducer
- S. Lithostar
- S. Lithostar Plus System C lithotriptor
- S. MRI unit
- S. Somatom DRH CT analyzer
- S. Somatom DRH CT analyzer unit
- S. Sonoline ultrasonography

sieving
- s. coefficient (SC)
- dextran s.
- s. effect
- s. function
- Keller hydrodynamic hypothesis of s.
- s. of solid food

sIgA
- secretory IgA

sigma
- S. 34 monoplace hyperbaric chamber
- s. rectum pouch

sigmoid
- s. colon
- s. colon carcinoma
- s. colon conduit
- s. colon reservoir
- s. colon volvulus
- s. conduit
- s. curve
- s. cystoplasty
- s. disease
- s. diverticulitis
- s. diverticulum
- s. enterocystoplasty
- s. flexure
- s. fold
- s. kidney
- s. loop
- s. loop reduction
- s. neobladder
- s. pouch

- s. ulcer
- s. valve

sigmoideae
- arteriae s.

sigmoidectomy
- hand-assisted laparoscopic s.

sigmoid-end colostomy
sigmoideum
- colon s.

sigmoid-loop rod colostomy
sigmoidoanal intussusception
sigmoidocele
sigmoidocystoplasty
sigmoidopexy
- endoscopic s.

sigmoidoproctostomy
sigmoidorectostomy
sigmoidoscope, sigmoscope
- ACMI T-915, TX-915 fiberoptic s.
- adult s.
- American ACMI flexible fiberoptic s.
- Boehm s.
- Buie s.
- disposable-sheath flexible s.
- ESI fiberoptic s.
- fiberoptic s.
- flexible s.
- Fujinon ES-200ER s.
- Fujinon FS-100ER s.
- Fujinon PRO-PC flexible fiberoptic s.
- Fujinon SIG-E2 fiberoptic s.
- Fujinon SIG-EK-series flexible fiberoptic s.
- Fujinon SIG-E-series flexible fiberoptic s.
- Fujinon SIG-ET-series flexible fiberoptic s.
- Kelly s.
- Lieberman s.
- Lloyd-Davis s.
- Montague s.
- Olympus CF-L-series flexible s.
- Olympus CF-OSF-series flexible s.
- Olympus CF100S s.
- Olympus OSF flexible s.
- Reichert FLPS-series flexible fiberoptic s.
- Reichert MS-series flexible fiberoptic s.
- Reichert SC-series flexible fiberoptic s.
- rigid s.
- semirigid s.
- sheathed flexible s.
- Vernon-David s.
- Vision System s.
- Welch Allyn flexible s.

S

sigmoidoscopy
  fiberoptic s.
  flexible s.
  s. table
sigmoidostomy
sigmoidotomy
sigmoidovesical fistula
sigmoidovesicostomy
  transverse retubularized s.
sigmoid-rectum pouch
sigmoscope (*var. of* sigmoidoscope)
sign
  Aaron s.
  accordion s.
  arrowhead s.
  auscultatory s.
  Ballance s.
  barber pole s.
  Battle s.
  beading s.
  Bergman s.
  Blatin s.
  blue dot s.
  Blumberg s.
  Boas s.
  bowler hat s.
  Boyce s.
  Brodie s.
  burning drops s.
  Carman s.
  Carman-Kirklin meniscus s.
  Carnett s.
  catheter coiling s.
  chain-of-lakes s.
  Chilaiditi s.
  Christmas tree s.
  Clark s.
  Claybrook s.
  closed eyes s.
  cobblestoning s.
  cobra-head s.
  coiled spring s.
  Cole s.
  colon cutoff s.
  colon single-stripe s.
  comblike redness s.
  comet s.
  Cope s.
  Courvoisier s.
  Cowen s.
  Cruveilhier s.
  Cruveilhier-Baumgarten s.
  cushion s.
  Dance s.
  Dew s.
  double bubble duodenal s.
  double duct s.
  double halo s.
  drooping lily s.

E s.
Earle s.
echo s.
Federici s.
flapping tremor s.
flush-tank s.
Fothergill s.
Fournier s.
Fraley s.
Frostberg reversed-3 s.
Gilbert s.
Gottron s.
Gowers s.
Grey Turner s.
Grocco s.
guarding s.
Guyon s.
Hampton s.
Haudek s.
heliotrope s.
Henning s.
histologic s.
Horn s.
Howship-Romberg s.
iliopsoas s.
inverted-V s.
Kantor string s.
Kehr s.
Kelly s.
Klemm s.
Lennhoff s.
lifting s.
ligature s.
4-lines s.
liver flap s.
Lloyd s.
lollipop tree s.
McBurney s.
McCormack gastric mucosal s.
McCort s.
Meltzer s.
meniscus s.
Mercedes Benz s.
Mexican hat s.
milk of calcium s.
moulage s.
multiple concentric rings s.
Murphy s.
Naclerio s.
naked fat s.
niche s.
obturator s.
s. of rising tide
peritoneal s.
Pfuhl s.
pillow s.
Pitres s.
Poppel s.
Prehn s.

pruning s.
pseudocholangiocarcinoma s.
pseudoparallel channel s.
psoas s.
puddle s.
pyloric string s.
rat-tail s.
rebound s.
red color s. (RCS)
red flag s.
red ring s.
reversed Mercedes Benz s.
Rigler s.
rim s.
Robertson s.
Roche s.
Rommelaere s.
Rosenbach s.
Rovighi s.
Rovsing s.
Russell s.
sawtooth appearance s.
scarf-ring s.
Sister Mary Joseph s.
snow-white duodenum s.
Stierlin s.
Stransky s.
Strauss s.
string s.
string-of-beads s.
string-of-pearls s.
Sumner s.
tail s.
tenting s.
Terry fingernail s.
tethered-bowel s.
Thornton s.
thread-and-streaks s.
thumbprinting s.
tissue rim s.
Toma s.
Trimadeau s.
Troisier s.
Turner s.
ureterocele drooping lily s.
vital s.'s
white ball s.
white nipple s.

Signa
S. Dress hydrocolloid dressing
S. Excite MRI system

signal
adenosine s.
adrenergic s.
beta-actin mRNA s.
s. peptide peptidase (SPP)
sodium s.
s. transducer and activator of
transcription 1 (Stat1)

s. transduction pathway
s. transduction process
transmembrane s.
weaker immunofluorescence s.

signaling
s. cascade
immune s.

signal-to-cutoff ratio

signet-ring
s.-r. cell
s.-r. cell carcinoma
s.-r. pattern of gastric carcinoma

significance
atypical glandular cells of unknown
s. (AGUS)
atypical squamous cells of
undetermined s. (ASCUS)
monoclonal gammopathy of
undetermined s. (MGUS)
prognostic s.
visible vessel s.

significant
s. clinical history
s. correlation
s. hydronephrosis
s. liver lesion
s. parameter estimate
s. reported complication
statistically s.

SIHC
surgically implanted hemodialysis
catheter

Silain-Gel

silastic
s. catheter
s. collar-reinforced stoma
s. indwelling ureteral stent
s. ring
s. ring vertical gastroplasty
s. silo reduction of gastroschisis
s. sling

Silber
S. testicular autotransplantation
technique
S. vasoepididymostomy

sildenafil
s. citrate
s. plus Doppler ultrasonography

silent
s. abdomen
s. aspiration
s. autonephrectomy
s. belch
s. gallstone
s. lupus nephritis
s. prostatism
s. stone
s. thrombosis
s. ulcer

S

silicate
- s. calculus
- s. urolithiasis

silicone
- s. balloon
- s. donut prosthesis
- s. elastomer band
- s. elastomer ring
- s. elastomer ring vertical gastroplasty (SRVG)
- s. microimplant
- particulate s.
- s. polymer
- s. pressure sensor device
- s. rubber Dacron cuffed catheter
- s. self-expanding prosthesis
- s. sizer

silicone-based oil
silicone-coated metallic self-expanding stent
silicone-covered self-expanding polyester stent
Silipos
- S. arthritic/diabetic gel sock
- S. soft-walk gel sock

Silitek Uropass stent
silk
- S. Bullet feeding tube
- s. jejunal tube
- s. ligature
- s. Mersilene suture
- S. Pill feeding tube
- s. pop-off suture
- s. seton
- S. Tip feeding tube
- s. traction suture

silodosin
Silon tent
silver
- s. catheter
- s. cell
- s. clip
- s. nephropathy
- s. nitrate
- s. probe
- s. stain
- s. stool

silver-coated stent
Silverman-Boeker needle
Silverman needle
Silybum marianum
Silymarin
SIM
- small-intestine mesentery
- SIM 2 catheter

Simaal Gel 2

simethicone
- aluminum hydroxide, magnesium hydroxide, and s.
- calcium carbonate and s.

simian
- s. strain
- s. virus 40 (SV40)

Similac PM 60/40 low-iron formula
similar psychometric properties
Simmons catheter
Simplastic catheter
simple
- s. cold storage preservation
- s. cystectomy
- S. Endoscopic Score for Crohn Disease (SES-CD)
- s. enterocele
- s. hydrocele
- s. mechanical obstruction
- s. nephrectomy
- s. renal cyst
- S. Soaps bland soap

simplex
- *Anisakis* s.
- exulceratio s.
- herpes s.
- herpesvirus s. (HVS)

simplified nocturnal home hemodialysis (SNHHD)
Simpson endoscope
Sims
- S. anoscope
- S. position
- S. rectal speculum

simulation skill
simulator
- flexible bronchoscopy s.
- heartbeating s.
- inanimate s.
- surgical s.
- validity of surgical s.
- virtual reality s.

Simulect
simultaneous
- s. bilateral extracorporeal shock waves
- s. bilateral percutaneous nephrolithotomies (SBPN)
- s. hemodialysis and hemofiltration
- s. Malone antegrade continent enema and Mitrofanoff procedures
- s. Malone antegrade continent enema and Mitrofanoff procedure using divided appendix
- s. pancreas and kidney transplant
- s. urethral cystometries

simvastatin
sincalide
Sinemet

sinensis
> *Clonorchis s.*
> *Opisthorchis s.*

Sinequan
Singer-Blom endoscopic tracheoesophageal puncture technique
single
> s. beta-actin mRNA species
> s. gamma wrap
> s. lumen
> s. midline calyceal infundibulum
> s. nucleotide polymorphism
> s. potential analysis of cavernous electrical activity
> s. stapling

single-action pumping system
single-cell keratinization
single-channel
> s.-c. colonoscope
> s.-c. in vivo light dosimeter
> s.-c. wire-guided sphincterotome

single-color direct immunofluorescence study
single-contrast
> s.-c. barium enema (SCBE)
> s.-c. radiography

single-dose
> s.-d. IV Timentin
> s.-d. packet

single-drug therapy
single-fiber
> s.-f. confocal microscopy
> s.-f. needle electromyography

single-layer continuous intestinal anastomosis
single-lens reflex camera
single-loop tourniquet
single-lumen Broviac silicone catheter
single-nephron
> s.-n. GFR
> s.-n. glomerular filtration rate (SNGFR)
> s.-n. glomerular transport

single-parameter
> s.-p. DNA
> s.-p. DNA analysis

single-pass
> s.-p. albumin dialysis (SPAD)
> s.-p. hemodialysis

single-pedicle
> gastric augment and s.-p. (GASP)

single-photon
> s.-p. emission computed tomography (SPECT)
> s.-p. emission computerized tomography (SPECT)

single-pigtail stent
single-puncture laparoscopy
single-shot voxel projection

single-stage total proctocolectomy
single-strand conformation polymorphism analysis
single-stripe colitis (SSC)
single-system ureterocele
single-use maximum-capacity radial jaw with needle
Singley
> S. intestinal forceps
> S. intestinal ring clamp

Singular Oval polypectomy snare
singultation
singultus, *pl.* **singultus**
sinister
> ductus hepaticus s.
> ductus lobi caudati s.

sinistra
> arteria gastrica s.
> arteria gastroomentalis s.
> flexura coli s.

sinistral portal hypertension
sink-trap malformation
sinoaortic
> s. baroreceptor
> s. denervation (SAD)

sinogram
sinus
> anal s.
> s. anales
> coronary s.
> draining s.
> s. excision
> Forssell s.
> perineal s.
> pilonidal s.
> piriform s.
> pleuroperitoneal s.
> prostatic s.
> rectal s.
> renal s.
> Rokitansky-Aschoff s.
> splenic s.
> subpubic s.
> s. tenderness
> s. tract
> urachal s.
> urogenital s.

sinusoid
> corporeal s.
> erectile s.
> hepatic s.
> liver s.

sinusoidal
> s. capillary pressure
> s. endothelial cell (SEC)
> s. endothelium
> s. endothelium cornucopia
> s. fibrosis
> s. lining cell

S

sinusoidal (*continued*)
    s. lymphocyte
    s. obstruction syndrome (SOS)
    s. wall
siphonage
Sipple syndrome
Sippy
    S. diet
    S. esophageal dilator
sipuleucel-T
Siroky
    S. nomogram
    S. nomogram for uroflowmetry
sirolimus
    s. monotherapy
    s. oral solution
    s. tablet
SIRS
    systemic inflammatory response syndrome
SIR-Spheres
Sister
    S. Mary Joseph lymph node
    S. Mary Joseph nodule
    S. Mary Joseph sign
site
    bleeding s.
    crypt-villus s.
    endoscopic biopsy s.
    entry s.
    estrogen binding s. (EBS)
    exit s.
    genomic s.
    injection s.
    internal ribosome entry s.
    s. specificity
    stoma s.
    vascular access s.
sitophobia
sitosterolemia
    beta s.
situ
    adenocarcinoma in s.
    bladder carcinoma in s.
    carcinoma in s. (CIS)
    in s.
    squamous cell carcinoma in s.
situation
    radiographic s.
situs
    s. inversus
    s. inversus viscerum
    s. perversus
sitz bath
Sitzmarks
    S. radiopaque marker in gelatin capsule
    S. test

Siurala gastritis classification
size
    inoculum s.
    kidney s.
    large needle s.
    normal penile s.
    spot s.
    uterine s.
sizer
    silicone s.
Sjögren syndrome
Sjöqvist method
skatole
Skelaxin
skeletal
    s. muscle disease
    s. radiography
skeletonize
Skene
    S. duct
    S. gland
skill
    minimal-access surgical s.
    simulation s.
skin
    anicteric s.
    s. atrophy
    s. bleeding time (SBT)
    s. crease
    s. dimpling
    s. disease
    dry s.
    s. graft
    s. graft imbibition phase
    s. graft inoculation phase
    s. graft neovagina
    icteric s.
    s. inlay urethroplasty
    jaundiced s.
    s. knife
    s. line
    nonicteric s.
    ostomy s.
    s. perfusion
    peristomal s.
    s. staple
    s. stapling
    s. sympathetic response
    s. tag
    s. tube
    s. turgor
    s. xanthoma
skin-CNS-bladder reflex
skinfold
    thickness of s.
    s. thickness test
skinny Chiba needle
skinny-needle biopsy

skip
    s. appendicitis
    s. area
    s. lesion
ski position
skirret
Skirrow
    S. agar plate
    S. medium
skirrowii
    Arcobacter s.
skullcap
SLA
    soluble liver antigen
slash pyelotomy
SLE
    systemic lupus erythematosus
SLED
    slow low-efficiency dialysis
    sustained low-efficiency dialysis
sleep enuresis
sleeve
    s. advancement
    Assura irrigation s.
    Bard irrigation s.
    Coloplast transparent irrigation s.
    ileal s.
    laparoscopic trocar s.
    Pneumo S.
    s. sensor
    Sur-Fit Natura irrigation s.
    s. technique
    Watzki s.
    Williams overtube s.
sleeve-type circumcision
slice
    coronal s.
slide
    gelatin-subbed s.
    guaiac-impregnated s.
    Hemoccult Sensa s.
    poly-l-lysine-coated glass s.
    s. system
slide-by view
sliding
    s. esophageal hiatal hernia
    s. filament model of contraction
    s. tube
SlimSIGHT gastrointestinal videoscope
sling
    AdVance male s.
    Advantage midurethral s.
    anterior vaginal wall s. (AVWS)
    autologous rectus fascia s.
    BioSling bioabsorbable urethral s.
    Brigham s.
    Burch-Cooper ligament s.
    buried vaginal wall s.
    Cooper ligament s.

    s. failure
    fascia lata suburethral s.
    FortaPerm surgical s.
    intestinal s.
    I-Stop midurethral s.
    Lynx midurethral s.
    lyophilized dura mater for pubovaginal s.
    Martius fascial s.
    Mersilene for pubovaginal s.
    midurethral s.
    Monarc urethral s.
    s. operation
    porcine dermis for pubovaginal s.
    s. procedure
    puboprostatic s.
    puborectalis s.
    pubourethral s.
    pubovaginal autologous fascial s.
    Raz anterior vaginal wall s.
    Raz 4-corner vaginal wall s.
    rectus fascia s.
    silastic s.
    Stratasis urethral s.
    suburethral s.
    Suspend s.
    triangular vaginal patch s.
    Vesica s.
sling-and-blanket technique
sling/mesh
    Surgisis s./m.
sling-ring complex
Slip-Coat tip
slippage
slipped
    s. fundoplication wrap
    s. Nissen fundoplication
    s. Nissen repair
slipper-tipped guidewire
slit
    Cheatle s.
    s. diaphragm
    dorsal s.
    s. lamp
    s. pore length density
SLM-8000 fluorescence spectrophotometer
Slo-bid
slotted
    s. anoscope
    s. instrument
    s. nerve clamp
    s. speculum
sloughed
    s. papilla
    s. urethra syndrome
sloughing of mucosa
slow
    s. bilirubin glucuronidation phenotype

slow (*continued*)
    s. colonic transit
    s. continuous ultrafiltration
      (SCUF)
    S. Fe
    s. low-efficiency dialysis (SLED)
    s. phasic contraction
    s. wave
Slow-K
slow-transit constipation (STC)
slow-twitch
    s.-t. oxidative
    s.-t. striated muscle fiber
slow-wave coupling
SLT
    Shiga-like toxin
    SLT contact MTRL laser
    SLT 7 laser fiber
sludge
    biliary s.
    gallbladder s.
slurry of stool
slush
    ice s.
    saline s.
SMA
    sequential multiple analyzer
    smooth muscle antibody
    superior mesenteric artery
      Doppler sonography of SMA
      SMA formula
      SMA spiral stent
small
    s. bowel (SB)
    s. dissecting sponge
    s. granule cell
    s. inflammatory polyp
    s. interfering ribonucleic acid
    s. intestine
    s. noncleaved-cell lymphoma
    s. polyp removal
    s. pseudocyst
    s. solitary renal calculus
    s. stomach syndrome
small-bowel
    s.-b. anastomosis
    s.-b. biopsy
    s.-b. continuity
    s.-b. enema
    s.-b. enteroclysis
    s.-b. enteroscopy (SBE)
    s.-b. erosion
    s.-b. followthrough (SBFT)
    s.-b. infarct
    s.-b. meal
    s.-b. obstruction (SBO)
    s.-b. shunt
    s.-b. thickening
    s.-b. transit time

    s.-b. transplantation
    s.-b. tube
small-caliber
    s.-c. duodenovideoscope
    s.-c. esophagogastroduodenoscopy
    s.-c. variable-stiffness colonoscope
Small-Carrion penile prosthesis
small-cell tumor
small-diameter endosonographic instrument
small-droplet fatty liver
small-duct primary sclerosing cholangitis
smaller gauge needle
SmallHand polypectomy snare
small-intestinal
    s.-i. Crohn disease
    s.-i. enterocyte
    s.-i. infarction
    s.-i. malignant lymphoma
    s.-i. membrane
    s.-i. stenosis
    s.-i. submucosa
    s.-i. ulcer
    s.-i. villus
small-intestine
    s.-i. bacterial overgrowth (SIBO)
    s.-i. leiomyosarcoma
    s.-i. mesentery (SIM)
    s.-i. trauma
SMA-portogram
SMART
    sperm microaspiration retrieval
      technique
    SMART anti-CD3
SmartCath esophageal balloon catheter
Smead-Jones closure
smear
    buccal s.
    duodenal s.
    KOH s.
    low-grade positive s.
    Papanicolaou s.
    potassium hydroxide s.
smegma praeputii
smegmatis
    Mycobacterium s.
SM-HCV Rapid test
smiley-face knotting technique
smiling incision
Smith
    S. electrode
    S. method of silver staining
    S. rectal retractor
    S. ring
    S. test
Smith-Boyce operation
Smith-Buie rectal retractor
Smith-Hodge pessary

smithii
    Methanobrevibacter s.
Smith-Lemli-Opitz syndrome
smoker's
    s. palate
    s. tongue
SmokEvac
smooth
    s. diet
    s. muscle
    s. muscle antibody (SMA)
    s. muscle immunologic study
    s. muscle isoform actin
    s. muscle motilin receptor
    s. muscle relaxant
    s. tissue forceps
    s. urethral sphincter
SMV
    superior mesenteric vein
    SMV thrombosis
SMX
    sulfamethoxazole
SMX-TMP, SMX/TMP
    sulfamethoxazole and trimethoprim
snail-headed catheter retriever
snakeskin mucosal pattern
**snake venom-converting enzyme-inhibiting
  action**
snap
    s. gauge
    s. gauge band
    s. gauge test
snap-frozen biopsy
Snap-Gauge
Snap-It lubricating jelly
snare
    barbed s.
    Captiflex polypectomy s.
    Captivator polypectomy s.
    s. cautery
    coaxial s.
    colorectal s.
    crescent s.
    diathermal s.
    Douglas rectal s.
    s. electrocoagulation
    electrosurgical s.
    endoscopic s.
    s. excision biopsy
    Frankfeldt rectal s.
    hexagon s.
    incarcerated s.
    lasso s.
    long-nosed retriever s.
    s. loop biopsy
    Nakao s. I, II
    Norwood rectal s.
    Olympus SD-5L semicircular s.
    open electrocautery s.

    oval s.
    s. polypectomy
    polypectomy s.
    Profile pediatric polypectomy s.
    rectal s.
    s. resection
    Rotator polypectomy s.
    Sensation Short Throw s.
    Singular Oval polypectomy s.
    SmallHand polypectomy s.
    standard endoscopic polypectomy s.
    UroSnare cystoscopic tumor s.
    Weston rectal s.
    wire s.
sneezewort
SNGFR
    single-nephron glomerular filtration rate
SNHHD
    simplified nocturnal home hemodialysis
Sn-mesoporphyrin
Snodgrass
    S. incised plate urethroplasty
    S. technique
Snowden-Pencer scissors
Snow procedure
snowstorm effect
snow-white duodenum sign
Sn-protoporphyrin
SNS
    sacral nerve stimulation
    SNS therapy
Snyder drain
soak
    perianal s.
soap
    Simple Soaps bland s.
soap-bubble nephrogram
soapsuds enema (SSE)
soap-sudsy appearance
soapy kidney
soar-crash effect
Soave
    S. abdominal pullthrough procedure
    S. endorectal pullthrough
    S. operation
Sober loop ureterostomy
sobria
    Aeromonas s.
society
    S. for Fetal Urology (SFU)
    International Continence S. (ICS)
    S. of American Gastrointestinal and
      Endoscopic Surgeons (SAGES)
sock
    polytetrafluoroethylene s.
    Silipos arthritic/diabetic gel s.
    Silipos soft-walk gel s.
SODA
    Severity of Dyspepsia Assessment

S

sodium

s. acid urate
acyclovir s.
s. anion diarrhea
s. azide
s. balance
s. bicarbonate
brequinar s.
butabarbital s.
Butisol S.
s. butyrate concentration
cefazolin s.
ceftriaxone s.
s. cellulose phosphate
cephapirin s.
s. channelopathy
s. chloride
s. citrate
s. citrate and potassium citrate
  mixture
s. cromoglycate
cromolyn s.
dalteparin s.
dantrolene s.
s. deficiency
s. deoxycholate
diclofenac s.
dietary s.
docusate s.
s. dodecyl sulfate (SDS)
s. dodecyl sulfate-polyacrylamide gel
  electrophoresis (SDS-PAGE)
Ecabet S.
s. electrolyte
enoxaparin s.
s. entry route
epoprostenol s.
ertapenem s.
estramustine phosphate s.
s. exchange
s. fluorescein (NaF)
s. flux
fractional excretion of s. (FENa)
s. homeostasis
s. hyaluronate
s. hyaluronate injection
s. iodipamide
s. iodipamide contrast medium
s. iothalamate
latamoxef s.
low s.
luminal s.
s. meclofenamate
s. meclofenamate-induced esophageal
  ulcer
mesalamine s.
s. methylglucamine diatrizoate
s. morrhuate
s. morrhuate injection

naproxen s.
s. nitroprusside
olsalazine s.
oxychlorosene s.
pantoprazole s.
s. pentosan polysulfate
pentosan polysulfate s.
peritubular s.
s. phosphate
s. phosphate-based laxative
s. phosphate dibasic anhydrous
s. phosphate monobasic monohydrate
s. picosulfate
s. picosulphate and magnesium
  citrate
piperacillin s.
s. polystyrene sulfonate
porfimer s.
s. pump
rabeprazole s.
s. reabsorption
renal s.
s. restriction
s. retention
s. signal
sterile ceftriaxone s.
sulbactam s.
s. taurocholate
s. tauroglycocholate
s. tetradecyl injection
s. tetradecyl sulfate
s. tetradecyl sulfate sclerosant
s. thiosulfate solution spray
s. transport
tyropanoate s.
Urovist S. 300
s. valproate
sodium-linked process
**sodium-lithium countertransporter
(SLC)**
sodium-loading test
sodium-wasting nephropathy
Soehendra
S. catheter dilator
S. catheter system
S. graduated dilating catheter
S. stent extractor
S. stent retrieval device
S. stent retriever
SOFA
Sepsis-Related Organ Failure
Assessment
SOFA score
**SofPulse noninvasive pulsed
electromagnetic therapy device**
soft
s. abdomen
s. balloon method for endoscopic
  ultrasound

s. bland diet
s. diverticuloscope
s. food dysphagia
S. Guard XL skin barrier
Modane S.
s. rubber string
s. stool
s. tissue
s. tissue mass
s. tissue stranding
s. x-ray film

softener
stool s.

SofTouch vacuum erection device
Softpatch
Impress S.

soft-tipped wire guide
software
Cytologic s.
SPOT mobile 3D ultrasound system
and s.
t-EASE s.
Un-Graph computer s.

soilage
peritoneal s.

soiling
colostomy s.
fecal s.

solani
Fusarium s.

solar fever
Solcia gastric dysplasia classification
solder
laser tissue-welding s.
protein s.

solid
s. and cystic tumors of pancreas
(SCTP)
s. bolus challenge
s. egg-white meal
s. emptying
s. evidence
s. food
s. food digestion
s. food dysphagia
s. sphere test
s. teratoma
s. tumor

solid-column esophagram
solid-phase
s.-p. extraction chromatography
s.-p. radioimmunoassay

solid-state
s.-s. esophageal manometry catheter
s.-s. pressure transducer

solifenacin
solitaire
cholesterol s.

solitarii (*pl. of* solitarius)

solitarius, *pl.* **solitarii**
folliculi lymphatici solitarii
nucleus s.
nucleus tractus s. (NTS)
nucleus tractus solitarii (NTS)

solitary
s. diverticulum
s. hepatic cyst
s. kidney
s. lower pole calculus
s. rectal ulcer syndrome
s. testis

solium
Taenia s.

SoloPass Percuflex biliary stent
SOLOS endoscopy clip-applying forceps
SOLO-Surg Colorectal self-retaining
retractor system
solubility
solubilization
micellar s.

solubilize
solubilized
s. HLA
s. human leukocyte antigen

Solu-Biloptin contrast medium
soluble
s. CD44 binding
s. egg antigen (SEA)
s. Fas (sFas)
s. liver antigen (SLA)
s. recombinant complement receptor
1
s. transferrin receptor (sTf-R)

Solu-Medrol
pulsed S.-M.

solute
s. diuresis
s. equilibrium
s. removal index
s. transport

solution
Adcon-P adhesion barrier s.
AIO parenteral s.
Albright s.
amino acid-based dialysate s.
Aminofusin L Forte amino acid s.
BA-EDTA s.
balanced electrolyte s.
balanced salt s. (BSS)
Balance lavage s.
barium sulfate s.
Belzer UW liver preservation s.
betaine anhydrous s.
bile acid-EDTA s.
Block-Ace s.
Bouin fixative s.
Bretschneider histidine tryptophan s.
buffer s.

S

solution (*continued*)
Burrow s.
Cidex activated dialdehyde s.
Cidex Plus s.
Collins indigo carmine s.
Collins intracellular electrolyte s.
colloid s.
colonic lavage s.
commercial dialysis s. (CDS)
crystalloid s.
Delflex peritoneal dialysis s.
Denhardt s.
diphosphate buffer s.
Domeboro s.
Earle s.
electrolyte flush s.
electrolyte lavage s.
electrolyte-polyethylene glycol lavage s.
Euro-Collins s.
Extraneal 7.5% peritoneal dialysis s.
ferumoxides injectable s.
formaldehyde s.
FreAmine amino acid s.
Gastrolyte oral s.
gluten s.
GoLYTELY s.
grit-free s.
Hank balanced salt s. (HBSS)
Hank buffer s.
Hartmann s.
HepatAmine amino acid s.
HEPES s.
Hibidil s.
Hollande s.
HSE s.
s. hybridization RNAse protection assay
hypertonic saline-epinephrine s.
iced lactated Ringer s.
icodextrin 7.5% peritoneal dialysis s.
Intergel adhesion prevention s.
Intergel irrigating s.
inulin s.
Krebs s.
Krebs-Ringer s.
Kristalose for oral s.
lactated Ringer s. (LRS)
lactulose s.
lavage s.
Liposyn II fat emulsion s.
LoSo Prep bowel cleansing s.
Lugol iodine s.
Lytren electrolyte s.
Mayer hematoxylin s.
Mefoxin-saline s.
Mitrofanoff s.
mucolytic-antifoam s.

normal saline s.
NTZ Long-Acting nasal s.
NutraPrep bowel cleansing s.
oral rehydration s. (ORS)
Pedialyte RS electrolyte s.
PEG-3500 s.
perfusate s.
phosphate-buffered saline s.
physiologic pH s.
physiologic salt s. (PSS)
podofilox s.
polyethylene glycol electrolyte lavage s. (PEG-ELS)
probenecid-containing s.
Rapamune oral s.
rehydrating s. (RS)
Resol electrolyte s.
Saccomanno s.
Sachs s.
Salivart s.
Salvanios pH 10 disinfectant s.
sclerosant s.
sclerosant-contrast s.
sclerosing s.
Shohl s.
sirolimus oral s.
Soyalac fat emulsion s.
Sporox disinfectant s.
Suby G s.
Synthamin amino acid s.
taurocholate s.
Tolerex feeding s.
Travamulsion fat emulsion s.
University of Wisconsin s.
UW s.
Vamin amino acid s.
warm saline s.
whole-gut lavage s.
Wisconsin s.
Y-type Dianeal peritoneal dialysis s.
solution-diluted India ink
Solutrast 300 contrast
Soluvite
solvent
s. drag
s. infusion
Nu-Hope cleaning s.
stone s.
solvent-dehydrated cadaveric fascia lata
Soma
somatic
s. allelic deletion
s. growth
s. nociceptive flexion reflex
s. pain
s. peripheral nerve
s. teniasis
somatization
somatointestinal reflex

somatomedin C
Somatome DRG CT technique
somatostatin
>s. analogue
>s. analogue octreotide
>s. analogue therapy
>antral s.
>s. cell
>s. infusion therapy
>s. mRNA-D-cell density ratio
>s. mRNA level
>s. peptide
>s. prevention
>s. receptor
>s. receptor scintigraphy (SRS)
>s. secretagogue
>s. stain

somatostatin-14, -28
somatostatinoma syndrome
somatotropin release-inhibiting factor (SRIF)
somatropin injection
somite
>müllerian duct, unilateral renal agenesis, and anomalies of cervicothoracic s.'s (MURCS)

Somogyi unit
Sonablate
>S. 200 system
>S. 500 ultrasound

Sonazoid
Sonde
>S. enteroscope
>S. enteroscopy

Song stent
sonicated albumin
Sonicath endoluminal ultrasound catheter
Sonne-Duval bacillus
Sonne dysentery
sonnei
>*Shigella s.*

Sonnenberg
>S. classification

Sonoblate ablation device
Sonocath ultrasound probe
sonoelasticity imaging
sonoelastrography
sonogram
>fatty meal s. (FMS)
>transverse s.

sonographic
>s. gallstone pattern
>s. layer

sonography
>amplitude-coded color Doppler s.
>catheter s.
>colonic transabdominal s. (CTAS)
>color-coded Doppler s.
>color-coded duplex s.

>3D s.
>duplex s.
>endoureteral ultrasound s.
>gray-scale s.
>high-frequency ultrasound probe s. (HFUPS)
>high-resolution endoluminal s. (HRES)
>intraaortic endovascular s.
>renal s.
>transabdominal hydrocolonic s.
>transrectal s.

sonography-guided aspiration
sonoguided biopsy
Sonoline SI-200/250 ultrasound imaging system
Sonolith
>S. Praktis
>S. Praktis portable lithotriptor

Sonoprobe endoscopic ultrasonography system
Sonotrode
>S. channel
>S. lithotriptor

sonourethrography
Sony Promavica still capture device
sorafenib tosylate
sorbent
>s. dialysate regeneration system
>s. hemodialysis

sorbitol
>s. dehydrogenase (SDH)
>s. diarrhea
>s. enema

sorbitol-MacConkey
>s.-M. agar
>s.-M. medium

sore
>canker s.
>pressure s.
>venereal s.

Soreson pressure transducer
sorter
>fluorescence-activated cell s. (FACS)

SOS
>Surgitek One-Step

sotalol
soterenol
Sotradecol sclerosant
souffle
>splenic s.

sound
>absent bowel s.'s
>active bowel s.'s
>apical s.
>auscultation of bowel .'s
>auscultatory s.
>Béniqúe s.
>breath s.'s

S

sound (*continued*)
    bronchial s.
    Campbell s.
    common duct s.
    crescendoing bowel s.'s
    Davis interlocking s.
    diminished bowel s.'s
    Dittel s.
    esophageal s.
    extra heart s.
    Goodwin s.
    Greenwald s.
    gurgling bowel s.'s
    Guyon s.
    high-pitched bowel s.'s
    hyperactive bowel s.'s
    hypoactive bowel s.'s
    Jewett s.
    Klebanoff common duct s.
    Le Fort s.
    low-pitched bowel s.'s
    McCrea s.
    metal s.
    musical bowel s.'s
    normoactive bowel s.'s
    (NABS)
    Otis s.
    positive bowel s.'s
    quiet bowel s.'s
    rumbling bowel s.'s
    scarce bowel s.'s
    succussion s.
    tinkling bowel s.'s
    van Buren s.
    Walther s.

sour
    s. brash
    s. stomach

source
    discrete bleeding s.
    endoscopic light s.
    s. of recurrence
    Olympus CLV10 fiberscope
      light s.
    Olympus CLV-U 20 endoscopic
      halogen light s.
    xenon light s.

South American trypanosomiasis
Southern
    S. blot
    S. blot analysis
    S. blot hybridization
    S. tsangshu
Souttar tube
soya-induced enteropathy
Soyalac
    S. fat emulsion
      solution
    S. formula

soy-based formula
soy protein sensitivity
SPA
    sperm penetration assay
space
    anorectal s.
    Bogros s.
    Bowman s.
    Courtney s.
    dead s.
    deep perineal s.
    deep postanal anorectal s.
    epidural s.
    extravascular s.
    intercellular s.
    intercostal s.
    intermediate s.
    intersphincteric anorectal s.
    ischiorectal anorectal s.
    Kiernan s.
    lateral fossa of preputial s.
    Lesgaft s.
    s. of Disse
    s. of Mall
    s. of Retzius
    perianal anorectal s.
    periglomerular s.
    perisinusoidal s.
    peritoneal s.
    preperitoneal s.
    presacral s.
    retroperitoneal s.
    retropubic s.
    retrorectal s.
    Retzius s.
    right anterior pararenal s.
    S. Saver volumetric pump
    subarachnoid s.
    subhepatic s.
    subperitoneal s.
    subphrenic s.
    subumbilical s.
    superficial perineal s.
    suprahepatic s.
    supralevator anorectal s.
    supraomental s.
    Traube semilunar s.
    vesicovaginal s.
3-space dissection
Spacemaker balloon dissector
space-occupying
    s.-o. disease
    s.-o. lesion
Space-OR flexible internal
  retractor
spacing
    third s.
SPAD
    single-pass albumin dialysis

span
>hepatic s.
>levator s.
>liver s.

Spanish chestnut

spansule

SPARC
>suprapubic approach to suburethral polypropylene
>SPARC sling system

sparfloxacin

sparing
>rectal s.

spark-gap shock wave generator

sparse
>s. inflammatory infiltrate
>s. polyposis

sparteine

spasm
>acid-provoked s.
>bladder s.
>cervical s.
>cricopharyngeal s.
>diffuse esophageal s. (DES)
>esophageal s.
>fecal paradoxical puborectalis s.
>glottic s.
>muscle s.
>rectal s.

spasmodic stricture

Spasmolin

spasmolytic

spastic
>s. bowel syndrome
>s. colon
>s. constipation
>s. esophagus
>s. gait
>s. ileus
>s. motor disorder
>s. paraparesis
>s. pelvic floor syndrome

spastica
>cholepathia s.
>dysphagia s.

spasticity

spatial
>s. change
>s. resolution

spatula
>Davis s.
>electrosurgical s.
>Haberer abdominal s.
>Pucci-Seed s.
>Reverdin abdominal s.
>Tuffier abdominal s.

spatulated overlap anastomosis

spatulation
>graft s.
>ureteral s.

spatula-tip laparoscopic electrode

Spearman
>S. rank
>S. rank correlation
>S. test

specialized
>s. columnar epithelium (SCE)
>s. intestinal metaplasia (SIM)

species
>*Cryptosporidium* s.
>gastrin mRNA s.
>reactive oxygen s.
>single beta-actin mRNA s.

specific
>s. activity
>antigen s.
>s. anti-Hp serology
>s. clinical parameter
>s. gastritis
>s. gravity test
>s. immunotherapy
>s. oligonucleotide
>s. organic acidopathy
>s. polymerase chain reaction (SP-PCR)
>s. red cell adherence test
>s. stone presentation
>s. urethritis

specificity
>DC locus allelic s.
>LKM s.
>site s.

specimen
>clean-catch urine s.
>clean-voided s. (CVS)
>culture of biopsy s.
>cytologic s.
>esophageal biopsy s.
>intraurethral swab s.
>multiple endoscopic biopsy s.'s
>negative core biopsy s.
>paraffin-embedded s.
>photomicrograph of colonoscopic biopsy s.
>s. retrieval
>s. trap
>yarn-collected s.

speck
>hemorrhagic s.

SPECT
>single-photon emission computed tomography
>single-photon emission computerized tomography
>SPECT scan

S

spectinomycin
spectometry
 time-of-flight mass s.
Spectracef
spectral
 s. analysis
 s. broadening
Spectramed transducer
spectrometer
 liquid scintillation s.
 Shimadzu RF-5301 PC s.
spectrometry
 gas isotope ratio mass s.
 laser desorption/ionization mass s.
spectrophotometer
 atomic absorbance s.
 Bilitec fiberoptic s.
 Genetics Systems microplate
  reader s.
 Hitachi F-2000 fluorescence s.
 IL 750 AA s.
 Perkin-Elmer 5000 atomic
  absorption s.
 reflectance s.
 SLM-8000 fluorescence s.
 Uvidec-77 s.
spectrophotometric analysis
spectrophotometry
 endoscopic reflectance s.
 reflectance s.
spectroscopy
 elastic scattering s.
 fluorescence correlation s.
  (FCS)
 Fourier transform infrared s.
 gas chromatography/mass s.
  (GC/MS)
 ^{1}H magnetic resonance s.
 infrared s.
 laser-induced fluorescence s.
  (LIFS)
 light-induced autofluorescence s.
 magnetic resonance s. (MRS)
 near-infrared Raman s.
 phosphorous-31 magnetic resonance
  s.
 proton magnetic resonance s.
 Raman s.
 reflectance s.
 steady-state autofluorescence s.
 x-ray photoelectron s.
Spectrum silicone Foley catheter
specula (pl. of speculum)
speculum, pl. specula
 Barr rectal s.
 Barr-Shuford rectal s.
 beveled s.
 Bodenhammer rectal s.

 Brinkerhoff rectal s.
 Chelsea-Eaton anal s.
 Cook rectal s.
 Czerny rectal s.
 David rectal s.
 Hinkle-James rectal s.
 Hirschmann s.
 Kelly rectal s.
 Killian rectal s.
 Martin-Davis rectal s.
 Mathews rectal s.
 Pennington rectal s.
 Pratt rectal s.
 rectal s.
 Sawyer rectal s.
 Sims rectal s.
 slotted s.
 Vernon-David rectal s.
Speedbander
Speedband SuperView ligator
Speed Lok soft stent
Spencer disease
Spence urethral diverticulum
 procedure
Spenco padding
SPEP
 serum protein electrophoresis
sperm, spermatozoon, pl. spermatozoa
 s. aspiration
 s. cryopreservation
 extracted ductal s.
 s. granuloma
 s. immunobead coincubation
 s. microaspiration retrieval technique
  (SMART)
 microsurgical extraction of ductal s.
  (MEDS)
 s. motility-inhibiting factor
 muzzled s.
 s. penetration assay (SPA)
 s. survival factor
 s. yield
spermacrasia
spermagglutination
Sperma-Tex preshaped mesh
spermatic
 s. abscess
 s. artery
 s. calculus
 s. cord
 s. cord anesthetic block
 s. cord leiomyosarcoma
 s. cord liposarcoma
 s. cord torsion
 s. fascia
 s. fistula
 s. plexus
 s. vein

s. vein ligation
s. vesicle
spermatica
chorda s.
spermaticus
funiculus s.
plexus s.
spermatid
spermatin
spermatoblast (*var. of* spermatogonium)
spermatocele, spermatocyst
alloplastic s.
autogenous s.
s. resection
spermatocelectomy
spermatocidal, spermicidal
s. jelly
spermatocide, spermicide
spermatocyst (*var. of* spermatocele)
spermatocystectomy
spermatocystitis
spermatocystotomy
spermatocytal
spermatocyte
primary s.
secondary s.
spermatocytic
spermatocytogenesis, spermatogeny,
spermatogenesis
spermatogenesis (*var. of*
spermatocytogenesis)
s. depression
spermatogenic, spermatogenous,
spermatopoietic
s. arrest
s. epididymitis
s. granulomatous orchitis
spermatogenous (*var. of* spermatogenic)
spermatogeny (*var. of* spermatocytogenesis)
spermatogone (*var. of* spermatogonium)
spermatogonium, spermatogone,
spermatoblast
s. dark type A
s. pale type A
s. type B
spermatogram
spermatoid
spermatology
spermatolysin
spermatolysis, spermolysis
spermatolytic, spermolytic
spermatopoietic (*var. of* spermatogenic)
spermatorrhea
spermatoschesis
spermatotoxin (*var. of* spermatoxin)
spermatoxin, spermatotoxin, spermotoxin
spermatozoa (*pl. of* spermatozoon)
spermatozoal, spermatozoan

spermatozoan (*var. of* spermatozoal)
spermatozoon (*var. of* sperm), *pl.*
spermatozoa
acrosome-reacted s.
s. concentration
s. cryopreservation
disordered acrosome reaction of s.
double-head s.
double-tail s.
s. motility
s. production
s. retrieval
s. volume
spermaturia (*var. of* semenuria)
SpermCheck test
spermectomy
spermia (*pl. of* spermium)
spermiation
spermicidal (*var. of* spermatocidal)
spermicide (*var. of* spermatocide)
spermidine
s. uptake
s. uptake activity
spermiduct
sperm-immunobead binding
spermine
s. NONOate
polyamine s.
spermiogenesis
spermium, *pl.* **spermia**
spermoblast
spermolith
spermolysis (*var. of* spermatolysis)
spermolytic (*var. of* spermatolytic)
spermophlebectasia
spermosphere
spermotoxic
spermotoxin (*var. of* spermatoxin)
SP-501 gastric lesion staging by
endoscopic ultrasonography
spherical reservoir
spheroplast
mycobacterial s.
sphincter
AMS double-cuff Silastic artificial
urinary s.
anal ileostomy with preservation of
s.
anorectal s.
artificial genitourinary s.
artificial urethral s. (AUS)
artificial urinary s. (AUS)
AS-800 artificial urinary s.
s. atony
biliary s.
Boyden s.
canine s.
cardiac s.

S

sphincter (*continued*)
   cardioesophageal s.
   choledochal s.
   s. contraction ring
   cricopharyngeal s.
   double-cuff urinary s.
   duodenojejunal s.
   s. dysfunction
   s. EMG
   esophageal s.
   external anal s. (EAS)
   external rectal s.
   external striated urethral s.
   s. function
   gastroesophageal s.
   Giordano s.
   Glisson s.
   Henle s.
   Hydroflex s.
   hypertensive lower esophageal s.
   (HLES)
   Hyrtl s.
   ileocecal s.
   incompetent s.
   inguinal s.
   internal anal s. (IAS)
   internal rectal s.
   intrinsic striated s.
   intrinsic urethral s.
   lesser esophageal s. (LES)
   long anal s.
   lower esophageal s. (LES)
   Lütkens s.
   Nélaton s.
   neoanal s.
   O'Beirne s.
   s. of Oddi
   s. of Oddi ablation
   s. of Oddi dysfunction
   s. of Oddi homogenate
   s. of Oddi manometry
   s. of Oddi pressure
   pancreatic duct s. (PDS)
   pancreaticobiliary s.
   pharyngoesophageal s.
   preprostatic s.
   prepyloric s.
   presumptive s.
   pyloric s.
   s. reaction
   s. reconstruction
   rectal s.
   s. repair
   Santorini s.
   servomechanism s.
   smooth urethral s.
   stomach s.
   striated detrusor s.
   striated urethral s.

   threshold of internal s.
   s. tone
   upper esophageal s. (UES)
   urethral s.
   urethrovaginal s.
   Wirsung s.
sphincteral achalasia
sphincterectomy
   endoscopic s.
sphincteric
   s. construction
   s. disobedience syndrome
   s. incontinence
   s. mechanism
   s. squeeze
sphincterismus
sphincteritis
sphincteroplasty
   endoscopic large-balloon s.
   overlapping s.
   pancreatic s.
   transduodenal s.
sphincteroscope
   Kelly s.
sphincteroscopy
sphincterotome
   Autotome rotatable s.
   bipolar s.
   Bitome bipolar s.
   Cotton s.
   DASH s.
   Demling-Classen s.
   Doubilet s.
   double-channel s.
   ERCP s.
   Fluorotome double-lumen s.
   long-nosed s.
   needle-knife s.
   needle-tipped s.
   Olympus s.
   open s.
   precut s.
   reverse s.
   rotating s.
   single-channel wire-guided s.
   Ultratome double-lumen s.
   Ultratome XL triple-lumen s.
   Wilson-Cook double-channel s.
   Wilson-Cook modified wire-guided
   s.
   wire-guided s.
sphincterotomy
   s. basket
   biliary endoscopic s.
   choledochal s.
   Doubilet s.
   endoscopic biliary s.
   endoscopic pancreatic duct s.
   Erlangen pull-type s.

external s.
guidewire s.
internal s.
lateral s.
minor papilla s.
Mulholland s.
multiple anal s.'s (MAS)
needle-knife endoscopic pancreatic s.
pancreatic duct s.
Parks partial s.
precut s.
pull-type s.
retrograde s.
stenosed s.
s. stenosis
stent-guided s.
transduodenal s.
transendoscopic s.
transurethral s.
urethral s.
zipper s.

sphincter-preserving operation (SPO)
sphincter-saving procedure
sphingolipid derivative
sphingomyelin
sphingomyelinase
acid s.

SPI
symptom problem index
spiculated appearance
spiculation on colon
spicule in profile
spider
s. angioma
arterial s.
colonic arterial s.
s. nevus
s. pelvis
s. telangiectasia
spiderweb appearance
spigelian hernia
spike
Monoscopy locking trocar with Woodford s.
s. potential
spike-burst
s.-b. electrical activity
s.-b. on electromyogram of colon
spiking fever
spillage
fecal s.
s. of tumor cells
tumor s.
spina bifida
spinach stool
spinal
s. anesthesia
s. cord compression
s. cord electric stimulation

s. cord injury (SCI)
s. cord injury without radiographic abnormality (SCIWORA)
s. cord necrosis
s. finding
s. hemangioblastoma
s. shock
s. stenosis
spindle
s. cell
s. cell nodule
s. colonic groove
spine
iliac s.
spin-echo
fat-suppressed s.-e. (FSSE)
half-Fourier acquisition single-shot turbo s.-e. (HASTE)
s.-e. T1-weighted MR image
Spinelli biopsy needle
spinning
spinning-top
s.-t. deformity of bladder
s.-t. urethra
spinobulbospinal
s. micturition reflex
s. micturition reflex inhibition
spinous
s. aspect
s. process
s. tenderness
spiral
s. bacterium
s. basket
s. computed tomography
s. computed tomography pneumocolon
s. CT
s. CT technique
s. fold
s. fold of cystic duct
s. gallstone forceps
intraprostatic s.
s. valve
s. valve of Heister
s. Z stent
spiralis
Trichinella s.
valvula s.
spiral-tip
s.-t. catheter
s.-t. Segura basket
spiramycin
SpiraStent ureteral stent
spirillar dysentery
spirochetal dysentery
spirochete
intestinal s.
spirochetosis

S

SpiroFlo prostate stent
spirometry
spironazide
spironolactone
    hydrochlorothiazide and s.
Spirozide
Spirulina Pacifica nutritional supplement
Spitzer-Weinstein syndrome
Spivack
    S. operation
    S. valve
SPK
    serum pyruvate kinase
    SPK transplantation
splanchnectopia
splanchnic
    s. afferent fiber
    s. AV fistula
    s. blood flow
    s. capillary pressure
    s. hyperemia
    s. nerve
    s. vasoconstriction
    s. vein
splanchnicectomy
    chemical s.
splanchnicus
    Bacteroides s.
splanchnocele
splanchnodiastasis
splanchnolith
splanchnopathy
splanchnoptosia (*var. of* splanchnoptosis)
splanchnoptosis, splanchnoptosia
splanchnotomy
splanchnotribe
splash
    succussion s.
S-plasty
spleen
    accessory s.
    s. index
    liver, kidneys, s. (LKS)
    s. tip
    trabeculae of s.
splenalgia
splenectomy
    incidental s.
splenic
    s. abscess
    s. agenesis syndrome
    s. angiogram
    s. anlage
    s. arterial embolization
    s. artery
    s. artery aneurysm (SAA)
    s. atrophy
    s. AV fistula
    s. avulsion

    s. capillary hemangiomatosis
    s. capsule
    s. dullness
    s. flexure
    s. flexure carcinoma
    s. flexure colonoscopy
    s. flexure syndrome
    s. function
    s. hilum
    s. injury
    s. laceration
    s. notch
    s. penetration
    s. perfusion measurement by dynamic CT scan
    s. portography
    s. pulp
    s. rupture
    s. sinus
    s. souffle
    s. tissue
    s. trauma
    s. vein
    s. vein obstruction (SVO)
    s. vein thrombosis
    s. venography
    s. venous blood flow
splenica
    arteria s.
    pulpa s.
splenicae
    trabeculae s.
splenici
    folliculi lymphatici s.
splenobronchial fistula
splenocele
splenocleisis
splenocolic ligament
splenodynia
splenogastric omentum
splenogonadal fusion
splenography
splenolaparotomy
splenomegalia (*var. of* splenomegaly)
splenomegaly, splenomegalia
    congenital s.
    congestive s.
    Egyptian s.
    fibrocongestive s.
    Gaucher s.
    hemolytic s.
    infectious s.
    infective s.
    myelophthisic s.
    siderotic s.
    spodogenous s.
    tropical s.
splenonephroptosis
splenopancreatic ligament

splenopathy
splenopexia (*var. of* splenopexy)
splenopexy, splenopexia
splenoportal
    s. hypertension
    s. venography
splenoportography
splenorenal
    s. angle
    s. artery bypass
    s. bypass graft
    s. bypass shunt
    s. ligament
    s. recess
    s. venous anastomosis
splenorrhagia
splenorrhaphy
splenosis
splice-cite mutation
splicing
    aberrant mRNA s.
    alternate mRNA s.
splinting of abdomen
splint/stent
    kidney internal s./s. (KISS)
split
    s. ileostomy
    s. overtube
    s. pelvis
    s. renal function
    s. renal function study
      (SRFS)
    s. renal function test
split-and-roll technique
split-beam coupler for TURP
split-cuff
    s.-c. nipple
    s.-c. nipple technique
split-liver
    s.-l. transplant
    s.-l. transplantation
split-nipple
    s.-n. technique
    s.-n. technique urinary diversion
split-sheath introducer
splitter
    Syn-Optics videoimage s.
split-thickness skin graft
splitting
    urea s.
SPN
    support parenteral nutrition
SPO
    sphincter-preserving operation
spodogenous splenomegaly
spondylitis
sponge
    absorbable gelatin s.
    cherry s.

    s. count
    s. dissector
    Endozime s.
    fibrin s.
    s. forceps
    gauze s.
    gelatin s.
    Ivalon s.
    lap s.
    laparotomy s.
    peanut s.
    polyvinyl alcohol s.
    Prosthex s.
    saline-moistened s.
    small dissecting s.
    s. stick
    s. tent
    Weck-Cel s.
sponge-holding forceps
spongiofibrosis
    periurethral s.
spongioplasty
spongiosal
spongiosi
    trabeculae corporis s.
    tunica albuginea corporis s.
spongiositis
spongiosum
    corpus s.
spongy pattern
spontaneous
    s. ascites filtration
    s. bacterial empyema
    s. bacterial peritonitis (SBP)
    s. cystometry
    s. cyst reabsorption
    s. dialytic ultrafiltration
    s. dissection
    s. fluctuation
    s. fragment passage
    s. heartburn
    s. partial elimination
    s. penile ischemic necrosis
    s. portosystemic shunt (SPSS)
    s. reactivation of hepatitis
    s. recanalization
    s. regression
    s. resolution
    s. rupture
    s. stone passage
spontaneously reducing intussusception
spoon
    Falk appendectomy s.
    s. forceps
    gall duct s.
    Mayo common duct s.
    s. retractor
    sharp s.
    Volkmann pancreatic calculus s.

S

spoon-tip laparoscopic electrode
Sporacidin disinfectant
sporadic
>s. dysentery
>s. gingival papilloma
>s. hollow visceral myopathy
>s. nonfamilial clear cell
>carcinoma

spore
>fungal s.

sporocyst
Sporothrix schenckii
Sporox disinfectant solution
sporozoite
sport sheath (SS)
sporulation
>coccidian s.

spot
>central s.
>cherry red s. (CRS)
>cold s.
>cotton-wool s. (CWS)
>dark s.
>S. endoscopic marker
>epigastric s.
>Fordyce s.
>gastric red s.
>hematocystic s. (HCS)
>hot s.
>hyperechoic s.
>Koplik s.
>S. mobile 3D ultrasound system
>and software
>mongolian s.
>Roth s.
>s. size

spout
>ileal s.

SPP
>signal peptide peptidase
>stannous pyrophosphate
>^{99m}Tc SPP

SP-PCR
>specific polymerase chain reaction

SPR
>static pressure release
>SPR Plus III low-air-loss system

Spratt curette
spray
>alginate s.
>DDAVP nasal s.
>Maalox s.
>Nascobal nasal s.
>Prevacare Total Solution skin care
>s.
>Quixil s.
>sodium thiosulfate solution s.
>thrombin s.

spray-fixed

spraying
>dye s.
>fibrin s.
>magnification endoscopy with acetic
>acid s.

spreader
>meatal s.
>pyloric s.

spreading fistulation
spring-loaded biopsy gun
spring-loaded-type biopsy instrument
spring-wire
>s.-w. coil
>s.-w. retractor

Sprinz-Dubin syndrome
Sprinz-Nelson syndrome
sprue
>celiac s.
>collagenous s.
>nontropical s.
>refractory s.
>subclinical s.
>tropical s.

SPSS
>spontaneous portosystemic shunt

SPT
>station pullthrough
>SPT technique

spun urine sediment
spur cell
spurge
>cypress s.

spuria
>hemospermia s.
>melena s.

spurious calculus
spurting blood
sputa (*pl. of* sputum)
sputum, *pl.* **sputa**
>s. aeruginosum
>green s.

SPV
>selective proximal vagotomy

SQMP
>subcutaneous morphine pump

squamocolumnar mucosal junction
squamous
>s. cell
>s. cell cancer
>s. cell carcinoma (SCC)
>s. cell carcinoma antigen
>s. cell carcinoma in situ
>s. cell papilloma
>s. epithelium

square knot
squeeze
>hot s.
>phasic fluctuation on s.
>s. pressure

s. pressure profile of anal sphincter
test
sphincteric s.
src-**homology**
s.-h. 2 (SH2)
s.-h. 2 domain
src **phosphorylation**
SRFS
split renal function study
SRH
stigmata of recent hemorrhage
SRIF
somatotropin release-inhibiting
factor
SRMD
stress-related mucosal disease
SRS
somatostatin receptor scintigraphy
SRVG
silicone elastomer ring vertical
gastroplasty
SRY **gene**
SS
sport sheath
Regulax SS
Uroplus DS, SS
Ssabanejew-Frank
S.-F. gastrostomy
S.-F. operation
SSBE
short-segment Barrett esophagus
SSC
single-stripe colitis
SSE
soapsuds enema
S3 segment
SSE2-L electrosurgical unit
S-shaped
S-s. body
S-s. ileal pouch-anal anastomosis
S-s. pouch
S-s. reservoir
SSI
symptom severity index
SSIS
side-to-side isoperistaltic
stricturotomy
S100 super family
St.
saint
St. John's wort
St. Mark pudendal electrode
stab
s. incision
s. wound
Stabiliplan orthovolt applicator
stability
detrusor muscle s.
structural s.

stabilization
percutaneous bladder neck s.
(PBNS)
Vesica percutaneous bladder neck s.
stabilizer
stable
s. face
microsatellite s.
stab-wound drain
staccato voiding
Stachrom AT III routine chromogenic
method
Stacke meatoplasty
stack-of-coins appearance
Stadol
2-stage
2-s. repair
2-s. triolein test
stage
s. B, C carcinoma
Dean s.
Dukes s.
Hoehn and Yahr s.
s. III papillary serous
cystadenocarcinoma
morphologic s.
Tanner s.
tumor s.
staged orchiopexy
stage-specific embryonic antigen
staghorn
s. calculus
s. stone
s. urolithiasis
staging
Ann Arbor cancer s.
Boden-Gibb tumor s.
clinicopathologic s.
endosonographic s.
Marshall and Tanner pubertal s.
neoplasm s.
neuroblastoma s.
s. of cancer
s. operation
operative s.
primary gastric lymphoma s.
Scheuer s.
Stanford s.
TNM system for tumor s.
transrectal ultrasound s.
tumor s.
stagnant
s. bile
s. loop syndrome
stain
19A2 s.
acid-Schiff s.
Alcian blue s.
anti-Schiff s.

S

stain (*continued*)
 argentaffin s.
 azan s.
 Bryan-Leishman s.
 carbol fuchsin s.
 chromogranin s.
 Congo red s.
 Diff-Quik s.
 elastin s.
 El-Zimaity triple s.
 eosin s.
 esterase s.
 Fite s.
 Fontana-Masson s.
 Fungi-Fluor chitin s.
 gastrin s.
 Genta s.
 Giemsa s.
 Glaxo s.
 glucagon s.
 Gram s.
 Grimelius silver s.
 Grocott methenamine silver s.
 Hale colloidal iron s.
 Hansel s.
 H&E s.
 hematologic s.
 hematoxylin and eosin s. (H&E
  stain)
 immunocytochemical s.
 immunohistochemical s.
 immunoperoxidase s.
 indigo carmine s.
 insulin s.
 Jones silver s.
 Ki-67 s.
 Kossa s.
 lead citrate s.
 Lendrum s.
 Lugol solution s.
 Mallory-Azan s.
 Martius scarlet blue s.
 Masson-Fontana s.
 Masson trichrome s.
 Mayer acid alum hematoxylin s.
 May-Grünwald-Giemsa s.
 methylene blue s.
 NADPH diaphorase s.
 oil red O s.
 Orcein s.
 pancreatic polypeptide s.
 Papanicolaou s.
 PAS s.
 periodic acid-Schiff s.
 periodic acid-Schiff-Alcian blue
  combination s.
 Perls s.
 peroxidase s.
 p53 immunohistochemical s.

 rhodamine s.
 RP3 s.
 saffron s.
 Schiff s.
 serotonin s.
 silver s.
 S-100 immunohistochemical s.
 somatostatin s.
 Steiner s.
 Sternheimer-Malbin s.
 Sudan black B fat s.
 Sudan-III s.
 sulfated mucin s.
 toluidine blue s.
 trichrome s.
 uranyl acetate s.
 vasoactive intestinal polypeptide s.
 VIP s.
 von Kossa s.
 Warthin-Starry silver s.
 Wright s.
 Wright-Giemsa s.
 Ziehl-Neelsen s.

staining
 Berlin blue s.
 BrDu s.
 cytokeratin s.
 cytoplasmic s.
 endoscopy with iodine s.
 ethidium bromide s.
 Feulgen s.
 Grimelius s.
 HMB — 45 s.
 immunoglobulin G4 s.
 immunohistochemical s.
 immunoperoxidase s.
 iodine s.
 lectin s.
 melan A s.
 MIB-1 s.
 perinuclear intracellular s.
 photomicrograph of specimen s.
 p53 nuclear s.
 S-100 s.
 Smith method of silver s.
 Steiner modification of
  Warthin-Starry s.
 vimentin s.
 vital s.

stainless
 s. steel mesh stent
 s. steel suture

stairstep air-fluid level

stalk
 polyp s.

Stamey
 S. classification
 S. colposuspension
 S. dorsal vein apical retractor

S. needle
S. needle bladder neck suspension
S. open-tip ureteral catheter
S. procedure
S. test
S. tube
S. urethrocystopexy
Stamey-Malecot catheter
**Stamey-Martius antiincontinence
 procedure**
Stamm
S. gastroplasty
S. gastrostomy
S. gastrostomy tube
stammering bladder
stand
Mayo s.
standard
s. acid reflux test (SART)
Aub-Dubois s.
s. colonoscope
s. duodenoscope
s. endoscopic polypectomy
 snare
s. ERCP catheter
s. fatty meal
s. hemodialysis
s. laparoscopy
s. measurement
s. orchiopexy
s. pyelolithotomy
s. radioenzymatic method
s. radiological test
s. silicone manometric assembly
s. transabdominal ultrasound
standardized
s. incidence ratio
s. instrument
Stanford
S. protocol
S. radical retropubic prostatectomy
S. staging
stanley
S. bacillus
Salmonella s.
stanniocalcin
stannous pyrophosphate (SPP)
stanolone
stanozolol
staphylococcal sepsis
Staphylococcus
S. *albus*
S. *aureus* (SA)
coagulase-negative S.
S. *epidermidis*
S. food poisoning
growth of coagulase-negative S.
S. *saprophyticus*
S. *viridans*

staple
absorbable s.
s. line dehiscence
metallic s.
polyglyconate s.
skin s.
stapled
s. closure
s. end-to-end ileoanal anastomosis
s. hemorrhoidectomy
s. intestinal anastomosis
s. pouch-anal anastomosis
s. stricturotomy
stapler
anvil portion of EEA s.
Auto Suture Multifire Endo
 GIA s.
Auto Suture Premium CEEA s.
CEEA s.
circular s.
double-headed P190 s.
s. doughnut
end-end s.
Endo-Babcock s.
Endo GIA suture s.
Endo hernia s.
Endopath EMS hernia s.
Ethicon CDH29 s.
Ethicon TLH30 s.
EZ vascular linear s.
GIA s.
hernia s.
ILA surgical s.
intraluminal s. (ILS)
laparoscopic s.
ligating and dividing s. (LDS)
linear s.
linear-array s.
PI-30 s.
PI-90 double-headed s.
PI surgical s.
PLC-50 linear s.
Poly GIA s.
Premium CEEA circular s.
Premium Plus CEEA disposable s.
ProTack s.
Proximate flexible linear s.
Proximate ILS circular s.
Proximate intraluminal s.
TA90-BN s.
TA30, TA55 s.
TL90 Ethicon s.
vascular s.
stapling
gastric s.
laparoscopic s.
single s.
skin s.
surgical s.

S

StAR
   steroidogenic acute regulatory
   StAR protein
star
   s. anise
   s. construction test
starch
   amylase-resistant s.
   (ARS)
   s. blocker
   s. granulomatous peritonitis
   wheat s.
Starck dilator
Starlix
Starr
   S. plication
   S. technique
stases (*pl. of* stasis)
stasis, *pl.* **stases**
   antral s.
   bile s.
   biliary s.
   s. cirrhosis
   s. esophagitis
   fecal s.
   gallbladder s.
   s. gallbladder
   gastric s.
   ileal s.
   intestinal s.
   s. liver
   pelvicalyceal s.
   postgastrectomy s.
   postsurgical gastric s.
   Roux limb s.
   s. syndrome
   s. ulceration
   urinary s.
   venous s.
stasis-induced ulceration
STAT!
   ImmunoCard S.
Stat1
   signal transducer and activator of
   transcription 1
state
   catecholamine excess s.
   S. end-to-end anastomosis
   hypercoagulable s.
   hypermetabolic s.
   hypogonadal s.
   neurohumoral excitation s.
   proliferating s.
   proteinuric s.
   sick euthyroid s.
   utopian s.
statement
   evidence-based position s.

Statham
   S. external transducer
   S. pressure transducer
   S. P23 strain gauge
statherin
static
   s. closure pressure
   s. cystogram
   s. cytophotometry
   s. image DNA cytometry
   s. pressure release (SPR)
station
   s. pullthrough (SPT)
   s. pullthrough esophageal manometry
      technique
statistic
   nonparametric Wilcoxon s.
   preliminary baseline descriptive s.
statistically significant
Stat Simple whole-blood antibody test
status
   apical biopsy s.
   s. evaluation
   fertility s.
   s. gastricus
   nutritional s.
   stone-free s.
   ureteroenteric s.
Stat-View computer program
Stauffer syndrome
stavudine
StayErec system
Stay-Put jejunal tube
stay suture
STC
   slow-transit constipation
STD
   sexually transmitted disease
STDS
   stone-tissue detection system
steady pain
steady-state autofluorescence spectroscopy
steakhouse syndrome
steal
   arterial s.
steam autoclave
stearrhea (*var. of* steatorrhea)
steatohepatitis
   nonalcoholic s. (NASH)
steatorrhea, stearrhea
   biliary s.
   idiopathic s.
   intestinal s.
   pancreatic s.
steatosis
   drug-induced s.
   hepatic s.
   macrovesicular s.

microvesicular s.
severe macrovesicular s.
toxic s.
Steblay nephritis
STEC
Shiga toxin-producing *Escherichia coli*
Stx 2-producing *Escherichia coli* strain
steely-hair disease
steerable
s. cystoscopy
s. nephroscope
Steers replicator
stegnosis
stegnotic
Steigmann-Goff
S.-G. endoscopic ligator kit
S.-G. endoscopic ligature overtube
Steinach operation
Steiner
S. modification of Warthin-Starry
staining
S. stain
Steinert
S. disease
S. myotonic dystrophy
Stein-Leventhal syndrome
Steinmann intestinal forceps
steinstrasse
Stelazine
stellate
s. cell
s. venule
stem cell
Stemetic
stemline
DNA s.
stem-loop structure
stenosed sphincterotomy
stenoses (*pl. of* stenosis)
stenosis, *pl.* **stenoses**
afferent limb nipple s.
ampullary s.
anal s.
anorectal s.
antral s.
aortic valvular s.
atherosclerotic renal artery s.
benign papillary s.
bile duct s.
canal s.
choledochoduodenal junctional s.
congenital esophageal s.
congenital hypertrophic pyloric s.
cystic duct s.
delayed ureteral anastomotic s.
diaphragmlike s.
distal esophageal s.
duodenal s.

esophageal s.
hypertrophic pyloric s. (HPS)
idiopathic hypertrophic pyloric s.
infantile hypertrophic pyloric s. (IHPS)
infundibular s.
infundibulopelvic s.
intestinal s.
luminal s.
malignant s.
meatal s.
s. of TIPS
pancreatic papillary s.
pancreatojejunostomy s.
papillary s.
preputial s.
pyloric s.
radiation s.
rectal s.
renal artery s.
short band s.
small-intestinal s.
sphincterotomy s.
spinal s.
stomal s.
transplant renal artery s. (TRAS)
tubular s.
unilateral renal artery s. (URAS)
ureteral reimplantation s.
ureteroileal s.
urethral s.
vesical neck s.
vesicoureteric s.
stenotic
s. cancer
s. lesion
s. shunt
s. stoma
Stenotrophomonas maltophilia
Stensen duct
stent
s. after ureteroscopy
Amsterdam biliary s.
s. and vent system
Angiomed blue s.
Angiomed Puroflex s.
antibiotic-coated s.
antireflux double-J s.
ASI prostatic s.
ASI Titan s.
Bard Memotherm colorectal s.
Beamer injection s.
biliary spiral Z s.
biliopancreatic diversion with
duodenal s.
Biofix s.
bioresorbable s.
BioSorb resorbable urology s.
Biostent biliary s.

S

stent (*continued*)

Black Beauty ureteral s.
Braun s.
Carson internal/external endopyelotomy s.
C-Flex Amsterdam s.
C-Flex ureteral s.
coil s.
colonic Z s.
common bile duct s.
conventional s.
Cook s.
Corinthian s.
Cotton-Huibregtse double-pigtail s.
Cotton-Leung biliary s.
covered biliary metal s.
Cragg Endopro System I s.
crutched stick-type biliary duct s.
Cysto Flex s.
s. deployment
Diamond s.
digestive-respiratory fistula s.
double-J indwelling catheter s.
double-J silicone s.
double-J Surgitek catheter s.
double-J ureteral s.
double-pigtail s.
DoubleStent biliary endoprosthesis s.
Dua antireflux s.
Elastalloy esophageal s.
Elgiloy s.
Eliminator biliary s.
Eliminator pancreatic s.
endobronchial s.
EndoCoil biliary s.
EndoCoil esophageal s.
endopyelotomy s.
endoscopic biliary s.
EsophaCoil self-expanding esophageal s.
esophageal I s.
esophageal Strecker s.
esophageal Z stent with Dua antireflux s.
s. exchange
expandable esophageal s. (EES)
expandable intrahepatic portacaval shunt s.
expandable metallic s.
Fader Tip ureteral s.
FerX-Ella antireflux s.
Firlit-Kluge s.
Flexima biliary s.
Flexxus endoscopic biliary s.
floating s.
forgotten s.
French double-J ureteral s.
s. funnel

Gianturco expandable self-expanding metallic biliary s.
Gianturco metal urethral s.
Gianturco-Rosch biliary Z s.
Gianturco-Rosch self-expandable Z s.
Gianturco-Roubin flexible coil s.
Gianturco Z s.
Gibbon indwelling ureteral s.
Greenen pancreatic s.
helical-ridged ureteral s.
Herculink Plus biliary s.
Heyer-Schulte s.
Horizon prostatic s.
Huibregtse biliary s.
hybrid metallic s.
Hydromer-coated polyurethane s.
Hydro Plus s.
ileal artery s.
s. incrustation
incrustation of s.
incrusted ureteral s.
indwelling ureteral s.
InStent EsophaCoil s.
internal biliary s.
intracholedochal s.
IntraCoil nitinol s.
intraesophageal s.
intraluminal silastic esophageal s.
intraprostatic s.
iridium 192-loaded s.
J-Maxx s.
large-bore double-pigtail s.
Lubri-Flex ureteral s.
Luminexx s.
magnetic internal ureteral s.
main pancreatic duct s.
Mardis soft s.
Megalink biliary s.
membrane-covered s.
Memotherm colorectal s.
Memotherm endoscopic biliary s.
Memotherm Flexx biliary s.
Memotherm nitinol s.
mesh s.
metallic biliary s.
metal Z s.
s. migration
modified Z s.
MPD s.
Multi-Flex s.
nephroureteral s.
nephrovesical s.
Nissenkorn s.
nitinol mesh s.
Niti-S s.
Oasis s.
Omnilink biliary s.
Palmaz balloon-expandable s.

Palmaz Blue s.
Palmaz Corinthian s.
Palmaz-Schatz biliary s.
pancreatic duct s.
s. patency
Percuflex Amsterdam s.
Percuflex biliary s.
Percuflex endopyelotomy s.
Percuflex Plus ureteral s.
percutaneous s.
pigtail biliary s.
polyethylene s.
Polyflex esophageal s.
polyurethane s.
polyurethane-covered metallic s.
Prostacoil s.
Prostakath urethral s.
prostatic s.
pyelovesical s.
Quadra-Coil ureteral s.
recanalization of clogged biliary s.
renal artery s.
Retromax endopyelotomy s.
Rusch s.
Schneider s.
self-expandable metallic s.
self-expanding biliary metal s.
self-expanding coil s.
self-expanding metallic s.
 (SEMS)
self-expanding plastic s. (SEPS)
self-retaining coil s.
SEM s.
shape memory alloy s.
Siegel s.
silastic indwelling ureteral s.
silicone-coated metallic
 self-expanding s.
silicone-covered self-expanding
 polyester s.
Silitek Uropass s.
silver-coated s.
single-pigtail s.
SMA spiral s.
SoloPass Percuflex biliary s.
Song s.
Speed Lok soft s.
spiral Z s.
SpiraStent ureteral s.
SpiroFlo prostate s.
stainless steel mesh s.
straight winged s.
Strecker s.
Surgitek Tractfinder ureteral s.
Surgitek Uropass s.
Tannenbaum s.
Teflon s.
thermoexpandable s.
thermosensitive s.

s. through wire mesh technique
Titan s.
titanium urethral s.
tracheobronchial Z s.
transhepatic biliary s.
transjugular portosystemic shunt s.
 (TIPSS)
transpapillary cystopancreatic s.
transpapillary insertion of
 self-expanding biliary metal s.
T-tube s.
Ultraflex Diamond s.
Ultraflex Microvasive s.
Ultraflex nitinol expandable
 esophageal s.
Ultraflex tracheobronchial s.
uncoated mesh s.
Universal s.
ureteral s.
urethral s.
UroCoil self-expanding s.
Uro-Guide s.
UroLume prostate s.
UroLume urethral s.
UroLume Wallstent s.
Urosoft s.
Urospiral urethral s.
U-tube s.
ViaDuct pancreatic s.
Vistaflex biliary s.
Wallstent covered SEM s.
whistle s.
Wilson-Cook French s.
Z s.
Za-Stent endoscopic biliary s.
Zilver biliary self-expanding s.
Zimmon biliary s.
stented ureteroscopic lithotripsy
stent-guided sphincterotomy
stent-induced pneumoperitoneum
stenting
 biliary s.
 s. catheter
 endoscopic pancreatic s. (EPS)
 endoscopic papillotomy and s.
 endoscopic retrograde biliary s.
 endovascular s.
 hilar bile duct s.
 indications for s.
 pancreatic transpapillary s.
 routine ureteral s.
 tumor s.
 ureteral s.
stent-related complication
2-step
 Aztec 2-s.
 2-s. orchiopexy
stepladder incision technique
steppage gait

stepping reflex
step-up shim
stepwise regression analysis
steradian (sr)
Sterapred
stercolith
stercoraceous, stercoral, stercorous
    s. abscess
    s. appendicitis
    s. colic
    s. diarrhea
    s. fistula
    s. formation
    s. perforation
    s. ulcer
    s. ulceration
    s. vomiting
    s. vomitus
stercoral (*var. of* stercoraceous)
stercoralis
    Strongyloides s.
stercoroma
stercorous (*var. of* stercoraceous)
stercus
Ste-20-related, proline-alanine-rich kinase (SPAK)
stereocilium
StereoGuide
    Lorad S.
stereomicroscopic view
sterile
    s. abscess
    s. ceftriaxone sodium
    s. cyst
    s. dressing
    s. pancreatic necrosis
    s. peritonitis
sterility
    absolute s.
    aspermatogenic s.
    chemotherapy-induced s.
    dysspermatogenic s.
    male s.
    normospermatogenic s.
    primary s.
    radiation-induced s.
    relative s.
    secondary s.
sterilization
    ETO s.
    gas s.
sterilize
sterilized
    autoclave s.
Steris automatic reprocessor
Steri-Strip
steri-stripped incision
sterna (*pl. of* sternum)
Sternberg paradigm

Sternheimer-Malbin stain
sternotomy scar
sternum, *pl.* sterna
    bowed s.
steroid
    adrenal s.
    anabolic s.
    s. foam enema
    high-dose pulse s.
    s. moiety
    s. receptor
    s. therapy
    s. withdrawal
steroid-dependent
    s.-d. Crohn disease
    s.-d. diet
    s.-d. idiopathic nephrosis
steroid-induced azoospermia
steroidogenic
    s. acute regulatory (StAR)
    s. acute regulatory protein
steroid-refractory
    s.-r. Crohn disease
    s.-r. diet
steroid-resistant
    s.-r. idiopathic nephrosis
    s.-r. nephrotic syndrome
    s.-r. rejection
steroid-responsive pancolitis
steroid-sensitive idiopathic nephrosis
sterol
stethoscope
    esophageal s.
Stetten intestinal clamp
Stevens-Johnson syndrome
Stewart crypt hook
Stewart-Treves syndrome
sTf-R
    soluble transferrin receptor
stick
    sponge s.
    s. tie
Stiegmann-Goff
    S.-G. Clearvue endoscopic ligator
    S.-G. endoscopic esophageal varices ligation technique
    S.-G. variceal ligator
Stierlin sign
Stifcore transbronchial aspiration needle
stiffening
    s. tube
    s. wire
stigma, *pl.* stigmas, stigmata
    endoscopic s.
    stigmata of recent hemorrhage (SRH)
    syphilitic s.
    Turner s.
stigmas (*pl. of* stigma)
stigmata (*pl. of* stigma)

stigmatic
stigmatism
stigmatization
still
    s. camera
    S. disease
Stille
    S. clamp
    S. elevator
    S. gallstone forceps
Stille-Barraya intestinal forceps
Stilphostrol
stimulant laxative
stimulated
    s. gastric secretion test
    s. gracilis neosphincter
    s. gracilis neosphincter technique
    s. graciloplasty
    s. release
    s. tube
stimulation
    adenyl cyclase s.
    anal electrical s.
    anocutaneous s.
    antigen s.
    central vagal nerve s.
    chronic low-frequency electrical s.
    chronic sacrospinal nerve s.
    cutaneous electrical field s.
    duodenal electrical s.
    electrogalvanic s. (EGS)
    extradural electrical s.
    s. fork
    gastric electrical s.
    hilum s.
    implantable gastric s. (IGS)
    interferential electrical s.
    interferon gamma s.
    intraoperative cavernous nerve s.
    intravaginal electrical s.
    magnetic s.
    mitogenic s.
    nociceptive s.
    peak acid output after pentagastrin
      s. (PAOPg)
    pelvic floor electrical s.
    penile vibratory s.
    percutaneous Stoller afferent nerve
      s. (PerQ SANS)
    s. probe
    rectal digital s.
    sacral nerve s. (SNS)
    S-CCK-Pz s.
    secretin s.
    spinal cord electric s.
    Stoller afferent nerve s. (SANS)
    s. test
    testosterone s.
    transcranial magnetic s. (TCMS)

    transcutaneous electrical nerve s.
      (TENS)
    transurethral electrical bladder s.
      (TEBS)
    vagal s.
    vaginal electrical s.
stimulator
    EGS 100 electrogalvanic s.
    electrogalvanic s.
    Grass S9 s.
    Nicolet SM-300 s.
    Transcend implantable gastric s.
    URYS 800 nerve s.
stimuli (*pl. of* stimulus)
stimulus, *pl.* **stimuli**
    external s.
    mitogenic s.
    osmotic s.
    symbolic s.
STING
    subureteric Teflon injection
    STING procedure
stinging nettle
stirrup
    Allen s.
    Lloyd-Davies s.
    pediatric s.
stitch
    baseball s.
    cobbler's s.
    Connell s.
    Gambee s.
    intersymphyseal s.
    lock s.
    marker s.
    tagging s.
    tilt s.
    Z s.
STK11 **gene**
stochastic knotting
Stockholm trial I, II
stoichiometry
    coupling s.
Stokvis
    S. disease
    S. test
Stokvis-Talma syndrome
Stoller
    S. afferent nerve stimulation
      (SANS)
    S. scoring system
Stoll test
stoma, *pl.* **stomas, stomata**
    abdominal s.
    anastomotic s.
    appendicoumbilical s.
    bowel s.
    s. cap
    concealed umbilical s.

S

stoma (*continued*)

    continent abdominal wall s.
    diverting s.
    dusky s.
    end s.
    endloop s.
    flush s.
    gastrointestinal s.
    Gomez horizontal gastroplasty with reinforced s.
    ileostomy s.
    Laws gastroplasty with silastic collar-reinforced s.
    loop s.
    maturing the s.
    Mitrofanoff catheterizable s.
    Mitrofanoff continent urinary s.
    nippled s.
    permanent s.
    prolapsed s.
    retracted s.
    rodless end-loop s.
    rosebud s.
    silastic collar-reinforced s.
    s. site
    stenotic s.
    Turnbull loop s.
    ureteral s.

stomach

    aberrant umbilical s.
    s. ache
    acid-suppressed s.
    adenomatous polyp of s.
    adenomyoepithelioma of s.
    anacidic s.
    angular notch of s.
    angulus of s.
    antrum of s.
    s. bed
    bilocular s.
    butterflies in s.
    s. calculus
    caliber-persistent artery of s.
    cardiac s.
    cardia of s.
    cascade s.
    cirrhosis of s.
    cup-and-spill s.
    curvature of s.
    dilation of s.
    distal blind s.
    drain-trap s.
    dumping s.
    functional disorder of s.
    fundus of s.
    granulocytic sarcoma of s.
    greater curvature of s.
    hourglass s.
    insufflation of s.

    intrathoracic s.
    s. lavage
    leather-bottle s.
    lesser curvature of s.
    middle s.
    mucous lake of s.
    s. neoplasm
    oblique fibers of s.
    s. pump
    s. reefing
    rugae of s.
    sclerotic s.
    sour s.
    s. sphincter
    thoracic s.
    trifid s.
    s. tube
    tympany of s.
    upset s.
    upside-down s.
    vascular coat of s.
    villous folds of s.
    watermelon s.
    water-trap s.

stomachache (*var. of* stomach ache)

stomachalgia

stomachodynia

Stomahesive

    S. paste
    S. skin barrier
    S. skin barrier wafer

stomal

    s. aperture
    s. bag
    s. duskiness
    s. invagination
    s. prolapse
    s. stenosis
    s. ulcer

stomalike channel

stomas (*pl. of* stoma)

stomata (*pl. of* stoma)

Stomate

    S. decompression tube
    S. extension tube

stomatitis

    aphthous s.
    herpetic s.

stomatoscopy

    diagnostic fiberoptic s.

stone

    ampullary s.
    s. and basket impaction
    artificial cystine s.
    bile duct s.
    biliary tract s.
    bilirubinate s.
    black faceted s.
    black pigment s.

bladder s.
branched s.
brown pigment s.
s. burden
calcium bilirubinate s.
calcium oxalate dihydrate s.
calcium oxalate monohydrate s.
carbonate apatite s.
CBD s.
cholesterol s.
S. clamp applier
s. clearance
s. comminution
common bile duct s. (CBDS)
complex s.
s. composition
S. Cone
S. Cone nitinol stone retrieval device
s. cup
cystic duct s.
cystine s.
s. disease
s. dislodger
endoscopic extraction of pancreatic duct s.
s. extraction
extraction of bile duct s.
extraction of pancreatic s.
s. former
s. fragmentation
gallbladder s.
genuine cystine s.
s. granuloma
s. granuloma formation
hepatic duct s.
hyperoxaluric s.
impacted ampullary s.
impacted ureteral s.
s. impactor
infection s.
S. intestinal clamp
intrahepatic s.
intraluminal s.
s. in urinary diversion
kidney s.
large common duct s.
large impacted ureteral s.
lower pole s.
s. management
s. maturation
metabolic s.
mulberry s.
multiple s.'s
noncalcified s.
nonstruvite s.
pancreatic duct s.
pelvic s.
periureteral s.

pigment s.
s. plaque
s. recognition system
s. recurrence rate
recurrent calcium-containing s.'s
renal s.
residual s.
s. retrieval balloon
s. retrieval basket
s. retriever
s. searcher
silent s.
s. solvent
staghorn s.
struvite s.
s. surgery
ureteral s.
uric acid s.
urinary s.
stonecrop
common s.
stone-forming patient
stone-free
s.-f. rate
s.-f. status
stone-grasping forceps
Stone-Holcombe intestinal clamp
stone-holding basket forceps
stonelike debris
stone-prevention program
StoneRisk
S. citrate test
S. cystine test
S. diagnostic monitoring kit
S. diagnostic profile
S. diagnostic test
S. profile test
stone-tissue
s.-t. detection system (STDS)
s.-t. recognition (STR)
s.-t. recognition system
stool
ability to form solid s.
acholic s.
s. antigen assay
bilious s.
black tarry s.
blood admixed with s.
blood in s.
blood on surface of s.
blood passed with s.
blood-streaked s.
bloody s.
brown s.
bulky s.
butter s.
caddy s.
s. chromatography
clay-colored s.

S

719

stool (*continued*)
    Clinitest-negative s.
    Clinitest-positive s.
    s. colonization
    s. color
    continent of s.
    s. culture
    currant jelly s.
    s. cytotoxin test
    dark s.
    diarrhea s.
    s. electrolyte
    s. electrolyte test
    s. elimination
    s. evacuation
    fatty s.
    floating s.
    foamy s.
    formed s.
    s. for occult blood
    s. for ova and parasites
    foul-smelling s.
    frank blood in s.
    frequency of s.
    Gram stain of s.
    green s.
    guaiac-negative s.
    guaiac-positive s.
    hard s.
    heme-negative s.
    heme-positive s.
    impacted s.
    s. incontinence
    lienteric s.
    liquid s.
    loose s.
    mahogany-colored s.
    malodorous s.
    maroon-colored s.
    melenic s.
    mucoid s.
    mucous s.
    mushy s.
    nonbloody s.
    oily s.
    s. osmolality test
    s. osmotic gap
    s. osmotic gap test
    pale s.
    palpable s.
    particulate s.
    passage of s.
    pea soup s.
    pelleted s.
    pencillike s.
    pipestem s.
    rabbit s.
    residual s.
    s. retention

    ribbon s.
    rice-water s.
    runny s.
    sago-grain s.
    s. sample
    scybalous s.
    semiformed s.
    semisolid s.
    silver s.
    slurry of s.
    soft s.
    s. softener
    spinach s.
    straining at s.
    tarry black s.
    s. toxin assay
    Trélat s.
    undigested food in s.
    unformed s.
    watery s.
    Wright stain of s.

stooling

stool-softening laxative

STOP
    selective tubal occlusion procedure

stopcock
    3-way s.

Stoppa
    S. operation
    S. repair

storage
    cold s.
    hypothermic s.

store
    hepatic glycogen s.
    iron s.
    liver iron s.
    liver protein s.

Storz
    S. cholangiograsper
    S. cystoscope
    S. esophagoscope
    S. minilaparoscope
    S. Modulith SL20
    S. multifunction valve trocar/cannula system
    S. nephroscope
    S. panendoscope
    S. resectoscope
    S. 27022 SK ureteroscope
    S. syringe
    S. urethrotome

STR
    stone-tissue recognition
    STR system

Strachan
    S. disease
    S. syndrome

Strachan-Scott syndrome

straddle injury
straight
    s. endoprosthesis
    s. intestine
    s. Maryland forceps
    s. mosquito clamp
    s. stent
    s. venule
    s. winged stent
straightener
    colonoscopy technique with external
    s.
    external s.
straightening maneuver
Straight-In
    S.-I. male sling system
    S.-I. surgical system
strain
    Bio-Tract proprietary s.
    Cowan 1 s.
    CR326 s.
    cystitis-causing s.
    eubacterial s.
    Helicobacter pylori cagA s.
    HM175 s.
    metronidazole-resistant s.
    precore mutant s.
    simian s.
    Stx 2-producing *Escherichia*
      coli s.
strain-gauge transducer
straining
    s. at stool
    defecatory s.
    excessive s.
    s. for urination
strand
    Billroth s.
    fibrin s.
    internodal s.
    intramembranous particle s.
stranding
    fascial s.
    hyperechoic s.
    mesenteric fat s.
    pericholecystic s.
    perinephric s.
    periureteral s.
    soft tissue s.
strangulated
    s. bowel
    s. bowel obstruction
    s. hemorrhoid
    s. hernia
    s. viscus
strangulation
    s. necrosis
    s. of bladder
stranguria (*var. of* strangury)

strangury, stranguria
S-transferase
Stransky sign
strap
    Allen s.
    Montgomery abdominal s.
Strassburg test
strata (*pl. of* stratum)
Stratagene SCS-96 thermocycler
Stratasis urethral sling
strategy
    antisense s.
    rational allocation s.
stratiform
Stratte needle holder
stratum, *pl.* **strata**
    s. malpighii
    submucous s.
Strauss sign
strawberry
    s. gallbladder
    s. hemangioma
straw-colored
    s.-c. ascites
    s.-c. fluid
streak
    erythematous s.
    s. gonad
    lymphangitic s.
    s. ovary
stream
    curve of s.
Strecker stent
Strelinger colon clamp
strength
    artery weld s.
    detrusor contraction s.
    double s. (DS)
    hemostatic bond s.
    masseter s.
    pelvic muscle s.
    tensile s.
streptavidin
    peroxidase-conjugated s.
streptavidin-biotin
streptococcal esophagitis
streptococci (*pl. of* streptococcus)
streptococcus, *pl.* **streptococci**
    S. agalactiae
    alpha-hemolytic s.
    anhemolytic s.
    beta-hemolytic s.
    S. bovis
    S. bovis bacteremia
    S. enteritis
    S. faecalis
    group B s. (GBS)
    hemolytic s.
    S. milleri

S

streptococcus (*continued*)
    nonhemolytic *S.*
    S. pyogenes
    S. salivarius
    S. sanguis
    S. thermophilus
    S. viridans
streptokinase
Streptomyces
    S. hygroscopicus
    S. misakiensis
    S. tsukubaensis
streptomycin nephropathy
streptozocin (*var. of* streptozotocin)
streptozotocin, streptozocin
streptozotocin-induced diabetes
  mellitus
stress
    s. cystogram
    s. erosion
    s. erythrocytosis
    s. gastritis
    s. hematuria
    s. incontinence type 0, I, II, III
    s. lesion
    oxidative s.
    s. protein
    s. relaxation
    surgical s.
    s. testing
    s. ulcer
    s. ulceration
    s. ulcer hemorrhage
    s. ulcer prophylaxis
    s. urethral pressure profile
    s. urinary incontinence (SUI)
stress-induced gastric ulceration
stress-related
    s.-r. erosive syndrome
    s.-r. mucosal disease (SRMD)
    s.-r. mucosal injury
Stresstein liquid feeding
stretch receptor
stretch-sensitive ion channel
Stretta
    S. catheter
    S. radiofrequency for GERD
      procedure
    S. system
stria, *pl.* **striae**
    striae distensae
    epidermal s.
    Looser-Milkman s.
striae (*pl. of* stria)
Striant buccal system
striated
    s. detrusor sphincter
    s. muscle innervation
    s. urethral sphincter

Strickler
    S. technique ureterocolonic
      anastomosis
    S. ureteral anastomosis
stricture
    anal s.
    anastomotic s.
    antral s.
    anular esophageal s.
    avascular s.
    benign bile duct s. (BBDS)
    benign biliary s.
    bile duct s.
    biliary tract s.
    bulbomembranous s.
    bulbourethral s.
    s. cannulation
    caustic s.
    cicatricial s.
    colorectal s.
    complete ureteral s.
    congenital ureteral s.
    congenital urethral s.
    contractile s.
    corrosive esophageal s.
    diaphragmlike s.
    distal esophageal s.
    ductal s.
    esophageal s.
    extrahepatic biliary s.
    filiform s.
    focal s.
    hourglass s.
    Hunner s.
    intestinal s.
    intrahepatic biliary s.
    intrinsic ureteral s.
    irritable s.
    left hepatic duct s.
    longitudinal esophageal s.
    malignant rectal s.
    membranous urethral s.
    nonsteroidal antiinflammatory
      drug-induced intestinal s.
    pancreatic duct s.
    pancreaticobiliary s.
    panurethral s.
    peptic esophageal s.
    postcholangitic s.
    postoperative s.
    posttraumatic posterior urethral s.
    s. prophylaxis
    pyloric s.
    radiation-induced ureteral s.
    rectal s.
    recurrent s.
    reflux-related s.
    ringlike s.
    severe ureteral s.

spasmodic s.
upper tract s.
ureteral s.
ureterocolic s.
ureteroenteric s.
ureteroileal s.
urethral s.
vas deferens s.
vesicoureteral anastomotic s.
vesicourethral anastomotic s.
strictured esophagus
strictureplasty (*var. of* stricturoplasty)
stricturoplasty, strictureplasty
Finney s.
Heineke-Mikulicz s.
isoperistaltic s.
Thal s.
stricturotomy
endoscopic s.
side-to-side isoperistaltic s. (SSIS)
stapled s.
stridor
strigosus
Ctenochaetus s.
string
s. guideline
s. method for treatment of penile
incarceration
s. operation
s. sign
soft rubber s.
swallowed s.
s. test
string-capsule endoscopy
string-of-beads
s.-o.-b. appearance
s.-o.-b. appearance of renal medial
fibroplasia
s.-o.-b. sign
string-of-pearls
s.-o.-p. appearance of gastric body
s.-o.-p. sign
strip
Ames Hemastix reagent s.
Bio-Gen urine test s.
s. biopsy
s. biopsy resection technique
DiaScreen 10 reagent s.
DisIntek reagent s.
ganglion-free muscle s.
Gore-Tex s.
HydraTrend urine test s.
PyloriTek reagent s.
s. resection
rhythm s.
roof s.
stripe
s. interstitial fibrosis
properitoneal flank s.

stripping
mucosal s.
urethral s.
stroke
saber s.
stroma, *pl.* **stromata**
fibroelastic connective tissue s.
fibrous s.
hyalinized s.
s. ovarii
prostate gland s.
stromal
s. invasion
s. tumor of unknown malignant
potential (STUMP)
stromata (*pl. of* stroma)
strong
s. association
s. clinical suspicion
S. Start chewable tablet
Strongyloides
S. stercoralis
S. venezuelensis
strongyloidiasis, strongyloidosis
disseminated s.
strongyloid infection
strongyloidosis (*var. of* strongyloidiasis)
strongyloma
strontium-89 chloride
Strovite Advance caplet
structural
s. effect of dietary salt
s. fatigue
s. property
s. stability
structure
biliary s.
cord s.
ductular s.
glandular s.
insular s.
malignant nuclear s.
mixed s.
nociceptive s.
seminiferous tubule peritubular s.
stem-loop s.
trabecular s.
undifferentiated s.
Strulle scissors
struma, *pl.* **strumae**
Hashimoto s.
s. ovarii
strumae (*pl. of* struma)
strumous bubo
strut
Mersilene s.
struvite
s. calculus
s. crystal formation

S

struvite (*continued*)
    s. stone
    s. urolithiasis
Stryker frame
STS
    serologic test for syphilis
    STS lithotripsy system
1st-stage repair
stuartii
    Providencia s.
Stucker bile duct dilator
studding
    omental s.
    peritoneal s.
Studer
    S. bladder substitute
    S. crossfolded ileal reservoir
    S. neobladder
    S. pouch
    S. pouch ileal neobladder
      procedure
    S. reservoir urinary diversion
studeri
    Bertiella s.
study
    AEC S.
    A28 immunologic s.
    American Endosonography Club s.
    antegrade contrast s.
    anti-DNA immunologic s.
    anti-ENA immunologic s.
    antihepatitis A-IgM immunologic s.
    antinuclear antibody immunologic
      s.
    anti-SSA immunologic s.
    anti-SSB immunologic s.
    barium s.
    bead-chain s.
    B12 immunologic s.
    bladder outlet kinesiologic s.
    bulb-tip retrograde s.
    Candida immunologic s.
    C3 immunologic s.
    cinefluorographic s.
    circulating immunocomplex
      immunologic s.
    Collaborative Transplant S. (CTS)
    colonic transit s.
    colonoscopic antegrade contrast
      enema s.
    colon transit marker s.
    colorectal physiologic s.
    colorectal transition s.
    congruent grade A s.
    dark adaptation s.
    detrusor muscle pressure-flow
      micturition s.
    diisopropyliminodiacetic acid
      enterogastroesophageal reflux s.

    DISIDA enterogastroesophageal
      reflux s.
    diuretic renal quantitative
      camera s.
    DNCB immunologic s.
    double-blind randomized s.
    dynamic urethral profile s.
    ESR immunologic s.
    European retrospective s.
    flow cytometric s.
    gene-blotting s.
    genitocerebral evoked potential s.
    HALT-C s.
    HBeAg immunologic s.
    HBsAg immunologic s.
    hematologic s.
    HLA typing immunologic s.
    HOPE s.
    24-hour ambulatory manometry s.
    24-hour intraesophageal pH s.
    IgA immunologic s.
    IgG immunologic s.
    IgM immunologic s.
    intestinal transit s.
    isotope s.
    kinetic gallbladder s.
    light micrographic s.
    luminal contrast s.
    MACH1 s.
    manometric s.
    marker transit s.
    microarray-based s.
    microperfusion s.
    mitochondrial immunologic s.
    molecular s.
    ^{99m}Tc-phytate liquid state esophageal
      transit s.
    multicenter s.
    Multicentre International Liver
      Tumor S. (MILTS)
    National Cooperative Dialysis S.
    nerve conduction s. (NCS)
    nuclear-tagged red blood cell
      bleeding s.
    Nurses' Health S. (NHS)
    observational followup s.
    one-session crossover s.
    ORCHID s.
    peak urinary flow s.
    perfusion s.
    phenotypic s.
    Physicians' Health S. I, II (PHS I,
      II)
    pilot s.
    polarographic s.
    positive secretin stimulation s.
    PPD immunologic s.
    pressure s.
    pressure-flow s. (PFS)

pressure-flow electromyography s.
pressure-flow micturition s.
prospective multicenter s.
radiologic s.
radionuclide transit s.
Ramipril Efficacy in Nephropathy s.
rectal barostat s.
rectosphincter manometric s.
REIN s.
renal function s. (RFS)
renal perfusion pressure-flow s.
retrograde contrast s.
retroperitoneal carbon dioxide
   insufflation s.
scintigraphic emptying s.
seroepidemiologic s.
single-color direct
   immunofluorescence s.
smooth muscle immunologic s.
split renal function s. (SRFS)
transurethral prostatic resection s.
Treponema immunofluorescence s.
T-tube s.
upper gastrointestinal barium
   roentgenographic s.
urodynamic flow s.
videoendoscopic swallowing s.
   (VESS)
videofluoroscopic swallow s.
   (VSS)
videofluorourodynamic s.
videourodynamic s.
voiding s.

Stühmer disease
STUMP
stromal tumor of unknown malignant
   potential
stump
appendiceal s.
blind s.
dehiscence of cystic s.
duodenal s.
funicular s.
gastric s.
s. invagination
s. ligation
polypectomy s.
rectal s.

Sturge-Weber syndrome
stuttering
s. priapism
urinary s.
s. urination

Stx
Shiga toxin
Stx 2-producing *Escherichia coli*
   (STEC)
Stx 2-producing *Escherichia coli*
   strain

stylet, stylette
bayonet s.
S. internal esophageal MRI coil
stylette (*var. of* stylet)
styloglossus muscle
stylohyoid muscle
stylopharyngeus muscle
S-type amylase
Stypven time test
subacute
s. abscess
s. atrophy of liver
s. cystitis
s. fatty liver of pregnancy
s. hepatic necrosis (SHN)
s. hepatitis
s. liver disease
s. liver failure (SALF)
s. nephritis
s. nonspecific peritonitis
subadventitial fibroplasia
subaponeurotic abscess
subarachnoid space
subareolar
subcapsular
s. hematoma
s. hemorrhage
s. hepatic abscess
s. nephrectomy
s. orchiectomy
subcarinal
s. lymph
s. node
subcecal appendix
subcholangiopancreatoscope
subchronic
s. atrophy of liver
s. sacral neuromodulation
subcitrate
colloidal bismuth s. (CBS)
subclavian
s. catheter
s. catheter insertion
s. position
s. vein
s. vein catheterization
subclinical
s. hepatic encephalopathy
   (SHE)
s. hepatitis
s. rejection
s. sprue
subcoronal hypospadias
subcostal
s. flank incision
s. margin
s. nerve
s. port
s. transperitoneal incision

S

subcutaneous
  s. EGF
  s. emphysema
  s. fat
  s. layer
  s. morphine pump (SQMP)
  s. penectomy
  s. tissue
  s. urinary diversion
subcuticular suture
subdeterminant
  hepatitis B surface antigen s.
subdiaphragmatic abscess
subendoscope
subendothelial deposit
subepididymal orchiectomy
subepithelial
  s. deposit
  s. hematoma of renal pelvis
  s. hemorrhage
subfascial endoscopic perforator surgery (SEPS)
subfertile
subfraction
  uremic serum s.
subfulminant liver failure
subglottic lesion
subgroup F adenovirus
subhepatic
  s. abscess
  s. area
  s. space
subinguinalis
  fossa s.
subinguinal microsurgical varicocelectomy
subjective
  s. improvement
  s. symptom
  s. vertigo
sublingual hyoscyamine
submassive hepatic necrosis
submucosa
  small-intestinal s.
submucosal
  s. arterial malformation
  s. artery
  s. calculus
  s. dissection
  s. endothelial angiodysplasia
  s. fat
  s. fibromuscular angiodysplasia
  s. gastric hemorrhage
  s. ileal lipoma
  s. mass
  s. saline injection
  s. saline injection technique
  s. tattoo
  s. Teflon injection
  s. thickening
  s. track
  s. upper gastrointestinal tract lesion
  s. vaginal muscle
  s. vaginal smooth musculofascial layer
  s. vascular dilation
  s. vascular malformation
  s. venous plexus
  s. wound
submucous
  s. cystitis
  s. layer
  s. plexus
  s. stratum
  s. ulcer
submuscular plexus
subparta
  ileus s.
subperitoneal
  s. abscess
  s. appendicitis
  s. fascia
  s. space
subphrenic
  s. abscess
  s. space
subpleural blanketing technique
subpubic sinus
Subrini penile prosthesis
subsalicylate
  bismuth s. (BSS)
subsaturation riboprobe concentration
subscapular
subsegmentectomy
  hepatic s.
subsequent
  s. diagnostic laparoscopy
  s. rejection episode
subserosal (*var. of* subserous)
subserous, subserosal
  s. calbindin
  s. disease
  s. fascia
  s. ganglion
  s. layer
  s. tunnel
subsigmoid fossa
substaging
  pathologic s.
substance
  s. abuse (SA)
  s. A
  caustic s.
  hepatic stimulatory s. (HSS)
  S. K
  noncholecystokinin s.
  ouabainlike s. (OLS)
  s. P

reducing s.
S. S
substantial regional difference
substernal region
substitute
graft s.
ileal orthotopic bladder s.
low-pressure bladder s.
Olestra fat s.
saliva s.
Studer bladder s.
substituted benzimidazole
substitution
bladder s.
colonic orthotopic bladder s.
ileal ureteral s.
orthotopic bladder s.
s. urethroplasty
substrate
copolymerized s.
narrow s.
s. oxidation
substratum
cell s.
subsymphysial epispadias
subtotal
s. colectomy
s. gastrectomy
s. gastric exclusion
s. pancreatectomy
s. villous atrophy (SVA)
subtraction angiography
subtrigonal cystectomy
subtunical venule
subtype
HBsAg s.
subtyping
HLA-DR2 s.
subumbilical space
subunit
beta s.
corticosteroid regulation of
amiloride-sensitive sodium channel s.
glutamylcysteine synthetase heavy s.
(GCS-HS)
transmembrane beta s.
subureteric Teflon injection (STING)
suburethral
s. component
s. epithelial inclusion cyst
s. rectus fascial sling procedure
s. sling
suburothelial
s. infiltrative cancer
s. nerve plexus
s. vascular bed
subvesical duct
subxiphoid
Suby G solution

subzonal insemination (SUZI)
succagogue
success
s. in retroflexion
s. of surgical treatment
succi (*pl. of* succus)
succimer
succinate
s. dehydrogenase
sumatriptan s.
succinylcholine
succorrhea
succulent mesenteric lymph node
succus, *pl.* **succi**
s. entericus
s. gastricus
s. pancreaticus
succussion
hippocratic s.
s. sound
s. splash
suck-and-cut
s.-a.-c. method
s.-a.-c. mucosectomy
s.-a.-c. technique
suck-and-ligate technique
sucker
tonsil s.
sucralfate
s. retention enema
s. therapy
sucrose
iron s.
s. tolerance test
sucrose-free (SF)
sucrose-isomaltase deficiency (SID)
suction
s. banding
s. biopsy
bulb s.
S. Buster catheter
s. channel
continuous NG s.
s. cylinder
s. drain
s. drainage
flexible dental s.
s. foot pedal
Gomco s.
Harris tube s.
lavage and s.
low intermittent s.
nasogastric s.
NG s.
s. oral brush
s. pump
s. tip
s. tube
Wangensteen s.

S

suction-coagulator
    Cameron-Miller s.-c.
suctioning
    intermittent s.
    rectal air s.
Suda classification type I, II, III of papilla
Sudan black B fat stain
Sudan-III stain
sudden
    s. expansion
    s. onset of pain
    s. valve prolapse
Sudeck
    S. atrophy
    S. critical point
sufentanil
sugar
    s. oxime
    s. test
Sugarbaker technique
Sugar-Free
    Citrucel S.-F.
Sugiura
    S. esophageal variceal transection
    S. esophageal varix procedure
    S. paraesophagogastric devascularization
SUI
    stress urinary incontinence
suis
    Trichuris s.
suite
    endoscopy s.
sulamserod HCl
sulbactam sodium
sulci (*pl. of* sulcus)
sulciform
sulcus, *pl.* **sulci**
    coronal s.
    costovertebral s.
    intersphincteric s.
    s. of umbilical vein
sulfa
sulfacytine
sulfadiazine
sulfamethizole
sulfamethoprim
sulfamethoxazole (SMX)
    s. and phenazopyridine
    s. and trimethoprim (SMX-TMP, SMX/TMP)
Sulfamylon
sulfanilamide
sulfasalazine enema
sulfasalazine-induced oxidative hemolysis
sulfasoxazole (*var. of* sulfisoxazole)
sulfate, sulphate
    atropine s.

    barium s.
    bleomycin s.
    dehydroepiandrosterone s. (DHAS)
    dermatan s.
    dextran sodium s. (DSS)
    ephedrine s.
    ferrous s.
    gentamicin s.
    hydrazine s.
    hyoscyamine s.
    pentosan s.
    protamine s.
    quinidine s.
    sodium dodecyl s. (SDS)
    sodium tetradecyl s.
    tetradecyl s.
sulfated
    s. glycoprotein-2 (SGP-2)
    s. lipid
    s. mucin stain
sulfate-reducing bacterium
sulfation
    tyrosine s.
Sulfatrim DS
sulfhydryl donor
sulfinpyrazone
sulfisoxazole, sulfasoxazole
    s. and phenazopyridine
sulfolithocholylglycine
sulfolithocholyltaurine
sulfomucin
    acidic s.
sulfonamide nephropathy
sulfonate
    mercaptoethane s.
    polystyrene sodium s.
    sodium polystyrene s.
sulfone syndrome
sulfosuccinate
sulfoxide
    dimethyl s. (DMSO)
sulfur, sulphur
    s. amino acid metabolism
    s. colloid (SC)
    s. colloid liver scan
sulfuric acid
sulglycotide
sulindac
Sulkowitch test
sulmarin
sulodexide
sulotroban
sulphate (*var. of* sulfate)
sulphonylurea
sulphur (*var. of* sulfur)
sulpiride
sumach
    sweet s.
sumatriptan succinate

Sumikoshi classification
summer
    s. cholera
    s. diarrhea
summit of bladder
Sumner
    S. method
    S. sign
sump
    s. drain
    s. nasogastric tube
    s. syndrome
    s. ulcer
Sumycin Oral
SUN
    serum urea nitrogen
sunitinib
superantigen
Super-Bright microsphere
SuperChar
Super-Cut scissors
superfibronectin
superficial
    s. abdominal ring
    s. bladder cancer
    s. bladder tumor
    s. depressed cancer
    s. esophageal carcinoma (SEC)
    s. extension
    s. fascia
    s. fluorescein
    s. gastric carcinoma
    s. gastritis
    s. inguinal pouch
    s. linear ulcer
    s. perineal aponeurosis
    s. perineal space
    s. trigonal muscle
superficialis
    arteria epigastrica s.
    colitis cystica s.
    esophagitis dissecans s.
    fascia penis s.
superficially spreading carcinoma
superimposed alcoholic hepatitis
superinfection
    delta hepatitis s.
    hepatitis D s.
superior
    s. aberrant ductule
    arteria epigastrica s.
    arteria mesenterica s.
    arteria rectalis s.
    ductulus aberrans s.
    s. duodenal fold
    s. extremity
    fascia diaphragmatis pelvis s.
    flexura duodeni s.
    s. hemorrhoidal artery

    s. hypogastric nerve plexus
    s. margin
    s. mesenteric angiography
    s. mesenteric arteriogram
    s. mesenteric artery (SMA)
    s. mesenteric artery syndrome
    s. mesenteric to renal artery
      saphenous vein bypass graft
    s. mesenteric vein (SMV)
    s. mesenterorenal bypass
    s. mesenterorenal bypass technique
    s. passive fixation
    plica duodenalis s.
    s. pubic ramotomy
    s. rectal vein
    s. rectal venous plexus
    s. vesical artery
supernatant
supernumerary kidney
superoxide
    s. dismutase
    extracellular s.
    s. production
    s. radical
Super PEG tube
supersaturated bile
supersaturation
    cystine s.
    relative s. (RSs)
    urine s.
superselective
    s. arteriography
    s. transcatheter embolization
    s. vagotomy
supination
supine position
supper
    fat-free s. (FFS)
supplement
    Arctic Omega fish oil s.
    Arginaid dietary s.
    caloric s.
    Cal Power calorie s.
    Casec calcium s.
    Case Power protein s.
    Dent s.
    Enrich protein and calorie s.
    food s.
    Hy-Cal calorie s.
    Impact nutritional s.
    keto acid-amino acid s.
    Maalox antacid/calcium s.
    Nepro diet s.
    Polycose glucose s.
    protein s.
    ProXeed dietary s.
    SAMe nutritional s.
    Spirulina Pacifica nutritional s.
    Travasorb MCT s.

S

supplementation
- calcium s.
- chronic intravenous s.
- citrate s.
- dietary L-arginine s.
- fish oil s.
- prostaglandin s.
- vitamin D s.

supplemented
- nonestrogen s.

support
- artificial hepatic s.
- bioartificial extracorporeal liver s. (BELS)
- bladder s.
- extracorporeal liver s.
- imaging bladder s.
- midurethral s.
- molecular extracorporeal liver s. (MELS)
- nutritional s.
- s. parenteral nutrition (SPN)
- psychological s.
- psychosexual s.
- ventilatory s.

supportive treatment

suppository
- alprostadil urethral s.
- B&O No. 15A, 16A C-II s.
- Canasa s.
- Compro s.
- FIV-ASA s.
- glycerin s.
- intraurethral prostaglandin s. (IPS)
- mesalamine rectal s.
- MUSE urethral s.
- prochlorperazine s.
- Proctocort s.
- rectal s.
- vaginal s.

suppression
- acid s.
- androgen s.
- cell-mediated s.
- hypothalamic s.
- immune s.
- metastasis s.
- s. treatment
- urinary tract infection s.

suppressive
- s. anuria
- s. maneuver

suppressor
- cellular tumor s.
- s. gene
- s. T cell

suppuration

suppurativa
- hidradenitis s.

suppurative
- s. appendicitis
- s. appendix
- s. cholangitis
- s. cortical nephritis
- s. gastritis

supraceliac aorta

supraclavicular

supracolic compartment

supracostal incision

supradiaphragmatic diverticulum

supraduodenal approach

Supra-Foley catheter

supragastric bursoscopy

supraglottic squamous cell carcinoma

suprahepatic
- s. abscess
- s. caval cuff
- s. space
- s. vena cava

suprahilar
- s. disease
- s. lymph node dissection

suprainguinal region

supralevator
- s. anorectal space
- s. pelvic exenteration
- s. perirectal abscess

Supramid suture

supraomental space

suprapapillary
- s. fistula
- s. Roux-en-Y duodenojejunostomy

supraphysiologic fundoplication

supraprostatectomy

suprapubic
- s. approach to suburethral polypropylene (SPARC)
- s. aspiration
- s. aspiration of bladder
- s. cystography
- s. cystostomy
- s. cystotomy
- s. cystotomy tract urethral atresia
- s. drainage
- s. lithotomy
- s. port
- s. prostatectomy
- s. puncture
- s. region
- s. tube

suprarenal
- s. area of liver
- s. gland
- s. Greenfield filter
- s. impression
- s. medulla
- s. plexus

suprarenale
  melasma s.
suprarenalectomy
suprarenalis
  cortex glandulae s.
  medulla glandulae s.
suprarenalism
suprarenalopathy
suprarenogenic syndrome
suprasphincteric fistula
supratrigonal cystectomy
supravesical urinary diversion
sural nerve graft
suramin
Sur-Catch NT stone retrieval basket
SureBite biopsy forceps
SureCath sterile intermittent catheter
Sure-Cut biopsy needle
Sureseal pressure bandage
Suretys
  S. incontinence briefs
  S. pants
  S. panty system
surface
  antimesenteric s.
  biomaterial s.
  bosselated s.
  colonic mucosal s.
  s. cooling
  s. cooling technique
  depression s.
  s. electrode
  s. epithelium
  s. membrane actin cytoskeleton
    complex
  s. nodularity
  s. nodule
  s. pelvic floor electromyography
  s. protein
  serosal s.
  s. thermometer
  urethral cooling s.
  ventral s.
surface-to-volume ratio
surfactant laxative
Surfak
Sur-Fit
  S.-F. auto-lock closed-end pouch
    with filter
  S.-F. minipouch
  S.-F. Natura closed-end pouch,
    opaque
  S.-F. Natura disposable convex
    insert
  S.-F. Natura flange cap
  S.-F. Natura flexible wafer and
    drainable pouch
  S.-F. Natura irrigation adapter
    faceplate

  S.-F. Natura irrigation sleeve
  S.-F. Natura irrigation sleeve tail
    closure
  S.-F. Natura loop ostomy rod
  S.-F. Natura night drainage
    container set
  S.-F. Natura night drainage
    container tubing
  S.-F. Natura opaque closed-end
    pouch with filter
  S.-F. Natura urostomy pouch
  S.-F. Natura Visi-Flow irrigation
    starter set
  S.-F. Natura Visi-Flow irrigator
  S.-F. pouch cover
  S.-F. stoma cap
Surgaloy suture
Surgenomic endoscope
surgeon
  colorectal s.
  genitourinary s.
  Society of American Gastrointestinal
    and Endoscopic S.'s (SAGES)
  urogynecologic s.
surgeon-endoscopist
surgeon's knot
surgery
  abdominal s.
  adrenal-sparing s.
  American Board of Colon and
    Rectal S.
  anal s.
  anorectal s.
  antireflux s.
  bariatric s.
  bench s.
  biliopancreatic obesity s.
  colorectal s. (CRS)
  complex reconstructive s.
  concomitant antireflux s.
  cytoreductive s.
  diagnostic s.
  dialysis access s.
  dysphagia after antireflux s.
  extracorporeal s.
  failed antireflux s.
  feminizing s.
  flank s.
  gastric bypass s. (GBS)
  hand-assisted laparoscopic s. (HALS)
  incontinence s.
  intestinal s.
  intracaval s.
  invasive s.
  invasiveness of s.
  jejunoileal bypass s.
  laparoscopic adrenal gland s.
  laparoscopic antireflux s. (LARS)
  laparoscopic colorectal cancer s.

S

surgery (*continued*)
    laser s.
    major GI s.
    minimal-access s.
    minimally invasive s.
    nephron-sparing s.
    nonbench s.
    open stone s.
    outcome equivalent to open s.
    palliative s.
    parenchyma-sparing s.
    Parietex composite mesh for
      hernia s.
    pelvic colonic s.
    penile reconstructive s.
    penile venous ligation s.
    PlasmaKinetic s.
    portosystemic shunt s.
    postchemotherapy s.
    posterior urethral valve s.
    primary perineal hypospadias s.
    radical s.
    radioimmunoguided s. (RIGS)
    reconstructive s.
    rectovaginal s.
    renal-sparing s.
    renovascular s.
    retrograde intrarenal s.
    retroperitoneal s.
    reversal of jejunoileal bypass s.
    salvage s.
    secondary s.
    sham s.
    stone s.
    subfascial endoscopic perforator s.
      (SEPS)
    systemic s.
    TAAA s.
    telerobotic-assisted laparoscopic s.
    thoracoabdominal aortic aneurysm s.
    transsexual s.
    ureteral reimplantation s.
    urologic s.
    vascular s.
    videoassisted thoracic s. (VATS)
    weight-reduction s.

surgical
    s. abdomen
    s. approach
    s. care
    s. cystogastrostomy
    s. decompression
    s. drain
    s. drape
    s. extirpation
    s. failure
    s. flap
    s. incision
    s. loupe

    s. portosystemic shunt
    s. procedure
    s. scissors
    s. simulation virtual reality
      laboratory
    s. simulator
    s. stapling
    s. stress
    s. therapy
    s. vagotomy

surgically implanted hemodialysis
** catheter (SIHC)**
Surgicel gauze
Surgilube lubricant
Surgi-PEG replacement gastrostomy
** feeding system**
Surgipro
    S. mesh
    S. suture
Surgisis
    S. Gold hernia repair graft
    S. sling/mesh
Surgitek
    S. button
    S. catheter
    S. Flexi-Flate II penile implant
    S. graduated cystoscope
    S. One-Step (SOS)
    S. One-Step percutaneous endoscopic
      gastrostomy
    S. Tractfinder ureteral stent
    S. Uropass stent
Surgitite ligating loop
Surgiwip suture ligature
Surpass
surreptitious vomiting
surrogate marker
surveillance
    s. colonoscopy
    s. cystogram
    endoscopic s.
    s. endoscopy
    Surveillance, Epidemiology, and End
      Results (SEER)
    s. program
    s. protocol
survey
    Digestive Health Status Instrument
      s.
    metabolic bone s.
    National Health and Nutrition
      Examination S. (NHANES)
    Rand Short Form-36 s.
    Third National Health and Nutrition
      Examination S. (NHANES III)
survival
    allograft s.
    s. analysis
    graft s.

improved graft s.
mean allograft s.
overall s.
progression-free s.
s. rate
renal allograft s.
Susano elixir
susceptibility
genetic s.
higher host s.
LDL s.
low-density lipoprotein s.
susceptible population
suspected blood indicator
Suspend sling
suspension
barium sulfate for s.
bladder neck s. (BNS)
Burch urethrovesical s.
charcoal s.
colloidal bismuth s.
Enecat CT concentrated rectal s.
EntroEase Dry powder for
oral s.
EntroEase oral radiopaque contrast
medium s.
extraperitoneal laparoscopic bladder
neck s. (ELBNS)
Formula EM oral s.
Gadolite oral s.
Gittes bladder neck s.
Gittes-Loughlin bladder neck s.
laparoscopic bladder neck s.
leuprolide acetate for injectable s.
Maalox Anti-Gas Extra-Strength oral
s.
Manchester-Fothergill uterine s.
modified Pereyra bladder neck s.
mycophenolate mofetil oral s.
needle bladder neck s.
Nephrox s.
nystatin s.
octreotide acetate for injectable s.
OK432 picibanil streptococcal s.
oral barium s.
percutaneous bladder neck s.
(PBNS)
Pereyra bladder neck s.
Prevacid Packet powder for oral s.
Raz bladder neck s.
Raz needle bladder s.
Raz 4-quadrant s.
Raz urethral s.
retropubic Lapides-Ball bladder
neck s.
Stamey needle bladder neck s.
triptorelin pamoate for injectable s.
urethral s.
vesicoureteral s.

vesicourethral s.
Young-Dees s.
suspensory
s. bandage
s. ligament
s. muscle
suspicion
strong clinical s.
Sustacal
S. HC liquid feeding
S. pudding
Sustagen liquid feeding
sustained
s. detrusor contraction
s. low-efficiency dialysis (SLED)
s. virologic response (SVR)
Sutent
suture
absorbable s.
Albert s.
Albert-Lembert s.
anastomotic s.
anchoring s.
Appolito s.
approximation s.
atraumatic s.
Bell s.
black silk s.
bolster s.
s. bridge
buried s.
button s.
cardinal s.
chain s.
chromic catgut s.
chromic gut s.
circular s.
Connell s.
continuous s.
corner s.
cotton s.
Cushing s.
s. cutter
Czerny s.
Czerny-Lembert s.
Dacron s.
dermal s.
Dermalene s.
Dermalon s.
Dexon s.
Dupuytren s.
Endoloop s.
Ethibond s.
Ethiflex s.
Ethilon s.
everting s.
s. fatigue
figure-of-8 s.
furrier s.

S

suture (*continued*)
- Gambee s.
- Gély s.
- Gould inverted mattress s.
- s. granuloma
- green Mersilene s.
- s. guide
- Gussenbauer s.
- Halsted interrupted mattress s.
- Halsted interrupted quilt s.
- heavy silk s.
- hemostatic s.
- horizontal mattress s.
- Horsley s.
- interrupted manual mucomucosal absorbable s.
- interrupted seromuscular s.
- intracuticular s.
- intradermal s.
- inverting s.
- Ivalon s.
- Jobert de Lamballe s.
- Kessler-Kleinert s.
- Lembert inverting seromuscular s.
- s. ligated
- s. ligature
- s. line
- s. line dehiscence
- s. line ulceration
- locking s.
- lock-stitch s.
- loop s.
- Marshall U-stitch s.
- s. material
- mattress s.
- Maxon s.
- Mersilene s.
- Monocryl s.
- monofilament absorbable s.
- monofilament nylon s.
- nonabsorbable s.
- over-and-over s.
- Parker-Kerr s.
- PDS Vicryl s.
- pericostal s.
- Perma-Hand silk s.
- plain catgut s.
- plain gut s.
- plication s.
- s. plication
- Polydek s.
- polydioxanone s. (PDS)
- polyglactin s.
- polyglecaprone 25 s.
- polyglycolic acid s.
- polyglyconate s.
- polypropylene s.
- pop-off s.
- primary s.
- Prolene s.
- pursestring s.
- quilted s.
- s. rectopexy
- s. rectopexy with sigmoid resection
- reinforcing s.
- relaxation s.
- retention s.
- running s.
- s. scissors
- secondary s.
- seromuscular Lembert s.
- silk Mersilene s.
- silk pop-off s.
- silk traction s.
- stainless steel s.
- stay s.
- subcuticular s.
- Supramid s.
- Surgaloy s.
- Surgipro s.
- swaged-on s.
- Teflon-coated Dacron s.
- Tevdek s.
- Tom Jones s.
- traction s.
- transition s.
- Tycron s.
- s. ulcer
- vascular s.
- vertical mattress s.
- vertical plication s.
- Vicryl s.
- Z s.

sutured hemorrhoidectomy

sutureless
- s. biofragmentable ring
- s. bowel anastomosis
- s. colostomy closure

suture-release needle

suturing
- s. time
- transoral endoscopic s.
- transvaginal s. (TVS)

SuturTek fascia closure device

suum
- *Ascaris* s.

SUZI
- subzonal insemination

SVA
- subtotal villous atrophy

SVG
- seminal vesiculography

SVO
- splenic vein obstruction

SVR
- sustained virologic response
- systemic vascular resistance

SVRI
systemic vascular resistance index
SW
shock wave
SW 480 cell
swab
urethral s.
Swabstick
CHG Maxi S.
swaged needle
swaged-on
s.-o. needle
s.-o. suture
swallow
s. apraxia
barium s.
dry s.
Gastrografin s.
Hypaque s.
ice-water s.
modified barium s. (MBS)
water-soluble contrast
esophageal s.
wet s.
swallowed string
swallowing
air s.
s. center
s. mechanism
4 phases of s.
s. reflex
s. threshold
Swan-Ganz
S.-G. pulmonary artery catheter
S.-G. thermodilution catheter
swan-neck
s.-n. deformity
s.-n. Missouri catheter
s.-n. pediatric Coil-Cath catheter
sweating
gustatory s.
sweat test
Swedish
S. adjustable gastric band
(SAGB)
S. Rectal Cancer Trial
Sween
S. Micro Guard powder
S. Peri-Care moisture barrier
ointment
S. Prep
S. 24 superior moisturizing skin
protectant cream
Sween-A-Peel skin barrier
sweep
duodenal s.
sweet
S. esophageal scissors
s. marjoram

s. orange
s. sumach
S. syndrome
swelling
cell s.
external s.
genital s.
lysosomal s.
popliteal s.
scrotal s.
testicular s.
uvular s.
Swenson
S. abdominal pullthrough
S. operation
S. papillotome
swimmer's itch
swim-up processing
Swiss
S. Lithoclast
S. Lithoclast lithotriptor
S. Lithoclast Master device
S. roll embedding technique
switch
duodenal s.
optic s.
swivel adapter
SWL
shock wave lithotripsy
swollen
s. tongue
s. turbinate
Swyer syndrome
Sydney
S. classification of gastritis
S. system
S. system gastritis classification
Syllact
sylvian fistula
Symadex
Symax Duotab
symbolic stimulus
Syme external urethrotomy
Symington body
Symlin
Symmetra I-125 brachytherapy seed
symmetric face movement
Symmetry endobipolar generator
sympathetic
s. chain
s. cystitis
s. enteroenteric inhibitory reflex
s. nervous system (SNS)
s. nervous system activity
s. projection
s. response to vasodilation
s. skin response
s. sphincter constrictor reflex
symphyseal (*var. of* symphysial)

symphyses (*gen. of* symphysis)
symphysial, symphyseal
    s. bar
symphysis, *gen.* **symphyses**
    s. ossium pubis
    pubic s.
    s. pubis
Symphytum
symptom
    alarm s.
    alcohol-induced gastrointestinal s.
    Bristol female lower urinary tract s.
    Candida s.
    S. Checklist-90R
    chronic functional gastrointestinal s.
    chronic prostatitis-like s.
    s. control
    dyspeptic s.
    extraesophageal s.
    s. free
    head s.
    incarceration s.
    intradialytic s.
    irritative s.
    lower urinary tract s. (LUTS)
    Medical Therapy of Prostatic S.'s
      (MTOPS)
    s. of chronic heartburn
    persistent s.
    postcibal s.
    s. problem index (SPI)
    prodromal s.
    reflux s.
    respiratory s.'s (RS)
    s. score
    s. sensitivity index
    s. severity index (SSI)
    subjective s.
    systematic progression of s.'s
    target s.
    tuberculosis s.
    unresponsive s.
    urgency-frequency s.'s
    urinary s.
    urologic s.
symptomatic
    s. benign prostatic hyperplasia
    s. benign prostatic hypertrophy
    s. fluid gain
    s. gallstone
    s. impotence
    s. varicocele
symptomatology
    chronic functional s.
    lower urinary tract s.
symptom-giving PGR
Syms tractor
Synalar Topical
Synalgos-DC capsule

synapse
    axoaxonic s.
synaptic transmission
synaptogenesis
synbiotic
synchondroseotomy
SynchroMed infusion system intraspinal
  catheter
Synchron automated analyzer
synchronous
    s. adenoma
    s. bladder reconstruction
    s. inferior cavography
    s. lesion
    s. neonatal torsion
    s. polyp
    s. superior cavography
    s. urinary tract infection
syncope
    defecation s.
syncytium
syndrome
    Aagenaes s.
    Aarskog s.
    Aarskog-Scott s.
    abdominal compartment s.
      (ACS)
    abdominal cutaneous nerve
      entrapment s.
    abdominal muscle deficiency s.
    acquired immunodeficiency s.
      (AIDS)
    acute flank pain s.
    acute nephritic s.
    acute urethral s.
    Adamantiades-Behçet s.
    Addison s.
    addisonian s.
    adrenogenital s.
    afferent loop s.
    Alagille s.
    Alagille-Watson s.
    Alcock s.
    Allemann s.
    Allen-Masters s.
    Alport s.
    Alstrom-Edwards s.
    Andersen s.
    androgen insensitivity s.
    androgenital s.
    anorexia-cachexia s.
    anterior abdominal wall s.
    anterior cord s.
    anterior rib impingement s.
    anterior spinal artery s.
    antiandrogen withdrawal s.
    anticardiolipin antibody s.
    antimüllerian derivative s.
    antiphospholipid s.

apparent mineral corticoid excess s.
apple-peel bowel s.
Arias s.
Asherson s.
asplenia s.
autoimmune deficiency s.
autosomal-recessive Alport s.
bacterial overgrowth s.
Bannayan-Ruvalcaba-Riley s.
Bannayan-Zonana s.
Banti s.
Bardet-Biedl s.
Barrett s.
Barsony-Polgar s.
Bartter s.
basal cell nevus s.
Bassen-Kornzweig s.
Baumgarten s.
Bazex s.
Bearn-Kunkel-Slater s.
Beckwith-Wiedemann s.
Behçet s.
bent nail s.
Bernard-Sergent s.
Bernard-Soulier s.
Bessauds-Hilmand-Augier s.
BHD s.
bilharzial bladder cancer s.
Birt-Hogg-Dube s.
Blatin s.
blind loop s. (BLS)
blue diaper s.
blue rubber bleb nevus s.
Boerhaave s.
Bouveret s.
bowel bypass s.
branchiootorenal s.
Brennemann s.
brown bowel s.
Budd s.
Budd-Chiari s. (BCS)
Bürger-Grütz s.
buried bumper s.
Burnett s.
burning mouth s. (BMS)
Byler s.
Bywaters s.
Cacchi-Ricci s.
cafe coronary s.
Canada-Cronkhite s.
carcinoid s.
Carignan s.
Caroli s.
Carpenter s.
Carter-Horsley-Hughes s.
cast s.
cat-eye s.
caudal regression s.
Cecil urethral stricture s.

celiac s.
cerebrohepatorenal s. (CHRS)
cerebrooculofacial s.
CHARGE s.
Cheek-Perry s.
Chilaiditi s.
Chinese restaurant s. (CRS)
cholestatic s.
cholesterol embolus s.
cholinergic s.
chronic intestinal ischemic s.
chronic intestinal
  pseudoobstruction s.
chronic pelvic pain s. (CPPS)
chronic prostate pain s. (CPPS)
chronic prostatitis/pelvic pain s.
chronic urethral s.
Cohen s.
colonic polyposis s.
colonic pseudoobstruction s.
colonic solitary ulcer s.
colorectal cancer s.
compression s.
congenital nephrotic s. (CNS)
Conn s.
constipation-predominant irritable
  bowel s.
Cooke-Apert-Gallais s.
Courvoisier-Terrier s.
couvade s.
Cowden s.
CREST s.
Crigler-Najjar s. type I, II
Cronkhite-Canada s.
CRST s.
crush s.
Cruveilhier-Baumgarten s.
Curran s.
Cushing medicamentosus s.
cyclic vomiting s. (CVS)
Danbolt-Closs s.
Debré-de Toni-Fanconi s.
Degos s.
Dejerine-Sottas s.
del Castillo s.
dengue shock s.
Denys-Drash s.
descending perineum s.
de Toni-Debré-Fanconi s.
de Toni-Fanconi-Debré s.
dialysis disequilibrium s. (DDS)
dialysis equilibrium s.
d. encephalopathy syndrome
diarrhea-predominant irritable bowel
  s.
diffuse alveolar hemorrhage s.
Diogenes s.
Down s.
Drash s.

S

syndrome (*continued*)

Dubin-Johnson s.
Dubin-Sprinz s.
Dubowitz s.
dumping s.
dyskinetic cilia s.
dysmetabolic s.
dysuria-pyuria s.
Eagle-Barrett s.
early dumping s.
Edwards s.
efferent loop s.
Ehlers-Danlos s.
empty sella s.
eosinophilic gastroenteritis s.
Epstein s.
Faber s.
faciodigital s.
familial atypical multiple-mole
  melanoma s.
familial chylomicronemia s.
familial polyposis s.
FAMM s.
Fanconi s.
Fanconi-de Toni-Debré s.
fatty liver and kidney s. (FLKS)
Fechtner s.
Felty s.
female urethral s.
fertile eunuch s.
fibromyalgia s.
Fiessinger-Leroy-Reiter s.
Fitz s.
Fitz-Hugh and Curtis s.
Flood s.
flulike s.
flushing s.
food protein-induced enterocolitis s.
  (FPIES)
Fraley s.
Fraser s.
frequency-urgency-pain s.
Friderichsen-Waterhouse s.
Fröhlich s.
functional bowel s.
G s.
Galloway-Mowat s.
Gardner s.
Gardner-Diamond s.
gas-bloat s.
Gasser s.
gasserian s.
gastrocardiac s.
gastrointestinal immunodeficiency s.
gastrojejunal loop obstruction s.
GAVE s.
gay bowel s.
Gee-Herter-Heubner s.
Gianotti-Crosti s.

Gilbert s.
Gilbert-Behçet s.
Gilbert-Dreyfus s.
Gitelman s.
glioma-polyposis s.
glucagonoma s.
Goldenhar s.
Goldston s.
Goodpasture s.
Gopalan s.
Gordon s.
Gorlin basal cell nevus s.
Gorlin-Chaudhry-Moss s.
Gowers s.
Guillain-Barré s. (GBS)
gynecomastia-aspermatogenesis s.
Hadefield-Clarke s.
Hadju-Cheney acroosteolysis s.
Hanot s.
Hanot-Chauffard s.
Hanot-Rössle s.
Hartnup s.
Hawes-Pallister-Landor s.
Heller-Nelson s.
HELLP s.
hematuria-dysuria s.
hemolytic-uremic s.
hemorrhagic fever with renal s.
hepatopulmonary s. (HPS)
hepatorenal s. (HRS)
hereditary flat adenoma s.
hereditary nonpolyposis colorectal
  cancer s.
Hermansky-Pudlak s.
Heyde s.
Hinman s.
Hinman-Allen s.
Hippel-Lindau s.
Holt-Oram s.
hormone-secreting tumor s.
Horner s.
Howel-Evans s.
HPRC s.
hungry bone s.
hyperammonemic s.
hyperdynamic s.
hypereosinophilia s.
hypertensive lower esophageal
  sphincter s.
hypoperistalsis s.
iatrogenic immunodeficiency s.
idiopathic hypereosinophilic s. (IHES)
idiopathic nephrotic s.
ileocecal s.
Imerslund s.
immotile cilia s.
impaired regeneration s.
infantile food protein-induced
  enterocolitis s.

infantile nephrotic s.
inflammatory bowel s. (IBS)
infrequent voider-lazy bladder s.
inhibitory s.
inspissated bile s.
inspissated sump s.
insulin resistance s.
intestinal polyposis-cutaneous
  pigmentation s.
intestinal stasis s.
irrigation-fluid absorption s.
irritable bowel s. (IBS)
irritable colon s.
irritable gut s.
irritable male s.
irritable pouch s.
isolated retained antrum s.
Ivemark s.
Jamaican vomiting s.
jejunal s.
Jeune s.
Job s.
Johanson-Blizzard s.
Joseph s.
juvenile polyposis s. (JPS)
Kallmann s.
Karroo s.
Kartagener s.
Kasabach-Merritt s.
Katayama s.
Kaufman s.
Kawasaki s.
Kearns-Sayre s.
Kimmelstiel-Wilson s.
Klinefelter s.
Klippel-Trenaunay-Weber s.
Koenig s.
Koro s.
Korsakoff s.
Kunkel s.
Labbe s.
Ladd s.
late dumping s.
Laubry-Soulle s.
Launois-Cléret s.
Laurence-Moon-Bardet-Biedl s.
Laurence-Moon-Biedl s.
lazy bladder s.
leaky gut s.
LEOPARD s.
Lesch-Nyhan s.
levator ani s.
Liddle s.
Lightwood s.
Lignac s.
Lignac-Fanconi s.
locker room s.
loin pain hematuria s. (LPHS)
Lowe s.

Lubb s.
Lucey-Driscoll s.
Luder-Sheldon s.
lymphadenopathy s.
lymphoproliferative s.
Lynch s. II
Mad Hatter s.
Maffucci s.
malabsorption s.
maldigestion-absorption s.
male Turner s.
malignant B-cell s.
malignant carcinoid s.
Mallory-Weiss s.
Maranon s.
Marchiafava-Micheli s.
Marfan s.
Marinesco-Sjögren s.
massive bowel resection s.
McArdle s.
McCune-Albright s.
Meckel s.
Meckel-Gruber s.
meconium plug s.
megacystic s.
megacystis-megaureter s.
megacystis-microcolon-intestinal
  hypoperistalsis s.
megasigmoid s.
MELAS s.
Melkersson-Rosenthal s.
MEN I s.
mesenteric steal s.
metastatic carcinoid s.
microscopic colitis s.
milk-alkali s.
Miller Fisher s.
mind-bladder s.
minimal-change nephrotic s.
minimal-lesion nephrotic s.
Mirizzi s.
mitochondrial neurogastrointestinal
  encephalomyopathy s.
Mosse s.
Muckle-Wells s.
mucocutaneous pigmentation of
  Peutz-Jeghers s.
mucosal prolapse s.
Muir-Torre s.
müllerian duct derivation s.
multiple endocrine neoplasia s.
  (MENS)
multiple hamartoma s.
multiple-organ failure s.
Munchausen s.
myoclonus-opsoclonus s.
narcotic bowel s.
necrolytic migratory erythema s.
nephritic s.

syndrome (*continued*)
    nephrotic s.
    nerve entrapment s.
    Neu-Laxova s.
    Nonnenbruch s.
    nutcracker s.
    obesity hypoventilation s. (OHS)
    Ochoa s.
    oculocerebrorenal s.
    s. of chloride depletion
    s. of inappropriate secretion of
      antidiuretic hormone (SIADH)
    s. of primary biliary cirrhosis
    Ogilvie s.
    Oldfield s.
    oligoteratoasthenozoospermia s.
    Opitz-Frias s.
    Ormond s.
    Osler II s.
    Osler-Weber-Rendu s.
    osmotic demyelination s.
    outlier s.
    ovarian hyperstimulation s.
    ovarian overstimulation s.
    ovarian remnant s.
    ovarian vein s.
    overlap s.
    pain-associated disability s.
    pain-predominant irritable bowel s.
    pancreatic cholera s.
    pancreaticohepatic s.
    paraneoplastic s.
    Paterson-Kelly s.
    Payr s.
    Pearson s.
    pelvic floor s.
    Pento-X s.
    pericolic membrane s.
    perihepatitis s.
    persistent müllerian duct s.
    Peutz-Jeghers s. (PJS)
    pharyngeal pouch s.
    Picchini s.
    pickwickian s.
    Pierre Robin s.
    Plummer-Vinson s.
    POEMS s.
    Polhemus-Schafer-Ivemark s.
    POLIP s.
    polyposis s.
    polysplenia s.
    postcholecystectomy s. (PCS)
    postcoagulation s.
    postcolonoscopy distention s.
    postenteritis s.
    postfundoplication s.
    postgastrectomy s.
    postpolypectomy coagulation s.
    postthrombotic s.

posttransurethral microwave
    thermotherapy prostatitis-like s.
post-TUMT prostatitis-like s.
postvagotomy s.
Potter s.
Prader-Willi s.
primary antiphospholipid s.
primary pseudoobstruction s.
pseudo-Cushing s.
pseudoobstruction s.
pseudopancreatic cholera s.
pseudoprune-belly s.
puborectalis s.
Rapunzel s.
refeeding s.
Reichmann s.
Reifenstein s.
Reiter s.
renal Fanconi-like s.
renal-hepatic steal s.
renal-ocular s.
renal-retinal s.
Rendu-Osler-Weber s.
reset osmostat s.
retained antrum s.
retained bladder s.
reuse s.
reversed anorexia s.
Reye s. (RS)
Richner-Hanhart s.
Rieger s.
right ovarian vein s.
Riley-Day s.
RMS s.
Roberts s.
Robinow s.
Roger s.
Rome I, II criteria for irritable
    bowel s.
Rosewater s.
Rothmund-Thomson s.
Rotor s.
Roux stasis s.
Rovsing s.
Rud s.
rudimentary testis s.
runting s.
Russell-Silver s.
Ruvalcaba-Myhre-Smith s.
Sandifer s.
Satoyoshi s.
Schmidt s.
Schultz s.
Schwartz-Jampel s.
SCO s.
sea-blue histiocyte s.
secondary pseudoobstruction s.
segmental colonic adenomatous
    polyposis s.

Senior-Loken s.
sepsis s.
Sertoli-cell-only s.
serum sicknesslike s.
sex reversal s.
short-bowel s.
short-gut s.
Shwachman s.
Shwachman-Diamond s.
Shy-Drager s.
sicca s.
sick cell s.
sinusoidal obstruction s.
Sipple s.
Sjögren s.
sloughed urethra s.
small stomach s.
Smith-Lemli-Opitz s.
solitary rectal ulcer s.
somatostatinoma s.
spastic bowel s.
spastic pelvic floor s.
sphincteric disobedience s.
Spitzer-Weinstein s.
splenic agenesis s.
splenic flexure s.
Sprinz-Dubin s.
Sprinz-Nelson s.
stagnant loop s.
stasis s.
Stauffer s.
steakhouse s.
Stein-Leventhal s.
steroid-resistant nephrotic s.
Stevens-Johnson s.
Stewart-Treves s.
Stokvis-Talma s.
Strachan s.
Strachan-Scott s.
stress-related erosive s.
Sturge-Weber s.
sulfone s.
sump s.
superior mesenteric artery s.
suprarenogenic s.
Sweet s.
Swyer s.
systemic inflammatory response s.
  (SIRS)
TAR s.
telangiectasia s.
terminal reservoir s.
testicular feminization s.
tethered-cord s.
thoracic endometriosis s.
Thorn salt-depletion s.
thrombocytopenia-absent radius s.
TINU s.
tissue matrix s.

Torres s.
Townes-Brocks s.
toxic shock s. (TSS)
transurethral resection s.
tremor-nystagmus-ulcer s.
triad s.
tropical diarrhea-malabsorption s.
  (TDMS)
Trousseau s.
tubulointerstitial nephritis and uveitis
  s.
tumor lysis s.
TUR s.
Turcot s.
Turner s.
Ullrich-Turner s.
uremic s.
urethral s.
urethritis s.
urge s.
VACTERL s.
vanished testis s.
vascular steal s.
VATER s.
venous leak s.
Verner-Morrison s.
vertebral, anal, cardiac,
  tracheoesophageal fistula, renal,
  limb s.
vertebral, anal, tracheoesophageal
  fistula, renal s.
Vinson s.
VIPoma s.
von Hippel-Lindau s. (vHL)
Vulcan s.
vulvar vestibulitis s.
WAGR s.
wasting s.
Waterhouse-Friderichsen s.
watery diarrhea, hypokalemia, and
  achlorhydria s.
Watson-Alagille s.
WDHA s.
3-week sulfasalazine s.
Weil s.
Weinstein s.
Welt s.
Wermer s.
Wernicke s.
Wernicke-Korsakoff s.
Whipple s.
Wiedemann-Beckwith s.
Williams s.
Wiskott-Aldrich s.
Wolfram s.
X-linked Alport s.
XX male s.
XYY male s.
Young s.

S

syndrome (*continued*)
    Youssef s.
    Zanca s.
    ZE s.
    Zellweger s.
    Zieve s.
    Zollinger-Ellison s.
synechia, *pl.* **synechiae**
    penile s.
synechiae (*pl. of* synechia)
synectenterotomy
Synectics
    S. computer program
    S. 6000 digital pH meter
    S. PC Polygraf 16HR
    S. visceral stimulator electronic
      barostat
Synectics-Dantec
    S.-D. Flo-Lab II uroflowmeter
    S.-D. UD10000 uroflowmeter
synergism
    in vitro s.
synergistic combination
Synergist vacuum erection device
synergy
Syn-Optics videoimage splitter
synorchidism, synorchism
synorchism (*var. of* synorchidism)
synoscheos
synovial fluid
Synthamin amino acid solution
synthase
    aldosterone s.
    citrate s.
    induced nitric oxide s. (iNOS)
    nitric oxide s.
syntheses (*pl. of* synthesis)
synthesis, *pl.* **syntheses**
    albumin s.
    apolipoprotein s.
    collagen s.
    dihydrotestosterone s.
    DNA s.
    eicosanoid s.
    focal collagen s.
    hepatocyte protein s.
    hormone-stimulated cAMP s.
    impaired lecithin s.
    mucosal prostaglandin s.
    prostaglandin s.
    prostanoid s.
    protein s.
    pyrimidine s.
    renin s.
    urea s.
synthesizer
    deoxyribonucleic acid s.
synthetase
    uroporphyrinogen s. (UROS)

synthetic
    s. 5-channel water-perfused motility
      catheter
    s. ^{13}C-urea
    s. mesh
    s. porcine secretin
    s. porcine secretin for injection
    s. vascular graft
Synthroid
syphilis
    anorectal s.
    gastric s.
    primary s.
    secondary s.
    serologic test for s. (STS)
    tertiary s.
syphilitic
    s. gastritis
    s. hepatitis
    s. inguinal adenitis
    s. nephritis
    s. stigma
syphiloma of Fournier
syringe
    Arrow Raulerson s.
    Asepto irrigation s.
    aspiration s.
    Fortuna s.
    LeVeen inflation s.
    Lewy s.
    Luer s.
    Luer-Lok s.
    motor s.
    Neisser s.
    piston-type s.
    s. shield
    Storz s.
    Toomey s.
    tuberculin s.
    Wolff s.
syringocele
    Cowper s.
syringoma
syrosingopine
syrup
    Calcidrine s.
    ipecac s.
    s. of glycyrrhiza
system
    Abbott Lifeshield needleless s.
    Ablatherm HIFU s.
    Adacolumn Apheresis S.
    Advantx digital s.
    Agile patency s.
    AJCC/UICC staging s.
    Aksys PHD s.
    Alimaxx-E esophageal stent s.
    alimentary s.
    Alliance II inflation s.

Alliance integrated inflation s.
Allient Sorbent hemodialysis s.
AlloMune s.
American Medical S.'s (AMS)
Amplatz TractMaster s.
AMS ProstaJect ethanol injection s.
Ancure abdominal aortic aneurysm s.
AneuRx stent graft s.
AngioJet rapid thrombectomy s.
AngioJet Rheolytic thrombectomy s.
Anodyne therapy s.
anomalous arrangement of pancreaticobiliary ductal s.
antigen-antibody s.
APACHE-II, -III scoring s.
AquaSens fluid monitoring s.
Arndorfer capillary perfusion s.
Arndorfer pneumohydraulic capillary infusion s.
Arrow UserGard injection cap s.
ASAP Stacker automated multisample biopsy s.
autofluorescent endoscopic s.
automatic titration s.
autonomic nervous s. (ANS)
Balthazar grading s.
Bard EndoCinch endoscopic suturing s.
Bard Urolase fiber laser s.
Baveno portal hypertensive gastropathy grading s.
Baxter Interline IV s.
Beamer injection stent s.
BELS s.
Bergkvist grading s.
BICAP hemostatic s.
bicarbonate buffer s.
BiliBlanket phototherapy s.
bioartificial extracorporeal liver support s.
BioLogic-DT s.
BioLogic-DTPF s.
Bitome bipolar s.
B-lymphocyte s.
Bookwalter retractor s.
Borrmann gastric cancer typing s. type I-IV
Boyarsky symptom scoring s.
Bravo Catheter-Free pH testing s.
Bridge Assurant biliary stent delivery s.
Bridge X3 renal stent s.
Browning and Parks continence grading s. category A, B, C, D
Bruel-Kjaer 1846 ultrasound s.
buffer s.
Caldwell needle/cannula Quick-Tap paracentesis s.

Can-Opt dual-lumen ERCP s.
CathTrack catheter locator s.
cell analysis s.
Cell Recovery S. (CRS)
Cell Soft s.
central nervous s. (CNS)
Ceralas PDT 633 diode laser s.
classification s.
Clave needleless s.
closed-suction drainage s.
Coban 2-layer compression s.
coculture s.
collecting s.
Colormate TLc BiliTest S.
Color Quad S.
Comhaire grading s.
computer-aided diagnostic s.
computer-controlled sedation infusion s.
computerized image analysis s.
ConMed biliary s.
Conseal 1-piece continent colostomy s.
contact-tip laser s.
Contrajet ERCP contrast delivery s.
Cool-tip RF ablation s.
core-cut s.
COSTART s.
cost-conscious healthcare s.
COX enzyme s.
CS-5 cryosurgical s.
CSM Stretta s.
C-Trak surgical guidance s.
cytochrome P450 enzyme s.
Dantec 12-channel Urocolor Video s.
Dantec Menuet s.
DASH s.
daughter endoscopic retrograde cholangiopancreatoscopy s.
da Vinci robotic s.
da Vinci surgical s.
Debioclip single-dose delivery s.
Dentsleeve pneumohydraulic perfusion s.
Desmet/Scheurer staging s.
digestive s.
Digitrapper Mark II pH monitoring s.
Dionex 2000 s.
Director guidewire s.
DNA sequencing s.
Doppler Quantum color flow s.
Dornier MPL 9000 electrohydraulic lithotriptor ultrasound focusing s.
double-antibody sandwich s.
double-balloon endoscopy s.
doxazosin gastrointestinal therapy s.
Drake-Willock delivery s.

S

system (*continued*)
    Drake-Willock peritoneal dialysis s.
    drug carrier s.
    dual-port s.
    ductal s.
    Dukes staging s.
    Dumon-Gilliard endoprosthesis s.
    duplex collecting s.
    Dynalink biliary self-expanding stent s.
    EdGr s.
    Edmondson grading s.
    e10 electrosurgery s.
    EndoCinch suturing s.
    endocrine s.
    Endo-Dop transendoscopic Doppler catheter probe s.
    endoscopic s.
    endoscopic video information s. (EVIS)
    enteric nervous s. (ENS)
    Enterra Therapy implantable neurostimulation s.
    ErecAid vacuum s.
    Esteem synergy ostomy s.
    EVIS EXERA video s.
    FastPack s.
    Fisher capillary s.
    Flexiflo Top-Fill enteral nutrition s.
    Flexi-Seal FMS fecal diversion and containment s.
    free-beam laser s.
    French Pharmacovigilance s.
    Fresenius volumetric dialysate balancing s.
    Fujinon SP-501 sonoprobe s.
    Fujinon videoendoscopy s.
    Garden prognostic s.
    GaSampler collection s.
    GastrograpH ambulatory pH monitoring s.
    gastrointestinal s. (GIS)
    gastrointestinal therapeutic s. (GITS)
    Gatekeeper reflux repair s.
    Gatta prognostic s.
    GERDcheck ambulatory esophageal pH monitoring s.
    Given diagnostic imaging s.
    Given videocapsule s.
    Gleason grading s.
    Grabstald Memorial staging s.
    Gynecare TVT support s.
    Gyrus endourology s.
    HandPort s.
    hemi-Kock s.
    hemodiadsorption s.
    HepatAssist liver support s.
    Hewlett-Packard IVUS imaging s.
    high-affinity low-capacity s.

    high-affinity sodium-dependent phosphate transport s.
    Hind-SITE 20/20 s.
    H+/K+-ATPase enzyme s.
    Hp Chek screening s.
    HP7754 pneumohydraulic capillary infusion s.
    human cytochrome P-450 enzyme s.
    Hybrid Capture s.
    hydraulic capillary infusion s.
    Hydra Vision Es urologic imaging s.
    Hydra Vision IV urology s.
    Hydra Vision Plus DR urologic imaging s.
    illumination s.
    immune s.
    Impact lithotriptor s.
    implantable gastric stimulation s.
    implantable neuromodulation s.
    IMx PSA s.
    InCare PRES 9300 s.
    Indigo LaserOptic treatment s.
    Indigo Optima laser s.
    InjecAid s.
    Innova home incontinence therapy s.
    InSIGHT manometry s.
    integrated automatic stone-tissue detection s.
    intensified radiographic imaging s. (IRIS)
    International Biomedical microcapillary infusion s.
    intracellular signaling s.
    intrarenal collecting s.
    IsoMed constant-flow infusion s.
    iterative bifid branching s.
    IVAC needleless IV s.
    Jackson staging s.
    Janus S. III
    Jewett staging s.
    Jewett-Strong s.
    Jewett-Whitmore cancer staging s.
    Johns Hopkins prostate cancer grading s.
    Joyce-Loebl Magiscan image analysis s.
    Kangaroo delivery s.
    kidney collecting s.
    Kleinert Safe and Dry panty and pad s.
    Kretz ultrasound s.
    KTP 532 laser s.
    KTP/YAG surgical laser s.
    LAGB s.
    Lambda Plus PDL 1, 2 laser s.
    Laparolift s.
    laparoscopic retraction s.

Laparoshield laparoscopic smoke filtration s.
Laser CHRP rigid fiberscope s.
LifeSite hemodialysis access s.
Lithostar Plus electromagnetic lithotriptor bidimensional x-ray focusing s.
liver dialysis s.
low-affinity high-capacity s.
low-compliance perfusion s.
low-pressure venous s.
Madsen-Iversen scoring s.
magnifying endoscopy with narrow-band image s.
Marlen Ultramax 1-piece disposable ostomy s.
Mayo grading s.
mechanical assist s.
MediClenze hygiene and water therapy s.
Mediflex MD-7 endoscopic video s.
Medstone IRIS s.
Medstone STS lithotripsy s.
MetaFluor s.
microsomal ethanol oxidizing s. (MEOS)
Microvasive biliary stent s.
Microvasive Ultraflex esophageal stent s.
mitochondrial ethanol oxidase s.
molecular adsorbent recirculating s. (MARS)
MOP-Videoplan morphometric s.
Morganstern aspiration/injection s.
mother-baby endoscope s.
mother-baby scope s.
mother endoscopic retrograde cholangiopancreatoscopy s.
Mui Scientific pressurized capillary infusion s.
Multipulse laser s.
Mycotrim triphasic culture s.
myeloperoxidase-H2O2-halide s.
NA+-linked cotransport s.
narrow-band imaging endoscopy s.
NA+ transport s.
Natura ostomy s.
needleless s.
Oasis tube s.
obstructed collecting s.
OEC-Diasonics 9400 fluoroscopy C-arm s.
Okuda staging s.
Olympus CLV-series fiberoptic s.
Olympus endoscopy s. (OES)
Olympus EVIS color computer chip s.
Olympus GF-UM3, -UM20 s.
Olympus MAJ363 FNA needle s.

Olympus OSP fluorescence measuring s.
Olympus videoendoscopy s.
Olympus videourology procedure s.
Omni-LapoTract support s.
One Action Stent Introduction S. (OASIS)
Opmilas 144 Plus laser s.
optic multichannel analyzer s.
Ortho Diagnostic S.
O'Sullivan scoring s.
oxybutynin transdermal s.
Oxytrol transdermal s.
Palco enuretic alarm s.
Palmaz Corinthian biliary stent and delivery s.
pancreaticobiliary ductal s.
P blood group s.
pelvicalyceal s.
Percutaneous Stoller Afferent Nerve Stimulation S.
Performa ultrasound s.
PerQ SANS s.
Personal Scanner TM 18 bedside real-time ultrasonography s.
pneumohydraulic capillary infusion s.
Polachrome slide s.
portable perfused manometric s.
portal venous s.
Precision office TUNA s.
Precision QID glucose monitoring s.
Precision SpeedTac transvaginal anchor s.
Precision Tack transvaginal anchor s.
Precision Twist transvaginal anchor s.
Prempree modification staging s.
probenecid-inhibited organic anion transport s.
Prolieve microwave therapy s.
Proscan ultrasound imaging s.
Prostalase laser s.
ProstaLund CoreTherm s.
Prostathermer prostatic hyperthermia s.
Prostatron microwave s.
Prostiva RF therapy s.
Pugh-Child scoring s.
Quick-Tap paracentesis s.
Raman spectroscopic s.
Ranson grading s.
Redy hemodialysis s.
Relay suture delivery s.
renal kallikrein-kinin s.
renal preservation-perfusion s.
renin-aldosterone s.
renin-angiotensin s. (RAS)

S

system (*continued*)

renin-angiotensin-aldosterone s. (RAAS)
reproductive s.
reticuloendothelial s.
Reuter suprapubic trocar and cannula s.
rod-lens s.
RX Herculink 14 biliary stent s.
RX Herculink Plus biliary stent s.
RX stent delivery s.
Sacks-Vine PEG s.
Safe and Dry panty and pad s.
Savary-Gilliard dilating s.
Secca radiofrequency s.
SeedNet cryotherapy s.
sentry s.
SF-9 baculovirus-insect cell s.
Signa Excite MRI s.
single-action pumping s.
slide s.
Soehendra catheter s.
SOLO-Surg Colorectal self-retaining retractor s.
Sonablate 200 s.
Sonoline SI-200/250 ultrasound imaging s.
Sonoprobe endoscopic ultrasonography s.
sorbent dialysate regeneration s.
SPARC sling s.
SPR Plus III low-air-loss s.
StayErec s.
stent and vent s.
Stoller scoring s.
stone recognition s.
stone-tissue detection s. (STDS)
stone-tissue recognition s.
Storz multifunction valve trocar/cannula s.
STR s.
Straight-In male sling s.
Straight-In surgical s.
Stretta s.
Striant buccal s.
STS lithotripsy s.
Suretys panty s.
Surgi-PEG replacement gastrostomy feeding s.
Sydney s.
sympathetic nervous s. (SNS)
Talent LPS endoluminal stent-graft s.
Targis microwave catheter-based s.
Technos ultrasound s.
telerobotic s.
terminal bifid branching s.
testosterone buccal s.
testosterone transdermal s. (TTS)

Therasonics lithotripsy s.
ThermoChem-HT s.
ThermoFlex s.
tissue-stone recognition s. (TSRS)
TMx-2000 BPH thermotherapy s.
Top Notch automated biopsy s.
transdermal therapeutic s. (TTS)
Transfix sutureless sling fixation s.
transvaginal suturing s.
tricomponent coaxial s.
triple-lumen perfused catheter s.
Truelove-Witts grading s.
TVS s.
UltraBag dialysis s.
UltraPak enteral closed feeding s.
Ultraseed s.
Ultra Twin bag s.
Ultra Y-set s.
UnDiet spray weight loss s.
United States Renal Data S. (USRDS)
Universal sheath s.
University of California at Los Angeles staging s.
Urgent PC sacral neuromodulation s.
Urocyte diagnostic cytometry s.
Uro-jet delivery s.
Urolab Janus S. III
Uro-Pak s.
Urotract x-ray s.
UroVive self-contained balloon s.
UroVysion ultrasound imaging s.
Vaccine Adverse Event Reporting S.
varix grading s. F1, F2, F3
Vet-Co vacuum s.
ViaCath computer-assisted robotic endoluminal s.
ViaCath endoluminal surgery s.
Virtual Biopsy s.
Visick gastric cancer grading s.
Vision Sciences Inc. flexible sigmoidoscope s.
VitalStim Therapy electrical stimulation s.
Vivonex Acutrol enteral feeding s.
Vocare bladder s.
V-sign single-ear sensory s.
Welch Allyn videoendoscopy s.
Whitmore-Jewitt prostate cancer classification s.
wireless M2A videocapsule s.
Wolf delivery s.
wolffian ductal s.
WuScope s.
Xillix LIFE-Lung s.
Y-set s.

Zeiss fluorescein filter s.
Zenith AAA endovascular graft s.
Zenith abdominal aortic aneurysm endovascular graft s.
Zieve s.
Z-stent esophageal endoprosthesis s.

systematic

s. progression of symptoms
s. sextant biopsy

systemic

s. amyloidosis
s. arterial pressure
s. *Candida*
s. duodenal sclerosis
s. effect
s. endotoxemia
s. hypertension
s. hypotension
s. inflammatory response syndrome (SIRS)
s. lupus erythematosus (SLE)
s. lupus erythematosus vasculitis
s. mast cell disease
s. mastocytosis
s. mercury intoxication
s. radiation therapy
s. sclerosis
s. surgery
s. vascular resistance (SVR)
s. vascular resistance index (SVRI)
s. venodilation

systolic

s. click
s. murmur

Szabo-Berci needle driver
Szabo test

S

T

T antigen
T bandage
T binder
T clamp
T connector
T drain
T effector cell
T fastener
T lymphocyte
T tube
T tubogram
T wave

TAAA

thoracoabdominal aortic aneurysm
TAAA surgery

tabes

t. dorsalis
t. mesaraica
t. mesenterica

tabetic

table

Aub-Dubois t.
Dornier Urotract cystoscopy t.
floating t.
Gerhardt t.
lithotripsy t.
Maquet endoscopy t.
Multifunctional Opus surgical t.
Partin t.
sigmoidoscopy t.
Urodiagnost x-ray t.

tablet

alosetron HCl t.
Asacol delayed-release t.
Body Fortress Natural
  Amino t.
Cal Carb 600 with Vitamin D
  antacid t.
Cal Carb 600 with Vitamin D
  dietary supplement t.
Chenix T.
Dairy Ease chewable t.
delayed-release t.
Hemocyte-F t.
Hemocyte Plus t.
hyoscyamine sulfate orally
  disintegrating t.
L-carnitine t.
Lotronex t.
Maalox Quick Dissolve
  chewable t.
Magsal t.
Monocal t.
mycophenolate mofetil t.

NuLev orally disintegrating t.
Nullo deodorant t.
Pantoloc t.
pantoprazole sodium
  delayed-release t.
Peptic Relief chewable t.
Protonix delayed-release t.
Rapamune t.
Renagel t.
sevelamer hydrochloride t.
sirolimus t.
Strong Start chewable t.
tegaserod maleate t.
Urex t.
Visicol t.
Vitelle Nesentials t.
Vitelle Nestrex t.
wax-matrix t.
Zelnorm t.

TA90-BN stapler

Tabs

Hydro-T T.
Urabeth T.

tabule

Mediplex Ultra t.

TAC

total abdominal colectomy

TACE

transarterial catheter embolization
transarterial chemoembolization
transcatheter arterial chemoembolization

tachygastria
tachykinin-bombesin family
tachykinin component
tachyphylaxis
tachypnea
tacked down
tacrolimus
tacrolimus-associated microangiopathy
tactile

t. feedback result
t. probe

Tactyl 1 glove
TACurea

timed average urea concentration

tadalafil
tadpolelike appearance
taenia (*var. of* tenia), *pl.* **taeniae**

T. saginata
T. solium

taenial (*var. of* tenial)
taeniasis (*var. of* teniasis)
taeniform (*var. of* teniform)
taenioides

Diphyllobothrium t.

tag
- edematous t.
- external skin t.
- hemorrhoidal t.
- H-shaped tilt t.
- perianal skin t.
- perineal skin t.
- sentinel t.
- skin t.

Tagamet HB
tagatose
tagged
- t. erythrocyte scintigraphy
- t. red blood cell bleeding scan

tagging
- fecal t.
- t. stitch

TAG-72 glycoprotein
tail
- t. of pancreas
- t. sign

2-tailed
- 2-t. Fisher test
- 2-t. McNemar test

tailgut cyst
tailing defect
Tait law
Takayasu arteritis
takedown
- bilateral ureterostomy t.
- t. of colostomy
- t. of pelvic sling procedure
- ostomy t.

taking down of adhesions
talc embolus
Talent LPS endoluminal stent-graft system
talin
TALT
- testicular adrenallike tissue

tamarind
Tamm-Horsfall
- T.-H. mucoprotein (THM)
- T.-H. protein (THP)

tamoxifen
tampon
- Corner t.
- t. tube

tamponade, tamponage
- balloon tube t.
- esophageal balloon t.
- esophagogastric balloon t. (EGBT)
- ferromagnetic t.
- Sengstaken-Blakemore t.
- tract t.

tamponage (*var. of* tamponade)
tamponment

tamsulosin HCl
Tanagho
- T. bladder flap urethroplasty
- T. bladder neck reconstruction

tandem
- t. colonoscopy
- T. thin-shaft transureteroscopic balloon dilation catheter
- T. XL triple-lumen ERCP cannula

Tandem-E PSA immunoenzymetric assay
Tandem-ERA PSA immunoenzymetric assay
Tandem-R
- T.-R assay kit
- T.-R PSA assay

tangential
- t. biopsy
- t. colonic submucosal injection

Tangier disease
tangle of hemorrhoidal veins
Tannenbaum stent
Tanner
- T. stage
- T. stomach devascularization operation

tannex
- bisacodyl t.

tannic acid
tansy
T138 antigen
tap
- abdominal t.
- peritoneal t.
- t. water enema

TAP gene
tape
- adhesive t.
- appendectomy t.
- Cath-Secure t.
- circular t.
- Coban t.
- lap t.
- laparotomy t.
- t. marker
- Mersilene t.
- Montgomery t.
- polyester-reinforced Dacron t.
- tension-free vaginal t. (TVT)
- transobturator t.
- Transpore t.
- umbilical t.

tapered
- t. common bile duct
- t. needle
- t. rubber bougie

tapered-tip
- t.-t. dilator
- t.-t. hydrophilic-coated push catheter

tapeworm
> beef t.
> *Cestoda* t.
> fish t.
> pork t.

TAPP
> transabdominal preperitoneal
> TAPP hernia repair

***TAP2* peptide transporter gene**

Taq polymerase

TAR
> thrombocytopenia-absent radius
> TAR syndrome

Tarceva

tarda
> *Edwardsiella* t.
> porphyria cutanea t. (PCT)

tardive
> forme t.

target
> t. appearance
> t. area
> t. cell
> t. hemocrit value
> t. lesion
> t. localization
> peritoneal dialysis creatinine
>   clearance t.
> t. symptom
> t. volume

targeted
> t. biopsy
> t. cryoablation device
> t. microwave thermotherapy

targeting
> selective t.

Targis microwave catheter-based system

Tarlov cyst

tarragon
> French t.

tarry black stool

tartrate
> antimony sodium t.
> metoprolol t.
> t. nephritis
> tolterodine t.
> trimeprazine t.

TA stapling device

taste perversion

TATA-binding protein (TBP)

TA30, TA55 stapler

tattoo
> colonic t.
> colonoscopic t.
> endoscopic 4-quadrant t.
> India ink t.
> submucosal t.

tattooing
> 4-quadrant t.

taurine
> t. cotransporter (TCT)
> t. cotransporter mRNA
> selenium-labeled homocholic acid
>   conjugated with t. (SeHCAT)

taurocholate
> sodium t.
> t. solution

taurocholic acid

tauroglycocholate
> sodium t.

taurolithocholate

Taut cystic duct catheter

taxis

Taxol

Taxoprexin DHA-paclitaxel

Taylor
> T. gastric balloon
> T. gastroscope

Tazicef

Tazidime

tazobactam

TBA
> total bile acid

T-bar retractor

TBW
> total body water

Tc
> technetium

TCCB
> transitional cell carcinoma of
>   bladder

TCD/CBDE
> transcystic duct/common bile duct
>   exploration

T-cell
> T-c. activation
> T-c. adhesion
> T-c. antigen receptor/CD3
>   complex
> T-c. crossmatch
> T-c. cytotoxic therapy
> T-c. depletion by elutriation
> T-c. epitope
> T-c. line
> T-c. lymphoma
> T-c. receptor (TCR, TcR)
> T-c. second messenger
> T-c. vaccination

T84 cell

T-cell-dependent mechanism

T-cell-specific protein

Tc-99m
> technetium-99m

TCMS
> transcranial magnetic stimulation

T-C needle holder

TCR, TcR
> T-cell receptor

T

TCT
taurine cotransporter
TCT mRNA
TDMS
tropical diarrhea-malabsorption
syndrome
TDx fluorescence polarization
immunoassay
TE
tracheoesophageal
TEA
tetraethylammonium
tea
bush t.
green t.
t. tree
Teale gorget
TEAP
transurethral ethanol ablation of
prostate
tear
capsular t.
diastatic serosal t.
t. duct
esophageal t.
gastric t.
Mallory-Weiss t.
mesenteric t.
mucosal t.
pharyngeal t.
pharyngoesophageal t.
serosal t.
teardrop
t. bladder
t. incision
t. poikilocyte
tearing
t. pain
t. through
t-EASE software
TEBS
transurethral electrical bladder
stimulation
TEC
transpapillary endoscopic
cholecystotomy
teceleukin and interferon alfa-2a
TechneScan MAG-3
technetium (Tc)
t. GSA
t. imaging
t. radionuclide scan
technetium-labeled
t.-l. autologous red blood cell
scan
t.-l. red blood cell scintigraphy
technetium-99m (^{99m}Tc, Tc-99m)
t.-9. diethylenetriamine pentaacetic
acid (^{99m}Tc-DPTA, ^{99m}Tc-DTPA)

t.-9. diethylenetriamine pentaacetic
acid scan
t.-9. diisopropyl iminodiacetic acid
t.-9. dimercaptosuccinic acid
scintigram
t.-9. Exametazime injection
t.-9. galactosyl-human serum
albumin (^{99m}Tc-GSA)
t.-9. HIDA scan
t.-9. macroaggregated albumin
(^{99m}Tc-MAA)
t.-9. mercaptoacetyltriglycine
isotope
t.-9. pertechnetate
t.-9. pyrophosphate-tagged RBC
t.-9. red cell scintigraphy
t.-9. sulfur colloid (^{99m}Tc SC)
t.-9. tin colloid
technic (*var. of* technique)
technical
t. advance
t. biomaterial
technically elaborate method
technique, technic
abdominal pressure t.
abdominal wall lift t.
anthrone colorimetric t.
antiperistaltic t.
antireflux ureteral implantation t.
aseptic t.
assisted reproductive t.
autosuture t.
avascular cuff t.
balloon catheter and basket
retrieval t.
band-and-snare t.
band-snare t.
Barcat distal hypospadias repair t.
Belt radical prostatectomy t.
bench surgical t.
bladder neck-preserving t.
blind t.
Brackin ureterointestinal anastomosis
t.
Bricker t.
bulking t.
Burhenne stone basket t.
buttonhole puncture t.
Campbell opening-wedge
thoracostomy t.
Cantwell-Ransley t.
Cape Town injection sclerotherapy
t.
capsule flap t.
cavernosal alpha blockade t.
cell separation t.
cephalotrigonal t.
clamshell t.
Cleveland Clinic t.

closed tubule fixation t.
Coffey ureterosigmoid transplant t.
Cohen cross-trigonal t.
colonic obstruction t.
combined endoscopic sandwich t.
continuous pullthrough t.
Coomassie brilliant blue t.
cup-patch ileocystoplasty t.
Davis t.
deflated lumen t.
Deisting t.
Denis Browne urethroplasty t.
de novo needle-knife t.
diagnostic t.
diathermy t.
direct fragmentation t.
double-balloon t.
double-folded cup-patch
  ileocystoplasty t.
double-staple t.
double stapling t. (DST)
dual-endoscope t.
Dufourmentel pilonidal cyst and
  sinus closure t.
Eisenberger t.
en bloc t.
endoscopic esophageal mucosal
  resection tube t.
endoscopic magnet-assisted
  nonsurgical t.
endoscopic rendezvous t.
end-to-side vasoepididymostomy t.
enuresis alarm t.
epididymal sperm procurement t.
esophageal banding t.
extra-anatomical renal
  revascularization t.
extraction balloon t.
extravesical bladder cuff t.
extravesical ureteral reimplantation
  t.
Fairley bladder washout localization
  t.
fan-shaped biopsy t.
Ferguson t.
finger fracture t.
flap t.
flip-flap t.
flow microsphere fluorescent
  immunoassay t.
full-bladder t.
full Monti t.
Gaur balloon distention t.
Gil-Vernet anti-vesicoureteral reflux
  t.
Gittes genitourinary t.
Glenn t.
Glenn-Anderson t.
Goldschmiedt t.

gold seed implantation t.
Goodwin-Hohenfellner ureteric
  reimplantation t.
Goodwin orthotopic ileal neobladder
  t.
Goodwin-Scott plastic reconstruction
  of prepuce t.
Graves t.
gravimetric t.
Grimelius t.
guidewire and minisnare t.
Hale colloidal iron t.
Hammock t.
Hartmann reconstruction t.
Hasson t.
Hauri penile revascularization t.
Heibronn t.
Hendren t.
Hippuran clearance t.
histocytochemical t.
Hofmeister t.
hot biopsy t.
hydrocelectomy plication t.
hydrogen gas clearance t.
immunoperoxidase staining t.
immunostaining t.
indirect immunolocalization t.
[111]In-leukocyte t.
interventional t.
intradermal tattooing t.
intramural incision t.
invagination t.
Jaboulay-Doyen-Winkleman hydrocele
  bottleneck t.
Jones-Politano t.
Kaliscinski ureteral folding t.
keystone anterior discectomy and
  fusion t.
King contrast venography t.
Kock t.
Kropp t.
laparoscopic colposuspension t.
LaRoque t.
laryngeal jack t.
laser-assisted tissue-welding t.
laser welding t.
lasso t.
lateral bending t.
lateral window t.
Latzko t.
lawn mower t.
2-layer latex and Marlex closure t.
2-layer open t.
Lazaro da Silva t.
Lazarus-Nelson peritoneal lavage t.
Leach dual-imaging surgical
  planning t.
Leadbetter and Clarke t.
Leadbetter tunneling t.

T

technique (*continued*)
Leadbetter ureteroplasty modification t.
LeDuc ureteral tunneling t.
Lich extravesical t.
Lich-Gregoire t.
lift-and-cut t.
3-loop t.
Lotheissen-McVay t.
Madden modified radical mastectomy t.
Marlex plug t.
Masson trichrome staining t.
Mathieu hypospadias repair t.
Meares-Stamey chronic prostatitis t.
membrane catheter t.
Menghini t.
Michal II t.
micropuncture t.
microtransducer t.
Mikulicz drain t.
miniperc t.
Mitchell t.
Mitrofanoff continent urinary diversion t.
modified Cantwell t.
modified Hassan open t.
modified Sacks-Vine push-pull t.
modified Thiersch-Duplay t.
modified Vest t.
Mohs microsurgery t.
morcellation t.
Moynihan t.
muscle-splitting t.
Myers bunching t.
nasovesicular catheter t.
needle-knife t.
Nesbit t.
Norfolk phalloplasty t.
t. of penile disassembly
onlay t.
onlay-tube-onlay urethroplasty t.
Orandi vascularized flap t.
over-the-wire t.
Palomo varicocele ligation t.
Paquin ureterocystoneostomy t.
patch clamp t.
pelviscopic clip ligation t.
perfusion hypothermia t.
Pippi Salle t.
pluck t.
Politano-Leadbetter t.
Pólya gastroduodenal anastomosis t.
Ponsky t.
prograde t.
pullthrough t.
push t.
push-pull T t.
quadrant-sampling t.

Quantikine quantitative immunoenzymatometric sandwich t.
Quartey pedicled penile flap urethroplasty t.
rapid pullthrough esophageal manometry t.
reconstruction t.
refining surgical t.
relaxation t.
rendezvous t.
retrograde t.
Rives-Stoppa incisional hernia repair t.
Roux-en-Y chimney surgical t.
RPT t.
Russell t.
Sacks-Vine t.
Saeed esophageal banding t.
safe-tract t.
salvage cytology t.
sandwich t.
Schoemaker-Billroth II t.
Seldinger t.
sextant t.
Silber testicular autotransplantation t.
Singer-Blom endoscopic tracheoesophageal puncture t.
sleeve t.
sling-and-blanket t.
smiley-face knotting t.
Snodgrass t.
Somatome DRG CT t.
sperm microaspiration retrieval t. (SMART)
spiral CT t.
split-and-roll t.
split-cuff nipple t.
split-nipple t.
SPT t.
Starr t.
station pullthrough esophageal manometry t.
stent through wire mesh t.
stepladder incision t.
Stiegmann-Goff endoscopic esophageal varices ligation t.
stimulated gracilis neosphincter t.
1st-line screening t.
strip biopsy resection t.
submucosal saline injection t.
subpleural blanketing t.
suck-and-cut t.
suck-and-ligate t.
Sugarbaker t.
superior mesenterorenal bypass t.
surface cooling t.
Swiss roll embedding t.
thermal therapy t.
Thomas nipple reconstruction t.

Thompson t.
T-pouch t.
transperineal ultrasonography t.
Traverso-Longmire
  pancreatoduodenectomy t.
tube-within-tube t.
tunneled t.
turn-and-suction biopsy t.
Turnbull temporary diverting
  ileostomy t.
Turner-Warwick and Ashken
  cecocystoplasty t.
ultrasound dilution t.
Ussing chamber t.
U-stitch reimplantation t.
ventral bending t.
videofluoroscopic t.
video transurethral resection t.
Vim-Silverman needle biopsy t.
VQ t.
VQQ t.
Wallace ureteroileal anastomosis t.
Wickham t.
xenon washout t.
Young-Dees genitourinary system t.
Young urinary bladder repair t.

Technoline anal bag
technological review
technology
computed tomography t.
cryoneedle t.
DNA microarray t.
endoscopic sewing machine t.
Equalizer bead t.
fiberoptic instrument t.
imaging t.
interactive video t. (IVT)
laser t.
lithotripsy t.
novel tissue ablation t.
polymerase chain reaction t.
vacuum erection t. (VET)
videographic tool t.
virtual reality t.

Technomed Sonolith 3000 lithotriptor
Technos ultrasound system
Techstar percutaneous closure device
teduglutide
teeth
carious t.
full-surface micromesh t.
interdigitating t.
TEF
thermic effect of feeding
tracheoesophageal fistula
Teflon
T. ERCP cannula
T. guiding catheter
T. injector

T. nasobiliary drain
T. nasobiliary tube
T. paste injection for incontinence
T. sheath
T. sling rectopexy
T. stent
Teflon-coated
T.-c. Dacron suture
T.-c. guidewire
Tegaderm
T. absorbent clear acrylic dressing
T. foam adhesive dressing
tegaserod
t. maleate
t. maleate tablet
Tegress endoscopic urethral implant
Tegretol
teicoplanin
Tektronix digital oscilloscope
tela, *pl.* **telae**
t. subserosa intestini tenuis
telae (*pl. of* tela)
telangiectasia
calcinosis cutis, Raynaud
  phenomenon, esophageal motility
  disorder, sclerodactyly, and t.
  (CREST)
calcinosis cutis, Raynaud
  phenomenon, sclerodactyly, and t.
  (CRST)
duodenal t.
gastrointestinal t.
hemorrhagic t.
hepatic t.
hereditary hemorrhagic t. (HHT)
Osler-Weber-Rendu t.
radiation t.
spider t.
t. syndrome
telangiectatic
t. angioma
t. vessel
telar vesical tenesmus
telbivudine
tele-endoscopy
telemanagement
home automated t. (HAT)
telemedicine
Telepaque contrast medium
**telerobotic-assisted laparoscopic
  surgery**
telerobotic system
telescope
forward-viewing t.
t. heater
Hopkins t.
Wolff t.
teletherapy
orthovoltage t.

T

television
t. camera
t. monitor
t. photography
Telfa dressing
Teline
tellurite resistance loci
telomerase
telomere length
telopeptide
TEM
transanal endoscopic microsurgery
transmission electron microscopy
TEM transanal endoscopy
temafloxacin
Temaril
temazepam
temperature
actual intraprostatic t.
core t.
hand t.
intraprostatic t.
laser t.
urethral t.
template
Mick prostate t.
Seyd-Neblett perineal t.
Tempo
temporary
t. end colostomy
t. endoprosthetic device
t. enteroscope
t. loop ileostomy
temporizing measure
temporomandibular arthritis
TEN
total enteral nutrition
Vivonex TEN
Tena pouch
tenatoprazole
Tenckhoff
T. 2-cuff catheter
T. peritoneal dialysis
catheter
tender
t. liver
t. thyroid
tenderness
adnexal t.
ballottement t.
bony t.
cervical motion t.
costochondral t.
costovertebral angle t.
(CVAT)
diffuse t.
exquisite t.
focal t.
frontal t.

generalized abdominal t.
localizing t.
palpation t.
paracervical t.
percussion t.
point t.
popliteal t.
rebound t.
rectal t.
salivary t.
scrotal t.
sinus t.
spinous t.
thyroid t.
uterine t.
tendinous
t. arch
t. arch of levator ani muscle
tendon
conjoined t.
perineal t.
t. xanthoma
tenesmic
tenesmus
rectal t.
telar vesical t.
Tenex
tenia, taenia, *pl.* **teniae**
t. coli
t. libera
t. mesocolica
t. of Valsalva
t. omentalis
teniae (*pl. of* tenia)
tenial, taenial
teniamyotomy
teniasis, taeniasis
somatic t.
teniform, taeniform
teniposide
Ten-K
Tenoretic
Tenormin
tenoxicam
TENS
transcutaneous electrical nerve
stimulation
TENS unit
tense ascites
tensile strength
Tensilon test
tensiometer
tension
t. pneumoperitoneum
t. pneumothorax
wall t.
tension-free
t.-f. anastomosis
t.-f. closure of abdominal cavity

t.-f. cystocele repair
t.-f. vaginal tape (TVT)
t.-f. vaginal tape procedure
tensor
t. fascia lata flap
t. veli palatini muscle
tensostat
tent
Silon t.
sponge t.
tenting
baseline t.
t. sign
Tenuate
tenuis
Corynebacterium t.
folliculi lymphatici solitarii
intestini t.
tela subserosa intestini t.
TEP
totally extraperitoneal
tracheoesophageal puncture
transesophageal endoscopic plication
TEP hernia repair
TEPA
thermic effect of physical
activity
Tepanil
tepoxalin
teratocarcinoma
teratogenesis
medication t.
teratogenic medicine
teratoma
anaplastic malignant t.
benign cystic t.
differentiated t.
gastric t.
immature t.
malignant t.
mature t.
ovarian t.
presacral t.
sacrococcygeal t.
solid t.
testicular t.
trophoblastic malignant t.
undifferentiated malignant t.
teratomatous
teratospermia
terazosin
terbutaline hepatitis
teres, *pl.* **teretes,** *gen.* **teretis**
fissura ligamenti teretis
fissure of ligamentum t.
ligamentum t.
teretes (*pl. of* teres)
terfenadine
terlipressin

term
Coding Systems for a Thesaurus of
Adverse Reaction T.'s (COSTART)
terminal
afferent t.
t. anuria vesical dialysis
t. bifid branching system
t. bile duct
t. colostomy
t. deoxynucleotide
transferase-mediated deoxyuridine
triphosphate
t. hematuria
t. ileal disease
t. ileal pouch
t. ileal resection
t. ileitis
t. ileostomy
t. ileum
t. ileum intubation (TII)
t. ileus
t. inner medullary collecting duct
t. repeat
t. reservoir syndrome
t. sedation
sensory nervous t.
t. uridine deoxynucleotide nick-end
labeling (TUNEL)
terminus
amino t.
duodenal t.
intrapapillary t.
terodiline
teroxirone
terrestrial organism
Terry fingernail sign
tert-**butyl ether**
tertiary
t. contraction
t. hyperparathyroidism (tHPT)
t. radicle
t. syphilis
tertium
Clostridium t.
Terumo
T. dialyzer
T. glidewire
T. hydrophilic guidewire
Terumo/Meditech guidewire
Terumo-Radiofocus hydrophilic
polymer-coated guidewire
Tesberg esophagoscope
TESE
testicular sperm extraction
Tesla
T. GE Signa whole-body scanner
T. Signa MR imager
Teslascan
tesmilifene

T

test

Abbott AxSYM antibody to hepatitis C virus lab t.
abnormal esophageal t.
Accu-Dx t.
acid clearance t. (ACT)
acidemia of stool t.
acid hemolysis t.
acidification of stool t.
acid perfusion t.
acid reflux t.
adrenocorticotropic hormone infusion t.
Advanced Care cholesterol t.
agglutination t.
air tightness t.
Albarran t.
Albustix t.
alcohol-use disorders identification t. (AUDIT)
alkaline phosphatase t.
alkalinization t.
Allen t.
ALT t.
Althausen t.
Ames t.
aminopyrine breath t.
Amplicor HBV monitor t.
Amplicor HCV RNA t.
AnemiaPro anemia screening t.
angiotensin II infusion t.
anorectal function t.
antiendomysial antibody t.
antigen stool detection t.
anti-Hu t.
antineuronal enteric antibody t.
anti-SLA t.
APC stool t.
APT-Downey alkali denaturation t.
argentaffin reaction t.
artificial erection t.
AST t.
Astra profile t.
Aura-Tek FDP t.
AxSYM free PSA t.
Baermann stool t.
balloon expulsion t.
Bard BTA t.
basal secretory flow rate t.
belt t.
bentiromide t.
bentonite flocculation t.
Bernstein acid perfusion t.
beta-2 t.
betazole stimulation t.
bethanechol t.
bile acid breath t.
bile acid tolerance t.
bile solubility t.

BiliChek t.
bilirubin t.
binder t.
Bio-Enzabead t.
biopsy urease t.
Biotel home screening t.
BioWhittaker assay t.
BladderScan t.
bladder tumor antigen t.
bolus challenge t.
Bonney t.
Bors ice water t.
Bourne t.
Boyden t.
Boyle and Goldstein saline t.
Bozicevich t.
t. breakfast
breath hydrogen excretion t.
breath pentane t.
Breslow-Day t.
BSFR t.
BSP t.
BTA STAT t.
BTA TRAK t.
BT-PABA t.
buckling t.
CA—19-9 t.
calcium infusion t.
Campylobacter t.
Campylobacter-like organism t. (CLOtest)
cancelling A's t.
captopril plasma renin activity t.
carbon-13 urea breath t. (^{13}C-UBT)
carbon-14 urea breath t. (^{14}C-UBT)
carbon-14 urinary excretion t.
Carnot t.
Casoni skin t.
catheterization t.
^{13}C-bicarbonate breath t.
CBP t.
^{13}C breath t.
C-cholylglycine breath excretion t.
CEA t.
cephalin-cholesterol flocculation t.
^{14}C-glycocholate breath t.
C-glycocholic acid breath t.
7C Gold urine t.
chew-and-spit t.
Chiron RIBA HCV t.
Choice2 t.
cholecystokinin t.
citrate t.
^{13}C-labeled cholesteryl octanoate breath t.
C-lactose t.
Clinitest stool t.
clomiphene t.

clonidine suppression t.
Coat-A-Count Free PSA IRMA t.
Cobas Amplicor HBV monitor t.
CO_2 breath t.
Cochran-Mantel-Haenszel t.
^{13}C-octanoic acid gastric emptying breath t.
C of Hosmer-Lemeshow ratio t.
Cohen t.
Colaris genetic susceptibility t.
Colaris molecular diagnostic t.
cold stress t.
ColoCARE fecal occult blood t.
colonic transit t.
ColorectAlert rectal mucus t.
combined intracavernous injection and stimulation t.
complement fixation t.
complete blood count t.
Coombs t.
copper-binding protein t.
cornflake esophageal motility t.
Cortrosyn stimulation t.
cosyntropin stimulation t.
cotton swab t.
cough stress t.
Cox-Mantel t.
CP t.
cracker t.
creatinine t.
C&S t.
CSF glutamine t.
^{14}C-triolein breath t.
culture and sensitivity t.
^{14}C urea breath t.
deferoxamine mesylate infusion t.
dexamethasone suppression t.
diabetes home screening t.
Diagnex Blue t.
differential renal function t.
differential ureteral catheterization t.
Dimension Free prostate-specific antigen Flex reagent cartridge t.
t. dinner
direct immunobead t.
direct immunofluorescence t. (DIF-test)
direct secretin endoscopic pancreatic function t.
Doppler flow t. (DFT)
Dreiling tube pancreatic function t.
duodenal secretin t. (DST)
D-xylose absorption t.
dye-exclusion t.
E t.
edrophonium t.
egg yolk-cobalamin absorption t. (EYCAT)
Einhorn string t.

Eitest MONO P-II t.
Ektachem slide t.
ELISA-1 t.
ELISA-2 t.
ELISA-3 t.
endomysial antibody t.
endoscopic gastrin t. (EGT)
Enzygnost anti-HIV 1+2 t.
Enzymun t.
ergonovine t.
erythrocyte sedimentation rate t.
esophageal acid infusion t.
esophageal function t.
Ez-*Helicobacter* blood t.
Fairley bladder washout t.
FDL t.
fecal alpha-1-antitrypsin t.
fecal fat t.
fecal leukocyte count t.
fecal occult blood t. (FOBT)
fingerprick latex agglutination t.
Fisher exact probability t.
Fisher 2-tailed exact t.
Fishman-Doubilet t.
FlexSure HP t.
FlexSure whole-blood t.
FloPoint t.
fluorescein dilaurate t.
fluorescein string t.
fluorescent treponemal antibody absorption t. (FTA-ABS)
FoodSCAN food allergy t.
Fouchet t.
Fowler-Stephens t.
Francis t.
FTA-ABS t.
gallbladder function t.
GAP t.
gastric accommodation t.
gastric emptying breath t. (GEBT)
gastric function t.
gastric secretory t.
gastrin stimulation t.
Gastroccult t.
gastrointestinal blood loss t.
Gerhardt t.
GGT t.
GGTP liver function t.
Ghedini-Weinberg serologic t.
Glahn t.
4-glass t.
glucose t.
Glucose Analyzer II t.
glutamine t.
glycopyrrolate t.
glycyltryptophan t.
Gmelin t.
gonadotropin-releasing hormone t.

test (*continued*)

graded esophageal balloon distention t.
Graham t.
Gram stain of stool t.
Griess t.
Gross t.
guaiac t.
Guenzberg t.
Ham t.
Hanger t.
Harrison spot t.
hatching t.
Hay t.
H2 breath t.
HCV DupliType t.
HCV ELISA t.
HCV QuantaSure Plus t.
heel tap t.
Helicobacter pylori breath excretion t.
Helicoblot 2.1 t.
Helisal rapid blood t.
Hematest t.
HemaWipe t.
heme t.
Hemoccult ICT fecal occult t.
Hemoccult II t.
Hemoccult Sensa t.
HemoQuant fecal blood t.
HemoSelect t.
Hepaplastin t.
hepatitis C virus DupliType t.
Heptimax hepatitis C viral load t.
Herzberg t.
Histalog stimulation t.
histamine t.
HM-CAP serological t.
Hoesch t.
Hollander t.
home screening t.
HomeSelect t.
24-hour ambulatory pH t.
72-hour fecal fat t.
24-hour gastric acidity t.
12-hour home pad t.
1-hour office pad t.
Howard t.
Hpfast rapid urease t.
HpSA t.
H. pylori SA t.
5-HT t.
human lymphocyte chromosomal aberration t.
Hunt t.
Hybritech Tandem PSA ratio t.
hydrochloric acid t.
hydrogen breath t.
ICA t.

ice-water t.
ICG t.
iliopsoas t.
immoCare fecal occult blood t.
immunoblot t.
ImmunoCard serum antibody t.
ImmunoCard STAT! Rotavirus t.
ImmunoCyt t.
immunodiffusion t.
immunofluorescent antibody t.
Immuno I complex PSA t.
immunologic fecal occult blood t. (IFOBT)
immunologic rapid urease t.
^{111}indium-labeled autologous leukocyte t.
InSure immunochemical fecal occult blood t.
intracavernous injection and stimulation t.
intraductal secretin t. (IDST)
intraesophageal acid t.
intraesophageal pH t.
intravenous secretin t.
Inutest t.
invasive diagnostic t.
Jacoby t.
Jaffe t.
Jaksch t.
Jatrox *Helicobacter pylori* t.
Jaworski t.
jejunal gas infusion t.
Jolles t.
Kapsinow t.
Kashiwado t.
Kato t.
Kelling t.
ketone body t.
KidneyScreen at Home t.
Kolmogorov-Smirnov t.
Krokiewicz t.
Kruskal-Wallis t.
Kveim t.
lactose tolerance t. (LTT)
lactulose breath t. (LBT)
lactulose-mannitol permeability t.
Lange t.
LAP t.
Lapides t.
last-generation serologic ELISA t.
latex fixation t.
LDH t.
LDL Direct t.
Leo t.
leucine aminopeptidase t.
leukocyte adherence inhibition t.
leukocyte alkaline phosphatase t.
leukocyte esterase t.
levulose t.

Ligat t.
lipase t.
litmus milk t.
liver function t.'s (LFT)
locally made rapid urease t.
  (LRUT)
log-rank t.
Lundh t.
Macdonald t.
Machado-Guerreiro t.
MacLean t.
magnetic susceptibility t.
Maly t.
Mann-Whitney rank sum t.
Mantel-Haenszel t.
Mardi t.
Marechal-Rosen t.
Marshall t.
Marshall-Bonney t.
Marshall-Marchetti t.
Masset t.
McNemar ascites t.
t. meal
measurement t.
Meltzer-Lyon t.
methyl red t.
metyrapone stimulation t.
Micral urine dipstick t.
1-minute endoscopy room t.
Mitscherlich t.
Mohr t.
monoethylglycinexylidide liver
  function t.'s
morphine-neostigmine t.
motility t.
Moynihan t.
Myers-Fine t.
Mylius t.
Nakayama t.
Nardi t.
N-benzoyl-L-tyrosyl-P-aminobenzoic
  acid excretion t.
NBT-PABA t.
Neubauer and Fischer t.
Neukomm t.
nitrite t.
nitrogen partition t.
nitrogen retention t.
NMP22 BladderChek t.
noninvasive diagnostic t.
noninvasive urodynamic t.
nonradioactive ^{13}C t.
Normotest t.
Nymox urinary t.
obturator t.
octanoic acid breath t.
omeprazole t.
O&P t.
Oresus Potentest t.

PABA t.
pad urinary incontinence t.
palmin t.
pancreatic secretory t.
Papanicolaou t.
paracetamol absorption t.
PAS t.
peak secretory flow rate t.
pentagastrin gastric secretory t.
pentagastrin infusion t.
pentagastrin provocative t.
pentagastrin stimulated analysis t.
Peptavlon stimulation t.
percutaneous pressure ureteral
  perfusion t.
perineal nerve terminal motor
  latency t.
periodic acid-Schiff t.
peripheral nerve evaluation t.
peritoneal equilibration t. (PET)
Pettenkofer t.
pH t.
Phadebas angiotensin-I t.
phenoltetrachlorophthalein t.
phentolamine t.
physiologic reflux t. (PRT)
pineapple t.
plasma renin activity captopril t.
PNE t.
POA t.
Posner attention t.
postage stamp penile tumescence t.
postcoital t.
post hoc t.
postural stimulation t. (PST)
posture t.
potassium sensitivity t. (PST)
PPD t.
PreGenPlus stool DNA t.
Premier Platinum HpSA t.
Prentice-Wilcoxon t.
Prostate Px clinical t.
proteinuria t.
Protocult t.
provocative t.
PSA4 prostate cancer t.
PSFR t.
psychometric t.
PyloriScreen t.
Pyloriset EIA-G t.
Pylori Stat assay t.
PyloriTek rapid urease t.
PYtest urea breath t.
Q-tip t.
qualitative fecal fat t.
quantitative fecal fat t.
Quick t.
QuickVue One-Step *H. pylori* t.
Quidel QuickVue *H. pylori* t.

T

test (*continued*)

Quinlan t.
Rabuteau t.
radioactive carbon-14 t.
radioallergosorbent t. (RAST)
radioimmunofocus inhibition t. (RIFIT)
radioisotope renal excretion t.
radioisotope renogram t.
rapid serum amylase t.
rapid urease t. (RUT)
Rapoport t.
recombinant immunoblot assay-2 t.
reducing substances t.
reflex HPV t.
Rehfuss t.
Reitan Trail-Making t.
Reitman-Frankel t.
renin stimulation t.
rhubarb t.
RIBA t.
RIBA-2 t.
rice-flour breath t.
Robinson-Kepler-Power water t.
rose bengal t.
Rosenbach-Gmelin t.
Rosenthal t.
Rotazyme t.
Saathoff t.
Sahli glutoid t.
Sahli-Nencki t.
saline continence t.
saline load t.
saline suppression t.
Salkowski-Schipper t.
Salomon t.
santonin t.
satiety t.
Saundby t.
scan t.
S-CCK-Pz t.
Scheffe-F t.
Schiff t.
Schilling t.
Schwartz t.
Scivoletto t.
secretin-CCK stimulation t.
secretin-pancreozymin stimulation t.
secretin provocation t.
secretin stimulation t.
SeHCAT t.
^{75}Se-labeled bile acid t.
semen analysis t.
serologic t.
serum amylase t.
serum bilirubin t.
serum creatinine t.
serum iron t.
serum protein t.

serum RIBA-2 t.
Sgambati reaction t.
SGOT t.
SGPT t.
sham feeding t.
Sitzmarks t.
skinfold thickness t.
SM-HCV Rapid t.
Smith t.
snap gauge t.
sodium-loading t.
solid sphere t.
Spearman t.
specific gravity t.
specific red cell adherence t.
SpermCheck t.
split renal function t.
squeeze pressure profile of anal sphincter t.
2-stage triolein t.
Stamey t.
standard acid reflux t. (SART)
standard radiological t.
star construction t.
Stat Simple whole-blood antibody t.
stimulated gastric secretion t.
stimulation t.
Stokvis t.
Stoll t.
StoneRisk citrate t.
StoneRisk cystine t.
StoneRisk diagnostic t.
StoneRisk profile t.
stool cytotoxin t.
stool electrolyte t.
stool osmolality t.
stool osmotic gap t.
Strassburg t.
string t.
Stypven time t.
sucrose tolerance t.
sugar t.
Sulkowitch t.
sweat t.
Szabo t.
2-tailed Fisher t.
2-tailed McNemar t.
Tensilon t.
Tes-Tape urine glucose t.
TIBC t.
tilt t.
Töpfer t.
Torquay t.
total fecal weight t.
total iron-binding capacity t.
Trail t.
Trail-Making T.
transferrin t.
transmucosal electrical potential t.

transvesical potassium sensitivity t.
triceps skinfold thickness t.
triolein C-14 breath t.
Trousseau t.
tuberculin t.
tubular reabsorption of phosphate t.
Tukey t.
Tuttle t.
t. type
Tyson t.
UBT breath t.
Udranszky t.
Uffelmann t.
ultrasound t.
Ultzmann t.
Uni-Gold *Helicobacter pylori* t.
uPM3 urine t.
urea breath t. (UBT)
urea nitrogen t.
urease t.
urecholine supersensitivity t.
uric acid t.
urinary nitrite t.
urine chloride t.
urine concentration t.
Uriscreen t.
van den Bergh t.
ViraPap HPV dot blot hybridization t.
vitamin A, B$_{12}$ absorption t.
Voges-Proskauer t.
von Jaksch t.
Wagner t.
washout t.
water-gurgle t.
water-load t.
water-nutrient t.
water-recovery t.
water-restriction t.
water-sipping t.
water-soluble contrast esophageal swallow t.
Watson-Schwartz t.
whiff t.
Whipple triad t.
Whitaker pressure-perfusion t.
Winckler t.
Witz t.
Woldman t.
Wolff-Junghans t.
Woolf t.
xylose absorption t.
xylose tolerance t.
Yang Pros-Check PSA t.
Z t.
Zappacosta t.
zona hamster egg t.
testalgia (*var. of* orchialgia)
Tes-Tape urine glucose test

testectomy (*var. of* orchiectomy)
testes (*pl. of* testis)
testicle
   maldescended t.
   nonpalpable t.
   retained t.
testicular
   t. abscess
   t. adenocarcinoma
   t. adenofibromyoma
   t. adenomatoid tumor vacuole
   t. adrenallike tissue (TALT)
   t. adrenal rest
   t. androgen-binding protein
   t. angioma
   t. artery
   t. biopsy
   t. cancer
   t. carcinoma
   t. cyst
   t. descent
   t. feminization syndrome
   t. fibroma
   t. Hodgkin disease
   t. hypothermia device
   t. implant
   t. interstitial fluid (TIF)
   t. leiomyoma
   t. leukemia
   t. lymphoma
   t. mass
   t. microlithiasis
   t. pain
   t. plexus
   t. prosthesis
   t. seminoma
   t. sperm extraction (TESE)
   t. swelling
   t. teratoma
   t. torsion
   t. tuberculosis
   t. tubular adenoma
   t. tubule
   t. tumor
testicularis
   plexus t.
testiculi (*pl. of* testiculus)
testiculus, *pl.* **testiculi**
Testim 1%
testing
   anorectal physiology t.
   breath alkane t.
   fecal DNA t.
   fecal occult blood t.
   histocompatibility t.
   lactose hydrogen breath t. (LHBT)
   multiple data t.
   nucleic acid t. (NAT)
   pad t.

T

testing (*continued*)
    penile injection t.
    pH-metric t.
    physiology t.
    provocative t.
    psychophysiologic t.
    RigiScan t.
    salivary t.
    sexual stimulation t.
    stress t.
    urea breath t.
    urodynamic t.
    viability t.
    vibrotactile stimulation t.
    videourodynamic t.
    visual sexual stimulation t.
testis, *pl.* **testes**
    abdominal t.
    aberratio t.
    adenocarcinoma of
      infantile t.
    albuginea t.
    appendix t.
    t. cancer
    t. carcinoid
    Cooper irritable t.
    descensus aberrans t.
    descensus paradoxus t.
    dorsum of t.
    dystopia transversa externa t.
    dystopia transversa interna t.
    ectopic t.
    femoral t.
    fibroma of t.
    free-floating t.
    fungus t.
    high t.
    interstitial cell tumor of t.
    inverted t.
    irritable t.
    lobuli t.
    mediastinum t.
    mottled t.
    movable t.
    obstructed t.
    peeping t.
    prosthetic t.
    pulpy t.
    retained t.
    rete t.
    retractile t.
    t. sarcoma
    septulum t.
    septum of t.
    solitary t.
    torsion of t.
    tunica albuginea t.
    tunica vaginalis t.
    undescended t.
    unilateral palpable right t.
    vanishing t.
testis-determining factor
testitis (*var. of* orchitis)
testitoxicosis
Testoderm
    T. patch
    T. TTS
testoid
testolactone
testopathy
testosterone
    basal t.
    t. buccal system
    t. cypionate
    t. deficiency
    t. enanthate
    free t.
    t. gel 1%
    t. patch
    t. plasma concentration
    t. propionate
    serum t.
    t. stimulation
    t. transdermal system (TTS)
    t. transdermal therapy
    undecenoate of t.
testosterone-binding globulin
testosterone-estrogen-binding globulin
testosterone-repressed prostate message-2 (TRPM-2)
testotoxicosis
Testred C-III
test-size orchidometer
test-yolk buffer cryopreservation agent
tetani
    Clostridium t.
tetanus globulin
tetany
    gastric t.
tether circulating leukocyte
tethered-bowel sign
tethered-cord
    t.-c. release
    t.-c. syndrome
tethered spinal cord
tethering of mucosa
tetracaine lozenge
Tetracap
tetrachloride
    carbon t.
tetracycline
    bismuth, metronidazole, t. (BMT)
    t. hydrochloride
    t. nephropathy
    ranitidine bismuth citrate,
      metronidazole, t. (RMT)
    t. sclerosis

tetracycline-induced spongiotic esophagitis
tetradecapeptide
tetradecyl sulfate
tetraethylammonium (TEA)
Tetragastrin-NS
tetrahydrocannabinol (THC)
tetrahydrochloride
    3′,3-diaminobenzidine t.
6-tetrahydropyridine
tetrahydrozoline
tetralogy
    Fallot t.
Tetram
tetramethyl ammonium chloride
(TEMAC)
tetrapalmitate
    maltose t.
tetraplegia
tetraploid cell
tetrapyrrol compound
tetrathiomolybdate
tetrazolium
    nitroblue t. (NBT)
tetrodotoxin (TTX)
tetrodotoxin-insensitive sodium
channel
tetroxide
    osmium t. (OsO4)
Teucrium chamaedrys
Tevdek suture
Tewameter MPA5 instrument
Texas-style 2-piece catheter
Texas trauma
texture
    heterogeneous t.
    homogeneous t.
tezacitabine
TFE-coated wire guide
TFF
    trefoil factor family 1–3
TF/UF
    tubular fluid:ultrafiltrate
TGF
    transforming growth factor
    tubuloglomerular feedback
      human recombinant TGF
TGF-alpha
    transforming growth factor alpha
TGF-beta
    transforming growth factor beta
TGF-beta-1
    transforming growth factor beta-1
      TGF-beta-1 gene
TGF-beta-2
    transforming growth factor beta-2
TGF-beta-3
    transforming growth factor beta-3
Th1
    T-helper type 1

Thal
    T. esophageal stricture repair
    T. esophagogastroscopy
    T. esophagogastrostomy
    T. fundic patch operation
    T. fundoplasty
    T. stricturoplasty
thalidomide
Thalitone
thallium
    t. imaging
    t. poisoning
thallium-201
thamuria
thaw-mount radioautography
Thaysen disease
THC
    tetrahydrocannabinol
    transhepatic cholangiogram
    transhepatic cholangiography
THE
    transhepatic embolization
The
    T. CURE Digestive Diseases
      Research Center
    T. Magic Foundation
Theis self-retaining retractor
thelia (*pl. of* thelium)
thelium, *pl.* **thelia**
T-helper
    T-h. precursor
    T-h. type 1 (Th1)
theophylline
    t. clearance
    t. ethylenediamine
    t. level
    t. olamine enema
    t. toxicity
theory
    Dieulafoy t.
    Freter t.
    hyperfiltration t.
    overflow t.
    peripheral arterial vasodilation t.
    set-point t.
TheraCLEC
TheraCys
Theradex
Theradigm-HBV
Theragyn
Theralax
therapeutic
    t. angiography
    t. colonoscopy
    t. concentrate (TC)
    t. endoscope
    t. endourology
    t. laparoscopy
    t. modality

T

therapeutic (*continued*)
    t. option
    t. pancreaticobiliary endoscopy
    t. plasmapheresis
    t. response
    t. side-viewing duodenoscope
    t. upper endoscopy
    t. value
therapia (*var. of* therapy)
therapy, therapia
    ablative laser t.
    acid suppression t. (AST)
    adjuvant drug t.
    adrenalin injection t.
    alarm t.
    alfa interferon t.
    alimentary t.
    alkaline citrate t.
    alpha-blocker t.
    alpha receptor blockade t.
    amoxicillin-tinidazole-ranitidine t.
    amphotericin B t.
    ampullary ablative t.
    androgen ablation t. (AAT)
    androgen deprivation t.
    androgen withdrawal endocrine t.
    antibiotic t.
    anticholinergic medicine t.
    anticoagulation t.
    antilymphocyte t.
    antimicrobial t.
    antioncogene t.
    antireflux t.
    antisecretory t.
    antitumor necrosis factor t.
    argon laser t.
    autolymphocyte t.
    aversion t.
    Aza-Pred t.
    azole t.
    balloon photodynamic t.
    beta-blocker t.
    bile acid t.
    biofeedback t.
    biologic response modifier t.
    bismuth-free triple t.
    bismuth triple t.
    bridging t.
    bright light t. (BLT)
    broad-spectrum t.
    bubble t.
    buprenorphine narcotic analgesic t.
    chemoradiation t. (CRT)
    cholestyramine t.
    CIFN t.
    clarithromycin triple t.
    coagulative laser t.
    combined chemoradiation t.
    conditioning t.

conformal radiation t.
continuous renal replacement t.
  (CRRT)
corticosteroid t.
cost effectiveness of t.
cost of t.
cytokine t.
cytolytic t.
debulking t.
dendritic cell t.
diclofenac analgesic t.
diet t.
dilation t.
diltiazem t.
3-dimensional conformal radiation t.
  (3DCRT)
dose-optimized t. (DOT)
doxycycline-metronidazole-bismuth
  subcitrate triple t.
drug t.
Emitasol nasal t.
endocrine t.
endoscopic Doppler
  ultrasound-guided injection t.
endoscopic hemoclip t.
endoscopic hemostatic t.
endoscopic injection t.
endoscopic laser t. (ELT)
endoscopic pancreatic t.
enterostomal t.
Enterra T.
enzyme replacement t.
eradication t.
erythropoietin t.
esophageal photodynamic t.
estrogen replacement t. (ERT)
ethanol injection t.
external-beam radiation t. (EBRT)
external vacuum t.
ex vivo liver-directed gene t.
fluid replacement t.
fluoroquinolone t.
flutamide t.
foscarnet t.
gamma globulin t.
gene t.
gene transfer t.
H2-antagonist t.
heat t.
heater probe t.
Helidac t.
hematoporphyrin derivative t.
hemofiltration t. (HFT)
hemostatic t.
highly active antiretroviral t.
  (HAART)
homeostatic t.
hormonal t.
H2-receptor antagonist t.

HydraLife oral rehydration t.
hydrocelectomy scleral t.
hydrostatic pressure t.
hyperbaric oxygen t. (HBOT)
hyperfractionated radiation t.
IFN alfa t.
IFN alfa-2b t.
image-guided t.
immunomodulatory gene t.
immunosuppressive t.
initial broad-spectrum t.
injection t.
instillation t.
intensity-modulated proton t. (IMPT)
intensity-modulated radiation t.
  (IMRT)
interferon alfa t.
interferon alfa-2b t.
intermittent calcitriol t.
intermittent hormone t.
International Association for
  Enterostomal T.
interstitial photodynamic t.
intracavernosal injection t. (ICIT)
intracavernous injection t.
intracavitary radiation boost t.
intracavitary topical t.
intracorporeal injection t.
intraoperative radiation t. (IORT)
IV fluid t.
ketoprofen analgesic t.
laser t.
laser interstitial thermal t. (LITT)
lifestyle t.
medical t.
metabolic t.
methyl-*tert*-butyl ether t.
metronidazole, amoxicillin,
  clarithromycin, *H. pylori*, 1-week
  t. (MACH1)
microwave t.
minimally invasive t.
monoclonal antibody t.
morphine narcotic analgesic t.
MTBE t.
m-tetrahydroxyphenyl chlorin
  photodynamic t.
Nd:YAG laser t.
negative-pressure wound t.
neoadjuvant androgen derivation t.
neoadjuvant hormonal ablation t.
neodymium:YAG laser t.
Nexium triple t.
nicotine t.
nonmyeloablative stem cell t.
nutritional t.
omeprazole t.
omeprazole-clarithromycin-
  amoxicillin t.

oral dissolution t.
oral rehydration t. (ORT)
OssaTron shock wave t.
palliative t.
pancreatic enzyme replacement t.
  (PERT)
pancreatic intraluminal radiation t.
Pariet t.
PEI t.
penile injection t.
penile vein occlusion t.
percutaneous embolization t.
percutaneous ethanol injection t.
periurethral injection t.
phosphate binder t.
photodynamic t. (PDT)
photoradiation t.
physiologic testosterone replacement
  t.
placebo t.
polidocanol injection t.
polyestradiol phosphate t.
porfimer sodium photodynamic t.
postoperative anticoagulation t.
posttransplant immunosuppression t.
PPI triple t.
preventive intravesical t.
Prevpac triple t.
probiotic t.
prokinetic t.
Protandim antioxidant t.
proton pump inhibition t.
psychosexual t.
pulsed-dye laser t.
quadruple t.
radiation t.
radionuclide t.
ranitidine t.
Rebetron combination t.
rehydration t.
renal replacement t.
rescue t.
resectional t.
resiniferatoxin t.
role of diet in t.
sacral nerve stimulation t.
saline injection t.
salvage t.
sandwich staghorn calculus t.
sclerosing t.
self-injection t.
sex t.
single-drug t.
SNS t.
somatostatin analogue t.
somatostatin infusion t.
steroid t.
sucralfate t.
surgical t.

T

therapy *(continued)*
systemic radiation t.
T-cell cytotoxic t.
testosterone transdermal t.
TheraSphere t.
thermal t.
thrombolytic t.
Trager t.
transcatheter arterial embolization t.
transpapillary t.
transurethral collagen injection t.
transvaginal t.
triple eradication t.
tumor suppressor gene t.
ultrasound-guided shock wave t.
universally accepted t.
unresponsiveness to standard t.
valproic acid t.
venesection t.
YAG laser t.
TheraSeed
Therasonics
T. lithotripsy system
T. lithotriptor
TheraSphere therapy
Theratope vaccine
Therevac Plus
Therevac-SB
Therma
T. Jaw disposable hot biopsy forceps
T. Jaw hot urologic forceps
thermal
t. ablation
t. blocking
t. burn
t. imaging
t. sphincteric reflex
t. therapy
t. therapy technique
thermally active method
TherMatrx
T. DOT
T. hyperthermia device
T. TMx-2000 device
Thermex-II transurethral prostate heating device
thermic
t. effect of feeding (TEF)
t. effect of physical activity (TEPA)
thermoablation
interstitial laser t.
transurethral hot-water balloon t.
ThermoChem-HT system
thermocoagulation
endoscopic heater probe t.
heater probe t.
heat probe t.

HP t.
KeyMed heater probe t.
laser t.
thermocoagulator
Olympus CD-Z-series heat probe t.
thermocycler
Stratagene SCS-96 t.
thermodisinfector
endoscopic t.
thermodynamic solubility product
thermoexpandable stent
ThermoFlex
T. system
T. thermotherapy unit
thermogenesis
adaptive t.
thermography
Primus transrectal t.
thermomechanical
thermometer
air t.
alcohol t.
Celsius t.
centigrade t.
Fahrenheit t.
gas t.
oral t.
rectal t.
surface t.
thermometry
magnetic resonance imaging t.
thermophilus
Streptococcus t.
thermoreceptor
thermosensitive stent
thermosensor
thermostable reverse transcriptase
thermotherapy
biologic predictor for treatment outcome of transurethral microwave t.
cooled catheter transurethral microwave t.
high-energy transurethral microwave t. (HE-TUMT)
low-energy transurethral microwave t. (LE-TUMT)
microwave t.
30-minute transurethral microwave t.
periurethral-transurethral microwave t. (P-TUMT)
targeted microwave t.
transurethral microwave t. (TUMT)
Urowave t.
water-induced t. (WIT)
Thermovac tissue pulverizer
Thermus
T. aquaticus
T. aquaticus DNA ligase

thetaiotaomicron
>*Bacteroides t.*

thiabendazole
thiacetazone
thiamine deficiency
thiazide diuretic
thiazide-induced hyponatremia
thiazolidinedione
thick
>t. adhesion
>t. ascending limb
>t. ascending limb of Henle
>t. bile

thickened gallbladder wall
thickening
>apical t.
>hypoechoic t.
>mediastinal t.
>plaquelike t.
>small-bowel t.
>submucosal t.
>wall t.

thick-loop transurethral resection of prostate
thickness
>esophageal wall t.
>mucous gel t.
>t. of skinfold
>triceps skinfold t.

thick-walled gallbladder
Thiersch
>T. anal incontinence operation
>T. anus procedure
>T. graft
>T. tube

Thiersch-Duplay
>T.-D. proximal tube urethroplasty procedure
>T.-D. repair
>T.-D. tube graft
>T.-D. tubularization
>T.-D. urethroplasty

thiethylperazine
thigh graft arteriovenous fistula
thimble bladder
thin
>t. adhesion
>t. basement membrane
>t. basement membrane disease
>Cutinova Hydro T.
>t. descending limb
>t. glomerular basement membrane disease

thin-layer chromatography (TLC)
thin-needle percutaneous cholangiogram
ThinPrep processor
thin-shave sectioning
thin-walled
>t.-w. diverticulum

>t.-w. gallbladder
>t.-w. vascular channel

thiocyanate
>guanidine t.

Thiola
thiol intermediate
thiopental
Thioplex
thiopropazate
thioridazine hydrochloride
thiosulfate-citrate-bile salts-sucrose agar
Thiosulfil
thiotepa
thiothixene
thiourea-resorcinol method
thiphenamil
thiram
third
>T. National Health and Nutrition Examination Survey (NHANES III)
>t. spacing

third-generation
>t.-g. cephalosporin
>t.-g. lithotriptor

thirst
>t. fever
>osmotic threshold for t.

Thiry fistula
Thiry-Vella fistula (TVF)
thistle
>blessed t.
>carline t.
>milk t.

THM
>Tamm-Horsfall mucoprotein

Thomas
>T. nipple reconstruction technique
>T. shunt

Thompson
>T. capsule flap pyeloplasty
>T. cleft lip repair procedure
>T. lithotrite
>T. technique

Thomsen-Friedenreich antigen
thoracic
>t. aortic pathology
>t. aortorenal bypass
>t. duct
>t. endometriosis syndrome
>t. esophagus
>t. fistula
>t. inlet
>t. kidney
>t. stomach

thoracoabdominal
>t. aortic aneurysm (TAAA)
>t. aortic aneurysm surgery
>t. collateral vein
>t. esophagogastrectomy

T

thoracoabdominal (*continued*)
    t. extrapleural approach
    t. incision
    t. intrapleural approach
    t. retroperitoneal lymphadenectomy
thoracolaparotomy
thoracoscopic transdiaphragmatic adrenalectomy
thoracotomy
    esophagectomy with t.
    t. scar
Thorazine
Thorek
    T. gallbladder aspirator
    T. gallbladder forceps
    T. gallbladder scissors
Thorek-Feldman gallbladder scissors
Thorek-Mixter gallbladder forceps
thorium
    colloidal t.
    t. dioxide
Thorn salt-depletion syndrome
Thornton sign
Thorotrast contrast medium
THP
    Tamm-Horsfall protein
tHPT
    tertiary hyperparathyroidism
thread-and-streaks sign
thread-locking device
threadworm
    nondisseminated
      intestinal t.
thready pulse
three-field
three-loop
three-pronged
three-way
threonine
threshold
    gastric mechanosensory t.
    median detection t. (MDT)
    t. of internal sphincter
    t. of rectal sensation
    pH t.
    t. potential (TP)
    swallowing t.
    urethral sensory t.
Th1 response
thrifty colon
thrive
    failure to t.
thrombectomy
thrombi (*pl. of* thrombus)
thrombin
    bovine t.
    t. spray
    topical bovine t.

thrombin-antithrombin
    t.-a. III
    t.-a. III complex
Thrombinar
Thrombin-JMI
thrombocytopenia
    heparin-induced t. (HIT)
thrombocytopenia-absent
    t.-a. radius (TAR)
    t.-a. radius syndrome
thrombocytopenic purpura
thrombocytosis
thromboelastography
thromboembolic
    t. disease
    t. event
thromboembolism
    venous t. (VTE)
thromboendarterectomy
    renal t.
Thrombogen
thrombolytic
    t. agent
    t. therapy
thrombomodulin
thrombophlebitis
    puerperal septic pelvic vein t.
thrombopoietin
thrombosed
    t. internal and external
      hemorrhoids
    t. pile
thromboses (*pl. of* thrombosis)
thrombosis, *pl.* **thromboses**
    arterial t.
    bilateral renal vein thromboses
    bland t.
    glomerular microvascular t.
    hepatic artery t. (HAT)
    hepatic vein t.
    inferior vena cava t.
    intracapillary t.
    intrarenal vascular t.
    intravascular t.
    mesenteric arterial t.
    mesenteric vein t. (MVT)
    nonocclusive mesenteric t.
    peripheral venous t.
    portal vein t. (PVT)
    renal artery t.
    renal vein t. (RVT)
    silent t.
    SMV t.
    splenic vein t.
    venous t.
thrombospondin
thrombotic
    t. lesion
    t. microangiopathy

t. risk factor
t. thrombocytopenic purpura (TTP)
thromboxane A$_2$ (TxA2)
thrombus, *pl.* **thrombi**
bile t.
mural t.
portal vein t.
retrocecalis tumor t.
t. tumor
white t.
through
tearing t.
through-and-through appearance
through-the-scope (TTS)
t.-t.-s. balloon
t.-t.-s. balloon dilation
t.-t.-s. balloon removal
t.-t.-s. bougie
t.-t.-s. catheter probe
t.-t.-s. dilator
t.-t.-s. injection needle
thrush
t. esophagitis
oral t.
thumbnail image
thumbprinting
t. of mucosa
t. sign
thymalfasin
thymi (*pl. of* thymus)
thymic
t. EC
t. hypoplasia
thymidine
thymidine-labeling index
Thymitaq
thymocyte NA+/H+ exchanger
Thymoglobulin
thymol crystal
Thymosin beta 4
thymoxamine
thymus, *pl.* **thymi, thymuses**
thymus-derived
t.-d. cell
t.-d. lymphocyte
thymuses (*pl. of* thymus)
thyreoideus impar plexus
thyroarytenoid muscle
thyroglobulin antibody (TGHA)
thyrohyoid muscle
thyroid
t. autoimmunity
t. disease
t. hormone
t. hormone response element (TRE)
t. hormone serum concentration
medullary carcinoma of t. (MCT)
t. microsomal antibody
t. nodule

tender t.
t. tenderness
thyroiditis
autoimmune t.
Hashimoto t.
thyroidization
thyroid-specific antibody
thyroid-stimulating hormone level
thyromegaly
thyroplasty
thyrotoxicosis
gestational t.
thyrotropin-releasing hormone
thyroxin (*var. of* thyroxine)
thyroxine, thyroxin
free t. (FT4)
thyroxine-binding globulin
TIBC
total iron-binding capacity
TIBC test
ticarcillin
tic douloureux of bladder
Tice
ticklish
ticlopidine
Ti-Cron (*var. of* Tycron)
ticrynafen-induced jaundice
tidal drainage
tide
sign of rising t.
tie
free t.
stick t.
Tycron t.
Tielle Plus hydropolymer dressing
tie-over dressing
TIF
testicular interstitial fluid
Tigan
tight
t. abdomen
t. junction membrane protein
t. junction permeability
t. Nissen repair
t. perirectal adhesion
tigroid appearance
tilt
t. stitch
t. test
Timberlake obturator
time
abdominopelvic orocecal transit t.
activated partial thromboplastin t. (aPTT, APTT)
activated thromboplastin t.
ascites euglobulin lysis t.
bleeding t.
calyceal filling t.
cancer doubling t.

time (*continued*)
    clotting t.
    coagulation t.
    cold ischemia t. (CIT)
    colonic transit t.
    dextrinizing t.
    t. domain ultrasound (TDU)
    doubling t.
    duration t.
    esophageal transit t.
    explosive doubling t.
    gastric bleeding t. (GBT)
    gastric emptying t. (GET)
    gastric transit t.
    intravaginal ejaculation latency t. (IELT)
    mean dissolution t. (MDT)
    mean input t. (MIT)
    mean resistance t. (MRT)
    mean transit t. (MTT)
    median operative t.
    nucleation t. (NT)
    operative t.
    orocecal transit t. (OCTT)
    partial thromboplastin t. (PTT)
    pH holding t.
    post-UUO t.
    preservation t.
    pro t.
    prothrombin t. (pro time, PT)
    prothrombin time/partial thromboplastin t. (PT/PTT)
    PSA doubling t.
    radionuclide esophageal emptying t.
    resection t.
    Russell viper venom t.
    shortened prep t.
    skin bleeding t.
    small-bowel transit t.
    suturing t.
    transit t.
    warm ischemia t.
time-activity curve
Timecaps
    Levsinex T.
time-concentration curve
timed
    t. average urea concentration (TACurea)
    t. voiding
time-dependent variable
Timentin
    double-dose IV T.
    single-dose IV T.
time-of-flight mass spectometry
timing of repair
Tim knot
timolol

timori
    Brugia t.
TIMP
    tissue inhibitor of metalloproteinase
TIMP-1
    tissue inhibitor of metalloproteinase-1
TIMP-2
    tissue inhibitor of metalloproteinase-2
TIN
    tubulointerstitial nephritis
tincture
    t. of belladonna
    t. of benzoin
Tindal
tinea
    t. cruris
    t. purpureum
    t. rubrum
tinidazole
tinkling bowel sounds
TINU
    tubulointerstitial nephritis and uveitis
    TINU syndrome
tinzaparin
tiopronin
tip
    Andrews suction t.
    atraumatic t.
    Buie rectal suction t.
    filiform t.
    Frazier suction t.
    oblique mucosectomy device t.
    occlusion of TIPS
    open-end flow-through radiopaque t.
    papillary t.
    TIPS procedure
    sharp-edged t.
    Slip-Coat t.
    spleen t.
    stenosis of TIPS
    suction t.
    tulip t.
    vessel t.
    villus t.
    weighted t.
TIPPB
    transperineal interstitial permanent prostate brachytherapy
TIPS, TIPSS
    transjugular intrahepatic portosystemic shunt
    occlusion of TIPS
    TIPS procedure
    stenosis of TIPS
Tis disease
Tisseel
    T. fibrin sealant
    T. fibrin sealant injection

tissue

acinar t.
t. adhesive
adipose t.
ampullary granulation t.
t. approximation
bronchus-associated lymphoepithelial
  t. (BALT)
chromaffin t.
cicatricial t.
t. coagulation
connective t.
t. culture
t. culture assay
t. cushion
t. damage
t. destruction result
t. expansion vaginoplasty
extraperitoneal t.
exuberant granulation t.
fatty t.
fibroadipose t.
fibrocollagenous t.
fibroelastic t.
fibrous t.
t. fixation
t. forceps
formalin-fixed t.
t. fusion
gastrointestinal-associated lymphoid t.
  (GALT)
t. glue
gut-associated lymphoepithelial t.
  (GALT)
gut-associated lymphoid t. (GALT)
hilar structure scar t.
t. inhibitor of metalloproteinase
  (TIMP)
t. inhibitor of metalloproteinase-1
  (TIMP-1)
t. inhibitor of metalloproteinase-2
  (TIMP-2)
t. kallikrein
lipomalike t.
lipomatous t.
t. manifestation
t. matrix syndrome
mesorectal t.
t. monomer
t. morcellator
mucosa-associated lymphoid t.
  (MALT)
t. necrosis
necrotic t.
neoplastic t.
noninflamed peripheral t.
nontarget t.
nonviable t.
paracancerous t.

paraffin-embedded t.
parenchymatous t.
periadventitial t.
perinephric t.
periprostatic t.
t. plasminogen activator (TPA, tPA)
t. polypeptide antigen
proliferation of prostatic t.
redundant sac t.
t. renewal
t. resistance
t. rim sign
t. sampling
sex accessory t.
soft t.
t. spectrum analyzer TS-200
splenic t.
subcutaneous t.
T. Tek-II cryostat
testicular adrenallike t. (TALT)
t. transglutaminase (tTG)
t. transglutaminase ELISA
treated t.
**TissueLink Floating Ball radiofrequency
  device**
TissueMend soft tissue repair matrix
tissue-specific gene expression
tissue-stone recognition system (TSRS)
tissue-type plasminogen activator
Titan
T. endoprosthesis
T. stent
titanium
t. clip
t. urethral stent
titanous chloride
titer
anti-HSV IgM Ab t.
antineutrophil cytoplasmic antibody
  t.
antistreptolysin-O t.
ELISA t.
endpoint dilution t.
IgE t.
IgG4 t.
IgM-HEV antibody t.
viral serologic t.
Titralac Plus
titratable acidity
**TJF-100, -130 large-channel
  duodenoscope**
TJF-10, -20 videoduodenoscope
TLA
transperitoneal laparoscopic
  adrenalectomy
TLB
transjugular liver biopsy
TLC
thin-layer chromatography

TLESR
transient lower esophageal sphincter relaxation
TL90 Ethicon stapler
TLN
transperitoneal laparoscopic nephrectomy
T-lymphocyte activation
T-lymphocyte-mediated cytotoxic reaction
TMC
transmural colitis
TMD
transmural drainage
TME
total mesorectal excision
TMPD
transmucosal potential difference
TMP-SMX
trimethoprim-sulfamethoxazole lomefloxacin TMP-SMX
3T3 murine fibroblast
TMx-2000 BPH thermotherapy system
TNF
tumor necrosis factor
TNF-alpha
tumor necrosis factor alpha
TNF-a. assay
TNF-a. gene
TNM
tumor, nodes, metastases
TNM classification
TNM classification of carcinoma
TNM system for tumor staging
TNTC
too numerous to count
toast
bananas, rice, cereal, applesauce, and t. (BRAT)
bananas, rice, cereal, applesauce, tea, and t. (BRATT)
tobacco dose exposure
tobramycin
tocainide hydrochloride
tocodynamometer
guard-ring t.
TODAY
Treatment Options for Type 2 Diabetes in Adolescents and Youth
Todd cirrhosis
toddler's diarrhea
toe
clubbing of fingers and t.'s
Tofranil, Tofranil-PM
toilet
peritoneal t.
tolazamide
tolazoline hydrochloride
tolbutamide-induced cholestasia

tolcapone
Toldt
line of T.
T. membrane
white line of T.
tolerability data
tolerance
glucose t.
oral t.
transplantation t.
tolerated
diet as t. (DAT)
toleration
maximal t.
Tolerex feeding solution
tolerogenic dendritic cell
tolevamer
toll-interleukin
t.-i. 1 receptor
t.-i. 1 receptor domain-containing adapter protein
toll-like receptor
tolmetin
tolnaftate
tolterodine
t. tartrate
t. tartrate capsule
toluidine
t. blue
t. blue stain
Tom
T. Jones closure
T. Jones suture
Toma sign
Tomenius gastroscope
Tomocat
tomodensitometric examination
tomodensitometry
computed t.
tomography
computed t. (CT)
computerized t. (CT)
contrast-enhanced computed t.
3-dimensional optical coherence t.
dual-phase helical computed t.
electron-beam computerized t. (EBCT)
endoscopic Doppler optical coherence t.
endoscopic optical coherence t.
F-18 fluorodeoxyglucose positron emission t.
18-fluorodeoxyglucose positron emission t.
helical computed t. (HCT)
noncontrast computerized t.
noncontrast helical computed t.
optic coherence t. (OCT)
positron emission t. (PET)

single-photon emission computed t. (SPECT)
single-photon emission computerized t. (SPECT)
spiral computed t.
ultrafast computerized t.
ultrasonic t.
unenhanced helical computed t.

Tonalin
tone
anal sphincter t.
bowel t.
cardiac sympathovagal t.
gastric t.
lower esophageal sphincter t.
pyloric t.
renovascular t.
sphincter t.

tongs
tongue
bifid t.
black hairy t.
t. deviation
fissured t.
geographic t.
hairy t.
t. movement
mucosal t.
t. of tumor
smoker's t.
swollen t.

tongue-shaped villus
tonic
t. contraction
t. neck

tonicity
low t.
plasma t.

Tonkaflo pump
tonometry
tonsil
t. clamp
t. forceps
orange-colored t.
t. sucker

tonsillar enlargement
tonsillectomy
tool
GERDyzer t.
prognostic t.

Toomey
T. evacuator
T. syringe

too numerous to count (TNTC)
toothed tissue forceps
TOPA
topical oropharyngeal anesthesia

Töpfer test
Top-Fill enteral feeding bag

topical
t. anesthetic
t. antibiotic
t. betamethasone
t. bovine thrombin
t. neuropathy
t. nifedipine
t. oropharyngeal anesthesia (TOPA)
Synalar T.
t. treatment
t. Xylocaine

Topicort cream
Topiglan
topiramate
Top Notch automated biopsy system
topogram
balloon t.

topography
scintigraphic balloon t.

topoisomerase I inhibitor
toposcopic catheter
topotecan
Toprol
Toradol
Torbot
T. cement
T. faceplate

Torecan
Torek
T. operation
T. orchiopexy

toremifene
tori (*pl. of* torus)
Toronto-Western catheter
torovirus
Torquay test
torque
t. catheter
translation of t.
t. vise
t. wire

torquing of scope
torrential hemorrhage
Torres syndrome
torsemide
torsion
adnexal t.
appendix testis t.
biliary tract t.
cryptorchidism t.
extravaginal t.
gallbladder t.
intravaginal t.
t. of appendage
t. of gallbladder
t. of testis
penile t.
perinatal t.
spermatic cord t.

torsion (*continued*)
    synchronous neonatal t.
    testicular t.
    ureteral t.
torso crease
torticollis
tortuous
    t. esophagus
    t. ureter
    t. venous ectasia
torulopsis
    T. glabrata
    t. infection
torus, *pl.* **tori**
    t. palatinus
    t. ureter
Toshiba
    T. ERVF 1A video floppy recorder
    T. Sal 38B real-time
      ultrasonography
    T. Sonolayer SSA250A transrectal
      ultrasonography
    T. TCE-M-series colonoscope
    T. videoendoscope
Tosoh assay
Tostrex
tosylate
    sorafenib t.
Totacillin
total
    t. abdominal colectomy (TAC)
    t. abdominal evisceration (TAE)
    t. anorectal reconstruction
    t. bilateral vagotomies
    t. bile acid (TBA)
    t. bilirubin
    t. body irradiation (TBI)
    t. body nitrogen (TBN)
    t. body water (TBW)
    t. bowel rest
    t. colonoscopy
    t. corrected incremental score
      (TCIS)
    t. cystectomy
    t. cystourethrectomy
    t. descent
    t. dose infusion
    t. enteral nutrition (TEN)
    t. fasting
    t. fecal weight test
    t. gastrectomy
    t. gastric wrap
    t. glutathione content
    t. hematuria
    t. hemolytic complement
    t. homocysteine (tHcy)
    t. homocysteine plasma concentration
    t. infarction
    t. internal reflection

    t. iron-binding capacity (TIBC)
    t. iron-binding capacity test
    t. lymphocytes
    t. lymphoid irradiation (TLI)
    t. measured renal cortex
    t. mesorectal excision (TME)
    t. pancreatectomy
    t. parenteral alimentation
    t. parenteral nutrition (TPN)
    t. parenteral nutrition line
    t. pelvic exenteration
    t. perineal prostatectomy
    t. peripheral parenteral nutrition
      (TPPN)
    t. peroral intraoperative enteroscopy
    t. predicted return
    t. prostatoseminal vesiculectomy
    t. protein
    t. protein concentration
    t. PSA (tPSA)
    t. scrotectomy
    t. serum prostatic acid phosphatase
      (TSPAP)
    t. slit pore length
    t. transurethral resection of prostate
      (T-TURP)
    t. urinary nitrogen (TUN)
    t. urogenital mobilization
totalis
    varicosis coli t.
totally
    t. extraperitoneal (TEP)
    t. extraperitoneal hernia repair
    t. stapled restorative proctocolectomy
      (TSRPC)
totipotent, totipotential
totipotential (*var. of* totipotent)
touch
    t. cytology
    T. preparation
Toupet
    T. antireflux procedure
    T. hemifundoplication
    T. partial posterior fundoplication
tour de maitre
tourniquet
    double-loop t.
    Dupuytren t.
    Gill renal t.
    t. occlusion
    Rumel t.
    single-loop t.
towel clip
Townes-Brocks syndrome
toxemia, toxicemia
    hepatic t.
    t. of pregnancy
toxic
    t. appearance

t. cirrhosis
t. colitis
t. diarrhea
t. dilation of bowel
t. dilation of colon
t. epidermal necrolysis (TEN)
t. gastritis
t. glomerulopathy
t. hepatitis
t. megacolon
t. metabolite
t. nephropathy
t. shock syndrome
t. steatosis
toxicemia (*var. of* toxemia)
toxicity
acetaminophen t.
acute hepatic t.
aluminum t.
ammonia t.
bleomycin t.
calcineurin inhibitor t.
chloroform t.
chlorzoxazone t.
cyclosporine t.
direct tubular t.
hyperbaric oxygen t.
octreotide-induced hepatic t.
potential t.
progressive t.
protein-mediated tubular t.
quality-adjusted time without symptoms or t. (Q-TWIST)
renal t.
theophylline t.
vitamin A t.
Toxicodendron dermatitis
toxicosis
toxicum
erythema t.
toxigenic
t. bacterium
t. diarrhea
toxin
t. A, B
albumin-bound t.
t. assay
botulinum t. (BTX, Botox)
botulinum toxin A (BTA)
cholera t.
Coley t.
cytoskeleton-altering t.
t. exposure
heat-labile t.
industrial t.
occupational t.

pertussin t.
secreted autotransporter t.
Shiga t. (Stx)
Shiga-like t. (SLT)
VacA t.
toxin-mediated intestinal secretion
Toxocara canis
toxocariasis
Toxoplasma
T. colitis
T. gondii
toxoplasmosis
TPA, tPA
12-O-tetradecanoylphorbol-13-acetate
tissue plasminogen activator
phorbol ester TPA
TP40 **gene**
TP53 **gene**
TPH
transrectal prostatic hyperthermia
*TP53***-mutated carcinoma**
TPN
total parenteral nutrition
TPN line
T-pouch
T-p. ileal neobladder
T-p. technique
TPPN
total peripheral parenteral nutrition
tPSA
total PSA
TP-400t pressure transducer
trabecula, *pl.* **trabeculae**
trabeculae corporis spongiosi
trabeculae corporum cavernosorum
trabeculae lienis
trabeculae of corpora cavernosa of penis
trabeculae of corpus spongiosum of penis
trabeculae of spleen
trabeculae splenicae
trabeculae (*pl. of* trabecula)
trabecular
t. bone fracture
t. sinusoidal pattern
t. structure
trabecularism
trabeculate
trabeculated bladder
trabeculation
detrusor muscle t.
t. of bladder dome
Trabucco double balloon catheter
trace-gas analysis
tracer
focal accumulation of t.
T. Hybrid wire guide
T. ST wire

T

tracheal
    t. bifurcation
    t. deviation
    t. ulceration
trachelocystitis
tracheobronchial
    t. aspiration
    t. malacia
    t. Z stent
tracheoesophageal (TE)
    t. fistula (TEF)
    t. junction
    t. puncture (TEP)
    t. septum
tracheostomy
Trach-Eze closed suction catheter
trachomatis
    Chlamydia t.
tracing
    Narco Bio-Systems MMS 200
      physiograph t.
    sexually transmitted disease contact
      t.
track
    horseshoe t.
    radial suture t.
    submucosal t.
Tracker catheter
tract
    aerodigestive t.
    alimentary t.
    allantoic t.
    benign mesothelioma of genital t.
    biliary t.
    digestive t.
    t. dilation
    double-contrast barium examination
      of upper gastrointestinal t. (DCGI)
    drilling t.
    fistula t.
    fistulous t.
    gastrocutaneous fistula t.
    gastrointestinal t. (GIT)
    genital t.
    genitourinary t.
    GI t.
    hepatic outflow t.
    ileal inflow t.
    ileal outflow t.
    infected t.
    intestinal t.
    intramural fistulous t.
    Lewis classification for vascular
      anomalies of gastrointestinal t.
    Moore classification for vascular
      anomalies of gastrointestinal t.
    needle t.
    nephrostomy t.
    nucleus of solitary t.

    ororespiratory t.
    outflow t.
    pancreaticobiliary t.
    perineal sinus t.
    portal t.
    sacrococcygeal pilonidal sinus t.
    safe gastrocutaneous fistula t.
    sinus t.
    t. tamponade
    transsphincteric fistula t.
    T-tube t.
    upper gastrointestinal t.
    urinary t.
    Z t.
traction
    caudal t.
    cephalad t.
    t. diverticulum
    enterocele t.
    postinflammatory t.
    t. suture
traction-type papillotome
tractor
    Lowsley t.
    Syms t.
    Young prostatic t.
trafficking
    leukocyte t.
    membrane t.
Trager therapy
Trail-Making Test
Trail test
trainer
    Personal EMG t.
training
    bladder t.
    endourological t.
    pelvic muscle t.
    pubococcygeal muscle t.
trait
    X-linked recessive t.
tramadol
tramazoline
tram-line calcification
Trandate
tranexamic
    t. acid
    t. acid enema
Tranilast
tranquilizer
transabdominal
    t. Burch urethrocystopexy
    t. cholangiography
    t. hydrocolonic sonography
    t. preperitoneal (TAPP)
    t. preperitoneal hernia repair
    t. scan
transactivator
    classical t.

transaminase
    glutamate pyruvate t. (GLPT)
    glutamic-oxaloacetic t. (GOT)
    glutamic-pyruvic t. (GPT)
    serum glutamic-oxaloacetic t.
      (SGOT)
    serum glutamic-pyruvic t. (SGPT)
transampullary
transanal
    t. anastomosis
    t. catheter
    t. drainage tube
    t. endoscopic microsurgery (TEM)
    t. endoscopic microsurgical resection
    t. excision
    t. ultrasonography
transaortic endarterectomy
transarterial
    t. catheter embolization (TACE)
    t. chemoembolization (TACE)
    t. perfusion cooling
transballoon cystometry
transblotting cell
transcapillary
    t. diffusion
    t. escape rate
    t. hydrostatic pressure gradient
transcarbamylase
    heterozygous ornithine t.
transcatheter
    t. arterial chemoembolization (TACE)
    t. arterial embolization therapy
    t. arterial infusion
    t. embolotherapy
    t. hepatic arterial embolization
    t. perfusion
    t. splenic arterial embolization
      (TSAE)
    t. treatment
    t. variceal embolization
transcellular
    t. absorption
    t. pathway
Transcend implantable gastric stimulator
transcoccygeal vesiculectomy
transcolonic endoscopy
transcranial magnetic stimulation
  (TCMS)
transcriptase
    avian myeloblastosis virus reverse t.
    t. polymerase chain reaction assay
    reverse t. (RT)
    thermostable reverse t.
transcription
    t. factor
    t. factor API
    reverse t.
    signal transducer and activator of t.
     1 (Stat1)

transcription-mediated amplification
  (TMA)
transcutaneous
    t. biopsy
    t. electrical nerve stimulation
      (TENS)
    t. nerve
    t. registration
    t. sacral neurostimulation
    t. sonogram endoscope
    t. ultrasonography
    t. ultrasound
    t. ultrasound imaging
transcystic duct/common bile duct
  exploration (TCD/CBDE)
transdermal
    t. oxybutynin for urinary
      incontinence
    t. therapeutic system (TTS)
Transderm-Nitro
transducer
    antral pressure t.
    bifocal multiplane rectal t.
    Bruel-Kjaer axial t.
    t. catheter
    curved-array t.
    Dantec Etude uroflow t.
    electromagnetic flow t.
    Elema-Siemens AB pressure t.
    external pressure t.
    GF-UM2, -UM3, -UM20
      radial-sector scan t.
    Gould pressure t.
    intracavitary t.
    linear-array t.
    LSC 7000 curved-array t.
    Nellcor Durasensor adult
      oxygen t.
    Olympus intracavity t.
    piezoelectric t.
    pressure t.
    Sensor Medics pressure t.
    Siemens Endo-P endodrectal t.
    solid-state pressure t.
    Soreson pressure t.
    Spectramed t.
    Statham external t.
    Statham pressure t.
    strain-gauge t.
    TP-400t pressure t.
    transrectal multiplane 3-dimensional
     t.
    ultrasound t.
    Unisensor strain-gauge t.
    volume displacement t.
transduction
    downstream signal t.
    t. pathway
    receptor and signal t.

T

transduodenal
    t. approach
    t. drainage
    t. endoscopic decompression
    t. injection
    t. sphincteroplasty
    t. sphincterotomy
transection, transsection
    t. and devascularization operation
    bladder t.
    esophageal t.
    high t.
    nerve t.
    Sugiura esophageal variceal t.
transendoscopic
    t. electrocoagulation
    t. laser photocoagulation
    t. sphincterotomy
    t. ultrasound
transepithelial tubular transport
transesophageal
    t. endoscopic plication (TEP)
    t. endoscopy
    t. ligation
    t. ligation of varix
transfected
transfection
transfemoral liver biopsy
transfer
    t. dysfunction
    t. dysphagia
    t. factor
    gamete intrafallopian t. (GIFT)
    unidirectional t.
transferase
    aspartate t.
    glucuronyl t.
    glutathione t.
transferrin
    t. receptor
    t. receptor 2
    t. saturation
    t. saturation level
    serum t.
    t. test
Transfix sutureless sling fixation system
transformary mass
transformation
    blastoid t.
    Eadie-Hofstee t.
    giant cell t.
    neoplastic t.
    nodular t.
    t. zone
transforming
    t. growth factor (TGF)
    t. growth factor alpha (TGF-alpha)
    t. growth factor beta (TGF-beta)

    t. growth factor beta-1 (TGF-beta-1)
    t. growth factor beta-2 (TGF-beta-2)
    t. growth factor beta-3 (TGF-beta-3)
transfuse
transfusion
    autologous t.
    blood t.
    donor-specific t. (DST)
    t. hepatitis
    intraoperative autologous t.
    t. nephritis
    peritoneal t.
    platelet t.
    postoperative autologous t.
    required t.
    type-specific blood t.
transfusional iron overload
transfusion-associated hepatitis
transfusion-related chronic liver disease
transfusion-transmitted virus (TTV)
transgastric
    t. cholangiogram
    t. drainage
    t. esophageal bougienage
    t. fine-needle aspiration biopsy
    t. ligation
    t. plication
transgastrostomic enteroscopy (TGE)
transgastrostomy
transgenesis
    mammalian t.
transglomerular hydrostatic filtration pressure
transglutaminase
    tissue t. (tTG)
trans-Golgi network
transhepatic
    t. antegrade biliary drainage procedure
    t. biliary drainage
    t. biliary stent
    t. catheterization
    t. cholangiogram (THC)
    t. cholangiography (TC, THC)
    t. embolization (THE)
    t. portacaval shunt
    t. portal venous sampling
    t. portography
    t. vascular resistance
transhiatal
    t. blunt esophagectomy
    t. radical esophagectomy
    t. resection
    t. simple esophagectomy
transient
    t. cholangitis
    t. discontinuation
    t. gastroparesis
    t. LES relaxation

t. lower esophageal sphincter relaxation (TLESR)
t. proteinuria
t. receptor potential vanilloid-5 (TRPV5)
t. relaxation of LES
transileostomy manometry
transilluminate
transillumination
kidney t.
transilluminator
UV t.
transistor
ion-sensitive field-effect t.
transit
bolus t.
delayed colonic t.
gastrointestinal t.
ileocolic t.
mean colonic t. (MCT)
slow colonic t.
t. time
whole-gut t.
transition
t. mutation
t. suture
t. zone index
t. zone volume
transitional
t. cell
t. cell cancer-associated (TCCA)
t. cell carcinoma
t. cell carcinoma of bladder (TCCB)
t. epithelium
t. feeding
t. zone
t. zone biopsy
transitory block
transjugular
t. intrahepatic portacaval shunt procedure
t. intrahepatic portosystemic shunt (TIPS, TIPSS)
t. liver biopsy (TLB)
t. portal venography
t. portosystemic shunt stent (TIPSS)
translation of torque
translocation
bacterial t.
translumbar inferior vena cava catheter
transluminal
t. pseudocyst drainage
t. ultrasonography
transmembrane
t. beta subunit
t. electrical potential difference

t. hydraulic pressure
t. protein
t. signal
transmesenteric plication
transmission
bloodborne t.
t. electron microscopy (TEM)
fecal t.
fecal-oral t.
horizontal t.
oral t.
real-time t.
synaptic t.
vertical t.
transmittable disease
transmitter
NANC inhibitory t.
nonadrenergic noncholinergic inhibitory t.
putative t.
transmucosal
t. electrical potential test
t. potential difference (TMPD)
transmural
t. approach
t. burn
t. colitis (TMC)
t. drainage (TMD)
t. endoscopy
t. fibrosis
t. hydrostatic pressure gradient
t. ileocolitis
t. inflammation
t. rejection
transnasal
t. bile duct catheterization
t. endoluminal ultrasonography
t. endoscopy
t. pancreaticobiliary drain
t. videogastroscope
transobturator tape
Transonics
T. laser-Doppler flowmeter
T. Systems flow probe
transoral endoscopic suturing
transpapillary
t. approach
t. biopsy
t. cannulation
t. catheterization
t. cystopancreatic stent
t. drain
t. drainage
t. endoscopic cholecystotomy (TEC)
t. endoscopic endoprosthesis
t. insertion of self-expanding biliary metal stent
t. therapy
transparent elastic band ligating device

transpeptidase
    gamma glutamyl t. (GGT, GGTP)
    glutamyl t. (GTP)
transperineal
    t. interstitial permanent prostate brachytherapy (TIPPB)
    t. palladium-103
    t. seed implant
    t. ultrasonography
    t. ultrasonography technique
    t. ultrasound-guided template biopsy
    t. vesiculectomy
transperitoneal
    t. anterior subcostal incision (TASI)
    t. laparoscopic adrenalectomy (TLA)
    t. laparoscopic nephrectomy (TLN)
    t. laparoscopic nephroureterectomy
    t. orchiopexy
    t. radical nephroureterectomy
    t. simple nephrectomy
transplant
    acute rejection of liver t.
    allogenic kidney t.
    auxiliary t.
    cadaveric intestinal t.
    cadaveric renal t.
    combined kidney and pancreas t. (CKPT)
    t. consideration
    Domino t.
    failed t.
    Gallie t.
    heart t.
    heart-kidney t.
    hypercholesterolemic cadaveric renal t.
    kidney t.
    liver t.
    living donor t.
    t. nephrectomy
    pancreas-kidney t.
    reduced liver t. (RLT)
    reduced-size liver t. (RSLT)
    t. rejection
    renal t.
    t. renal artery stenosis (TRAS)
    simultaneous pancreas and kidney t.
    split-liver t.
    xenograft t.
transplantation
    ABO-incompatible living donor kidney t.
    anhepatic stage of liver t.
    t. antigen
    auxiliary heterotopic liver t. (AHLT)
    auxiliary partial orthotopic liver t. (APOLT)
    auxiliary partial orthotopic living donor t.

cadaveric renal t.
chronic rejection after renal t.
en bloc kidney t.
ex vivo bench surgery with renal t.
future role of target of rapamycin inhibitors in renal t.
heart t.
hemopoietic cell t.
hepatocyte t.
infection after renal t.
kidney t.
liver t.
living donor liver t. (LDLT)
nonmyeloablative allogeneic peripheral blood stem cell t.
organ t.
orthotopic liver t. (Olt, OLT, OLTx)
pancreas t.
pancreatic islet cell t. (PICT)
pancreaticoduodenal t.
piggyback liver t.
renal t.
small-bowel t.
SPK t.
split-liver t.
t. tolerance
transplantectomy
transplanted cancer
Transpore tape
transport
    active t.
    t. aminoaciduria
    BD ProbeTec urine preservative t.
    bolus t.
    cation t.
    chyme t.
    condition of impaired sodium t.
    convective t.
    diffusive t.
    fluid t.
    glucose t.
    lymphatic t.
    nephron t.
    peritoneal membrane t.
    peritoneal solute t.
    retinoid t.
    single-nephron glomerular t.
    sodium t.
    solute t.
    transepithelial tubular t.
    urine t.
transporter
    divalent metal t. 1 (DMT1)
    glucose t.
    low-affinity t.
    multispecific organic anion t.
    polarized glucose t.
    putative anion t.
    serotonin reuptake t.

transporterlike
 zinc-iron regulated t. (ZIRTL)
transposition
 buttonhole preputial t.
 gastric t.
 gluteus maximus t.
 ileocecal segment t.
 penoscrotal t.
 portacaval t. (PCT)
transpubic incision
transpyloric
 t. feeding
 t. tube
transrectal
 t. multiplane 3-dimensional
  transducer
 t. probe
 t. prostatic hyperthermia (TPH)
 t. prostatic ultrasonography
 t. scan
 t. sonography
 t. ultrasonography (TRUS)
 t. ultrasonography-guided biopsy
 t. ultrasound (TRUS)
 t. ultrasound scanning (TRUS)
 t. ultrasound staging
 t. vasography
transscrotal
transsection (*var. of* transection)
transseptal orchiopexy
transsexual surgery
transsphincteric
 t. anal fistula
 t. fistula tract
transthoracic
 t. esophagectomy
 t. resection of esophageal carcinoma
transthyretin
transtubular potassium gradient (TTKG)
transudative ascites
transureteropyelocutaneous ureterostomy
transureteropyelostomy
transureteroureteral anastomosis
transureteroureterostomy (TUU)
transurethral
 t. ablative prostatectomy
 t. balloon dilation
 t. balloon laserthermia prostatectomy
 t. catheter
 t. collagen injection therapy
 t. cutaneous ureterostomy
 t. electrical bladder stimulation
  (TEBS)
 t. electrovaporization
 t. electrovaporization of prostate
  (TUVP, TVP, TUEVP)
 t. endoscopic manipulation
 t. ethanol ablation of prostate
  (TEAP)

 t. evaporation of prostate (TUEP)
 t. grooving of prostate
 t. hot-water balloon thermoablation
 t. incision (TUI)
 t. incision of bladder neck (TUIBN)
 t. incision of prostate (TUIP)
 t. laser incision of prostate
 t. microwave thermotherapy (TUMT)
 t. microwave thermotherapy
  functional result
 t. needle ablation (TUNA)
 t. needle ablation of prostate
 t. prostatic resection study
 t. rectal ultrasound
 t. resection (TUR)
 t. resection of bladder (TURB)
 t. resection of bladder tumor
  (TURBT)
 t. resection of prostate (TURP)
 t. resection of prostate functional
  result
 t. resection syndrome
 t. resectoscope
 t. sphincterotomy
 t. ultrasound-guided laser-induced
  prostatectomy (TULIP)
 t. unroofing
 t. ureterorenoscopy (URS)
 t. vaporization of prostate (TUVP)
 t. vaporization-resection of prostate
  (TUVRP)
transvaginal
 t. bone anchor
 t. Burch procedure
 t. enterocele repair
 t. mesh cystocele repair
 t. sacrospinous colpopexy
 t. suturing (TVS)
 t. suturing system
 t. therapy
 t. trocar
 t. ultrasound (TVUS, TVU)
 t. urethrolysis
transvenous
 t. liver biopsy
 t. perfusion
transversa
 plica vesicalis t.
transversalis fascia
transverse
 t. colectomy
 t. colon
 t. colostomy
 t. colostomy effluent
 t. duodenotomy
 t. fissure
 t. folds of rectum
 t. image
 t. loop

T

transverse (*continued*)
  t. loop rod colostomy
  t. process
  t. resection
  t. retubularized ileovesicostomy
  t. retubularized sigmoidovesicostomy
  t. semilunar skin incision
  t. sonogram
  t. testicular ectopia
  t. ulceration
  t. umbilical line
  t. vaginal septum
  t. view
transversion mutation
transversostomy
transversourethralis
transversum
  colon t.
transversus
  t. abdominis muscle
  t. perinei muscle
transvesical
  t. laparoscopic approach
  t. laparoscopic detachment
  t. potassium sensitivity test
  t. scan
  t. vesiculectomy
Transwell cell culture
Tranxene
tranylcypromine
trap
  Endodynamics suction polyp t.
  specimen t.
trapezoid method
trapped
  t. basket
  t. penis
  t. penis after circumcision
  t. prostate gland
trapping
  penoscrotal t.
TRAS
  transplant renal artery stenosis
Tratner catheter
Traube semilunar space
trauma
  autoerotic rectal t.
  bile duct t.
  birth t.
  bladder t.
  blunt abdominal t.
  blunt liver t.
  blunt pancreatic t.
  colonic t.
  colorectal t.
  diaphragmatic hernia t.
  duodenal t.
  esophageal t.
  external t.

foreign body t.
functional t.
gallbladder t.
gastric t.
hepatic t.
homosexual rectal t.
iatrogenic pancreatic t.
liver t.
management of adult urinary
  tract t.
t. of gallbladder
pancreatic t.
penetrating abdominal t.
penetrating pancreatic t.
penetrating penile t.
penile t.
perineal impact t.
rectal t.
renal t.
scrotal t.
small-intestine t.
splenic t.
Texas t.
TraumaCal enteral feeding
Traum-Aid HBC enteral feeding
traumatic
  t. appendicitis
  t. corporeal venoocclusive
    dysfunction
  t. diaphragmatic hernia
  t. grasping forceps
  t. inflammation
  t. lesion
  t. locking grasper
  t. masturbation
  t. orchitis
  t. proctitis
  t. renal mass
  t. rupture
Travamulsion fat emulsion solution
Travasol amino acid
Travasorb
  T. Hepatic Diet
  T. HN powdered feeding
  T. MCT liquid feeding
  T. MCT supplement
  T. Renal Diet
  T. STD liquid feeding
traveler's
  t. chemoprophylaxis
  t. diarrhea
Traverso-Longmire
  pancreatoduodenectomy technique
tray
  Curity irrigation t.
  Urine Meter Foley t.
trazodone
treated tissue
treating physician

treatment
    acorn t.
    add-back t.
    adjuvant t.
    alfa interferon t.
    alpha-blocker t.
    alternate-day t.
    amoxicillin-clavulanate t.
    amoxicillin-omeprazole t.
    anabolic steroid t.
    anoplasty t.
    anti-*Helicobacter pylori* t.
    antihypertensive t.
    t. balloon
    behavioral t.
    BrachySeed prostate cancer t.
    t. channel
    cholecystectomy t.
    chronic anoplasty t.
    conventional t.
    corticosteroid t.
    CyPat t.
    dialytic t.
    downregulation after furosemide t.
    endoscopic t.
    endovascular t.
    esophageal dilation t.
    t. failure
    famotidine maintenance t.
    first-line t.
    fixed and dynamic urethral
      compression t.
    foscarnet t.
    Gelfoam particle transarterial
      embolization t.
    glucocorticoid t.
    hemangioma laser t.
    initial t.
    interferon t.
    intracavernosal injection t.
    intralesional t.
    intraprostatic temperature-guided t.
    KTP/Nd:YAG laser t.
    lipiodol transarterial embolization t.
    lower energy t.
    maintenance t.
    mercury bougienage t.
    microwave nonsurgical t.
    Milligan-Morgan technique for
      hemorrhoid t.
    minimally invasive t.
    mitomycin transarterial
      embolization t.
    t. morbidity
    Murphy t.
    neoadjuvant antiandrogenic t.
    Ochsner t.
    t. of bladder cancer
    t. of neurogenic refractory urge

    t. of nonspecific inflammatory injury
    t. of renal calculus
    t. of rhabdomyosarcoma
    T. Options for Type 2 Diabetes in
      Adolescents and Youth (TODAY)
    oxandrolone t.
    pharmacologic t.
    photocoagulation t.
    Plummer t.
    preoperative tumor t.
    prophylactic antibiotic t.
    ProstaLund feedback t.
    prostatic thermal t.
    ProstRcision t.
    t. protocol
    rectovaginal surgical t.
    self-bougienage t.
    serotonin antagonist t.
    sham t.
    shock wave t.
    success of surgical t.
    supportive t.
    suppression t.
    topical t.
    transcatheter t.
    t. with rapamycin

tree
    apple t.
    biliary t.
    cannulation of biliary t.
    chaste t.
    cotton t.
    Croton lechleri t.
    fringe t.
    hepatobiliary t.
    t. of heaven
    pancreatic t.
    pancreaticobiliary t.
    phylogenetic t.
    tea t.

trefoil
    t. deformity
    t. domain
    t. factor
    t. factor family 1—3 (TFF)
    t. peptide

trehalose

Treitz
    T. arch
    T. fossa
    T. hernia
    ligament of T.

Trélat stool

Trelex mesh

Trelstar
    T. Depot
    T. LA

tremor
    resting t.

tremor-nystagmus-ulcer syndrome
trench nephritis
Trendelenburg
    T. gait
    T. position
Trental
trephine biopsy
Treponema
    T. immunofluorescence study
    T. pallidum
treprostinil
tretinoin
Treves
    T. fold
    plane of T.
Trexall
triad
    Andersen t.
    Borchardt t.
    Charcot t.
    Currarino t.
    Dieulafoy t.
    hepatic t.
    Meltzer t.
    t. of adenoma sebaceum, epilepsy,
      and mental retardation
    t. of Rigler
    portal t.
    Quincke t.
    radiographic t.
    t. syndrome
    Whipple t.
triaditis
    portal t.
trial
    T. AG
    aggressive therapeutic t.
    AIPRI t.
    angiotensin-converting enzyme
      inhibition in progressive renal
      insufficiency t.
    t. antacid
    antihypertensive and lipid-lowering
      treatment to prevent heart attack t.
      (ALLHAT)
    Antioxidant Polyp Prevention T.
    calcitriol t.
    CHARM t.
    cisapride-functional dyspepsia t.
    clinical t.
    direct-current electrotherapy t.
    domperidone-functional dyspepsia t.
    Medical Therapy of Prostatic
      Symptoms t.
    Modification of Diet in Renal
      Disease t.
    MTOPS t.
    multicenter prospective t.
    placebo-controlled t.

    prospective clinical t.
    prospective multicenter
      randomized t.
    prospective randomized controlled t.
    Prostate Cancer Intervention Versus
      Observation T. (PCIVOT, PIVOT)
    published comparative t.
    recent clinical t.
    Stockholm t. I, II
    Swedish Rectal Cancer T.
    T. Using Medicinal Microbiotic
      Yogurt (TUMMY)
    Vioxx Gastrointestinal Outcomes
      Research t.
    t. without catheter (TWOC)
triamcinolone cream
Triamonide 40
triamterene
    t. calculus
    hydrochlorothiazide and t.
    t. urolithiasis
triangle
    anal t.
    Calot t.
    cardiohepatic t.
    Charcot t.
    cystohepatic t.
    digastric t.
    femoral t.
    gastrinoma t.
    T. gelatin-sealed sling material
    Grynfeltt t.
    Henke t.
    Hesselbach t.
    inguinal t.
    Killian t.
    Labbe t.
    Lesgaft t.
    Livingston t.
    lumbocostoabdominal t.
    mesenteric t.
    t. of doom
    t. of pain
    Petit t.
    Scarpa t.
    urogenital t.
triangle-tipped knife
triangular
    t. ligament
    t. vaginal patch sling
triangulation stapling method
triazolam
tricarboxylic
    t. acid (TCA)
    t. acid cycle
triceps
    t. skinfold thickness
    t. skinfold thickness test
trichilemmoma

Trichinella
> *T. paupae*
> *T. pseudospiralis*
> *T. spiralis*

trichinelliasis (*var. of* trichinosis)
trichinellosis (*var. of* trichinosis)
trichiniasis (*var. of* trichinosis)
trichinosis, trichinelliasis, trichinellosis, trichiniasis
trichiura
> *Trichuris t.*

trichlormethiazide
trichloroacetic acid (TCA)
trichloroethylene
trichobezoar
trichocyst
trichomonal balanitis
Trichomonas
> *T. hominis*
> *T. vaginalis* (TV)

trichomoniasis
> vaginal t.

trichomycosis
trichophagia
trichophytobezoar
Trichophyton
> *T. mentagrophytes*
> *T. rubrum*

Trichosporon
> *T. beigelii*
> *T. capitatum*

Trichostrongylus
trichrome
> Masson t.
> t. stain

trichuriasis
Trichuris
> *T. muris*
> *T. suis*
> *T. trichiura*

tricitrate
trickle perfusion
TriClip endoscopic clipping device
triclosan 0.1%
tricomponent coaxial system
tricyclamol
tricyclic antidepressant
tridecapeptide
tridihexethyl chloride
Tridrate bowel preparation
triene
> macrocyclic t.

triethylenethiophosphoramide
trifid stomach
trifluoperazine
triflupromazine
trifurcation variant
trigeminy
Trigesic

trigger
> rectal feedback t.
> urethral feedback t.
> t. voiding

triggering
> R-wave t.

triglyceride
> t. enzyme deficiency
> long-chain t. (LCT)
> medium-chain t. (MCT)
> serum t.
> VLDL t.

triglyceride-rich
> t.-r. lipoprotein (TRL)
> t.-r. protein

trigona (*pl. of* trigonum)
trigonal plate
trigone
> bladder t.
> deep t.
> fascia of urogenital t.

trigonitis
trigonotome
trigonum, *pl.* **trigona**
> t. vesicae

trihexyphenidyl
trihydrate
> amoxicillin t.

trihydrocoprostanic acid (TCA)
trihydroxy salt
triiodobenzene
Trilafon
trilobar
> t. hyperplasia
> t. hypertrophy

Trilogy low-profile balloon dilation catheter
TriLyte
Trimadeau sign
Trimazide
Trimedyne
> T. Flex MAX fiber
> T. holmium laser
> T. Optilase 1000 device

trimeprazine tartrate
trimer
trimetaphan
trimethidinium
trimethobenzamide
trimethoprim (TMP)
> sulfamethoxazole and t. (SMX-TMP, SMX/TMP)

trimethoprim-sulfamethoxazole (TMP-SMX)
> t.-s. DS

trimethylsilyl ether
trimetrexate glucuronate
Trimox
Trimpex

T

Trinalin Repetabs
trinitrate
glyceryl t.
Trinovin
Trinsicon
triolein C-14 breath test
triopathy
trioxide
antimony t.
tripelennamine
tripeptide
disaccharide t.
triphasic cystometric curve
triphosphatase
adenosine t. (ATPase)
hydrogen adenosine t.
1,4,5-triphosphate
inositol 1,4,5-t. (IP$_3$)
triphosphate
adenosine t. (ATP)
guanosine t. (GTP)
inositol t.
terminal deoxynucleotide
transferase-mediated deoxyuridine t.
triple
t. eradication therapy
t. intussusception
t. rubber band ligation
triple-balloon probe
triple-lobe hepatectomy
triple-loop pouch
triple-lumen
t.-l. manometry catheter
t.-l. perfused catheter system
t.-l. Sengstaken-Blakemore tube
triple-phosphate crystal
triplet
neurofilament protein t.
triple-voiding cystography
triplication
triploid cell
tripod
t. grasper
t. grasping forceps
triprolidine
**triptorelin pamoate for injectable
suspension**
trip wire
triradiate cecal fold
trisegmentectomy
Tris HCl
tris(hydroxymethyl)aminomethane
trisilicate
aluminum hydroxide and magnesium
t.
magnesium t.
trismus presentation
trisodium
mangafodipir t.

trisomy 13, 18, 21
Tritec
Triticum
Triton tumor
TRL
triglyceride-rich lipoprotein
trocar
accessory t.
Beardsley cecostomy t.
Campbell t.
conical t.
Cook urologic t.
t. cystostomy
disposable t.
ensheathing t.
Ethicon t.
gallbladder t.
Hasson t.
Landau t.
Ochsner gallbladder t.
Origin t.
pyramidal t.
transvaginal t.
**3-trocar technique for laparoscopic
cholecystectomy**
trochanter
troglitazone
Troisier
T. ganglion
T. node
T. sign
troleandomycin
Trombovar
tromethamine
carboprost t.
fosfomycin t.
ketorolac t.
Tronolane
Tropheryma whipplei
trophic
t. change
t. lesion
trophoblastic malignant teratoma
trophozoite
amebic t.
t. form
tropical
t. calcific pancreatitis (TCP)
t. diarrhea
t. diarrhea-malabsorption syndrome
(TDMS)
t. mesangiocapillary
glomerulonephritis
t. nephropathy
t. spastic paraparesis
t. splenomegaly
t. sprue
tropicalis
Candida t.

tropomyosin
troponin
>   baseline t. T
trospium hydrochloride
trota
>   *Aeromonas t.*
Trousseau
>   T. esophageal bougie
>   T. syndrome
>   T. test
Troutman rectus forceps
trovafloxacin
Trovan/Zithromax Compliance Pak
TRPM-2
>   testosterone-repressed prostate
>   message-2
TRPV5
>   transient receptor potential
>   vanilloid-5
Tru-cut, Trucut
>   T.-C. biopsy needle
>   T.-C. needle biopsy
Trucut (*var. of* Tru-Cut)
Truelove-Witts
>   T.-W. grading system
>   T.-W. index
trumpet
>   nasal t.
truncal
>   t. vagotomy
>   t. vagotomy and gastroenterostomy
>   t. vagotomy and pyloroplasty
trunci (*pl. of* truncus)
truncus, *pl.* **trunci**
>   t. celiacus
>   trunci intestinales
trunk
>   bicarotid t.
>   celiac t.
>   lumbosacral t.
>   portal t.
TRUS
>   transrectal ultrasonography
>   transrectal ultrasound
>   transrectal ultrasound scanning
truss
Tru Taper Ethalloy needle
Trypan blue-stained cell
Trypanosoma
>   *T. congolense*
>   *T. cruzi*
>   *T. rhodesiense*
trypanosomiasis
>   American t.
>   Rhodesian t.
>   South American t.
trypsin
>   bovine t.
>   t. inhibitor

trypsinization
trypsinogen, trypsogen
>   t. activation peptide
>   immunoreactive t. (IRT)
trypsogen (*var. of* trypsinogen)
tryptic soy broth
tryptophan
>   t. hydroxylase 1
>   t. metabolism
TSAE
>   transcatheter splenic arterial
>   embolization
tsangshu
>   Southern t.
TSC
>   tuberous sclerosis complex
TSPAP
>   total serum prostatic acid
>   phosphatase
TSRPC
>   totally stapled restorative
>   proctocolectomy
TSRS
>   tissue-stone recognition system
tsukubaensis
>   *Streptomyces t.*
TTC
>   T-tube cholangiogram
tTG
>   tissue transglutaminase
>   IgA tTG
T-1/2 time of gastric emptying
TTKG
>   transtubular potassium gradient
TT-3 needle
TTP
>   thrombotic thrombocytopenic purpura
TTS
>   testosterone transdermal system
>   through-the-scope
>   transdermal therapeutic system
>   TTS balloon dilation
>   TTS dilator
>   Testoderm TTS
T-tube
>   T-t. cholangiogram (TTC)
>   T-t. cholangiography
>   T-t. drain
>   T-t. drainage
>   T-t. stent
>   T-t. study
>   T-t. tract
>   T-t. tract choledochofiberoscopy
>   T-t. tract choledochoscopy
T-TURP
>   total transurethral resection of prostate
TTV
>   transfusion-transmitted virus
tuaminoheptane

T

tubal
- t. ectopic pregnancy
- t. infertility
- t. ligation

tube
- Abbott t.
- Abbott-Miller t.
- Abbott-Rawson double-lumen gastrointestinal t.
- Adson suction t.
- All-Silicone Side-Eye EPT feeding t.
- Anderson gastric t.
- Argyle chest t.
- Argyle-Salem sump t.
- ascites drainage t.
- aspiration and dissection t.
- Aspisafe nasogastric t.
- Atkinson silicone rubber t.
- Axiom double sump t.
- Baker intestinal decompression t.
- Baker jejunostomy t.
- Bard gastrostomy feeding t.
- Bard PEG t.
- Bilbao-Dotter t.
- Blakemore t.
- Blakemore-Sengstaken t.
- Bower PEG t.
- Boyce modification of Sengstaken-Blakemore t.
- Broncho-Cath double-lumen endotracheal t.
- Buie rectal suction t.
- button-type G t.
- Caluso PEG gastrostomy t.
- Cantor t.
- castlike t.
- Cattell T t.
- t. cecostomy
- Celestin esophageal t.
- Celestin latex rubber t.
- chest t.
- COBED t.
- collecting t.
- conical centrifuge t.
- Cope loop nephrostomy t.
- Corflo enteral feeding t.
- Corflo PEG t.
- Corpak feeding t.
- Corpak weighted-tip self-lubricating t.
- Council-tip t.
- cuffed endotracheal t.
- cystostomy t.
- Davol colon t.
- Davol feeding t.
- decompression t.
- t. decompression
- Dennis colorectal t.
- Dennis intestinal t.
- Diamond t.
- digestive t.
- direct percutaneous jejunostomy t.
- Dobbhoff gastrectomy feeding t.
- Dobbhoff gastric decompression t.
- Dobbhoff PEG t.
- double-lumen t.
- DPJ t.
- drainage t.
- Dreiling t.
- dual percutaneous gastrostomy t.
- Dumon-Gilliard prosthesis pushing t.
- duodenal t.
- Duo-Tube feeding t.
- Edlich gastric lavage t.
- endoscopic gastrostomy t.
- endothelial t.
- endotracheal t. (ET, ETT)
- Endo-Tube nasojejunal feeding t.
- t. enlargement
- EnteraFlo feeding t.
- enteroclysis t.
- t. enteroscope
- t. enterostomy
- EntriStar feeding t.
- EntriStar polyurethane PEG t.
- Eppendorf t.
- esophageal t.
- t. esophagram
- Ethox feeding t.
- Ewald t.
- fallopian t.
- t. feeding
- feeding gastrostomy t.
- Ferrein t.
- Flexiflo Inverta-PEG t.
- Flexiflo stoma-creator t.
- Flexiflo Stomate low-profile gastrostomy t.
- Flexiflo tungsten weighted feeding t.
- Flexiflo Versa-PEG t.
- Flow-Thru feeding t.
- Frazier suction t.
- Frederick-Miller t.
- French T t.
- G t.
- gastric aspiration t.
- gastric augment and single-pedicle t.
- gastric lavage t.
- gastrostomy t. (GT, G-tube)
- Gilman-Abrams gastric t.
- Glasser gastrostomy t.
- Gomco suction t.
- Gott t.
- t. graft
- guttered T t.

Haldane-Priestly t.
Harris t.
Hodge intestinal decompression t.
insertion t.
J t.
jejunal feeding t.
jejunostomy t. (J-tube)
K t.
Kangaroo gastrostomy t.
Kaslow intestinal t.
Kehr T t.
Keofeed II feeding t.
Killian suction t.
large-bore gastric lavage t.
t. leakage
Levin t.
Linton-Nachlas t.
long intestinal t.
4-lumen t.
Malecot gastrostomy t.
Malecot nephrostomy t.
marked t.
Medena t.
mediastinal t.
Medina t.
Medoc-Celestin pulsion t.
mercury-weighted t.
metal-weighted silastic feeding t.
MIC gastroenteric t.
MIC gastrostomy t.
MIC-Key G gastrostomy t.
MIC-Key J gastrostomy t.
MIC-TJ transgastric jejunal t.
t. migration
Mikulicz gastrostomy t.
Miller-Abbott intestinal t.
Minnesota t.
Mitrofanoff t.
modified Minnesota t.
Montgomery salivary bypass t.
Moss G t.
Moss gastrostomy t.
Moss Mark IV t.
Mousseau-Barbin prosthetic t.
myringotomy t.
Nachlas gastrointestinal t.
nasobiliary t. (NBT)
nasocystic drainage t.
nasoduodenal feeding t.
nasoenteric feeding t.
nasogastric t. (NGT)
nasogastric feeding t.
nasoileal t.
nasojejunal feeding t.
negative-pressure t.
negative-pressure-controlled t.
nephrostomy t.
nephrotomy t.
NJ feeding t.

Nuport PEG t.
Nyhus-Nelson gastric decompression
  and jejunal feeding t.
Olympus 1-Step Button gastrostomy
  t.
orogastric Ewald t.
oropharyngeal t.
t. overgrowth
Panda gastrostomy feeding t.
Paul-Mixter t.
pediatric feeding t.
pediatric nasogastric t.
Pedi PEG t.
Pee Wee low-profile gastrostomy t.
PEG t.
PEG-400 t.
PEJ t.
percutaneous endoscopic gastrostomy
  and jejunal extension t. (PEG-JET)
percutaneous endoscopic placement
  of jejunal t.
photomultiplier t.
pigtail nephrostomy t.
t. placement
pleural t.
polyethylene t.
Poole suction t.
postpyloric feeding t.
Proctor-Livingston t.
pusher t.
Quinton t.
Radius enteral feeding t.
rectal t.
Rehfuss duodenal t.
Rehfuss stomach t.
t. removal
t. replacement
Replogle t.
Rubin t.
Rubin-Quinton small-bowel biopsy
  t.
Ryle t.
Sacks-Vine feeding gastrostomy t.
Sacks-Vine PEG t.
Salem duodenal sump t.
Salem sump double-lumen polyvinyl
  t.
Sandoz balloon replacement t.
Sandoz Caluso PEG t.
Sandoz feeding/suction t.
S-B t.
Schachowa spiral t.
Sengstaken-Blakemore t.
Shiner t.
Silk Bullet feeding t.
silk jejunal t.
Silk Pill feeding t.
Silk Tip feeding t.
skin t.

T

tube (*continued*)
    sliding t.
    small-bowel t.
    Souttar t.
    Stamey t.
    Stamm gastrostomy t.
    Stay-Put jejunal t.
    stiffening t.
    stimulated t.
    stomach t.
    Stomate decompression t.
    Stomate extension t.
    suction t.
    sump nasogastric t.
    Super PEG t.
    suprapubic t.
    T t.
    tampon t.
    Teflon nasobiliary t.
    Thiersch t.
    transanal drainage t.
    transpyloric t.
    triple-lumen Sengstaken-Blakemore t.
    Vacutainer t.
    venting percutaneous gastrostomy t.
    Vivonex Moss t.
    Wangensteen suction t.
    Willscher t.
    Wilson-Cook nasobiliary t.
    Wilson-Cook NJFT-series feeding t.
    wire-guided J t.
    Wookey skin t.
    woven Dacron t.
    Wurbs-type nasobiliary t.
    Yankauer suction t.
    Young-Dees t.
tubed
    t. free skin graft
    t. groin flap
    t. urethroplasty
tube-fed patient
tubeless lithotriptor
tubercle
    pubic t.
tubercular, tuberculated
    t. diarrhea
    t. involvement
tuberculated (*var. of* tubercular)
tuberculin
    t. syringe
    t. test
tuberculocele
tuberculoid
tuberculoma
    cavitating t.
tuberculosis (TB, TBC)
    adrenal t.
    bladder t.
    colonic t.

    duodenal t.
    esophageal t.
    gastric t.
    genital t.
    genitourinary t.
    ileocecal t.
    intestinal t.
    miliary t.
    Mycobacterium t.
    t. of kidney and bladder
    penile t.
    peritoneal t.
    t. polyp
    primary t.
    prostatic t.
    renal t.
    segmental colonic t.
    t. symptom
    testicular t.
    ureteral t.
    urethral t.
tuberculous
    t. colitis
    t. enteritis
    t. gastritis
    t. ileocolitis
    t. infectious esophagitis
    t. nephritis
    t. peritonitis
    t. prostatitis
tuberosity
    ischial t.
    omental t.
tuberous
    t. sclerosis
    t. sclerosis angiomyolipoma
    t. sclerosis complex (TSC)
    t. sclerosis gene TS1
    t. sclerosis gene TS2
tube-within-tube technique
tubi (*pl. of* tubus)
tubing
    t. clamp
    large-bore Tygon t.
    Nu-Hope t.
    polyvinyl t.
    shunt t.
    Sur-Fit Natura night drainage
      container t.
    Tygon venovenous bypass t.
    Y-connecting t.
tubogram
    T t.
tubular
    t. adenoma of Pick
    t. atrophy
    t. basement membrane (TBM)
    t. carcinoma
    t. cell desquamation

t. cell dysfunction
t. colonic duplication
t. damage
t. diuresis
t. epithelial cell
t. epithelial cell injury
t. excretory mass
t. fluid flow
t. fluid:ultrafiltrate (TF/UF)
t. iron accumulation
t. ischemia
t. maximal (Tm)
t. morphologic injury
t. narrowing and sacculation
t. necrosis
t. nephropathy
t. obstruction
t. polyp
t. proteinuria
t. reabsorption of phosphate test
t. reabsorption of phosphorus
t. regeneration
t. resorption
t. sodium handling
t. sodium reabsorption
t. stenosis
t. vertical gastroplasty

tubularization
bladder neck t.
Thiersch-Duplay t.

tubularized
t. bladder neck reconstruction
t. cecal flap
t. incised plate
t. incised plate urethroplasty

tubule
Albarran t.
Bellini t.
collecting t.
connecting t.
cortical collecting t. (CCT)
distal t.
distal convoluted t. (DCT)
epididymal t.
epithelium-lined t.
Ferrein t.
Henle t.
human proximal t.
immunostaining of transversely
sectioned t.
isolated cortical t. (ICT)
lumen of seminiferous t.
mesonephric t.
metanephric t.
nonischemic t.
proximal convoluted t. (PCT)
proximal straight t. (PST)
renal t.
seminiferous t.

sex cord tumors with annular t.'s
(SCTAT)
testicular t.
urine-collecting t.
uriniferous t.
uriniparous t.

tubuli (*pl. of* tubulus)
tubulin
tubulitis
mild t.

tubulocystic
tubulogenesis
vitronectin-inhibiting HGF-induced t.

tubulogenic
tubuloglomerular
t. feedback (TGF)
t. feedback mechanism

tubulointerstitial
t. disease
t. fibrosis
t. inflammation
t. injury
t. nephritis (TIN)
t. nephritis and uveitis (TINU)
t. nephritis and uveitis syndrome
t. nephropathy
t. rejection

tubulointerstitium
tubulopathy
cyclosporine t.

tubuloreticular inclusion (TRI)
tubulorrhexis
tubulosaccular
tubulose (*var. of* tubulous)
tubulotoxic effect
tubulous, tubulose
tubulovesicle
tubulovillous
t. adenoma
t. lesion
t. polyp

tubulus, *pl.* **tubuli**
tubus, *pl.* **tubi**
t. digestorius

tuck
dorsal tunical t.

Tucker
T. esophagoscope
T. spindle-shaped dilator

Tucks ointment
TUEP
transurethral evaporation of prostate

TUEVP
transurethral electrovaporization of
prostate

Tuffier
T. abdominal retractor
T. abdominal spatula
T. operation

T

793

tuft
>   t. adhesion
>   glomerular t.
>   sclerotic t.
>   vascular t.

tufting disease

TUI
>   transurethral incision

TUIBN
>   transurethral incision of bladder neck

TUIP
>   transurethral incision of prostate

Tukey test

TULIP
>   transurethral ultrasound-guided laser-induced prostatectomy

tulip tip

tumefaction
>   mesenteric t.

tumescence, turgescence
>   t. monitoring
>   nocturnal penile t. (NPT)
>   penile t.

TUMMY
>   Trial Using Medicinal Microbiotic Yogurt

tumor
>   abdominal desmoid t.
>   t. ablation
>   Abrikosov t.
>   adenomatoid t.
>   adnexal t.
>   adrenal cortex estrogen-secreting t.
>   adrenal cortex testosterone-secreting t.
>   adrenal gland metastatic t.
>   adrenal rest t.
>   alcohol injection of t.
>   ampullary t.
>   anaplastic Wilms t.
>   t. angiogenesis
>   angiomatoid t.
>   benign t.
>   bifurcation t.
>   bilateral renal t.'s
>   bilateral Wilms t.'s
>   biliary tract t.
>   bismuth t.
>   bladder t. (BT)
>   bladder nonepithelial t.
>   bladder yolk sac t.
>   bleeding t.
>   Bolande t.
>   branch duct-type t.
>   Brenner t.
>   burned-out t.
>   Buschke-Löwenstein t.
>   t. cachexia

carcinoid t.
Castleman t.
celiac t.
t. cell
t. cell lysis
chemotherapy of primary t.
chromophobe cell t.
colorectal t.
core of t.
cystic Wilms t.
t. debulking
depressed t.
dermatologic t.
desmoid t.
diagnosis of testicular t.
diploid t.
t. displacement
duct-ectatic t.
duodenal t.
embryonal t.
encapsulated carcinoid t.
t. encapsulation
enterochromaffin-like gastric carcinoid t. (ECLoma)
epithelial t.
esophageal t.
extracapsular t.
fecal t.
focal t.
t. focus
focus of t.
gastric carcinoid t.
gastrin-secreting nonbeta islet cell t.
gastroenteropancreatic t.
gastrointestinal autonomic nerve t.
gastrointestinal stromal t. (GIST)
germ cell t.
gestational trophoblastic t.
glomus t.
glycoprotein-producing t.
t. grade
t. grading
granular cell t.
granulosa cell t.
granulosa-theca cell t.
Grawitz t.
gritty t.
hepatic t.
high-grade t.
histopathologic nature of t.
hypersecreting t.
t. infiltration
inflammatory myofibroblastic t.
ingrowth of t.
internist t.
intraabdominal desmoid t.
intracaval t.
intractable t.

intraductal mucin-producing t.
intraductal papillary t. (IPT)
intraductal papillary and mucinous t.'s
intraductal papillary-mucinous t. (IPMT)
intramesenteric desmoid t.
intraparenchymal t.
islet cell t.
juxtaglomerular apparatus t.
kidney ossifying t.
Klatskin t.
Krukenberg t.
Leydig cell t.
t. location
luteinized granulosa-theca cell t.
lymphoid t.
t. lysis syndrome
malignant mesenchymal t.
t. marker
MCF-7 t.
mediastinal t.
mediastinum germ cell t.
metachronous t.
mixed germ cell t.
mixed germ cell-sex cord stromal t.
mucin-hypersecreting t.
mucinous cystic t.
mucinous pancreatic t.
mucin-producing t.
multifocal bladder t.
myogenic t.
t. necrosis
t. necrosis factor (TNF)
t. necrosis factor alpha (TNF-alpha)
t. necrosis factor-alpha assay
neuroendocrine t.
neurogenic t. (NET)
4-nitroquinolin-1-oxide-induced t. (4NOQ)
t., nodes, metastases (TNM)
nonaneuploid t.
non-B islet cell t.
nonfunctional pituitary t.
noninvasive t.
nonsecreting pituitary t.
nonseminomatous germ cell t. (NSGCT)
notification of t.
null cell t.
t. overgrowth
pancreatic islet cell t.
pancreatic polypeptide-secreting t. (PPoma)
paratesticular t.
paraumbilical vein t. (PUVT)
parenchymatous t.
t. peak systolic velocity
periampullary duodenal t.

persistent postmolar gestational trophoblastic t.
polypoid t.
prepubertal testicular t. (PPTT)
presacral t.
primary staging of testicular t.
primitive neuroectodermal t.
t. probe
t. proliferative index
rectal carcinoid t. (RCT)
rectal myogenic t.
renin-secreting juxtaglomerular cell t.
retroperitoneal t.
rhabdoid Wilms t.
ruptured hepatic t.
sacrococcygeal region germ cell t.
secondary t.
t. seeding
semipedunculated t.
Sertoli cell t.
sex cord-mesenchyme t.
shaggy t.
solid t.
t. spillage
t. stage
t. staging
t. stenting
superficial bladder t.
t. suppressor gene
t. suppressor gene therapy
testicular t.
thrombus t.
tongue of t.
transurethral resection of bladder t. (TURBT)
Triton t.
upper GI submucosal t.
upper tract urothelial t.
ureteral t.
urethral t.
urothelial t.
t. vaccine
vasoactive intestinal peptide-secreting t. (VIPoma)
vasoactive intestinal polypeptide t. (VIPoma)
villous t.
virilizing t.
von Recklinghausen t.
Wilms t.
yolk sac t.
Zollinger-Ellison t.
tumoral calcinosis
tumor-associated antigen (TAA)
tumor-bearing segment
tumor-derived angiogenic inhibitor
tumorigenesis
t. activity
colorectal t.

tumorigenic
tumor-infiltrating lymphocyte (TIL)
tumorlet
    Wilms t.
tumorous
    t. epithelium
    t. pseudopodia
tumor-rejection antigen
Tums
TUMT
    transurethral microwave thermotherapy
    cooled catheter TUMT
    TUMT functional result
    high-energy TUMT
    low-energy TUMT
    30-minute TUMT
TUN
    total urinary nitrogen
TUNA
    transurethral needle ablation
tunable
    t. dye laser lithotripsy
    t. pulsed-dye laser
tunic, tunica
    t. cyst
    epididymal t.
    fibrous t.
    mucous t.
    muscular t.
    t. of spermatic cord
    pharyngeal t.
    pharyngobasilar t.
    proper t.
tunica (*var. of* tunic), *pl.* **tunicae**
    t. adventitia
    t. albuginea
    t. albuginea corporis spongiosi
    t. albuginea corporum cavernosorum
    t. albuginea cyst
    t. albuginea ovarii
    t. albuginea plication
    t. albuginea testis
    t. fibrosa
    t. mucosa
    t. muscularis
    t. propria
    t. replacement
    t. serosa
    t. spongiosa urethrae feminae
    t. vaginalis blanket wrap
    t. vaginalis testis
    t. vasculosa
tunicae (*pl. of* tunica)
tunnel
    t. creation
    cross-trigonal t.
    t. disease
    extravesical seromuscular t.
    t. infection

    retropancreatic t.
    subserous t.
    ureteral t.
    t. vision
    Witzel feeding jejunostomy t.
tunneled
    t. technique
    t. technique urinary diversion
tunneler
    Davol t.
Tuohy-Borst
    T.-B. adapter
    T.-B. connector
TUR
    transurethral resection
    TUR syndrome
    videomonitored TUR
Turapy device
TURB
    transurethral resection of bladder
turbid
    t. bile
    t. peritoneal fluid
turbidity
    urinalysis t.
    urine t.
turbinate
    swollen t.
turbo spin-echo sequence
TURBT
    transurethral resection of bladder tumor
turbulent flow
Türck zone
Turcot syndrome
TUR-Cue photometer
turgescence (*var. of* tumescence)
turgor
    skin t.
turista
Turkel punch
turmeric
turn-and-suction
    t.-a.-s. biopsy technique
    t.-a.-s. method
Turnbull
    T. colostomy
    T. end-loop ileostomy
    T. loop stoma
    T. ostomy operation
    T. temporary diverting ileostomy
      technique
Turner
    T. sign
    T. stigma
    T. syndrome
Turner-Warwick
    T.-W. and Ashken cecocystoplasty
      technique
    T.-W. incision

T.-W. inlay
T.-W. needle
T.-W. operation
T.-W. stone forceps
T.-W. urethroplasty
TURP
transurethral resection of prostate
bipolar TURP
direct-beam coupler for TURP
TURP functional result
split-beam coupler for TURP
turpentine enema
Turrell-Wittner rectal forceps
Tuttle test
TUU
transureteroureterostomy
TUVP
transurethral vaporization of prostate
TUVRP
transurethral vaporization-resection of prostate
TVF
Thiry-Vella fistula
TVS
transvaginal suturing
TVS system
TVT
tension-free vaginal tape
TVT procedure
TVUS, TVU
transvaginal ultrasound
Tween 20
T1-weighted image (T1WI)
T2-weighted image (T2WI)
T1WI
T1-weighted image
T2WI
T2-weighted image
Twinheads shock wave lithotriptor
twin-pulse shock wave release
Twinrix
T. IM injection
T. vaccine
twisted beta-pleated sheet fibril
TWOC
trial without catheter
two-layer
two-stage
two-step
two-tailed
TxA2
thromboxane A_2
TxA2 receptor antagonist
Tycron, Ti-Cron
T. suture
T. tie
Tygon venovenous bypass tubing

Tylenol
tylosis
t. palmaris
t. palmaris et plantaris
Tylox
tymazoline
tympanites
false t.
uterine t.
tympanitic
t. abdomen
t. abscess
t. dullness
t. resonance
tympany
abdominal t.
t. of stomach
type
t. A, B antral gastritis
t. 1, 2 autoimmune hepatitis
autoimmune polyglandular syndrome t. 1
biomaterial t.
blood t.
t. C cirrhosis
t. C, D ulcer
cell t.
chronic-continuous t.
complement receptor t. 1 (CR1)
t. 2 diabetes mellitus
diffuse vasculitis of polyarteritis nodosa t.
DR1 HLA-DRB tissue t.
DR2 1501 HLA-DRB tissue t.
DR2 1502 HLA-DRB tissue t.
DR2 1601 HLA-DRB tissue t.
DR2 1602 HLA-DRB tissue t.
DR3 HLA-DRB tissue t.
DR4 HLA-DRB tissue t.
DR7 HLA-DRB tissue t.
DR9 HLA-DRB tissue t.
DRw8 HLA-DRB tissue t.
DRw10 HLA-DRB tissue t.
DRw11 HLA-DRB tissue t.
DRw12 HLA-DRB tissue t.
DRw13 HLA-DRB tissue t.
DRw14 HLA-DRB tissue t.
hepatitis t. 1
IGV t. 1, 2
t. II cryoglobulinemia
t. III cholangiocarcinoma
t. III glycogenosis
t. I, II pseudohypoaldosteronism
t. I interferon
t. I mesangiocapillary glomerulonephritis
t. IV amyloidosis
phage t.

T

type (*continued*)
    t. 3 serotonin receptor
     antagonist
    test t.
    T-helper t. 1 (Th1)
typed blood
type-specific blood transfusion
typhi
    Salmonella t.
typhimurium
    Salmonella t.
    Salmonella t. R5
typhlectasis
typhlectomy
typhlenteritis (*var. of* typhlitis)
typhlitis, typhlenteritis
    neutropenic t.
typhlodicliditis
typhloempyema
typhlolithiasis
typhlomegaly
typhlopexia (*var. of* typhlopexy)
typhlopexy, typhlopexia
typhlorrhaphy
typhlostenosis
typhlostomy
typhlotomy
typhloureterostomy

typhoid
    abdominal t.
    t. fever
typing
    HLA t.
    HLA-DQ t.
    HLA-DR DNA t.
    molecular t.
tyramine
tyremesis
tyropanoate
    t. contrast medium
    t. sodium
tyrosine
    t. kinase activity
    t. kinase growth-factor receptor
    peptide t.
    t. phosphorylation
    t. protein kinase
    t. sulfation
tyrosinemia
    hereditary t.
tyrosinuria
tyrosis
TyRx bioresorbable polymer mesh
Tyshak catheter
Tyson test
Tzyeka

UA
    urinalysis
UA/C
    urinary albumin to creatinine
        UA/C ratio
UBG
    urobilinogen
ubiquitination
UBM
    urothelial basement membrane
UBT
    urea breath test
        UBT breath test
        ^{14}C UBT
UC
    ulcerative colitis
UCB
    unconjugated bilirubin
UCHL-1 monoclonal antibody
UCLA
    University of California at Los
        Angeles
        UCLA catheterization pouch
UCP
    ultrasound catheter probe
UCPP
    urethral closure pressure profile
UDC
    ursodeoxycholate
UDCA
    ursodeoxycholic acid
UDI
    Urogenital Distress Inventory
UDP
    uridine 5′-diphosphate
        UDP glucuronyltransferase
UDPGT
    uridine diphosphate
        glucuronosyltransferase
        UDPGT deficiency
Udranszky test
UES
    upper esophageal sphincter
UESL
    undifferentiated embryonal sarcoma of
        liver
UESR
    upper esophageal sphincter
        relaxation
UF
    ultrafiltration
Uffelmann test
UFT/leucovorin calcium
UGI
    upper gastrointestinal

UGI endoscope
UGI endoscopy
UGIB
    upper gastrointestinal bleeding
UGIE
    upper gastrointestinal endoscopy
UGIH
    upper GI hemorrhage
UIBC
    unbound iron-binding capacity
UICC
    Union Internationale Contre le Cancer
        UICC tumor classification
UJ13A nuclear isotope bone scan
UKM
    urea kinetic modeling
UKTSSA
    United Kingdom Transplant Support
    Service Authority
ulcer
        acid-peptic u.
        active duodenal u.
        agranulocytic u.
        Allingham u.
        amebic u.
        anastomotic u.
        anastomotic-stomal u.
        anterior duodenal u.
        anterior wall antral u.
        antral u.
        antroduodenal u.
        aphthoid u.
        aphthous u.
        apical duodenal u.
        Barrett u.
        u. base
        bear claw u.
        u. bed
        benign gastric u.
        bladder u.
        bleeding u.
        Bouveret u.
        Bouveret-Duguet u.
        bulbar peptic u.
        Cameron u.
        cecal u.
        cervical u.
        chronic u.
        CMV-related u.
        coalescent u.
        u. collar
        collar-buttonlike u.
        colonic u.
        colorectal u.
        complication of benign gastric u.

U

ulcer (*continued*)
- corneal u.
- u. crater
- Crohn duodenal u.
- Cruveilhier u.
- Curling u.
- Cushing u.
- Cushing-Rokitansky u.
- cysteamine-induced duodenal u.
- decubitus u.
- Dieulafoy u.
- distention u.
- drug-induced u.
- duodenal u.
- duodenal ulceroinflammatory u.
- u. duodenum
- u. dyspepsia
- elusive u.
- esophageal u.
- Fenwick-Hunner u.
- flat u.
- focal colonic mucosal u.
- Forrest classification of gastroduodenal u.
- gastric u.
- gastroduodenal double u.
- general peptic u.
- genital u.
- giant gastric u. (GGU)
- giant peptic u.
- greater curvature u.
- healed u.
- herpetic u.
- Hunner u.
- idiopathic esophageal u. (IEU)
- indolent radiation-induced rectal u.
- intractable u.
- jejunal u.
- juxtapyloric u.
- kissing u.'s
- Kocher dilation u.
- lesser curvature u.
- linear-array gastric u.
- linear gastric u.
- longitudinal u.
- malignant u.
- Mann-Williamson u.
- marginal u.
- Martorell hypertensive u.
- mucosal gastric u.
- nonhealing u.
- open u.
- oral u.
- Palmer acid test for peptic u.
- penetrating u.
- peptic u.
- perforated acid peptic u.
- perforating u.
- perineal u.

- phantom u.
- postbulbar duodenal u.
- posterior duodenal u.
- postligation u.
- postsurgical recurrent u.
- prepyloric gastric u.
- punched-out u.
- punctate u.
- pyloric channel u.
- rake u.
- rectal u.
- recurrent u.
- refractory duodenal u.
- reserpine-induced u.
- Rokitansky-Cushing u.
- rose thorn u.
- round u.
- sea anemone u.
- secondary jejunal u.
- serpiginous u.
- sigmoid u.
- silent u.
- small-intestinal u.
- sodium meclofenamate-induced esophageal u.
- stercoraceous u.
- stomal u.
- stress u.
- submucous u.
- sump u.
- superficial linear u.
- suture u.
- type C, D u.
- vaginal u.
- u. vessel
- virgin u.
- V-shaped u.
- u. with heaped-up edge

ulcera (*pl. of* ulcus)

ulcerating
- u. adenocarcinoma
- u. carcinoma

ulceration
- anal u.
- anastomotic u.
- ASA-induced gastric u.
- CMV-associated u.
- CMV-induced esophageal u.
- collar-button u.
- duodenal u.
- esophageal u.
- fissurelike u.
- flat polycyclic u.
- gastric u.
- labial u.
- linear u.
- linear-array u.
- necrotic u.
- patchy colonic u.

pouch u.
punched-out u.
radiation-induced u.
serpiginous u.
stasis u.
stasis-induced u.
stercoraceous u.
stress u.
stress-induced gastric u.
suture line u.
tracheal u.
transverse u.

ulcerative
u. colitis (UC)
u. enteritis
u. gastritis
u. jejunitis
u. jejunitis jejunocecostomy
u. lymphoma
u. proctitis
u. reflux esophagitis

ulcerlike dyspepsia
ulcerogenic fistula
ulcer-prone personality
ulcus, *pl.* **ulcera**
Uldall subclavian hemodialysis catheter
Ulex europeus I antigen
Ullrich-Turner syndrome
ultimate fistula formation
Ultra
U. Twin bag system
U. Y-set system

UltraBag dialysis system
UltraCision harmonic laparoscopic cutting shears
ultradian rhythm
ultrafast
u. computerized tomography
u. MRI

Ultrafem pants
ultrafiltrate
glomerular u.
plasma u.

ultrafiltration (UF)
u. coefficient
continuous arteriovenous u. (CAVU)
dialytic u.
extracorporeal u. (ECU)
glomerular u.
u. hemodialyzer
hydrostatic u.
slow continuous u. (SCUF)
spontaneous dialytic u.

Ultraflex
U. Diamond stent
U. esophageal prosthesis
U. Microvasive stent

U. nitinol expandable esophageal stent
U. tracheobronchial stent

ultrahigh-magnification endoscopy
UltraKlenz skin cleanser
Ultralente insulin
ultraline
U. fiber
U. laser

ultralow anastomosis
ultralow-volume sclerotherapy
UltraPak enteral closed feeding system
Ultraseed system
Ultrase MT20, MT24
ultrasmall superparamagnetic iron oxide
ultrasonic
u. aspirator and dissector
u. cytoreduction
u. diagnosis
u. dissection
u. endoscope
u. fragmentation
u. lithotresis
u. lithotripsy
u. lithotriptor
u. lithotriptor probe
u. oscillating bur
u. scalpel
u. tactile sensor
u. tomography

ultrasonogram
renal u.

ultrasonographic finding
ultrasonography (US)
abdominal u.
bladder u.
B-mode u.
catheter probe-assisted endoluminal u. (CP-EUS)
color Doppler u.
contrast-enhanced endoscopic u. (CE-EUS)
contrast-enhanced transabdominal u.
3-dimensional endoscopic u.
Doppler u.
ejaculatory duct u.
endoluminal rectal u. (ELUS)
endoscopic u. (EUS)
endoscopic color Doppler u.
u. estimate
EUS-AD gastric lesion staging by endoscopic u.
EUS-M gastric lesion staging by endoscopic u.
EUS-SM gastric lesion staging by endoscopic u.
gray-scale u.
high-frequency probe u.
high-intensity focused u.

U

ultrasonography (US) (*continued*)
    high-resolution u.
    intraductal u. (IDUS)
    intraoperative u. (IOUS)
    intraportal endovascular u. (IPEUS)
    intrarectal u.
    laparoscopic contact u. (LCU)
    pelvic u.
    penile duplex u.
    pharmacoduplex u.
    prenatal u.
    real-time u. (RUS)
    rectal endoscopic u. (REUS)
    secretin u.
    sex assignment by fetal u.
    Siemens Sonoline u.
    sildenafil plus Doppler u.
    SP-501 gastric lesion staging by
      endoscopic u.
    Toshiba Sal 38B real-time u.
    Toshiba Sonolayer SSA250A
      transrectal u.
    transanal u.
    transcutaneous u.
    transluminal u.
    transnasal endoluminal u.
    transperineal u.
    transrectal u. (TRUS)
    transrectal prostatic u.
ultrasonography/angiography
    Doppler u.
ultrasound (US)
    abdominal u.
    u. ablation
    u. basket extraction
    BladderScan u.
    u. bone analyzer
    u. catheter probe (UCP)
    catheter probe u.
    colonoscopic endoluminal u.
    colorectal endoluminal u.
    compression u.
    condom catheter endoscopic u.
    u. dilution technique
    3-dimensional linear endoscopic u.
    Doppler u.
    dual-plane catheter-based u.
    endoanal u. (EAUS)
    endoluminal ureteral u.
    endorectal u. (ERUS)
    u. endoscope
    endoscopic u. (EUS)
    u. gastrointestinal fiberscope
    gray-scale u.
    high-frequency intraluminal u.
    high-intensity focused u.
    hydrogen peroxide u.
    intraductal u. (IDUS)
    intraluminal u. (ILUS)

    intravascular u. (IVUS)
    laparoscopic u. (LUS)
    laparoscopic intracorporeal u. (LICU)
    piezoelectrically generated u.
    power Doppler u.
    pulsed Doppler u.
    quantitative u. (QUS)
    real-time gallbladder u.
    u. scan
    soft balloon method for endoscopic
      u.
    Sonablate 500 u.
    standard transabdominal u.
    u. test
    time domain u.
    transcutaneous u.
    u. transducer
    transendoscopic u.
    transrectal u. (TRUS)
    transurethral rectal u.
    transvaginal u. (TVUS, TVU)
    u. wand
ultrasound-assisted
    u.-a. PEG placement
    u.-a. percutaneous endoscopic
      gastrostomy
ultrasound-guided
    u.-g. anterior subcostal liver biopsy
    u.-g. laser
    u.-g. shock wave therapy
    u.-g. systematic sextant biopsy
ultrastiff wire
ultrastructural basket-weave change
UltraTag RBC kit
ultrathin
    u. araldite section
    u. endoscope
    u. endoscopy
    u. esophagoduodenoscopy (UT-EGD)
    u. needle brachytherapy-style
      delivery renal application
    u. pancreatoscope
Ultratome
    U. double-lumen sphincterotome
    Microvasive U.
    U. XL triple-lumen sphincterotome
ultraviolet (UV)
    u. irradiation
    u. light C
Ultravist 300
Ultrex
    U. cylinder
    U. Plus penile prosthesis
Ultroid
Ultzmann test
umami taste receptor
umbilical
    u. artery
    u. cord

u. disorder
u. fissure
u. fistula
u. granuloma
u. hernia
u. hernia rupture
u. ligament
u. port
u. port grasper
u. portography
u. region
u. scissors
u. tape
u. vein catheterization
u. vein recanalization

umbilicalis
plica u.

umbilicated angioma
umbilication
umbilici (*pl. of* umbilicus)
umbilicoplasty
umbilicovesical fascia
umbilicus, *pl.* **umbilici**
everted u.
Richet fascia u.

umbrella
Mobin-Uddin u.

UN
urea nitrogen

Unasyn
unbanded gastroplasty
unbound iron-binding capacity
(UIBC)
UNC
urine net charge

uncentrifuged urine
unciform pancreas
uncinate
u. process
u. process of pancreas

uncoated mesh stent
uncomplicated
u. appendectomy
u. cystitis
u. urinary tract infection (UUTI)

unconjugated
u. bilirubin (UCB)
u. hyperbilirubinemia

unconscious incontinence
uncorrected
u. maternal morbidity
u. reflux morbidity

uncoupling
actual gastric myoelectric u.

undecapeptide
amino-terminal u.

undecenoate of testosterone
underactivity
detrusor muscle u.

underdosing
nephron u.

underfilling
arterial u.

underlying
u. chronic renal insufficiency
u. muscularis propria

undersurface of liver
underwater spark gap
underwear
Prevail protective u.

undescended testis
UnDiet spray weight loss system
undifferentiated
u. adenoma
u. cell
u. embryonal sarcoma of liver
(UESL)
u. malignant teratoma
u. structure

undigested food in stool
undiversion
urinary u.

unenhanced
u. helical computed tomography
u. helical CT

unequal calf diameter
unexplained finding
unextractable gallstone
unfavorable infundibular width
unfolded protein response
unformed stool
Un-Graph computer software
ungual fibroma
unguliformis
unicameral cyst
unicornuate uterus
unidirectional transfer
Uni-Flate 1000 penile prosthesis
uniformis
Bacteroides u.

uniform loading
Uni-Gold *Helicobacter pylori* **test**
unilateral
u. fused kidney
u. megaureter
u. nephrectomy
u. palpable right testis
u. periorbital emphysema
u. renal artery stenosis (URAS)
u. renal hypoplasia
u. renin production
u. subcostal incision
u. ureteral calculus
u. ureteral obstruction (UUO)

unilobular cirrhosis
unilocular
u. hydatid disease
u. ovarian cyst

U

uninhibited
  u. neurogenic bladder
  u. overactive bladder
union
  anomalous pancreaticobiliary u.
    (APBU)
  anomalous pancreaticobiliary ductal
    u. (APBDU)
  U. Internationale Contre le Cancer
    (UICC)
unipapillary kidney
uniplanar imaging
unipolar
  u. glass electrode
  u. neuron
unique esophageal feature
Unisensor strain-gauge transducer
unit
  amylase u.
  arbitrary u.
  biceps femoris musculocutaneous u.
  Bodansky u.
  Bovie electrocoagulation u.
  Cameron electrosurgical u.
  Cameron-Miller electrocoagulation u.
  Century bicarbonate dialysis control
    u.
  colony-forming u. (CFU)
  crypt-villus u.
  densitometric u.
  Diasonics DRF ultrasound u.
  duodenal cluster u.
  electrosurgical u.
  ERBE electrocautery u.
  Erbotom F2 electrocoagulation u.
  good performance u.
  GPL u.
  gracilis musculocutaneous u.
  Grass SIU5A stimulation isolation
    u.
  HemoTherapies liver dialysis u.
  Hounsfield u. (HU)
  image-processing u.
  international androgen u.
  Karmen u.
  KeyMed u.
  King-Armstrong u.
  liver dialysis u.
  u. of packed red blood cells
    (UPRBC)
  Olympus heater probe u.
  Osmo reverse osmosis u.
  Proscan ultrasound u.
  QAD1 sonography u.
  real-time sonographic u.
  Siemens MRI u.
  Siemens Somatom DRH CT
    analyzer u.
  Somogyi u.

SSE2-L electrosurgical u.
TENS u.
ThermoFlex thermotherapy u.
UroCystom u.
Valleylab E3B cautery u.
Valleylab SSE-2 cautery u.
Unitary inflatable penile prosthesis
United
  U. Kingdom Transplant Support
    Service Authority (UKTSSA)
  U. Max-E drainable pouch
  U. Network for Organ Sharing
    (UNOS)
  U. Ostomy Association (UOA)
  U. Ostomy irrigation set
  U. Skin Prep
  U. States Renal Data System
    (USRDS)
  U. Surgical Bongort Lifestyle
    pouch
  U. Surgical convex insert
  U. Surgical Featherlite ileostomy
    pouch
  U. Surgical Hypalon faceplate
  U. Surgical Seal-Tite gasket
  U. Surgical Shear Plus drainable
    pouch
  U. Surgical Soft Secure pouch
  U. XL 14 skin barrier
univariate analysis
universal
  U. esophagoscope
  U. gastroscope
  U. sheath
  U. sheath system
  U. stent
universale
  angiokeratoma corporis diffusum u.
universally accepted therapy
university
  U. of California at Los Angeles
    (UCLA)
  U. of California at Los Angeles
    staging system
  U. of Wisconsin (UW)
  U. of Wisconsin preservation fluid
  U. of Wisconsin solution
unobstructed patient
UNOS
  United Network for Organ Sharing
unreconstructable obstructive azoospermia
unrelenting
  u. diarrhea
  u. pain
unrelieved pain
unremitting pain
unresectable hepatocellular carcinoma
unresolved urinary tract infection
unresponsiveness to standard therapy

unresponsive symptom
unrest
>peristaltic u.

unroofing
>u. of diverticulum
>transurethral u.

unsaturated fatty acid
unsensitized transplant recipient
unsporulated coccidian
unstable
>u. bladder
>u. colon
>u. urethra

unsteady gait
untethering procedure
untranslated region
unweighted
UOA
>United Ostomy Association

UPEP
>urine protein electrophoresis

UPJ
>ureteropelvic junction

uPM3 urine test
U-pouch construction
UPP
>urethral pressure profile
>urethral pressure profilometry

upper
>u. alimentary endoscopy
>u. arm flap
>u. endoscopy and colonoscopy
>u. esophageal sphincter (UES)
>u. esophageal sphincter relaxation
>(UESR)
>u. gastrointestinal (UGI)
>u. gastrointestinal angioma
>u. gastrointestinal barium
>roentgenographic study
>u. gastrointestinal bleeding
>(UGIB)
>u. gastrointestinal endoscopy
>(UGIE)
>u. gastrointestinal panendoscopy
>u. gastrointestinal procedure
>u. gastrointestinal tract
>u. GI endoscope
>u. GI hemorrhage (UGIH)
>u. GI series
>u. GI submucosal tumor
>u. GI tract foreign body
>U. Hands retractor
>u. midclavicular line
>u. motor neuron
>u. tract dilation
>u. tract disease
>u. tract stricture
>u. tract transitional cell carcinoma
>u. tract urothelial tumor

>u. ureter
>u. urinary tract calculus

UPRBC
>unit of packed red blood cells

upregulation of monocyte
chemoattractant protein-1 gene
cytoplasm of cells
Uprima
upsaliensis
>*Campylobacter u.*

upset stomach
upside-down stomach
upstream pancreatic duct
upstroke
>delayed u.

uptake
>glucose u.
>hepatic u.
>^{3}H-thymidine u.
>spermidine u.

URA
>urethral resistance factor

Urabeth Tabs
urachal
>u. abscess
>u. adenocarcinoma
>u. anomaly
>u. cyst
>u. cyst excision
>u. disorder
>u. diverticulum
>u. fistula
>u. sinus

urachus
>patent u.

uracil/tegafur
uragogue
uranyl
>u. acetate
>u. acetate stain

URAS
>unilateral renal artery stenosis

urate
>u. calculus
>u. crystal
>monosodium u.
>u. nephropathy
>sodium acid u.

uraturia
urea
>u. adequacy
>u. breath test (UBT)
>u. breath testing
>u. channel
>u. clearance
>u. cycle
>u. distribution volume
>hepatic u.
>u. hydrolysis

urea (*continued*)
  u. kinetic modeling (UKM)
  u. kinetics
  Kt/V u.
  u. nitrogen (UN)
  u. nitrogen test
  percent reduction in u. (PRU)
  u. permeability
  plasma u.
  u. reduction ratio (URR)
  u. splitting
  u. splitting organism
  u. synthesis
urea-derived cyanate
urea-impermeable membrane
urealyticum
  Ureaplasma u.
Ureaplasma
  U. urealyticum
  U. urethritis
urease
  cytoplasmic u.
  mucosal u.
  u. test
urease-positive bacterium
urease-producing bacterium
urecchysis
urecholine supersensitivity test
uredema, uroedema
Urelief
uremia, urinemia
  extrarenal u.
  retention u.
uremic
  u. acidosis
  u. breath
  u. cardiomyopathy
  u. colitis
  u. encephalopathy
  u. gastritis
  u. gastrointestinal lesion
  u. medullary cystic
    disease
  u. PMN
  u. pruritus
  u. serositis
  u. serum subfraction
  u. syndrome
ureolyticus
  Bacteroides u.
ureter
  abdominal u.
  aberrant u.
  bifid u.
  circumcaval u.
  u. contractility
  u. creep
  dilemma of distal u.
  distal u.

  u. duplication anomaly
  ectopic u.
  en bloc u.
  extraperitoneal excision of lower 1/3
    of u.
  ileal u.
  impassable u.
  u. implantation
  intramural u.
  juxtavesical u.
  left u.
  lower u.
  middle u.
  pelvic u.
  postcaval u.
  retrocaval u.
  retroiliac u.
  right u.
  tortuous u.
  torus u.
  upper u.
ureteral, ureteric
  u. anastomosis
  u. atony
  u. bladder augmentation
  u. bud
  u. calcification
  u. calculus
  u. calculus in pregnancy
  u. *Candida*
  u. carcinoma
  u. catheterization
  u. colic
  u. dissection
  u. diverticulum
  u. ectopia
  u. electromyography
  u. encasement
  u. hernia
  u. injury
  u. jet
  u. jet into bladder
  u. meatoscopy
  u. meatotomy
  u. muscle cell
  u. neocystostomy
  u. obstruction
  u. occlusion balloon catheter
  u. orifice
  u. patch procedure
  u. peristalsis second messenger
  u. plexus
  u. pressure
  u. reimplantation
  u. reimplantation stenosis
  u. reimplantation surgery
  u. retrieval net
  u. ridge
  u. schistosomiasis

u. scoping basketing
u. spatulation
u. split-cuff nipple
u. stent
u. stenting
u. stent placement
u. stoma
u. stoma removal
u. stone
u. stricture
u. torsion
u. tuberculosis
u. tumor
u. tunnel
ureteralgia
uretercystoscope
ureterectasia
ureterectomy
distal u.
segmental u.
ureteric (*var. of* ureteral)
uretericus
plexus u.
ureteritis
u. cystica
u. glandularis
ureterocalicostomy
ureterocele
u. cobra-head deformity
u. drooping lily sign
ectopic u.
intravesical u.
orthotopic u.
u. prolapse
single-system u.
ureterocelectomy
ureterocelorraphy
ureterocervical
ureterocolic
u. fistula
u. stricture
ureterocolonic anastomosis
ureterocolostomy, ureterosigmoidostomy
ileocecal u.
Mainz-type u.
Maydl u.
ureterocutaneostomy
ureterocutaneous fistula
ureterocystanastomosis
ureterocystoneostomy
ureterocystoplasty
ureterocystoscope
ureterocystostomy
ureteroduodenal
ureteroendoscopic disconnection
ureteroendoscopy
ureteroenteric
u. status
u. stricture

ureteroenteroanastomosis
ureteroenterostomy
ureterogram
bulb-tip retrograde u.
ureterography
ureteroheminephrectomy
ureterohydronephrosis
ureteroileal
u. anastomosis
u. neocystostomy
u. stenosis
u. stricture
ureteroileocecoproctostomy
ureteroileoneocystostomy
ureteroileostomy
Bricker u.
ureteroinfundibuloplasty
ureterointestinal
u. anastomosis
u. implantation
ureterolith
ureterolithiasis
ureterolithotomy
laparoscopic u.
ureterolysis
combined u.
extravesical u.
intravesical u.
laparoscopic u.
Lich-Gregoire u.
Pacquin u.
Politano-Leadbetter u.
ureteromeatotomy
ureteroneocystostomy
Cohen u.
Glenn-Anderson u.
u. herniation
Leadbetter-Politano u.
modified Lich-Gregoir u.
Politano-Leadbetter u.
reoperative u.
ureteroneopyelostomy,
  ureteropyeloneostomy
ureteronephrectomy
ureteronephrosis
ureteropathy
ureteropelvic
u. fungus ball
u. junction (UPJ)
u. junction obstruction
u. junction obstruction
  repair
u. ligament
u. region
ureteropelvioneostomy (*var. of*
ureteropyelostomy)
ureteropelvioplasty (*var. of*
ureteropyeloplasty)
Culp u.

U

ureteroplasty
  ileal patch u.
ureteroproctostomy, ureterorectostomy
ureteropyelitis
ureteropyelogram
  retrograde u.
ureteropyelography (*var. of* pyelography)
ureteropyeloneostomy (*var. of*
  ureteroneopyelostomy, ureteropyelostomy)
ureteropyelonephritis
ureteropyelonephrostomy
ureteropyeloplasty, ureteropelvioplasty
  Culp-DeWeerd u.
  Foley Y-type u.
  Foley Y-V u.
  Scardino u.
  Scardino-Prince u.
ureteropyeloscope
  Karl Storz flexible u.
ureteropyeloscopy
  flexible u.
ureteropyelostomy, ureteropelvioneostomy,
  ureteropyeloneostomy
ureteropyosis
ureterorectostomy (*var. of*
  ureteroproctostomy)
ureterorenal reflux
ureterorenoscope procedure sheath
ureterorenoscopy
  flexible u.
  transurethral u.
ureterorrhagia
ureterorrhaphy
ureteroscope
  Circon-ACMI MR-6, MR-9 u.
  flexible u.
  Gautier u.
  Micro-6 u.
  offset-lens u.
  Olympus URF type P2 flexible u.
  Panoview rod-lens u.
  rigid u.
  semirigid fiberoptic u.
  u. sheath
  Storz 27022 SK u.
  Wolf u.
  working-port u.
ureteroscopic
  u. approach
  u. endopyelotomy
  u. intracorporeal electrohydraulic
    lithotripsy
ureteroscopy
  rigid u.
  role of u.
  stent after u.
ureterosigmoid anastomosis
ureterosigmoidostomy (*var. of*
  ureterocolostomy)

ureterostegnosis (*var. of* ureterostenosis)
ureterostenoma (*var. of* ureterostenosis)
ureterostenosis, ureterostegnosis,
  ureterostenoma
ureterostomy
  cutaneous loop u.
  Davis intubated u.
  end-cutaneous u.
  high cutaneous loop u.
  high-loop cutaneous u.
  low-loop cutaneous u.
  pelvic u.
  retroperitoneal cutaneous u.
  Sober loop u.
  transureteropyelocutaneous u.
  transurethral cutaneous u.
ureterotome
  optic u.
ureterotomy
  Davis intubated u.
  intubated u.
ureterotrigonoenterostomy
ureterotubal anastomosis
ureteroureteral anastomosis
ureteroureterostomy
ureterouterine fistula
ureterovaginal fistula
ureterovesical
  u. junction (UVJ)
  u. obstruction
ureterovesicoplasty
  Leadbetter-Politano u.
ureterovesicostomy
urethra, *pl.* **urethrae**
  accessory phallic u.
  anterior u.
  AS-800 male bulbous u.
  u. blowout injury
  bulbar u.
  bulbomembranous u.
  bulbus urethrae
  compressor u.
  devastated u.
  u. duplication
  u. feminina
  fixed drain pipe u.
  fossa navicularis urethrae
  fossa of male u.
  hemispherium bulbi urethrae
  intrinsic striated muscle of u.
  isthmus u.
  labium urethrae
  lacuna of u.
  membranous u.
  u. muliebris
  native u.
  patent u.
  pendulous u.
  penile u.

posterior u.
preprostatic u.
prostatic u.
septum bulbi urethrae
short u.
spinning-top u.
unstable u.
u. virilis
urethrae (*pl. of* urethra)
urethral
  u. abscess
  u. apoplexy
  u. artery
  u. arthritis
  u. atresia
  u. calculus
  u. cancer
  u. carcinoma
  u. caruncle
  u. catheterization
  u. catheter movement
  u. closure mechanism
  u. closure pressure (UCP)
  u. closure pressure profile (UCPP)
  u. cooling
  u. cooling surface
  u. crest
  u. cyst
  u. dilation
  u. discharge
  u. diverticulectomy
  u. diverticulum
  u. electrical conductance
  u. feedback trigger
  u. fistula
  u. gland
  u. hemangioma
  u. hematuria
  u. hemi-Kock
  u. hypermobility
  u. lacuna
  u. meatus
  u. obstruction
  u. occlusion
  u. plate
  u. plate division
  u. plug
  u. pressure measurement
  u. pressure profile (UPP)
  u. pressure profilometry (UPP)
  u. prolapse
  u. pseudodiverticulum
  u. pseudotumor
  u. reconstruction complication
  u. resistance
  u. resistance factor (URA)
  u. sarcoidosis
  u. self-channelization
  u. sensory threshold

u. sphincter
u. sphincterotomy
u. stenosis
u. stent
u. stent prosthesis
u. stricture
u. stripping
u. surgical reconstruction
u. suspension
u. swab
u. syndrome
u. temperature
u. tuberculosis
u. tumor
u. valve
u. vein
urethralgia
urethralis
  anulus u.
  crista u.
urethrameter
urethratresia
urethrectomy
urethremorrhagia (*var. of* urethrorrhagia)
urethremphraxis, urethrophraxis
Urethrin
urethrism, urethrismus, urethrospasm
urethrismus (*var. of* urethrism)
urethritis
  acute u.
  atrophic u.
  chlamydia u.
  u. cystica
  u. glandularis
  gonococcal u.
  gonorrheal u.
  gouty u.
  u. granulosa
  hypoestrogenic u.
  mycoplasma u.
  nongonococcal u.
  nonspecific u. (NSU)
  u. orificii externi
  u. petrificans
  polypoid u.
  prophylactic u.
  specific u.
  u. syndrome
  Ureaplasma u.
  u. venerea
urethrobalanoplasty
urethroblennorrhea
urethrocavernous fistula
urethrocele
urethrocutaneous fistula
urethrocystitis
urethrocystocele
urethrocystography
urethrocystometrography

U

urethrocystometry
urethrocystopexy, urethropexy
    Gittes u.
    laparoscopic Burch u.
    Lapides-Ball u.
    Marshall-Marchetti-Krantz u.
    Stamey u.
    transabdominal Burch u.
urethrocystoscopy
urethrodetrusor facilitative reflex
urethrodynia
urethrogram
    ascending u.
    retrograde u. (RUG)
urethrograph
urethrography
    positive-pressure u. (PPUG)
    retrograde u. (RUG)
urethrohymenal fusion
urethrolysis
    retropubic u.
    transvaginal u.
urethromeatal erythema
urethrometer
urethrometry
urethropelvic ligament
urethropenile
urethroperineal
urethroperineoscrotal
urethropexy (*var. of* urethrocystopexy)
urethrophraxis (*var. of* urethremphraxis)
urethrophyma
urethroplasty
    anastomotic u.
    augmented anastomotic u.
    buccal mucosal substitution u.
    Cantwell-Ransley u.
    Cecil u.
    long-term outcome of u.
    modified Young u.
    one-stage u.
    onlay bulbar u.
    onlay island flap u.
    patch graft u.
    pedicled penile skin u.
    pedicle flap u.
    Schwartz-Pregenzer u.
    skin inlay u.
    Snodgrass incised plate u.
    substitution u.
    Tanagho bladder flap u.
    Thiersch-Duplay u.
    tubed u.
    tubularized incised plate u.
    Turner-Warwick u.
    ventral patch u.
urethroprostatic
urethrorectal fistula
urethrorrhagia, urethremorrhagia

urethrorrhaphy
urethrorrhea
urethroscope
    Robertson TM u.
urethroscopic
urethroscopy
    retropubic u.
urethroscrotal
urethrospasm (*var. of* urethrism)
urethrosphincteric
    u. guarding reflex
    u. inhibitory reflex
    u. recruitment reflex
urethrostaxis
urethrostenosis
urethrostomy
    perineal u.
urethrotome
    u. knife
    Otis u.
    Sachse u.
    Storz u.
urethrotomy
    core-through optical u.
    direct-vision internal u. (DVIU)
    endoscopic optical u.
    external u.
    internal u.
    Otis u.
    perineal u.
    Sachse u.
    Syme external u.
urethrotrigonitis
urethrovaginal
    u. fistula
    u. septum
    u. sphincter
urethrovesical
    u. anastomosis
    u. junction
urethrovesicopexy
uretic
Urex tablet
urge
    u. incontinence
    u. syndrome
    u. to defecate
    treatment of neurogenic refractory u.
    u. urinary incontinence (UUI)
urgency
    defecatory u.
    u. incontinence
    motor u.
    sensory u.
    urinary u.
urgency-frequency symptom
urgent
    u. colonoscopy
    U. PC sacral neuromodulation system

uric
- u. acid
- u. acid calculus
- u. acid crystal
- u. acid infarct
- u. acid level
- u. acid nephropathy
- u. acid shower
- u. acid stone
- u. acid test
- u. acid urolithiasis

uricaciduria

uricometer

uricosuria

uricosuric

Uricult dipslide

uridine
- u. 5′-diphosphate (UDP)
- u. diphosphate glucuronosyltransferase (UDPGT)
- u. diphosphate glucuronosyltransferase deficiency
- u. phosphorylase
- u. rescue

Uridium

Uri-Drain male incontinence device

uridyltransferase
- galactose-1 — phosphate u.

Urifon-Forte

Urigen

Uri-Kit culture kit

Urimar-T

Urimax

urinable

urinacidometer

urinae
- accelerator u.
- ardor u.
- detrusor u.
- incontinentia u.

urinal
- condom u.
- Millie female u.
- Uro-Tex McGuire male u.
- Ursec u.

urinalysis (UA)
- chemical u.
- u. color
- u. dipstick
- midstream u.
- u. pH
- u. sediment microscopy
- u. specific gravity
- u. turbidity

urinaria
- vesica u.

urinariae
- fundus vesicae u.

urinarius
- meatus u.

urinary
- u. abscess
- u. acidity
- u. albumin to creatinine (UA/C)
- u. alkalinization
- u. amylase
- u. anion gap
- u. ascites
- u. bicarbonate
- u. bilirubin
- u. bladder
- u. cachexia
- u. calcium
- u. calculus
- u. catecholamine
- u. catheterization
- u. cGMP level
- u. chloride
- u. chloride excretion
- u. citrate
- u. composition
- u. concentration
- u. conduit
- u. continence
- u. continence reflex
- u. continuity
- u. control urethral insert
- u. cortisol
- u. crystal
- u. cyclic AMP
- u. cyst
- u. dribbling
- u. exertional incontinence
- u. extravasation
- u. extraversion
- u. fibronectin
- u. flow
- u. frequency
- u. glucose
- u. glycosaminoglycan excretion
- u. hesitancy
- u. incontinence episode
- u. indican
- u. intestinal diversion
- u. kallikrein
- u. kallikrein excretion
- u. ketone
- u. leukocyte esterase
- u. lithiasis
- u. lithogenesis
- u. marker protein
- u. 3-methylhistidine
- u. nitrite test
- u. obstruction
- u. output
- u. oxalate
- u. oxalate excretion

urinary (*continued*)
  u. pH
  u. protein excretion
  u. protein-urinary creatinine ratio
  u. reconstruction
  u. retention
  u. sand
  u. schistosomiasis
  u. sediment
  u. sediment cast
  u. sodium excretion (UNaV)
  u. specific gravity
  u. stasis
  u. stone
  u. stress incontinence (USI)
  u. stuttering
  u. symptom
  u. tract
  u. tract anomaly
  u. tract disease
  u. tract 4-glass evaluation
  u. tract infection (UTI)
  u. tract infection suppression
  u. tract reconstruction-augmentation
    cystoplasty
  u. trypsin inhibitor (UTI)
  u. trypsinogen activation
    peptide
  u. umbilical fistula
  u. undiversion
  u. urea nitrogen excretion
  u. urgency
  u. urobilinogen
urination
  precipitant u.
  straining for u.
  stuttering u.
urine
  u. acidification
  anemic u.
  u. ascites
  barium sediment in u.
  Bence Jones u.
  u. bilirubin
  black u.
  u. chloride test
  chylous u.
  u. color
  u. composition
  concentrated u.
  u. concentration
  u. concentration test
  crude u.
  u. culture
  u. cytokine analysis
  u. cytology
  dark concentrated u.
  diabetic u.
  u. dipstick

dyspeptic u.
u. extravasation
febrile u.
u. flow rate
u. glitter cell
gouty u.
hyperosmotic u.
hypoosmotic u.
U. Meter Foley tray
midstream specimen of u.
  (MSU)
milky u.
nebulous u.
nervous u.
u. net charge (UNC)
u. osmolality
u. osmolarity (Uosm)
postvoid dribbling of u.
postvoid residual u.
u. protein electrophoresis
  (UPEP)
residual u.
u. sample
u. specific gravity
u. supersaturation
u. transport
u. turbidity
uncentrifuged u.
u. urea nitrogen (UUN)
u. urobilinogen (UU)
voided u.
urine-based enzyme-linked
  immunosorbent assay
urine-collecting tubule
urinemia (*var. of* uremia)
urine-plasma ratio
uriniferous
  u. pseudocyst
  u. tubule
uriniparous tubule
urinocryoscopy
urinogenous, urogenous
urinoglucosometer
urinology (*var. of* urology)
urinoma
urinometer, urometer
urinometry
urinosexual
urinous abscess
Uriscreen test
Urised
Urisedamine
UriSite urine collection kit
Urispas
Uri-Three culture kit
Urizole
uroanthelone
Urobak
urobilin complex

urobilinogen (UBG)
    fecal u.
    urinary u.
    urine u. (UU)
urobilinogenuria (*var. of* urobilinuria)
urobilinuria, urobilinogenuria
Uro-Bond skin adhesive
Urocam videocamera
Urocath external catheter
urocele, uroscheocele
urocheras (*var. of* uropsammus)
urochezia
urochrome
urochromogen
Urocit
Urocit-K
uroclepsia
UroCoil self-expanding stent
urocortin
urocrisia (*var. of* urocrisis)
urocrisis, urocrisia
urocriterion
urocyanogen
urocyst
Urocystin
urocystitis
UroCystom unit
Urocyte diagnostic cytometry system
urocytogram
urodeum
Urodiagnost x-ray table
urodialysis
urodochium
urodynamic
    u. assessment
    u. catheter
    u. dysfunction
    u. evaluation
    u. flow study
    u. investigation
    u. obstruction
    u. parameter
    u. testing
urodynamically
urodynamics
    ambulatory u.
urodynia
urodysfunction
uroedema (*var. of* uredema)
uroenterone
uroepithelial glycoid receptor
uroerythrin
uroflavin
uroflometer (*var. of* uroflowmeter)
uroflow
    u. index
    peak u.
uroflowmeter, uroflometer
    Dantec Urodyn 1000 u.

    Drake u.
    Synectics-Dantec Flo-Lab II u.
    Synectics-Dantec UD10000 u.
uroflowmetry
    Bristol nomogram for u.
    home u.
    Siroky nomogram for u.
urofuscin
urofuscohematin
urogastrone
urogenital
    u. abnormality
    u. diaphragm
    U. Distress Inventory (UDI)
    u. fistula
    u. mobilization
    u. prolapse
    u. region
    u. sinus
    u. sinus anomaly
    u. sinus mobilization
    u. sphincter muscle
    u. triangle
urogenous (*var. of* urinogenous)
    u. pyelitis
Urogesic
uroglaucin
Urografin 290 contrast medium
urogram
    constant infusion excretory u.
      (CIXU)
    excretory u.
    intravenous u. (IVU)
    retrograde u.
urograph
    Disa 5500 u.
urography
    antegrade u.
    cystoscopic u.
    descending u.
    excretory u. (EXU)
    high-dose intravenous u.
    intravenous u. (IVU)
    magnetic resonance u. (MRU)
    percutaneous antegrade u.
    retrograde u.
    1-shot intravenous u.
Uro-Guide stent
urogynecologic surgeon
urogynecologist
urogynecology
urohematin
urohematonephrosis
urohematoporphyrin
urohypertensin
Uro-jet delivery system
urokinase plasminogen activator
urokinetic
Uro-KP-Neutral

urokymography
Urolab Janus System III
Urolase
    Bard U.
    U. laser
    U. neodymium:YAG laser fiber
Urolene Blue
urolith
urolithiasis
    ammonium acid urate u.
    asymptomatic u.
    calcium oxalate u.
    calcium phosphate u.
    cystine u.
    dihydroxyadenine u.
    iatrogenic u.
    u. in childhood
    magnesium ammonium
      phosphate u.
    matrix u.
    miscellaneous u.
    pediatric u.
    recurrent calcium u. (RCU)
    silicate u.
    staghorn u.
    struvite u.
    triamterene u.
    uric acid u.
    xanthine u.
urolithic
urolithology
urolithotomy
urologic, urological
    u. aspect
    u. condition
    u. disease
    u. drug compendium
    u. intervention
    u. surgery (URS)
    u. symptom
    u. system cancer
urological (*var. of* urologic)
urologist
    general practice u.
urology, urinology, uronology
    Brief Male Sexual Function
      Inventory for U.
    u. clinic
    geriatric u.
    laparoscopic surgery in pediatric u.
    laparoscopy in pediatric u.
    pediatric u.
    perinatal u.
    u. set
    Society for Fetal U. (SFU)
Uroloop
UroLume
    U. endoprosthesis
    U. Endourethral Wallstent prosthesis

    U. prostate stent
    U. urethral prosthesis
    U. urethral stent
    U. Wallstent
    U. Wallstent stent
urolutein
Uro-Mag
Uromat dilation
UroMax II high-pressure balloon
  catheter
uromelanin
urometer (*var. of* urinometer)
uromodulin gene
uromucoid
uronate
    glycosaminoglycan u. (GAGUA)
    macromolecular u. (MMUA)
uroncus
uronephrosis
uronic acid-rich protein
uronology (*var. of* urology)
urononcometry
uronophile
uronoscopy (*var. of* uroscopy)
Uro-Pak system
uropathogen
uropathogenic bacterium
uropathologist
uropathy
    chronic obstructive u.
    congenital u.
    obstructive u.
    positional obstructive u.
uropenia
uropepsinogen
urophanic
urophein
urophosphometer
uroplania
Uroplus DS, SS
uropoiesis
uropoietic
uropontin
uroporphyria
uroporphyrinogen
    u. decarboxylase (UROD)
    u. synthetase (UROS)
uropsammus, urocheras
uropterin
uropyonephrosis
uropyoureter
Uroquid-Acid
uroradiology
    diagnostic u.
    interventional u.
urorectal septum
urorhythmography
urorubin
urorubrohematin

UROS
>uroporphyrinogen synthetase
>UROS infuser

Uro-San Plus external catheter
uroscheocele (*var. of* urocele)
uroschesis
uroscopy, uronoscopy
urosemiology
urosepsin
urosepsis
uroseptic
UroSnare cystoscopic tumor snare
Urosoft stent
urospectrin
Urospiral urethral stent
urostalagmometry
urostealith calculus
urostomy
Uro-Tex McGuire male urinal
urothelial
>u. augmentation
>u. basement membrane (UBM)
>u. cancer
>u. carcinoma
>u. dysplasia
>u. mucosa
>u. neoplasm
>u. tumor

urothelium
>seromuscular enterocystoplasty lined with u. (SELU)

urotherapy
Urotract x-ray system
uroureter
Urovac bladder evacuator
Urovist
>U. Cysto
>U. Meglumine
>U. Sodium 300

UroVive self-contained balloon system
UroVysion
>U. assay
>U. ultrasound imaging system

Urowave thermotherapy
uroxanthin
Uroxatral
URR
>urea reduction ratio

Ursec urinal
ursi
>*Diphyllobothrium u.*

Ursinus Inlay-Tabs
Urso 250
ursodeoxycholate (UDC)
ursodeoxycholic acid (UDCA)
ursodiol
urticarial, urticarious
>u. fever
>u. reaction

urticaria pigmentosa
urticarious (*var. of* urticarial)
URYS 800 nerve stimulator
US
>ultrasonography
>ultrasound

U.S. Army double-ended retractor
use
>long-term catheter u.

USG
>urine specific gravity

U-shaped skin flap
USI
>urinary stress incontinence

USRDS
>United States Renal Data System

Ussing
>U. chamber
>U. chamber technique

U-stitch reimplantation technique
UT-EGD
>ultrathin esophagoduodenoscopy

uteri (*pl. of* uterus)
uterine
>u. artery
>u. colic
>u. coring
>u. enlargement
>u. fibroid
>u. lateral fusion defect
>u. rupture
>u. size
>u. tenderness
>u. tympanites

utero
>hydronephrosis in u.

uterocele
uterolysis
>laparoscopic u.

uterosacral ligament
uteroscope
uterus, *pl.* **uteri**
>anteflexed u.
>anteverted u.
>bicornuate u.
>descensus uteri
>u. didelphys
>double u.
>duplicate u.
>enlarged u.
>gravid u.
>u. masculinus
>pregnant u.
>preservation of u.
>retroflexed u.
>retroverted u.
>unicornuate u.

U

UTI
    urinary tract infection
    urinary trypsin inhibitor
utopian state
utricle
       prostatic u.
utriculi (*pl. of* utriculus)
utriculitis
utriculocele
utriculus, *pl.* **utriculi**
    u. masculinus
    u. prostaticus
    u. vestibuli
U-tube stent
U-turn maneuver
UU
    urine urobilinogen
UUI
    urge urinary incontinence
UUN
    urine urea nitrogen
UUO
    unilateral ureteral
      obstruction
UUTI
    uncomplicated urinary tract
      infection

UV
    ultraviolet
      UV transilluminator
uva-ursi
uveitides (*pl. of* uveitis)
uveitis, *pl.* **uveitides**
      tubulointerstitial nephritis and u.
        (TINU)
UV-Flash ultraviolet germicidal exchange device
Uvidec-77 spectrophotometer
UVJ
    ureterovesical junction
uvomorulin
uvula, *pl.* **uvulae**
      Lieutaud u.
      u. of bladder
      u. vesicae
uvulae (*pl. of* uvula)
uvular
      u. deviation
      u. swelling
uvularis
UW
      University of Wisconsin
      UW solution
Uzara

V

V sign of Naclerio

VAB

vinblastine, actinomycin D, bleomycin

VAB6

vincristine, actinomycin, bleomycin,
cisplatinum, Cytoxan
VAB6 chemotherapy protocol

VABES

vasoablative endothelial sarcoma

VAC

vincristine, Adriamycin,
cyclophosphamide

VacA

vacuolating toxin gene A
VacA cytotoxin
VacA toxin

vaccination

T-cell v.

vaccine

V. Adverse Event Reporting System
BCG v.
ChronVac DNA v.
DCVax-Prostate v.
edible v.
GRNVAC1 v.
GVAX pancreatic cancer v.
Helivax v.
hepatitis A inactivated hepatitis B
  recombinant v.
hepatitis B virus v. (HBVV)
irradiated tumor v.
JT1001 prostate cancer v.
mucosal v.
OraVax v.
rhesus rotavirus-tetravalent v.
  (RRV-TV)
rotavirus tetravalent v.
Theratope v.
tumor v.
Twinrix v.
yeast-recombinant hepatitis B v.

vaccine-preventable hepatitis (VPH)

VAC GranuFoam silver dressing

VACTERL

vertebral, anal, cardiac,
tracheoesophageal fistula, renal, limb
VACTERL syndrome

vacuolar

v. H+-ATPase
v. nephrosis

vacuolar-type proton pump
immunocytochemistry

vacuolating

v. toxin gene A (VacA)

v. toxin gene A cytotoxin

vacuolation, vacuolization

vacuole

pinocytosis v.
testicular adenomatoid tumor v.

vacuolization (*var. of* vacuolation)

isometric tubular v.

Vacutainer

V. bag
V. bottle
V. tube

vacuum

v. constriction device (VCD)
v. constriction erection
v. entrapment device
v. erection device (VED)
v. erection technology
v. extraction device
v. tumescence device

VAD

vincristine, Adriamycin, dexamethasone

vagal

v. efferent outflow
v. input neuron
v. preganglionic neuron
v. stimulation

vagina, *pl.* **vaginae**

atrophic v.
high-ending v.
passage of flatus per v.
rhabdomyosarcoma of v.
septate v.

vaginae (*pl. of* vagina)

vaginal

v. atresia
v. bleeding
v. *Candida*
v. celiotomy
v. cone
v. cone biopsy
v. cone for pelvic floor exercise
v. construction
v. cuff
v. cuff cellulitis
v. cutback
v. descent
v. discharge
v. electrical stimulation
v. estrogen deficiency
v. eversion
v. fistula
v. fistula cup
v. flap
v. flap reconstruction and
  pubovaginal sling procedure

V

vaginal (*continued*)
    v. foreign body
    v. hiatus
    v. inflammation
    v. lithotomy
    v. mass
    v. morcellation
    v. mucosa
    v. needle suspension procedure
    v. prolapse
    v. repair
    v. suppository
    v. trichomoniasis
    v. ulcer
    v. vesicostomy
    v. wall approach
    v. wall sling procedure
vaginalis
    Gardnerella v.
    patent processus v.
    processus v.
    Trichomonas v.
    vestigium processus v.
vaginalitis
vaginate
vaginectomy
vaginoplasty
    cutback-type v.
    posterior flap v.
    tissue expansion v.
vaginoscopy
vaginosis
    bacterial v.
vaginourethroplasty
vagosympathetic balance
vagotomy
    v. and pyloroplasty (V&P)
    bilateral v.'s
    hemigastrectomy and v.
      (H&V)
    highly selective v. (HSV)
    laparoscopic v.
    laser laparoscopic v.
    medical v.
    parietal cell v. (PCV)
    proximal gastric v. (PGV)
    pyloroplasty and v. (P&V)
    Roux-en-Y procedure with v.
    selective proximal v. (SPV)
    superselective v.
    surgical v.
    total bilateral v.'s
    truncal v.
vagovagally mediated receptive
  relaxation
vagus nerve
Val10003
    valine

valaciclovir (*var. of* valacyclovir)
valacyclovir, valaciclovir
Valcyte
Val-d-Cytosine
valdecoxib
valerian
valethamate bromide
valganciclovir
validity of surgical simulator
valine (Val10003)
Valium
vallate papilla
vallecula, *pl.* **valleculae**
valleculae (*pl. of* vallecula)
vallecular
    v. dysphagia
    v. pooling
Valleylab
    V. E3B cautery unit
    V. II generator
    V. SSE-2 cautery unit
    V. SSE-2L generator
V-alpha gene
Valpin 50
valproate
    sodium v.
valproic
    v. acid
    v. acid hepatotoxicity
    v. acid therapy
Valsalva
    V. leak-point pressure (VLPP)
    V. leak-point pressure concept
    V. maneuver
    V. ratio
    tenia of V.
valsalviana
    dysphagia v.
Valtrac BAR
valuable additional parameter
value
    F v.
    negative predictive v.
    positive predictive v. (PPV)
    predictive v.
    reference v.
    target hemocrit v.
    therapeutic v.
valva, *pl.* **valvae**
    v. ileocecalis
valvae (*pl. of* valva)
valve
    v. ablation
    Amussat v.
    anal v.
    anterior urethral v.
    antireflux v.
    Ball v.

Bauhin v.
Benchekroun hydraulic ileal v.
v. bladder
blunting of v.
Braune v.
competent ileocecal v.
continent v.
esophageal v. (ESV)
esophageal Z stent with Dua
  antireflux v.
failed nipple v.
flap v.
frenulum of ileocolic v.
gastroesophageal flap v.
Gerlach v.
gonadal vein v.
Heister v.
Holter v.
Houston v.
ileal intestinal antireflux v.
ileal nipple v.
ileocecal intestinal antireflux v.
incompetent ileocecal v.
intestinal antireflux v.
intussuscepted nipple v.
Kock nipple v.
Kohlrausch v.
LeVeen v.
lipomatous ileocecal v.
Lopez enteral v.
Mitrofanoff v.
modified ileocecal v.
Morgagni v.
nipple v.
nonintussuscepted v.
v. of Bauhin
v. of colon
v. of Guérin
v. of Houston
v. of Kerckring
v. of Macalister
v. of Varolius
posterior urethral v. type I-IV
  (PUV)
v. prolapse
Quinton single-port scissors v.
rectal v.
scissors v.
Setguard antireflux v.
sigmoid v.
spiral v.
Spivack v.
urethral v.
valved
v. rectum
v. voice prosthesis
valvotomy, valvulotomy
rectal v.

valvula (*var. of* valvule), *pl.* **valvulae**
Amussat v.
v. fossae navicularis
v. processus vermiformis
v. spiralis
valvulae (*pl. of* valvula)
v. anales
v. conniventes
valvular heart disease
valvule, valvula
valvulectomy
valvulotomy (*var. of* valvotomy)
Vamin amino acid solution
van
v. Andel dilating catheter
v. Bogaert disease
v. Buren disease
v. Buren sound
V. de Kamer fecal fat procedure
v. den Bergh disease
v. den Bergh reaction
v. den Bergh test
v. Hees Activity Index (VHAI)
v. Hook operation
V. Slyke formula
v. Sonnenberg gallbladder
  catheter
v. Sonnenberg sump drain
Vanceril inhaler
Vancocin HCl
Vancoled
vancomycin hydrochloride
vancomycin/nalidixic acid agar
vancomycin-resistant enterococcus
  (VRE)
vanillacetic acid (VLA)
vanilloid-5
transient receptor potential v.-5
  (TRPV5)
vanilloid agent
vanillylmandelic acid (VMA)
vanished testis syndrome
vanishing
v. cancer phenomenon
v. gonad
v. testis
Vanquish analgesic caplet
Vansil
Vantin
vapor
V. Cut loop
v. pressure osmometer
vaporization
benign prostatic hyperplasia
  transurethral v.
contact laser v.
laser v.
VaporTome

V

VaporTrode electrode
Vaqta
Varco gallbladder forceps
vardenafil HCl
variability
variable
    v. nuclear crowding
    time-dependent v.
variable-stiffness
    v.-s. endoscope
    v.-s. enteroscope
Varian
    V. brachytherapy
    V. gas chromatography
variance
    geographic v.
    hypovolemic v.
    isovolemic v.
    Kruskal-Wallis analysis of v.
variant
    DLG5 gene v.
    kidney v.
    SEN virus v. D (SENV-D)
    SEN virus v. H (SENV-H)
    trifurcation v.
    Wilms tumor clear cell sarcoma v.
    Wilms tumor multilocular cyst v.
    Wilms tumor rhabdomyosarcoma v.
variation
    coefficient of v.
    diurnal v.
    intraprostatic characteristic v.
    phasic-free tone v.
Varibar oral contrast medium
variceal
    v. banding
    v. band ligation
    v. bleeding
    v. column
    v. decompression
    v. hemorrhage
    v. ligator
    v. pressure
    v. pressure measuring device
    v. sclerosant
    v. sclerosis
    v. sclerotherapy
    v. sclerotherapy in esophagus
    v. size inclusion criteria
    v. wall
varicella-zoster
    v.-z. infection
    v.-z. virus (VZV)
varices (*pl. of* varix)
varicocele
    v. embolization
    v. repair
    symptomatic v.

varicocelectomy
    inguinal v.
    laparoscopic v.
    microsurgical inguinal v.
    Palomo v.
    retroperitoneal v.
    scrotal v.
    subinguinal microsurgical v.
Varicoscreen
varicosis coli totalis
varicosity
variegate
    v. coproporphyria
    v. porphyria
Variject needle
varioliform
    v. gastritis
    v. gastropathy
varioliformis
    gastritis v.
variolosa
    orchitis v.
VariSeed 7.0 software computer program
varix, *pl.* **varices**
    actively bleeding v.
    alcoholic v.
    anorectal v.
    bar-type esophageal v.
    bleeding gastric v. (BGV)
    blue v.
    colonic v.
    common bile duct v.
    downhill esophageal v.
    duodenal v.
    ectopic v.
    EEA stapling of v.
    endoscopic band ligation of v.
    esophageal v.
    esophagogastric v.
    familial colonic v.
    fundal v.
    fundic v.
    gallbladder v.
    gastric v.
    gastroesophageal v. type 1, 2
    v. grading system F1, F2, F3
    idiopathic v.
    ileal v.
    isolated gastric v. type 1, 2 (IGV)
    jejunal v.
    v. ligation
    mesenteric v.
    obliterated v.
    v. of colon
    Okuda transhepatic obliteration of v.
    paraesophageal v.
    percutaneous transhepatic obliteration
      of esophageal v.

peristomal v.
radius of v.
rectal v.
rectosigmoid v.
transesophageal ligation of v.
Varolius
valve of V.
VAS
vascular
vasectomy
vas, *pl.* **vasa, vasorum**
v. aberrans
v. afferens glomerulus
vasa afferentia
v. deferens
v. deferens obstruction
v. deferens secretion
v. deferens stricture
v. efferens glomerulus
vasa recta
vasa recta bundle
vasa vasorum
vasa (*pl. of* vas)
vasalgia
vasal pedicle orchiopexy
Vas-Cath
Vasclip alternative to vasectomy
vascopressin
hydroosmotic action of v.
vascular (VAS)
v. abnormality
v. access
v. access complication
v. access failure
v. access graft (VAG)
v. access site
v. anastomosis
v. bruit
v. cachexia
v. cecal fold
v. cell adhesion molecule-1 (VCAM-1)
v. cirrhosis
v. clamp
v. coat of stomach
v. collateral network
v. compromise
v. disease
v. ectasia
v. endothelial cell marker
v. endothelial growth factor (VEGF)
v. hemangioma
v. injury
v. insufficiency
v. invasion
v. laceration
v. laceration repair

v. lamina
v. lesion
v. malformation
v. malformation of bladder
v. neoplasia
v. nephritis
v. nephropathy
v. parameter
v. pattern
v. pedicle
v. permeability factor (VPF)
v. permeation of tumor cell
v. plasminogen activator (v-PA)
v. plexus
v. rejection
v. renal mass
v. smooth muscle
v. smooth muscle cell (VSMC)
v. stapler
v. steal syndrome
v. surgery
v. suture
v. tuft
vascularity
vascularization
intraprostatic v.
vasculature
appearance of normal colon v.
intraprostatic v.
kidney v.
preglomerular v.
v. responsiveness
vasculitic
v. lesion
v. neuropathy
vasculitis
allergic v.
ANCA-associated systemic v.
antineutrophilic cytoplasmic autoantibody-small vessel v. (ANCA-SVV)
extrarenal v.
leukocytoclastic v.
lymphocytic v.
mesenteric v.
necrotizing bowel v.
renal v.
rheumatoid v.
systemic lupus erythematosus v.
visceral v.
vasculogenic impotence
vasculopathy
acute renal transplant v.
noncerebral v.
portal hypertensive intestinal v. (PHIV)
vasculosa
tunica v.

V

vasculum aberrans
vasectomized
vasectomy (VAS)
    Casale v.
    crossover v.
    no-scalpel v.
    open-ended v.
    percutaneous v.
    v. reversal
    reversible v.
    Vasclip alternative to v.
Vaseline gauze
vasiform
vasitis nodosa
vasoablative endothelial sarcoma (VABES)
vasoactive
    v. drug
    v. intestinal peptide (VIP)
    v. intestinal peptide distribution
    v. intestinal peptide-secreting tumor (VIPoma)
    v. intestinal polypeptide (VIP)
    v. intestinal polypeptide binding
    v. intestinal polypeptide immunoreactivity (VIP-IR)
    v. intestinal polypeptide stain
    v. intestinal polypeptide tumor (VIPoma)
    v. peptide-cytokine interaction
vasoconstriction
    afferent arteriolar v.
    baroreceptor-mediated mesenteric arterial v.
    radiocontrast-induced renal v.
    reflex splanchnic v.
    renal v.
    splanchnic v.
vasoconstrictor peptide
vasocutaneous fistula
vasodilatation (*var. of* vasodilation)
vasodilation, vasodilatation
    endothelium-dependent v.
    v. of portasystemic collateral
    peripheral v.
    renal v.
    sympathetic response to v.
vasodilator
    renal v.
vasoepididymography
vasoepididymostomy
    ASSI end-to-end v.
    Goldstein Microspike approximator clamp for v.
    Silber v.
vasoformative
vasography
    fine-needle v.

    percutaneous v.
    transrectal v.
vasoligation
Vasomax
vasomotor disorder
vasoorchidostomy
vasopressin
    arginine v. (AVP)
    fetal arginine v.
    v. infusion
    neonatal arginine v.
    v. type 2 receptor
    v. with nitroglycerin
vasopressinase
vasopressin-induced cAMP
vasopuncture
vasorelaxation
vasoresection
vasorrhaphy
vasorum (*pl. of* vas)
vasosection (*var. of* vasotomy)
vasospasm
vasospasmolytic
vasospastic
vasostomy
Vasotec
vasotomy, vasosection
vasovagal reflex
vasovasostomy
    Goldstein Microspike approximator clamp for v.
    multiple v.'s
vasovasotomy
    cross v.
vasovesiculectomy
vasovesiculitis
vasovesiculography
Vasoxyl
vastus lateralis muscle flap
vater
    ampulla of V.
    invaginating ampulla of V.
    papilla of V.
VATER
    vertebral, anal, tracheoesophageal fistula, renal
        VATER syndrome
VATS
    videoassisted thoracic surgery
Vattikuti Institute prostatectomy
vault
    rectal v.
Vaxcel dialysis catheter
V-beta gene
VBG
    vertical banded gastroplasty
VCAM-1
    vascular cell adhesion molecule-1

VCD
    vacuum constriction device
       Dacomed Catalyst VCD
       Mission VCD
       Osbon ErecAid VCD
       Pos-T-Vac VCD
VCG
    voiding cystogram
VCUG
    vesicoureterogram
    voiding cystourethrogram
    voiding cystourethrography
VDD
    vincristine, Adriamycin, dexamethasone
VDRL
    Venereal Disease Research
      Laboratory
V-echinocandin
Vectastain ABC kit
Vectibix
vector
    amplitude-acrophase v.
    bacterial v.
    V. volume measurement
vectorial delivery
Vectra hemodialysis access graft
vecuronium
VED
    vacuum erection device
      Mission VED
Veetids
VEFG
    vascular endothelial growth
     factor
vegetable
    allium v.
    cruciferous v.
vegetans
    pyostomatitis v.
vegetarian diet
vegetative lesion
veil
    Jackson v.
vein, vena
    aberrant obturator v.
    accessory saphenous v.
    adrenal v.
    arcuate v.
    arterialization of portal v.
    azygos v.
    bladder v.
    Burow v.
    cardinal v.
    cavernosal v.
    cavernous transformation of portal v.
     (CTPV)
    circumflex v.
    common iliac v.
    crural v.

deep dorsal v. (DDV)
dilated v.
dorsal v.
esophageal collateral v. (ECV)
external spermatic v.
extrahepatic portal v.
gastric v.
gonadal v.
gubernacular v.
hepatic v.
idiopathic myointimal hyperplasia of
  mesenteric v.
iliac v.
inferior adrenal v.
inferior mesenteric v.
inferior rectal v.
interlobar v.
internal iliac v.
internal pudendal v.
Krukenberg v.
left hepatic v.
lumbar v.
mesenteric v.
middle hepatic v. (MHV)
middle rectal v.
muscularization of v.
obturator v.
omental v.
palisade-type v.
pancreaticoduodenal v.
paraesophageal collateral v.
paraumbilical v.
v. patch
periesophageal collateral v.
peripheral acinar v.
peritoneal v.
periurethral v.
portal v.
pudendal v.
rectal v.
renal v.
v. retractor
Retzius v.
right hepatic v.
Ruysch v.
sacral v.
saphenous v.
shunt index via inferior
  mesenteric v.
shunt index via superior
  mesenteric v.
spermatic v.
splanchnic v.
splenic v.
subclavian v.
sulcus of umbilical v.
superior mesenteric v. (SMV)
superior rectal v.
tangle of hemorrhoidal v.'s

V

vein (*continued*)
thoracoabdominal collateral v.
urethral v.
vesical v.
Velban
Velban, actinomycin D, bleomycin
Velban, actinomycin D, bleomycin,
platinum
cisplatin, methotrexate, V. (CMV)
Velcade
Vella fistula
velocimetry
laser Doppler v.
velocity
angular v.
dorsal nerve conduction v.
v. measurement
portal vein blood flow v.
portal venous v. (PVV)
prostate-specific antigen v.
(PSAV)
tumor peak systolic v.
velopharyngeal insufficiency (VPI)
Velosef
Velpeau hernia
vena (v), *pl.* **venae**
v. cava
v. cava hiatus
venae cavernosae penis
v. marginalis epididymis of
Haberer
venacavogram
venacavography
venae (*pl. of* vena)
venerea
urethritis v.
venereal
v. bubo
v. disease
V. Disease Research Laboratory
(VDRL)
v. proctocolitis
v. sore
v. wart
venereum
lymphogranuloma v. (LGV)
papilloma v.
veneris
mons v.
venesection therapy
venezuelensis
Strongyloides v.
venipuncture
peripheral v.
venlafaxine
venodilation
nitrate-induced v.
systemic v.
Venofer

venogenic impotence
venogram
hepatic v.
renal v.
weeping willow appearance on v.
venography
adrenal v.
hepatic v.
pedal control v.
renal v.
splenic v.
splenoportal v.
transjugular portal v.
venoocclusive
v. disease of liver
v. dysfunction
v. liver disease
venoperitoneostomy
venosi
fissura ligamenti v.
venosum
fissure of ligamentum v.
ligamentum v.
venosus
plexus v.
venous
v. blood sample
v. circulation
v. ectasia
v. engorgement
v. invasion
v. leakage
v. leak impotence
v. leak syndrome
v. outflow obstructive disease
v. pattern
v. pooling
v. stasis
v. thromboembolism (VTE)
v. thrombosis
v. web
v. web disease
venovenous
v. access
v. bypass
v. continuous hemodialysis
v. hemofiltration
venter propendens
ventilation
mechanical v.
ventilatory support
venting
v. percutaneous gastrostomy
(VPG)
v. percutaneous gastrostomy tube
Ventolin
ventral
v. apron prepuce
v. bending technique

v. bud
v. celiotomy
v. chronic calcific pancreatitis
v. hernia
v. herniorrhaphy
v. meatotomy
v. mesogastrium
v. patch urethroplasty
v. posteroinferior (VPI)
v. sacral rootlet
v. surface
v. transperitoneal laparoscopic
approach
ventralis
ventricle
ventricular canal
ventriculare
corpus v.
ventricularis
fundus v.
ventriculi (*pl. of* ventriculus)
ventriculoperitoneal (VP)
v. shunt
ventriculus, *pl.* **ventriculi**
anadenia ventriculi
corpus ventriculi
descensus ventriculi
fundus ventriculi
polyposis ventriculi
ventrocystorrhaphy
ventroscopy
ventrotomy
ventrum
v. of penis
v. penis flap
venula (*var. of* venule), *pl.*
 venulae
venulae rectae renis
venulae (*pl. of* venula)
venular
venule, venula
collecting v.
hepatic v.
portal v.
stellate v.
straight v.
subtunical v.
VePesid, ifosfamide with mesna rescue,
 Platinol (VIP)
vera
hemospermia v.
melena v.
polycythemia v. (PCV)
verapamil
Veratrum alkaloid
Veregen
Veress
V. cannula
V. needle

verge
anal v.
Vergon
veritas
in vivo v.
vermicular
v. appendage
v. colic
v. movement
vermicularis
Enterobius v.
vermiform
v. appendix
v. body
vermiformis
ostium appendicis v.
valvula processus v.
verminous
v. appendicitis
v. colic
v. ileus
Vermox
Verner-Morrison syndrome
Vernon-David
V.-D. proctoscope
V.-D. rectal speculum
V.-D. sigmoidoscope
verruca vulgaris
verruciform xanthoma
verrucose, verrucous
verrucous (*var. of* verrucose)
v. carcinoma
v. gastritis
Versabran
Modane V.
Versant HCV RNA qualitative assay
Versa-PEG gastrostomy kit
VersaPulse
V. PowerSuite dual-wavelength laser
V. PowerSuite holmium laser
V. Select laser
Versed
vertebra, *pl.* **vertebrae**
vertebrae (*pl. of* vertebra)
vertebral
v., anal, cardiac, tracheoesophageal
fistula, renal, limb (VACTERL)
v., anal, cardiac, tracheoesophageal
fistula, renal, limb syndrome
v., anal, tracheoesophageal fistula,
renal (VATER)
v., anal, tracheoesophageal fistula,
renal syndrome
vertex, *pl.* **vertices**
v. of urinary bladder
vertical
v. banded gastroplasty (VBG)
v. fold
v. mattress suture

V

vertical (*continued*)
    v. midline incision
    v. plication suture
    v. reduction rectoplasty
    v. ring gastroplasty (VRG)
    v. silastic ring gastroplasty
    v. transmission
    v. vesicomyotomy (VVM)
vertices (*pl. of* vertex)
vertigo
    gastric v.
    objective v.
    subjective v.
verum
    diverticulum ilei v.
verumontanitis
verumontanum
very
    v. late activation (VLA)
    v. low calorie diet (VLCD)
    v. low density lipoprotein (VLDL)
    v. low density lipoprotein
      cholesterol
vesica, *pl.* **vesicae**
    v. biliaris
    bullous edema vesicae
    ectopia vesicae
    endometriosis vesicae
    v. fellea
    v. ileale pouch
    malacoplakia vesicae
    V. percutaneous bladder neck
      stabilization
    V. percutaneous bladder neck
      suspension kit
    v. prostatica
    V. sling
    V. sling procedure
    trigonum vesicae
    v. urinaria
    uvula vesicae
vesicae (*pl. of* vesica)
vesical
    v. artery
    v. calculus
    v. compliance
    v. diverticulectomy
    v. diverticulum
    v. exstrophy
    v. external sphincter dyssynergia
    v. fibrosis
    v. fistula
    v. hematuria
    v. leak point pressure (VLPP)
    v. ligament
    v. lithotomy
    v. neck
    v. neck resistance
    v. neck stenosis

    v. plexus
    v. prostatism
    v. schistosomiasis
    v. vein
vesicalis
    anus v.
    plexus v.
vesical-sacral-sphincter loop
Vesicare
vesicle
    brush-border membrane v. (BBMV)
    endocytotic v.
    Golgi v.
    v. hernia
    leiomyoma of seminal v.
    metanephric v.
    prechylomicron transport v.
    seminal v.
    spermatic v.
vesicoamniotic shunt
vesicoanal reflex
vesicocavernous
vesicocele
vesicocervical
vesicoclysis
vesicocolic, vesicocolonic
    v. fistula
vesicocolonic (*var. of* vesicocolic)
vesicocutaneous fistula
vesicoenteric fistula
vesicofixation
vesicoileal reflux
vesicointestinal
    v. fistula
    v. reflex
vesicolithiasis
vesicomyectomy
vesicomyotomy
    circular v. (CVM)
    vertical v. (VVM)
vesicopelvic fascia
vesicoperineal
vesicoprostatic
    v. calculus
    v. plexus
vesicopubic
vesicopustule
vesicorectal fistula
vesicorectostomy
vesicorenal
vesicosalpingovaginal fistula
vesicosigmoid
vesicosigmoidostomy
vesicosphincteric dyssynergia
vesicospinal
vesicostomy
    Blocksom v.
    Casale v.
    continent v.

cutaneous v.
Lapides v.
preputial continent v.
Rink modification of Casale
  continent catheterizable v.
vaginal v.
vesicotomy
vesicoumbilical fistula
vesicourachal diverticulum
vesicoureteral
v. anastomotic stricture
v. reflux (VUR)
v. regurgitation
v. suspension
vesicoureteric
v. reflux
v. stenosis
vesicoureterogram (VCUG)
vesicourethral
v. anastomosis
v. anastomotic stricture
v. canal
v. reflux
v. reflux and renal
  dysplasia
v. suspension
vesicouterina
excavatio v.
vesicouterine
v. fistula
v. pouch
vesicouterinum
cavum v.
vesicouterovaginal
vesicovaginal
v. fistula (VVF)
v. Holter
v. lithotomy
v. space
vesicovaginorectal fistula
vesicovaginostomy
vesicula, *pl.* **vesiculae**
v. bilis
v. seminalis
vesiculae (*pl. of* vesicula)
vesicular stomatitis virus (VSV)
vesiculase
vesiculectomy
prostatoseminal v.
retrovesical v.
total prostatoseminal v.
transcoccygeal v.
transperineal v.
transvesical v.
vesiculitis
vesiculobullous disorder
vesiculocavernous
vesiculodeferential artery
vesiculogram

vesiculography
seminal v. (SVG)
vesiculoprostatitis
vesiculotomy
seminal v.
vesiculotubular
vesiculotympanitic resonance
Vespore disinfectant
Vesprin
VESS
videoendoscopic swallowing study
VESS chair
vessel
accessory v.
blood v.
caliber-persistent v.
capsular blood v.
chyliferous v.
cremasteric v.
v. dilator
dysmorphic v.
ectatic v.
feeding v.
gastroepiploic blood v.
gonadal v.
hypogastric v.
hypoplastic blind-ending spermatic v.
ileal blood v.
ileocolic v.
internal spermatic v.
lacteal v.
lymphatic v.
mesocolonic v.
nonbleeding visible v.
palisade v.
pudendal v.
replaced hepatic v.
serosal blood v.
telangiectatic v.
v. tip
ulcer v.
visible ulcer v.
vestibular gland
vestibularis
anus v.
vestibule
laryngeal v.
vestibuli
utriculus v.
vestibulourethral
vestige
vestigial
vestigium processus vaginalis
vest-over-pants
v.-o.-p. hernia repair
v.-o.-p. herniorrhaphy
vetch
common kidney v.
Vet-Co vacuum system

Vezien abdominal scissors
Vfend
V-flap meatoplasty
VFR
    voiding flow rate
VGE
    viral gastroenteritis
VHAI
    van Hees Activity Index
VHL
    von Hippel-Lindau
      VHL gene
Viabil biliary endoprosthesis
viability
    intestinal v.
    v. testing
ViaCath
    V. computer-assisted robotic
      endoluminal system
    V. endoluminal surgery system
ViaDuct pancreatic stent
Viadur
Viagra
    esprolol plus V.
    PT141 with V.
vial
    Port-A-Germ anaerobic transport v.
    scintillation v.
Vibramycin
Vibrio
    V. alginolyticus
    V. cholerae
    V. cholerae biotype *albensis*
    V. cholerae biotype *eltor*
    V. cholerae biotype *Proteus*
    V. cholera O1
    V. cholera O139
    V. eltor
    V. fetus infection
    V. fluvialis
    V. furnissii
    V. hollisae
    V. metschnikovii
    V. parahaemolyticus
    V. vulnificus
vibriocidal
vibrotactile stimulation testing
Vickers M85a microdensitometer
Vicodin
Vicryl
    V. mesh
    V. suture
VID
    vitellointestinal duct
Vidal operation
vidarabine
video
    v. headset
    V. Image Processor

    v. monitor
    v. pill
    v. pressure flow electromyography
    v. push enteroscope
    v. recorder
    v. small-bowel enteroscopy
    v. timer
    v. transurethral resection technique
videoassisted thoracic surgery (VATS)
videocamera
    PillCam ESO v.
    Urocam v.
videocapsule
    v. endoscopy
    v. enteroscopy
    Given M2A endoscopic v.
videocholangioscope
videocholangioscopy
videocolonoscope
    EVE Fujinon v.
    forward-viewing v.
    Fujinon EC7-CM2 v.
    Fujinon EVC-M v.
    Olympus CF100TL v.
    Olympus CF-1T100L v.
    Olympus CF-TL-series
      forward-viewing v.
    Olympus EVIS v.
    Olympus PCF-130L v.
    Welch Allyn v.
videoconverter
    sequential v.
videocystourethrography
videodensitometry
videoduodenoscope
    Fujinon ED7-XU2 v.
    Fujinon EVD-XL v.
    Fujinon 310XU v.
    Olympus JF-series v.
    Olympus JF-V-series v.
    Olympus JT-series v.
    side-viewing v.
    TJF-10, -20 v.
videoechoendoscope
    large-channel curvilinear v.
videoelectroscope
    Fujinon CEG-FP-series v.
videoendoscope
    double-channel v.
    Fujinon UGI-FP-series v.
    infrared v.
    JF-200 side-viewing v.
    Olympus EVIS 140Q v.
    Olympus GF-series v.
    Olympus GIF-series double-channel
      therapeutic v.
    Olympus GIF-SQ-series v.
    Olympus GIF-T-series v.
    Olympus GIF-200Z v.

Olympus JF-series v.
Olympus Q200 v.
Olympus SSIF-series v.
Olympus XQ-200, XQ-230 v.
Pentax EC-series v.
Pentax FD-series v.
Toshiba v.
Welch Allyn v.
videoendoscopic swallowing study (VESS)
videoendoscopy
dynamic fluorescence v.
Lugol-combined upper gastrointestinal v.
zoom v.
videoenteroscope
Olympus SIF-M-series v.
Olympus SIF-SW-series v.
Olympus SIG-100L v.
Olympus SSIF-series v.
Olympus XSIF-series v.
videoesophagoscopy
videoesophagram
videofluoroscopic
v. swallow study (VSS)
v. technique
videofluoroscopy
videofluorourodynamic study
videogastroscope
Fujinon 400-series super image v.
Olympus GIF-XQ200 v.
Olympus GIF-XQ230 v.
Olympus GIF-XQ240 v.
Pentax EG-2900 v.
transnasal v.
videographic tool technology
videoinstrument
XQ v.
videolaparoscope
EL2-LS2 flexible v.
flexible v.
videolaryngoscope
Kantor-Berci v.
videolaseroscopy-cholecystectomy
videomonitored TUR
videoprocessor
real-time v.
videoproctography
videoresectoscope
Richard Wolf v.
videoscope
CV-1 v.
SlimSIGHT gastrointestinal v.
videosigmoidoscope
Pentax FS-series flexible fiberoptic v.
videothorascopic
videourodynamic
v. evaluation

v. study
v. testing
Vienna classification of Crohn disease
view
en face v.
longitudinal v.
postevacuation v.
retroflexed v.
slide-by v.
stereomicroscopic v.
transverse v.
vigabatrin
VIGOR
Vioxx Gastrointestinal Outcomes Research
VIGOR trial
vigorous achalasia
villi (*pl. of* villus)
villiferous
villoglandular
v. adenoma
v. polyp
villose (*var. of* villous)
villous, villose
v. arteritis
v. arthritis
v. atrophy
v. coat of small intestine
v. colorectal adenoma
v. effacement
v. epithelium
v. folds of stomach
v. papilloma
v. polyp
v. tumor
villous-tip cell
villus, *pl.* **villi**
v. cell
colonic v.
duodenal v.
fingerlike v.
intestinal v.
jejunal v.
leaflike v.
ridged convoluted v.
small-intestinal v.
v. tip
tongue-shaped v.
vimentin staining
Vim-Silverman
V.-S. biopsy needle
V.-S. needle biopsy technique
V.-S. technique for liver biopsy
vinblastine
v., actinomycin D, bleomycin cisplatin, methotrexate, v. (CMV)
doxorubicin, bleomycin sulfate, v. (ABV)
methotrexate, cisplatin, v. (MCV)

Vincent curtsy
vincristine
>v., actinomycin, bleomycin, cisplatinum, Cytoxan (VAB6)
>v., Adriamycin, cyclophosphamide (VAC)
>v., Adriamycin, dexamethasone (VAD, VDD)

Vindelov method flow cytometry analysis
vine
>chocolate v.

vinorelbine
Vinson syndrome
Viokase
violaceous
violation
>scrotal v.

violet
>gentian v.

violin-string adhesion
Vioxx Gastrointestinal Outcomes Research (VIGOR)
VIP
>vasoactive intestinal peptide
>vasoactive intestinal polypeptide
>VePesid, ifosfamide with mesna rescue, Platinol
>voluntary interruption of pregnancy
>VIP antiserum
>VIP stain

VIP-IR
>vasoactive intestinal polypeptide immunoreactivity

VIPoma
>vasoactive intestinal peptide-secreting tumor
>vasoactive intestinal polypeptide tumor
>VIPoma syndrome

Virag
>V. injector
>V. operation

viral
>v. cholangitis
>v. colitis
>v. culture
>v. cystitis
>v. diarrhea
>v. dysentery
>v. enteritis
>v. gastritis
>v. gastroenteritis (VGE)
>v. glycoprotein
>v. hemorrhagic fever
>v. hepatitis
>v. hepatitis marker
>v. hepatitis type A, B
>v. inclusion body

>v. infection
>v. membrane fusion
>v. oncoprotein
>v. replication
>v. serologic titer

Viramidine
ViraPap HPV dot blot hybridization test
Virazole
Virchow sentinel node
Virchow-Troisier node
viremia
>hepatitis C v.

virgin
>v. lymphocyte
>v. ulcer

viridans
>alpha *Streptococcus v.*
>*Staphylococcus v.*
>*Streptococcus v.*

virile
>membrum v.
>v. reflex

virilis
>crista urethralis v.
>urethra v.

virilism
>adrenal v.

virilization
virilizing tumor
Virilon
virion
>HBV v.

virological
virology
virtual
>V. Biopsy system
>v. colonoscopy Side Fire APC probe
>v. cystoscopy
>v. endoscopy
>v. enteroscopy
>v. focus shock wave
>v. nephroureteroscopy
>v. reality simulator
>v. reality technology
>V. Vision
>V. Vision audiovisual system for EGD and colonoscopy

virucidal agent
virulence
>encoding v.
>enhanced v.
>v. factor

virulent diarrhea
Virulizin
virus
>v. A, B hepatitis

adenoassociated v. (AAV)
Aichi v.
antibody to hepatitis A v. (anti-HAV)
antibody to hepatitis C v. (anti-HCV)
antibody to hepatitis D v. (anti-HDV)
blood-borne v.
delta v.
dengue v.
encephalomyocarditis v.
Epstein-Barr v. (EBV)
esophageal condyloma v.
Guillian-Barré virus C/hepatitis G v. (GBV-C/HGV)
Hawaii v.
hepatitis A v. (HAV)
hepatitis B v. (HBV)
hepatitis B-like DNA v.
hepatitis C v. (HCV)
hepatitis D v. (HDV)
hepatitis delta v.
hepatitis E v. (HEV)
hepatitis G v. (HGV)
herpes simplex v. (HSV)
herpes zoster v. (HZV)
human immunodeficiency v. (HIV)
human T-cell leukemia v. type I (HTLV-1, HTLV-I)
human T-cell lymphotrophic v. type I, II
IgM-hepatitis E v. (IgM-HEV)
influenza v.
live attenuated v.
v. load
Manchester v.
Marburg v.
molluscum contagiosum v. (MCV)
mother-to-infant transmission of hepatitis C v.
neutropic v.
Norwalk v.
Norwalk-like v. (NLV)
recombinant capsid protein of Norwalk v. (rNV)
Rous sarcoma v.
Sapporo v.
SEN v.
v. shedding
simian v. 40
transfusion-transmitted v. (TTV)
varicella-zoster v. (VZ)
vesicular stomatitis v. (VSV)
viruslike
v. action (VLA)
v. particle
viscera (*pl. of* viscus)

visceral
v. angiography
v. arteriography
v. dysfunction
v. hyperalgesia
v. hypersensitivity
v. ischemia
v. larva migrans
v. leishmaniasis
v. muscle
v. neuropathy
v. pain
v. peritoneum
v. traction reflex
v. vasculitis
visceralgia
visceralis
fascia pelvis v.
viscerimotor (*var. of* visceromotor)
visceromegaly
visceromotor, viscerimotor
visceroparietal
visceroperception score
visceroptosia (*var. of* visceroptosis)
visceroptosis, visceroptosia
viscerosensory reflex
viscerotomy
viscerotrophic
viscerotropic
viscerum
situs inversus v.
viscid bile
viscidosis
viscoelastic
v. collagen fiber
v. gel
viscoelasticity
bladder v.
viscometer
viscosity
plasma v.
semen v.
viscous
v. bile
v. lidocaine
v. lidocaine premedication
v. Xylocaine gargle
viscus, *pl.* **viscera**
abdominal v.
hollow v.
intraabdominal v.
intraperitoneal v.
perforated v.
strangulated v.
vise
torque v.

V

visible
  v. abdominal distention
  v. peristalsis
  v. ulcer vessel
  v. vessel significance
visible-light lithotripsy
Visicath endoscope
Visick
  V. dysphagia classification
  V. gastric cancer grading system
Visicol tablet
Visilex mesh
visilizumab
vision
  direct v.
  V. Sciences Inc. (VSI)
  V. Sciences Inc. flexible
    sigmoidoscope system
  V. System EndoSheath
  V. System sigmoidoscope
  tunnel v.
  Virtual V.
Visiport device
Visken
Vistaflex biliary stent
Vistaril
Vistide
visual
  v. endoscopically controlled laser
  v. evoked potential
  v. laser ablation
  v. laser ablation of prostate (VLAP)
  v. laser-assisted prostatectomy
    (VLAP)
  v. sexual stimulation testing
visualization
  enhanced v.
  improved v.
vital
  V. HN feeding
  v. signs
  v. staining
**VitalStim Therapy electrical stimulation
  system**
vitamin
  v. A, B_{12} absorption test
  v. A, D deficiency
  v. A toxicity
  v. B_6
  v. B_{12}
  v. B_{12} malabsorption
  v. C
  v. D-binding protein
  v. D-dependent calbindin-D9k
  v. D receptor
  v. D resistance
  v. D supplementation
  v. E
  fat-soluble v.

  v. K2
  Maxisal with v. C
  water-soluble v.
Vitaneed
  V. feeding
  V. tube-feeding formula
Vitaxin
Vitelle
  V. Irospan
  V. Nesentials tablet
  V. Nestrex tablet
vitelline
  v. duct
  v. duct anomaly
vitellointestinal
  v. cyst
  v. duct (VID)
vitiligo
vitro
  in v.
**vitronectin-inhibiting HGF-induced
  tubulogenesis**
Vitros
  V. Immunodiagnostic Products
    HBsAg confirmatory kit
  V. Immunodiagnostic Products
    HBsAg reagent pack and
    calibrator
Vittaforma corneae
Vivactil
viverrini
  Opisthorchis v.
vividialysis
vividiffusion
vivo
  ex v.
  in v. (IV)
Vivonex
  V. Acutrol enteral feeding system
  V. HN powdered feeding
  V. Moss tube
  V. TEN
  V. TEN feeding
VLA
  vanillacetic acid
  very late activation
  viruslike action
VLAP
  visual laser ablation of prostate
  visual laser-assisted prostatectomy
VLCD
  very low calorie diet
VLDL
  very low density lipoprotein
  VLDL cholesterol
  VLDL triglyceride
VLPP
  Valsalva leak-point pressure
  vesical leak point pressure

VMA
vanillylmandelic acid
VMC
von Meyenburg complex
vocal cord
Vocare bladder system
Vogel operation
Voges-Proskauer test
voided
v. urine
v. volume
voiding
alarm clock v.
v. biofeedback
classic high-pressure low-flow v.
v. cystogram (VCG)
v. cystometrography
v. cystometry
v. cystourethrogram (VCUG)
v. cystourethrography (VCUG)
v. diary
dysfunctional v.
v. dysfunction classification
v. dysfunction role of prostate stem
cell antigen
v. flow rate (VFR)
fractionated v.
good v.
incomplete v.
v. initiation
orthotopic v.
v. parameter
v. pressure
reflex v.
staccato v.
v. study
timed v.
trigger v.
v. urethral pressure measurement
(VUPM)
v. urine cytology (VUC)
Voillemier point
volar
Volhard-Fahr method
Volhard nephritis
Volkmann
V. operation
V. pancreatic calculus spoon
V. rake retractor
V. spoon for pancreatic calculus
voltage
RMS v.
root mean square v.
voltage-dependent anion channel
voltage-gated channel
Voltaren
volume
bladder v.
v. displacement transducer

drain v.
effective arterial blood v. (EABV)
emptying delta v.
v. expansion
extracellular fluid v. (ECFV, EFV)
fiber bundle v.
flow v.
functional hepatic v.
gallbladder v.
gastric v.
interstitial v.
intragastric v.
intraperitoneal v.
intravascular v.
liver v.
maximum tolerable v. (MTV)
mean corpuscular v.
mean prostatic v.
mean renal v.
v. of distribution
v. overload
pelvic ileal reservoir v.
plasma v.
prostate v.
prostatic v.
renal v.
v. replacement
residual urine v. (RUV)
semen v.
spermatozoon v.
target v.
transition zone v.
urea distribution v.
voided v.
weight-based peritoneal exchange v.
volumetric data
voluminous hiatus hernia
voluntarily stopping eating and drinking
(VSED)
voluntary
v. guarding
v. interruption of pregnancy (VIP)
v. sphincter contraction
volunteer
normal asymptomatic v.
volvulated Meckel diverticulum
volvulus
cecal v.
colonic v.
gastric v.
idiopathic v.
intestinal v.
mesenteroaxial gastric v.
midgut v.
v. neonatorum
nongangrenous sigmoid v.
v. of colon
Onchocerca v.
organoaxial gastric v.

V

volvulus (*continued*)
    v. reduction
    secondary v.
    sigmoid colon v.
vomica
    nux v.
vomit
    Barcoo v.
    bilious v.
    black v.
    coffee-grounds v.
vomiting, vomition
    bilious v.
    v. center
    chemotherapy-induced v.
    concealed v.
    cyclic v.
    diarrhea and v. (D&V)
    dry v.
    epidemic v.
    episodic v.
    erotic v.
    explosive v.
    fecal v.
    hysterical v.
    intractable v.
    ipecac-induced v.
    nausea and v. (N&V)
    nervous v.
    periodic v.
    perioperative v.
    pernicious v.
    persistent v.
    postoperative v.
    postprandial v.
    posttussive v.
    profuse v.
    projectile v.
    psychogenic v.
    recurrent bouts of v.
    retention v.
    Rhodes Inventory of Nausea and V.
    self-induced v.
    stercoraceous v.
    surreptitious v.
    winter v.
vomition (*var. of* vomiting)
vomitive (*var. of* vomitory)
vomito negro
vomitory, vomitive
vomiturition (*var. of* retching)
vomitus
    Barcoo v.
    bile-stained v.
    black v.
    bloody v.
    bright red v.
    coffee-grounds v.

    v. cruentes
    feculent v.
    v. marinus
    v. matutinus
    v. niger
    nonbilious v.
    stercoraceous v.
von
    v. Ebner gland
    v. Gierke disease
    v. Haberer-Finney anastomosis
    v. Hansemann cell
    v. Hippel-Lindau (VHL)
    v. Hippel-Lindau cerebellar hemangioblastomatosis
    v. Hippel-Lindau disease
    v. Hippel-Lindau gene
    v. Hippel-Lindau syndrome (vHL)
    v. Jaksch test
    v. Kossa stain
    v. Kupffer cell
    v. Mering reflex
    v. Meyenburg complex (VMC)
    v. Petz clamp
    v. Petz suture clip
    v. Petz suturing apparatus
    v. Recklinghausen disease
    v. Recklinghausen gastric neurofibroma
    v. Recklinghausen neurofibromatosis
    v. Recklinghausen tumor
    v. Rokitansky disease
    v. Willebrand disease
    v. Willebrand factor
voracious appetite
voriconazole
Voronoff operation
V&P
    vagotomy and pyloroplasty
VP
    ventriculoperitoneal
VP16, VP-16
    etoposide
VPG
    venting percutaneous gastrostomy
VPH
    vaccine-preventable hepatitis
VPI
    velopharyngeal insufficiency
    ventral posteroinferior
      ColoScreen VPI
      VPI nonadhesive open-end pouch
VP4 protein conservation
V8 protease
VP shunt
VQQ technique
VQ technique
VRE
    vancomycin-resistant enterococcus

VRG
vertical ring gastroplasty
VSED
voluntarily stopping eating and drinking
V-shaped ulcer
VSI
Vision Sciences Inc.
V-sign single-ear sensory system
VSL#3 probiotic
VSS
videofluoroscopic swallow study
VSV
vesicular stomatitis virus
VTE
venous thromboembolism
VTR-300 enteral feeding pump
VTU-1 vacuum erection device
VUC
voiding urine cytology
Vulcan syndrome
vulgaris
acne v.
pemphigus v.
Proteus v.
verruca v.
vulgatus
Bacteroides v.
vulnificus
Vibrio v.
vulva, *pl.* **vulvae**
rima v.

vulvae (*pl. of* vulva)
vulval (*var. of* vulvar)
vulvar, vulval
v. carcinoma
v. vestibulitis syndrome
vulvitis
vulvoplasty
vulvorectal fistula
vulvovaginal
v. anus
v. candidiasis (VVC)
vulvovaginoplasty
Williams v.
VUPM
voiding urethral pressure measurement
VUR
vesicoureteral reflux
VVC
vulvovaginal candidiasis
VVF
vesicovaginal fistula
VVF repair
VVM
vertical vesicomyotomy
VX950 protease inhibitor
V-Y
V-Y plasty
V-Y sliding skin graft
Vygon Nutricath S catheter
Vysis UroVysion DNA probe assay
VZV
varicella-zoster virus

V

Wacker Sil-Gel 604 silicone cement
wafer
    w. ash
    Stomahesive skin barrier w.
Waffle bariatric seat cushion
Wagner test
WAGR
    Wilms tumor, aniridia, genitourinary
    abnormalities, and mental retardation
    WAGR syndrome
wait-and-see approach
wake reflex
Waldenström macroglobulinemia
Waldeyer
    W. fascia
    pelvic colon of W.
    W. sheath
Wales rectal bougie
Walker gallbladder retractor
walking stick phenomenon
wall
    abdominal w.
    anterior abdominal w.
    bowel w.
    capillary w.
    colonic w.
    esophageal w.
    gallbladder w.
    gas-forming organism in bowel w.
    glomerular capillary w. (GCW)
    hydrocele w.
    midabdominal w.
    pharyngeal w.
    posterior abdominal w.
    sinusoidal w.
    w. tension
    thickened gallbladder w.
    w. thickening
    variceal w.
Wallace
    W. anastomosis
    W. technique urinary diversion
    W. ureteroileal anastomosis
    technique
Wallstent
    W. covered SEM stent
    W. delivery device
    W. endoprosthesis
    W. esophageal prosthesis
    UroLume W.
Wallstent-I
Walsh
    W. procedure
    W. radical retropubic prostatectomy
    W. surgical modification

Walther
    W. dilator
    W. sound
Waltz endoscopic lithotriptor
wand
    ultrasound w.
wandering
    w. gallbladder
    w. liver
Wangensteen
    W. anastomosis clamp
    W. colostomy
    W. drain
    W. drainage
    W. incision
    W. operation
    W. suction
    W. suction apparatus
    W. suction tube
Wappler
    W. cystoscope with microlens optics
    W. microlens cystourethroscope
warfarin
warfarin-associated subcapsular
  hematoma
warm
    w. ischemia
    w. ischemia time
    w. saline solution
war nephritis
Warren splenorenal shunt
wart
    anal w.
    cervical w.
    exophytic w.
    genital w.
    intraanal w.
    perianal w.
    venereal w.
Warthin-Starry
    W.-S. method
    W.-S. silver stain
wash
    povidone-iodine w.
washer
    Olympus Europe ETD automated
    endoscope w.
washing
    bladder w.
    w. catheter
washout
    w. cannula
    w. factor
    high rectal w.
    mucosal w.

W

washout (*continued*)
    w. pyelography
    seminal tract w.
    w. test
Wassilieff disease
wastage
    pregnancy w.
waste
    w. nitrogen excretion
    nitrogenous w.
wastebasket
    w. diagnosis
    w. pouchitis
wasting
    muscle w.
    renal sodium w.
    w. syndrome
water
    w. avens
    w. balance
    body w.
    w. brash
    w. channel
    contamination of w.
    w. cushion lithotriptor
    w. cystometry
    degassed w.
    w. diuresis
    w. dock
    w. excretion
    fecal contamination of w.
    w. germander
    w. immersion
    insensible loss of w.
    w. loading
    w. permeability
    w. pot perineum
    w. probe
    total body w. (TBW)
watercress
water-displacing balloon
water-filled balloon sheath
water-gurgle test
Waterhouse-Friderichsen syndrome
water-induced thermotherapy (WIT)
water-infusion esophageal manometry catheter
watering-can
    w.-c. perineum
    w.-c. scrotum
water-jet dissection
water-load test
water-losing nephritis
watermelon
    w. cecum
    w. colon
    w. rectum
    w. stomach

water-nutrient test
water-perfused catheter
Waterpik
    endoscopic W.
    W. lavage
water-recovery test
water-restriction test
watershed area
water-sipping test
water-soluble
    w.-s. bilirubin
    w.-s. contrast
    w.-s. contrast enema
    w.-s. contrast esophageal swallow
    w.-s. contrast esophageal swallow test
    w.-s. contrast medium
    w.-s. vitamin
Waterston aorto-to-right-pulmonary artery closure method
water-trap stomach
watery
    w. diarrhea
    w. diarrhea, hypokalemia, and achlorhydria (WDHA)
    w. diarrhea, hypokalemia, and achlorhydria syndrome
    w. diarrhea, hypokalemia, and hypovolemia (WDHH)
    w. diarrhea with hypokalemic alkalosis (WDHA)
    w. stool
Watson
    W. capsule
    W. capsule biopsy
Watson-Alagille syndrome
Watson-Schwartz test
wattage
Watzki sleeve
Waugh-Clagett
    W.-C. operation
    W.-C. pancreatoduodenostomy
wave
    abdominal fluid w.
    w. analyzer
    clustered w.'s (CW)
    clustered jejunal w.'s
    double-peaked w.
    duodenal pressure w.
    extracorporeal shock w.
    flipped T w.
    fluid w.
    focused shock w.
    mechanical stress w.
    peristaltic w.
    piezoelectric shock w.
    primary peristaltic w.
    propulsive w.

pyloric pressure w.
real focus shock w.
secondary peristaltic w.
shock w. (SW)
simultaneous bilateral extracorporeal
  shock w.'s
slow w.
T w.
virtual focus shock w.

waveform
blend w.
coagulase w.
cut w.
electrical w.
low-pulsatility arterial w.

waveguide
quartz w.

wavelength
wavenumber, wave number
waveshape
Wavicide disinfectant
wax-matrix
w.-m. slow-release form
w.-m. tablet

wax-tipped bougie
3-way
3-w. irrigating catheter
3-w. stopcock

WBC
white blood cell
WBC band
WBC basophil
WBC differential
elevated WBC
WBC immature form
WBC leukocyte
WBC lymphocyte
WBC monocyte
WBC neutrophil

WCE
wireless capsule endoscopy

WDHA
watery diarrhea, hypokalemia, and
  achlorhydria
watery diarrhea with hypokalemic
  alkalosis
WDHA syndrome

WDHH
watery diarrhea, hypokalemia, and
  hypovolemia

weaker immunofluorescence signal
weakness
extremity w.
proximal muscle w.

weaning brash
web
antral w.
duodenal w.

endoscopic resection of antral w.
esophageal w.
hepatic w.
intestinal w.
mucosal w.
postcricoid w.
venous w.

Webb-Balfour abdominal retractor
webbed penis
webbing
penoscrotal w.

Weber-Christian disease
Weck
W. clip
W. high-flow laparoflator

Weck-Cel sponge
weddellite calculus
wedge
W. electrosurgical resection device
W. loop
w. pressure
w. resection

wedged
w. hepatic venous pressure (WHVP)
w. retrograde portography

weed
jewel w.

3-week sulfasalazine syndrome
1-week therapy
weeping willow appearance on venogram
Weerda endoscope
Wegener granulomatosis
Weibel-Palade
W.-P. body
W.-P. granule

Weigert-Meyer
W.-M. law
W.-M. rule

weighing
gravimetric w.

weight
actual w. (AW)
actual body w. (ABW)
body w. (BW)
desirable body w. (DBW)
dry w. (DW)
Femina vaginal w.
w. gain
ideal body w. (IBW)
kidney w.
w. loss
w. loss with hyperphagia
low molecular w. (LMW)
molecular w. (mol wt)
seminal vesicle w.
W. Watchers diet

weight-based peritoneal exchange volume
weighted tip

W

weight-reduction surgery
Weil
    W. disease
    W. syndrome
Weinberg
    W. modification of pyloroplasty
    W. vagotomy retractor
Weinstein syndrome
Weiss reaction
Weitlaner retractor
Welch
    W. Allyn flexible sigmoidoscope
    W. Allyn videocolonoscope
    W. Allyn videoendoscope
    W. Allyn videoendoscopy system
welchii
    Clostridium w.
Welchol
weld
    laser tissue w.
welding
    chromophore-enhanced laser w.
    laser tissue w.
well
    W. operation for rectal prolapse
    quadruplicate w.
well-defined anatomical entry criteria
well-differentiated
    w.-d. adenoma
    w.-d. papillary mesothelioma
Wellferon
well-known virulence factor
well-matched organ
Wells posterior rectopexy
Welt syndrome
Werdnig-Hoffman disease
Wermer syndrome
Wernicke
    W. encephalopathy
    W. syndrome
Wernicke-Korsakoff syndrome
Wesson perineal retractor
Westcott tenotomy scissors
Western
    W. blot
    W. blot analysis
    W. diet
Weston rectal snare
Westphal
    W. gall duct forceps
    W. hemostat
Westphal-Strümpell disease
wet
    w. colostomy
    w. swallow
Wexler retractor
WGTS
    whole-gut transit scintigraphy
Wharton duct

wheal
wheat
    w. amylase inhibitor
    w. gliadin
    w. gluten
    w. starch
Wheeless method
Wheelhouse operation
whewellite calculus
whiff test
Whipple
    W. bacillus
    W. disease
    W. operation
    W. pancreaticoduodenostomy
    W. pancreatic resection
    W. pancreatoduodenectomy
    W. pancreatoduodenostomy
    pylorus-preserving W. (PPW)
    W. radical pancreatoduodenectomy
      procedure
    W. syndrome
    W. triad
    W. triad test
whipplei
    Tropheryma w.
whipworm infection
whistle stent
whistle-tip ureteral catheter
Whitaker
    W. hook
    W. perfusion pressure
    W. pressure-perfusion test
white
    w. anococcygeal line
    w. atrophy
    w. ball sign
    w. bile
    w. blood cell (WBC)
    w. blood cell blast
    w. blood cell cast
    w. blood cell count
    w. blood count differential
    w. daisy
    w. diarrhea
    w. hellebore
    w. light endoscopy
    w. line of Toldt
    w. nipple sign
    W. operation
    w. patch
    w. soft petrolatum
    w. thrombus
    w. willow
Whitehead
    W. deformity
    W. gastritis classification
    W. operation
whitish exudate

Whitmore
  W. bag
  W. classification of prostate cancer
Whitmore-Jewitt prostate cancer classification system
WHO
  World Health Organization
  WHO gastric carcinoma classification
whole
  w. blood
  w. body cooling
  w. crypt mitotic count
whole-blood
  w.-b. clearance
  w.-b. trough level
whole-cell oxygen consumption
whole-grain
  rye w.-g.
whole-gut
  w.-g. irrigation
  w.-g. lavage solution
  w.-g. transit
  w.-g. transit scintigraphy (WGTS)
whole-kidney fractional excretion
WHVP
  wedged hepatic venous pressure
Wickham
  W. retractor
  W. technique
wide
  w. albumin gradient ascites
  w. elliptical anastomosis
  w. pubic diastasis
wide-angled loupe
wide-lumen stapled anastomosis
wide-mouth sac
widening
  mediastinal w.
width
  infundibular w.
  red cell distribution w.
  unfavorable infundibular w.
Wiedemann-Beckwith syndrome
wild
  w. cherry
  w. mint
  w. yam
Wilkie disease
Wilkins-Chalgren agar
Wilkinson abdominal retractor
Willauer thoracic scissors
Williams
  W. intestinal forceps
  W. needle
  W. overtube sleeve
  W. syndrome
  W. varix injection overtube
  W. vulvovaginoplasty

Willis
  antrum of W.
  W. pancreas
  W. pouch
willow
  white w.
Willscher
  W. catheter
  W. tube
Wilms
  W. tumor
  W. tumor angiography
  W. tumor, aniridia, genitourinary abnormalities, and mental retardation (WAGR)
  W. tumor capsule invasion
  W. tumor clear cell sarcoma variant
  W. tumorlet
  W. tumor multilocular cyst variant
  W. tumor recurrence
  W. tumor rhabdomyosarcoma variant
  W. tumor tubuloglomerular pattern
Wilpowr Oral
Wilson
  W. disease
  W. muscle
Wilson-Cook
  W.-C. dilating balloon
  W.-C. double-channel sphincterotome
  W.-C. endoprosthesis
  W.-C. esophageal balloon
  W.-C. feeding tube kit
  W.-C. fine-needle aspiration catheter
  W.-C. French stent
  W.-C. gastric balloon
  W.-C. ligator band
  W.-C. mechanical lithotriptor
  W.-C. modified wire-guided sphincterotome
  W.-C. nasobiliary tube
  W.-C. NJFT-series feeding tube
  W.-C. papillotome
  W.-C. plastic prosthesis
  W.-C. prosthesis introducer
  W.-C. Protector guidewire
  W.-C. Quantum TTC esophageal balloon dilation catheter
  W.-C. 6-shooter
  W.-C. 10-shooter
  W.-C. THSF-series guidewire
  W.-C. Tracer guidewire
Wiltek papillotome
Winckler test
wind
  w. colic
  w. sock appearance
window
  gastric w.
  mesenteric w.

W

window (*continued*)
    w. of Deaver
    peritoneal w.
    zinc selenide w.
windowed esophageal balloon
winged
    w. catheter
    w. steel needle
2-wing Malecot drain
4-wing Malecot drain
wink
    anal w.
    w. reflex
Winkleman procedure
Winslow
    foramen of W.
    W. pancreas
winter
    w. acidosis
    w. gastroenteritis
    W. priapism repair procedure
    W. shunt
    W. shunt for priapism
    w. vomiting
wintergreen
    round-leafed w.
wire
    bypass w.
    cesium-137 w.
    Cope w.
    cutting w.
    diathermy w.
    w. electrode
    Extra Stiff Amplatz w.
    hydrophilic w.
    Ir-192 w.
    J w.
    lead w.
    memory w.
    monofilament snare w.
    needle-knife w.
    nitinol w.
    Pathfinder w.
    protector plus w.
    Roadrunner w.
    safety w.
    w. snare
    stiffening w.
    torque w.
    Tracer ST w.
    trip w.
    ultrastiff w.
wire-guided
    w.-g. balloon-assisted endoscopic biliary stent exchange
    w.-g. cytology
    w.-g. hydrostatic balloon
    w.-g. J tube
    w.-g. metal spiral retrieval device

    w.-g. placement
    w.-g. polyvinyl bougie
    w.-g. sphincterotome
wireless
    w. capsule endoscope
    w. capsule endoscopy (WCE)
    w. M2A videocapsule system
    w. pH monitoring
wire-loop
    w.-l. connector
    w.-l. lesion
Wire-Wrap
wiring
    jaw w.
Wirsung
    canal of W.
    W. dilation
    duct of W.
    W. sphincter
Wirthlin splenorenal clamp
Wisconsin
    W. solution
    University of W. (UW)
Wishbone Omni-Track retractor
Wiskott-Aldrich syndrome
Wistar-Kyoto heart
WIT
    water-induced thermotherapy
witch hazel
withdrawal
    w. of cyclosporine
    steroid w.
Witzel
    W. closure
    W. duodenostomy
    W. enterostomy
    W. enterostomy catheter
    W. feeding jejunostomy tunnel
    W. gastrostomy
    W. jejunostomy
    W. pneumatic dilator
Witz test
Wnt/wingless signaling pathway
Woldman test
Wolf
    W. delivery system
    W. lithotrite
    W. percutaneous universal nephroscope
    W. Piezolith 2300 lithotripsy device
    W. Piezolith lithotriptor
    W. resectoscope
    W. rigid panendoscope
    W. Sonolith lithotriptor
    W. ureteroscope
Wolfe miniscope
Wolff
    duct of W.

W. syringe
W. telescope

wolffi

corpus W.
ductus W.

wolffian

w. duct
w. ductal system

Wolff-Junghans test
Wolf-Henning gastroscope
Wolf-Knittlingen gastroscope
Wolfram syndrome
Wolf-Schindler semiflexible gastroscope
Wolfson

W. gallbladder retractor
W. intestinal clamp

Wolinella
Wolman

W. disease
W. xanthomatosis

Womack portal systemic shunting procedure
Women's Gentle Laxative
Wood

W. lamp
W. operation

wooden

w. belly
w. resonance

Woodward

W. esophagogastroscopy
W. esophagogastrostomy

Wookey skin tube
wool ball
Woolf

W. method
W. test

work

neuromodulation w.

working-port ureteroscope
working sheath
workstation

Dornier MFL 5000 urological w.

World Health Organization (WHO)
worm

bilharzial w.
bladder w.
w. colic
herring w.
kidney w.

wormwood
wort

St. John's w.

wound

anal w.
w. approximation
aseptic w.

w. closure
w. contact dressing
w. dehiscence
w. drainage
w. healing
w. healing disorder
w. hematoma
w. infection
open w.
penetrating w.
renal stab w.
septic w.
stab w.
submucosal w.

woven Dacron tube
W pelvic ileal pouch
W-pouch configuration
wrap

antireflux w.
double gracilis w.
floppy Nissen fundic w.
gamma split-sling w.
gastric fundus w.
Kerlix w.
Nissen fundoplication w.
rectus fascial w.
single gamma w.
slipped fundoplication w.
total gastric w.
tunica vaginalis blanket w.

wrapping

fat w.
omental w.

Wright

W. stain
W. stain of stool

Wright-Giemsa stain
writer

laser w.

W-shaped

W-s. forceps
W-s. ileal pouch-anal anastomosis
W-s. pouch

W-stapled

W-s. ileal neobladder
W-s. urinary reservoir

WTI **gene**
Wuchereria bancrofti
Wurbs-type nasobiliary tube
WuScope system
Wyamine
Wyamycin E, S
Wyanoids Relief Factor
Wylie

W. hypogastric clamp
W. splanchnic retractor

Wymox

W

Xanax
xanthelasma
xanthic calculus
xanthine
  x. calculus
  x. dehydrogenase (XDH)
  x. oxidase
  x. oxidation
  x. oxidoreductase activity
  x. urolithiasis
xanthinuria, xanthiuria, xanthuria
xanthiuria (*var. of* xanthinuria)
xanthogranuloma
  juvenile x.
xanthogranulomatous
  x. cholecystitis
  x. cystitis
  x. pyelonephritis (XGP)
xanthoma
  bladder x.
  x. cell
  gastric x.
  planar x.
  skin x.
  tendon x.
  verruciform x.
xanthomatosis
  biliary hypercholesterolemia x.
  cerebrotendinous x.
  familial hypercholesteremic x.
  gastric x.
  Wolman x.
Xanthomonas maltophilia
xanthuria (*var. of* xanthinuria)
Xatral OD
Xc
  reactance
Xc/R
  reactance and resistance
    Xc/R ratio
XDH
  xanthine dehydrogenase
Xenaderm ointment
Xenical
xenoantigen
xenobiotic
  x. absorption
  x. glutathione conjugate
  x. pump
xenograft
  x. rejection
  x. sling procedure
  x. transplant
xenon
  x. lamp

  x. light source
  x. washout technique
xenopi
  Mycobacterium x.
xenoreactive antibody
xenotransplantation
Xeroform gauze
xerophthalmia (X)
xerostomia
xerotica
  balanitis x.
XGP
  xanthogranulomatous pyelonephritis
Xifaxan
Xillix LIFE-Lung system
xiphisternum
xiphoid appendix
xiphoid-to-pubis midline abdominal
  incision
xiphoid-to-umbilicus incision
XL
  extended release
    Ash Split Cath XL
    Ditropan XL
    Flomaxtra XL
    Procardia XL
XL1-blue cell
X-linked
  X-l. Alport syndrome
  X-l. chronic granulomatous disease
    (X-CGD)
  X-l. hypophosphatemia
  X-l. infantile agammaglobulinemia
  X-l. recessive NDI
  X-l. recessive nephrolithiasis
    (XRN)
  X-l. recessive trait
XL784 renal damage marker
Xpeedior catheter
X-Prep
  X-P. bowel preparation
  Senokot X-P.
XQ videoinstrument
XR
  extended release
    Cipro XR
    Pyridorin XR
x-ray
  x-r. analysis
  x-r. crystallography
  x-r. diffractometry
  x-r. photoelectron spectroscopy
XRN
  X-linked recessive nephrolithiasis
Xtrax DNA commercial extraction kit

X

XX male syndrome
xylene
Xylocaine
 X. jelly
 topical X.
 X. topical anesthetic

xylometazoline
xylose
 x. absorption test
 x. tolerance test
Xyotax
XYY male syndrome

Y
Y adapter
YAG
yttrium-aluminum-garnet
YAG 1064
YAG laser
Laserscope YAG 1064
YAG laser therapy
yam
wild y.
Yang
Y. needle
Y. polyclonal assay
Y. Pros-Check PSA assay
Y. Pros-Check PSA test
Y. PSA radioimmunoassay
Yang-Monti
Y.-M. conduit
Y.-M. ileovesicostomy
Y.-M. principle
Yangtze Valley fever
Yankauer
Y. esophagoscope
Y. suction tube
yarn-collected specimen
yarrow
Yates correction
Y-connecting tubing
yeast
y. balanitis
brewer's y.
y. overgrowth
y. saccharomyces
y. strain mannan
yeast-recombinant hepatitis B vaccine
Yellolax
yellow
y. atrophy of liver
y. gentian
y. nodule
y. phosphorus hepatotoxicity
Yeoman rectal biopsy forceps
Yeoman-Wittner rectal forceps
yerba santa
Yersinia
Y. enteritis
Y. enterocolitica
Y. enterocolitica colitis
Y. frederiksenii
Y. intermedia
Y. kristensenii
Y. pestis
Y. pseudotuberculosis
yersiniosis

yield
diagnostic y.
sperm y.
Yocon
yoghurt (*var. of* yogurt)
yogurt, yoghurt
Activia y.
Trial Using Medicinal Microbiotic Y. (TUMMY)
yohimbine hydrochloride
Yohimex
yokogawai
Metagonimus y.
yolk
y. sac
y. sac carcinoma
y. sac tumor
York-Mason repair of postoperative rectoprostatic-urethral fistula procedure
Yoshi-864 antineoplastic alkylating agent
Young
Y. cystoscope
Y. enucleator
Y. epispadias repair
Y. intestinal forceps
Y. needle holder
Y. operation
Y. prostatic retractor
Y. prostatic tractor
Y. syndrome
Y. urinary bladder repair technique
Young-Dees
Y.-D. bladder neck reconstruction
Y.-D. bladder neck repair
Y.-D. bladder neck repair procedure
Y.-D. genitourinary system technique
Y.-D. suspension
Y.-D. tube
Young-Dees-Leadbetter
Y.-D.-L. bladder neck reconstruction
Y.-D.-L. operation
Youssef syndrome
youth
maturity-onset diabetes of y. (MODY)
Treatment Options for Type 2 Diabetes in Adolescents and Y. (TODAY)
yo-yo weight fluctuation phenomenon
Y-plasty
Foley Y-p.
Schweizer-Foley Y-p.

Y-port connector
Y-set system
Y-shaped incision
yttrium-90 (^{90}Y)
yttrium-aluminum-garnet (YAG)
  y.-a.-g. laser
Y-type Dianeal peritoneal dialysis
  solution

yucca
  Adams Needle y.
Yu-Holtgrewe prostatic retractor
Y-V
  Y-V anoplasty
  Y-V meatotomy
  Y-V plasty
  Y-V sliding skin graft

Z

Z line
Z stent
Z stitch
Z suture
Z test
Z tract
Zachary Cope-DeMartel clamp
zacopride
Zacutex
Zadaxin
zafirlukast
Zagam
Zahn

anomaly of Z.
Z. infarct
zalcitabine
Zamboni fixative
Zanca syndrome
Zanosar
zanoterone
Zantac

Z. EFFERdose
Z. GELdose
Zappacosta test
Zaroxolyn
Za-Stent endoscopic biliary stent
ZE

Zollinger-Ellison
ZE cap
ZE syndrome
zebra

z. body
Z. exchange guidewire
Zebrax
zedoary
Zefazone
Zegerid
Zeiss

Z. Axiophot microscope
Z. fluorescein filter system
Z. IDO3 phase-contrast microscope
Z. morphomate M30
Z. S9 electron microscope
Zellweger syndrome
Zelmac
Zelnorm tablet
Zenapax
Zenith

Z. AAA endovascular graft system
Z. abdominal aortic aneurysm endovascular graft system
Zenker

Z. diverticulum

Z. leiomyoma
Z. pouch
Zeppelin clamp
Zestril
Zeta probe nylon filter
zidovudine
Ziehen-Oppenheim
Ziehl-Neelsen stain
Zieve

Z. syndrome
Z. system
zileuton
Zilver biliary self-expanding stent
Zimmon

Z. biliary stent
Z. papillotome/sphincterotome
zinc

bacitracin z.
z. colic
z. deficiency
z. finger
z. selenide window
zinc-iron regulated transporterlike (ZIRTL)
zinc-requiring enzyme
Ziox ointment
zipper

leucine z.
z. sphincterotomy
Zipser penile clamp
ZIRTL

zinc-iron regulated transporterlike
ZIRTL sequence
Zixoryn
Z-Med catheter
Zocor
Zoladex implant
zoledronic

z. acid
z. acid for injection
Zolicef
Zollinger-Ellison (ZE)

Z.-E. syndrome
Z.-E. tumor
zomepirac
Zometa for injection
zona, *pl.* **zonae**

z. fasciculata
z. glomerulosa
z. hamster egg test
z. pellucida
z. reticularis
zonae (*pl. of* zona)
zonal gastritis

zone
    abdominal z.
    adrenal cortex z.
    anal transitional z. (ATZ)
    border z.
    calcified z.
    claudin-2-positive z.
    cooled antenna z.
    electric z.
    epigastric z.
    hemorrhoidal z.
    high-pressure z.
    hyperemic border z.
    hypogastric papillary z.
    nephrogenic z.
    peripheral z.
    portal z.
    prostate gland peripheral z.
    prostate gland periurethral z.
    prostate gland transition z.
    prostate-specific antigen density of transition z. (PSA-TZ)
    rugae z.
    transformation z.
    transitional z.
    Türck z.
zonisamide
zonula, *pl.* **zonulae**
    z. occludens
zonulae (*pl. of* zonula)
zoom videoendoscopy

Zoon
    balanitis of Z.
    Z. erythroplasia
zoonotic foodborne pathogen
zoospermia
Zorbtive powder for subcu injection
zoster
    herpes z.
Zovirax
Z-plasty anastomosis
Z-stent esophageal endoprosthesis system
Z-type deformity
Zuckerkandl
    organ of Z.
Zuelzer-Ogden
Zyderm
Zyflamend
Zygomycetes
zygomycosis
zygote
Zyloprim
Zymase
zymogen
    z. granule
    laboratory z.
zymogenic cell
zymosan
    opsonized z.
Zypan
ZZ phenotype

Contents: The Appendices

Anatomical Illustrations

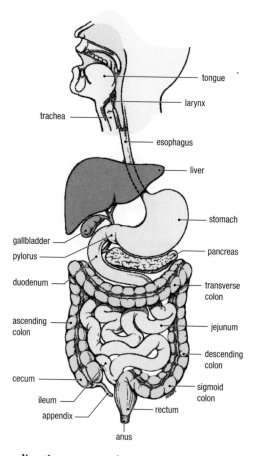

digestive organs and associated structures

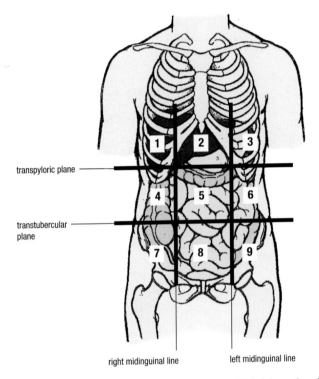

transpyloric plane

transtubercular
plane

right midinguinal line   left midinguinal line

abdominal regions: (1) right hypochondriac; (2) epigastric; (3) left hypochondriac; (4) right
lateral (lumbar); (5) umbilical; (6) left lateral (lumbar); (7) right iliac; (8) hypogastric
(suprapubic); (9) left iliac

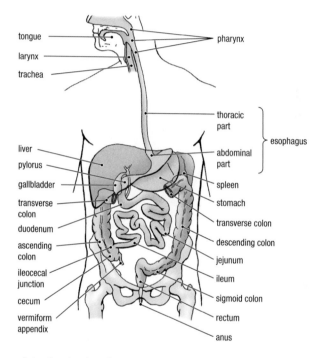

tongue

larynx

trachea

pharynx

thoracic
part

esophagus

liver

pylorus

gallbladder

transverse
colon

duodenum

ascending
colon

ileocecal
junction

cecum

vermiform
appendix

abdominal
part

spleen

stomach

transverse colon

descending colon

jejunum

ileum

sigmoid colon

rectum

anus

small and large intestine in situ: diagrammatic orientation drawing of the digestive system, extending from the lips to the anus

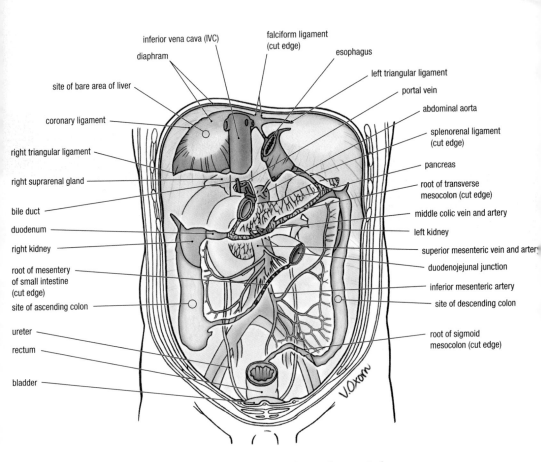

small and large intestine, arteries, and mesenteries

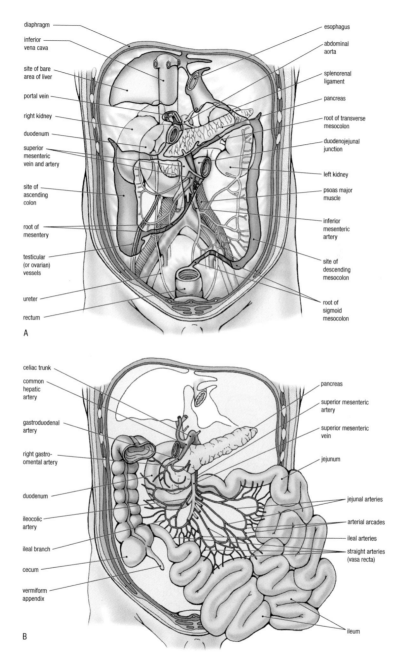

arterial supply and mesentery of the intestine: (A) arterial supply to the large intestine. The roots (cut) of mesocolon of transverse and sigmoid and mesentery of the jejunum and ileum are also illustrated; (B) arterial supply and venous drainage of the small intestine. The superior mesenteric artery (SMA) supplies the jejunoileum, and the superior mesenteric vein (SMV) draws blood from the intestine into the portal vein

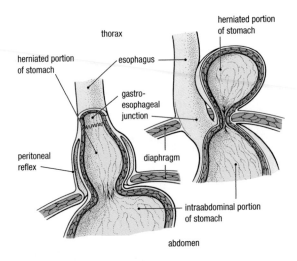

sliding esophageal and paraesophageal hernias: in sliding esophageal hernias (left), the upper stomach and the cardioesophageal junction slide in and out of the thorax; in paraesophageal hernias (right), all or part of the stomach pushes through the diaphragm next to the gastroesophageal junction

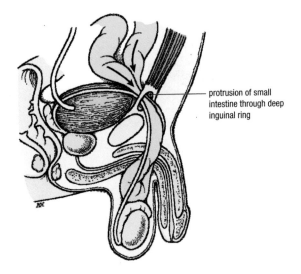

indirect inguinal hernia

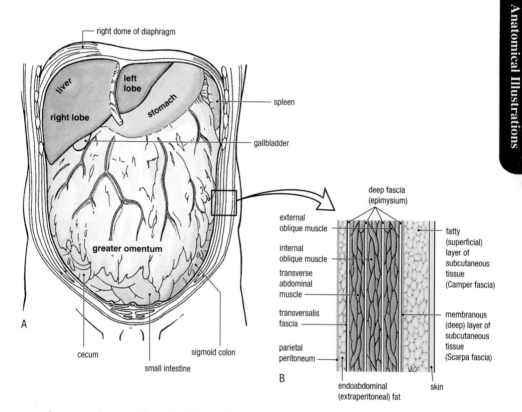

layers of the anterolateral abdominal wall: (A) orientation drawing, anterior view. The anterior abdominal wall is cut away. Most of the intestine is covered by the greater omentum; (B) longitudinal section showing the layers of the inferior part of the wall

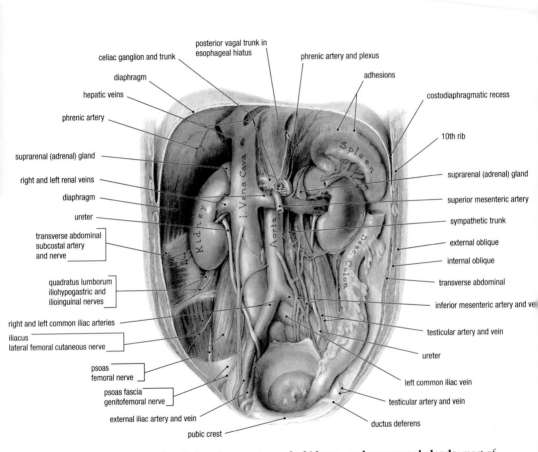

posterior abdominal wall showing great vessels, kidneys, and suprarenal glands: most of the fascia has been removed. The ureter crosses the external iliac artery just beyond the common iliac bifurcation, and the testicular vessels cross anterior to the ureter and join the ductus deferens (vas deferens) to enter the inguinal canal. Note that the renal arteries are not seen because they lie posterior to the renal veins. Note also that the left renal vein is compressed between the aorta posteriorly and the superior mesenteric artery (SMA), which bears the weight of the intestine

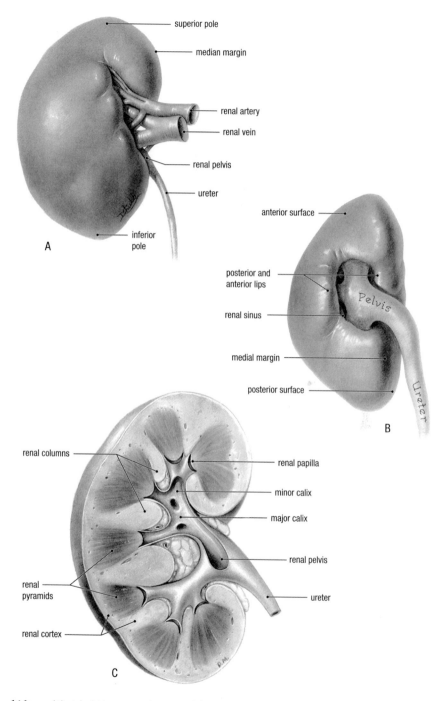

kidney: (A) right kidney, anterior view; (B) sinus of kidney, anteromedial view; (C) kidney, coronal view

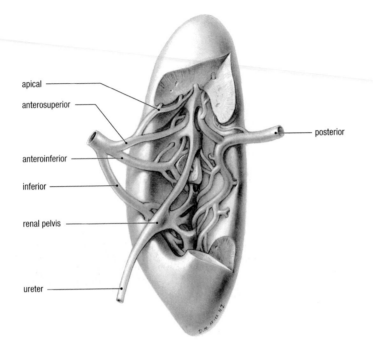

branches of renal artery within renal sinus, medial view

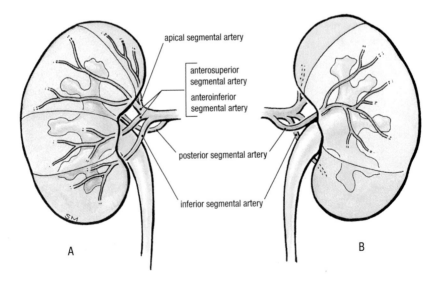

segmental arteries: (A) anterior view; (B) posterior view

A **hemodialysis**

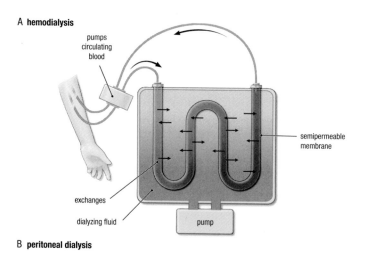

pumps circulating blood

semipermeable membrane

exchanges

dialyzing fluid

pump

B **peritoneal dialysis**

dialysis fluid

peritoneal cavity

blood vessels in peritoneal membrane

C **principles of dialysis**

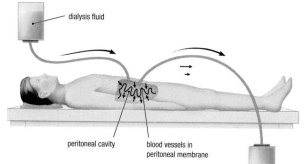

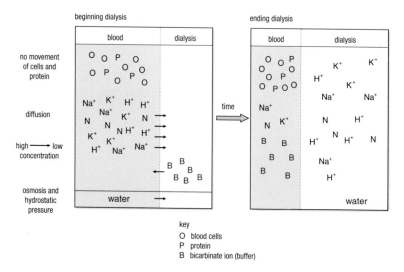

beginning dialysis

ending dialysis

blood | dialysis

no movement of cells and protein

diffusion

high — low concentration

osmosis and hydrostatic pressure

water

time

blood | dialysis

water

key
O blood cells
P protein
B bicarbinate ion (buffer)

dialysis or artificial kidney: (A) hemodialysis; (B) peritoneal dialysis; (C) principles of dialysis

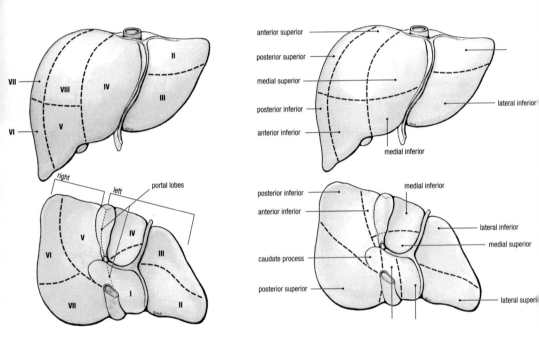

segments of liver: each of the lobes is divided into segments that can be numerically identified, as shown (left)

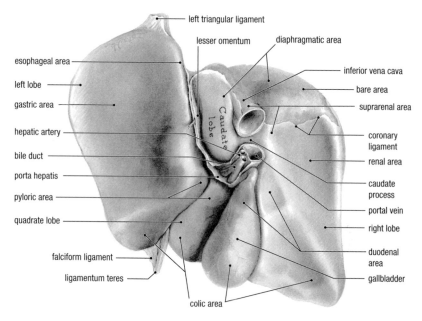

inferior and posterior surfaces of liver

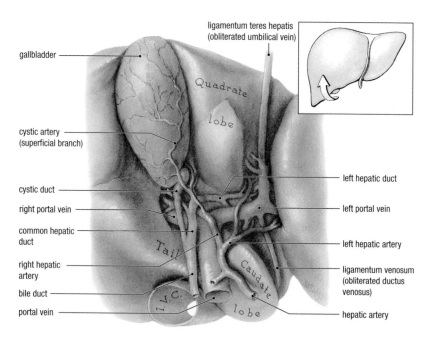

porta hepatic and cystic artery, posterior view

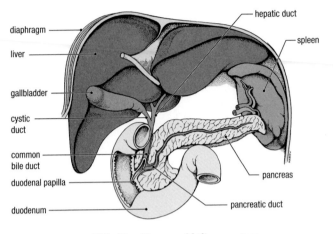

gallbladder, liver, and biliary system

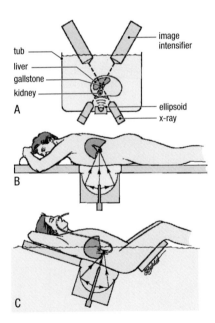

extracorporeal shock wave lithotripsy: (A) gallbladder stone is localized by imaging; shock waves are generated in ellipsoid reflector and transmitted through water to stone; (B) positioning of patient for treatment of stones located in gallbladder; fluid-filled bag is recessed in table and transmits shock waves from generator to patient's skin; (C) positioning of patient for treatment of stones located in common bile duct; the patient is partially submerged in a water bath; nasobiliary tube is used to introduce contrast material to permit visualization and localization of stone and to decompress biliary tree

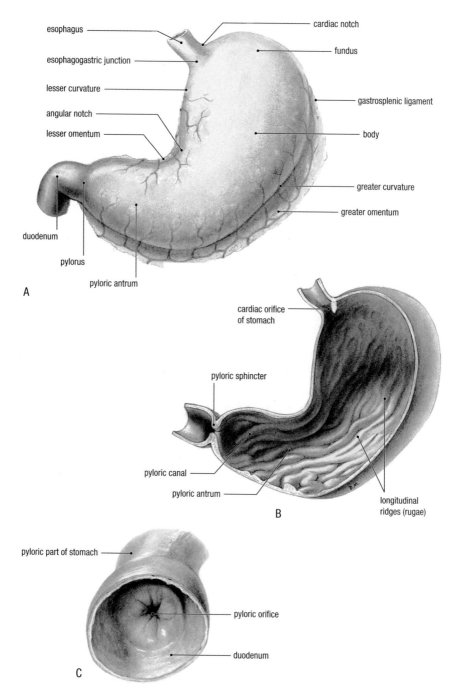

esophagus

esophagogastric junction

lesser curvature

angular notch

lesser omentum

duodenum

pylorus

pyloric antrum

A

cardiac notch

fundus

gastrosplenic ligament

body

greater curvature

greater omentum

cardiac orifice
of stomach

pyloric sphincter

pyloric canal

pyloric antrum

B

longitudinal
ridges (rugae)

pyloric part of stomach

pyloric orifice

duodenum

C

stomach: (A) external surface, anterior view; (B) internal surface (mucous membrane), anterior wall removed; (C) pylorus, viewed from the duodenum

A17

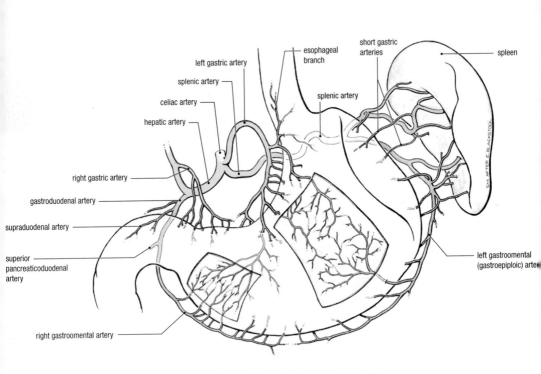

arteries of stomach and spleen, anterior view

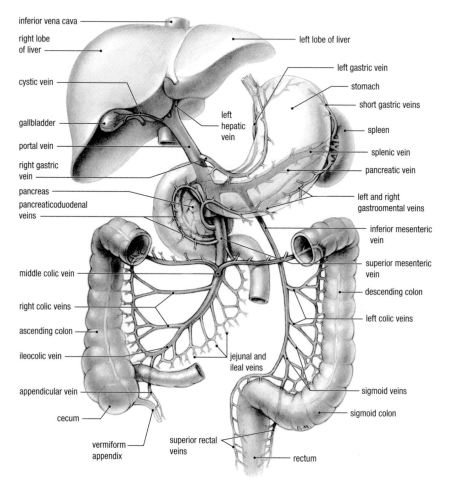

inferior vena cava

right lobe
of liver

left lobe of liver

left gastric vein

cystic vein

stomach

short gastric veins

gallblader

left
hepatic
vein

spleen

portal vein

splenic vein

right gastric
vein

pancreatic vein

pancreas

left and right
gastroomental veins

pancreaticoduodenal
veins

inferior mesenteric
vein

superior mesenteric
vein

middle colic vein

descending colon

right colic veins

left colic veins

ascending colon

ileocolic vein

jejunal and
ileal veins

appendicular vein

sigmoid veins

cecum

sigmoid colon

vermiform
appendix

superior rectal
veins

rectum

portal venous system, anterior view

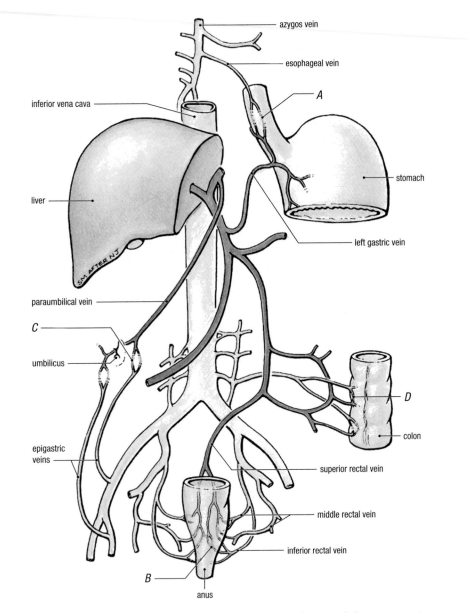

azygos vein

esophageal vein

A

inferior vena cava

stomach

liver

left gastric vein

paraumbilical vein

C

umbilicus

D

colon

epigastric veins

superior rectal vein

middle rectal vein

inferior rectal vein

B

anus

portacaval system, anterior view: portal tributaries are shown in dark gray; systemic tributaries and communicating veins are shown in light gray; sites of anastomosis: *A, B, C,* and *D*

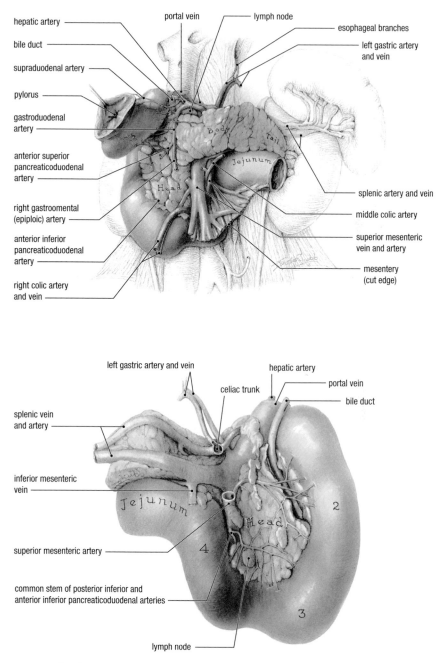

hepatic artery

portal vein

lymph node

esophageal branches

left gastric artery and vein

bile duct

supraduodenal artery

pylorus

gastroduodenal artery

anterior superior pancreaticoduodenal artery

right gastroomental (epiploic) artery

anterior inferior pancreaticoduodenal artery

right colic artery and vein

Body

Tail

Jejunum

Head

splenic artery and vein

middle colic artery

superior mesenteric vein and artery

mesentery (cut edge)

left gastric artery and vein

hepatic artery

celiac trunk

portal vein

bile duct

splenic vein and artery

inferior mesenteric vein

superior mesenteric artery

common stem of posterior inferior and anterior inferior pancreaticoduodenal arteries

lymph node

Jejunum

Head

2

4

3

duodenum and pancreas: anterior view (top); posterior view (bottom)

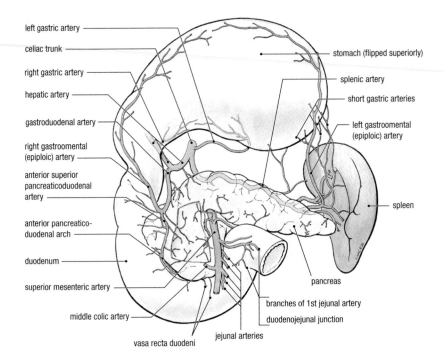

left gastric artery

celiac trunk

right gastric artery

hepatic artery

gastroduodenal artery

right gastroomental (epiploic) artery

anterior superior pancreaticoduodenal artery

anterior pancreatico-duodenal arch

duodenum

superior mesenteric artery

middle colic artery

vasa recta duodeni

jejunal arteries

stomach (flipped superiorly)

splenic artery

short gastric arteries

left gastroomental (epiploic) artery

spleen

pancreas

branches of 1st jejunal artery

duodenojejunal junction

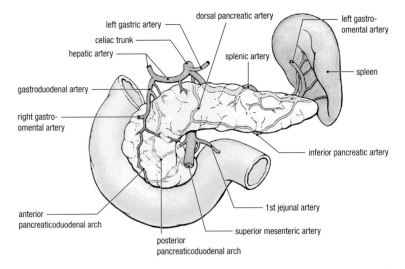

left gastric artery

celiac trunk

hepatic artery

gastroduodenal artery

right gastro-omental artery

anterior pancreaticoduodenal arch

dorsal pancreatic artery

splenic artery

posterior pancreaticoduodenal arch

1st jejunal artery

superior mesenteric artery

left gastro-omental artery

spleen

inferior pancreatic artery

blood supply to the pancreas, duodenum, and spleen, anterior views: celiac trunk and superior mesenteric artery (top); pancreatic and pancreaticoduodenal arteries (bottom)

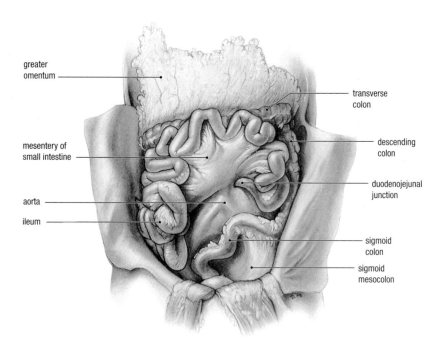

greater omentum

transverse colon

mesentery of small intestine

descending colon

duodenojejunal junction

aorta

ileum

sigmoid colon

sigmoid mesocolon

descending and sigmoid colon and mesentery of small intestine

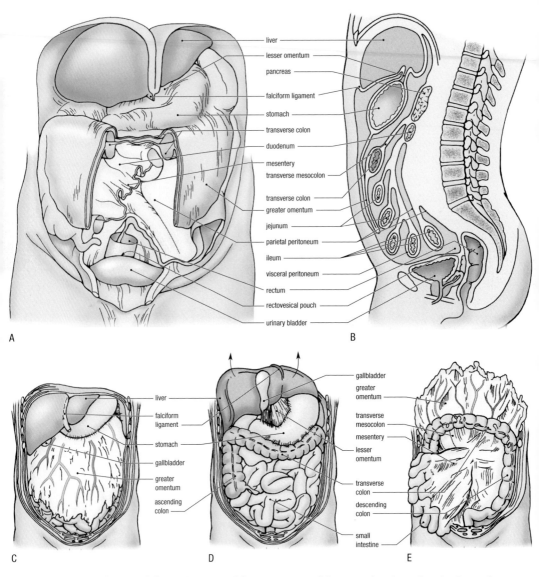

principal parts of the peritoneum: (A) anterior view of the opened peritoneal cavity. Parts of the greater omentum, transverse colon, and small intestine have been cut away to reveal deep structures and the layers of the mesenteric structures. The mesentery of the jejunum and ileum (small intestine) and sigmoid mesocolon have been cut close to their parietal attachments; (B) sagittal section of the abdominopelvic cavity of a male, showing the relationships of the peritoneal attachments; (C) the greater omentum is shown in its "normal" position covering most of the abdominal viscera; (D) the lesser omentum, attaching the liver to the lesser curvature of the stomach, is shown by reflecting the liver and gallbladder superiorly. The greater omentum has been removed from the greater curvature of the stomach to reveal the intestines; (E) the greater omentum has been reflected superiorly and the small intestine has been retracted to the right side to reveal the mesentery of the small intestine

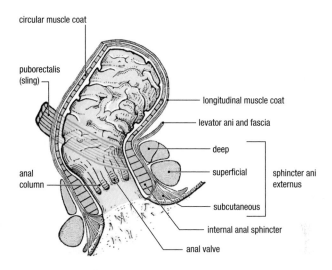

rectum, anal canal, and anal sphincter

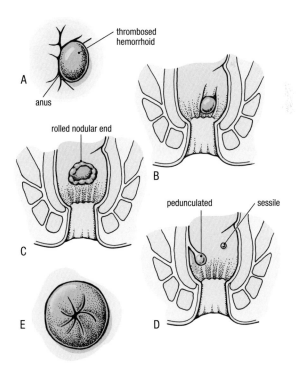

anal and rectal masses: (A) external hemorrhoid; (B) internal hemorrhoid; (C) rectal tumor; (D) rectal polyps; (E) rectal prolapse

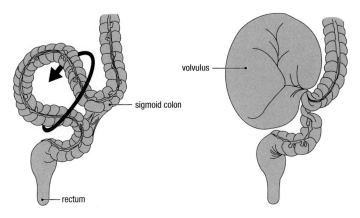

volvulus of sigmoid colon: the unattached loop of bowel twists (left image), causing the bowel lumen to become obstructed (right image), which leads to the inability of stool to pass and compression of the blood supply to the looped bowel segment

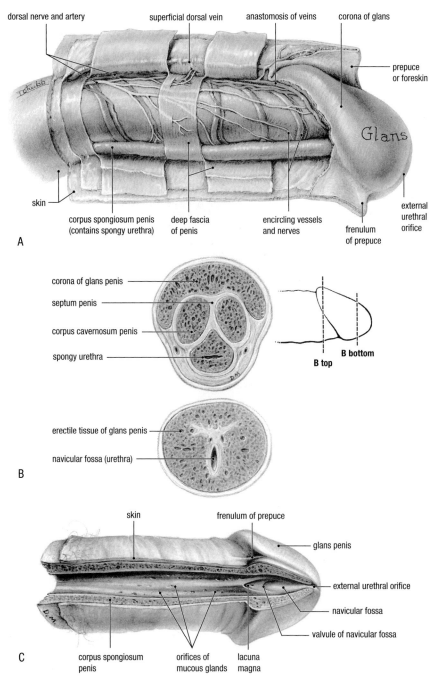

penis: (A) lateral view; (B) transverse sections; (C) spongy urethra, interior

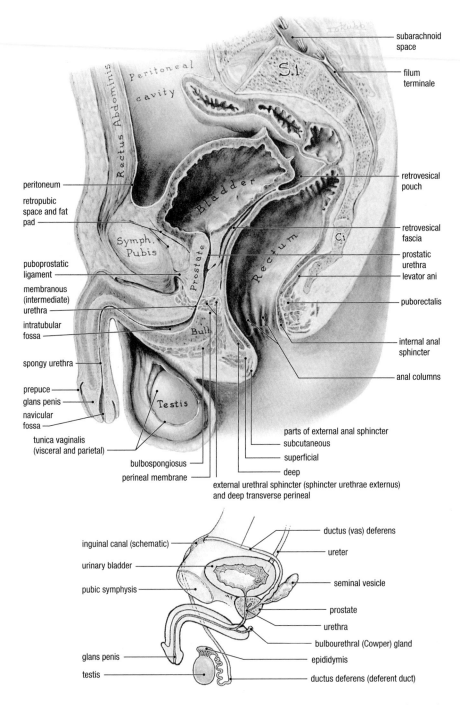

subarachnoid space

filum terminale

retrovesical pouch

retrovesical fascia

prostatic urethra

levator ani

puborectalis

internal anal sphincter

anal columns

peritoneum

retropubic space and fat pad

puboprostatic ligament

membranous (intermediate) urethra

intratubular fossa

spongy urethra

prepuce

glans penis

navicular fossa

tunica vaginalis (visceral and parietal)

bulbospongiosus

perineal membrane

parts of external anal sphincter

subcutaneous

superficial

deep

external urethral sphincter (sphincter urethrae externus) and deep transverse perineal

ductus (vas) deferens

ureter

seminal vesicle

prostate

urethra

bulbourethral (Cowper) gland

epididymis

ductus deferens (deferent duct)

inguinal canal (schematic)

urinary bladder

pubic symphysis

glans penis

testis

male pelvis: median section (top); overview of urogenital system, median section (bottom)

A28

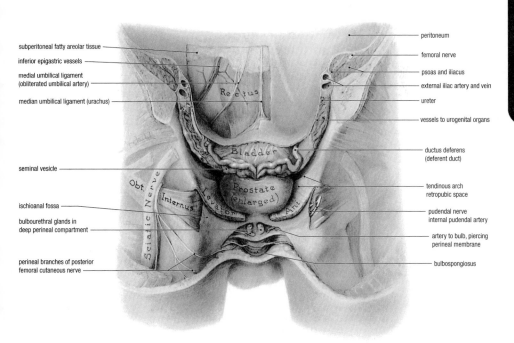

subperitoneal fatty areolar tissue

inferior epigastric vessels

medial umbilical ligament
(obliterated umbilical artery)

median umbilical ligament (urachus)

seminal vesicle

ischioanal fossa

bulbourethral glands in
deep perineal compartment

perineal branches of posterior
femoral cutaneous nerve

peritoneum

femoral nerve

psoas and iliacus

external iliac artery and vein

ureter

vessels to urogenital organs

ductus deferens
(deferent duct)

tendinous arch
retropubic space

pudendal nerve
internal pudendal artery

artery to bulb, piercing
perineal membrane

bulbospongiosus

Rectus

Bladder

Prostate
(enlarged)

Obt.

Internus

Sciatic Nerve

Levator

Ani

male pelvis, view of anterior portion from behind

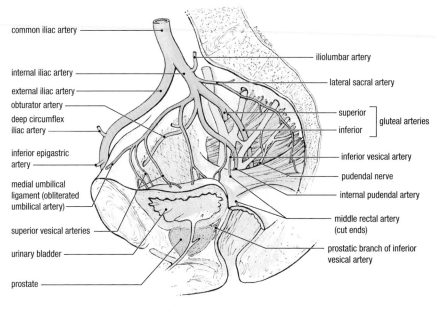

common iliac artery

internal iliac artery

external iliac artery

obturator artery

deep circumflex
iliac artery

inferior epigastric
artery

medial umbilical
ligament (obliterated
umbilical artery)

superior vesical arteries

urinary bladder

prostate

iliolumbar artery

lateral sacral artery

superior
inferior } gluteal arteries

inferior vesical artery

pudendal nerve

internal pudendal artery

middle rectal artery
(cut ends)

prostatic branch of inferior
vesical artery

arteries of the pelvis: male pelvis, median section

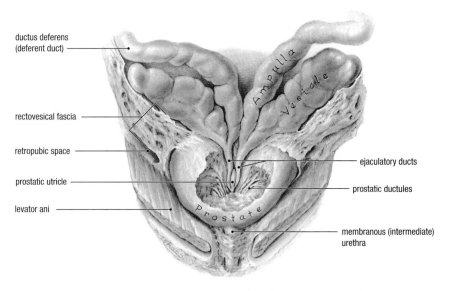

ductus deferens
(deferent duct)

rectovesical fascia

retropubic space

prostatic utricle

levator ani

ejaculatory ducts

prostatic ductules

membranous (intermediate)
urethra

prostate, posterior view

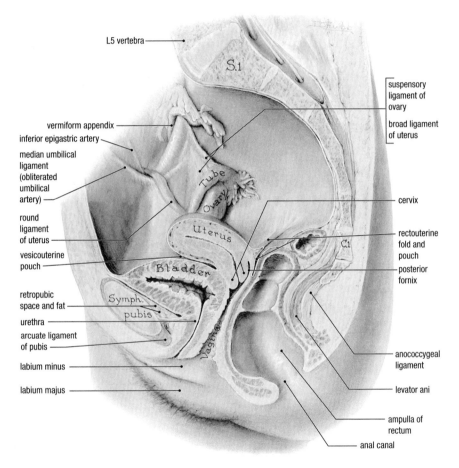

L5 vertebra

S.1

suspensory ligament of ovary

broad ligament of uterus

vermiform appendix

inferior epigastric artery

median umbilical ligament (obliterated umbilical artery)

Tube

Ovary

cervix

round ligament of uterus

Uterus

rectouterine fold and pouch

vesicouterine pouch

C1

posterior fornix

Bladder

retropubic space and fat

Symph. pubis

urethra

arcuate ligament of pubis

Vagina

anococcygeal ligament

labium minus

labium majus

levator ani

ampulla of rectum

anal canal

female pelvis, median section

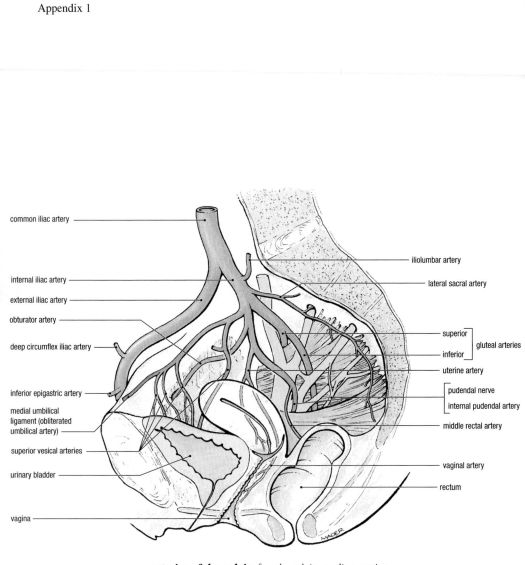

common iliac artery

iliolumbar artery

internal iliac artery

lateral sacral artery

external iliac artery

obturator artery

deep circumflex iliac artery

superior ⎤
         ⎥ gluteal arteries
inferior ⎦

uterine artery

inferior epigastric artery

⎡ pudendal nerve
⎣ internal pudendal artery

medial umbilical
ligament (obliterated
umbilical artery)

middle rectal artery

superior vesical arteries

urinary bladder

vaginal artery

rectum

vagina

MADER

arteries of the pelvis: female pelvis, median section

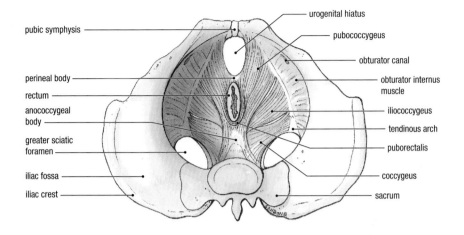

pubic symphysis

urogenital hiatus

pubococcygeus

obturator canal

perineal body

rectum

anococcygeal body

greater sciatic foramen

iliac fossa

iliac crest

obturator internus muscle

iliococcygeus

tendinous arch

puborectalis

coccygeus

sacrum

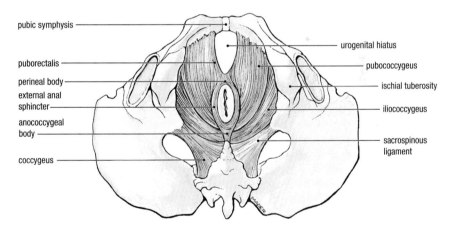

pubic symphysis

puborectalis

perineal body

external anal sphincter

anococcygeal body

coccygeus

urogenital hiatus

pubococcygeus

ischial tuberosity

iliococcygeus

sacrospinous ligament

muscles of pelvic walls and floors: superior view (top) and inferior view (bottom)

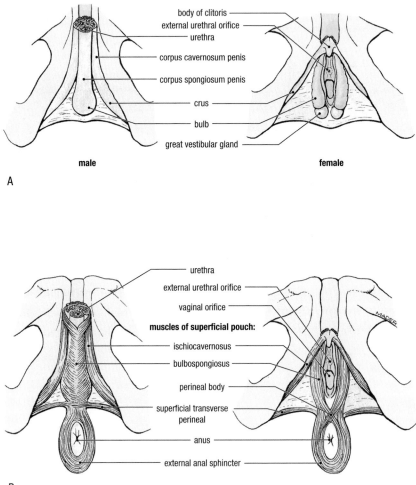

male and female perineum, inferior views: (A) crura and bulb of penis and clitoris; (B) muscles of superficial perineal compartment

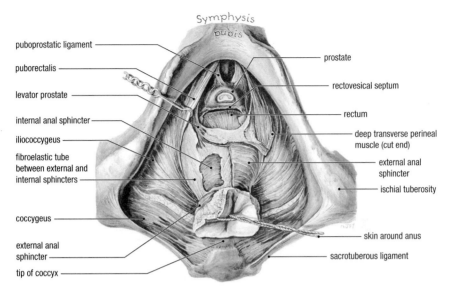

dissection of male perineum: levator ani and coccygeus muscles, and exposure of prostate, inferior view

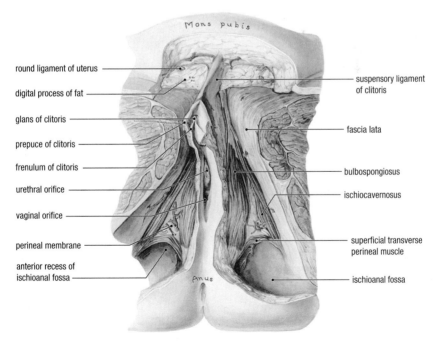

female perineum, inferior view

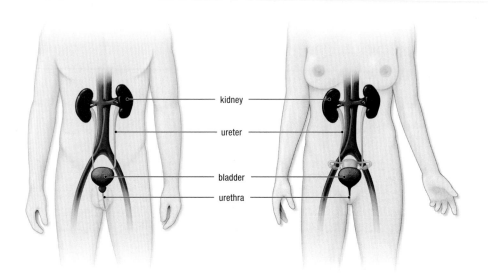

A **anterior view**

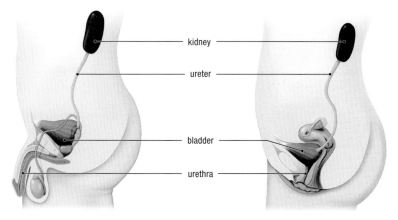

B **lateral view**

components of the urinary system in men and women: (A) anterior view; (B) lateral view

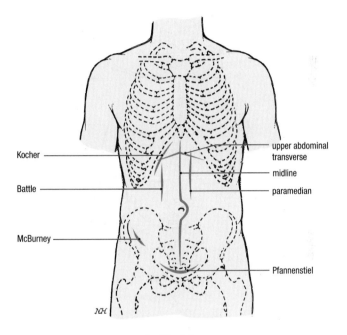

Kocher

Battle

McBurney

upper abdominal transverse

midline

paramedian

Pfannenstiel

surgical incisions

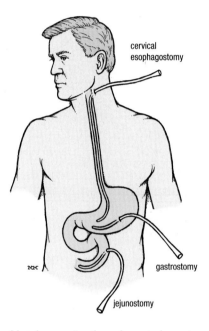

cervical
esophagostomy

gastrostomy

jejunostomy

enterostomy tubes: flexible tubes passing through surgical openings into selected portions of
the gastrointestinal tract, providing access for liquid food

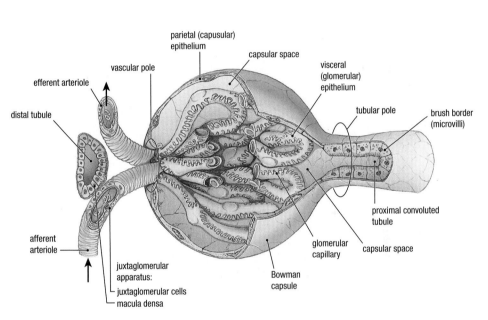

parietal (capusular)
epithelium

capsular space

vascular pole

visceral
(glomerular)
epithelium

efferent arteriole

tubular pole

brush border
(microvilli)

distal tubule

afferent
arteriole

proximal convoluted
tubule

juxtaglomerular
apparatus:

glomerular
capillary

capsular space

juxtaglomerular cells

Bowman
capsule

macula densa

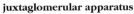

juxtaglomerular apparatus

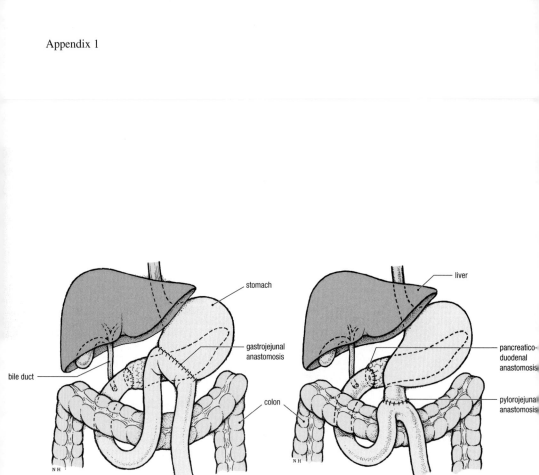

pancreatoduodenectomy: excision of all or part of the pancreas together with the duodenum and usually the distal stomach; Whipple operation (left); pylorus-saving Whipple procedure (right)

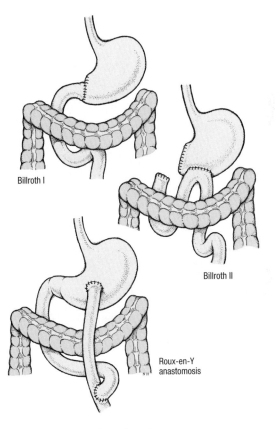

Billroth I

Billroth II

Roux-en-Y
anastomosis

gastroenterostomy

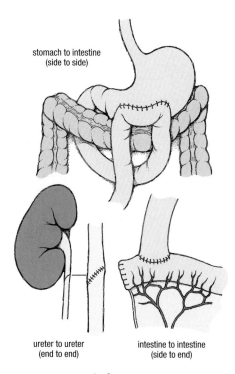

stomach to intestine
(side to side)

ureter to ureter
(end to end)

intestine to intestine
(side to end)

surgical anastomoses

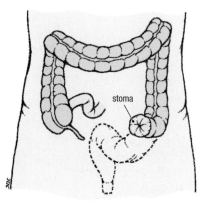

colostomy: stoma opens on anterior abdominal wall

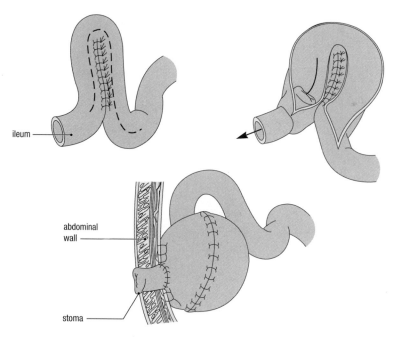

three-part illustration showing section of intestine undergoing procedure for creating a continent ileostomy: bowel segment anastomosed (top); pouch is formed (center); pouch shown in place with stoma (bottom)

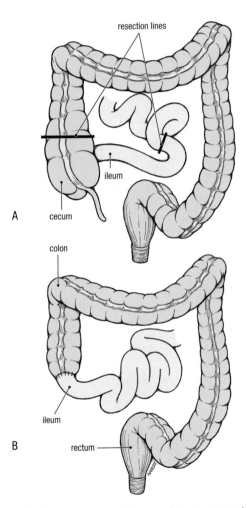

ileocolostomy: (A) diseased portions of ileum and cecum resected; (B) resected ends
anastomosed

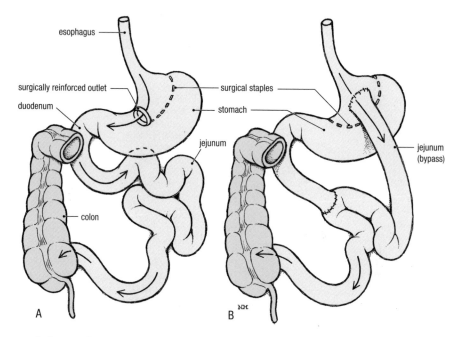

esophagus

surgically reinforced outlet

duodenum

surgical staples

stomach

jejunum

colon

jejunum (bypass)

A

B

surgical procedures to control morbid obesity: (A) vertical banded gastroplasty; (B) gastric bypass (gastrojejunostomy). In both procedures, the reduction in gastric capacity leads to early satiety and, thus, favors consumption of smaller meals

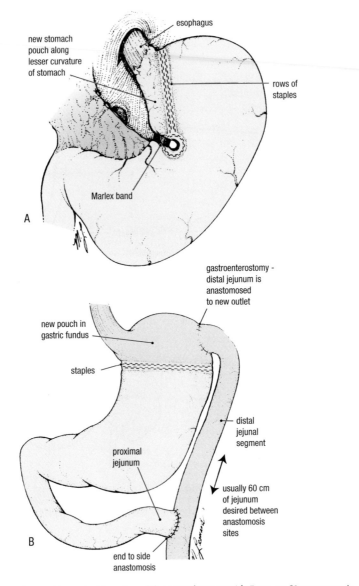

esophagus

new stomach
pouch along
lesser curvature
of stomach

rows of
staples

Marlex band

A

gastroenterostomy -
distal jejunum is
anastomosed
to new outlet

new pouch in
gastric fundus

staples

distal
jejunal
segment

proximal
jejunum

usually 60 cm
of jejunum
desired between
anastomosis
sites

B

end to side
anastomosis

(A) gastroplasty with vertical banding; (B) gastric bypass with Roux-en-Y anastomosis

Normal Lab Values

Tests	Conventional Units	SI Units
albumin		
serum		
adult	3.5–5.2 g/dL	35–52 g/L
urine		
qualitative	negative	negative
quantitative	50–80 mg/24 h.	50–80 mg/24 h.
CSF	10–30 mg/dL	100–300 mg/dL
*bilirubin		
serum		
adult		
conjugated	0.0–0.3 mg/dL	0–5 μmol/L
unconjugated	0.1–1.1 mg/dL	1.7–19 μmol/L
delta	0–0.2 mg/dL	0–3 μmol/L
total	0.2–1.3 mg/L	3–22 μmol/L
neonates		
conjugated	0–0.6 mg/dL	0–10 μmol/L
unconjugated	0.6–10.5 mg/dL	10–180 μmol/L
total	1.5–12 mg/dL	1.7–180 μmol/L
urine, qualitative	negative	negative
calcium, urine		
low calcium diet	50–150 mg/24 h	1.25–3.75 mmol/24 h
usual diet; trough	100–300 mg/24 h	2.50–7.50 mmol/24 h
catecholamines, urine		
dopamine	65–400 μg/24 h	425–2610 nmol/24 h
epinephrine	0–20 μg/24 h	0–109 nmol/24 h
norepinephrine	15–80 μg/24 h	89–473 nmol/24 h
*creatinine clearance, serum or		
plasma and urine		
male	94–140 mL/min/1.73 m^2	0.91–1.35 mL/s/m^2
female	72–110 mL/min/1.73 m^2	0.69–1.06 mL/s/m^2

(continued)

Normal Lab Values

Tests	Conventional Units	SI Units
cyclic AMP		
plasma (EDTA)		
male	4.6–8.6 ng/mL	14–26 nmol/L
female	4.3–7.6 ng/mL	13–23 nmol/L
urine, 24 h	0.3–3.6 mg/d or	100–723 μmol/d or
	0.29–2.1 mg/g creatinine	100–723 μmol/mol creatinine
cystine or cysteine, urine, qualitative	negative	negative
hemoglobin (Hb)		
males	14.0–18.0 g/dL	2.17–2.79 mmol/L
females	12.0–16.0 g/dL	1.86–2.48 mmol/L
newborn	17.0–23.0 g/dL	2.64–3.57 mmol/L
children (varies with age)	11.2–16.5 g/dL	1.74–2.56 mmol/L
hemoglobin, fetal	≥ 1 y old: <2% of total Hb	≥ 1 y old: <0.02% of total Hb
*lipase, serum	23–300 U/L (37°C)	0.39–5.1 μkat/L (37°C)
magnesium		
serum	1.3–2.1 mEq/L	0.65–1.07 mmol/L
	1.6–2.6 mg/dL	16–26 mg/L
pH		
blood, arterial	7.35–7.45	7.35–7.45
urine	4.6–8.0 (depends on diet)	same
phosphorus, urine	0.4–1.3 g/24 h	12.9–42 mmol/24 h
porphobilinogen, urine		
qualitative	negative	negative
quantitative	<2.0 mg/24 h	<9 μmol/24 h
porphyrins, urine		
coproporphyrin	34–230 μg/24 h	52–351 nmol/ 24 h
uroporphyrin	27–52 μg/24 h	32–63 nmol/ 24 h

Tests	Conventional Units	SI Units
potassium		
urine, 24 h	25–125 mmol/d; (depends on diet)	25–125 mmol/d; (depends on diet)
*prostate-specific antigen (PSA), serum		
male	<4.0 ng/mL	<4.0 µg/L
*protein, serum		
total	6.4–8.3 g/dL	64–83 g/L
albumin	3.9–5.1 g/dL	39–51 g/L
globulin		
α_1	0.2–0.4 g/dL	2–4 g/L
α_2	0.4–0.8 g/dL	4–8 g/L
β	0.5–1.0 g/dL	5–10 g/L
γ	0.6–1.3 g/dL	6–13 g/L
urine		
qualitative	negative	negative
quantitative	50–80 mg/24 h (at rest)	50–80 mg/24 h (at rest)
sodium		
urine, 24 h	40–220 mEq/d (depends on diet)	40–220 mmol/d (depends on diet)
urea nitrogen, serum	6–20 mg/dL	2.1–7.1 mmol urea/L
urea nitrogen/creatinine ratio, serum	12:1 to 20:1	48–80 urea/creatinine mole ratio
*uric acid		
serum, enzymatic		
male	4.5–8.0 mg/dL	0.27–0.47 mmol/L
female	2.5–6.2 mg/dL	0.15–0.37 mmol/L
child	2.0–5.5 mg/dL	0.12–0.32 mmol/L
urine	250–750 mg/24 h (with normal diet)	1.48–4.43 mmol/24 h (with normal diet)
urobilinogen, urine	0.1–0.8 EU/2 h 0.5–4.0 EU/d	0.1–0.8 EU/2 h 0.5–4.0 EU/d
vitamin B_{12}, serum	110–800 pg/mL	81–590 pmol/L

*Test values are method dependent.

Appendix 3
Herbs Used to Treat GI & GU Conditions

Herb	Condition
acacia	Mild laxative for occasional constipation.
African plum	Benign prostatic hyperplasia.
alder buckthorn	See *buckthorn bark.*
aloe	Short-term treatment of occasional constipation.
angelica root	Loss of appetite, peptic discomforts such as mild spasms of the gastrointestinal tract, feeling of fullness, and flatulence.
artichoke leaf	Liver dysfunction, bloating, nausea, and impairment of digestion. Also used as a lipid-lowering agent.
asparagus root	Irrigation therapy for inflammatory diseases of the urinary tract and for prevention of kidney stones. Also used as a diuretic and laxative.
Bael tree	Amebic dysentery, diarrhea, intestinal worms, irritable bowel syndrome and inflammatory condition of bowels.
Banyan tree	Nausea, diarrhea and bloody dysentery.
basil	Reduction of gas, resolution of stomach cramps and constipation.
bilberry fruit	Nonspecific, acute diarrhea and local therapy for mild inflammation of the mucous membranes of the mouth and throat.
black elder	Hemorrhoids.
blessed thistle	Loss of appetite, dyspepsia, and for the increase of gastric juice secretion.
Boerhaavia	Urinary tract infections and kidney problems.

Herb	Condition
boldo leaf	Mild dyspepsia and spastic gastrointestinal complaints, gallstones, liver ailments and cystitis.
bottlebrush	See *horsetail*.
box holly	See *butcher's broom*.
brewer's yeast/Hansen CBS 5926	Symptomatic treatment of acute diarrhea. Prophylactic and symptomatic treatment of traveler's diarrhea and diarrhea occurring while tube feeding.
bromelain	In combination with pancreatic extracts of titrated trypsin. Also used as treatment for dyspepsia symptoms and exocrine hepatic insufficiency.
buckthorn bark	Stool softener.
butcher's broom	Itching and burning of hemorrhoids.
camphor	Intestinal worms.
cascara	Stool softener for occasional constipation.
cascara sagrada bark	See *cascara*.
cassia (cassia cinnamon)	See *Chinese cinnamon bark*.
catnip	Used as a tea for treatment of diarrhea.
cayenne	Healing effect on ulcers. Also used in treatment of stomach aches, cramps, gas, indigestion, loss of appetite, and diarrhea.
cranberry	Treatment of urinary tract infection.
ceylon cinnamon	See *cinnamon bark*.
chamomile flower	Used internally for treatment of digestive ailments such as dyspepsia, epigastric bloating, impaired digestion, and flatulence. Used externally for irritation of the mouth and gums, and for hemorrhoids.

(continued)

Herbs Used to Treat GI & GU

Herb	Condition
Chinese cinnamon bark	Loss of appetite, gastrointestinal tract spasm, nausea, diarrhea, bloating, flatulence, colic and dyspepsia.
chittem bark	See *cascara.*
cinnamon bark	Loss of appetite, dyspeptic complaints such as mild spastic conditions of the gastrointestinal tract, bloating and flatulence.
coriander seed/fruit	Dyspeptic complaints and loss of appetite.
couch grass	Cystitis, urethritis, prostatitis, enlarged prostate gland, kidney stones and gravel, and enuresis and nervous incontinence. Healing action on the mucosa of the bladder and associated organs.
cumin	Seeds useful in treatment of abdominal colic, flatulence, intestinal worms, dysentery, diarrhea, indigestion, inflammatory bowel, renal calculus, gonorrhea, obstruction of urine, nausea and vomiting.
dandelion	Loss of appetite, dyspepsia, constipation, cholecystitis, and prevention of renal gravel.
dandelion root	Disturbances in bile flow, stimulation of diuresis, loss of appetite, and dyspepsia.
devil's claw root	Loss of appetite and dyspepsia.
dill weed	Stomach and intestinal spasm, flatulence, and colic. Also used to stimulate appetite and as a diuretic.
echinacea herb/root	Administered orally in supportive therapy for infections of the urinary tract.
fennel oil/seed	Dyspepsia, fullness and flatulence.
fenugreek seed	Anorexia, dyspepsia and gastritis.

Herb	Condition
flaxseed/flax	Chronic constipation, colon damage from laxative abuse, irritable colon and diverticulitis. Mucilage for gastritis and enteritis.
frangula	See *buckthorn bark*.
gentian root	Loss of appetite, fullness and flatulence.
ginger	Prophylaxis of nausea and vomiting associated with motion sickness, postoperative nausea, and seasickness.
goldenrod/European goldenrod	Irrigation therapy for inflammatory diseases of the lower urinary tract, urinary calculi, and kidney gravel. Prophylaxis for urinary calculi and kidney gravel.
goldenseal	Stomach and intestines such as irritable bowel syndrome, colitis, ulcers and gastritis. Also used in elimination of internal parasites.
holy thistle	See *blessed thistle*
horehound/white horehound	Loss of appetite, bloating and flatulence.
horsetail	Inflammation of the lower urinary tract, renal gravel, and urinary and prostatic disease
huckleberry	See *bilberry fruit*.
hydrangea	Inflamed or enlarged prostate, urinary calculus with gravel and cystitis, and acute nephritis.
juniper berry/common juniper	Bladder and kidney conditions.
lemon balm/common balm	Gastrointestinal complaints.
licorice root	Gastric or duodenal ulcers.
linseed	See *flaxseed/flax*.

(continued)

Herbs Used to Treat GI & GU

Herb	Condition
marshmallow root	Used internally for gastroenteritis, peptic and duodenal ulceration, common and ulcerative colitis, and enteritis. Used topically as a mouthwash or gargle for inflammation of the mouth and pharynx.
melissa	See *lemon balm.*
milk thistle fruit/St. Mary's thistle	Chronic inflammatory liver disease and hepatic cirrhosis.
mint oil	Flatulence. Also used in treatment of gastrointestinal and gallbladder disorders.
oak bark	Nonspecific, acute diarrhea and local treatment of mild inflammation of the genital and anal area.
orange peel/bitter orange peel	Loss of appetite, and dyspeptic ailments.
onion	Loss of appetite.
parsley herb/root	Flushing out the urinary tract to prevent and treat kidney gravel. Also used in treatment of dysuria and flatulent dyspepsia.
peppermint leaf	Spastic complaints of the gastrointestinal tract, gallbladder, and bile ducts.
peppermint oil	Spastic discomfort of the upper gastrointestinal and bile duct, and irritable bowel syndrome.
pomelo	Mild laxative for occasional constipation. Also used as a digestive aid, for appetite stimulation, and treatment of abdominal colic, worms, vomiting and nausea
psyllium seed	Bulk-forming laxative used for treatment of chronic and temporary constipation, irritable bowel syndrome, and constipation related to duodenal ulcer or diverticulitis. Also used as a stool softener after anorectal surgery and for patients with hemorrhoids.

Herb	Condition
pumpkin seed	Irritable bladder and micturition problems of benign prostatic hyperplasia stages 1 and 2, functional disorders of the bladder, difficult urination, childhood enuresis nocturna, and irritable bladder. Also used to eliminate tapeworms.
rhubarb root	Short-term treatment of occasional constipation.
rye pollen	Treatment of outflow tract obstruction due to benign prostatic hyperplasia.
sacred bark	See *cascara*.
sage leaf	Dyspeptic symptoms and stomatitis.
saw palmetto berry	Urinary problems in benign prostatic hyperplasia stages 1 and 2. Also used in treatment of testicular atrophy and prostatic enlargement.
senna leaf/fruit	Short-term treatment of occasional constipation.
shave grass	See *horsetail*.
slippery elm	Crohn disease and ulcerative colitis.
South African star grass	Benign prostatic hyperplasia.
sparrow grass	See *asparagus root*.
stinging nettle herb/leaf	Irrigation therapy for inflammatory diseases of the lower urinary tract. Also used in prevention and treatment of kidney gravel.
stone root	Treatment and prevention of stones in the urinary tract and gallbladder. Also used in treatment of intestinal and bowel disease, kidney stones and hemorrhoids.
sweet balm	See *lemon balm*.
sweet flag	Constipation, atonic dyspepsia, flatulence and colic.

(continued)

Herbs Used to Treat GI & GU

Herb	Condition
turmeric root	Treatment of acid, and flatulent or atonic dyspepsia.
uva ursi leaf	Inflammatory disorders of the efferent urinary tract.
wild gentian	See *gentian root.*
witch hazel	External hemorrhoids.
whortleberry	See *bilberry fruit.*
yarrow	Mild spastic discomforts of the gastrointestinal tract.
yellow gentian	See *gentian root.*
yohimbine	Erectile dysfunction.

Sample Reports

BILATERAL VASECTOMY

PREOPERATIVE DIAGNOSIS: Requested vasectomy for family planning.

POSTOPERATIVE DIAGNOSIS: Requested vasectomy for family planning.

PROCEDURE PERFORMED: Bilateral vasectomy.

INDICATIONS: This 44-year-old dentist is absolutely aware of the pros and cons of vasectomy, including the possibility of spontaneous recanalization in 1:1000, formation of antibodies against the sperm and the risk of sperm granuloma in 1:10, and he comes in today for the procedure. He declines having any sedation in preparation for the procedure, as he is scheduled to work this evening, and he is aware of the fact that he could develop a little more swelling and accepts that.

PROCEDURE: Through a single incision close to the median raphe, bilateral vasectomy was carried out using Xylocaine 1% with adrenaline. A portion of the vas from both the right and left side was submitted for histopathology. On the right side, we took a portion of vas from the convoluted end of the vas. The left side was done on the straight portion. The ends were doubly ligated and bent back using 3-0 chromic, and the skin was closed with interrupted 5-0 plain.

The procedure was very well tolerated. He was given a prescription for Tylenol 3 to take on a p.r.n. basis. He was instructed to have a semen sample tested in 3 months' time and to continue using alternative contraception methods until that time. The semen sample should be negative.

CYSTOSCOPY

PREOPERATIVE DIAGNOSIS: Transitional cell tumors of the urinary bladder; last exam 1 year ago.

POSTOPERATIVE DIAGNOSIS: Negative cystoscopy.

SURGERY PERFORMED: Cystoscopy.

INDICATIONS FOR PROCEDURE: The patient is a 75-year-old gentleman. It is now 4 years since his last bladder tumor resection, and he has been asymptomatic. Unfortunately, he still smokes from time-to-time. He is on anticoagulants, and he has been well maintained.

PROCEDURE: Today, in the lithotomy position, he was prepped and draped. His urethra was lubricated, and using a flexible cystoscope we could identify that the urethra was perfectly normal. The prostatic urethra was wide open, and on entering the bladder the mucosa was perfectly stable with the exception of mild trabeculation. No other abnormalities were noted.

Urine was sent for cytology and C&S, and this gentleman will return for followup cystoscopy in 1 year's time. Rectal examination confirmed the prostate capsule to be no more than 10-15 g, benign in consistency. His prostatic urethra was wide open. He left the outpatient department in satisfactory condition and will return in 1 year.

CYSTOSCOPY AND CONSULTATION

PREOPERATIVE DIAGNOSES: Recurrent urinary tract infections that have been particularly troublesome for the last 2 years and history of increased urinary frequency and nocturia for perhaps a longer period of time.

POSTOPERATIVE DIAGNOSES: Severe urethritis and a multitude of inflammatory polyps around the bladder neck, superficial varicose veins in the base of the bladder which could cause significant problems with hematuria, squamous metaplasia in the distal third of the trigone and a significantly diminished functional bladder capacity of 250 mL.

PROCEDURE PERFORMED: Cystoscopy and consultation.

INDICATIONS: The patient is a 34-year-old female who had no urinary tract infections until about 2 years ago. She states at that time she started to have real problems and began taking low-dose antibiotics with suppression of the symptoms. Unfortunately, soon after she stopped the medications, her symptoms returned. She did not want to be on long-term antibiotics, so she decided to take an antibiotic for only 5 days, thinking she could tolerate her bladder problems; however, her bladder symptoms have become increasingly more troublesome. She had a terrible experience after a previous bladder examination, with bleeding and severe pain for 5 days, so she is understandably apprehensive about having her bladder examined again today.

She has had significant problems with dysfunctional bleeding with menstrual cycles, often going 3-4 months between menstrual periods. She needs to take birth control pills, and withdrawal of the pill is what eventually leads to a menstrual period. One suspects the possibility of polycystic ovary syndrome, as she appears to have a body habitus for that condition. She is taking Nexium and hyoscine, and she also has irritable bowel syndrome. She states for the past 2 years she has been under a great deal of stress. Her grandmother had to be relocated to a nursing home, and apparently the patient was her primary caregiver.

On examination the patient has a body mass index close to 45. Her abdomen is soft. There is no visceromegaly, hernias or masses, but she states she experiences intermittent lower abdominal pain and pain in the left lower quadrant.

The perineum is very small, making it difficult to visualize the urethra, but we managed to get a #17 scope into the bladder and collect approximately 5-6 mL of urine, which was a true residual that she had today, and this was sent for C&S. Careful examination of the bladder revealed presence of superficial and quite prominent varicose veins in the floor of the bladder close to the trigone. The ureteral orifices were normal. There was significant squamous metaplasia in the distal urethra and in the trigone, and there was evidence of numerous inflammatory polyps all around the bladder neck. Her functional bladder capacity was diminished to 250 mL, and that is why she has been experiencing urinary frequency, but this has been going on for a lot longer than infections. She has actually been urinating 3 or 4 times per night for the last 10 years, and she is now having some problems with urgency to the point of incontinence. This could certainly be improved with an anticholinergic.

I suspect the patient has an immune incompetence that leads her to have more recurrent infections. The perineum is very tiny. Her hormonal imbalance is also aggravating these problems. Meticulous perineal hygiene is recommended. It is difficult to get a clean-catch urine specimen from this patient. She will require some Flagyl for the next 10 nights to eliminate any possibility of bacterial overgrowth in the vagina that could get into the urethra. The uterus seems to be descended at least to a first-degree prolapse, and I suspect this also has something to do with her body size; however, we did not identify any adnexal masses. There are no abnormalities in the fornices, but the base of the bladder is sensitive to palpation after the bladder has been decompressed. No doubt she will benefit from taking some doxycycline to try to eliminate the inflammatory changes in the urethra, bladder neck and trigone. This should penetrate the biofilm better than most of the antibiotics; however, she most likely will get a yeast overgrowth even though she states she has never had a yeast infection in her life. The Flagyl hopefully will prevent that. We would like her husband to take this medication as well, as mycoplasma or Ureaplasma could be a cofactor in passing this infection back and forth. We will recommend getting a proper gynecological assessment, as she may well have polycystic ovaries, and this could make her more susceptible to infections. She states she is not quite sure if she will ever have any children, and she plans to discuss that with the gynecologist. She may be a candidate for taking Macrobid on days that she has intercourse, as this will prevent bacterial contamination and may eliminate the need for long-term systemic antibiotics. In view of the significant changes in her bladder, she may also benefit from intravesical silver nitrate therapy if symptoms do not improve. The examination was well tolerated, and the patient left the outpatient department in satisfactory condition.

CYSTOSCOPY AND CONSULTATION – 2

PREOPERATIVE DIAGNOSIS: Persistent microscopic hematuria in a gentleman who has mild renal insufficiency and a history of bilateral infections in his knees that required intravenous antibiotics for methicillin-resistant Staphylococcus.

POSTOPERATIVE DIAGNOSIS: Normal knees, no draining sinuses, and no discomfort in his joints. Evidence of congestion in the prostatic urethra with fragile superficial veins in the prostatic fossa resulting in his microhematuria.

INDICATIONS: The patient is a 70-year-old gentleman who has been found to have renal insufficiency. His creatinine is in the neighborhood of 180 mmol/L and has actually been well maintained. He has a history of hypertension for which he has been taking a diuretic as well as Inderal. He has had a lot of problems with his knees, had surgery twice, and he was found to have a methicillin-resistant staphylococcal infection. After receiving intravenous antibiotics for several weeks, this completely resolved, and he has been doing very well. He has had no evidence of recurrent disease. This gentleman unfortunately has atherosclerosis that causes some renal insufficiency, and he has persistent microhematuria. For this reason, he is coming in today for assessment of his lower urinary tract. He seems to have a good sense of humor.

On examination, this is a 70-year-old gentleman who appears his stated age. He wears glasses, multifocals. His abdomen is soft with no visceromegaly, hernias or masses. The extremities reveal surgical scars on both knees from prior knee replacements. The incisions are lateral to the midline on both knees, and apparently this was done electively by the surgeon because of the previous infection the patient had. He has been very lucky in that his knees are functioning remarkably well. There is no evidence of peripheral edema, and the pulses are satisfactory.

PROCEDURE: In the lithotomy position, the patient was prepped and draped. The urethra was lubricated, and under direct vision a #17 Olympus scope was introduced. The distal urethra was normal. The membranous urethra was working well, and the prostatic urethra was only discretely compromised by a trilobar prostatic hypertrophy with a very fragile mucosa that leads to bleeding; I suspect this can be easily corrected by using Avodart. This will decrease the volume of his prostate and also decrease the tendency to bleed from the mucosa of the urothelium. The patient has a normal bladder with mild trabeculation. The rest of the bladder appeared entirely normal.

IMPRESSION: We are very confident that we are dealing with benign microscopic hematuria from turbulent flow in the prostatic urethra. This should improve significantly with Avodart, and he can stay on this medication for an indefinite period of time. I have taken the liberty of giving the patient a prescription for 6 months, and he may have it renewed by his family physician if he is doing well. The patient was also given a prescription for Cipro 250 mg twice a day for the next 10 days to cover the instrumentation of the urinary tract. The exam was well tolerated, and the patient left the outpatient department in satisfactory condition.

CYSTOSCOPY AND CONSULTATION – 3

PREOPERATIVE DIAGNOSIS: Neurogenic bladder with episodes of urinary retention in a gentleman who has been suffering from multiple sclerosis for the last 18 years.

POSTOPERATIVE DIAGNOSIS: Apical prostatic tissue, worse on the left side than the right, completely obstructing the prostatic urethra, and aggravated by constipation and intermittent urinary retention.

OPERATION PERFORMED: Cystoscopy and consultation.

PREAMBLE: The patient is a very pleasant but most unfortunate 64-year-old male who has been troubled with MS for at least 18 years. He has also had a surgical bypass procedure done approximately 5 years ago. He has psoriasis which is managed remarkably well. He also has a significant footdrop in his left foot and ambulates in a wheelchair. He has been on an interferon program for at least 2 years, and it has decreased the rate of recurrence of acute flare-ups of his MS.

On exam today, the patient is a pleasant 64-year-old gentleman who gets around with a wheelchair fairly well and who enjoys a very good sense of humor. He has been having a lot of trouble with urinary retention, and this is occurring every time he develops constipation. He has been doing quite well with his bowels since he started taking antibiotics for a recent episode of pneumonia. Lactulose in the past has not worked very well for him. He has never used a bowel program or bowel routine, as we use in quadriplegics or paraplegics, consisting of a Dulcolax every morning after breakfast and Metamucil on a daily basis. This will be worthwhile trying to see if that can improve his bowel routine.

On examination of his abdomen, he has significant patches of psoriasis around his umbilicus and the right and left upper quadrants. His penis is circumcised, and he has no significant psoriasis in his perineum. The testicles are normally descended, most likely atrophic, and the spermatic cords were normal. The left leg has significant wasting, and there is a surgical scar in the medial aspect of his leg from having had the saphenous vein harvested for bypass surgery. He is wearing a brace on his left foot for a footdrop from his MS.

The patient was placed in the lithotomy position and prepped and draped. The urethra was anesthetized with Xylocaine 2%, and under direct vision we were able to advance the Olympus flexible cystoscope. He had urinated just before the exam, and he states he has been urinating as many as 20 times a day but only very small amounts. We confirmed that he had at least 250 mL residual. His bladder appeared quite trabeculated, confirming he has been obstructed, with complete intraurethral prostatic outlet obstruction by mostly apical prostatic tissue, and more tissue on the left side than on the right. Therefore, if he does not respond to alpha-blocker treatment such as Flomax 1-2 a day, he will be considered a candidate for transurethral resection that will relieve the obstruction, and then the spasticity of the bladder can be treated aggressively with anticholinergics. At the moment, the obstruction is significant enough that the anticholinergics will make his residuals larger and make his problems worse.

Rectal examination is normal, although the sphincter tone is somewhat weak, but the rectum is empty, and his prostatic bed is approximately 20 g in size and benign.

We will continue the patient on his current antibiotic program. We do not want to add or change medications unless the urine culture grows something different, but he did not appear to be infected today. The patient was instructed to take 1-2 Flomax a day, to use a Dulcolax suppository after breakfast every morning and to take Metamucil twice a day. Hopefully, this regimen will significantly improve his bowel and bladder function. However, if significant improvement is not achieved, he will be evaluated for transurethral resection.

CYSTOSCOPY AND EXAMINATION

PREOPERATIVE DIAGNOSES: Urinary frequency and urgency with significant lack of control.

POSTOPERATIVE DIAGNOSES: Evidence of dysfunctional voiding with a diminished functional bladder capacity of 400 mL, and chronic urethrotrigonitis, but we could not demonstrate any evidence of stress incontinence. Possible pelvic mass requiring ultrasound assessment.

SURGERY PERFORMED: Cystoscopy and examination.

INDICATIONS: The patient was admitted to the hospital with a depressive illness and is now much improved. She is scheduled to have breast reduction surgery next week and is excited about that, as her back has been really sore, and the breasts are really getting in her way. She has had persistent urinary problems for several years. In 2000 she had a hysterectomy and since then has had progressive symptoms of urinary frequency as well as what sounds like urinary incontinence. In an attempt to determine the etiology of her symptoms, she comes today for cystoscopy.

PROCEDURE: In the lithotomy position, the patient was prepped and draped. She had urinated about 20 minutes before the examination. A 17 scope was introduced into the bladder. She was found to have approximately 100 mL of urine in the bladder, so it was uncertain if she empties the bladder completely or not. She appeared to have a good closure pressure of the urethra and the bladder neck. There were some inflammatory changes noted in the urethra suggestive of an ascending bacterial infection, and the trigone was covered with squamous metaplasia. The ureteral orifices were normal. The bladder capacity was diminished to 400 mL, and there was an extrinsic pressure mass in the dome of her bladder, which was not the uterus but perhaps the bowel or possibly an adnexal mass. Her bladder was emptied.

On pelvic exam, at the vault of the vagina she appeared to have a fixed mass, just slightly to the left of the midline. This will require assessment with an ultrasound. She will need a transvaginal ultrasound to make sure we do not overlook the possibility of ovarian remnant syndrome. Although she had a hysterectomy with bilateral salpingo-oophorectomy, it is still possible she may have something there. This did not appear to be stool. Her stool has been much better since her hospitalization. She has had a bowel routine. Today we could not demonstrate any evidence of stress incontinence. Her bladder seemed to be emptying reasonably well, and no hypermotility of the bladder neck was observed.

At this time, we think her symptoms will be best managed with medications, and she will be started on Zithromax 250 mg a day for a period of 10 days, use vaginal cream for 10 nights and switch the Detrol to Bentyl 10-20 mg 4 times a day if needed. Hopefully this will alleviate her symptoms. If long-term relief is not obtained, further studies will be considered.

GASTRIC BYPASS

PREOPERATIVE DIAGNOSIS: Morbid obesity.

POSTOPERATIVE DIAGNOSIS: Morbid obesity.

PROCEDURE PERFORMED: Gastric bypass.

INDICATIONS: The patient is a morbidly obese woman who has undergone a successful preoperative workup and appropriate counseling in preparation for bariatric surgery.

FINDINGS: The patient has a few adhesions from previous pelvic surgery. She also has a bit of an abnormal abdominal wall, in that she previously had an abdominoplasty including what looked like plication of the linea alba.

DESCRIPTION OF PROCEDURE: With the patient under general endotracheal anesthesia and prepped and draped in the usual manner, a vertical midline xiphoid-to-umbilicus incision was made.

The abdomen was explored, and the adhesions inside the abdomen were taken down with careful blunt and sharp dissection. The bare area along the lesser omentum was opened, and the left side of the GE junction was dissected out to explore the lesser peritoneal sac from the top and from the right side. A 40-mm dilator was passed into the stomach, and the anvil of a Premium curved EEA 31-mm stapler was passed up through the posterior aspect of the lesser sac, through the posterior and anterior gastric walls, and the 2 parts of the stapler joined and fired, 9 cm down from the GE junction. A GIA 100 stapler was then passed alongside the dilator, closed and fired. The dilator was removed, and the lower end of the proximal gastric pouch was then formed by dividing what was left with a GIA 55. The staple lines were oversewn with interrupted figure-of-eight sutures of 3-0 silk.

The Roux-en-Y limbs were then fashioned with an 80 × 80-cm pattern, and enteroenterostomy was fashioned with a GIA 55 stapler and 3-0 PDS. Suture of 3-0 PDS was also used to close the mesenteric defect.

The proximal limb was brought through the mesenteric window created in the transverse mesocolon and was brought up in a retrocolic, retrogastric fashion to lay against the proximal gastric pouch. The inferior staple line was removed from the proximal gastric pouch, and an end-to-side anastomosis was done on the anterior mesenteric side of the Roux-en-Y loop. PDS 3-0 running sutures were used to effect this anastomosis, and reinforcing stitches were also placed. The mesenteric window at the transverse mesocolon was approximated with 3-0 silk, and the abdomen was sponge cleaned. The fascia was closed with running #2 Prolene, and the skin was closed with staples after irrigating the subcutaneous tissue.

The patient tolerated the procedure well, and there were no complications. All counts were correct.

GASTROSCOPY

PREOPERATIVE DIAGNOSIS: Previous marginal ulcer.

POSTOPERATIVE DIAGNOSIS: Awaiting pathology.

SURGERY PERFORMED: Gastroscopy.

INDICATIONS: The patient is a pleasant older gentleman who had a previous gastrojejunostomy for treatment of ulcer disease. He has had a lot of problems with abdominal pain. He has been on Carafate since July when we last gastroscoped him and determined the marginal ulceration. He says he is considerably better at this time.

DESCRIPTION OF PROCEDURE: The patient underwent IV sedation with 5 mg of midazolam, and subsequently was prepped with oropharyngeal benzocaine spray. The flexible gastroscope was inserted into the oropharynx and was advanced under direct vision into the esophagus, stomach and duodenum. Biopsies were taken in the antrum, and the scope was retroflexed before being removed.

FINDINGS: The patient had a normal esophagus down to the squamocolumnar junction at 40 cm from the teeth. There were no hiatal hernias, strictures, varices or neoplasm. The cardia, fundus and body of the stomach appeared normal, but there was a lot of retained food, so the anatomy could not be well defined. The anastomosis was somewhat narrower than it had appeared with the previous endoscopy, but there was no visible ulceration. It was, however, extremely friable.

The patient tolerated the procedure well, and there were no complications. Sponge and instrument counts were correct.

LAPAROTOMY, CREATION OF TRANSVERSE LOOP COLOSTOMY

PREOPERATIVE DIAGNOSIS: Large bowel obstruction.

POSTOPERATIVE DIAGNOSES: Large bowel obstruction secondary to pelvic mass involving sigmoid colon, uterus and possibly left ovary.

OPERATION PERFORMED: Laparotomy with creation of transverse loop colostomy.

INDICATIONS: This is a 58-year-old female who gives a 2-week history of abdominal pain and distention. She has had vague symptoms and was investigated with a CT scan, Gastrografin enema and an attempt at flexible sigmoidoscopy, results of which all gave the suggestion of a rectosigmoid mass; however, the etiology was impossible to identify. At flexible sigmoidoscopy, we were unable to manipulate the scope beyond 25 cm. A discussion of the case was held with my colleague at an outside hospital. Stenting was discussed; however, given the patient's current findings, he felt stent placement would most likely not be successful and recommended proceeding with laparotomy.

PROCEDURE: Informed consent was obtained. The patient had been started on IV antibiotics, Ancef and Flagyl, and an NG tube and Foley catheter were placed. She was given a general anesthetic, intubated and placed supine on the OR table. She had pneumatic compression stockings applied for DVT prophylaxis. She was prepped and draped in the usual fashion.

A skin incision was made from just above the umbilicus down to her lower abdomen with a scalpel. Dissection through the subcutaneous tissue and fascia was done with cautery. The peritoneum was entered sharply. Upon entering the peritoneal cavity, there was a moderate amount of ascites which was sent for cytology.

A laparotomy was performed. She had loops of small bowel that were mildly dilated. Her colon was significantly dilated. Examination of her pelvis revealed a large pelvic mass in her sigmoid colon, adherent to the left sidewall and possibly involving the uterus and left ovary. The mass was very fixed. There was no evidence of peritoneal spread or involvement. Examination of the liver showed no abnormalities. Given the nature of this mass, it was felt we should de-function her and further assess for the best possible treatment. We elected to proceed with a transverse loop colostomy.

A site was created just superior to the umbilicus on the left side, and we created our colostomy site through the rectus muscle bringing out the transverse colon. A transverse colostomy bridge was placed under the colon. We then proceeded with closing the abdominal cavity with a single layer of fascial closure using 1 PDS. The skin was stapled. We then opened the transverse colon with cautery and sutured this in place with interrupted 3-0 PDS. Using suction we were able to decompress a part of the large bowel; however, stool certainly was significantly solid. Tegaderm and colostomy bag were applied.

The patient had minimal blood loss and left the OR for recovery in stable condition. Sponge, needle and instrument counts were reported to be correct.

LEFT GROIN EXPLORATION WITH FEMORAL HERNIA REPAIR

PREOPERATIVE DIAGNOSIS: Recurrent left inguinal hernia.

POSTOPERATIVE DIAGNOSIS: Small left femoral hernia.

OPERATION PERFORMED: Exploration of left groin and left femoral hernia repair with interrupted Prolene sutures.

INDICATIONS: This is a 21-year-old female who presents with a left groin lump with some discomfort. She states it becomes more prominent with heavy lifting. She had bilateral inguinal hernias repaired 15 years ago. On examination she does have a reducible bulge inferior to the inguinal ligament. I have discussed with her that this defect is very small; however, she does wish to proceed with surgery and is aware of the potential risks, including chronic pain and paresthesias as well as recurrence.

PROCEDURE: Informed consent was obtained. The patient was brought to the operating room and given a general anesthetic. She received Ancef 1 g IV on call. She was prepped and draped in the usual manner and placed supine on the OR table.

A skin incision was made in the previous groin incision with a scalpel. Dissection through subcutaneous tissue and scar tissue was performed with cautery. We then opened the external oblique aponeurosis. The round ligament was identified to the internal ring, and there was no evidence of hernia. We then opened the posterior wall after we retracted internal oblique muscles and conjoined tendon. This revealed a very small defect at the femoral canal. There was a small amount of preperitoneal fat through this defect. We repaired the femoral canal with interrupted 0 Prolene sutures. Marcaine 0.25%, a total of 20 mL, was infiltrated in this area and also in the pubic tubercle area.

We then proceeded with closing the external oblique aponeurosis with 0 Vicryl using continuous running stitch. Again Marcaine 0.25% with epinephrine was infiltrated. Scarpa fascia was closed with interrupted 2-0 Vicryl, and the skin was closed with 4-0 Monocryl subcuticular sutures with a continuous running stitch. Steri-Strips and an all-in-one dressing were applied.

The patient tolerated the procedure well and left the operating room for recovery in stable condition. Sponge, needle and instrument counts were correct.

RIGHT INDIRECT INGUINAL HERNIA REPAIR WITH PROLENE PLUG AND PATCH

PREOPERATIVE DIAGNOSIS: Right inguinal hernia.

POSTOPERATIVE DIAGNOSIS: Right indirect inguinal hernia.

OPERATION PERFORMED: Repair of right indirect inguinal hernia with medium-sized Prolene plug and patch.

INDICATIONS: The patient is a 35-year-old male who presents with a right inguinal hernia which is increasing in size and causing him discomfort. He is requesting that it be repaired.

PROCEDURE: Informed consent was obtained. The patient was given a general anesthetic, placed supine on the OR table, and prepped and draped in the usual manner. He received Ancef I g IV on call. A skin incision was made in the right lower quadrant with a scalpel. Dissection through the subcutaneous tissue and Scarpa fascia was done with cautery. The external oblique aponeurosis was identified and cleared. We mobilized the spermatic cord at the pubic tubercle, as the external oblique aponeurosis was quite attenuated. The external oblique aponeurosis was opened for a short distance at the lateral side of the external inguinal ring. We identified the ilioinguinal nerve, and this was preserved as much as possible, given there was so much stretching of the external oblique aponeurosis.

A large indirect inguinal hernia sac was identified, and this was separated from the spermatic cord as well as associated lipoma. We opened the hernia sac to ensure that there were no contents. We then performed a high ligation at the internal inguinal ring using 2-0 Vicryl, and the hernia sac was removed. The posterior inguinal wall was very attenuated. The internal inguinal ring was reinforced with a medium-sized Prolene patch, and this was sutured superiorly to conjoined tendon with interrupted 2-0 Prolene and inferiorly to the shelving edge of the inguinal ligament. We then reinforced the posterior wall with a Prolene patch. This was sutured medially to the pubic tubercle, again with 2-0 Prolene, superiorly to conjoined tendon and inferiorly to the shelving edge of the inguinal ligament. We fastened the tails of the Prolene around the spermatic cord, and this was sutured in place. The spermatic cord was returned to its normal anatomical position.

We then closed the external oblique aponeurosis with 2-0 Vicryl. A total of 20 mL of Marcaine 0.25% with epinephrine was infiltrated. Scarpa fascia was closed with interrupted 4-0 Vicryl, and the skin was closed with continuous running 4-0 Vicryl subcuticular stitch. Steri-Strips were applied to the wound, and a sterile dressing was applied.

The patient tolerated the procedure well and left the operating room for recovery in stable condition. Sponge, needle and instrument counts were correct.

TRANSURETHRAL RESECTION OF BLADDER TUMOR

PREOPERATIVE DIAGNOSIS: Renal failure with gross hematuria.

POSTOPERATIVE DIAGNOSIS: Invasive transitional cell carcinoma of bladder.

OPERATION PROPOSED: Cystoscopy and bilateral retrograde pyelograms.

OPERATION PERFORMED: Transurethral resection of bladder tumor.

PROCEDURE: Following general anesthetic, the patient was placed in the lithotomy position, limbs well-padded, and prepped and draped in routine fashion. An indwelling Foley catheter was removed. A 21 scope was passed under direct vision.

FINDINGS: The anterior urethra was normal. The prostate was not obstructing. Within the bladder, however, there was a large exophytic invasive tumor involving the entire trigone, primarily on the left side extending up to about the 2-o'clock position on the left lateral wall. There was a separate tumor on the back wall on the right side of the bladder that was quite sessile.

After ensuring that INR was satisfactory and there was blood available, transurethral resection of the bulk of this tumor was carried out. A large number of fragments were removed, and the tumor was clearly invasive into the detrusor muscle. At the end of the procedure, all fragments were irrigated free, and a 24 three-way irrigating catheter was inserted. With the CBI running, returns were clear.

Rectal examination was performed, again revealing a benign prostate, but above the prostate there was still a residual mass within the bladder suggesting that this is in fact invasive disease and likely the reason that he has obstructed ureters. By the end of the procedure, we were finally able to visualize the left ureteric orifice, having resected it, and hopefully this will drain resulting in stabilization of his creatinine and eliminating the need for further dialysis.

The patient returned to postoperative recovery in satisfactory condition. Sponge, needle and instrument counts were correct.

UMBILICAL HERNIA REPAIR

PREOPERATIVE DIAGNOSIS: Umbilical hernia.

POSTOPERATIVE DIAGNOSIS: Umbilical hernia.

SURGERY PERFORMED: Repair of umbilical hernia with Prolene suture.

INDICATIONS: This is a 21-year-old female who developed an umbilical hernia during her last pregnancy. She has had increasing discomfort from this and is requesting that it be repaired.

PROCEDURE: Informed consent was obtained. Clindamycin 300 mg IV in case mesh was administered, and the patient was prepped and draped in the usual fashion.

A skin incision was made just below the umbilicus with a scalpel. Dissection was performed with cautery down to the fascia. We then proceeded with dissecting around the umbilicus with a snap. The umbilicus was separated from the hernia with cautery.

There was some preperitoneal fat present, and this was reduced. The umbilical defect was less than 0.5 cm and easily approximated with 3 interrupted Prolene sutures. We then cleared the posterior side of the umbilicus and sutured the umbilicus down to the fascia with interrupted 2-0 Vicryl stitch. The skin was closed with 4-0 Vicryl subcuticular stitch. A total of 20 mL of Marcaine 0.25% was infiltrated. Steri-Strips were applied around the wound, followed by application of fluff gauze and Cover-Roll.

The patient tolerated the procedure well and left the operating room for recovery in stable condition. Sponge, needle and instrument counts were correct.

Appendix 5

Common Terms by Procedure

BILATERAL VASECTOMY

3-0 chromic
Adrenaline
antibodies
doubly ligated
granuloma
histopathology
interrupted 5-0 plain
median raphe
recanalization
semen sample
Tylenol 3
vas
Xylocaine

CYSTOSCOPY

bladder mucosa
bladder tumor resection
C&S (culture and sensitivity)
cystoscope
cytology
lithotomy position
prostate capsule
rectal exam
trabeculation
transitional cell tumor
urethra
urinary bladder
urine

CYSTOSCOPY AND CONSULTATION

#17 scope
adnexal mass
antibiotic
anticholinergic
bacterial overgrowth
biofilm
bladder
bladder neck
C&S (culture and sensitivity)
cystoscopy
doxycycline
Flagyl
fornix
functional bladder capacity
hematuria
hernia
incontinence
inflammatory polyp
intravesical silver nitrate
long-term antibiotic
Macrobid
mass
mycoplasma
nocturia
perineal hygiene
perineum
polycystic ovary syndrome
polyp
prolapse
squamous metaplasia
trigone
Ureaplasma
ureteral orifice
urethra
urethritis
urgency
urinary frequency
urinary tract infection
uterus
vagina
varicose vein
visceromegaly
yeast overgrowth

CYSTOSCOPY AND CONSULTATION – 2

#17 Olympus scope
atherosclerosis
Avodart

Cipro
creatinine
diuretic
hernia
hypertension
Inderal
lithotomy position
mass
membranous urethra
methicillin-resistant *Staphylococcus* (MRSA)
microhematuria
microscopic hematuria
mucosa
peripheral edema
prostate
prostatic fossa
prostatic hypertrophy
prostatic urethra
pulse
renal insufficiency
trabeculation
turbulent flow
urethra
urinary tract
urothelium
visceromegaly

CYSTOSCOPY AND CONSULTATION – 3

abdomen
alpha-blocker treatment
anticholinergic
bladder
constipation
cystoscopy
Dulcolax
Flomax
lactulose
lithotomy position
Metamucil
neurogenic bladder
obstruction
Olympus flexible cystoscope

prostatic bed
prostatic outlet obstruction
prostatic urethra
rectal examination
rectum
spasticity
sphincter tone
transurethral resection (TUR)
urethra
urinary retention
urine culture
Xylocaine

CYSTOSCOPY AND EXAMINATION

17 scope
adnexal mass
bacterial infection
Bentyl
bladder
bladder capacity
bladder neck
bowel
cystoscopy
Detrol
dysfunctional voiding
functional bladder capacity
hypermotility
lithotomy position
mass
ovarian remnant syndrome
squamous metaplasia
stool
stress incontinence
transvaginal ultrasound
trigone
ultrasound
ureteral orifice
urethra
urethrotrigonitis
urgency
urinary frequency
urinary incontinence
urine

Common Terms by Procedure

uterus
vagina
Zithromax

LEFT GROIN EXPLORATION WITH FEMORAL HERNIA REPAIR

2-0 Vicryl
4-0 Monocryl subcuticular suture
all-in-one (AIO) dressing
Ancef
cautery
conjoined tendon
dissection
external oblique aponeurosis
femoral canal
femoral hernia
groin incision
hernia
inguinal hernia
inguinal ligament
internal oblique muscle
Marcaine
preperitoneal fat
Prolene suture
pubic tubercle
round ligament
Scarpa fascia
Steri-Strips
subcutaneous tissue
supine
Vicryl

GASTROSCOPY

abdominal pain
anastomosis
antrum
benzocaine
Carafate
cardia
duodenum
endoscopy
esophagus
flexible gastroscope

fundus
gastrojejunostomy
gastroscopy
hiatal hernia
IV sedation
marginal ulcer
midazolam
neoplasm
oropharynx
scope
squamocolumnar junction (SCJ)
stomach
stomach
stricture
ulceration
varices

LAPAROTOMY, CREATION OF TRANSVERSE LOOP COLOSTOMY

1 PDS
3-0 PDS
abdomen
abdominal pain
Ancef
antibiotics
ascites
cautery
colon
colostomy
colostomy bag
colostomy bridge
cytology
dissection
distention
DVT (deep venous thrombosis)
    prophylaxis
fascia
Flagyl
flexible sigmoidoscopy
Foley catheter
Gastrografin enema
laparotomy

large bowel
large bowel obstruction
liver
mass
NG (nasogastric) tube
ovary
peritoneal
peritoneal cavity
peritoneum
pneumatic compression stockings
rectosigmoid
rectus muscle
sidewall
sigmoid colon
stool
subcutaneous tissue
Tegaderm
transverse colon
transverse loop
umbilicus
uterus

RIGHT INDIRECT INGUINAL HERNIA REPAIR WITH PROLENE PLUG AND PATCH

2-0 Prolene
2-0 Vicryl
4-0 Vicryl
Ancef
anesthetic
Cautery
conjoined tendon
dissection
external inguinal ring
external oblique aponeurosis
hernia sac
high ligation
ilioinguinal nerve
indirect inguinal hernia
inguinal hernia
inguinal ligament
internal inguinal ring

lipoma
Marcaine
patch
Prolene patch
Prolene plug
pubic tubercle
Scarpa fascia
spermatic cord
sterile dressing
Steri-Strips
supine

TRANSURETHRAL RESECTION OF BLADDER TUMOR

21 scope
bladder
CBI (continuous bladder irrigation)
creatinine
cystoscopy
detrusor muscle
dialysis
exophytic
Foley catheter
gross hematuria
lithotomy position
prostate
renal failure
retrograde pyelogram
sessile
three-way irrigating catheter
transitional cell carcinoma
transurethral resection (TUR)
trigone
tumor
ureter
urethra

UMBILICAL HERNIA REPAIR

2-0 Vicryl
4-0 Vicryl
cautery
Clindamycin

Cover-Roll
dissection
fascia
fluff gauze
Marcaine

preperitoneal fat
Prolene suture
Steri-Strips
umbilical hernia
umbilicus

Appendix 6

Drugs by Indication

ABDOMINAL DISTENTION (POSTOPERATIVE)
Hormone, Posterior Pituitary
Pitressin(R) [US]
Pressyn(R) [Can]
Pressyn(R) AR [Can]
vasopressin

ABETALIPOPROTEINEMIA
Vitamin, Fat Soluble
Alph-E [US-OTC]
Alph-E-Mixed [US-OTC]
Aquasol A(R) [US]
Aquasol E(R) [US-OTC]
Aquavit-E(R) [US-OTC]
d-Alpha-Gems(TM) [US-OTC]
E-Gems(R) [US-OTC]
E-Gems Elite(R) [US-OTC]
E-Gems Plus(R) [US-OTC]
Ester-E(TM) [US-OTC]
Gamma E-Gems(R)
   [US-OTC]
Gamma-E Plus [US-OTC]
High Gamma Vitamin E
   Complete(TM) [US-OTC]
Key-E(R) [US-OTC]
Key-E(R) Kaps [US-OTC]
Palmitate-A(R) [US-OTC]
vitamin A
vitamin E

ACHALASIA
Adrenergic Agonist Agent
Brethine(R) [US]
Bricanyl(R) [Can]
terbutaline
Calcium Channel Blocker
Adalat(R) XL(R) [Can]
Adalat(R) CC [US]
Afeditab(TM) CR [US]

Apo-Nifed(R) [Can]
Apo-Nifed PA(R) [Can]
Nifediac(TM) CC [US]
Nifedical(TM) XL [US]
nifedipine
Novo-Nifedin [Can]
Nu-Nifed [Can]
Procardia(R) [US/Can]
Procardia XL(R) [US]
Vasodilator
Apo-ISDN(R) [Can]
Cedocard(R)-SR [Can]
Coronex(R) [Can]
Dilatrate(R)-SR [US]
Gen-Nitro [Can]
Isochron(TM) [US]
Isordil(R) [US]
isosorbide dinitrate
Minitran(TM) [US/Can]
Nitrek(R) [US]
Nitro-Bid(R) [US]
Nitro-Dur(R) [US/Can]
nitroglycerin
Nitrol(R) [Can]
Nitrolingual(R) [US]
NitroQuick(R) [US]
Nitrostat(R) [US/Can]
NitroTime(R) [US]
Novo-Sorbide [Can]
PMS-Isosorbide [Can]
Rho-Nitro [Can]
Transderm-Nitro(R) [Can]
Trinipatch(R) 0.2 [Can]
Trinipatch(R) 0.4 [Can]
Trinipatch(R) 0.6 [Can]

ACHLORHYDRIA
Gastrointestinal Agent, Miscellaneous
glutamic acid

ALPHA1-ANTITRYPSIN DEFICIENCY (CONGENITAL)

Antitrypsin Deficiency Agent
  alpha1-proteinase inhibitor
  Aralast [US]
  Prolastin(R) [US/Can]
  Zemaira(R) [US]

AMEBIASIS

Amebicide
  Apo-Metronidazole(R) [Can]
  Diodoquin(R) [Can]
  Flagyl(R) [US/Can]
  Flagyl ER(R) [US]
  Flagyl(R) I.V. RTU(TM) [US]
  Florazole(R) ER [Can]
  Humatin(R) [US/Can]
  iodoquinol
  MetroCream(R) [US/Can]
  MetroGel(R) [US/Can]
  MetroGel-Vaginal(R) [US]
  MetroLotion(R) [US]
  metronidazole
  Nidagel(TM) [Can]
  Noritate(R) [US/Can]
  paromomycin
  Trikacide [Can]
  Vandazole(TM) [US]
  Yodoxin(R) [US]
Antibiotic, Miscellaneous
  Apo-Metronidazole(R) [Can]
  Flagyl(R) [US/Can]
  Flagyl ER(R) [US]
  Flagyl(R) I.V. RTU(TM) [US]
  Florazole(R) ER [Can]
  MetroCream(R) [US/Can]
  MetroGel(R) [US/Can]
  MetroGel-Vaginal(R) [US]
  MetroLotion(R) [US]
  metronidazole
  Nidagel(TM) [Can]
  Noritate(R) [US/Can]
  Trikacide [Can]

  Vandazole(TM) [US]
Antiprotozoal
  Apo-Metronidazole(R) [Can]
  Flagyl(R) [US/Can]
  Flagyl ER(R) [US]
  Flagyl(R) I.V. RTU(TM) [US]
  Florazole(R) ER [Can]
  MetroCream(R) [US/Can]
  MetroGel(R) [US/Can]
  MetroGel-Vaginal(R) [US]
  MetroLotion(R) [US]
  metronidazole
  Nidagel(TM) [Can]
  Noritate(R) [US/Can]
  Trikacide [Can]
  Vandazole(TM) [US]

AMMONIACAL URINE

Urinary Acidifying Agent
  K-Phos(R) Original [US]
  potassium acid phosphate

AMMONIA INTOXICATION

Ammonium Detoxicant
  Acilac [Can]
  Apo-Lactulose(R) [Can]
  Constulose(R) [US]
  Enulose(R) [US]
  Generlac [US]
  Kristalose(TM) [US]
  lactulose
  Laxilose [Can]
  PMS-Lactulose [Can]

AMYLOIDOSIS

Mucolytic Agent
  Acetadote(R) [US]
  acetylcysteine
  Acetylcysteine Solution [Can]
  Mucomyst(R) [Can]
  Parvolex(R) [Can]

ANEMIA

Anabolic Steroid
  Anadrol(R) [US]
  oxymetholone

Androgen
  Deca-Durabolin(R) [Can]
  Durabolin(R) [Can]
  nandrolone
Antineoplastic Agent
  cyclophosphamide
  Cytoxan(R) [US/Can]
  Procytox(R) [Can]
Colony-Stimulating Factor
  Aranesp(R) [US/Can]
  darbepoetin alfa
  epoetin alfa
  Epogen(R) [US]
  Eprex(R) [Can]
  Procrit(R) [US]
Electrolyte Supplement, Oral
  Apo-Ferrous Gluconate(R) [Can]
  Apo-Ferrous Sulfate(R) [Can]
  Dexferrum(R) [US]
  Dexiron(TM) [Can]
  Femiron(R) [US-OTC]
  Feosol(R) [US-OTC]
  Feratab(R) [US-OTC]
  Fer-Gen-Sol [US-OTC]
  Fergon(R) [US-OTC]
  Fer-In-Sol(R) [US-OTC/Can]
  Fer-Iron(R) [US-OTC]
  Ferodan(TM) [Can]
  Ferretts [US-OTC]
  Ferrex 150 [US-OTC]
  Ferro-Sequels(R) [US-OTC]
  ferrous fumarate
  ferrous gluconate
  ferrous sulfate
  Hemocyte(R) [US-OTC]
  Hytinic(R) [US-OTC]
  INFeD(R) [US]
  Infufer(R) [Can]
  Ircon(R) [US-OTC]
  iron dextran complex
  Nephro-Fer(R) [US-OTC]
  Niferex(R) [US-OTC]
  Niferex(R) 150 [US-OTC]
  Novo-Ferrogluc [Can]

Nu-Iron(R) 150 [US-OTC]
Palafer(R) [Can]
polysaccharide-iron complex
Slow FE(R) [US-OTC]
Immunosuppressant Agent
  antithymocyte globulin (equine)
  Atgam(R) [US/Can]
  cyclosporine
  Gengraf(R) [US]
  Neoral(R) [US/Can]
  Restasis(R) [US]
  Rhoxal-cyclosporine [Can]
  Sandimmune(R) [US]
  Sandimmune(R) I.V. [Can]
  Sandoz-Cyclosporine [Can]
Iron Salt
  iron sucrose
  Venofer(R) [US/Can]
Recombinant Human Erythropoietin
  Aranesp(R) [US/Can]
  darbepoetin alfa
Vitamin
  Fero-Grad 500(R) [US-OTC]
  ferrous sulfate and ascorbic acid
Vitamin, Water Soluble
  Apo-Folic(R) [Can]
  cyanocobalamin
  folic acid
  Nascobal(R) [US]
  Twelve Resin-K [US]

ANESTHESIA (GENERAL)
Barbiturate
  Brevital(R) [Can]
  Brevital(R) Sodium [US]
  methohexital
General Anesthetic
  Amidate(R) [US/Can]
  Compound 347(TM) [US]
  desflurane
  Diprivan(R) [US/Can]
  enflurane
  Ethrane(R) [US]
  etomidate

Forane(R) [US]
halothane
isoflurane
Ketalar(R) [US/Can]
ketamine
Ketamine Hydrochloride Injection,
USP [Can]
propofol
sevoflurane
Sevorane(TM) [Can]
Suprane(R) [US/Can]
Terrell(TM) [US]
Ultane(R) [US]

ASCARIASIS
Anthelmintic
albendazole
Albenza(R) [US]

ASCITES
Diuretic, Loop
Apo-Furosemide(R) [Can]
bumetanide
Bumex(R) [US/Can]
Burinex(R) [Can]
Demadex(R) [US]
Edecrin(R) [US/Can]
ethacrynic acid
furosemide
Furosemide Injection, USP [Can]
Furosemide Special [Can]
Lasix(R) [US/Can]
Lasix(R) Special [Can]
Novo-Semide [Can]
torsemide
Diuretic, Miscellaneous
Apo-Chlorthalidone(R) [Can]
Apo-Indapamide(R) [Can]
chlorthalidone
Gen-Indapamide [Can]
indapamide
Lozide(R) [Can]
Lozol(R) [US/Can]
metolazone
Mykrox(R) [Can]

Novo-Indapamide [Can]
Nu-Indapamide [Can]
PMS-Indapamide [Can]
Thalitone(R) [US]
Zaroxolyn(R) [US/Can]
Diuretic, Potassium Sparing
Aldactone(R) [US/Can]
Novo-Spiroton [Can]
spironolactone
Diuretic, Thiazide
Apo-Hydro(R) [Can]
Aquatensen(R) [Can]
chlorothiazide
Diuril(R) [US/Can]
Enduron(R) [Can]
hydrochlorothiazide
methyclothiazide
Microzide(TM) [US]
Novo-Hydrazide [Can]
PMS-Hydrochlorothiazide
[Can]

BARTTER SYNDROME
Nonsteroidal Antiinflammatory Drug
(NSAID)
Advil(R) [US-OTC/Can]
Advil(R) Children's [US-OTC]
Advil(R) Infants' [US-OTC]
Advil(R) Junior [US-OTC]
Advil(R) Migraine [US-OTC]
Apo-Ibuprofen(R) [Can]
Apo-Indomethacin(R) [Can]
ElixSure(TM) IB [US-OTC]
Genpril(R) [US-OTC]
Ibu-200 [US-OTC]
ibuprofen
Indocid(R) P.D.A. [Can]
Indocin(R) [US/Can]
Indocin(R) I.V. [US]
Indocin(R) SR [US]
Indo-Lemmon [Can]
indomethacin
Indotec [Can]
I-Prin [US-OTC]

Midol(R) Cramp and Body Aches
[US-OTC]
Motrin(R) [US]
Motrin(R) Children's [US-OTC/Can]
Motrin(R) IB [US-OTC/Can]
Motrin(R) Infants' [US-OTC]
Motrin(R) Junior Strength [US-OTC]
NeoProfen(R)
Novo-Methacin [Can]
Novo-Profen [Can]
Nu-Ibuprofen [Can]
Nu-Indo [Can]
Proprinal [US-OTC]
Rhodacine(R) [Can]
Ultraprin [US-OTC]

BEHÇET SYNDROME

Immunosuppressant Agent
Alti-Azathioprine [Can]
Apo-Azathioprine(R) [Can]
Azasan(R) [US]
azathioprine
cyclosporine
Gen-Azathioprine [Can]
Gengraf(R) [US]
Imuran(R) [US/Can]
Neoral(R) [US/Can]
Novo-Azathioprine [Can]
Restasis(R) [US]
Rhoxal-cyclosporine [Can]
Sandimmune(R) [US]
Sandimmune(R) I.V. [Can]
Sandoz-Cyclosporine [Can]

BENIGN PROSTATIC HYPERPLASIA (BPH)

Alpha-Adrenergic Blocking Agent
alfuzosin
Alti-Doxazosin [Can]
Alti-Terazosin [Can]
Apo-Doxazosin(R) [Can]
Apo-Prazo(R) [Can]
Apo-Terazosin(R) [Can]
Cardura(R) [US]

Cardura-1(TM) [Can]
Cardura-2(TM) [Can]
Cardura-4(TM) [Can]
Cardura(R) XL [US]
doxazosin
Flomax(R) [US/Can]
Flomax(R) CR [Can]
Gen-Doxazosin [Can]
Hytrin(R) [US/Can]
Minipress(R) [US/Can]
Novo-Doxazosin [Can]
Novo-Prazin [Can]
Novo-Terazosin [Can]
Nu-Prazo [Can]
Nu-Terazosin [Can]
PMS-Terazosin [Can]
prazosin
tamsulosin
terazosin
Uroxatral(TM) [US]
Xatral [Can]
Antiandrogen
finasteride
Propecia(R) [US/Can]
Proscar(R) [US/Can]
Antineoplastic Agent, Anthracenedione
Avodart(TM) [US/Can]
dutasteride

BLADDER IRRIGATION

Antibacterial, Topical
acetic acid

BOTULISM

Immune Globulin
BabyBIG(R) [US]
botulism immune globulin
(intravenous-human)

BOWEL CLEANSING

Electrolyte Supplement, Oral
Fleet(R) Accu-Prep(R) [US-OTC]
Fleet Enema(R) [Can]
Fleet(R) Phospho-Soda(R)
[US-OTC]

Fleet(R) Phospho-Soda(R) Oral
    Laxative [Can]
OsmoPrep(TM) [US]
sodium phosphates
Visicol(R) [US]
Laxative
castor oil
Citro-Mag(R) [Can]
Colyte(R) [US/Can]
Fleet(R) Accu-Prep(R) [US-OTC]
Fleet Enema(R) [Can]
Fleet(R) Phospho-Soda(R) [US-OTC]
Fleet(R) Phospho-Soda(R) Oral
    Laxative [Can]
GoLYTELY(R) [US]
Klean-Prep(R) [Can]
magnesium citrate
NuLYTELY(R) [US]
OsmoPrep(TM) [US]
PegLyte(R) [Can]
polyethylene glycol-electrolyte
    solution
Purge(R) [US-OTC]
sodium phosphates
TriLyte(TM) [US]
Visicol(R) [US]
Laxative, Bowel Evacuant
HalfLytely(R) and Bisacodyl [US]
polyethylene glycol-electrolyte
    solution and bisacodyl
Laxative, Stimulant
HalfLytely(R) and Bisacodyl [US]
polyethylene glycol-electrolyte
    solution and bisacodyl

BOWEL STERILIZATION
Aminoglycoside (Antibiotic)
Neo-Fradin(TM) [US]
neomycin
Neo-Rx [US]

BRUCELLOSIS
Antibiotic, Aminoglycoside
    streptomycin
Antitubercular Agent
    streptomycin
Tetracycline Derivative
Adoxa(TM) [US]
Alti-Minocycline [Can]
Apo-Doxy(R) [Can]
Apo-Doxy Tabs(R) [Can]
Apo-Minocycline(R) [Can]
Apo-Tetra(R) [Can]
Declomycin(R) [US/Can]
demeclocycline
Doryx(R) [US]
Doxy-100(R) [US]
Doxycin [Can]
doxycycline
Doxytec [Can]
Dynacin(R) [US]
Gen-Minocycline [Can]
Minocin(R) [US/Can]
minocycline
Monodox(R) [US]
myrac(TM) [US]
Novo-Doxylin [Can]
Novo-Minocycline [Can]
Nu-Doxycycline [Can]
Nu-Tetra [Can]
oxytetracycline
Periostat(R) [US/Can]
Rhoxal-minocycline [Can]
Sandoz-Minocycline [Can]
Solodyn(TM) [US]
Sumycin(R) [US]
Terramycin(R) [Can]
tetracycline
Vibramycin(R) [US]
Vibra-Tabs(R) [US/Can]

CACHEXIA
Antineoplastic Agent
Apo-Megestrol(R) [Can]
Megace(R) [US/Can]
Megace(R) ES [US]
Megace(R) OS [Can]
megestrol
Nu-Megestrol [Can]

CANDIDIASIS
Antifungal Agent, Systemic
  AmBisome(R) [US/Can]
  amphotericin B liposomal
Antifungal/Corticosteroid
  nystatin and triamcinolone
Echinocandin
  anidulafungin
  Eraxis(TM) [US]

CELIAC DISEASE
Antacid
  Alcalak [US-OTC]
  Alka-Mints(R) [US-OTC]
  Apo-Cal(R) [Can]
  Calcarb 600 [US-OTC]
  Calci-Chew(R) [US-OTC]
  Calci-Mix(R) [US-OTC]
  Calcite-500 [Can]
  calcium carbonate
  Cal-Gest [US-OTC]
  Cal-Mint [US-OTC]
  Caltrate(R) [Can]
  Caltrate(R) 600 [US-OTC]
  Caltrate(R) Select [Can]
  Children's Pepto [US-OTC]
  Chooz(R) [US-OTC]
  Florical(R) [US-OTC]
  Maalox(R) Quick Dissolve [US-OTC]
  Mylanta(R) Children's [US-OTC]
  Nephro-Calci(R) [US-OTC]
  Nutralox(R) [US-OTC]
  Os-Cal(R) [Can]
  Os-Cal(R) 500 [US-OTC]
  Oysco 500 [US-OTC]
  Oyst-Cal 500 [US-OTC]
  Rolaids(R) Softchews [US-OTC]
  Titralac(TM) [US-OTC]
  Titralac(TM) Extra Strength
    [US-OTC]
  Tums(R) [US-OTC]
  Tums(R) E-X [US-OTC]
  Tums(R) Extra Strength Sugar Free
    [US-OTC]

Tums(R) Smoothies(TM) [US-OTC]
Tums(R) Ultra [US-OTC]
Electrolyte Supplement, Oral
  Alcalak [US-OTC]
  Alka-Mints(R) [US-OTC]
  Apo-Cal(R) [Can]
  Apo-Ferrous Gluconate(R) [Can]
  Apo-Ferrous Sulfate(R) [Can]
  Calcarb 600 [US-OTC]
  Calci-Chew(R) [US-OTC]
  Calci-Mix(R) [US-OTC]
  Calcite-500 [Can]
  Cal-Citrate(R) 250 [US-OTC]
  calcium carbonate
  calcium citrate
  calcium glubionate
  calcium lactate
  Cal-Gest [US-OTC]
  Cal-Mint [US-OTC]
  Caltrate(R) [Can]
  Caltrate(R) 600 [US-OTC]
  Caltrate(R) Select [Can]
  Children's Pepto [US-OTC]
  Chooz(R) [US-OTC]
  Citracal(R) [US-OTC]
  Femiron(R) [US-OTC]
  Feosol(R) [US-OTC]
  Feratab(R) [US-OTC]
  Fer-Gen-Sol [US-OTC]
  Fergon(R) [US-OTC]
  Fer-In-Sol(R) [US-OTC/Can]
  Fer-Iron(R) [US-OTC]
  Ferodan(TM) [Can]
  Ferretts [US-OTC]
  Ferro-Sequels(R) [US-OTC]
  ferrous fumarate
  ferrous gluconate
  ferrous sulfate
  Florical(R) [US-OTC]
  Hemocyte(R) [US-OTC]
  Ircon(R) [US-OTC]
  Maalox(R) Quick Dissolve [US-OTC]
  Mylanta(R) Children's [US-OTC]
  Nephro-Calci(R) [US-OTC]

Nephro-Fer(R) [US-OTC]
Novo-Ferrogluc [Can]
Nutralox(R) [US-OTC]
Os-Cal(R) [Can]
Os-Cal(R) 500 [US-OTC]
Osteocit(R) [Can]
Oysco 500 [US-OTC]
Oyst-Cal 500 [US-OTC]
Palafer(R) [Can]
Rolaids(R) Softchews [US-OTC]
Slow FE(R) [US-OTC]
Titralac(TM) [US-OTC]
Titralac(TM) Extra Strength
 [US-OTC]
Tums(R) [US-OTC]
Tums(R) E-X [US-OTC]
Tums(R) Extra Strength Sugar Free
 [US-OTC]
Tums(R) Smoothies(TM)
 [US-OTC]
Tums(R) Ultra [US-OTC]
Vitamin
 Fero-Grad 500(R) [US-OTC]
 ferrous sulfate and ascorbic acid
Vitamin, Fat Soluble
 AquaMEPHYTON(R) [Can]
 Konakion [Can]
 Mephyton(R) [US/Can]
 phytonadione

CHOLELITHIASIS

Gallstone Dissolution Agent
 Actigall(R) [US]
 Urso(R) [Can]
 Urso 250(TM) [US]
 ursodiol
 Urso(R) DS [Can]
 Urso Forte(TM) [US]

CHOLESTASIS

Vitamin, Fat Soluble
 AquaMEPHYTON(R) [Can]
 Konakion [Can]
 Mephyton(R) [US/Can]
 phytonadione

CIRRHOSIS

Bile Acid Sequestrant
 cholestyramine resin
 Novo-Cholamine [Can]
 Novo-Cholamine Light [Can]
 PMS-Cholestyramine [Can]
 Prevalite(R) [US]
 Questran(R) [US]
 Questran(R) Light [US]
 Questran(R) Light Sugar Free [Can]
Chelating Agent
 Cuprimine(R) [US/Can]
 Depen(R) [US/Can]
 penicillamine
Immunosuppressant Agent
 Alti-Azathioprine [Can]
 Apo-Azathioprine(R) [Can]
 Azasan(R) [US]
 azathioprine
 Gen-Azathioprine [Can]
 Imuran(R) [US/Can]
 Novo-Azathioprine [Can]
Vitamin D Analog
 Calciferol(TM) [US]
 Drisdol(R) [US/Can]
 ergocalciferol
 Ostoforte(R) [Can]
Vitamin, Fat Soluble
 AquaMEPHYTON(R) [Can]
 Aquasol A(R) [US]
 Konakion [Can]
 Mephyton(R) [US/Can]
 Palmitate-A(R) [US-OTC]
 phytonadione
 vitamin A

COLITIS (ULCERATIVE)

5-Aminosalicylic Acid Derivative
 Alti-Sulfasalazine [Can]
 Asacol(R) [US/Can]
 Asacol(R) 800 [Can]
 Azulfidine(R) [US]
 Azulfidine(R) EN-tabs(R) [US]
 balsalazide

Canasa(TM) [US]
Colazal(R) [US]
Dipentum(R) [US/Can]
mesalamine
Mesasal(R) [Can]
Novo-5 ASA [Can]
olsalazine
Pendo-5 ASA [Can]
Pentasa(R) [US/Can]
Quintasa(R) [Can]
Rowasa(R) [US/Can]
Salazopyrin(R) [Can]
Salazopyrin En-Tabs(R) [Can]
Salofalk(R) [Can]
sulfasalazine
Sulfazine [US]
Sulfazine EC [US]
Antiinflammatory Agent
balsalazide
Colazal(R) [US]

COLONIC EVACUATION
Laxative
Alophen(R) [US-OTC]
Apo-Bisacodyl(R) [Can]
Bisac-Evac(TM) [US-OTC]
bisacodyl
Bisacodyl Uniserts(R) [US-OTC]
Carter's Little Pills(R) [Can]
Correctol(R) Tablets [US-OTC]
Doxidan(R) (reformulation) [US-OTC]
Dulcolax(R) [US-OTC/Can]
Femilax(TM) [US-OTC]
Fleet(R) Bisacodyl Enema [US-OTC]
Fleet(R) Stimulant Laxative [US-OTC]
Gentlax(R) [Can]
Modane Tablets(R) [US-OTC]
Veracolate [US-OTC]

CONDYLOMA ACUMINATUM
Antiviral Agent

interferon alfa-2b and ribavirin
Rebetron(R) [US]
Biological Response Modulator
Alferon(R) N [US/Can]
interferon alfa-2a
interferon alfa-2b
interferon alfa-2b and ribavirin
interferon alfa-n3
Intron(R) A [US/Can]
Rebetron(R) [US]
Roferon-A(R) [US/Can]
Immune Response Modifier
Aldara(TM) [US/Can]
imiquimod
Keratolytic Agent
Condyline(TM) [Can]
Condylox(R) [US]
Podocon-25(R) [US]
Podofilm(R) [Can]
podofilox
podophyllum resin
Wartec(R) [Can]

CONSTIPATION
Ammonium Detoxicant
Acilac [Can]
Apo-Lactulose(R) [Can]
Constulose(R) [US]
Enulose(R) [US]
Generlac [US]
Kristalose(TM) [US]
lactulose
Laxilose [Can]
PMS-Lactulose [Can]
Antacid
Dulcolax(R) Milk of Magnesia [US-OTC]
Mag-Caps [US-OTC]
MagGel(TM) [US-OTC]
magnesium hydroxide
magnesium oxide
Mag-Ox(R) 400 [US-OTC]

Phillips'(R) Milk of Magnesia
[US-OTC]
Uro-Mag(R) [US-OTC]
Gastrointestinal Agent, Miscellaneous
Equalactin(R) [US-OTC]
FiberCon(R) [US-OTC]
Fiber-Lax(R) [US-OTC]
Konsyl(R) Fiber Tablets [US-OTC]
Phillips'(R) Fibercaps [US-OTC]
polycarbophil
Laxative
Acilac [Can]
Alophen(R) [US-OTC]
Apo-Bisacodyl(R) [Can]
Apo-Lactulose(R) [Can]
Bisac-Evac(TM) [US-OTC]
bisacodyl
Bisacodyl Uniserts(R) [US-OTC]
Black Draught Tablets [US-OTC]
Carter's Little Pills(R) [Can]
castor oil
Citrucel(R) [US-OTC]
Citrucel(R) Fiber Shake [US-OTC]
Citrucel(R) Fiber Smoothie
[US-OTC]
Colace(R) Adult/Children
Suppositories [US-OTC]
Colace(R) Infant/Children
Suppositories [US-OTC]
Constulose(R) [US]
Correctol(R) Tablets [US-OTC]
Doxidan(R) (reformulation)
[US-OTC]
Dulcolax(R) [US-OTC/Can]
Dulcolax(R) Milk of Magnesia
[US-OTC]
Enulose(R) [US]
Equalactin(R) [US-OTC]
Evac-U-Gen [US-OTC]
ex-lax(R) [US-OTC]
ex-lax(R) Maximum Strength
[US-OTC]
Femilax(TM) [US-OTC]
Fiberall(R) [US]

FiberCon(R) [US-OTC]
Fiber-Lax(R) [US-OTC]
Fibro-XL [US-OTC]
Fibro-Lax [US-OTC]
Fleet(R) Accu-Prep(R) [US-OTC]
Fleet(R) Babylax(R) [US-OTC]
Fleet(R) Bisacodyl Enema
[US-OTC]
Fleet Enema(R) [Can]
Fleet(R) Glycerin Suppositories
[US-OTC]
Fleet(R) Glycerin Suppositories
Maximum Strength [US-OTC]
Fleet(R) Liquid Glycerin
Suppositories [US-OTC]
Fleet(R) Phospho-Soda(R)
[US-OTC]
Fleet(R) Phospho-Soda(R) Oral
Laxative [Can]
Fleet(R) Stimulant Laxative
[US-OTC]
Fletcher's(R) Castoria(R)
[US-OTC]
Generlac [US]
Genfiber(R) [US-OTC]
Gentlax(R) [Can]
glycerin
Hydrocil(R) Instant [US-OTC]
Konsyl(R) [US-OTC]
Konsyl-D(R) [US-OTC]
Konsyl(R) Easy Mix [US-OTC]
Konsyl(R) Fiber Tablets [US-OTC]
Konsyl(R) Orange [US-OTC]
Kristalose(TM) [US]
lactulose
Laxilose [Can]
Mag-Caps [US-OTC]
MagGel(TM) [US-OTC]
magnesium hydroxide
magnesium hydroxide and mineral oil
magnesium oxide
magnesium sulfate
Mag-Ox(R) 400 [US-OTC]
Metamucil(R) [US-OTC/Can]

Metamucil(R) Plus Calcium
[US-OTC]
Metamucil(R) Smooth Texture
[US-OTC]
methylcellulose
Modane(R) Bulk [US-OTC]
Modane Tablets(R) [US-OTC]
Natural Fiber Therapy [US-OTC]
OsmoPrep(TM) [US]
Perdiem(R) Overnight Relief
[US-OTC]
Phillips'(R) M-O [US-OTC]
Phillips'(R) Fibercaps [US-OTC]
Phillips'(R) Milk of Magnesia
[US-OTC]
PMS-Lactulose [Can]
polycarbophil
psyllium
Purge(R) [US-OTC]
Reguloid(R) [US-OTC]
Sani-Supp(R) [US-OTC]
Senexon(R) [US-OTC]
senna
Senna-Gen(R) [US-OTC]
Sennatural(TM) [US-OTC]
Senokot(R) [US-OTC]
Serutan(R) [US-OTC]
sodium phosphates
sorbitol
Uni-Senna [US-OTC]
Uro-Mag(R) [US-OTC]
Veracolate [US-OTC]
Visicol(R) [US]
Laxative, Osmotic
GlycoLax(TM) [US]
MiraLax(TM) [US]
polyethylene glycol 3350
Laxative, Stimulant
docusate and senna
Peri-Colace(R) (reformulation)
[US-OTC]
Senokot-S(R) [US-OTC]
Stool Softener
Apo-Docusate-Sodium(R) [Can]

Colace(R) [US-OTC/Can]
Colax-C(R) [Can]
Diocto(R) [US-OTC]
docusate
docusate and senna
Docusoft-S(TM) [US-OTC]
DOK(TM) [US-OTC]
DOS(R) [US-OTC]
D-S-S(R) [US-OTC]
Dulcolax(R) Stool Softener
[US-OTC]
Enemeez(R) [US-OTC]
Fleet(R) Sof-Lax(R) [US-OTC]
Genasoft(R) [US-OTC]
Novo-Docusate Calcium [Can]
Novo-Docusate Sodium [Can]
Peri-Colace(R) (reformulation)
[US-OTC]
Phillips'(R) Stool Softener Laxative
[US-OTC]
PMS-Docusate Calcium [Can]
PMS-Docusate Sodium [Can]
Regulex(R) [Can]
Selax(R) [Can]
Senokot-S(R) [US-OTC]
Silace [US-OTC]
Soflax(TM) [Can]
Surfak(R) [US-OTC]

CONSTIPATION (CHRONIC IDIOPATHIC)
Gastrointestinal Agent, Miscellaneous
Amitiza(TM) [US]
lubiprostone

CROHN DISEASE
5-Aminosalicylic Acid Derivative
Alti-Sulfasalazine [Can]
Asacol(R) [US/Can]
Asacol(R) 800 [Can]
Azulfidine(R) [US]
Azulfidine(R) EN-tabs(R) [US]
Canasa(TM) [US]
Dipentum(R) [US/Can]

mesalamine
Mesasal(R) [Can]
Novo-5 ASA [Can]
olsalazine
Pendo-5 ASA [Can]
Pentasa(R) [US/Can]
Quintasa(R) [Can]
Rowasa(R) [US/Can]
Salazopyrin(R) [Can]
Salazopyrin En-Tabs(R) [Can]
Salofalk(R) [Can]
sulfasalazine
Sulfazine [US]
Sulfazine EC [US]
Monoclonal Antibody
infliximab
Remicade(R) [US/Can]

CRYPTORCHIDISM

Gonadotropin
chorionic gonadotropin (human)
Humegon(R) [Can]
Novarel(R) [US]
Pregnyl(R) [US]
Profasi(R) HP [Can]

CYSTINURIA

Chelating Agent
Cuprimine(R) [US/Can]
Depen(R) [US/Can]
penicillamine

CYSTITIS (HEMORRHAGIC)

Antidote
mesna
Mesnex(R) [US/Can]
Uromitexan [Can]

DIABETIC GASTRIC STASIS

Gastrointestinal Agent, Prokinetic
Apo-Metoclop(R) [Can]
metoclopramide
Metoclopramide Hydrochloride
Injection [Can]
Nu-Metoclopramide [Can]
Reglan(R) [US]

DIARRHEA

Antidiarrheal
Apo-Loperamide(R) [Can]
attapulgite
Diamode [US-OTC]
Diarr-Eze [Can]
Diasorb(R) [US-OTC]
difenoxin and atropine
diphenoxylate and atropine
Imodium(R) [Can]
Imodium(R) A-D [US-OTC]
kaolin and pectin
Kao-Paverin(R) [US-OTC]
Kaopectate(R) [Can]
K-Pek II [US-OTC]
Lomotil(R) [US/Can]
Lonox(R) [US]
Loperacap [Can]
loperamide
Motofen(R) [US]
Novo-Loperamide [Can]
PMS-Loperamine [Can]
Rho(R)-Loperamine [Can]
Riva-Loperamine [Can]
Gastrointestinal Agent, Miscellaneous
Bacid(R) [US-OTC/Can]
bismuth subgallate
bismuth subsalicylate
Children's Kaopectate(R)
(reformulation) [US-OTC]
Colo-Fresh(TM) [US-OTC]
Culturelle(R) [US-OTC]
Diotame(R) [US-OTC]
Dofus [US-OTC]
Equalactin(R) [US-OTC]
Fermalac [Can]
FiberCon(R) [US-OTC]
Fiber-Lax(R) [US-OTC]
Flora-Q(TM) [US-OTC]
Kala(R) [US-OTC]
Kaopectate(R) [US-OTC]
Kaopectate(R) Extra Strength
[US-OTC]
Konsyl(R) Fiber Tablets [US-OTC]

Lactinex(TM) [US-OTC]
Lactobacillus
Lacto-Bifidus [US-OTC]
Lacto-Key [US-OTC]
Lacto-Pectin [US-OTC]
Lacto-TriBlend [US-OTC]
Megadophilus(R) [US-OTC]
MoreDophilus(R) [US-OTC]
Pepto-Bismol(R) [US-OTC]
Pepto-Bismol(R) Maximum Strength
    [US-OTC]
Phillips'(R) Fibercaps [US-OTC]
polycarbophil
Superdophilus(R) [US-OTC]
Laxative
    Equalactin(R) [US-OTC]
    FiberCon(R) [US-OTC]
    Fiber-Lax(R) [US-OTC]
    Konsyl(R) Fiber Tablets [US-OTC]
    Phillips'(R) Fibercaps [US-OTC]
    polycarbophil
Somatostatin Analog
    octreotide
    Octreotide Acetate Injection [Can]
    Octreotide Acetate Omega [Can]
    Sandostatin(R) [US/Can]
    Sandostatin LAR(R) [US/Can]

DIARRHEA (BACTERIAL)

Aminoglycoside (Antibiotic)
    Neo-Fradin(TM) [US]
    neomycin
    Neo-Rx [US]
Antiprotozoal
    Alinia(R) [US]
    nitazoxanide

DIARRHEA (BILE ACIDS)

Bile Acid Sequestrant
    cholestyramine resin
    Novo-Cholamine [Can]
    Novo-Cholamine Light [Can]
    PMS-Cholestyramine [Can]
    Prevalite(R) [US]
    Questran(R) [US]

Questran(R) Light [US]
Questran(R) Light Sugar Free [Can]

DIARRHEA (CRYPTOSPORIDIAL)

Amebicide
    Humatin(R) [US/Can]
    paromomycin

DIARRHEA (TRAVELER'S)

Antibiotic, Miscellaneous
    rifaximin
    Xifaxan(TM) [US]
Gastrointestinal Agent, Miscellaneous
    bismuth subsalicylate
    Children's Kaopectate(R)
        (reformulation) [US-OTC]
    Colo-Fresh(TM) [US-OTC]
    Diotame(R) [US-OTC]
    Kaopectate(R) [US-OTC]
    Kaopectate(R) Extra Strength
        [US-OTC]
    Pepto-Bismol(R) [US-OTC]
    Pepto-Bismol(R) Maximum Strength
        [US-OTC]

DIVERTICULITIS

Amebicide
    Apo-Metronidazole(R) [Can]
    Flagyl(R) [US/Can]
    Flagyl ER(R) [US]
    Flagyl(R) I.V. RTU(TM) [US]
    Florazole(R) ER [Can]
    MetroCream(R) [US/Can]
    MetroGel(R) [US/Can]
    MetroGel-Vaginal(R) [US]
    MetroLotion(R) [US]
    metronidazole
    Nidagel(TM) [Can]
    Noritate(R) [US/Can]
    Trikacide [Can]
    Vandazole(TM) [US]
Aminoglycoside (Antibiotic)
    AKTob(R) [US]
    Alcomicin(R) [Can]

Diogent(R) [Can]
Garamycin(R) [Can]
Gentak(R) [US]
gentamicin
Gentamicin Injection, USP [Can]
PMS-Tobramycin [Can]
SAB-Gentamicin [Can]
Sandoz-Tobramycin [Can]
TOBI(R) [US/Can]
tobramycin
Tobramycin Injection, USP [Can]
Tobrex(R) [US/Can]
Antibiotic, Miscellaneous
Alti-Clindamycin [Can]
Apo-Clindamycin(R) [Can]
Apo-Metronidazole(R) [Can]
Azactam(R) [US/Can]
aztreonam
Cleocin(R) [US]
Cleocin HCl(R) [US]
Cleocin Pediatric(R) [US]
Cleocin Phosphate(R) [US]
Cleocin T(R) [US]
Clindagel(R) [US]
ClindaMax(TM) [US]
clindamycin
Clindamycin Injection, USP
   [Can]
Clindesse(TM) [US]
Clindets(R) [US]
Clindoxyl(R) [Can]
Dalacin(R) C [Can]
Dalacin(R) T [Can]
Dalacin(R) Vaginal [Can]
Evoclin(TM) [US]
Flagyl(R) [US/Can]
Flagyl ER(R) [US]
Flagyl(R) I.V. RTU(TM) [US]
Florazole(R) ER [Can]
MetroCream(R) [US/Can]
MetroGel(R) [US/Can]
MetroGel-Vaginal(R) [US]
MetroLotion(R) [US]
metronidazole

Nidagel(TM) [Can]
Noritate(R) [US/Can]
Novo-Clindamycin [Can]
Taro-Clindamycin [Can]
Trikacide [Can]
Vandazole(TM) [US]
Antiprotozoal
Apo-Metronidazole(R) [Can]
Flagyl(R) [US/Can]
Flagyl ER(R) [US]
Flagyl(R) I.V. RTU(TM) [US]
Florazole(R) ER [Can]
metronidazole
Nidagel(TM) [Can]
Noritate(R) [US/Can]
Trikacide [Can]
Vandazole(TM) [US]
Carbapenem (Antibiotic)
imipenem and cilastatin
Primaxin(R) [US/Can]
Primaxin(R) I.V. [Can]
Cephalosporin (Second Generation)
cefoxitin
Mefoxin(R) [US]
Penicillin
ampicillin
ampicillin and sulbactam
Apo-Ampi(R) [Can]
Novo-Ampicillin [Can]
Nu-Ampi [Can]
piperacillin and tazobactam sodium
Tazocin(R) [Can]
ticarcillin and clavulanate potassium
Timentin(R) [US/Can]
Unasyn(R) [US/Can]
Zosyn(R) [US]

DUODENAL ULCER
Antacid
calcium carbonate and simethicone
Dulcolax(R) Milk of Magnesia
   [US-OTC]
Gas Ban(TM) [US-OTC]
magaldrate and simethicone

Mag-Caps [US-OTC]
MagGel(TM) [US-OTC]
magnesium hydroxide
magnesium oxide
Mag-Ox(R) 400 [US-OTC]
Phillips'(R) Milk of Magnesia
[US-OTC]
Titralac(R) Plus [US-OTC]
Uro-Mag(R) [US-OTC]
Antibiotic, Macrolide Combination
Hp-PAC(R) [Can]
lansoprazole, amoxicillin, and
clarithromycin
Prevpac(R) [US/Can]
Antibiotic, Penicillin
Hp-PAC(R) [Can]
lansoprazole, amoxicillin, and
clarithromycin
Prevpac(R) [US/Can]
Gastric Acid Secretion Inhibitor
AcipHex(R) [US/Can]
Apo-Omeprazole(R) [Can]
lansoprazole
Losec(R) [Can]
Losec MUPS(R) [Can]
omeprazole
Pariet(R) [Can]
Prevacid(R) [US/Can]
Prevacid(R) SoluTab(TM) [US]
Prilosec(R) [US]
Prilosec OTC(TM) [US-OTC]
rabeprazole
Gastrointestinal Agent, Gastric or
Duodenal Ulcer Treatment
Carafate(R) [US]
Novo-Sucralate [Can]
Nu-Sucralate [Can]
PMS-Sucralate [Can]
sucralfate
Sulcrate(R) [Can]
Sulcrate(R) Suspension Plus
[Can]
Gastrointestinal Agent, Miscellaneous
Hp-PAC(R) [Can]

lansoprazole, amoxicillin, and
clarithromycin
Prevpac(R) [US/Can]
Histamine H2 Antagonist
Alti-Ranitidine [Can]
Apo-Cimetidine(R) [Can]
Apo-Famotidine(R) [Can]
Apo-Famotidine(R) Injectable
[Can]
Apo-Nizatidine(R) [Can]
Apo-Ranitidine(R) [Can]
Axid(R) [US/Can]
Axid(R) AR [US-OTC]
BCI-Ranitidine [Can]
cimetidine
CO Ranitidine [Can]
famotidine
Famotidine Omega [Can]
Gen-Cimetidine [Can]
Gen-Famotidine [Can]
Gen-Nizatidine [Can]
Gen-Ranidine [Can]
nizatidine
Novo-Cimetidine [Can]
Novo-Famotidine [Can]
Novo-Nizatidine [Can]
Novo-Ranidine [Can]
Nu-Cimet [Can]
Nu-Famotidine [Can]
Nu-Nizatidine [Can]
Nu-Ranit [Can]
Pepcid(R) [US/Can]
Pepcid(R) AC [US-OTC/Can]
Pepcid(R) I.V. [Can]
PMS-Cimetidine [Can]
PMS-Nizatidine [Can]
PMS-Ranitidine [Can]
ranitidine
Ranitidine Injection, USP [Can]
Rhoxal-ranitidine [Can]
Riva-Famotidine [Can]
Sandoz-Ranitidine [Can]
Tagamet(R) [US]
Tagamet(R) HB [Can]

Tagamet(R) HB 200 [US-OTC]
Ulcidine [Can]
Zantac(R) [US/Can]
Zantac 75(R) [US-OTC/Can]
Zantac 150(TM) [US-OTC]
Zantac(R) EFFERdose(R) [US]

DYSURIA

Analgesic, Urinary
AZO-Gesic(R) [US-OTC]
AZO-Standard(R) [US-OTC]
Baridium(R) [US-OTC]
Phenazo(TM) [Can]
phenazopyridine
Pyridium(R) [US]
ReAzo [US-OTC]
Uristat(R) [US-OTC]
UTI Relief(R) [US-OTC]
Antispasmodic Agent, Urinary
Apo-Flavoxate(R) [Can]
flavoxate
Urispas(R) [US/Can]

ENURESIS

Antidepressant, Tricyclic (Tertiary Amine)
Apo-Imipramine(R) [Can]
imipramine
Novo-Pramine [Can]
Tofranil(R) [US/Can]
Tofranil-PM(R) [US]
Antispasmodic Agent, Urinary
Apo-Oxybutynin(R) [Can]
Ditropan(R) [US/Can]
Ditropan(R) XL [US/Can]
Gen-Oxybutynin [Can]
Novo-Oxybutynin [Can]
Nu-Oxybutyn [Can]
oxybutynin
Oxytrol(R) [US/Can]
PMS-Oxybutynin [Can]
Uromax(R) [Can]
Vasopressin Analog, Synthetic
Apo-Desmopressin(R) [Can]
DDAVP(R) [US/Can]

desmopressin acetate
Minirin(R) [Can]
Octostim(R) [Can]
Stimate(TM) [US]

ERECTILE DYSFUNCTION (ED)

Androgen
Android(R) [US]
Methitest(TM) [US]
methyltestosterone
Testred(R) [US]
Virilon(R) [US]
Miscellaneous Product
Aphrodyne(R) [US]
PMS-Yohimbine [Can]
Yocon(R) [US/Can]
yohimbine
Phosphodiesterase (Type 5) Enzyme Inhibitor
Cialis(R) [US/Can]
Levitra(R) [US/Can]
Revatio(TM) [US]
sildenafil
tadalafil
vardenafil
Viagra(R) [US/Can]

EROSIVE ESOPHAGITIS

Proton Pump Inhibitor
esomeprazole
Nexium(R) [US/Can]

ERYTHROPOIETIC PROTOPORPHYRIA (EPP)

Vitamin, Fat Soluble
A-Caro-25(R) [US]
B-Caro-T(TM) [US]
beta-carotene
Lumitene(TM) [US]

ESOPHAGEAL VARICES

Hormone, Posterior Pituitary
Pitressin(R) [US]
Pressyn(R) [Can]

Pressyn(R) AR [Can]
vasopressin

Sclerosing Agent
Ethamolin(R) [US]
ethanolamine oleate
sodium tetradecyl
Sotradecol(R) [US]
Trombovar(R) [Can]

Variceal Bleeding (Acute)
Agent
somatostatin (Canada only)
Stilamin(R) [Can]

ESOPHAGITIS

Gastric Acid Secretion Inhibitor
Apo-Omeprazole(R) [Can]
lansoprazole
Losec(R) [Can]
Losec MUPS(R) [Can]
omeprazole
Prevacid(R) [US/Can]
Prevacid(R) SoluTab(TM) [US]
Prilosec(R) [US]
Prilosec OTC(TM) [US-OTC]

FAMILIAL ADENOMATOUS POLYPOSIS

Nonsteroidal Antiinflammatory Drug
(NSAID), COX-2 Selective
Celebrex(R) [US/Can]
Celecoxib

GAG REFLEX SUPPRESSION

Local Anesthetic
Americaine(R) [US-OTC]
benzocaine
benzocaine, butyl aminobenzoate,
tetracaine, and benzalkonium
chloride
Benzodent(R) [US-OTC]
Cepacol(R) Dual Action Maximum
Strength [US-OTC]
dyclonine
Hurricaine(R) [US]

Orabase(R) with Benzocaine
[US-OTC]
Orajel(R) Maximum Strength
[US-OTC]
tetracaine
Zilactin(R)-B [US-OTC/Can]

GAS PAINS

Antiflatulent
Alamag Plus [US-OTC]
Aldroxicon I [US-OTC]
Aldroxicon II [US-OTC]
Almacone(R) [US-OTC]
Almacone Double Strength(R)
[US-OTC]
aluminum hydroxide, magnesium
hydroxide, and simethicone
calcium carbonate and simethicone
Diovol Plus(R) [Can]
Equalizer Gas Relief [US-OTC]
Gas-X(R) [US-OTC]
Gas-X(R) Extra Strength
[US-OTC]
Gas-X(R) Maximum Strength
[US-OTC]
GasAid [US-OTC]
Gas Ban(TM) [US-OTC]
Gelusil(R) [US-OTC/Can]
Genasyme(R) [US-OTC]
Infantaire Gas Drops [US-OTC]
Maalox(R) [US-OTC]
Maalox(R) Max [US-OTC]
magaldrate and simethicone
Mi-Acid(TM) [US-OTC]
Mi-Acid(TM) Maximum Strength
[US-OTC]
Mintox Extra Strength [US-OTC]
Mintox Plus [US-OTC]
Mylanta(R) Double Strength [Can]
Mylanta(R) Extra Strength [Can]
Mylanta(R) Gas [US-OTC]
Mylanta(R) Gas Maximum Strength
[US-OTC]
Mylanta(R) Liquid [US-OTC]

Mylanta(R) Maximum Strength
Liquid [US-OTC]
Mylanta(R) Regular Strength [Can]
Mylicon(R) Infants [US-OTC]
Ovol(R) [Can]
Phazyme(R) [Can]
Phazyme(R) Quick Dissolve
[US-OTC]
Phazyme(R) Ultra Strength
[US-OTC]
simethicone
Titralac(R) Plus [US-OTC]

GASTRIC ULCER

Antacid
calcium carbonate and simethicone
Dulcolax(R) Milk of Magnesia
[US-OTC]
Gas Ban(TM) [US-OTC]
magaldrate and simethicone
Mag-Caps [US-OTC]
MagGel(TM) [US-OTC]
magnesium hydroxide
magnesium oxide
Mag-Ox(R) 400 [US-OTC]
Phillips'(R) Milk of Magnesia
[US-OTC]
Titralac(R) Plus [US-OTC]
Uro-Mag(R) [US-OTC]
Histamine H2 Antagonist
Alti-Ranitidine [Can]
Apo-Cimetidine(R) [Can]
Apo-Famotidine(R) [Can]
Apo-Famotidine(R) Injectable [Can]
Apo-Nizatidine(R) [Can]
Apo-Ranitidine(R) [Can]
Axid(R) [US/Can]
Axid(R) AR [US-OTC]
BCI-Ranitidine [Can]
cimetidine
CO Ranitidine [Can]
famotidine
Famotidine Omega [Can]
Gen-Cimetidine [Can]

Gen-Famotidine [Can]
Gen-Nizatidine [Can]
Gen-Ranidine [Can]
nizatidine
Novo-Cimetidine [Can]
Novo-Famotidine [Can]
Novo-Nizatidine [Can]
Novo-Ranidine [Can]
Nu-Cimet [Can]
Nu-Famotidine [Can]
Nu-Nizatidine [Can]
Nu-Ranit [Can]
Pepcid(R) [US/Can]
Pepcid(R) AC [US-OTC/Can]
Pepcid(R) I.V. [Can]
PMS-Cimetidine [Can]
PMS-Nizatidine [Can]
PMS-Ranitidine [Can]
ranitidine
Ranitidine Injection, USP [Can]
Rhoxal-ranitidine [Can]
Riva-Famotidine [Can]
Sandoz-Ranitidine [Can]
Tagamet(R) [US]
Tagamet(R) HB [Can]
Tagamet(R) HB 200 [US-OTC]
Ulcidine [Can]
Zantac(R) [US/Can]
Zantac 75(R) [US-OTC/Can]
Zantac 150(TM) [US-OTC]
Zantac(R) EFFERdose(R) [US]
Prostaglandin
Apo-Misoprostol(R) [Can]
Cytotec(R) [US]
misoprostol
Novo-Misoprostol [Can]

GASTRITIS

Antacid
Alamag [US-OTC]
aluminum hydroxide and magnesium
hydroxide
Diovol(R) [Can]
Diovol(R) Ex [Can]

Gelusil(R) Extra Strength [Can]
Mylanta(TM) [Can]
Rulox [US-OTC]
Histamine H2 Antagonist
Alti-Ranitidine [Can]
Apo-Cimetidine(R) [Can]
Apo-Ranitidine(R) [Can]
BCI-Ranitidine [Can]
cimetidine
CO Ranitidine [Can]
Gen-Cimetidine [Can]
Gen-Ranidine [Can]
Novo-Cimetidine [Can]
Novo-Ranidine [Can]
Nu-Cimet [Can]
Nu-Ranit [Can]
PMS-Cimetidine [Can]
PMS-Ranitidine [Can]
ranitidine
Ranitidine Injection, USP [Can]
Rhoxal-ranitidine [Can]
Sandoz-Ranitidine [Can]
Tagamet(R) [US]
Tagamet(R) HB [Can]
Tagamet(R) HB 200 [US-OTC]
Zantac(R) [US/Can]
Zantac 75(R) [US-OTC/Can]
Zantac 150(TM) [US-OTC]
Zantac(R) EFFERdose(R) [US]

GASTROESOPHAGEAL REFLUX DISEASE (GERD)

Cholinergic Agent
bethanechol
Duvoid(R) [Can]
Myotonachol(R) [Can]
PMS-Bethanechol [Can]
Urecholine(R) [US]
Gastric Acid Secretion Inhibitor
AcipHex(R) [US/Can]
Apo-Omeprazole(R) [Can]
lansoprazole
Losec(R) [Can]
Losec MUPS(R) [Can]

omeprazole
Pariet(R) [Can]
Prevacid(R) [US/Can]
Prevacid(R) SoluTab(TM) [US]
Prilosec(R) [US]
Prilosec OTC(TM) [US-OTC]
rabeprazole
Gastrointestinal Agent, Prokinetic
Apo-Metoclop(R) [Can]
cisapride
metoclopramide
Metoclopramide Hydrochloride
Injection [Can]
Nu-Metoclopramide [Can]
Propulsid(R) [US]
Reglan(R) [US]
Histamine H2 Antagonist
Alti-Ranitidine [Can]
Apo-Cimetidine(R) [Can]
Apo-Famotidine(R) [Can]
Apo-Famotidine(R) Injectable [Can]
Apo-Nizatidine(R) [Can]
Apo-Ranitidine(R) [Can]
Axid(R) [US/Can]
Axid(R) AR [US-OTC]
BCI-Ranitidine [Can]
cimetidine
CO Ranitidine [Can]
famotidine
Famotidine Omega [Can]
Gen-Cimetidine [Can]
Gen-Famotidine [Can]
Gen-Nizatidine [Can]
Gen-Ranidine [Can]
nizatidine
Novo-Cimetidine [Can]
Novo-Famotidine [Can]
Novo-Nizatidine [Can]
Novo-Ranidine [Can]
Nu-Cimet [Can]
Nu-Famotidine [Can]
Nu-Nizatidine [Can]
Nu-Ranit [Can]
Pepcid(R) [US/Can]

Pepcid(R) AC [US-OTC/Can]
Pepcid(R) I.V. [Can]
PMS-Cimetidine [Can]
PMS-Nizatidine [Can]
PMS-Ranitidine [Can]
ranitidine
Ranitidine Injection, USP [Can]
Rhoxal-ranitidine [Can]
Riva-Famotidine [Can]
Sandoz-Ranitidine [Can]
Tagamet(R) [US]
Tagamet(R) HB [Can]
Tagamet(R) HB 200 [US-OTC]
Ulcidine [Can]
Zantac(R) [US/Can]
Zantac 75(R) [US-OTC/Can]
Zantac 150(TM) [US-OTC]
Zantac(R) EFFERdose(R) [US]
Proton Pump Inhibitor
Panto(TM) IV [Can]
Pantoloc(R) [Can]
pantoprazole
Protonix(R) [US/Can]

GASTROINTESTINAL STROMAL TUMOR (GIST)

Antineoplastic Agent, Tyrosine Kinase
  Inhibitor
  sunitinib
  Sutent(R) [US]
Vascular Endothelial Growth Factor
  (VEGF) Inhibitor
  sunitinib
  Sutent(R) [US]

GIARDIASIS

Amebicide
  Apo-Metronidazole(R) [Can]
  Flagyl(R) [US/Can]
  Flagyl ER(R) [US]
  Flagyl(R) I.V. RTU(TM) [US]
  Florazole(R) ER [Can]
  Humatin(R) [US/Can]
  MetroCream(R) [US/Can]

MetroGel(R) [US/Can]
MetroGel-Vaginal(R) [US]
MetroLotion(R) [US]
metronidazole
Nidagel(TM) [Can]
Noritate(R) [US/Can]
paromomycin
Trikacide [Can]
Vandazole(TM) [US]
Anthelmintic
  albendazole
  Albenza(R) [US]
Antiprotozoal
  Apo-Metronidazole(R) [Can]
  Flagyl(R) [US/Can]
  Flagyl ER(R) [US]
  Flagyl(R) I.V. RTU(TM) [US]
  Florazole(R) ER [Can]
  MetroCream(R) [US/Can]
  MetroGel(R) [US/Can]
  MetroGel-Vaginal(R) [US]
  MetroLotion(R) [US]
  metronidazole
  Nidagel(TM) [Can]
  Noritate(R) [US/Can]
  Trikacide [Can]
  Vandazole(TM) [US]

GONORRHEA

Antibiotic, Miscellaneous
  spectinomycin
Antibiotic, Quinolone
  gatifloxacin
  Tequin(R) [Can]
  Zymar(TM) [US/Can]
Antibiotic, Topical
  Apo-Tetra(R) [Can]
  Nu-Tetra [Can]
  Sumycin(R) [US]
  tetracycline
Cephalosporin (Second Generation)
  Apo-Cefuroxime(R) [Can]
  cefoxitin
  Ceftin(R) [US/Can]

cefuroxime
Mefoxin(R) [US]
ratio-Cefuroxime [Can]
Zinacef(R) [US/Can]
Cephalosporin (Third Generation)
ceftriaxone
Rocephin(R) [US/Can]
Quinolone
Apo-Ciproflox(R) [Can]
Apo-Oflox(R) [Can]
Apo-Ofloxacin(R) [Can]
Ciloxan(R) [US/Can]
Cipro(R) [US/Can]
Cipro(R) XL [Can]
ciprofloxacin
Cipro(R) XR [US]
CO Ciprofloxacin [Can]
Floxin(R) [US/Can]
Gen-Ciprofloxacin [Can]
Novo-Ciprofloxacin [Can]
Novo-Ofloxacin [Can]
Ocuflox(R) [US/Can]
ofloxacin
PMS-Ciprofloxacin [Can]
PMS-Ofloxacin [Can]
Proquin(R) XR [US]
RAN(TM)-Ciprofloxacin [Can]
ratio-Ciprofloxacin [Can]
Rhoxal-ciprofloxacin [Can]
Sandoz-Ciprofloxacin [Can]
Taro-Ciprofloxacin [Can]
Tetracycline Derivative
Adoxa(TM) [US]
Apo-Doxy(R) [Can]
Apo-Doxy Tabs(R) [Can]
Apo-Tetra(R) [Can]
Doryx(R) [US]
Doxy-100(R) [US]
Doxycin [Can]
doxycycline
Doxytec [Can]
Monodox(R) [US]
Novo-Doxylin [Can]
Nu-Doxycycline [Can]
Nu-Tetra [Can]
Periostat(R) [US/Can]
Sumycin(R) [US]
tetracycline
Vibramycin(R) [US]
Vibra-Tabs(R) [US/Can]

GRAM-NEGATIVE INFECTION

Aminoglycoside (Antibiotic)
AKTob(R) [US]
Alcomicin(R) [Can]
amikacin
Amikacin Sulfate Injection, USP [Can]
Amikin(R) [US/Can]
Diogent(R) [Can]
Garamycin(R) [Can]
Gentak(R) [US]
gentamicin
Gentamicin Injection, USP [Can]
kanamycin
Kantrex(R) [US/Can]
PMS-Tobramycin [Can]
SAB-Gentamicin [Can]
Sandoz-Tobramycin [Can]
TOBI(R) [US/Can]
tobramycin
Tobramycin Injection, USP [Can]
Tobrex(R) [US/Can]
Antibiotic, Carbapenem
ertapenem
Invanz(R) [US/Can]
Antibiotic, Miscellaneous
Apo-Nitrofurantoin(R) [Can]
Azactam(R) [US/Can]
aztreonam
colistimethate
Coly-Mycin(R) M [US/Can]
Furadantin(R) [US]
Macrobid(R) [US/Can]
Macrodantin(R) [US/Can]
nitrofurantoin
Novo-Furantoin [Can]

Antibiotic, Quinolone
  gatifloxacin
  Iquix(R) [US]
  Levaquin(R) [US/Can]
  levofloxacin
  Novo-Levofloxacin [Can]
  Quixin(TM) [US]
  Tequin(R) [Can]
  Zymar(TM) [US/Can]
Carbapenem (Antibiotic)
  imipenem and cilastatin
  meropenem
  Merrem(R) [Can]
  Merrem(R) I.V. [US]
  Primaxin(R) [US/Can]
  Primaxin(R) I.V. [Can]
Cephalosporin (First Generation)
  Ancef(R) [US]
  Apo-Cefadroxil(R) [Can]
  Apo-Cephalex(R) [Can]
  Biocef(R) [US]
  cefadroxil
  cefazolin
  cephalexin
  cephalothin
  Duricef(R) [US/Can]
  Keflex(R) [US]
  Keftab(R) [Can]
  Novo-Cefadroxil [Can]
  Novo-Lexin [Can]
  Nu-Cephalex [Can]
Cephalosporin (Second Generation)
  Apo-Cefaclor(R) [Can]
  Apo-Cefuroxime(R)
    [Can]
  Ceclor(R) [Can]
  cefaclor
  cefoxitin
  cefpodoxime
  cefprozil
  Ceftin(R) [US/Can]
  cefuroxime
  Cefzil(R) [US/Can]
  Mefoxin(R) [US]

Novo-Cefaclor [Can]
Nu-Cefaclor [Can]
PMS-Cefaclor [Can]
Raniclor(TM) [US]
ratio-Cefuroxime [Can]
Vantin(R) [US/Can]
Zinacef(R) [US/Can]
Cephalosporin (Third Generation)
  Cedax(R) [US]
  Cefizox(R) [US/Can]
  cefotaxime
  ceftazidime
  ceftibuten
  ceftizoxime
  ceftriaxone
  Claforan(R) [US/Can]
  Fortaz(R) [US/Can]
  Rocephin(R) [US/Can]
  Tazicef(R) [US]
Cephalosporin (Fourth Generation)
  cefepime
  Maxipime(R) [US/Can]
Macrolide (Antibiotic)
  Akne-Mycin(R) [US]
  Apo-Azithromycin(R)
    [Can]
  Apo-Erythro Base(R) [Can]
  Apo-Erythro E-C(R) [Can]
  Apo-Erythro-ES(R) [Can]
  Apo-Erythro-S(R) [Can]
  A/T/S(R) [US]
  azithromycin
  Biaxin(R) [US/Can]
  Biaxin(R) XL [US/Can]
  clarithromycin
  CO Azithromycin [Can]
  Diomycin(R) [Can]
  E.E.S.(R) [US/Can]
  Erybid(TM) [Can]
  Eryc(R) [US/Can]
  Eryderm(R) [US]
  Erygel(R) [US]
  EryPed(R) [US]
  Ery-Tab(R) [US]

Erythrocin(R) [US]
erythromycin
erythromycin and sulfisoxazole
GMD-Azithromycin [Can]
Novo-Azithromycin [Can]
Novo-Rythro Estolate [Can]
Novo-Rythro Ethylsuccinate
  [Can]
Nu-Erythromycin-S [Can]
PCE(R) [US/Can]
Pediazole(R) [US/Can]
PMS-Azithromycin [Can]
PMS-Erythromycin [Can]
ratio-Azithromycin [Can]
ratio-Clarithromycin [Can]
Romycin(R) [US]
Sandoz-Azithromycin [Can]
Sans Acne(R) [Can]
Theramycin Z(R) [US]
Zithromax(R) [US/Can]
Zmax(TM) [US]
Penicillin
  Alti-Amoxi-Clav [Can]
  amoxicillin
  amoxicillin and clavulanate
    potassium
  Amoxil(R) [US]
  ampicillin
  ampicillin and sulbactam
  Apo-Amoxi(R) [Can]
  Apo-Amoxi-Clav(R) [Can]
  Apo-Ampi(R) [Can]
  Apo-Pen VK(R) [Can]
  Augmentin(R) [US/Can]
  Augmentin ES-600(R) [US]
  Augmentin XR(TM) [US]
  Bicillin(R) L-A [US]
  Bicillin(R) C-R [US]
  Bicillin(R) C-R 900/300 [US]
  carbenicillin
  Clavulin(R) [Can]
  Gen-Amoxicillin [Can]
  Geocillin(R) [US]
  Lin-Amox [Can]

Novamoxin(R) [Can]
Novo-Ampicillin [Can]
Novo-Clavamoxin [Can]
Novo-Pen-VK [Can]
Nu-Amoxi [Can]
Nu-Ampi [Can]
Nu-Pen-VK [Can]
penicillin V potassium
penicillin G benzathine
penicillin G benzathine and penicillin
  G procaine
penicillin G procaine
Pfizerpen-AS(R) [Can]
PHL-Amoxicillin [Can]
piperacillin
piperacillin and tazobactam sodium
Piperacillin for Injection, USP [Can]
pivampicillin (Canada only)
PMS-Amoxicillin [Can]
Pondocillin(R) [Can]
ratio-Aclavulanate [Can]
Tazocin(R) [Can]
Ticar(R) [US]
ticarcillin
ticarcillin and clavulanate potassium
Timentin(R) [US/Can]
Unasyn(R) [US/Can]
Veetids(R) [US]
Wycillin(R) [Can]
Zosyn(R) [US]
Quinolone
  Apo-Ciproflox(R) [Can]
  Apo-Norflox(R) [Can]
  Apo-Oflox(R) [Can]
  Apo-Ofloxacin(R) [Can]
  Ciloxan(R) [US/Can]
  Cipro(R) [US/Can]
  Cipro(R) XL [Can]
  ciprofloxacin
  Cipro(R) XR [US]
  CO Ciprofloxacin [Can]
  CO Norfloxacin [Can]
  Floxin(R) [US/Can]
  Gen-Ciprofloxacin [Can]

norfloxacin
Norfloxacine(R) [Can]
Noroxin(R) [US/Can]
Novo-Ciprofloxacin [Can]
Novo-Norfloxacin [Can]
Novo-Ofloxacin [Can]
Ocuflox(R) [US/Can]
ofloxacin
PMS-Ciprofloxacin [Can]
PMS-Norfloxacin [Can]
PMS-Ofloxacin [Can]
Proquin(R) XR [US]
RAN(TM)-Ciprofloxacin [Can]
ratio-Ciprofloxacin [Can]
Rhoxal-ciprofloxacin [Can]
Riva-Norfloxacin [Can]
Sandoz-Ciprofloxacin [Can]
Taro-Ciprofloxacin [Can]
Sulfonamide
Apo-Sulfatrim(R) [Can]
Apo-Sulfatrim(R) DS [Can]
Apo-Sulfatrim(R) Pediatric [Can]
Bactrim(TM) [US]
Bactrim(TM) DS [US]
erythromycin and sulfisoxazole
Gantrisin(R) [US]
Novo-Soxazole [Can]
Novo-Trimel [Can]
Novo-Trimel D.S. [Can]
Nu-Cotrimox [Can]
Pediazole(R) [US/Can]
Septra(R) [US]
Septra(R) DS [US]
Septra(R) Injection [Can]
sulfadiazine
sulfamethoxazole and trimethoprim
sulfisoxazole
Sulfizole(R) [Can]
Tetracycline Derivative
Adoxa(TM) [US]
Alti-Minocycline [Can]
Apo-Doxy(R) [Can]
Apo-Doxy Tabs(R) [Can]
Apo-Minocycline(R) [Can]

Apo-Tetra(R) [Can]
Doryx(R) [US]
Doxy-100(R) [US]
Doxycin [Can]
doxycycline
Doxytec [Can]
Dynacin(R) [US]
Gen-Minocycline [Can]
Minocin(R) [US/Can]
minocycline
Monodox(R) [US]
myrac(TM) [US]
Novo-Doxylin [Can]
Novo-Minocycline [Can]
Nu-Doxycycline [Can]
Nu-Tetra [Can]
oxytetracycline
Periostat(R) [US/Can]
Rhoxal-minocycline [Can]
Sandoz-Minocycline [Can]
Solodyn(TM) [US]
Sumycin(R) [US]
Terramycin(R) [Can]
tetracycline
Vibramycin(R) [US]
Vibra-Tabs(R) [US/Can]

HEARTBURN
Antacid
Alcalak [US-OTC]
Alka-Mints(R) [US-OTC]
Apo-Cal(R) [Can]
Calcarb 600 [US-OTC]
Calci-Chew(R) [US-OTC]
Calci-Mix(R) [US-OTC]
Calcite-500 [Can]
calcium carbonate
calcium carbonate and simethicone
Cal-Gest [US-OTC]
Cal-Mint [US-OTC]
Caltrate(R) [Can]
Caltrate(R) 600 [US-OTC]
Caltrate(R) Select [Can]
Children's Pepto [US-OTC]

Chooz(R) [US-OTC]
famotidine, calcium carbonate, and
magnesium hydroxide
Florical(R) [US-OTC]
Gas Ban(TM) [US-OTC]
Maalox(R) Quick Dissolve
[US-OTC]
Mylanta(R) Children's [US-OTC]
Nephro-Calci(R) [US-OTC]
Nutralox(R) [US-OTC]
Os-Cal(R) [Can]
Os-Cal(R) 500 [US-OTC]
Oysco 500 [US-OTC]
Oyst-Cal 500 [US-OTC]
Pepcid(R) Complete [US-OTC/Can]
Rolaids(R) Softchews [US-OTC]
Titralac(TM) [US-OTC]
Titralac(TM) Extra Strength
[US-OTC]
Titralac(R) Plus [US-OTC]
Tums(R) [US-OTC]
Tums(R) E-X [US-OTC]
Tums(R) Extra Strength Sugar Free
[US-OTC]
Tums(R) Smoothies(TM) [US-OTC]
Tums(R) Ultra [US-OTC]
Histamine H2 Antagonist
Apo-Cimetidine(R) [Can]
cimetidine
famotidine, calcium carbonate, and
magnesium hydroxide
Gen-Cimetidine [Can]
Novo-Cimetidine [Can]
Nu-Cimet [Can]
Pepcid(R) Complete [US-OTC/Can]
PMS-Cimetidine [Can]
Tagamet(R) [US]
Tagamet(R) HB [Can]
Tagamet(R) HB 200 [US-OTC]
Proton Pump Inhibitor
Panto(TM) IV [Can]
Pantoloc(R) [Can]
pantoprazole
Protonix(R) [US/Can]

HELICOBACTER PYLORI

Amebicide
Apo-Metronidazole(R) [Can]
Flagyl(R) [US/Can]
Flagyl ER(R) [US]
Flagyl(R) I.V. RTU(TM) [US]
Florazole(R) ER [Can]
MetroCream(R) [US/Can]
MetroGel(R) [US/Can]
MetroGel-Vaginal(R) [US]
MetroLotion(R) [US]
metronidazole
Nidagel(TM) [Can]
Noritate(R) [US/Can]
Trikacide [Can]
Vandazole(TM) [US]
Antibiotic, Miscellaneous
Apo-Metronidazole(R) [Can]
Flagyl(R) [US/Can]
Flagyl ER(R) [US]
Flagyl(R) I.V. RTU(TM) [US]
Florazole(R) ER [Can]
MetroCream(R) [US/Can]
MetroGel(R) [US/Can]
MetroGel-Vaginal(R) [US]
MetroLotion(R) [US]
metronidazole
Nidagel(TM) [Can]
Noritate(R) [US/Can]
Trikacide [Can]
Vandazole(TM) [US]
Antidiarrheal
bismuth subsalicylate, metronidazole,
and tetracycline
Helidac(R) [US]
Antiprotozoal
Apo-Metronidazole(R) [Can]
Flagyl(R) [US/Can]
Flagyl ER(R) [US]
Flagyl(R) I.V. RTU(TM) [US]
Florazole(R) ER [Can]
MetroCream(R) [US/Can]
MetroGel(R) [US/Can]
MetroGel-Vaginal(R) [US]

MetroLotion(R) [US]
metronidazole
Nidagel(TM) [Can]
Noritate(R) [US/Can]
Trikacide [Can]
Vandazole(TM) [US]
Gastrointestinal Agent, Miscellaneous
bismuth subsalicylate
Children's Kaopectate(R)
(reformulation) [US-OTC]
Colo-Fresh(TM) [US-OTC]
Diotame(R) [US-OTC]
Kaopectate(R) [US-OTC]
Kaopectate(R) Extra Strength
[US-OTC]
Pepto-Bismol(R) [US-OTC]
Pepto-Bismol(R) Maximum Strength
[US-OTC]
Macrolide (Antibiotic)
Biaxin(R) [US/Can]
Biaxin(R) XL [US/Can]
clarithromycin
ratio-Clarithromycin [Can]
Penicillin
amoxicillin
Amoxil(R) [US]
Apo-Amoxi(R) [Can]
Gen-Amoxicillin [Can]
Lin-Amox [Can]
Novamoxin(R) [Can]
Nu-Amoxi [Can]
PHL-Amoxicillin [Can]
PMS-Amoxicillin [Can]
Tetracycline Derivative
Apo-Tetra(R) [Can]
Nu-Tetra [Can]
Sumycin(R) [US]
Tetracycline

HEMORRHOIDS

Adrenal Corticosteroid
Anucort-HC(R) [US]
Anusol-HC(R) [US]
Anusol(R) HC-1 [US-OTC]

Cortenema(R) [Can]
Corticool(R) [US-OTC]
Cortifoam(R) [US/Can]
Hemril(R)-30 [US]
hydrocortisone (rectal)
Preparation H(R) Hydrocortisone
[US-OTC]
Proctocort(R) [US]
ProctoCream(R) HC [US]
Procto-Kit(TM) [US]
Procto-Pak(TM) [US]
Proctosert [US]
Proctosol-HC(R) [US]
Proctozone-HC(TM) [US]
Tucks(R) Anti-Itch
[US-OTC]
Anesthetic/Corticosteroid
Analpram-HC(R) [US]
Enzone(R) [US]
Epifoam(R) [US]
Pramosone(R) [US]
Pramox(R) HC [Can]
pramoxine and hydrocortisone
ProctoFoam(R)-HC [US/Can]
Zone-A(R) [US]
Zone-A Forte(R) [US]
Astringent
Dickinson's(R) Witch Hazel
[US-OTC]
Preparation H(R) Cleansing Pads
[Can]
Preparation H(R) Medicated Wipes
[US-OTC]
T.N. Dickinson's(R) Hazelets
[US-OTC]
Tucks(R) [US-OTC]
witch hazel
Local Anesthetic
Americaine(R) [US-OTC]
Americaine(R) Hemorrhoidal
[US-OTC]
Ametop(TM) [Can]
benzocaine
dibucaine

Foille(R) [US-OTC]
HDA(R) Toothache [US-OTC]
Hurricaine(R) [US-OTC]
Pontocaine(R) [US/Can]
Pontocaine(R) Niphanoid(R)
 [US]
pramoxine
Prax(R) [US-OTC]
ProctoFoam(R) NS [US-OTC]
tetracaine
Thorets [US-OTC]
Trocaine(R) [US-OTC]
Tronolane(R) [US-OTC]
Tucks(R) Hemorrhoidal
 [US-OTC]

HEPATIC CIRRHOSIS

Diuretic, Potassium Sparing
 amiloride
 Apo-Amiloride(R) [Can]

HEPATITIS A

Immune Globulin
 BayGam(R) [Can]
 GannaSTAN(TM) S/D [US]
 immune globulin (intramuscular)
Vaccine
 hepatitis A inactivated and hepatitis B
  (recombinant) vaccine
 Twinrix(R) [US/Can]
Vaccine, Inactivated Virus
 Avaxim(R) [Can]
 Avaxim(R)-Pediatric [Can]
 Havrix(R) [US/Can]
 hepatitis A vaccine
 VAQTA(R) [US/Can]

HEPATITIS B

Antiretroviral Agent, Non-nucleoside
 Reverse Transcriptase Inhibitor
 (NNRTI)
 adefovir
 Hepsera(TM) [US]
Antiretroviral Agent, Reverse
 Transcriptase Inhibitor (Nucleoside)

Baraclude(TM) [US]
 entecavir
Antiviral Agent
 Epivir(R) [US]
 Epivir-HBV(R) [US]
 Heptovir(R) [Can]
 interferon alfa-2b and ribavirin
 lamivudine
 Rebetron(R) [US]
 3TC(R) [Can]
Biological Response Modulator
 interferon alfa-2b
 interferon alfa-2b and ribavirin
 Intron(R) A [US/Can]
 Rebetron(R) [US]
Immune Globulin
 BayHep B(R) [Can]
 HepaGam B(TM) [US]
 hepatitis B immune globulin
 HyperHep B(R) [Can]
 HyperHEP B(TM) S/D [US]
 Nabi-HB(R) [US]
Vaccine
 hepatitis A inactivated and hepatitis B
  (recombinant) vaccine
 Twinrix(R) [US/Can]
Vaccine, Inactivated Virus
 Comvax(R) [US]
 Engerix-B(R) [US/Can]
 Haemophilus B conjugate and
  hepatitis B vaccine
 hepatitis B vaccine
 Recombivax HB(R) [US/Can]

HEPATITIS C

Antiviral Agent
 interferon alfa-2b and ribavirin
 Pegasys(R) RBV [Can]
 Pegetron(TM) [Can]
 peginterferon alfa-2b and ribavirin
  (Canada only)
 Rebetron(R) [US]
Biological Response Modulator
 interferon alfa-2b

interferon alfa-2b and ribavirin
Intron(R) A [US/Can]
Rebetron(R) [US]
Interferon
Infergen(R) [US]
interferon alfacon-1
Pegasys(R) [US/Can]
Pegasys(R) RBV [Can]
Pegetron(TM) [Can]
peginterferon alfa-2a
peginterferon alfa-2b
peginterferon alfa-2b and ribavirin
(Canada only)
PEG-Intron(R) [US/Can]

HEREDITARY TYROSINEMIA
4-Hydroxyphenylpyruvate Dioxygenase
Inhibitor
nitisinone
Orfadin(R) [US]

HERPES SIMPLEX
Antiviral Agent
acyclovir
Apo-Acyclovir(R) [Can]
Cytovene(R) [US/Can]
famciclovir
Famvir(R) [US/Can]
foscarnet
Foscavir(R) [US/Can]
ganciclovir
Gen-Acyclovir [Can]
Nu-Acyclovir [Can]
ratio-Acyclovir [Can]
SAB-Trifluridine [Can]
Sandoz-Trifluridine [Can]
trifluridine
Viroptic(R) [US/Can]
Vitrasert(R) [US/Can]
Zovirax(R) [US/Can]
Antiviral Agent, Topical
Abreva(R) [US-OTC]
docosanol

HERPES ZOSTER
Analgesic, Topical
ArthriCare(R) for Women Extra
Moisturizing [US-OTC]
ArthriCare(R) for Women
Multi-Action [US-OTC]
ArthriCare(R) for Women Silky Dry
[US-OTC]
Capsagel(R) [US-OTC]
capsaicin
Capzasin-HP(R) [US-OTC]
Capzasin-P(R) [US-OTC]
Zostrix(R) [US-OTC/Can]
Zostrix(R)-HP [US-OTC/Can]
Antiviral Agent
acyclovir
Apo-Acyclovir(R) [Can]
famciclovir
Famvir(R) [US/Can]
Gen-Acyclovir [Can]
Nu-Acyclovir [Can]
ratio-Acyclovir [Can]
valacyclovir
Valtrex(R) [US/Can]
Zovirax(R) [US/Can]
Vaccine
Zostavax(R) [US]
zoster vaccine

HIATAL HERNIA
Antacid
calcium carbonate and simethicone
Gas Ban(TM) [US-OTC]
magaldrate and simethicone
Titralac(R) Plus [US-OTC]

HICCUPS
Phenothiazine Derivative
chlorpromazine
Largactil(R) [Can]
Novo-Chlorpromazine
[Can]

H. INFLUENZAE
Toxoid

diphtheria, tetanus toxoids, and
acellular pertussis vaccine and
Haemophilus influenzae b
conjugate vaccine
TriHIBit(R) [US]
Vaccine, Inactivated Bacteria
ActHIB(R) [US/Can]
diphtheria, tetanus toxoids, and
acellular pertussis vaccine and
Haemophilus influenzae b
conjugate vaccine
Haemophilus B conjugate
vaccine
HibTITER(R) [US]
PedvaxHIB(R) [US/Can]
TriHIBit(R) [US]
Vaccine, Inactivated Virus
Comvax(R) [US]
Haemophilus B conjugate and
hepatitis B vaccine

HISTOPLASMOSIS

Antifungal Agent
Amphocin(R) [US]
amphotericin B (conventional)
Apo-Ketoconazole(R)
[Can]
Fungizone(R) [Can]
itraconazole
ketoconazole
Ketoderm(R) [Can]
Nizoral(R) [US]
Nizoral(R) A-D [US-OTC]
Novo-Ketoconazole [Can]
Sporanox(R) [US/Can]

HOOKWORMS

Anthelmintic
albendazole
Albenza(R) [US]
Combantrin(TM) [Can]
mebendazole
Pamix(TM) [US-OTC]
Pin-X(R) [US-OTC]
pyrantel pamoate

Reese's(R) Pinworm Medicine
[US-OTC]
Vermox(R) [Can]

HUMAN PAPILLOMAVIRUS (HPV) TYPES 6, 11, 16, 18

Vaccine
Gardasil(R) [US]
papillomavirus (Types 6, 11, 16, 18)
recombinant vaccine

HYDATIDIFORM MOLE (BENIGN)

Prostaglandin
Cervidil(R) [US/Can]
dinoprostone
Prepidil(R) [US/Can]
Prostin E2(R) [US/Can]

HYPERACIDITY

Antacid
Alamag [US-OTC]
Alamag Plus [US-OTC]
Alcalak [US-OTC]
Aldroxicon I [US-OTC]
Aldroxicon II [US-OTC]
Alenic Alka Tablet [US-OTC]
Alka-Mints(R) [US-OTC]
Almacone(R) [US-OTC]
Almacone Double Strength(R)
[US-OTC]
ALternaGel(R) [US-OTC]
aluminum hydroxide
aluminum hydroxide and magnesium
carbonate
aluminum hydroxide and magnesium
hydroxide
aluminum hydroxide and magnesium
trisilicate
aluminum hydroxide, magnesium
hydroxide, and simethicone
Amphojel(R) [Can]
Apo-Cal(R) [Can]
Basaljel(R) [Can]
Brioschi(R) [US-OTC]

Calcarb 600 [US-OTC]
Calci-Chew(R) [US-OTC]
Calci-Mix(R) [US-OTC]
Calcite-500 [Can]
calcium carbonate
calcium carbonate and magnesium
  hydroxide
calcium carbonate and simethicone
Cal-Gest [US-OTC]
Cal-Mint [US-OTC]
Caltrate(R) [Can]
Caltrate(R) 600 [US-OTC]
Caltrate(R) Select [Can]
Children's Pepto [US-OTC]
Chooz(R) [US-OTC]
Dermagran(R) [US-OTC]
Diovol(R) [Can]
Diovol(R) Ex [Can]
Diovol Plus(R) [Can]
Dulcolax(R) Milk of Magnesia
  [US-OTC]
Florical(R) [US-OTC]
Gas Ban(TM) [US-OTC]
Gaviscon(R) Extra Strength
  [US-OTC]
Gaviscon(R) Liquid [US-OTC]
Gaviscon(R) Tablet [US-OTC]
Gelusil(R) [US-OTC/Can]
Gelusil(R) Extra Strength [Can]
Genaton Tablet [US-OTC]
Maalox(R) [US-OTC]
Maalox(R) Max [US-OTC]
Maalox(R) Quick Dissolve [US-OTC]
magaldrate and simethicone
Mag-Caps [US-OTC]
MagGel(TM) [US-OTC]
magnesium hydroxide
magnesium oxide
Mag-Ox(R) 400 [US-OTC]
Mi-Acid(TM) [US-OTC]
Mi-Acid(TM) Double Strength
  [US-OTC]
Mi-Acid(TM) Maximum Strength
  [US-OTC]

Mintox Extra Strength [US-OTC]
Mintox Plus [US-OTC]
Mylanta(TM) [Can]
Mylanta(R) Children's [US-OTC]
Mylanta(R) Double Strength [Can]
Mylanta(R) Extra Strength [Can]
Mylanta(R) Gelcaps(R) [US-OTC]
Mylanta(R) Liquid [US-OTC]
Mylanta(R) Maximum Strength
  Liquid [US-OTC]
Mylanta(R) Regular Strength [Can]
Mylanta(R) Supreme [US-OTC]
Mylanta(R) Ultra [US-OTC]
Nephro-Calci(R) [US-OTC]
Neut(R) [US]
Nutralox(R) [US-OTC]
Os-Cal(R) [Can]
Os-Cal(R) 500 [US-OTC]
Oysco 500 [US-OTC]
Oyst-Cal 500 [US-OTC]
Phillips'(R) Milk of Magnesia
  [US-OTC]
Rolaids(R) [US-OTC]
Rolaids(R) Extra Strength [US-OTC]
Rolaids(R) Softchews [US-OTC]
Rulox [US-OTC]
sodium bicarbonate
Titralac(TM) [US-OTC]
Titralac(TM) Extra Strength
  [US-OTC]
Titralac(R) Plus [US-OTC]
Tums(R) [US-OTC]
Tums(R) E-X [US-OTC]
Tums(R) Extra Strength Sugar Free
  [US-OTC]
Tums(R) Smoothies(TM) [US-OTC]
Tums(R) Ultra [US-OTC]
Uro-Mag(R) [US-OTC]

HYPERAMMONEMIA

Ammonium Detoxicant
  Acilac [Can]
  Ammonul(R) [US]
  Apo-Lactulose(R) [Can]

Constulose(R) [US]
Enulose(R) [US]
Generlac [US]
Kristalose(TM) [US]
lactulose
Laxilose [Can]
PMS-Lactulose [Can]
sodium phenylacetate and sodium
    benzoate

HYPERURICEMIA

Enzyme
Elitek(TM) [US]
Fasturtec(R) [Can]
rasburicase
Uricosuric Agent
Apo-Sulfinpyrazone(R) [Can]
Benuryl(TM) [Can]
Nu-Sulfinpyrazone [Can]
probenecid
sulfinpyrazone
Xanthine Oxidase Inhibitor
allopurinol
Aloprim(TM) [US]
Apo-Allopurinol(R) [Can]
Novo-Purol [Can]
Zyloprim(R) [US/Can]

HYPOGONADISM

Androgen
Andriol(R) [Can]
Androderm(R) [US/Can]
AndroGel(R) [US/Can]
Android(R) [US]
Andropository [Can]
Delatestryl(R) [US/Can]
Depotest(R) 100 [Can]
Depo(R)-Testosterone [US]
Everone(R) 200 [Can]
First(R) Testosterone [US]
First(R) Testosterone MC [US]
Methitest(TM) [US]
methyltestosterone
Striant(R) [US]
Testim(R) [US]

Testopel(R) [US]
testosterone
Testred(R) [US]
Virilon(R) [US]
Virilon(R) IM [Can]
Diagnostic Agent
Factrel(R) [US]
gonadorelin
Lutrepulse(TM) [Can]
Estrogen and Androgen Combination
Estratest(R) [US/Can]
Estratest(R) H.S. [US]
estrogens (esterified) and
    methyltestosterone
Syntest D.S. [US]
Syntest H.S. [US]
Estrogen Derivative
Alora(R) [US]
Cenestin(R) [US]
Climara(R) [US/Can]
Delestrogen(R) [US]
Depo(R)-Estradiol [US/Can]
Esclim(R) [US]
Estrace(R) [US/Can]
Estraderm(R) [US/Can]
estradiol
Estradot(R) [Can]
Estrasorb(TM) [US]
Estratab(R) [Can]
Estring(R) [US/Can]
EstroGel(R) [US/Can]
estrogens (conjugated A/synthetic)
estrogens (conjugated/equine)
estrogens (esterified)
estropipate
Femring(TM) [US]
Femtrace(R) [US]
Gynodiol(R) [US]
Menest(R) [US/Can]
Menostar(TM) [US/Can]
Oesclim(R) [Can]
Ogen(R) [US/Can]
Ortho-Est(R) [US]
Premarin(R) [US/Can]

Sandoz-Estradiol Derm 50 [Can]
Sandoz-Estradiol Derm 75 [Can]
Sandoz-Estradiol Derm 100 [Can]
Vagifem(R) [US/Can]
Vivelle(R) [US]
Vivelle-Dot(R) [US]
Gonadotropin
  Factrel(R) [US]
  gonadorelin
  Lutrepulse(TM) [Can]

HYPOKALEMIA
Diuretic, Potassium Sparing
  Aldactone(R) [US/Can]
  amiloride
  Apo-Amiloride(R) [Can]
  Dyrenium(R) [US]
  Novo-Spiroton [Can]
  spironolactone
  triamterene
Electrolyte Supplement, Oral
  Apo-K(R) [Can]
  Effer-K(TM) [US]
  Glu-K(R) [US-OTC]
  K-10(R) [Can]
  Kaon-Cl-10(R) [US]
  Kaon-Cl(R) 20 [US]
  Kay Ciel(R) [US]
  K-Dur(R) [Can]
  K-Dur(R) 10 [US]
  K-Dur(R) 20 [US]
  K-Lor(R) [US/Can]
  Klor-Con(R) [US]
  Klor-Con(R) 8 [US]
  Klor-Con(R) 10 [US]
  Klor-Con(R)/25 [US]
  Klor-Con(R) M [US]
  Klor-Con(R)/EF [US]
  K-Lyte(R) [US]
  K-Lyte(R)/Cl [Can]
  K-Lyte(R) DS [US]
  K-Phos(R) MF [US]
  K-Phos(R) Neutral [US]
  K-Phos(R) No. 2 [US]

K+ Potassium [US]
K-Tab(R) [US]
microK(R) [US]
microK(R) 10 [US]
Micro-K Extencaps(R) [Can]
Neutra-Phos(R) [US-OTC]
Neutra-Phos(R)-K [US-OTC]
Phos-NaK [US]
Phospha 250(TM) Neutral [US]
potassium acetate
potassium acetate, potassium
  bicarbonate, and potassium citrate
potassium bicarbonate
potassium bicarbonate and potassium
  chloride
potassium bicarbonate and potassium
  citrate
potassium chloride
potassium gluconate
potassium phosphate
potassium phosphate and sodium
  phosphate
Roychlor(R) [Can]
Rum-K(R) [US]
Slo-Pot [Can]
Slow-K(R) [Can]
Tri-K(R) [US]
Uro-KP-Neutral(R) [US]

INFERTILITY (FEMALE)
Antigonadotropic Agent
  Antagon(R) [US/Can]
  ganirelix
  Orgalutran(R) [Can]
Anti-Parkinson Agent
  Apo-Bromocriptine(R) [Can]
  bromocriptine
  Parlodel(R) [US/Can]
  PMS-Bromocriptine [Can]
Ergot Alkaloid and Derivative
  Apo-Bromocriptine(R) [Can]
  bromocriptine
  Parlodel(R) [US/Can]
  PMS-Bromocriptine [Can]

Gonadotropin
  chorionic gonadotropin (human)
  Humegon(R) [Can]
  Menopur(R) [US]
  menotropins
  Novarel(R) [US]
  Pregnyl(R) [US]
  Profasi(R) HP [Can]
  Repronex(R) [US/Can]
Ovulation Stimulator
  Clomid(R) [US/Can]
  clomiphene
  follitropin alfa
  follitropin beta
  Gonal-f(R) [US/Can]
  Milophene(R) [Can]
  Serophene(R) [US/Can]
Progestin
  Crinone(R) [US/Can]
  Prochieve(TM) [US]
  progesterone
  Prometrium(R) [US/Can]

INFERTILITY (MALE)

Gonadotropin
  chorionic gonadotropin (human)
  Humegon(R) [Can]
  Menopur(R) [US]
  menotropins
  Novarel(R) [US]
  Pregnyl(R) [US]
  Profasi(R) HP [Can]
  Repronex(R) [US/Can]

INFLAMMATORY BOWEL DISEASE

5-Aminosalicylic Acid Derivative
  Alti-Sulfasalazine [Can]
  Asacol(R) [US/Can]
  Asacol(R) 800 [Can]
  Azulfidine(R) [US]
  Azulfidine(R) EN-tabs(R) [US]
  Canasa(TM) [US]
  Dipentum(R) [US/Can]

  mesalamine
  Mesasal(R) [Can]
  Novo-5 ASA [Can]
  olsalazine
  Pendo-5 ASA [Can]
  Pentasa(R) [US/Can]
  Quintasa(R) [Can]
  Rowasa(R) [US/Can]
  Salazopyrin(R) [Can]
  Salazopyrin En-Tabs(R) [Can]
  Salofalk(R) [Can]
  sulfasalazine
  Sulfazine [US]
  Sulfazine EC [US]

INFLUENZA

Antiviral Agent
  amantadine
  Endantadine(R) [Can]
  Flumadine(R) [US/Can]
  PMS-Amantadine [Can]
  rimantadine
  Symmetrel(R) [US/Can]
Antiviral Agent, Inhalation Therapy
  Relenza(R) [US/Can]
  zanamivir
Antiviral Agent, Oral
  oseltamivir
  Tamiflu(R) [US/Can]
Vaccine, Inactivated Virus
  Fluarix(TM) [US]
  fluMist(R) [US]
  Fluviral S/F(R) [Can]
  Fluvirin(R) [US]
  Fluzone(R) [US]
  influenza virus vaccine
  Vaxigrip(R) [Can]

INFLUENZA A

Antiviral Agent
  amantadine
  Endantadine(R) [Can]
  Flumadine(R) [US/Can]
  PMS-Amantadine [Can]

rimantadine
Symmetrel(R) [US/Can]

INTERSTITIAL CYSTITIS
Analgesic, Urinary
Elmiron(R) [US/Can]
pentosan polysulfate sodium
Urinary Tract Product
dimethyl sulfoxide
Dimethyl Sulfoxide Irrigation, USP
[Can]
Kemsol(R) [Can]
Rimso(R)-50 [US/Can]

IRRITABLE BOWEL SYNDROME (IBS)
Anticholinergic Agent
Apo-Chlorax(R) [Can]
AtroPen(R) [US]
atropine
Atropine-Care(R) [US]
Bentyl(R) [US]
Bentylol(R) [Can]
clidinium and chlordiazepoxide
dicyclomine
Dioptic's Atropine Solution [Can]
Donnatal(R) [US]
Donnatal Extentabs(R) [US]
Formulex(R) [Can]
hyoscyamine, atropine, scopolamine,
and phenobarbital
Isopto(R) Atropine [US/Can]
Librax(R) [US/Can]
Lomine [Can]
propantheline
Riva-Dicyclomine [Can]
Sal-Tropine(TM) [US]
Antispasmodic Agent, Gastrointestinal
Apo-Trimebutine(R) [Can]
Modulon(R) [Can]
trimebutine (Canada only)
Gastrointestinal Agent, Miscellaneous
Dicetel(R) [Can]
pinaverium (Canada only)

5-HT3 Receptor Antagonist
alosetron
Lotronex(R) [US]
Serotonin 5-HT4 Receptor Agonist
tegaserod
Zelnorm(R) [US/Can]

KIDNEY STONE
Alkalinizing Agent
citric acid, sodium citrate, and
potassium citrate
Cytra-3 [US]
K-Citra(R) [Can]
Polycitra(R) [US]
Polycitra(R)-LC [US]
potassium citrate
Urocit(R)-K [US]
Chelating Agent
Cuprimine(R) [US/Can]
Depen(R) [US/Can]
penicillamine
Electrolyte Supplement, Oral
K-Phos(R) MF [US]
K-Phos(R) Neutral [US]
K-Phos(R) No. 2 [US]
Neutra-Phos(R) [US-OTC]
Neutra-Phos(R)-K [US-OTC]
Phos-NaK [US]
Phospha 250(TM) Neutral [US]
potassium phosphate
potassium phosphate and sodium
phosphate
Uro-KP-Neutral(R) [US]
Irrigating Solution
citric acid, magnesium carbonate, and
glucono-delta-lactone
Renacidin(R) [US]
Urinary Tract Product
Calcibind(R) [US/Can]
cellulose sodium phosphate
Thiola(R) [US/Can]
tiopronin
Xanthine Oxidase Inhibitor
allopurinol

Aloprim(TM) [US]
Apo-Allopurinol(R) [Can]
Novo-Purol [Can]
Zyloprim(R) [US/Can]

LACTOSE INTOLERANCE
Nutritional Supplement
Dairyaid(R) [Can]
Lactaid(R) Fast Act [US-OTC]
Lactaid(R) Original [US-OTC]
lactase
Lactrase(R) [US-OTC]

MALABSORPTION
Trace Element
Iodopen(R) [US]
Molypen(R) [US]
M.T.E.-4(R) [US]
M.T.E.-5(R) [US]
M.T.E.-6(R) [US]
M.T.E.-7(R) [US]
Multitrace(TM)-4 [US]
Multitrace(TM)-4 Neonatal
[US]
Multitrace(TM)-4 Pediatric
[US]
Multitrace(TM)-5 [US]
Neotrace-4(R) [US]
Pedtrace-4(R) [US]
P.T.E.-4(R) [US]
P.T.E.-5(R) [US]
Selepen(R) [US]
trace metals
Vitamin, Fat Soluble
Aquasol A(R) [US]
Palmitate-A(R) [US-OTC]
vitamin A

MALNUTRITION
Caloric Agent
total parenteral nutrition
Electrolyte Supplement, Oral
Anuzinc [Can]
Orazinc(R) [US-OTC]
Rivasol [Can]

Zincate(R) [US]
zinc sulfate
Intravenous Nutritional Therapy
total parenteral nutrition
Nutritional Supplement
Carnation Instant Breakfast(R)
[US-OTC]
Citrotein(R) [US-OTC]
Criticare HN(R) [US-OTC]
cysteine
Ensure(R) [US-OTC]
Ensure Plus(R) [US-OTC]
glucose polymers
Isocal(R) [US-OTC]
Magnacal(R) [US-OTC]
Microlipid(TM) [US-OTC]
Moducal(R) [US-OTC]
nutritional formula, enteral/oral
Osmolite(R) HN [US-OTC]
Pedialyte(R) [US-OTC]
Polycose(R) [US-OTC]
Portagen(R) [US-OTC]
Pregestimil(R) [US-OTC]
Propac(TM) [US-OTC]
Soyalac(R) [US-OTC]
Vital HN(R) [US-OTC]
Vitaneed(TM) [US-OTC]
Vivonex(R) [US-OTC]
Vivonex(R) T.E.N. [US-OTC]
Trace Element
Iodopen(R) [US]
Molypen(R) [US]
M.T.E.-4(R) [US]
M.T.E.-5(R) [US]
M.T.E.-6(R) [US]
M.T.E.-7(R) [US]
Multitrace(TM)-4 [US]
Multitrace(TM)-4 Neonatal [US]
Multitrace(TM)-4 Pediatric [US]
Multitrace(TM)-5 [US]
Neotrace-4(R) [US]
Pedtrace-4(R) [US]
P.T.E.-4(R) [US]
P.T.E.-5(R) [US]

Selepen(R) [US]
trace metals
zinc chloride
Vitamin
ADEKs [US-OTC]
Advanced NatalCare(R) [US]
A-Free Prenatal [US]
AllanFol RX [US]
Aminate Fe-90 [US]
Cal-Nate(TM) [US]
Centrum(R) [US-OTC]
Centrum(R) Kids Jimmy Neutron(R)
Complete [US-OTC]
Centrum(R) Kids Jimmy Neutron(R)
Extra C [US-OTC]
Centrum(R) Kids Rugrats(TM)
Complete [US-OTC]
Centrum(R) Kids Rugrats(TM) Extra
C [US-OTC]
Centrum(R) Kids Rugrats(TM) Extra
Calcium [US-OTC]
Centrum(R) Performance(TM)
[US-OTC]
Centrum(R) Silver(R) [US-OTC]
Chromagen(R) OB [US]
Citracal(R) Prenatal Rx [US]
Duet(R) [US]
Duet(TM) DHA [US]
Flintstones(R) Complete [US-OTC]
Flintstones(R) Plus Calcium
[US-OTC]
Flintstones(R) Plus Extra C
[US-OTC]
Flintstones(R) Plus Iron [US-OTC]
Folbee [US]
Folgard(R) [US-OTC]
folic acid, cyanocobalamin, and
pyridoxine
Foltx(R) [US]
Geriation [US-OTC]
Geritol Complete(R) [US-OTC]
Geritol Extend(R) [US-OTC]
Geritol(R) Tonic [US-OTC]
Glutofac(R)-MX [US]

Glutofac(R)-ZX [US]
Gynovite(R) Plus [US-OTC]
Hemocyte Plus(R) [US]
Hi-Kovite [US-OTC]
Iberet(R) [US-OTC]
Iberet(R)-500 [US-OTC]
Infuvite(R) Adult [US]
Infuvite(R) Pediatric [US]
KPN Prenatal [US]
Monocaps [US-OTC]
Multiret Folic 500 [US]
M.V.I. Adult(TM) [US]
M.V.I(R) Pediatric [US]
My First Flintstones(R) [US-OTC]
NataChew(TM) [US]
NataFort(R) [US]
NatalCare(R) GlossTabs(TM) [US]
NatalCare(R) PIC [US]
NatalCare(R) PIC Forte [US]
NatalCare(R) Plus [US]
NatalCare(R) Rx [US]
NatalCare(R) Three [US]
NataTab(TM) CFe [US]
NataTab(TM) FA [US]
NataTab(TM) Rx [US]
Nestabs(R) CBF [US]
Nestabs(R) FA [US]
Nestabs(R) RX [US]
Niferex(R)-PN [US]
Niferex(R)-PN Forte [US]
NutriNate(R) [US]
OB-20 [US]
Obegyn(R) [US]
Ocuvite(R) [US-OTC]
Ocuvite(R) Extra(R) [US-OTC]
Ocuvite(R) Lutein [US-OTC]
Olay(R) Vitamins Complete
Women's [US-OTC]
Olay(R) Vitamins Complete
Women's 50+[US-OTC]
Olay(R) Vitamins Even Complexion
[US-OTC]
One-A-Day(R) 50 Plus Formula
[US-OTC]

One-A-Day(R) Active Formula [US-OTC]
One-A-Day(R) Carb Smart [US-OTC]
One-A-Day(R) Cholesterol Plus(TM) [US-OTC]
One-A-Day(R) Essential Formula [US-OTC]
One-A-Day(R) Kids Bugs Bunny and Friends Complete [US-OTC]
One-A-Day(R) Kids Bugs Bunny and Friends Plus Extra C [US-OTC]
One-A-Day(R) Kids Extreme Sports [US-OTC]
One-A-Day(R) Kids Scooby-Doo! Complete [US-OTC]
One-A-Day(R) Kids Scooby-Doo! Fizzy Vites [US-OTC]
One-A-Day(R) Kids Scooby-Doo! Plus Calcium [US-OTC]
One-A-Day(R) Maximum Formula [US-OTC]
One-A-Day(R) Men's Formula [US-OTC]
One-A-Day(R) Today [US-OTC]
One-A-Day(R) Weight Smart [US-OTC]
One-A-Day(R) Women's Formula [US-OTC]
Optivite(R) P.M.T. [US-OTC]
Poly-Vi-Flor(R) [US]
Poly-Vi-Flor(R) With Iron [US]
Poly-Vi-Sol(R) [US-OTC]
Poly-Vi-Sol(R) with Iron [US-OTC]
PreCare(R) [US]
PreCare(R) Conceive(TM) [US]
PreCare(R) Prenatal [US]
Prenatal 1-A-Day [US]
Prenatal AD [US]
Prenatal H [US]
Prenatal MR 90 Fe(TM) [US]
Prenatal MTR with Selenium [US]
Prenatal Plus [US]
Prenatal Rx 1 [US]

Prenatal U [US]
Prenatal Z [US]
Prenate Elite(TM) [US]
Prenate GT(TM) [US]
PreserVision(R) AREDS [US-OTC]
PreserVision(R) Lutein [US-OTC]
Quintabs [US-OTC]
Quintabs-M [US-OTC]
Replace [US-OTC]
Replace with Iron [US-OTC]
Repliva 21/7(TM) [US]
Soluvite-F [US]
StrongStart(TM) [US]
Strovite(R) Forte [US]
Stuart Prenatal(R) [US-OTC]
Tricardio B [US]
Trinate [US]
Tri-Vi-Flor(R) [US]
Tri-Vi-Flor(R) with Iron [US]
Tri-Vi-Sol(R) [US-OTC]
Tri-Vi-Sol(R) with Iron [US-OTC]
T-Vites [US-OTC]
Ultra Freeda Iron Free [US-OTC]
Ultra Freeda with Iron [US-OTC]
Ultra NatalCare(R) [US]
Unicap M(R) [US-OTC]
Unicap Sr(R) [US-OTC]
Unicap T(TM) [US-OTC]
Viactiv(R) Multivitamin [US-OTC]
Vicon Forte(R) [US]
Vitaball(R) [US-OTC]
Vitaball(R) Wild 'N Fruity [US-OTC]
Vitacon Forte [US]
vitamins (multiple/injectable)
vitamins (multiple/oral)
vitamins (multiple/pediatric)
vitamins (multiple/prenatal)
Xtramins [US-OTC]
Vitamin, Fat Soluble
Alph-E [US-OTC]
Alph-E-Mixed [US-OTC]
Aquasol A(R) [US]
Aquasol E(R) [US-OTC]
Aquavit-E(R) [US-OTC]

d-Alpha-Gems(TM) [US-OTC]
E-Gems(R) [US-OTC]
E-Gems Elite(R) [US-OTC]
E-Gems Plus(R) [US-OTC]
Ester-E(TM) [US-OTC]
Gamma E-Gems(R) [US-OTC]
Gamma-E Plus [US-OTC]
High Gamma Vitamin E
   Complete(TM) [US-OTC]
Key-E(R) [US-OTC]
Key-E(R) Kaps [US-OTC]
Palmitate-A(R) [US-OTC]
vitamin A
vitamin E
Vitamin, Water Soluble
  Allbee(R) C-800 [US-OTC]
  Allbee(R) C-800 + Iron [US-OTC]
  Allbee(R) with C [US-OTC]
  Aminoxin(R) [US-OTC]
  Apatate(R) [US-OTC]
  Betaxin(R) [Can]
  Diatx(TM) [US]
  DiatxFe(TM) [US]
  Gevrabon(R) [US-OTC]
  NephPlex(R) Rx [US]
  Nephrocaps(R) [US]
  Nephron FA(R) [US]
  Nephro-Vite(R) [US]
  Nephro-Vite(R) Rx [US]
  pyridoxine
  Stresstabs(R) B-Complex [US-OTC]
  Stresstabs(R) B-Complex + Iron
   [US-OTC]
  Stresstabs(R) B-Complex + Zinc
   [US-OTC]
  Surbex-T(R) [US-OTC]
  thiamine
  Trinsicon(R) [US]
  vitamin B complex combinations
  Z-Bec(R) [US-OTC]

MAPLE SYRUP URINE DISEASE

Vitamin, Water Soluble

Betaxin(R) [Can]
thiamine

MASTOCYTOSIS

Histamine H2 Antagonist
  Alti-Ranitidine [Can]
  Apo-Cimetidine(R) [Can]
  Apo-Famotidine(R) [Can]
  Apo-Famotidine(R) Injectable [Can]
  Apo-Ranitidine(R) [Can]
  BCI-Ranitidine [Can]
  cimetidine
  CO Ranitidine [Can]
  famotidine
  Famotidine Omega [Can]
  Gen-Cimetidine [Can]
  Gen-Famotidine [Can]
  Gen-Ranidine [Can]
  Novo-Cimetidine [Can]
  Novo-Famotidine [Can]
  Novo-Ranidine [Can]
  Nu-Cimet [Can]
  Nu-Famotidine [Can]
  Nu-Ranit [Can]
  Pepcid(R) [US/Can]
  Pepcid(R) AC [US-OTC/Can]
  Pepcid(R) I.V. [Can]
  PMS-Cimetidine [Can]
  PMS-Ranitidine [Can]
  ranitidine
  Ranitidine Injection, USP [Can]
  Rhoxal-ranitidine [Can]
  Riva-Famotidine [Can]
  Sandoz-Ranitidine [Can]
  Tagamet(R) [US]
  Tagamet(R) HB [Can]
  Tagamet(R) HB 200 [US-OTC]
  Ulcidine [Can]
  Zantac(R) [US/Can]
  Zantac 75(R) [US-OTC/Can]
  Zantac 150(TM) [US-OTC]
  Zantac(R) EFFERdose(R) [US]
Mast Cell Stabilizer
  Apo-Cromolyn(R) [Can]

Crolom(R) [US]
cromolyn sodium
Gastrocrom(R) [US]
Intal(R) [US/Can]
Nalcrom(R) [Can]
NasalCrom(R) [US-OTC]
Nu-Cromolyn [Can]
Opticrom(R) [US/Can]

MECONIUM ILEUS
Mucolytic Agent
Acetadote(R) [US]
acetylcysteine
Acetylcysteine Solution [Can]
Mucomyst(R) [Can]
Parvolex(R) [Can]

NAUSEA
Anticholinergic Agent
Buscopan(R) [Can]
Isopto(R) Hyoscine [US]
Scopace(TM) [US]
scopolamine derivatives
Tebamide(TM) [US]
Tigan(R) [US/Can]
Transderm-V(R) [Can]
Transderm Scŏp(R) [US]
trimethobenzamide
Antiemetic
Aloxi(R) [US]
aprepitant
dronabinol
droperidol
Emend(R) [US]
Emetrol(R) [US-OTC]
Especol(R) [US-OTC]
Formula EM [US-OTC]
fructose, dextrose, and phosphoric
acid
Inapsine(R) [US]
Kalmz [US-OTC]
Marinol(R) [US/Can]
Nausea Relief [US-OTC]
palonosetron
Phenadoz(TM) [US]

Phenergan(R) [US/Can]
promethazine
Promethegan(TM) [US]
Tebamide(TM) [US]
Tigan(R) [US/Can]
trimethobenzamide
Antihistamine
Apo-Dimenhydrinate(R) [Can]
Children's Motion Sickness Liquid
[Can]
Diclectin(R) [Can]
dimenhydrinate
Dinate(R) [Can]
doxylamine and pyridoxine (Canada
only)
Dramamine(R) [US-OTC]
Gravol(R) [Can]
Jamp(R) Travel Tablet [Can]
Nauseatol [Can]
Novo-Dimenate [Can]
SAB-Dimenhydrinate [Can]
Gastrointestinal Agent, Prokinetic
Apo-Metoclop(R) [Can]
metoclopramide
Metoclopramide Hydrochloride
Injection [Can]
Nu-Metoclopramide [Can]
Reglan(R) [US]
Phenothiazine Derivative
Apo-Perphenazine(R) [Can]
Apo-Prochlorperazine(R) [Can]
chlorpromazine
Compazine(R) [Can]
Compro(TM) [US]
Largactil(R) [Can]
Novo-Chlorpromazine [Can]
Nu-Prochlor [Can]
perphenazine
Phenadoz(TM) [US]
Phenergan(R) [US/Can]
prochlorperazine
promethazine
Promethegan(TM) [US]
Stemetil(R) [Can]

Selective 5-HT3 Receptor Antagonist
  Aloxi(R) [US]
  granisetron
  Kytril(R) [US/Can]
  ondansetron
  palonosetron
  Zofran(R) [US/Can]
  Zofran(R) ODT [US/Can]
Vitamin
  Diclectin(R) [Can]
  doxylamine and pyridoxine (Canada
    only)

NEPHROLITHIASIS
Alkalinizing Agent
  K-Citra(R) [Can]
  potassium citrate
  Urocit(R)-K [US]

NEPHROPATHIC CYSTINOSIS
Urinary Tract Product
  Cystagon(R) [US]
  cysteamine

NEPHROTIC SYNDROME
Adrenal Corticosteroid
  Apo-Dexamethasone(R) [Can]
  Apo-Prednisone(R) [Can]
  Aristocort(R) [US/Can]
  Aristospan(R) [US/Can]
  Betaject(TM) [Can]
  betamethasone (systemic)
  Bubbli-Pred(TM) [US]
  Celestone(R) [US]
  Celestone(R) Soluspan(R)
    [US/Can]
  Cortef(R) [US/Can]
  corticotropin
  cortisone acetate
  Decadron(R) [US]
  Depo-Medrol(R) [US/Can]
  Dexamethasone Intensol(R) [US]
  dexamethasone (systemic)
  Dexasone(R) [Can]

DexPak(R) TaperPak(R) [US]
Diodex(R) [Can]
Diopred(R) [Can]
H.P. Acthar(R) Gel [US]
Hydeltra T.B.A.(R) [Can]
hydrocortisone (systemic)
Kenalog(R) [US/Can]
Kenalog-10(R) [US]
Kenalog-40(R) [US]
Medrol(R) [US/Can]
methylprednisolone
Novo-Prednisolone [Can]
Novo-Prednisone [Can]
Oracort [Can]
Orapred(R) [US]
Pediapred(R) [US/Can]
PMS-Dexamethasone [Can]
prednisolone (systemic)
prednisone
Prednisone Intensol(TM) [US]
Prelone(R) [US]
Sab-Prenase [Can]
Solu-Cortef(R) [US/Can]
Solu-Medrol(R) [US/Can]
Sterapred(R) [US]
Sterapred(R) DS [US]
triamcinolone (systemic)
Winpred(TM) [Can]
Antihypertensive Agent, Combination
  Aldactazide(R) [US]
  Aldactazide 25(R) [Can]
  Aldactazide 50(R) [Can]
  Apo-Triazide(R) [Can]
  Dyazide(R) [US]
  hydrochlorothiazide and
    spironolactone
  hydrochlorothiazide and triamterene
  Maxzide(R) [US]
  Maxzide(R)-25 [US]
  Novo-Spirozine [Can]
  Novo-Triamzide [Can]
  Nu-Triazide [Can]
  Penta-Triamterene HCTZ [Can]
  Riva-Zide [Can]

Antineoplastic Agent
chlorambucil
cyclophosphamide
Cytoxan(R) [US/Can]
Leukeran(R) [US/Can]
Procytox(R) [Can]
Diuretic, Loop
Apo-Furosemide(R) [Can]
bumetanide
Bumex(R) [US/Can]
Burinex(R) [Can]
Demadex(R) [US]
furosemide
Furosemide Injection, USP
[Can]
Furosemide Special [Can]
Lasix(R) [US/Can]
Lasix(R) Special [Can]
Novo-Semide [Can]
torsemide
Diuretic, Miscellaneous
Apo-Chlorthalidone(R)
[Can]
Apo-Indapamide(R) [Can]
chlorthalidone
Gen-Indapamide [Can]
indapamide
Lozide(R) [Can]
Lozol(R) [US/Can]
metolazone
Mykrox(R) [Can]
Novo-Indapamide [Can]
Nu-Indapamide [Can]
PMS-Indapamide [Can]
Thalitone(R) [US]
Zaroxolyn(R) [US/Can]
Diuretic, Thiazide
Apo-Hydro(R) [Can]
Aquatensen(R) [Can]
chlorothiazide
Diuril(R) [US/Can]
Enduron(R) [Can]
hydrochlorothiazide
methyclothiazide

Microzide(TM) [US]
Novo-Hydrazide [Can]
PMS-Hydrochlorothiazide
[Can]
Immunosuppressant Agent
Alti-Azathioprine [Can]
Apo-Azathioprine(R) [Can]
Azasan(R) [US]
azathioprine
cyclosporine
Gen-Azathioprine [Can]
Gengraf(R) [US]
Imuran(R) [US/Can]
Neoral(R) [US/Can]
Novo-Azathioprine [Can]
Restasis(R) [US]
Rhoxal-cyclosporine [Can]
Sandimmune(R) [US]
Sandimmune(R) I.V. [Can]
Sandoz-Cyclosporine [Can]

NEPHROTOXICITY (CISPLATIN-INDUCED)
Antidote
amifostine
Ethyol(R) [US/Can]

NEUROGENIC BLADDER
Antispasmodic Agent, Urinary
Apo-Oxybutynin(R) [Can]
Ditropan(R) [US/Can]
Ditropan(R) XL [US/Can]
Gen-Oxybutynin [Can]
Novo-Oxybutynin [Can]
Nu-Oxybutyn [Can]
oxybutynin
Oxytrol(R) [US/Can]
PMS-Oxybutynin [Can]
Uromax(R) [Can]

NOCTURIA
Antispasmodic Agent, Urinary
Apo-Flavoxate(R) [Can]
flavoxate
Urispas(R) [US/Can]

ORGAN REJECTION
Immunosuppressant Agent
  daclizumab
  Zenapax(R) [US/Can]

ORGAN TRANSPLANT
Immunosuppressant Agent
  basiliximab
  CellCept(R) [US/Can]
  cyclosporine
  Gengraf(R) [US]
  muromonab-CD3
  mycophenolate
  Myfortic(R) [US/Can]
  Neoral(R) [US/Can]
  Orthoclone OKT(R) 3 [US/Can]
  Prograf(R) [US/Can]
  Protopic(R) [US/Can]
  Rapamune(R) [US/Can]
  Restasis(R) [US]
  Rhoxal-cyclosporine [Can]
  Sandimmune(R) [US]
  Sandimmune(R) I.V. [Can]
  Sandoz-Cyclosporine [Can]
  Simulect(R) [US/Can]
  sirolimus
  tacrolimus

OSTOMY CARE
Protectant, Topical
  A and D(R) Original [US-OTC]
  Baza(R) Clear [US-OTC]
  Sween Cream(R) [US-OTC]
  vitamin A and vitamin D

OVERACTIVE BLADDER
Anticholinergic Agent
  darifenacin
  Detrol(R) [US/Can]
  Detrol(R) LA [US/Can]
  Enablex(R) [US/Can]
  Sanctura(TM) [US]
  solifenacin
  tolterodine
  Trosec [Can]
  trospium
  Unidet(R) [Can]
  VESIcare(R) [US]

PAIN (ANOGENITAL)
Anesthetic/Corticosteroid
  Analpram-HC(R) [US]
  Enzone(R) [US]
  Epifoam(R) [US]
  Pramosone(R) [US]
  Pramox(R) HC [Can]
  pramoxine and hydrocortisone
  ProctoFoam(R)-HC [US/Can]
  Zone-A(R) [US]
  Zone-A Forte(R) [US]
Local Anesthetic
  Americaine(R) [US-OTC]
  Americaine(R) Hemorrhoidal
    [US-OTC]
  benzocaine
  dibucaine
  dyclonine
  Foille(R) [US-OTC]
  Hurricaine(R) [US-OTC]
  Mycinettes(R) [US-OTC]
  Nupercainal(R) [US-OTC]
  Pontocaine(R) [US/Can]
  Pontocaine(R) Niphanoid(R) [US]
  pramoxine
  Prax(R) [US-OTC]
  ProctoFoam(R) NS [US-OTC]
  tetracaine
  Trocaine(R) [US-OTC]
  Tronolane(R) [US-OTC]
  Tucks(R) Hemorrhoidal [US-OTC]

PANCREATIC EXOCRINE INSUFFICIENCY
Enzyme
  Cotazym(R) [Can]
  Creon(R) [US]
  Creon(R) 5 [Can]
  Creon(R) 10 [Can]
  Creon(R) 20 [Can]

Creon(R) 25 [Can]
ku-zyme(R) HP [US]
Lipram 4500 [US]
Lipram-CR [US]
Lipram-PN [US]
Lipram-UL [US]
Palcaps [US]
Pancrease(R) [Can]
Pancrease(R) MT [US/Can]
Pancrecarb MS(R) [US]
pancrelipase
Pangestyme(TM) CN [US]
Pangestyme(TM) EC [US]
Pangestyme(TM) MT [US]
Pangestyme(TM) UL [US]
Panocaps [US]
Panocaps MT [US]
Panokase(R) [US]
Panokase(R) 16 [US]
Plaretase(R) 8000 [US]
Ultracaps MT [US]
Ultrase(R) [US/Can]
Ultrase(R) MT [US/Can]
Viokase(R) [US/Can]

PANCREATIC EXOCRINE INSUFFICIENCY (DIAGNOSTIC)

Diagnostic Agent
SecreFlo(TM) [US]
secretin

PARALYTIC ILEUS (PROPHYLAXIS)

Gastrointestinal Agent, Stimulant
dexpanthenol
Panthoderm(R) [US-OTC]

PEPTIC ULCER

Amebicide
Apo-Metronidazole(R) [Can]
Flagyl(R) [US/Can]
Flagyl ER(R) [US]
Flagyl(R) I.V. RTU(TM) [US]
Florazole(R) ER [Can]

MetroCream(R) [US/Can]
MetroGel(R) [US/Can]
MetroGel-Vaginal(R) [US]
MetroLotion(R) [US]
metronidazole
Nidagel(TM) [Can]
Noritate(R) [US/Can]
Trikacide [Can]
Vandazole(TM) [US]
Antibiotic, Miscellaneous
Apo-Metronidazole(R) [Can]
Flagyl(R) [US/Can]
Flagyl ER(R) [US]
Flagyl(R) I.V. RTU(TM) [US]
Florazole(R) ER [Can]
MetroCream(R) [US/Can]
MetroGel(R) [US/Can]
MetroGel-Vaginal(R) [US]
MetroLotion(R) [US]
metronidazole
Nidagel(TM) [Can]
Noritate(R) [US/Can]
Trikacide [Can]
Vandazole(TM) [US]
Anticholinergic Agent
Anaspaz(R) [US]
Apo-Chlorax(R) [Can]
AtroPen(R) [US]
atropine
Atropine-Care(R) [US]
Cantil(R) [Can]
clidinium and chlordiazepoxide
Cystospaz(R) [US/Can]
Dioptic's Atropine Solution [Can]
Donnatal(R) [US]
Donnatal Extentabs(R) [US]
glycopyrrolate
hyoscyamine
hyoscyamine, atropine, scopolamine,
    and phenobarbital
Hyosine [US]
Isopto(R) Atropine [US/Can]
Levbid(R) [US]
Levsin(R) [US/Can]

Levsinex(R) [US]
Levsin/SL(R) [US]
Librax(R) [US/Can]
mepenzolate
methscopolamine
NuLev(TM) [US]
Pamine(R) [US/Can]
Pamine(R) Forte [US]
propantheline
Robinul(R) [US]
Robinul(R) Forte [US]
Sal-Tropine(TM) [US]
Symax SL [US]
Symax SR [US]
Antiprotozoal
Apo-Metronidazole(R) [Can]
Flagyl(R) [US/Can]
Flagyl ER(R) [US]
Flagyl(R) I.V. RTU(TM) [US]
Florazole(R) ER [Can]
MetroCream(R) [US/Can]
MetroGel(R) [US/Can]
MetroGel-Vaginal(R) [US]
MetroLotion(R) [US]
metronidazole
Nidagel(TM) [Can]
Noritate(R) [US/Can]
Trikacide [Can]
Vandazole(TM) [US]
Gastric Acid Secretion Inhibitor
Apo-Omeprazole(R) [Can]
lansoprazole
lansoprazole and naproxen
Losec(R) [Can]
Losec MUPS(R) [Can]
omeprazole
Prevacid(R) [US/Can]
Prevacid(R) NapraPAC(TM) [US]
Prevacid(R) SoluTab(TM) [US]
Prilosec(R) [US]
Prilosec OTC(TM) [US-OTC]
Gastrointestinal Agent, Gastric or
Duodenal Ulcer Treatment
Carafate(R) [US]

Novo-Sucralate [Can]
Nu-Sucralate [Can]
PMS-Sucralate [Can]
sucralfate
Sulcrate(R) [Can]
Sulcrate(R) Suspension Plus [Can]
Gastrointestinal Agent, Miscellaneous
bismuth subsalicylate
Children's Kaopectate(R)
(reformulation) [US-OTC]
Colo-Fresh(TM) [US-OTC]
Diotame(R) [US-OTC]
Kaopectate(R) [US-OTC]
Kaopectate(R) Extra Strength
[US-OTC]
Pepto-Bismol(R) [US-OTC]
Pepto-Bismol(R) Maximum Strength
[US-OTC]
Histamine H2 Antagonist
Alti-Ranitidine [Can]
Apo-Cimetidine(R) [Can]
Apo-Famotidine(R) [Can]
Apo-Famotidine(R) Injectable [Can]
Apo-Nizatidine(R) [Can]
Apo-Ranitidine(R) [Can]
Axid(R) [US/Can]
Axid(R) AR [US-OTC]
BCI-Ranitidine [Can]
cimetidine
CO Ranitidine [Can]
famotidine
Famotidine Omega [Can]
Gen-Cimetidine [Can]
Gen-Famotidine [Can]
Gen-Nizatidine [Can]
Gen-Ranidine [Can]
nizatidine
Novo-Cimetidine [Can]
Novo-Famotidine [Can]
Novo-Nizatidine [Can]
Novo-Ranidine [Can]
Nu-Cimet [Can]
Nu-Famotidine [Can]
Nu-Nizatidine [Can]

Nu-Ranit [Can]
Pepcid(R) [US/Can]
Pepcid(R) AC [US-OTC/Can]
Pepcid(R) I.V. [Can]
PMS-Cimetidine [Can]
PMS-Nizatidine [Can]
PMS-Ranitidine [Can]
ranitidine
Ranitidine Injection, USP [Can]
Rhoxal-ranitidine [Can]
Riva-Famotidine [Can]
Sandoz-Ranitidine [Can]
Tagamet(R) [US]
Tagamet(R) HB [Can]
Tagamet(R) HB 200 [US-OTC]
Ulcidine [Can]
Zantac(R) [US/Can]
Zantac 75(R) [US-OTC/Can]
Zantac 150(TM) [US-OTC]
Zantac(R) EFFERdose(R) [US]
Macrolide (Antibiotic)
Biaxin(R) [US/Can]
Biaxin(R) XL [US/Can]
clarithromycin
ratio-Clarithromycin [Can]
Penicillin
amoxicillin
Amoxil(R) [US]
Apo-Amoxi(R) [Can]
Gen-Amoxicillin [Can]
Lin-Amox [Can]
Novamoxin(R) [Can]
Nu-Amoxi [Can]
PHL-Amoxicillin [Can]
PMS-Amoxicillin [Can]

PERIANAL WART
Immune Response Modifier
Aldara(TM) [US/Can]
imiquimod

PINWORMS
Anthelmintic
Combantrin(TM) [Can]
mebendazole

Pamix(TM) [US-OTC]
Pin-X(R) [US-OTC]
pyrantel pamoate
Reese's(R) Pinworm Medicine
[US-OTC]
Vermox(R) [Can]

PROCTITIS
5-Aminosalicylic Acid Derivative
Asacol(R) [US/Can]
Asacol(R) 800 [Can]
Canasa(TM) [US]
mesalamine
Mesasal(R) [Can]
Novo-5 ASA [Can]
Pendo-5 ASA [Can]
Pentasa(R) [US/Can]
Quintasa(R) [Can]
Rowasa(R) [US/Can]
Salofalk(R) [Can]

PROCTOSIGMOIDITIS
5-Aminosalicylic Acid Derivative
Asacol(R) [US/Can]
Asacol(R) 800 [Can]
Canasa(TM) [US]
mesalamine
Mesasal(R) [Can]
Novo-5 ASA [Can]
Pendo-5 ASA [Can]
Pentasa(R) [US/Can]
Quintasa(R) [Can]
Rowasa(R) [US/Can]
Salofalk(R) [Can]

PROSTATITIS
Sulfonamide
Apo-Sulfatrim(R) [Can]
Apo-Sulfatrim(R) DS [Can]
Apo-Sulfatrim(R) Pediatric [Can]
Bactrim(TM) [US]
Bactrim(TM) DS [US]
Novo-Trimel [Can]
Novo-Trimel D.S. [Can]
Nu-Cotrimox [Can]

Septra(R) [US]
Septra(R) DS [US]
Septra(R) Injection [Can]
sulfamethoxazole and trimethoprim

PROTEIN UTILIZATION
Dietary Supplement
l-lysine
Lysinyl [US-OTC]

PROTOZOAL INFECTIONS
Amebicide
Apo-Metronidazole(R) [Can]
Flagyl(R) [US/Can]
Flagyl ER(R) [US]
Flagyl(R) I.V. RTU(TM) [US]
Florazole(R) ER [Can]
MetroCream(R) [US/Can]
MetroGel(R) [US/Can]
MetroGel-Vaginal(R) [US]
MetroLotion(R) [US]
metronidazole
Nidagel(TM) [Can]
Noritate(R) [US/Can]
Trikacide [Can]
Vandazole(TM) [US]
Antibiotic, Miscellaneous
Apo-Metronidazole(R) [Can]
Flagyl(R) [US/Can]
Flagyl ER(R) [US]
Flagyl(R) I.V. RTU(TM) [US]
Florazole(R) ER [Can]
MetroCream(R) [US/Can]
MetroGel(R) [US/Can]
MetroGel-Vaginal(R) [US]
MetroLotion(R) [US]
metronidazole
Nidagel(TM) [Can]
Noritate(R) [US/Can]
Trikacide [Can]
Vandazole(TM) [US]
Antiprotozoal
Apo-Metronidazole(R) [Can]
Flagyl(R) [US/Can]
Flagyl ER(R) [US]

Flagyl(R) I.V. RTU(TM) [US]
Florazole(R) ER [Can]
MetroCream(R) [US/Can]
MetroGel(R) [US/Can]
MetroGel-Vaginal(R) [US]
MetroLotion(R) [US]
metronidazole
NebuPent(R) [US]
Nidagel(TM) [Can]
Noritate(R) [US/Can]
Pentam-300(R) [US]
pentamidine
Trikacide [Can]
Vandazole(TM) [US]

PYELONEPHRITIS
Antibiotic, Carbapenem
ertapenem
Invanz(R) [US/Can]
Antibiotic, Quinolone
gatifloxacin
Tequin(R) [Can]
Zymar(TM) [US/Can]

RENAL ALLOGRAFT REJECTION
Immunosuppressant Agent
antithymocyte globulin (rabbit)
Thymoglobulin(R) [US]

RENAL COLIC
Analgesic, Nonnarcotic
Acular(R) [US/Can]
Acular LS(TM) [US/Can]
Acular(R) PF [US]
Apo-Ketorolac(R) [Can]
Apo-Ketorolac Injectable(R)
[Can]
ketorolac
Ketorolac Tromethamine Injection,
USP [Can]
Novo-Ketorolac [Can]
ratio-Ketorolac [Can]
Toradol(R) [US/Can]
Toradol(R) IM [Can]

Anticholinergic Agent
  Donnatal(R) [US]
  Donnatal Extentabs(R) [US]
  hyoscyamine, atropine, scopolamine,
    and phenobarbital
Nonsteroidal Antiinflammatory Drug
  (NSAID)
  Acular(R) [US/Can]
  Acular LS(TM) [US/Can]
  Acular(R) PF [US]
  Apo-Ketorolac(R) [Can]
  Apo-Ketorolac Injectable(R) [Can]
  ketorolac
  Ketorolac Tromethamine Injection,
    USP [Can]
  Novo-Ketorolac [Can]
  ratio-Ketorolac [Can]
  Toradol(R) [US/Can]
  Toradol(R) IM [Can]

ROUNDWORMS
Anthelmintic
  Combantrin(TM) [Can]
  mebendazole
  Pamix(TM) [US-OTC]
  Pin-X(R) [US-OTC]
  pyrantel pamoate
  Reese's(R) Pinworm Medicine
    [US-OTC]
  Vermox(R) [Can]

SALIVATION (EXCESSIVE)
Anticholinergic Agent
  Anaspaz(R) [US]
  AtroPen(R) [US]
  atropine
  Buscopan(R) [Can]
  Cantil(R) [Can]
  Cystospaz(R) [US/Can]
  glycopyrrolate
  hyoscyamine
  Hyosine [US]
  Isopto(R) Hyoscine [US]
  Levbid(R) [US]
  Levsin(R) [US/Can]

  Levsinex(R) [US]
  Levsin/SL(R) [US]
  mepenzolate
  NuLev(TM) [US]
  Robinul(R) [US]
  Robinul(R) Forte [US]
  Sal-Tropine(TM) [US]
  Scopace(TM) [US]
  scopolamine derivatives
  Symax SL [US]
  Symax SR [US]

STOMATITIS
Local Anesthetic
  Cĕpacol(R) Dual Action Maximum
    Strength [US-OTC]
  dyclonine
  Sucrets(R) [US-OTC]
Skin and Mucous Membrane Agent
  Gelclair(R) [US]
  maltodextrin
  Multidex(R) [US-OTC]
  OraRinse(TM) [US-OTC]

SYPHILIS
Antibiotic, Miscellaneous
  chloramphenicol
  Chloromycetin(R) [Can]
  Chloromycetin(R) Sodium Succinate
    [US]
  Chloromycetin(R) Succinate [Can]
  Diochloram(R) [Can]
  Pentamycetin(R) [Can]
Penicillin
  Bicillin(R) L-A [US]
  penicillin G benzathine
  penicillin G (parenteral/aqueous)
  penicillin G procaine
  Pfizerpen(R) [US/Can]
  Pfizerpen-AS(R) [Can]
  Wycillin(R) [Can]
Tetracycline Derivative
  Adoxa(TM) [US]
  Apo-Doxy(R) [Can]
  Apo-Doxy Tabs(R) [Can]

Apo-Tetra(R) [Can]
Doryx(R) [US]
Doxy-100(R) [US]
Doxycin [Can]
doxycycline
Doxytec [Can]
Monodox(R) [US]
Novo-Doxylin [Can]
Nu-Doxycycline [Can]
Nu-Tetra [Can]
Periostat(R) [US/Can]
Sumycin(R) [US]
tetracycline
Vibramycin(R) [US]
Vibra-Tabs(R) [US/Can]

TAPEWORM INFESTATION
Amebicide
Humatin(R) [US/Can]
paromomycin

TENESMUS
Analgesic, Narcotic
belladonna and opium
B&O Supprettes(R) [US]

THREADWORM (NONDISSEMINATED INTESTINAL)
Antibiotic, Miscellaneous
ivermectin
Stromectol(R) [US]

ULCER (DUODENAL)
Proton Pump Inhibitor
Panto(TM) IV [Can]
Pantoloc(R) [Can]
pantoprazole
Protonix(R) [US/Can]

ULCER (GASTRIC)
Proton Pump Inhibitor
Panto(TM) IV [Can]
Pantoloc(R) [Can]
pantoprazole
Protonix(R) [US/Can]

UPPER GASTROINTESTINAL MOTILITY DISORDERS
Dopamine Antagonist
Alti-Domperidone [Can]
Apo-Domperidone(R) [Can]
Dom-Domperidone [Can]
domperidone (Canada only)
FTP-Domperidone Maleate [Can]
Motilium(R) [Can]
Novo-Domperidone [Can]
Nu-Domperidone [Can]
RAN(TM)-Domperidone [Can]
ratio-Domperidone [Can]

URINARY BLADDER SPASM
Anticholinergic Agent
propantheline

URINARY RETENTION
Antispasmodic Agent, Urinary
Apo-Oxybutynin(R) [Can]
Ditropan(R) [US/Can]
Ditropan(R) XL [US/Can]
Gen-Oxybutynin [Can]
Novo-Oxybutynin [Can]
Nu-Oxybutyn [Can]
oxybutynin
Oxytrol(R) [US/Can]
PMS-Oxybutynin [Can]
Uromax(R) [Can]
Cholinergic Agent
bethanechol
Duvoid(R) [Can]
Myotonachol(R) [Can]
neostigmine
PMS-Bethanechol [Can]
Prostigmin(R) [US/Can]
Urecholine(R) [US]

URINARY TRACT INFECTION
Antibiotic, Carbacephem
Lorabid(R) [US/Can]
loracarbef

Antibiotic, Miscellaneous
  Apo-Nitrofurantoin(R) [Can]
  Apo-Trimethoprim(R) [Can]
  Azactam(R) [US/Can]
  aztreonam
  Dehydral(R) [Can]
  fosfomycin
  Furadantin(R) [US]
  Hiprex(R) [US/Can]
  Macrobid(R) [US/Can]
  Macrodantin(R) [US/Can]
  Mandelamine(R) [US/Can]
  methenamine
  Monurol(TM) [US/Can]
  nitrofurantoin
  Novo-Furantoin [Can]
  Primsol(R) [US]
  Proloprim(R) [US]
  trimethoprim
  Urasal(R) [Can]
  Urex(R) [US/Can]
  Vancocin(R) [US/Can]
  vancomycin
Antibiotic, Quinolone
  gatifloxacin
  Iquix(R) [US]
  Levaquin(R) [US/Can]
  levofloxacin
  Novo-Levofloxacin [Can]
  Quixin(TM) [US]
  Tequin(R) [Can]
  Zymar(TM) [US/Can]
Antibiotic, Urinary Antiinfective
  Atrosept(R) [US]
  Dolsed(R) [US]
  methenamine, phenyl salicylate,
    atropine, hyoscyamine, benzoic
    acid, and methylene blue
  UAA(R) [US]
  Uridon Modified(R) [US]
  Urised(R) [US]
  Uritin(R) [US]
Cephalosporin (First Generation)
  Ancef(R) [US]

Apo-Cefadroxil(R) [Can]
Apo-Cephalex(R) [Can]
Biocef(R) [US]
cefadroxil
cefazolin
cephalexin
cephalothin
Duricef(R) [US/Can]
Keflex(R) [US]
Keftab(R) [Can]
Novo-Cefadroxil [Can]
Novo-Lexin [Can]
Nu-Cephalex [Can]
Cephalosporin (Second Generation)
  Apo-Cefaclor(R) [Can]
  Apo-Cefuroxime(R) [Can]
  Ceclor(R) [Can]
  cefaclor
  cefoxitin
  cefpodoxime
  cefprozil
  Ceftin(R) [US/Can]
  cefuroxime
  Cefzil(R) [US/Can]
  Mefoxin(R) [US]
  Novo-Cefaclor [Can]
  Nu-Cefaclor [Can]
  PMS-Cefaclor [Can]
  Raniclor(TM) [US]
  ratio-Cefuroxime [Can]
  Vantin(R) [US/Can]
  Zinacef(R) [US/Can]
Cephalosporin (Third Generation)
  Cedax(R) [US]
  Cefizox(R) [US/Can]
  cefotaxime
  ceftazidime
  ceftibuten
  ceftizoxime
  ceftriaxone
  Claforan(R) [US/Can]
  Fortaz(R) [US/Can]
  Rocephin(R) [US/Can]
  Tazicef(R) [US]

Cephalosporin (Fourth Generation)
  cefepime
  Maxipime(R) [US/Can]
Genitourinary Irrigant
  neomycin and polymyxin B
  Neosporin(R) G.U. Irrigant [US]
  Neosporin(R) Irrigating Solution
    [Can]
Irrigating Solution
  citric acid, magnesium carbonate, and
    glucono-delta-lactone
  Renacidin(R) [US]
Penicillin
  Alti-Amoxi-Clav [Can]
  amoxicillin
  amoxicillin and clavulanate
    potassium
  Amoxil(R) [US]
  ampicillin
  ampicillin and sulbactam
  Apo-Amoxi(R) [Can]
  Apo-Amoxi-Clav(R) [Can]
  Apo-Ampi(R) [Can]
  Apo-Cloxi(R) [Can]
  Apo-Pen VK(R) [Can]
  Augmentin(R) [US/Can]
  Augmentin ES-600(R) [US]
  Augmentin XR(TM) [US]
  Bicillin(R) L-A [US]
  Bicillin(R) C-R [US]
  Bicillin(R) C-R 900/300 [US]
  carbenicillin
  Clavulin(R) [Can]
  cloxacillin
  dicloxacillin
  Dycill(R) [Can]
  Gen-Amoxicillin [Can]
  Geocillin(R) [US]
  Lin-Amox [Can]
  nafcillin
  Nallpen(R) [Can]
  Novamoxin(R) [Can]
  Novo-Ampicillin [Can]
  Novo-Clavamoxin [Can]

Novo-Cloxin [Can]
Novo-Pen-VK [Can]
Nu-Amoxi [Can]
Nu-Ampi [Can]
Nu-Cloxi [Can]
Nu-Pen-VK [Can]
oxacillin
Pathocil(R) [Can]
penicillin V potassium
penicillin G benzathine
penicillin G benzathine and penicillin
  G procaine
penicillin G (parenteral/aqueous)
penicillin G procaine
Pfizerpen(R) [US/Can]
Pfizerpen-AS(R) [Can]
PHL-Amoxicillin [Can]
piperacillin
piperacillin and tazobactam sodium
Piperacillin for Injection, USP [Can]
pivampicillin (Canada only)
PMS-Amoxicillin [Can]
Pondocillin(R) [Can]
ratio-Aclavulanate [Can]
Riva-Cloxacillin [Can]
Tazocin(R) [Can]
Ticar(R) [US]
ticarcillin
ticarcillin and clavulanate potassium
Timentin(R) [US/Can]
Unasyn(R) [US/Can]
Unipen(R) [Can]
Veetids(R) [US]
Wycillin(R) [Can]
Zosyn(R) [US]
Quinolone
  Apo-Norflox(R) [Can]
  Apo-Oflox(R) [Can]
  Apo-Ofloxacin(R) [Can]
  CO Norfloxacin [Can]
  Floxin(R) [US/Can]
  norfloxacin
  Norfloxacine(R) [Can]
  Noroxin(R) [US/Can]

Novo-Norfloxacin [Can]
Novo-Ofloxacin [Can]
ofloxacin
PMS-Norfloxacin [Can]
PMS-Ofloxacin [Can]
Riva-Norfloxacin [Can]
Sulfonamide
Apo-Sulfatrim(R) [Can]
Apo-Sulfatrim(R) DS [Can]
Apo-Sulfatrim(R) Pediatric [Can]
Bactrim(TM) [US]
Bactrim(TM) DS [US]
Gantrisin(R) [US]
Novo-Soxazole [Can]
Novo-Trimel [Can]
Novo-Trimel D.S. [Can]
Nu-Cotrimox [Can]
Septra(R) [US]
Septra(R) DS [US]
Septra(R) Injection [Can]
sulfadiazine
sulfamethoxazole and trimethoprim
sulfisoxazole
Sulfizole(R) [Can]
Urinary Tract Product
acetohydroxamic acid
Atrosept(R) [US]
Dolsed(R) [US]
Lithostat(R) [US/Can]
methenamine, phenyl salicylate,
atropine, hyoscyamine, benzoic
acid, and methylene blue
UAA(R) [US]
Uridon Modified(R) [US]
Urised(R) [US]
Uritin(R) [US]

VASOACTIVE INTESTINAL PEPTIDE-SECRETING TUMOR (VIP)

Somatostatin Analog
octreotide
Octreotide Acetate Injection [Can]
Octreotide Acetate Omega [Can]

Sandostatin(R) [US/Can]
Sandostatin LAR(R) [US/Can]

VENEREAL WARTS

Biological Response Modulator
Alferon(R) N [US/Can]
interferon alfa-n3

VOMITING

Anticholinergic Agent
Buscopan(R) [Can]
Isopto(R) Hyoscine [US]
Scopace(TM) [US]
scopolamine derivatives
Tebamide(TM) [US]
Tigan(R) [US/Can]
Transderm-V(R) [Can]
Transderm Scŏp(R) [US]
trimethobenzamide
Antiemetic
Aloxi(R) [US]
Apo-Hydroxyzine(R) [Can]
aprepitant
Atarax(R) [Can]
dronabinol
droperidol
Emend(R) [US]
hydroxyzine
Hydroxyzine Hydrochloride
Injection, USP [Can]
Inapsine(R) [US]
Marinol(R) [US/Can]
Novo-Hydroxyzin [Can]
palonosetron
Phenadoz(TM) [US]
Phenergan(R) [US/Can]
PMS-Hydroxyzine [Can]
promethazine
Promethegan(TM) [US]
Tebamide(TM) [US]
Tigan(R) [US/Can]
trimethobenzamide
Vistaril(R) [US/Can]
Antihistamine
Apo-Dimenhydrinate(R) [Can]

Apo-Hydroxyzine(R) [Can]
Atarax(R) [Can]
Children's Motion Sickness Liquid
[Can]
Diclectin(R) [Can]
dimenhydrinate
Dinate(R) [Can]
doxylamine and pyridoxine (Canada
only)
Dramamine(R) [US-OTC]
Gravol(R) [Can]
hydroxyzine
Hydroxyzine Hydrochloride
Injection, USP [Can]
Jamp(R) Travel Tablet [Can]
Nauseatol [Can]
Novo-Dimenate [Can]
Novo-Hydroxyzin [Can]
PMS-Hydroxyzine [Can]
SAB-Dimenhydrinate [Can]
Vistaril(R) [US/Can]
Phenothiazine Derivative
Apo-Perphenazine(R) [Can]
Apo-Prochlorperazine(R) [Can]
chlorpromazine
Compazine(R) [Can]
Compro(TM) [US]
Largactil(R) [Can]
Novo-Chlorpromazine [Can]
Nu-Prochlor [Can]
perphenazine
Phenadoz(TM) [US]
Phenergan(R) [US/Can]
prochlorperazine
promethazine
Promethegan(TM) [US]
Stemetil(R) [Can]
Selective 5-HT3 Receptor Antagonist
Aloxi(R) [US]
palonosetron
Vitamin
Diclectin(R) [Can]
doxylamine and pyridoxine (Canada
only)

WHIPWORMS
Anthelmintic
mebendazole
Vermox(R) [Can]

ZOLLINGER-ELLISON SYNDROME
Antacid
calcium carbonate and simethicone
Dulcolax(R) Milk of Magnesia
[US-OTC]
Gas Ban(TM) [US-OTC]
magaldrate and simethicone
Mag-Caps [US-OTC]
MagGel(TM) [US-OTC]
magnesium hydroxide
magnesium oxide
Mag-Ox(R) 400 [US-OTC]
Phillips'(R) Milk of Magnesia
[US-OTC]
Titralac(R) Plus [US-OTC]
Uro-Mag(R) [US-OTC]
Gastric Acid Secretion Inhibitor
AcipHex(R) [US/Can]
Apo-Omeprazole(R) [Can]
lansoprazole
Losec(R) [Can]
Losec MUPS(R) [Can]
omeprazole
Pariet(R) [Can]
Prevacid(R) [US/Can]
Prevacid(R) SoluTab(TM) [US]
Prilosec(R) [US]
Prilosec OTC(TM) [US-OTC]
rabeprazole
Histamine H2 Antagonist
Alti-Ranitidine [Can]
Apo-Cimetidine(R) [Can]
Apo-Famotidine(R) [Can]
Apo-Famotidine(R) Injectable [Can]
Apo-Ranitidine(R) [Can]
BCI-Ranitidine [Can]
cimetidine
CO Ranitidine [Can]

famotidine
Famotidine Omega [Can]
Gen-Cimetidine [Can]
Gen-Famotidine [Can]
Gen-Ranidine [Can]
Novo-Cimetidine [Can]
Novo-Famotidine [Can]
Novo-Ranidine [Can]
Nu-Cimet [Can]
Nu-Famotidine [Can]
Nu-Ranit [Can]
Pepcid(R) [US/Can]
Pepcid(R) AC [US-OTC/Can]
Pepcid(R) I.V. [Can]
PMS-Cimetidine [Can]
PMS-Ranitidine [Can]
ranitidine
Ranitidine Injection, USP
 [Can]
Rhoxal-ranitidine [Can]
Riva-Famotidine [Can]
Sandoz-Ranitidine [Can]
Tagamet(R) [US]
Tagamet(R) HB [Can]
Tagamet(R) HB 200 [US-OTC]
Ulcidine [Can]

Zantac(R) [US/Can]
Zantac 75(R) [US-OTC/Can]
Zantac 150(TM) [US-OTC]
Zantac(R) EFFERdose(R) [US]
Laxative
 Dulcolax(R) Milk of Magnesia
  [US-OTC]
 Mag-Caps [US-OTC]
 MagGel(TM) [US-OTC]
 magnesium hydroxide
 magnesium oxide
 Mag-Ox(R) 400 [US-OTC]
 Phillips'(R) Milk of Magnesia
  [US-OTC]
 Uro-Mag(R) [US-OTC]
Prostaglandin
 Apo-Misoprostol(R) [Can]
 Cytotec(R) [US]
 misoprostol
 Novo-Misoprostol [Can]

ZOLLINGER-ELLISON SYNDROME (DIAGNOSTIC)

Diagnostic Agent
 SecreFlo(TM) [US]
 secretin

GI & GU Common Organs & Associated Structures

GASTROINTESTINAL

anus
appendix
ascending colon
cecum
descending colon
duodenum
esophagus
gallbladder
ileocecal junction
ileum
jejunum
large intestine
larynx
liver
pancreas
pharynx
pylorus
rectum
salivary gland
sigmoid colon
small intestine
spleen
stomach
tongue
trachea
transverse colon

GENITOURINARY

bulbourethral gland
deferent duct
epididymis
fallopian tube
glans penis
inguinal canal
kidney
labia majus
labia minus
navicular fossa
ovary
pelvis
posterior fornix
prostate
pubic symphysis
renal pelvis
renal sinus
retropubic space
seminal vesicle
testis
ureter
urethra
urinary bladder
uterus
vagina
vesicouterine pouch